Encyclopedia of Pathology

Series Editor
J. H. J. M. van Krieken

The scope of this 15–20-volume set encompasses the entire field of pathology ranging from general pathological terms to specific diseases to diagnostic methods. Published as print edition and online version (eReference) in the Springer Reference Program each topical volume sticks out by clearly and homogenously structured entries. A team of international experts guarantee that the essays and definitions are scientifically sound. The A–Z format of each topical volume allows readers to quickly and easily find the information they need. The major advantage of the encyclopedia is the way it makes relevant information available not only to pathologists but also to all clinicians and researchers of the neighboring disciplines working together with pathologists who occasionally might wish to look up terms online.

More information about this series at http://www.springer.com/series/14876

Fátima Carneiro • Paula Chaves
Arzu Ensari
Editors

Pathology of the Gastrointestinal Tract

With 480 Figures and 26 Tables

Springer

Editors
Fátima Carneiro
Faculty of Medicine of Porto University
Centro Hospitalar São João and
Ipatimup/i3S
Porto, Portugal

Paula Chaves
Serviço de Anatomia Patológica
Instituto Português de Oncologia de
Lisboa de Francisco Gentil
Lisbon, Portugal

Faculdade de Ciências da Saúde
Universidade da Beira Interior
Covilhã, Portugal

Arzu Ensari
Department of Pathology
Ankara University Medical School
Sihhiye, Ankara, Turkey

ISBN 978-3-319-40559-9 ISBN 978-3-319-40560-5 (eBook)
ISBN 978-3-319-40561-2 (print and electronic bundle)
DOI 10.1007/978-3-319-40560-5

Library of Congress Control Number: 2017936962

Printed on acid-free paper

This Springer imprint is published by Springer Nature
The registered company is Springer International Publishing AG
The registered company address is: Gewerbestrasse 11, 6330 Cham, Switzerland

Dedicated to Els, Lotte, Bas and Wouter who are my inspiration

J.H.J.M. van Krieken

Series Preface

When Denis Diderot started the first encyclopedia in the eighteenth century, it was a groundbreaking and timely event. It was the time of the Enlightenment, and knowledge was seen as something which was to be spread to many and to build upon by creating new knowledge. His ambition was to bring all available knowledge together in one series of books so that every person who could read has access to all there is to know. Nowadays, in a time of easily accessible knowledge, the question is whether there is still need of an encyclopedia. It is obvious that the amount of knowledge is such that it is not possible to bring it all together in one encyclopedia. One may argue that the Internet is the encyclopedia of today, but that misses an important point of Diderot, a point that is probably even more valid today. He created a team that valued information and selected what was worth to be presented in the encyclopedia. He recognized that science is not a democratic process where the majority decides what is true and valuable, but rather a growing body of knowledge in which radical ideas from individuals may bring about huge changes, even though most would reject these new ideas in the beginning. Indeed, the Internet lacks such authority and it is not easy to select valuable information from nonsense, especially when one is not an expert in a certain field.

It is therefore that an encyclopedia is only as good as the team that creates it. It goes without saying the team that is responsible for the *Encyclopedia of Pathology* consists of recognized experts in the field. Pathology is a growing medical discipline in which the amount of information is probably already more than that the whole encyclopedia of Diderot contained. For experts in subspecialties within pathology, it is already almost impossible to keep an overview on new developments and to select relevant from less relevant new information. There are plenty of textbooks for every disease group, and scientific literature is available for most pathologists through PubMed or Google Scholar. What is lacking is a systematic overview of what we know in an alphabetical order, easily accessible to all. The *Encyclopedia of Pathology* fills that gap. It is written by experts with the general pathologist in mind and also specialist from other disciplines. It will consist of a series of volumes on subspecialties, and when it is completed there will be an online version combining these. Yearly updates from the online version is foreseen and readers are welcome to provide suggestions for improvement. These will be judged by the editorial team in order to keep the encyclopedia authoritative yet using the expertise of many.

Finally, it is my hope that the encyclopedia will grow into a reliable body of knowledge in pathology, enabling communication through a common language, and that it will grow and adapt to new developments.

Nijmegen, The Netherlands J.H.J.M. van Krieken
April 2017

Volume Preface

Knowledge in all fields of science is expanding very rapidly together with advances in technology allowing easy access to publications. The reader has a whole variety of options ranging from published hardcover books placed on the bookshelves to online articles accessible via the Internet. The major advantage of the *Encyclopedia of Pathology* (published as print edition and online version) is its structure, providing alphabetically arranged entries, each of which with a detailed description of a specific pathological disease entity, allowing the readers to quickly and easily find the information they need.

This encyclopedia volume covers the complete field of the pathology of the gastrointestinal (GI) tract and is organized in two sections: Upper Gastrointestinal Pathology and Lower Gastrointestinal Pathology. More than 200 entries/key terms related to various GI disorders ranging from developmental abnormalities, infectious diseases, and inflammatory conditions to neoplastic processes have been entered by more than 75 authors, all experienced and/or interested in GI pathology. Each entry consists of a brief definition and clinical and histopathologic features of the entity accompanied with gross and microscopic photographs, tables, and figures. An average of five references was also provided for each entry. In order to facilitate the search function, key terms were highlighted and activated so that "clicking" would be possible to search through the entries.

We sincerely hope that the volume will help the pathologist to get basic information related to the search term which would ideally prompt the reader to search for more. As the GI team including the editors and the authors, we would like to share our great enthusiasm for GI pathology with the readers.

Porto, Portugal — Fátima Carneiro
Lisbon, Portugal — Paula Chaves
Ankara, Turkey — Arzu Ensari

Acknowledgments

Pathologists serve everyday new patients based on the knowledge collected in this encyclopedia gained over more than a century from other patients and pathologists. I am therefore feeling a deep gratitude to all of them. I also like to thank all who have contributed to the large amount of items but especially to the editors who had the difficult task to select and collect, evaluate, and approve.

J.H.J.M. van Krieken

As the editorial team we would like to express our gratitude to the authors who have contributed to this volume of *Encyclopedia of Pathology*. It was a great amount of work for the authors who all have wholeheartedly contributed to the completion of this encyclopedia. Their meticulous efforts made it possible to have an extensive overview of GI pathology. We, as editors, would therefore like to thank the team of international experts who have accepted the challenge to collaborate in this initiative with their enthusiasm and great interest in GI pathology. They have spent countless hours drafting, revising, and finalizing their entries. We hope that you have enjoyed this time and have gained as much from your contribution as the reader pathologists will benefit from your work.

Fátima Carneiro
Paula Chaves
Arzu Ensari

Editors Biography

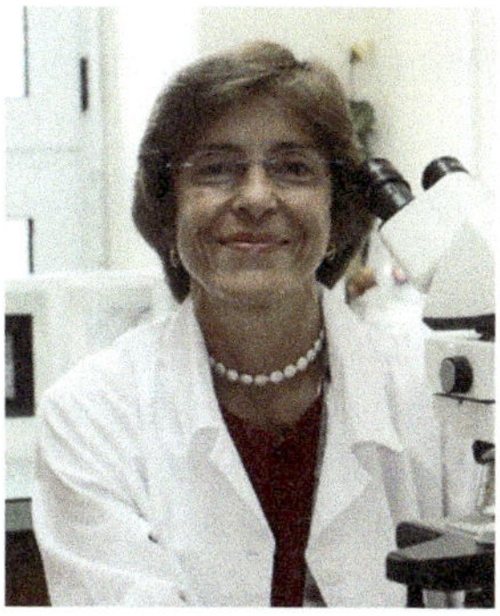

Fátima Carneiro Faculty of Medicine of Porto University, Centro Hospitalar São João and Ipatimup/i3S, Porto, Portugal

Fátima Carneiro, M.D., Ph.D., is Full Professor of Pathology (Medical Faculty of Porto), Head of Department of Anatomic Pathology (Centro Hospitalar São João), and Senior Researcher at Ipatimup/i3S. She is past president of the European Society of Pathology (ESP), chair of the Advisory Board of the ESP, coordinator of the Portuguese Network of Tumour Banks, member of Council of the International Gastric Cancer Association, and fellow of the European Academy of Cancer Sciences. She was delegate of Portugal to the Committee for the FP7 specific program "Cooperation" of the European Commission and is a member of the Scientific Advisory Board of the ERA-NET on translational cancer research (TRANSCAN). She is coauthor of more than 300 peer-reviewed publications ("h factor": 57 – Scopus, accessed April 2017) and 28 book chapters, including books issued by the WHO (*Pathology and Genetics of Tumours of the Digestive System*, 3rd Edition, 2000, and *WHO Classification of Tumours of the Digestive System*, 4th Edition, 2010), the UICC (*Comprehensive Tumour Terminology Handbook*, 2001), and the IARC (*World Cancer Report* 2014). She is one of the editors of the WHO Blue Book on "Tumours of the Digestive System" and section editor of the *Encyclopedia of Pathology*. Her field of specialization is gastrointestinal pathology. Her research is directed towards the understanding of the etiopathogenesis and molecular pathology of gastric carcinoma, in the sporadic and hereditary settings, with a particular interest in hereditary diffuse gastric cancer (HDGC).

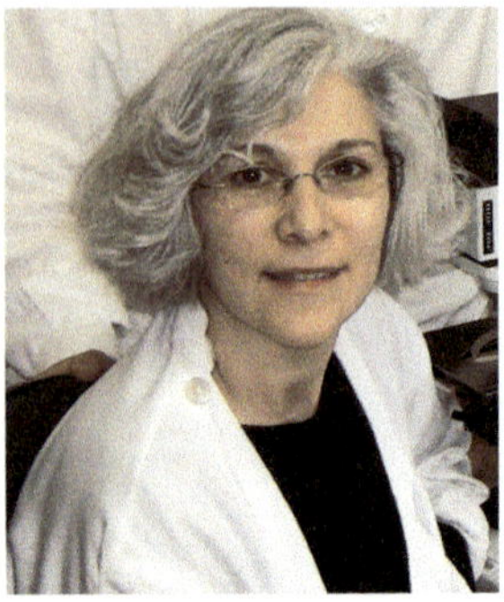

Paula Chaves Instituto Português de Oncologia de Lisboa – EPE, Lisboa, Portugal

Faculdade de Ciências da Saúde, Universidade da Beira Interior, Covilhã, Portugal

Paula Chaves, M.D., Ph.D., is Full Professor of Pathology at the Faculdade de Ciências da Saúde, Universidade da Beira Interior, Covilhã, and Head of the research center of the Instituto Português de Oncologia de Lisboa, EPE, where she is the Group Leader of the digestive pathology group. She is Senior Pathologist and responsible for the histopathology laboratory of the Department of Pathology, at the Instituto Português de Oncologia de Lisboa, EPE. She is coauthor of more than 100 peer-reviewed publications and 8 book chapters. Her field of specialization is gastrointestinal pathology, and her main area of research as PI of the Barrett's esophagus study group of the Instituto Português de Oncologia de Lisboa, EPE, is the cellular differentiation of Barrett's esophagus epithelium, its control, and its relationship with malignant progression to esophageal adenocarcinoma.

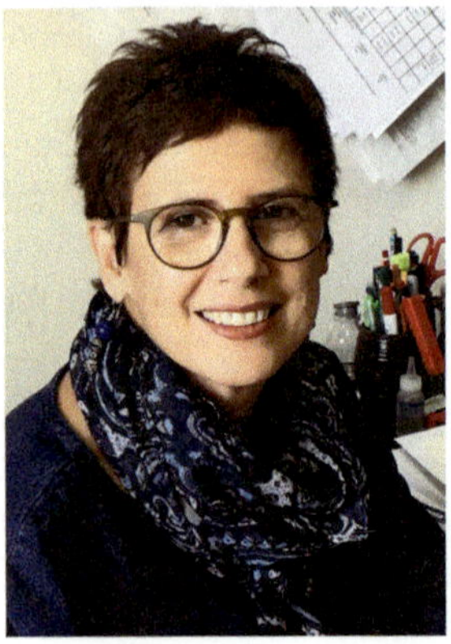

Arzu Ensari finished her pathology training in Ankara in 1991 and went to UK for a Ph.D. on "Cellular and Molecular Pathology of Gluten Sensitivity" under the supervision of Dr. Michael N. Marsh between 1991 and 1994. She worked with Dr. Yo Kato (Japan) for 3 months in 1995 on GI cancer and precursor lesions. Following her return to the department she started to do GI pathology. In 2008 she worked in Toronto, Canada, as a visiting professor with Professor Robert Riddell mainly on IBD. Dr. Ensari was the former chair of the GI pathology working group of ESP. She is a faculty member of EScoP GI pathology working team. Dr. Ensari is currently working as a full-time Professor in the Department of Pathology, Ankara University Medical School. Dr. Ensari has published many articles and book chapters in the field of GI pathology with particular interest in malabsorption, IBD, polyps, and colorectal cancer.

Series Editor Biography

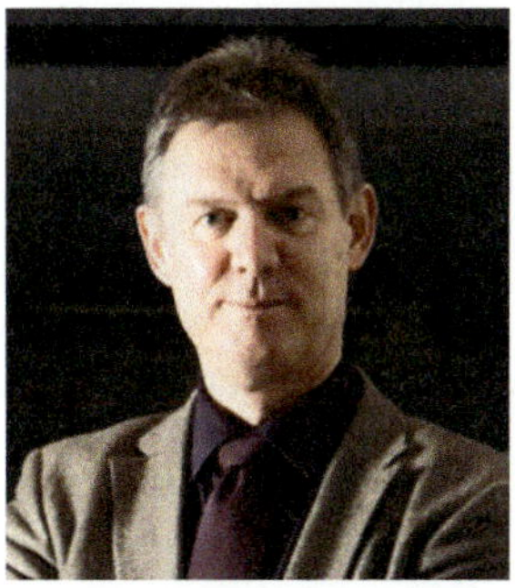

J.H.J.M. van Krieken is a pathologist with special expertise in the fields of hematopathology and the pathology of the gastrointestinal tract. He was professor for tumor pathology since 1999 and kept from 2005 to 2015 the chair of pathology at the Radboud University Nijmegen Medical Centre in Nijmegen. He furthermore served as chairman of the Board of the Oncology Institute of the Radboud University Nijmegen from 2008 to 2016. Since 2016, he is the rector magnificus (vice chancellor) of the Radboud University.

He was the treasurer/secretary of the European Association for Hematopathology from 2000 to 2008, from 2003 to 2011 the treasurer, from 2013 to 2015 the president of the European Society for Pathology (ESP), and from 2015 to 2017 the past-president of the ESP. Furthermore, he coordinates the ESP quality assessment program and is the chair of IQNpath. He is (co) author of more than 500 papers in peer-reviewed journals (H-index 79), has written chapters in books on pathology and oncology, is editor of a Dutch textbook on oncology, and serves on the editorial board of the *American Journal of Surgical Pathology*, is managing editor of *Virchows Archiv*, and is the chief editor of the *Journal of Hematopathology*. Since 2011, he is member of the German Academy of Sciences Leopoldina, and since 2014 of Academia Europea and Honorary Fellow of the Royal Society of Pathology of Great Britain and Ireland.

Contributors

Ana Afonso Serviço de Anatomia Patológica, Hospital Cuf Descobertas e IPOLFG, E.P.E Parque das Nações, Lisbon, Portugal

Andreia Albuquerque Serviço de Gastrenterologia, Centro Hospitalar de São João, Porto, Portugal

Raquel Almeida Institute of Molecular Pathology and Immunology of the University of Porto (IPATIMUP), Porto, Portugal

Faculty of Medicine, University of Porto, Porto, Portugal

Helena Baldaia Serviço de Anatomia Patológica, Centro Hospitalar de São João, Porto, Portugal

Francisco Baldaque-Silva Centro Hospitalar de São João, Alameda Professor Hernani Monteiro, Porto, Portugal

Rita Barros Institute of Molecular Pathology and Immunology of the University of Porto (IPATIMUP), Porto, Portugal

Gabriel Becheanu Department of Pathology, Fundeni Clinical Institute, Carola Davila University of Medicine and Pharmacy, Bucharest, Romania

Iva Brcic Institute of Pathology, Medical University of Graz, Graz, Austria

Maria José Brito Serviço Anatomia Patológica, Hospital Garcia de Orta, Almada, Portugal

Rita Canas Marques Serviço de Anatomia Patológica, Instituto Português de Oncologia de Lisboa de Francisco Gentil and Faculdade de Ciências Médicas, Universidade Nova de Lisboa, Lisbon, Portugal

Fátima Carneiro Faculty of Medicine of Porto University, Centro Hospitalar São João and Ipatimup/i3S, Porto, Portugal

Denis Chatelain Service d'Anatomie Pathologique, Centre Hospitalier et Universitaire du Nord, Amiens, France

Paula Chaves Serviço de Anatomia Patológica, Instituto Português de Oncologia de Lisboa de Francisco Gentil, Lisbon, Portugal

Faculdade de Ciências da Saúde, Universidade da Beira Interior, Covilhã, Portugal

Janice Mary Chicarino Coelho Fundação Oswaldo Cruz (Fiocruz) Instituto de Pesquisa Clínica Evandro Chagas, Rio de Janeiro, Brasil

Joaninha Costa Rosa Serviço de Anatomia Patológica, Instituto Português de Oncologia de Lisboa Francisco Gentil, Lisbon, Portugal

J. Alberto Pereira da Silva Serviço de Reumatologia, Hospital de S. Maria, Lisbon, Portugal

Francisco Ferro de Beça Department of Pathology, Centro Hospitalar de São João, Porto, Portugal

Faculty of Medicine of the University of Porto, Porto, Portugal

IPATIMUP – Institute of Pathology and Molecular Immunology of the University of Porto, Porto, Portugal

Susana Mão de Ferro Department of Gastroenterology, IPOLFG, E.P.E., Lisbon, Portugal

Gert De Hertogh Department of Pathology, Pathologische Ontleedkunde, UZ Leuven, Leuven, Belgium

Mário Ferraz de Oliveira Serviço Anatomia Patológica, Centro Hospitalar Lisboa Central EPE, Lisbon, Portugal

Mário Dinis-Ribeiro Serviço de Gastrenterologia, Portuguese Oncology Institute, Porto, Portugal

Instituto Português de Oncologia (IPO - Porto), Cintesis (FMUP-UP), Porto, Portugal

Başak Doğanavşargil Department of Pathology, Ege University Medical School, Bornova, Izmir, Turkey

Ann Driessen Department of Pathology, University Hospital Antwerp, Edegem, Belgium

Maastricht University Medical Centre, Maastricht, The Netherlands

Özgür Ekinci Department of Pathology, Gazi University, Ankara, Turkey

Arzu Ensari Department of Pathology, Ankara University Medical School, Sihhiye, Ankara, Turkey

Sibel Erdamar Department of Pathology, Cerrahpasa Medical College, Istanbul, Turkey

Cevriye Cansiz Ersöz Department of Pathology, Ankara University Medical School, Sihhiye, Ankara, Turkey

Sandra Faias Instituto Português de Oncologia de Lisboa Francisco Gentil, E.P.E., Lisbon, Portugal

Liesbeth Ferdinande Department of Pathology, Ghent University Hospital, Ghent, Belgium

Catarina Fidalgo Instituto Português de Oncologia de Lisboa Francisco Gentil, E.P.E., Lisbon, Portugal

Ceu Figueiredo Department of Pathology, Faculty of Medicine of the University of Porto, Institute of Molecular Pathology and Immunology of the University of Porto (IPATIMUP), Porto, Portugal

Jean-François Fléjou Faculté de Médecine Pierre et Marie Curie, Service d'Anatomie et Cytologie Pathologiques, Hôpital Saint-Antoine, Paris, France

Isabel Fonseca Serviço de Anatomia Patológica, Instituto Português de Oncologia Francisco Gentil – Lisboa, Lisbon, Portugal

Faculdade de Medicina de Lisboa, Instituto de Anatomia Patológica, Lisbon, Portugal

Ricardo Fonseca Serviço de Anatomia Patológica, Instituto Português de Oncologia de Lisboa Francisco Gentil, Lisboa, Portugal

Maria Gabriela Gasparinho Instituto Português de Oncologia de Lisboa Francisco Gentil, Lisboa, Portugal

Instituto de Anatomia Patológica da Faculdade de Ciências da Saúde da Universidade da Beira Interior, Covilhã, Portugal

Karel Geboes Department of Pathology, N. Goormaghtig Institute, University Gent, Gent, Belgium

Department of Pathology, KU Leuven, Leuven, Belgium

Armagan Gunal Department of Pathology, Gulhane Military Medical Academy, Etlik, Ankara, Turkey

Tiago Henriques-Coelho Department of Paediatrics, University of Porto, Porto, Portugal

Anne Jouret-Mourin Department of Pathology, Cliniques Universitaires St. Luc, UCL, Brussels, Belgium

Saba Kiremitci Department of Pathology, Ankara University Medical School, Sihhiye, Ankara, Turkey

Ayca Kirmizi Department of Pathology, Ankara University Medical School, Sihhiye, Ankara, Turkey

Ana Lagos Department of Gastroenterology, IPOLFG, E.P.E., Lisbon, Portugal

Cord Langner Institute of Pathology, Medical University of Graz, Graz, Austria

Gregory Y. Lauwers Department of Pathology, Massachusetts General Hospital, Harvard Medical School, Boston, MA, USA

Jason T. Lewis Division of Anatomic Pathology, Department of Laboratory Medicine and Pathology, Mayo Clinic, Jacksonville, FL, USA

Wen-Yih Liang Department of Pathology, Taipei Veterans General Hospital, Taipei, Taiwan

Ana Isabel Lopes Unidade de Gastrenterologia Pediátrica, Departamento de Pediatria, Faculdade de Medicina de Lisboa, Hospital Universitário de Santa Maria/CHLN, Lisbon, Portugal

José Manuel Lopes Faculty of Medicine of the University of Porto and Institute of Molecular Pathology and Immunology of the University of Porto, Porto, Portugal

Guilherme Macedo Centro Hospitalar de São João, Alameda Professor Hernani Monteiro, Porto, Portugal

Manuela Mafra Centro Hospitalar Lisboa Central-H.S.J, Lisbon, Portugal

Ricardo Marcos-Pinto Serviço de Gastrenterologia, Portuguese Oncology Institute, Porto, Portugal

Centro Hospitalar do Porto, Instituto de Ciências Biomédicas Abel Salazar (ICBAS-UP), Cintesis (FMUP-UP), Porto, Portugal

Ivanir Martins Serviço de Anatomia Patológica, Instituto Nacional do Cancer Rio de Janeiro, Rio de Janeiro, RJ, Brasil

Andrzej Mróz Department of Gastroenterology and Hepatology, Histopathology Unit, Medical Center for Postgraduate Education, Warsaw, Poland

Luis Novais Neurogastroenterology and Gastrointestinal Motility Laboratory, CEDE-Faculty of Medical Sciences, New University of Lisbon, Lisbon, Portugal

Paula Borralho Nunes Hospital Cuf Descobertas and Escola Superior de Tecnologia da Saúde de Lisboa and Instituto de Anatomia Patológica, Faculdade de Medicina da, Universidade de Lisboa, Lisboa, Portugal

Erdener Özer Department of Pathology, Dokuz Eylül University School of Medicine, Izmir, Turkey

Bruno Pereira Instituto Português de Oncologia de Lisboa Francisco Gentil, E.P.E., Lisbon, Portugal

Servico de Gastrenterologia, Hospital Amato Lusitano, ULS de Castelo Branco, Castelo Branco, Portugal

António Dias Pereira Instituto Português de Oncologia de Lisboa Francisco Gentil, E.P.E., Lisbon, Portugal

Pedro Pimentel-Nunes Serviço de Gastrenterologia, Portuguese Oncology Institute, Porto, Portugal

Instituto Português de Oncologia (IPO - Porto), Cintesis (FMUP-UP), Porto, Portugal

Rafaela L. Rego Departamento de Diagnóstico Laboratorial – Serviço de Anatomia Patológica, Instituto Portugues de Oncologia Lisboa Francisco Gentil, IPOLFG, E.P.E, Lisbon, Portugal

Elisabete Rios Department of Pathology, Centro Hospitalar de São João, Porto, Portugal

Faculty of Medicine of the University of Porto, Porto, Portugal

IPATIMUP – Institute of Pathology and Molecular Immunology of the University of Porto, Porto, Portugal

Ari Ristimäki Division of Pathology, Haartman Institute and Genome-Scale Biology, Research Programs Unit, HUSLAB/Helsinki University Central Hospital and University of Helsinki, Helsinki, Finland

Susana Rodrigues Serviço de Gastrenterologia, Centro Hospitalar de São João, Alameda Professor Hernani Monteiro, Porto, Portugal

Isadora Rosa Instituto Português de Oncologia de Lisboa Francisco Gentil, E.P.E., Lisboa, Portugal

Xavier Sagaert Department of Pathology, University Hospitals KU Leuven, Leuven, Belgium

Ozgul Sagol Department of Pathology, Dokuz Eylul University Medical School, Inciralti, Izmir, Turkey

Berna Savaş Department of Pathology, Ankara University Medical School, Ankara, Turkey

Miguel Serrano Department of Gastroenterology, IPOLFG, E.P.E., Lisbon, Portugal

Namrata Setia Department of Pathology, Massachusetts General Hospital, Boston, MA, USA

Maria Sotiropoulou Department of Pathology, Alexandra Hospital, Athens, Attica, Greece

Ana Berta Sousa Departamento de Pediatria, Faculdade de Medicina de Lisboa, Serviço de Genética Médica, Hospital Universitário de Santa Maria/CHLN, Lisbon, Portugal

Magali Svrcek Hôpital Saint-Antoine, Service d'Anatomie Pathologique, AP-HP, Hôpitaux Universitaires de l'Est Parisien, Paris, France

Alexandra Thiel Division of Pathology, Haartman Institute and Genome-Scale Biology, Research Programs Unit, HUSLAB/Helsinki University Central Hospital and University of Helsinki, Helsinki, Finland

Wilhermo Torres Departamento de Patologia, Universidade Federal Fluminense, Rio de Janeiro, Brasil

Chella R. S. van der Post Department of Pathology, Radboud University Medical Center, Nijmegen, The Netherlands

J. Han van Krieken Department of Pathology, Radboud University Medical Center, Nijmegen, The Netherlands

Filipe Vilas-Boas Centro Hospitalar de São João, Alameda Professor Hernani Monteiro, Porto, Portugal

Xiaogang Wen Centro hospitalar de Vila Nova de Gaia/Espinho, Institute of Molecular Pathology and Immunology of the University of Porto, Porto, Portugal

A

Abdominal Adhesions

Maria Sotiropoulou
Department of Pathology, Alexandra Hospital, Athens, Attica, Greece

Synonyms

Pelvic adhesions; Synechiae

Definition

Peritoneal adhesions can be defined as fibrous bands between two parts of organs or tissues or both which are normally separated. These fibrous bands develop as part of healing processes that occur after any tissue disturbance such as surgery, infection, trauma, or radiation. The abdomen and pelvis are the two most common locations of adhesions.

Adhesions are rarely congenital and more commonly acquired, of which abdominal-pelvic surgery is the most common cause. Less common causes are intraperitoneal infections or abdominal trauma. Congenital adhesions arise during physiological organogenesis, like the frequently observed attachment of the sigmoid colon to the left pelvic wall, or can be traced back to abnormal embryonal development of the abdominal cavity. These are usually asymptomatic and are diagnosed incidentally. Patients who undergo abdominal or pelvic surgery are prone to develop post-operative adhesions in a percentage estimated to 93%. It was found that all patients who had undergone an abdominal surgery developed one to more than ten adhesions. The extent of adhesions depends on the type and magnitude of surgery, possible complications, and intraoperative foreign bodies such as glove, powder, suture materials etc. Pelvic adhesions usually occur from cesarean section or hysterectomy and may involve any organ of the pelvis such as the uterus, ovaries, fallopian tubes, or bladder. Endometriosis and pelvic inflammatory disease are the second leading cause of pelvic adhesions that frequently involve the area around the fallopian tube. Other inflammatory processes such as appendicitis, acute cholecystitis, acute diverticulosis, and Crohn's disease are also implicated in the formation of adhesions.

In any peritoneal surface, damage (operative trauma, infection, foreign bodies, desiccation, irradiation, allergic reaction, or chemical injury) induces a series of biochemical-molecular biologic cascades involving elements such as peritoneal fluid, neutrophils, macrophages, and mesothelial cells. Peritoneal repair and adhesion development occur through the major pathways of fibrolytic system, extracellular matrix deposition, growth factors, cell adhesion molecules and cytokines via angiogenesis, apoptosis, proliferation, and re-mesothelialization. In any surgery trauma can occur from various mechanisms, notably

F. Carneiro et al. (eds.), *Pathology of the Gastrointestinal Tract*, Encyclopedia of Pathology,
DOI 10.1007/978-3-319-40560-5

cutting, abrasion, ischemia, etc. Bleeding and vascular permeability with leakage elicit post-traumatic inflammatory response with the release of proinflammatory cytokines and complement activation. Fibrinogen from exudate fluid converts to fibrin with activation of the coagulation cascade. Fibrin is a tacky substance and causes adjacent organs or injured serosal surfaces to coalesce. Fortunately, under normal circumstances fibrin matrix is transient and becomes absorbed due to activation of the fibrolytic system (proteases).

If fibrinolysis does not occur or is impaired, the fibrin matrix becomes more organized by the ingrowth of collagen-secreting fibroblasts. In addition to fibrinolysis there are also inhibitors to prevent excessive fibrin deposition and degradation. Tissue plasminogen activator (tPA) and urokinase-like plasminogen activator (uPA) are capable of converting plasminogen to plasmin which is a protease degradating various molecules such as fibrin. Moreover, there are two groups of plasminogen activator inhibitors (PAI) which intervene to improve fibrinolysis. In case which there is peritoneal injury or ischemia, peritoneal fibrinolysis is depressed, the most widely accepted pathway leading to adhesion formation.

Clinical Features

- **Incidence**
  The incidence of intraperitoneal adhesions after general abdominal surgeries ranges from 67% to 93% and rises up to 97% following open gynecologic procedures. In autopsy studies of patients who had laparotomies in their history, the incidence is 70–90%. Adhesions are also present in 10.4% of individuals who have never had abdominal surgery.
- **Age**
  Adhesions occur at any age depending on the type of previous surgery.
- **Sex**
  Adhesion are more common in women (with racial predisposition in blacks than Caucasians) than men (1:1,8).
- **Site**
  The greater omentum is involved in 80% of post-operative intra-abdominal adhesions and the bowel in only around 50% (the small bowel with a higher incidence). Ovarian and fallopian tube adhesions can be demonstrated in over 90% of the patients after gynecological adnexal surgery.
- **Treatment**
  The aim of treatment is to prevent the adhesion formation. Careful and gentle tissue handling, removal of intraperitoneal blood clots, and meticulous hemostasis can minimize the adhesion production. Agents such as sodium citrate, heparin, olive oil, liquid paraffin, ACTH, pepsin, and amniotic fluid have been used in prevention with no satisfactory results. Non-steroidal anti-inflammatory drugs (NSAIDs) and corticosteroids have been also tested for their ability to prevent adhesions, but their effectiveness is controversial due to complications. Barriers are the most promising group of agents in preventing the surgically induced adhesions. Surgical release of adhesions (adhesiolysis) is the only effective treatment applied by two common techniques, laparoscopy and laparotomy. Laparoscopic surgery has the theoretical advantage of inducing adhesions in a minor degree.
- **Outcome**
  Surgical removal of adhesions has a good outcome in the majority of patients. Unfortunately, in about 11–21% of cases, the adhesions will reform after surgery.

Macroscopy

Thin or thick adhesive bands between loops of small bowel, or other organs, omentum, or abdominal wall are observed. The trapped bowel segment shows ischemic features, with dark-red dilated, edematous, and sometimes thin wall.

Microscopy

Adhesions historically have been thought to consist of avascular scar tissue but instead are highly cellular, vascularized, dynamic, and regenerating structures containing well-developed arterioles, venules, and capillaries. In early adhesions there are fibroblasts, inflammatory cells, and macrophages in a fibrous matrix. In a high percentage of patients having recent surgeries, both suture and starch granulomas with foreign body multinucleate cells are observed. Later the "mature" adhesion becomes a highly organized cellular structure containing arterioles, venules, capillaries, adipose tissue, and smooth muscle clusters in some areas displaying fibrosis. It seems that nerve fibers, with both myelinated and non-myelinated axons, are present in many patients, with increased incidence in those with malignancy. Endometriosis-related adhesions contain more inflammatory cells and tissue edema than post-surgical and post-infectious ones.

Immunophenotype

There are not specific immunohistochemical markers in adhesions.

Molecular Studies

Specific cytokines and growth factors are responsible for upregulating the expression of genes which interfere with their produced proteins in adhesion creation. Transforming growth factor beta (TGF-b), a cytokine, contributes to a decrease in peritoneal fibrolytic capacity by local regulation of PAI-1. The role of interleukin-1 (IL-1) chiefly and IL-1b secondarily interplay in pathophysiology of adhesion formation by stimulating the release of PAI-1 in human mesothelial cells. Substance P (SP), a neuropeptide which can be found in peritoneal fluid and affect the expression of intercellular adhesion molecules (intercellular adhesion molecule, ICAM-1; vascular cell adhesion molecule, VCAM-1), and TGF-b seem to play a central role. The mRNA levels of the neurokinin-1 (NK-1) receptor and SP are significantly increased in peritoneal adhesions very early after surgery.

Differential Diagnosis

Sclerosing peritonitis can be differentiated from adhesions by discrete plaque or continuous sheets involving hepatic, splenic, diaphragmatic, or rarely small bowel peritoneum. Differential diagnosis from desmoplastic mesothelioma may also be difficult in a small biopsy specimen.

References and Further Reading

Arung, W., Meurisse, M., & Detry, O. (2011). Pathophysiology and prevention of postoperative peritoneal adhesions. *World Journal of Gastroenterology, 17*(41), 4545–4553.

Becker, G., & Stucchi, A. (2004). Intra-abdominal adhesion prevention: Are we getting any closer? *Annals of Surgery, 240*, 202–204.

Bruggeman, D., Tchartchian, G., et al. (2010). Intra-abdominal adhesions. *Deutsches Ärzteblatt International, 107*(44), 769–775.

Ellis, H., Moran, B. G., Thomson, J. N., et al. (1999). Adhesion-related hospital readmissions after abdominal and pelvic surgery: A retrospective cohort study. *Lancet, 353*, 1476–1480.

Liakakos, T., Thomakos, N., Paul, F., Dervenis, C., & Young, R. (2001). Peritoneal adhesions: Etiology, pathophysiology and clinical significance. *Digestive Surgery, 18*, 260–273.

Abetalipoproteinemia

Arzu Ensari
Department of Pathology, Ankara University Medical School, Sihhiye, Ankara, Turkey

Synonyms

Bassen-Kornzweig syndrome

Definition

Abetalipoproteinemia (ABL) is a rare, autosomal recessive lipid storage disorder resulting from defective lipid assembly within the intestinal mucosa. It is characterized by the absence of apolipoprotein B (apoB-48 and apoB-100) an essential component of chylomicrons and VLDL, respectively, responsible for the transport of dietary fat from the small bowel lumen into the circulation. The defect is attributed to defective lipid transfer from the membrane of the endoplasmic reticulum to apoB due to mutations in the gene encoding a microsomal triglyceride transfer protein (MTTP). As a result, apoB-containing lipoproteins, namely, chylomicrons, and low-density and very low-density lipoproteins are absent from the patient's bloodstream. Lipid profile reveals low total cholesterol and triglyceride levels. Infants present with failure to thrive, diarrhea, and steatorrhea. Malabsorption of fat-soluble vitamins leads to neuromuscular impairment including poor muscle coordination, difficulty with balance and movement (ataxia), and retinitis pigmentosa (due to deficiency of vitamin A) later in life.

Clinical Features

- **Incidence**
  It is a very rare disorder affecting less than 1:1,000,000 individuals.
- **Age**
  Many ABL patients present in the second to fourth decades, while a few others present in the first and sixth decades.
- **Sex**
  No sex predilection for abetalipoproteinemia has been noted.
- **Site**
  Although ABL is a systemic disorder, the small intestinal mucosa is the main affected site where defective fat absorption takes place.
- **Treatment**
  Treatment consists of a low fat diet and replacement of fat-soluble vitamins involving large amounts of vitamin E which helps the body restore and produce lipoproteins. A low fat diet has been shown to improve steatorrhea associated with fat malabsorption and allow absorption of other nutrients essential for growth and development. Neuromuscular symptoms are usually treated with physiotherapy or occupational therapy. Dietary restriction of triglycerides has also been useful.
- **Outcome**
  Treatment with fat-soluble vitamins, may delay symptoms, but large majority of the patients progress. Before the use of high-dose oral fat-soluble vitamin treatment, many ABL patients developed neurological complications before the second decade and some did not survive past the third decade.

Macroscopy

Endoscopy reveals diffuse granular white mucosa. No other specific gross findings have been reported for ABL.

Microscopy

Duodenal biopsies show normal villous morphology with lipid vacuolization of surface enterocytes showing intact brush border (Fig. 1). Because the epithelial cells of the bowel lack the ability to place fats into chylomicrons, lipids accumulate at the surface of the cell, interfering with the functions that are necessary for proper absorption. The distribution of vacuolization corresponding to lipid droplets is heterogeneous as fat-filled enterocytes in the villus tip are

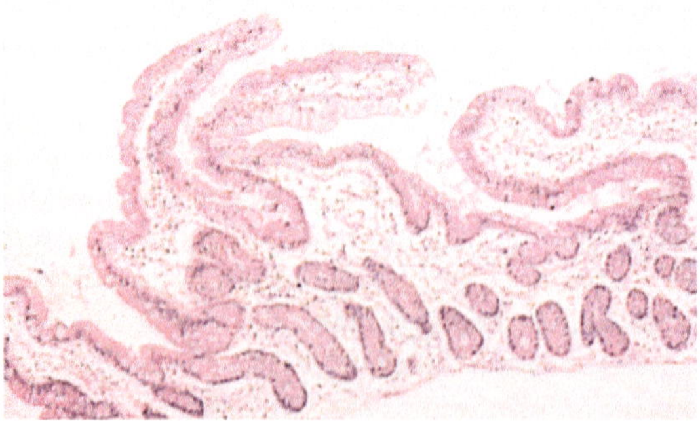

Abetalipoproteinemia, Fig. 1 Duodenal mucosa with preserved villus architecture and vacuolization of the surface enterocytes (H&E; ×100)

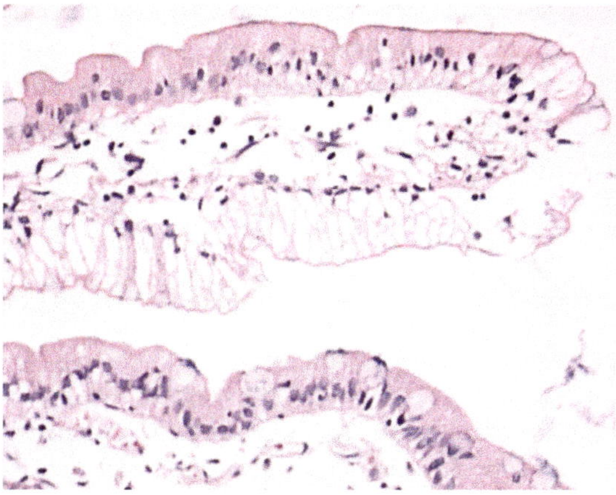

Abetalipoproteinemia, Fig. 2 Vacuolization of surface enterocytes (H&E; ×200)

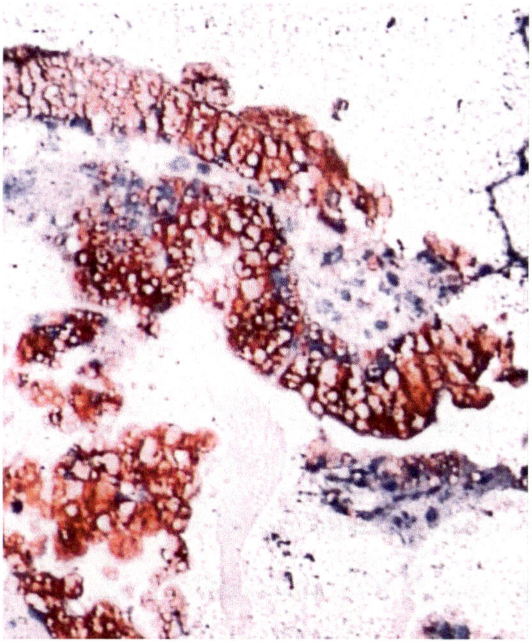

Abetalipoproteinemia, Fig. 3 Presence of lipid in the vacuolated enterocytes (Oil Red O stain; ×200)

associated with normal enterocytes in the crypts (Fig. 2). The lipid in the enterocytes may be demonstrated by histochemical lipid stains such as Oil Red O (Fig. 3) and Sudan Black. However, one would need fresh tissue to perform the former while the latter works well on paraffin-embedded tissue. Electron microscopy shows numerous vacuoles in the cytoplasm of the enterocytes. There is juxtaposition of intercellular membranes lacking lipid molecules. This disorder may also result in fat accumulation in the liver (hepatic steatosis).

Immunophenotype

There is no distinctive immunophenotypic feature of ABL.

Molecular Features

Mutation in microsomal triglyceride transfer protein, MTTP, located in 4q22–q24 in ABL has been reported.

Differential Diagnosis

Many genetic disorders cause defects in apoB synthesis among which three main causes of familial hypocholesterolemia are included: hypobetalipoproteinemia (HBL), abetalipoproteinemia (ABL), and chylomicron retention disease (CRD) or Anderson's disease. In HBL apoB on chromosome 2 is mutated leading to protein truncation in apoB. The phenotype is usually milder than ABL. SAR1B gene, which is involved in chylomicron transport from the ER to the Golgi, is mutated in CRD. Histological abnormality is identical in all three diseases characterized by lipid accumulation in surface enterocytes of duodenal mucosa.

Similar but less striking findings in the small intestinal mucosa can be seen in individuals who have ingested a fat-containing meal before endoscopy. Long fasting may also cause similar vacuolization in the enterocytes. In celiac disease, surface epithelium may show vacuolization; however these are usually less striking than those of ABL, and additional features including villous abnormalities and IELosis help to differentiate the two diseases.

References and Further Reading

Abumrad, N. A., & Davidson, N. O. (2012). Role of gut in lipid homeostasis. *Physiological Reviews, 9*, 1061–1085.

Berriot-Varoqueaux, N., Aggerbeck, L. P., Samson-Bouma, M., & Wetterau, J. R. (2000). The role of the microsomal triglygeride transfer protein in abetalipoproteinemia. *Annual Review of Nutrition, 20*, 663–697.

Khatun, I., Walsh, M. T., & Hussain, M. M. (2013). Loss of both phospholipid and triglyceride transfer activities of microsomal triglyceride transfer protein in abetalipoproteinemia. *Journal of Lipid Research, 54*, 1541–1549.

Pautler, D., Easley, D., & Pohl, J. F. (2008). Abetalipoproteinemia. *Journal of Pediatric Gastroenterology and Nutrition, 46*, 355–360.

Peretti, N., Sassolas, A., Roy, C. C., Deslalndres, C., Charcosset, M., Castagnetti, J., et al. (2010). Guidelines for the diagnosis and management of chylomicron retention disease based on a review of literature and the experience of two centers. *Orphanet Journal of Rare Diseases, 5*, 1–24.

Achalasia, Esophagus

Luis Novais[1] and Paula Chaves[2,3]
[1]Neurogastroenterology and Gastrointestinal Motility Laboratory, CEDE-Faculty of Medical Sciences, New University of Lisbon, Lisbon, Portugal
[2]Serviço de Anatomia Patológica, Instituto Português de Oncologia de Lisboa de Francisco Gentil, Lisbon, Portugal
[3]Faculdade de Ciências da Saúde, Universidade da Beira Interior, Covilhã, Portugal

Synonyms

Primary achalasia

Definition

Achalasia is an esophageal disorder of unknown cause characterized by aperistalsis of esophagus body and impaired relaxation of the lower esophageal sphincter (LES).

The most common symptoms for achalasia presentation are dysphagia, regurgitation, weight loss, chest pain, and pulmonary symptoms such as cough. The dysphagia to solids is present in nearly all achalasia patients and to liquids present in two-thirds of patients. The onset of the dysphagia is usually gradual; initially, the dysphagia may be primarily for solids; however, by the time of clinical presentation, nearly all patients complain of dysphagia for solids and liquids while eating and drinking, especially cold beverages. Regurgitation is found in 60–90% of achalasia patients. It usually occurs shortly after a meal or while recumbent. Undigested food is regurgitated. Chest pain is found in one-third of achalasia patients. It is retrosternal and is typical of noncardiac chest pain. Pain is precipitated by eating. Chest pain occurs in some patients, primarily at night, and is especially seen in patients with milder disease when the esophagus is minimally dilated. Heartburn is a frequent symptom in achalasia, probably related to retention of acid beverages such as carbonated or fruit drinks and the production of lactic acid from retained food in a dilated esophagus. It is not associated with episodes of gastroesophageal acid reflux by ambulatory pH monitoring or combined multichannel intraluminal impedance and pH (MIII-pH).

Diagnosis of achalasia is made correctly if a systematic approach is made; it requires radiographic, manometric, and endoscopic esophageal evaluation. Early cases of achalasia may be misdiagnosed because screening barium X-ray studies fail to reveal esophageal dilation and peristalsis is not evaluated or endoscopy is used as the only test for the patient presenting with dysphagia. Barium esophagram with fluoroscopy is the best initial diagnostic test. Essential features are bird's beak narrowing of the LES with incomplete opening and loss of primary peristalsis. The esophagus is usually dilated and sometimes tortuous, does not empty, retains food and saliva, and produces an air–fluid level at the top of the barium column. Fluoroscopy always shows a lack of peristalsis, replaced by to-and-fro movement in the supine position. Timed barium swallow assesses esophageal emptying of barium in the upright position over 5 min. This technique has been shown to be a simple and reproducible method for objective assessment of esophageal function before and after treatment of achalasia and correlates with the patients' symptoms.

Esophageal manometry is the gold standard for diagnosing achalasia; it is required to establish the diagnosis of achalasia and must be done in any patient before pneumatic dilation or surgical myotomy is planned.

Essential features are aperistalsis and abnormal LES relaxation. Abnormal LES relaxation is seen in all achalasia patients; about 70–80% have absent or incomplete LES relaxation with wet swallows, while the remainder will have complete but shortened LES relaxation. A new technique, the high-resolution esophageal manometry (HRM) allows a better evaluation of esophageal body function and a more careful study of LES and esophagogastric junction relaxation using the integrated relaxation pressure – IRP (Fig. 1). HRM has improved the sensitivity of manometry for detecting achalasia and greatly helped in making the diagnosis of achalasia. As reported by a group from the Northwestern University of Chicago, three patterns of achalasia are described: Type I, impaired relaxation with esophageal dilation and negligible esophageal pressurization; Type II, pan-esophageal pressurization; and Type III, spastic contractions of the distal esophageal segment (Figs. 2, 3, and 4).

Endoscopy is necessary to rule out pseudo-achalasia secondary to malignancies at the esophagogastric junction. A typical endoscopy in an achalasia patient is a dilated and tortuous esophagus. It is not uncommon to find retained food debris and secretions in the esophagus. The LES remains closed with air insufflations and appears puckered. The endoscope usually passes into the stomach with gentle pressure. The gastroesophageal junction (GEJ) and gastric cardia are carefully examined for evidence of tumors. Other techniques such as endoscopic ultrasound (EUS) and computed tomography (CT) scan may be

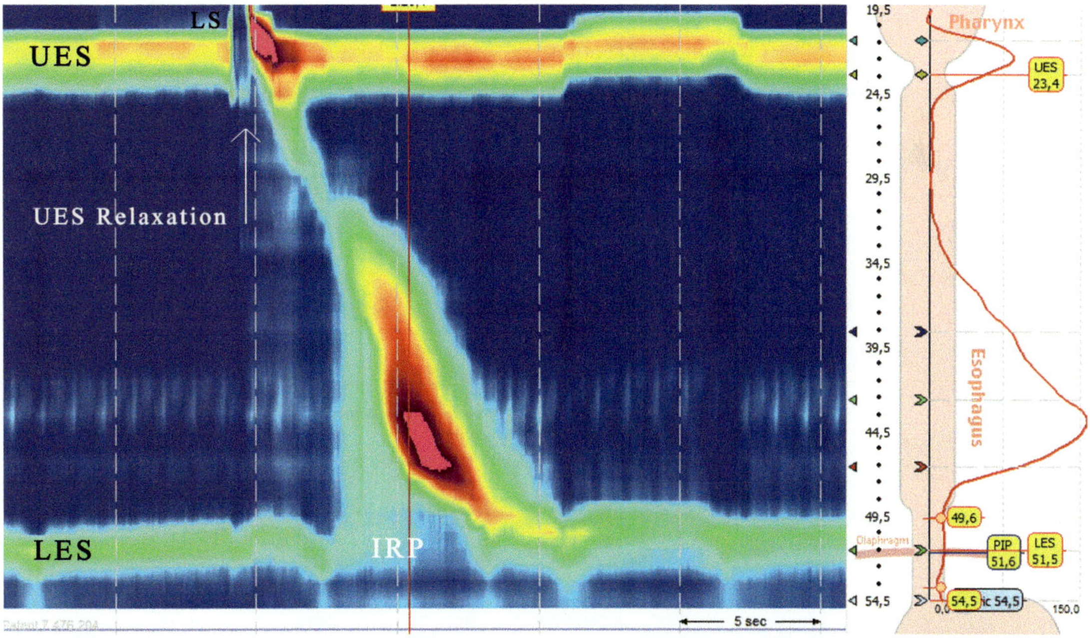

Achalasia, Esophagus, Fig. 1 Normal esophageal high-resolution manometry tracing. The wet swallow initiates a progressive peristaltic contraction. The LES relaxes completely to the gastric baseline. Normal IRP. (Neurogastroenterology and Gastrointestinal Motility Laboratory. CEDE – Faculty of Medical Sciences New University of Lisbon, Portugal). *UES* upper esophageal sphincter, *LES* lower esophageal sphincter, *IRP* integrated relaxation pressure

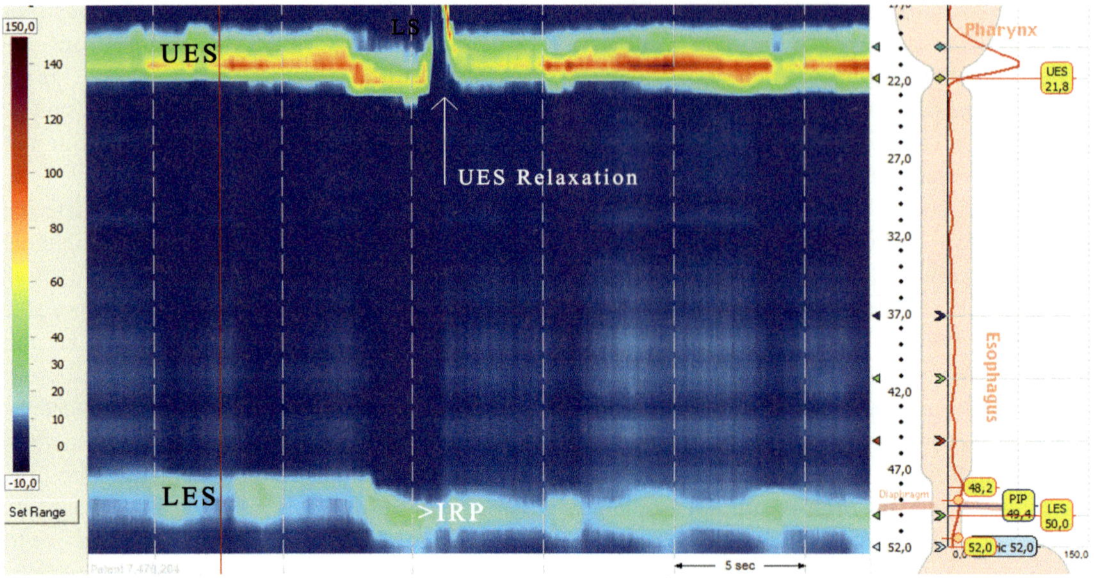

Achalasia, Esophagus, Fig. 2 Achalasia subtypes by esophageal high-resolution manometry. Type I: Classic achalasia (Neurogastroenterology and Gastrointestinal Motility Laboratory. CEDE – Faculty of Medical Sciences New University of Lisbon, Portugal). *UES* upper esophageal sphincter, *LES* lower esophageal sphincter, *IRP* integrated relaxation pressure

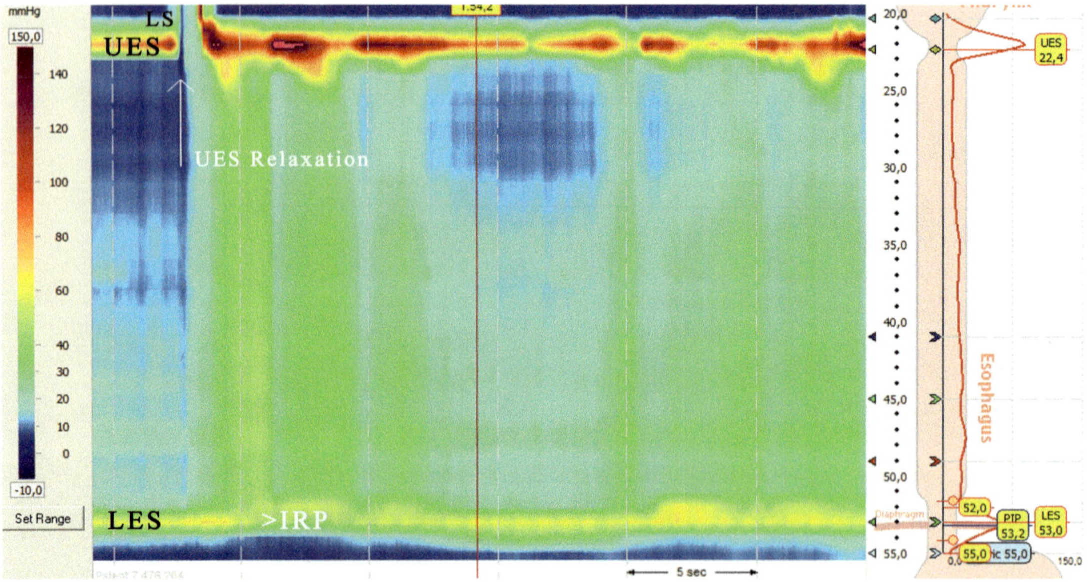

Achalasia, Esophagus, Fig. 3 Achalasia subtypes by esophageal high-resolution manometry. Type II: Classic achalasia with compression (Neurogastroenterology and Gastrointestinal Motility Laboratory. CEDE – Faculty of Medical Sciences New University of Lisbon, Portugal). *UES* upper esophageal sphincter, *LES* lower esophageal sphincter, *IRP* integrated relaxation pressure

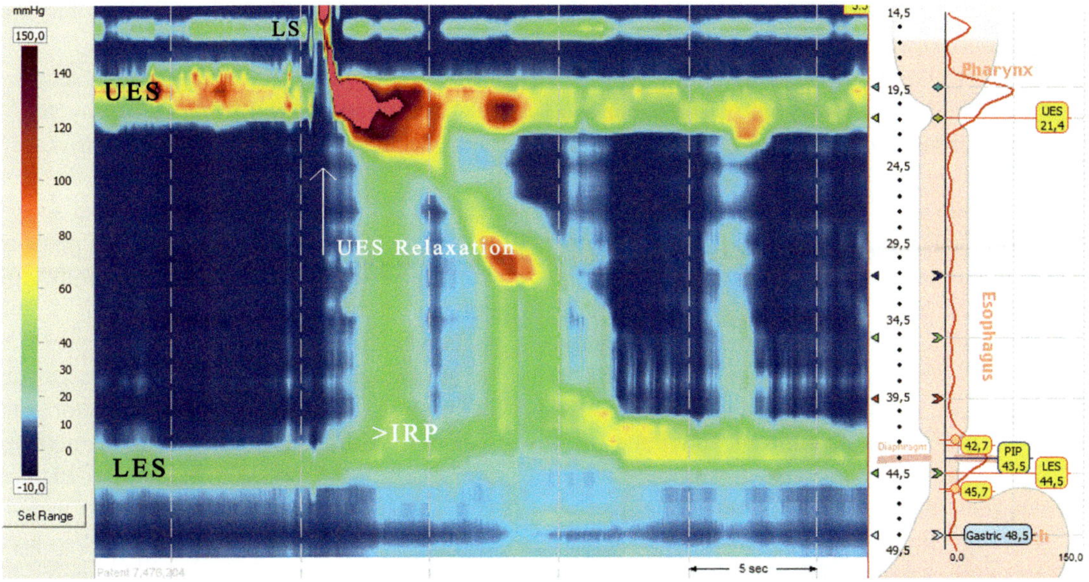

Achalasia, Esophagus, Fig. 4 Achalasia subtypes by esophageal high-resolution manometry. Type III: Spastic achalasia (Neurogastroenterology and Gastrointestinal Motility Laboratory. CEDE – Faculty of Medical Sciences New University of Lisbon, Portugal). *UES* upper esophageal sphincter, *LES* lower esophageal sphincter, *IRP* integrated relaxation pressure

helpful in evaluating the patient with suspected pseudoachalasia.

Clinical Features

- **Incidence**
  The incidence of achalasia is about 0.5 cases per 100,000 population per year, with a prevalence of approximately 10 cases per 100,000 population.
- **Age**
  Achalasia can occur at any age, with the peak incidence between 30 and 60 years of age. In children, it can be part of the Triple A syndrome, characterized by achalasia, alacrima, and adrenocorticotropic hormone-resistant adrenal insufficiency.
- **Sex**
  Achalasia occurs with equal frequency in men and women.
- **Site**
  Achalasia is confined to the esophagus.
- **Treatment**
  No treatment reverses the degeneration of inhibitory neurons of achalasia. Treatment is directed at reducing LES basal pressure so that hydrostatic forces of the ingested foods permit transit into the stomach. The goal is to reduce the pressure sufficiently to allow transit without leading to an inordinate amount of gastroesophageal reflux. Treatment options include pneumatic dilation, surgical cardiomyotomy (Heller), botulinum toxin injection, and medical therapy. Recently, a new approach of endoscope myotomy was presented. The disruption of the LES gradient is best accomplished by pneumatic dilation or surgical myotomy and, less effectively, by pharmacologic agents.

  Pneumatic dilation aims at disrupting the LES by forceful dilation using air-filled noncompliant polyethylene balloons available in 3 diameters (3.0, 3.5, and 4.0 cm). A 3.0 cm balloon is usually used for initial dilation. With the recurrence of symptoms, repeat dilations are performed in a stepwise graded fashion using larger-sized balloons. The balloon is positioned over a guide wire using either endoscopic or fluoroscopic control across the LES. The balloon is then inflated until the balloon waist (formed by the LES) is obliterated. The pressure applied is usually 7–12 psi of air, held for 15–60 s.

Surgical therapy (Heller myotomy) consists of anterior myotomy across the LES, which is performed either laparoscopically (abdominal approach) or open (transthoracic approach). The circular muscle fibers are divided down to the level of the mucosa, and the myotomy extends to several centimeters above the LES and <1 cm onto the stomach. Anti-reflux surgery (Dor fundoplication) is usually performed concomitantly.

Botulinum toxin injection inhibits acetylcholine release from nerve terminals, thereby blocking excitatory effects of the cholinergic neurons. It is injected by an endoscope through a sclerotherapy needle into the LES; a total dose of 100 units is divided into 25 unit aliquots, one in each quadrant of the sphincter. This can be performed on patients who are high risk for pneumatic dilation or surgical myotomy, such as the elderly or those with other comorbidities. Botox markedly improves symptoms in approximately 75% of achalasia patients. However, symptoms recur in more than 50% of patients within 6 months. Those responding to the first injection, the response decreases with further injections.

The most common medical therapies used to decrease LES pressure are nitrates and calcium channel blockers. Nitrates increase the nitric oxide concentration in smooth muscle cells, which subsequently increases cyclic guanosine monophosphatase (GMP) levels and results in muscle relaxation. Calcium is necessary for esophageal smooth muscle contractions, and its action is blocked by calcium antagonist.

- **Outcome**

  Because pathophysiological changes of achalasia, aperistalsis of esophagus body and impaired relaxation of the LES, could not be rectified by any therapeutic measures, the treatment usually aims at the temporary or persistent reduction of LES pressure. Treatments with greatest durability involve mechanical disruption of the LES: surgical myotomy and pneumatic dilation. Esophageal myotomy lowers LES pressure more consistently than pneumatic dilation. Partial return of peristalsis is reported in a small percentage of patients after pneumatic dilation and in up to 20% of patients after myotomy.

  Pneumatic dilation decreases LES pressure by 39–68%. Over time, LES pressure seems to increase to a varying degree. Predictor risk factors for relapse after pneumatic dilation are young age (<40 years), male, single dilation with a 3.0 cm balloon, posttreatment LES pressure >10–15 mmHg, poor esophageal emptying on timed barium swallow, and Type I and III pattern on high-resolution manometry. Complications after pneumatic dilation are reported. The most serious complication from pneumatic dilation is esophageal perforation, with an overall rate in experienced hands and with the new Rigiflex balloon dilators of 1.9% (range 0–16%). Treatment may be conservative with antibiotics and total parenteral nutrition, or surgical repair through a thoracotomy may be required. Other minor complications include chest pain (15% of patients), aspiration pneumonia, hematemesis, fever, esophageal mucosal tear, and hematoma. Complications of gastroesophageal reflux disease (esophagitis, peptic stricture, and Barrett's esophagus) are rare after pneumatic dilation, but 15–35% of patients have heartburn, responding to proton pump inhibitors. Over a third of achalasia patients treated with pneumatic dilation will experience symptom recurrence during a 4–6-year period of follow-up. Long-term remission can be achieved in virtually all of these patients treated by repeated pneumatic dilation according to an "on demand" strategy, based on symptom recurrence.

  Esophageal myotomy lowers LES pressure more consistently than pneumatic dilation. Depending on the distal extent of the myotomy onto the cardia, LES pressure is lowered by 55–75%, with the remaining residual pressure usually being less than 10 mmHg. Myotomy lowers intraesophageal pressure and solid esophageal emptying studies are improved. Younger patients, especially men, and patients with higher LES pressures may benefit most from primary surgery. Patients who fail pneumatic dilation or Botox treatment can be successfully treated with surgical myotomy, but repeated Botox injections significantly hinder the dissection of the submucosal plane, leading to a high percentage of mucosal perforations of the operations. Recurrence of dysphagia after a laparoscopic Heller myotomy is usually the result of an incomplete myotomy, particularly on the gastric side, esophageal scarring, obstruction by the fundoplication, megaesophagus, or complications of severe GERD, including esophagitis or peptic stricture.

Pneumatic dilation versus Heller myotomy has been compared in multiple studies, including randomized studies. Recently, an achalasia trial involving five European countries randomized 94 patients to Rigiflex pneumatic dilation (3.0 and 3.5 cm) and 106 to laparoscopic Heller myotomy with Dor fundoplication. After 2 years of follow-up, both treatments had comparable success rates: 92% for pneumatic dilation and 87% for laparoscopic myotomy. Barium swallow emptying and LES pressures were similar for both groups. Four perforations occurred after pneumatic dilations, compared to 11 perioperatively recognized perforations (1 converted to open operation) during laparoscopic Heller myotomy.

The choice between treatment options should be based on achalasia patients (patient age, patient surgical risk), randomized comparative studies, local medical centers (gastroenterologists with expertise in pneumatic dilation and surgeons in laparoscopic cardiomyotomy), and patient option.

Patients with long-standing achalasia have a small risk for developing an esophageal cancer over that of the general population. Risk factors for achalasia patients are male, older patients, long-standing disease, and megaesophagus. There are no guidelines of Endoscopy Societies that recommend routine endoscopy surveillance for squamous cell cancer in achalasia.

Macroscopy

The most striking macroscopic aspect of primary achalasia is the dilation of the esophageal body associated to impaired relaxation of the LES. The thickness of the esophageal wall may be normal, thicker than normal owing to muscular hypertrophy, or thinned in result of esophageal dilation. The mucosal lining may be unaffected, but it is usually damaged as a consequence of stasis and retained food debris. During endoscopy macroscopic evidence of inflammation or ulceration may be found.

Microscopy

The histologic picture usually confirms the macroscopic findings of esophageal dilation with or without hypertrophy of the muscular layers. The myenteric ganglia are usually absent from the esophageal body but may be reduced in number in the LES. Esophagitis, with or without ulceration, is usually present and *Candida esophagitis* is a frequent complication.

Immunophenotype

Not applicable

Molecular Features

Not applicable

Differential Diagnosis

Various disorders with similar manometric and radiologic features similar to achalasia should be considered in making a diagnosis of achalasia (Table 1). The most common disorders mimicking primary achalasia are malignancies and Chagas

Achalasia, Esophagus, Table 1 Secondary causes of achalasia

Malignancies (pseudoachalasia) involving the gastroesophageal junction (GEJ):
Adenocarcinoma (breast, gastric, lung, prostate)
Esophageal squamous cell carcinoma
Lymphoma (gastric, esophageal)
Esophageal lymphangioma
Malignancies (pseudoachalasia) remote from the GEJ:
Brainstem metastasis
Hodgkin's disease
Hepatocellular carcinoma
Gastric adenocarcinoma
Poorly differentiated lung carcinoma
Reticular cell carcinoma
Peritoneal mesothelioma
Retroperitoneal B-cell lymphoma
Nonmalignant esophageal infiltrative disorders:
Amyloidosis
Leiomyomatosis
Eosinophilic esophagitis
Sarcoidosis
Sphingolipidosis (Anderson–Fabry's disease)
Miscellaneous:
Chagas disease
Congenital lower esophageal diaphragmatic web
Diabetes mellitus
Familial adrenal insufficiency with alacrima
Multiple endocrine neoplasia type IIb
Pancreatic pseudocyst
Post-vagotomy
Laparoscopy Nissen fundoplication
Laparoscopic banding operative for obesity

disease, with the disorders being rare case reports. Tumors cause pseudoachalasia by encircling or compressing the distal esophagus or infiltrating the esophageal myenteric plexus and impairing inhibitory LES innervation. Clinical features that suggest malignancy are age, short duration of symptoms, and excessive weight loss. Barium studies could reveal findings of secondary achalasia: an eccentric, nodular, or shoulder segment of distal esophageal narrowing; narrowed distal esophageal segment that was longer 3 and 5 cm; and a minimal degree of esophageal dilation of 4 cm or less. Esophagogastroduodenoscopy (EGD) findings include mucosal ulcerations or nodularity, reduced compliance of the GEJ, or the inability to pass the endoscope into the stomach. EGD with biopsies results in the diagnosis of pseudoachalasia in most patients. EUS is helpful in selected patients. Computed tomography (CT) scan could show marked (>1 cm) and/or asymmetric esophageal wall thickening but usually find only nondiagnostic features unless massive tumor involvement is present.

References and Further Reading

Boeckxstaens, G. E., Annese, V., des Varannes, S. B., et al. (2010). The European achalasia trial: A randomized multi-centre trial comparing endoscopic pneumodilation and laparoscopic myotomy as primary treatment of idiopathic achalasia. *Gastroenterology, 138*(Suppl. 1), S53.

Bredenoord, A. J., Fox, M., Kahrilas, P. J., Pandolfino, J. E., Schizer, W., Smouth, A. J. P. M., & The International High Resolution Manometry Working Group. (2012). Chicago classification criteria of esophageal motility disorders defined in high resolution esophageal pressure topography. *Neurogastroenterology and Motility, 24*(Suppl 1), 57–65.

Eckardt, A. J., & Eckardt, V. F. (2009). Current clinical approach to achalasia. *World Journal of Gastroenterology, 15*, 3969–3975.

Pandolfino, J. E., Kwiatek, M. A., Nealis, T., Bulsiewicz, W., Post, J., & Kahrilas, P. J. (2008). Achalasia: A new clinically relevant classification by high-resolution manometry. *Gastroenterology, 135*, 1526–1533.

Richter, J. E., & Roberts, J. R. (2012). The esophagus. In J. E. Richter, & D. O. Castell (Eds.), *Achalasia* (5th ed., pp. 257–301). Blackwell Publishing Ltd.

Acute Gastritis

Chella R. S. van der Post[1] and
Fátima Carneiro[2]
[1]Department of Pathology, Radboud University Medical Center, Nijmegen, The Netherlands
[2]Faculty of Medicine of Porto University, Centro Hospitalar São João and Ipatimup/i3S, Porto, Portugal

Synonyms

Acute erosive gastritis; Acute erosive gastropathy; Acute hemorrhagic gastritis; Stress gastritis

Definition

Acute gastritis is a broad term referring to many disorders that may induce acute inflammatory changes in the gastric mucosa. Distinguished are acute hemorrhagic gastritis and acute infectious gastritis. In this entry the emphasis is especially on acute hemorrhagic gastritis, clinically characterized by a sudden onset of symptoms and rapid resolution after the underlying etiological mechanisms or agents (either chemical or physical) have been corrected. The different etiologies share the same general clinical presentation; however, they differ in their own unique histologic pattern with or without hemorrhage and erosive changes.

Acute gastritis is mostly associated with the intake of large doses of aspirin or other nonsteroidal anti-inflammatory drugs (NSAIDs), excess alcohol, or ischemic injury following major trauma. In many cases the etiology remains unknown. Generally, acute gastritis arises when there is an acute imbalance between mucosal injury and repair mechanisms. Mucosal irritants such as acid, pepsin, bile salts, NSAIDs, alcohol, and other chemicals cause injury. Mucoprotective factors include gastric mucus, tissue prostaglandins, intramural pH, bicarbonates, epidermal growth factors, mucosal blood flow, and the regenerative ability of gastric mucosa. The injury starts with direct irritant reaction of chemical agents and leads to mucosal erosion, necrosis, and hemorrhage. Additional injury is caused by acid, pepsin, and bile salts that gain entry resulting from the disrupted mucosal barrier. Suppression of acid secretion with proton pump inhibitors can reduce the severity of mucosal damage and facilitates mucosal healing.

Clinical Features

The symptoms in patients with acute gastritis range from abdominal discomfort to clinically alarming manifestations associated with massive bleeding or gastric perforation. Patients often present with acute gastroenteritis-like illness with burning epigastric pain, nausea, vomiting, hematemesis, melena, and occult bleeding. Patients with gastritis induced by aspirin or other NSAIDs may present with hypochromic, microcytic anemia caused by undetected chronic bleeding.

- **Incidence**
  The exact incidence of acute gastritis is unknown. Most often symptoms will be treated without histological confirmation. The majority of patients within intensive care units develop mucosal ulcers and around 20% develop overt bleeding with up to 5% leading to life-threatening bleeding. Studies have found acute hemorrhagic gastritis as the cause of upper GI bleeding in 6–34% of cases.
- **Age**
  Patients are mostly older, above 60 years, but acute gastritis can develop at any age.
- **Sex**
  No sex predilection.
- **Site**
  Stress-related ulcers develop in the fundus and corpus; NSAID-related erosions and alcoholic binge-related damage are centered in the antrum.
- **Treatment**
  Treatment should be targeted to identify and stop the offending agent. The patient may need to be stabilized using intravenous fluids and blood transfusion, H2 blockers, proton pump inhibitors, and prostaglandin analogues. Surgical intervention may be needed for stopping massive bleeding in approximately 5% of cases.
- **Outcome**
  Most cases have an uneventful course with full recovery within a short period. The outcome is greatly variable and depends on the etiologic agent involved and underlying illness of the patient. Patients with aspirin- or alcohol-induced injury usually make a quick recovery, whereas hypoperfusion-related gastritis (stress ulcer) is associated with greater morbidity and mortality. The overall mortality of acute hemorrhagic gastritis may reach up to 50% in seriously ill patients. Treatment with proton pump inhibitors or antacids has proven useful prophylactically in patients using NSAIDs.

Macroscopy

Acute gastritis is characterized grossly by hyperemic edematous mucosa with dark erosions, redness, and widespread petechial hemorrhages in any portion of the stomach or regions of confluent mucosal or submucosal bleeding. Sometimes aphthous ulcerations and rarely perforation are observed. The picture may change rapidly so that 24–48 h after bleeding has stopped the mucosa may appear normal. The pattern of distribution is related to the cause, with gastrotoxic substances as NSAIDs and ethanol causing mucosal damage predominantly in the antrum, while stress-related ulcers more often are located in the corpus or fundus region.

Microscopy

Histological findings depend on the biopsy interval. Frequent observed histological changes are dilation and congestion of mucosal capillaries, edema, interstitial hemorrhage within the lamina propria, mucosal sloughing, superficial erosions with fibrin, and usually mild neutrophilic infiltrate (Fig. 1). Regenerative changes are seen in the preexistent mucosa with elongation and tortuosity of foveolae (Fig. 2). Other regenerative features associated with healing are increased proliferation with prominent mitotic activity, hyperchromatic nuclei, prominent nucleoli, amphophilic cytoplasm, and mucin depletion. These changes should not be mistaken for dysplasia or malignancy.

Ethanol/Medicines/Drugs/Corrosive Substances

Gastric mucosal damage related to various substances and drugs is more and more commonly recognized.

- Alcohol causes direct damage to the gastric mucosa, and the amount of injury is related to the alcohol concentration obtained. Features of alcohol-induced injury range from hyperemia and petechia to necrosis and severe hemorrhage.
- Acute upper gastrointestinal bleeding with diffuse hemorrhagic and necrotic gastritis and duodenitis is described in patients using cocaine (benzoylmethylecgonine). Cocaine has systemic effects on the nervous system mediated by alterations in synaptic transmission, and activation of the sympathetic nervous system may produce intense vasoconstriction leading to ischemia and necrosis in the gastrointestinal tract.
- Aspirin and other NSAIDs may induce acute gastritis. Identified risk factors include advanced age, history of ulcer, concomitant use of corticosteroids, high doses or combined use of NSAIDs, concomitant administration of

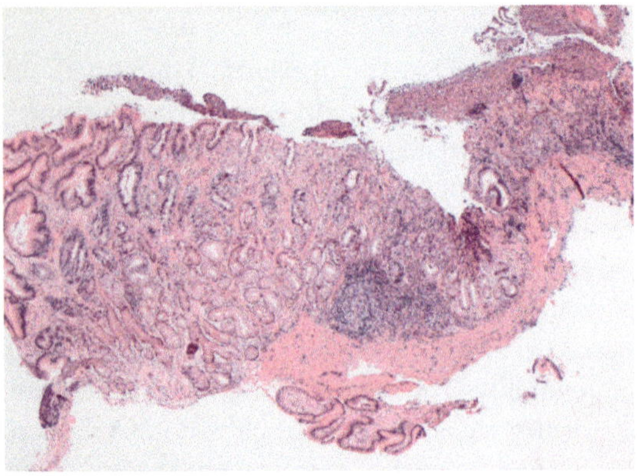

Acute Gastritis, Fig. 1 Superficial necrosis with congestion and fibrinopurulent exudate

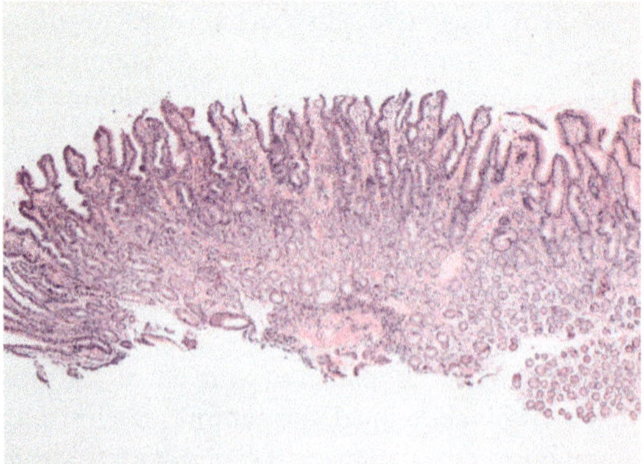

Acute Gastritis, Fig. 2 Regenerative changes with elongation and tortuosity of foveolae and mild lymphocytic inflammatory infiltrate

anticoagulants, and serious systemic disorder. Mucosal injury is initiated topically by the acidic properties of aspirin and other NSAIDs. The systemic effects of NSAIDs are largely the effect of their cyclooxygenase-inhibiting action inhibiting endogenous prostaglandin synthesis. Prostaglandin inhibition, in turn, leads to decreases in mucosal blood flow, epithelial proliferation, epithelial mucus, and secretion of bicarbonate that have protective roles on the mucosal surface. This leads to impairment in mucosal resistance and permits injury by endogenous irritants including acid, pepsin, and bile salts as well as by exogenous factors such as NSAIDs, concomitant use of ethanol, and other noxious agents. The spectrum of NSAID-related gastroduodenal injury includes subepithelial hemorrhage, erosions, and ulcerations.

– Iron pills give mucosal changes through local corrosive effects. The mechanism of injury is unclear, but it is possible that the physiological transport channels of iron are overrun and oxygen metabolites secondary to ferrous and ferric iron metabolism mediate the mucosal damage. In biopsies necrosis is seen with golden brown pigments that can be highlighted by an iron stain.
– Gastric mucosal calcinosis refers to the presence of small, pink, and calcified crystals found beneath the surface epithelium of the antrum. This is seen in posttransplant patients or chronic renal failure patients and is caused by either aluminum-containing antacids or sucralfate.
– Colchicine, used to treat a variety of medical conditions (mainly gout), leads to gastrointestinal mucosal changes when this alkaloid reaches toxic levels in patients with renal failure or impaired hepatic function. Reported histologic features in the gastric antrum and duodenum include metaphase mitoses, crypt apoptotic bodies, epithelial pseudostratification, and loss of polarity. Recognition is important since colchicine toxicity which can be fatal is undiagnosed clinically.
– Erosive or ulcerative lesions with a typical mosaic pattern of kayexalate crystals may be observed in patients using kayexalate. The cation-exchange resin kayexalate (sodium polystyrene sulfonate) is administered in a suspension with hypertonic sorbitol to patients with renal failure to treat hyperkalemia. The acute damage in the gastrointestinal tract is probably caused by the hyperosmotic action of sorbitol.
– Various chemotherapeutic agents can induce acute gastritis. In biopsies obtained from oncologic patients ulceration and striking epithelial atypia may be observed in epithelial cells, but also in stromal and endothelial cells with polymorphic nuclei and prominent nucleoli. There is usually low proliferation and a history of (recent) chemotherapy. However, it may be very difficult to differentiate between chemo-induced changes and (recurrence of) malignancy.
– Radiation therapy for upper abdominal malignancy or bone marrow radiation can induce gastric mucosal injury. Early changes involve nuclear karyorrhexis and cytoplasmic eosinophilia of the gastric pit epithelium, followed by edema, congestion, and erosion with fibrin deposition. The superficial necrosis and lamina propria hyalinization with vascular thrombi can mimic ischemic gastritis.
– Uncommonly the accidental or suicidal ingestion of corrosive substances (acid and alkali ingestion) may lead to erosive esophagitis and acute gastric injury.

Stress Ulcer

Acute gastritis is observed in patients in critical condition. Changes are mediated by ischemia related to shock with hypotension, decreased gastric mucosal blood flow, vasoconstriction, and reperfusion injury with release of free oxygen radicals. Patients occasionally exhibit both gastric and duodenal ulcers, and deep ulceration can even cause perforation of the stomach. Stress ulcers and erosions, long known to occur in severely burned persons (Curling ulcer), commonly result in bleeding, which is occasionally severe. Trauma to the central nervous system, either accidental or surgical (Cushing ulcer) is another cause of stress ulcer. Injury to the brain can lead to increased acid secretion in the stomach, presumably as a result of increased vagal tone. Severe trauma, postoperative stage, especially accompanied by shock, sepsis, and incapacitation from many debilitating chronic diseases also predispose to the development of ulcerative acute hemorrhagic gastritis. Microcirculatory changes in the stomach induced by shock or sepsis suggest that ischemic injury may contribute to the development of acute hemorrhagic gastritis. Certain types of prolonged psychological stresses have also been reported to produce erosive lesions in the stomach and duodenum.

Infectious Agents Associated with Acute Infectious Gastritis

Infection with *Helicobacter pylori* almost never elicits an acute inflammatory gastritis. Acquiring of infection with *H. pylori* is often at child age, and asymptomatic *H. pylori*-associated gastritis at later age is typically a chronic active gastritis with superficial diffuse lymphoplasmacytic and (focal) active neutrophilic infiltrate. Infectious agents causing acute inflammation can be viruses, including Cytomegalovirus characterized by focal, enlarged endothelial, stromal, or epithelial cells with owl's-eye intranuclear inclusions or intracytoplasmic inclusion bodies; herpesvirus showing epithelial cells with ground-glass nuclei and eosinophilic intranuclear inclusions surrounded by a clear halo; and Epstein-Barr virus characterized by enlarged lymph nodes. Emphysematous and acute suppurative (phlegmonous) gastritis can be caused by bacterial infections, including streptococci, *E. coli*, enterobacteria or other Gram-negative bacilli, and *Staphylococcus aureus*. Other rare infectious agents of acute inflammatory gastritis, often associated with underlying AIDS, are *Mycobacterium tuberculosis*, *actinomycosis*, *syphilis*, fungi including *Candida*, and parasitic infections such as *cryptosporidiosis, Strongyloides stercoralis*, and *anisakiasis*.

Immunophenotype

Not applicable.

Molecular Features

Not applicable.

Differential Diagnosis

- Chronic active *Helicobacter pylori*-associated gastritis and peptic ulcer are sometimes difficult to separate from acute gastritis. Features more in favor of acute hemorrhagic gastritis include relatively minimal active inflammatory infiltrate, but abundant edema, hemorrhage, patchy necrosis, and reactive epithelial changes. In extreme cases, penetrating ulcers are associated with necrosis extending through to the serosa. In most cases, there is only mild neutrophilic and mononuclear inflammation. Healing is usually complete within a few days.
- Other causes of upper gastrointestinal bleeding include bleeding from esophageal varices and Mallory-Weiss tear.
- Regenerative features can raise suspicion of dysplasia or adenocarcinoma. Features favoring true dysplastic changes include surface nuclear stratification and atypia, hyperchromasia, intestinal metaplasia, and increased mitoses.
- Commonly seen are hemorrhagic changes in biopsies due to biopsy forceps trauma; this should not be mistaken for acute hemorrhagic gastritis. In these biopsies there is no accompanying injury such as regenerative changes, necrosis, or inflammation.

References and Further Reading

Chamberlain, C. E. (1993). Acute hemorrhagic gastritis. *Gastroenterology Clinics of North America, 22*(4), 843–873.

Iacobuzio-Donahue, C. A., Lee, E. L., Abraham, S. C., Yardley, J. H., & Wu, T. T. (2001). Colchicine toxicity: Distinct morphologic findings in gastrointestinal biopsies. *The American Journal of Surgical Pathology, 25*(8), 1067–1073.

Kodali, V. P., & Gordon, S. C. (1995). Gastrointestinal hemorrhage secondary to crack cocaine. *Gastrointestinal Endoscopy, 41*(6), 604–605.

Laine, L., & Weinstein, W. M. (1988). Histology of alcoholic hemorrhagic "gastritis": A prospective evaluation. *Gastroenterology, 94*(6), 1254–1262.
Lauwers, G. Y., Fujita, H., Nagata, K., & Shimizu, M. (2010). Pathology of non-*Helicobacter pylori* gastritis: Extending the histopathologic horizons. *Journal of Gastroenterology, 45*(2), 131–145.
Srivastava, A., & Lauwers, G. Y. (2007). Pathology of non-infective gastritis. *Histopathology, 50*(1), 15–29.
Wolfe, M. M., Lichtenstein, D. R., & Singh, G. (1999). Gastrointestinal toxicity of nonsteroidal anti-inflammatory drugs. *The New England Journal of Medicine, 340*(24), 1888–1899.

Adenoacanthoma

Helena Baldaia
Serviço de Anatomia Patológica, Centro Hospitalar de São João, Porto, Portugal

Synonyms

Adenocarcinoma with squamous metaplasia

Definition

Adenoacanthomas are adenocarcinomas which contain foci of benign-appearing squamous metaplasia (Fenoglio-Preiser et al. 2008a). The literature is somewhat obscure on the subject of adenoacanthomas as this designation was previously used to refer to carcinomas with combined glandular and squamous components, regardless of the appearance (benign or malignant) of the squamous component. As such, much of the literature concerning adenoacanthomas actually describes adenosquamous carcinomas.

The origin of the squamous epithelium is subject to debate. Some authors believe that adenoacanthomas may arise from adenomas with squamous morules or squamous metaplasia (Fenoglio-Preiser et al. 2008a). A common view on the origin of neoplasias with glandular and squamous components in the colon is that they arise from direct stimulation, by repeated mucosal trauma, of uncommitted basal cells that are capable of differentiating into glandular and squamous cells (Ngo et al. 1999).

Clinical Features

- **Incidence**
  Adenoacanthomas in the gastrointestinal (GI) tract are very rare. Actually, some authors report that all forms of gastric cancer that express a squamous phenotype probably amount to less than 0.5% of gastric carcinomas. Also, adenoacanthomas account for less than 0.2% of all colonic malignancies (Fenoglio-Preiser et al. 2008b).
- **Age**
  There does not seem to exist a difference in the age spectrum regarding adenoacanthomas in relation to other adenocarcinomas (Frizelle et al. 2001).
- **Sex**
  There is no gender predilection.
- **Site**
  Adenoacanthomas have been described throughout the GI tract, in the esophagus, stomach and colon. There are some reports of adenoacanthomas occurring in the gallbladder and pancreas (Redston 2009).
- **Treatment**
  Treatment modalities do not differ from other adenocarcinomas, depending on site and stage (Redston 2009).
- **Outcome**
  The natural history of adenoacanthomas is similar to pure adenocarcinomas (Redston 2009).

Macroscopy

Adenoacanthomas are not grossly distinctive (Fenoglio-Preiser et al. 2008a). They can appear as ulcerating, polypoid or infiltrative lesions that reflect the adenocarcinoma component which is the predominant feature in these tumors.

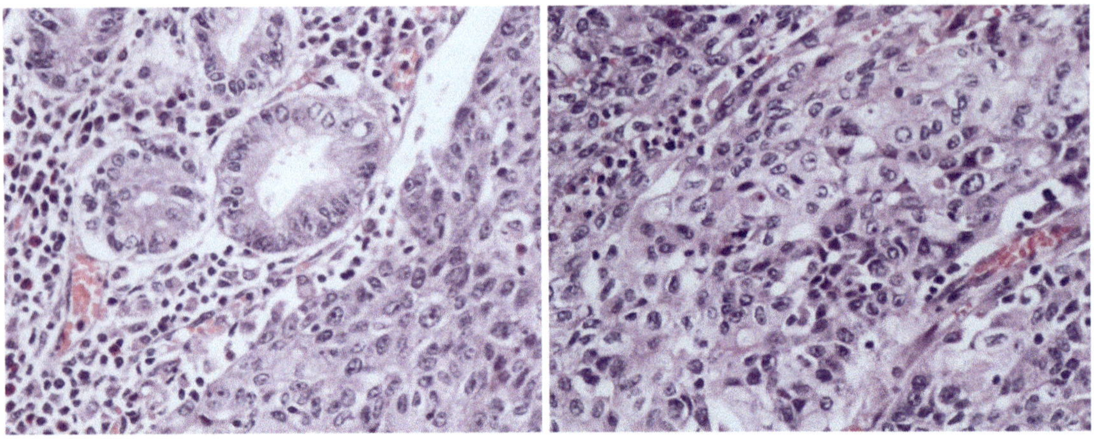

Adenoacanthoma, Fig. 1 Gastric adenocacanthoma. Adenocarcinoma tubules mixed with squamoid morules

Microscopy

Adenoacanthomas are composed of a predominant adenocarcinoma component with tubules and trabeculae of neoplastic mucin secreting cells. These are infiltrative, and show variable degrees of atypia and mitotic activity. Intermingled with the glandular component there are squamous morules, well differentiated, with frequent keratinization (Fig. 1). The squamous component does not show prominent atypical features or mitotic activity and is, on the contrary, very benign appearing and bland (Fenoglio-Preiser et al. 2008b).

Immunophenotype

Adenoacanthomas stain with keratins. The glandular and squamous components of the tumors have an immunophenotype that corresponds to their line of differentiation. The squamous component stains frequently with high molecular weight keratins. One study reported on CD44 as a marker of squamous differentiation in adenosquamous neoplasms (Ylagan et al. 2000).

Kreyberg histochemical method stains differently mucin containing adenocarcinoma cells and the squamous component.

Molecular Features

Particular molecular features of adenoacanthomas of the GI tract have not yet been published.

Differential Diagnosis

Adenoacanthomas must be distinguished from adenosquamous carcinomas, since the latter are frequently associated with a less favourable outcome (Fenoglio-Preiser et al. 2008b). Adenosquamous carcinomas are composed by glandular and prominent squamous malignant components with variable degrees of atypia and differentiation.

References and Further Reading

Fenoglio-Preiser, C. M., Noffsinger, A. E., Stemmermann, G. N., Lantz, P. E., & Isaacson, P. G. (2008a). Epithelial neolasms of the stomach. In J. McGouh & J. Pine (Eds.), *Gastrointestinal pathology an atlas and text* (p. 258). Philadelphia: Lippincott Williams & Wilkins.

Fenoglio-Preiser, C. M., Noffsinger, A. E., Stemmermann, G. N., Lantz, P. E., & Isaacson, P. G. (2008b). Epithelial neoplasms of the colon. In J. McGouh & J. Pine (Eds.), *Gastrointestinal pathology an atlas and text* (p. 981). Philadelphia: Lippincott Williams & Wilkins.

Frizelle, F. A., Hobday, K. S., Batts, K. P., & Nelson, H. (2001). Adenosquamous and squamous carcinoma of the colon and upper rectum: A clinical and histopathologic study. *Diseases of the Colon and Rectum, 44*(3), 341–346.

Ngo, N., Villamil, C., Macauley, W., & Cole, S. R. (1999). Adenosquamous carcinoma of the small intestine. Report of a case and review of the literature. *Archives of Pathology & Laboratory Medicine, 123*(8), 739–742.

Redston, M. (2009). Epithelial neoplasms of the large intestine. In R. Odze & J. Goldblum (Eds.), *Surgical pathology of the GI tract, liver, biliary tract and pancreas*. Philadelphia: Saunders.

Ylagan, L. R., Scholes, J., & Demopoulos, R. (2000). Cd44: A marker of squamous differentiation in adenosquamous neoplasms. *Archives of Pathology & Laboratory Medicine, 124*(2), 212–215.

Adenocarcinoma, Upper Gastrointestinal Tract

Chella R. S. van der Post[1] and Fátima Carneiro[2]
[1]Department of Pathology, Radboud University Medical Center, Nijmegen, The Netherlands
[2]Faculty of Medicine of Porto University, Centro Hospitalar São João and Ipatimup/i3S, Porto, Portugal

Definition

The World Health Organization (WHO) has defined "adenocarcinoma" as "a malignant epithelial tumor with glandular differentiation" (WHO 2010). Esophageal adenocarcinomas arise primarily in the lower third of the esophagus from Barrett's mucosa. Heterotopic gastric mucosa in the upper esophagus, mucosal, and submucosal glands can also give rise to adenocarcinomas of the esophagus. In the stomach, the most frequent site of "non-cardia" gastric cancer is the distal antro-pyloric region. In contrast to distal esophageal adenocarcinomas, there has been a steady decline in incidence of gastric (non-cardia) carcinoma over the last 15 years.

Adenocarcinoma of the esophagus, gastroesophageal junction (GEJ), and proximal stomach share many characteristics and risk factors. The incidence is increasing in high-resource countries; there is a high male:female ratio; and a higher incidence among whites and groups with higher socioeconomic status has been reported. In the last WHO classification, adenocarcinomas of the esophagus, gastroesophageal junction, and proximal stomach are described in separate chapters; however, since there are no universally accepted and clearly reproducible landmarks that identify the GEJ with precision, the origin of the tumor extending from the GEJ is often arbitrary. There is not a separate classification or grading system for tumors of the GEJ, but an attempt must be made to classify them into esophagus and gastric carcinomas. The seventh edition of the *AJCC Cancer Staging Manual* (TNM classification) stages them as

> Carcinomas whose epicenter is located in the lower thoracic esophagus, GEJ, or within the proximal 5 cm of the stomach that extend into the GEJ or esophagus are staged as esophageal adenocarcinomas. Tumors with an epicenter in the stomach >5 cm distal to the GEJ or within 5 cm of the GEJ but not extending into the GEJ or esophagus are staged as primary gastric carcinomas. (WHO 2010)

Barrett's esophagus has been identified as the most important precursor lesion and risk factor of developing adenocarcinoma. It results from metaplastic replacement of the normal squamous esophageal epithelium by columnar epithelium. Intestinal metaplasia of the esophagus can develop when the squamous esophageal epithelium is replaced by columnar epithelium during the process of healing after repetitive injury and is typically associated with gastroesophageal reflux disease (GERD). Intestinal metaplasia around the tumor can be detected in most patients with esophageal adenocarcinoma. Patients with Barrett's esophagus have at least a 20-fold increased risk of developing esophageal adenocarcinoma. For more information about Barrett's mucosa, the reader is referred to the entry "Barrett's esophagus." There is a three- to sixfold excess risk of developing esophageal adenocarcinoma among overweight persons. Obesity predisposes to hiatus hernia and GERD; however, a body mass index >25 itself seems to be an independent risk factor. Especially abdominal obesity is associated with malignant transformation; the factors released by centrally deposited fat may have an effect on the process of metaplasia transforming to dysplasia. Other identified predisposing factors for the development of esophageal adenocarcinoma include male gender, white race, smoking, and alcohol consumption. In countries with an increase in GERD and esophageal cancer, there has been a decrease in incidence of *H. pylori* infection. The hypochlorhydria associated with *H. pylori* and ammonia production from urea by the bacteria may protect the lower esophagus by changing the content of the gastric juice (Allum et al. 2011; Bosman et al. 2012).

Gastric cancer has a complex pathogenesis, in which several factors are involved including a familial risk and environmental factors, with the strongest known risk factor being chronic gastritis induced by *H. pylori* infection. In 1994, the WHO classified *H. pylori* as a class I carcinogen based mainly on epidemiological evidence for its role in the pathogenesis of gastric adenocarcinoma. Several bacterial virulence factors define the malignant potential of each *H. pylori* strain. *H. pylori* strains expressing all three genes CagA, VacA, and BabA are associated with the highest risk of developing gastric cancer.

Esophageal adenocarcinomas have typically a papillary and/or tubular growth pattern. Gastric carcinomas are divided into five main categories according to the WHO classification. These are termed tubular, papillary, mucinous, poorly cohesive (including signet ring cell type), and mixed carcinomas. For more detailed information of tubular, papillary, mucinous, and signet ring cell carcinoma of the stomach, the reader is referred to these separate entries. Besides adenocarcinoma and squamous carcinoma of the esophagus and the five main categories of gastric carcinomas, other uncommon histological variants represent less than 5% of upper gastrointestinal carcinomas. These include adenosquamous carcinoma, adenoid cystic carcinoma, mucoepidermoid carcinoma, hepatoid adenocarcinoma, carcinoma with lymphoid stroma, carcinosarcoma, parietal cell carcinoma, malignant rhabdoid tumor, undifferentiated carcinoma, mixed adenoneuroendocrine carcinomas, choriocarcinoma, embryonal carcinoma, and pure gastric yolk sac tumor (WHO 2010). Clinical and histological features of some of these uncommon histological upper gastrointestinal carcinomas are discussed beneath the section "Microscopy."

Clinical Features

Clinical manifestations of esophageal cancer include dysphagia, heartburn, retrosternal pain, and loss of body weight irrespective of histological subtype. Gastric cancer often presents with loss of appetite, epigastric pain, nausea, melena, and loss of body weight.

- **Incidence**
  The incidence and prevalence of esophageal adenocarcinoma has risen during the last decades of the twentieth century in developed countries and is the fastest growing cause of cancer mortality. An estimated 456,000 esophageal cancer cases and 400,000 deaths occurred in 2012. A large proportion are squamous cell carcinomas, especially in Asian countries. Esophageal adenocarcinoma is now relatively common in Europe and the USA, while it remains rare in Africa, Asia and Latin America. Most adenocarcinomas of the esophagus arise in the setting of Barrett's esophagus, and often areas of dysplastic Barrett mucosa will be found near the carcinoma. Barrett's esophagus affects approximately 2% of the population in developed countries and is strongly associated with GERD. In developing countries this incidence is increasing. The incidence of esophageal adenocarcinoma was estimated at 1–5 per 100,000 individuals per year in Europa and North America. The countries with the highest incidence are the United Kingdom, Australia, the Netherlands and the USA. There have been parallel increases in adenocarcinoma of the gastric cardia, which now accounts for approximately 50% of all gastric cancers. The incidence of non-cardia carcinoma of the stomach has been declining the last 15 years; however the absolute rate

continues to rise, presumably due to the advancing age of the global population. A total of 952,000 new gastric cancer cases and 723,000 deaths are estimated to have occurred in 2012. Gastric cancer (GC) is the fifth leading cause of cancer globally and ranks third in terms of cancer-related mortality. Over 70% of new cases and death occur in developing countries. The highest incidence rates are in Eastern Asia, Eastern Europe and Latin America. Uncommon histological variants represent less than 5% of upper gastrointestinal carcinomas, while exact incidence numbers are not known of every histological subtype (Ferlay et al. 2013).

- **Age**
  Incidences of esophageal and gastric cancer increase progressively with age and are rare in persons younger than 30 years. The peak age group is between 50 and 60 years of age, and this seems to be the same for the more uncommon histological variant of upper gastrointestinal carcinoma.
- **Sex**
  In both gastric and esophageal adenocarcinoma, men are more affected than women; the male to female ratio varies between 2:1 and 12:1 (Allum et al. 2011; Ferlay et al. 2013; Parkin, Bray, Ferlay, & Pisani, 2005).
- **Site**
  Esophageal adenocarcinomas arise primarily in the lower third of the esophagus in a segment of columnar-lined esophagus. It develops most commonly in the distal region of Barrett's mucosa with intestinal metaplasia. Heterotopic gastric mucosa in the upper esophagus, mucosal, and submucosal glands can also give rise to adenocarcinomas of the esophagus. In the stomach, the most frequent site of "noncardia" gastric cancer is the distal antro-pyloric region.
- **Treatment**
  Esophageal Cancer

  Endoscopic mucosal resection is indicated for early, well-, or moderately differentiated cancer (T1N0) and mucosal dysplasia. There are now consistent reports indicating a 5-year disease-free survival of 95% and a low morbidity rate. Localized therapy can result in the development of metachronous cancer in up to 30% of patients with Barrett's esophagus. This recurrence rate can be reduced by ablation of the remaining Barrett's epithelium.

  Preoperative neoadjuvant chemotherapy and radiotherapy followed by local esophagectomy is the preferred treatment in advanced esophageal adenocarcinoma. Preoperative chemoradiation improves long-term survival over surgery alone. Chemotherapy regimen includes cisplatin and 5-fluorouracil (5-FU). The location, extent of the proposed lymphadenectomy, patient factors, and the experience of the surgeon should determine the operative approach. The operative strategy should ensure that adequate longitudinal and radial resection margins are achieved with lymphadenectomy appropriate to the location. Palliative options include brachytherapy and/or chemotherapy to provide symptom relief in inoperable or metastatic esophageal cancer. Esophageal intubation with a self-expanding stent is the treatment of choice for firm stenosing tumors (Allum et al. 2011).

  Gastric Cancer

  Radical surgery represents the standard form of curative therapy aiming to excise the primary tumor with clear longitudinal and circumferential margins. Early, limited gastric mucosal cancer can be treated with endoscopic mucosal or submucosal dissection. Advanced carcinomas should be treated according to the location, distally by subtotal gastrectomy and proximally by total gastrectomy. Cardia tumors should be treated by transhiatal extended total gastrectomy or esophagogastrectomy. The extent of lymphadenectomy should be tailored to the age and fitness of the patient together with the location and stage of the cancer. The distal pancreas, spleen, and splenic nodes should be removed only when there is direct invasion and still a chance of a curative procedure in patients with carcinoma of the proximal stomach. In a palliative setting, limited gastric resection or a stent in patients with gastric outlet obstruction can be considered. Perioperative (neoadjuvant and adjuvant) combination chemotherapy conveys a significant survival benefit and is a standard of care. Accepted perioperative regimens are ECF (epirubicin, cisplatin, and 5-FU) or ECX (epirubicin, cisplatin, and capecitabine); trastuzumab in combination with cisplatin/fluoropyrimidine should be considered for patients with *ERBB2/HER2-neu*-positive gastric carcinoma (Allum et al. 2011).

- **Outcome**
  Prognosis is dependent on whether the intent is curative or palliative, and this depends on the depth of mural invasion and the presence of lymph node or distant metastases. Furthermore, for surgery, there is a strong relationship between lower hospital mortality and increasing surgeon experience and institutional patient volumes.

  Esophageal carcinoma is often diagnosed at a late stage, despite the established association with the precursor Barrett's esophagus. Up to 50–60% of patients develop invasive adenocarcinoma within 3–5 years of a diagnosis of high-grade dysplastic esophageal epithelium. In Barrett's esophagus, there is often duplication of the muscularis mucosae. Cancers infiltrating between the inner and outer muscularis mucosae are considered to be intramucosal cancer, but they have a higher frequency of angiolymphatic invasion and lymph node metastases compared with those that are limited to the original lamina propria.

  The prognosis of early gastric cancer is good; however, this is predominantly seen in Asian countries, owing to active screening programs. In Western countries, approximately 80–90% of patients are diagnosed at an advanced stage with high recurrence rates after curative intent therapy. The prognosis for advanced gastric cancer remains poor, with reported 1-year and 5-year survival rates of 42% and 24%, respectively.

Macroscopy

Esophageal carcinomas usually arise in the distal third of the esophagus. Endoscopically early-stage carcinoma is difficult to assess and to distinguish from high-grade dysplasia which is often multicentric present. Early-invasive carcinomas are often small, flat, depressed, whitish lesions. Advanced adenocarcinoma is often seen as an axial, tight stenosis in the distal third of the esophagus with a polypoid tumor. Since preoperative neoadjuvant chemotherapy and radiotherapy is the preferred treatment in advanced esophageal adenocarcinoma, followed by local esophagectomy, pathologists increasingly face resection specimens without macroscopically identifiable carcinoma.

The growth pattern of advanced gastric carcinoma is commonly described according to the Borrmann classification, subdividing polypoid (type I), fungating (type II), ulcerating (type III), and diffusely infiltrating (type IV) growth patterns. Most common are the fungating and ulcerating type and associated with an intestinal-type carcinoma histologically. Diffuse carcinomas show the diffusely infiltrating growth pattern or linitis plastica in advanced stage. Mucinous adenocarcinomas have a gelatinous aspect.

Microscopy

Esophageal adenocarcinomas appear as other adenocarcinomas and are composed of irregular glands with a tubular or papillary growth pattern. Most adenocarcinomas are well or moderately differentiated with well-formed glands (intestinal type, according to the Laurén classification). Glandular structures are only slightly formed in poorly differentiated adenocarcinomas and absent in undifferentiated tumors. A minority of cases is of the diffuse type with signet ring cells. Sometimes there are scattered endocrine cells, Paneth cells, or leaks of mucin. Subclassifying of esophageal adenocarcinomas has no practical, therapeutic, or prognostic value.

Early carcinomas in Barrett's esophagus are mostly well- or moderately differentiated carcinomas. Poorly differentiated carcinomas are rare. The distinction between high-grade dysplasia and early invasive (intramucosal) carcinoma remains difficult. Features of invasive carcinoma include a syncytial growth pattern,

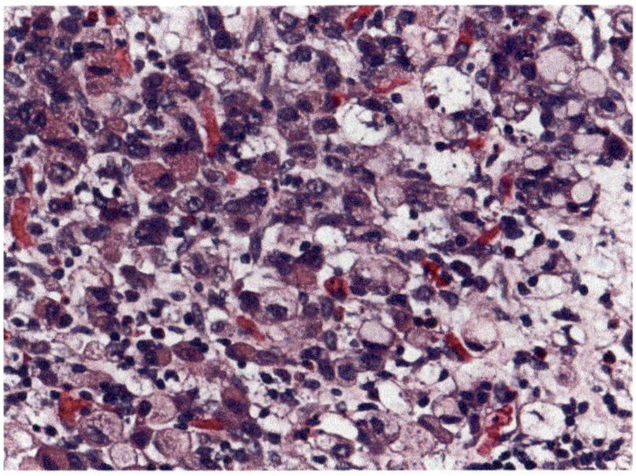

Adenocarcinoma, Upper Gastrointestinal Tract, Fig. 1 Poorly cohesive carcinoma composed of a combined cellular infiltrate with classic signet ring cells and more pleomorphic cells (H&E, original magnification 400×)

micro-glands, and single cells in the lamina propria and irregular cells with prominent nucleoli. Current information in literature regarding the risk for regional lymphogenic metastatic spread identify low-risk and high-risk groups based on histological evaluation (Stolte and Dostler 2012).

Gastric carcinomas are often subdivided into intestinal or diffuse carcinomas (with the Laurén classification) or tubular, papillary, mucinous, poorly cohesive, and mixed carcinomas according to the WHO classification (see also these separate entries for more information). Tubular adenocarcinoma is composed of dilated, irregular tubules of varying diameter surrounded by desmoplastic stroma. Papillary adenocarcinoma is characterized by exophytic projections lined by cuboidal neoplastic cells. Mucinous adenocarcinoma shows more than 50% extracellular mucin with irregular neoplastic glands and/or scattered signet ring cells in these mucin leaks. Poorly cohesive carcinomas are composed of isolated pleomorphic cells often combined with classic signet ring cells (Fig. 1). A tumor predominantly more than 50% or exclusively composed of signet ring cells is defined as a signet ring cell carcinoma. Mixed carcinomas are composed of a mixture of tubular/papillary and poorly cohesive histological components.

Other Upper Gastrointestinal Adenocarcinomas

Mucoepidermoid carcinoma, which is characterized by a mixture of mucus-secreting glandular, intermediate, and epidermoid/squamous cells, is the most common malignant neoplasm of salivary glands but relatively uncommon in the esophagus. Mucoepidermoid carcinomas are most often found in the middle and lower third of the thoracic esophagus, with a median length of 5.0 cm. Macroscopically, mucoepidermoid carcinoma is indistinguishable from pure squamous cell carcinoma. The origin of primary esophageal mucoepidermoid carcinoma is believed to arise from the esophageal gland cells or ductal cells. This is supported by the embryological similar origin of the esophageal and salivary glands. The location of the tumor is often submucosal. However, there is also evidence that the tumor originates from squamous epithelial cells, since mucoepidermoid carcinomas of the esophagus have a different behavior compared to the counterparts of the salivary glands. And most mucoepidermoid carcinomas also show metaplastic changes in surrounding squamous epithelium. The diagnosis of primary mucoepidermoid carcinoma of the esophagus is prone to be misdiagnosed by endoscopic biopsy (Chen et al. 2011). Periodic acid-Schiff (PAS) and alcian blue stains are positive in the mucus and mucus-secreting cells. In the squamous regions, there are intercellular bridges, dyskeratotic cells, and pearl keratinization. Primary esophageal mucoepidermoid carcinoma is rare, accounting for less than 1% of all cases of primary esophageal carcinoma. The median survival time of patients with mucoepidermoid carcinoma reported by Chen et al. was 29.0 months (95% confidence interval 20.0–38.0). The 1- and 5-year overall survival rates were 80.6% and 25.8%, respectively. Also in other reports the survival rates are lower than for patients with squamous cell carcinoma, maybe caused by its clinicopathological aggressive behavior. Lymph node metastasis and operation type are independent prognostic factors; adjuvant radiotherapy has probably little effect.

Adenosquamous carcinomas have a slight predominance of the middle thoracic esophagus.

Macroscopically the tumor presents often as ulcerative and infiltrating. Mean diameter is 3.5 cm. Adenosquamous carcinoma of the esophagus and stomach contains mixed elements of infiltrating squamous cell carcinoma and adenocarcinoma. The WHO states that adenosquamous carcinoma has a significant squamous carcinomatous part intermingled with tubular adenocarcinoma. The Japanese Society for esophageal diseases has defined adenosquamous carcinoma as a combination of at least 20% of each subtype. The squamous cell carcinoma is usually the predominant component of the tumor. Adenocarcinoma can be more often identified in the deeper portions of the tumor, while squamous cell carcinoma dominates in the mucosa. In preoperative biopsies the tumor is therefore often misnamed as a squamous cell carcinoma. In the esophagus, the adenocarcinoma component may originate from the esophageal glands and their ducts; however, in the underlying esophageal glands, there was no cellular atypia in the series of Yachida et al. Also in rats that do not have esophageal submucosal glands, adenosquamous carcinoma can be induced. Therefore it is most likely that glandular differentiation in the deep part of adenosquamous tumors originates from the covering squamous epithelium (Yachida et al. 2004). Adenosquamous carcinoma is distinguished from mucoepidermoid carcinoma by the presence of marked nuclear pleomorphism, occasional keratin pearls, and the anatomical separation of the two components within the tumor. Esophageal adenosquamous carcinoma has an incidence of less than 1% of all cases of primary esophageal carcinomas. Yachida et al. reported a better outcome for patients with adenosquamous carcinoma compared to squamous cell carcinoma or adenocarcinoma, with 5-year survival rate of 63.6%. This is probably due to their smaller size and lower stage at presentation. Adenosquamous carcinoma of the stomach is very rare, accounting for fewer than 0.5% of all gastric cancers.

Adenoid cystic carcinoma is most often found in the minor salivary glands (60%); other sites of occurrence include the tracheobronchial tree, breast, lacrimal gland, female genital tract, and esophagus. Esophageal adenoid cystic carcinoma accounts for 0.1% of esophageal malignancies. Adenoid cystic carcinomas present as a fungating or polypoid mass rather than an ulcerative or infiltrative growth pattern. They have most frequently been reported in the middle third of the esophagus (63%). It probably arises from esophageal glands. The irregular glands contain two main cell types: duct-lining epithelial cells and myoepithelial cells; their growth pattern is cribriform, tubular, or basaloid/solid. Nests of cells with cylindromatous microcystic spaces characterize the cribriform pattern. In the tubular subtype, inner epithelial and outer myoepithelial cells line well-formed ducts and tubules with central lumina. These are filled with hyaline mucoid material. The solid or basaloid type consists of sheets of uniform basaloid cells lacking tubular or microcystic formation. The basaloid type (also called basaloid squamous cell carcinoma) has a worse prognosis. The presence of associated squamous carcinoma in situ is a strong argument for basaloid carcinoma. Immunohistochemical positive stains including epithelial membrane antigen, CEA, and keratin stains are focally positive, especially in cells around tubular and cribriform structures. Solid areas stain with S100 antibodies. The 5-year survival of adenoid cystic carcinoma is approximately 35%. Eighty to ninety percent of patients with adenoid cystic carcinoma in the salivary glands die within 10–15 years. Adenoid cystic carcinoma is known to be a slowly growing epithelial tumor in the salivary glands. Spread to the lymph nodes is uncommon; however, distant spread to lungs, liver, and bones is frequent. Its clinical behavior is characterized by a high rate of local recurrence and distant metastasis even after aggressive surgical treatment (Na et al. 2007).

Hepatoid adenocarcinoma can originate in different organs, for instance, the stomach, gallbladder, colon, lung, and urinary bladder; however, the majority originates in the stomach and reported incidence among gastric adenocarcinoma cases ranged from 0.3% to 1%. Clinical features include old age (mean 65 years), male gender (male:female ratio is 2.3:1), aggressive clinical course, poor survival, and frequent metastasis including the lymph nodes, liver, and lung.

An important finding is elevated serum alpha-fetoprotein (AFP), which is measurable in most patients and ranged in literature from less than 1.0 to 475,000 ng/mL. Hepatoid adenocarcinoma is composed of large polygonal eosinophilic hepatocyte-like neoplastic cells with a trabecular or glandular growth pattern. The polygonal cells may also be arranged in solid nests or sheets with scattered large pleomorphic or multinucleated giant cells. Distinguishing between hepatoid adenocarcinoma and hepatocellular carcinoma is important for therapeutic strategies and prognostic factors. However, due to similar clinicopathological features, it may be impossible to make this distinction, especially when liver and gastric tumors are found simultaneously. A panel of immunohistochemical stains can help in the differentiation. In favor of hepatoid adenocarcinoma are positive staining of AFP, CEA, CK18, CK19, pancytokeratin stain AE1/AE3, CK7, CDX-2, α1-antitrypsin stain, CD10, and glypican-3 (GPC-3). Promising seems to be PLUNC staining in hepatoid adenocarcinoma, which is reported negative in hepatocellular carcinoma. Especially positive staining of Hep Par 1 is more in favor of hepatocellular carcinoma. Bile and PAS-positive and diastase-resistant intracytoplasmic eosinophilic globules can be observed in hepatoid gastric carcinoma (Su et al. 2013).

Parietal cell carcinoma or oncocytic adenocarcinoma of the stomach is a well- to moderately differentiated tubular adenocarcinomas and consists of cells with eosinophilic, finely granular cytoplasm resembling parietal cells of gastric fundic mucosa. On ultrastructural examination these cells have numerous mitochondria, intracytoplasmic secretory canaliculi, and cytoplasmic tubulovesicles. Tumor cells are strongly positive with antimitochondrial antibody stains. Parietal cell carcinoma is very rare, with only few case reports in literature. It has been suggested that these tumors have a better prognosis than usual gastric adenocarcinoma (Takubo et al. 2002).

Gastric cancers with germ cell tumor components are uncommon and consist purely or of a mixture of adenocarcinoma with choriocarcinoma, yolk sac tumor, or embryonal carcinoma. Primary gastric chorioadenocarcinoma is characterized by an elevated serum beta-human chorionic gonadotropin (ß-HCG) which causes symptoms as morning sickness and gynecomastia. Macroscopically these tumors are hemorrhagic, highly vascular, and exophytic. The tumor consists of gastric adenocarcinoma cells with glandular differentiation and a choriocarcinomatous component of malignant cytotrophoblast and syncytiotrophoblast cells that shows positive immunohistochemical staining for ß-HCG. Less than 25% of cases are pure choriocarcinoma. Due to a mixture of adenocarcinoma and choriocarcinomatous component, gastric choriocarcinoma is often misdiagnosed as adenocarcinoma on biopsies. Intratumoral hemorrhage, necrosis, and vascular invasion are often observed (Dye et al. 2005; Kobayashi et al. 2005; Shastri et al. 2011). Gastric carcinomas with yolk sac components are sporadically reported and have a poor prognosis due to widespread metastases at the time of presentation. Yolk sac tumor has the features of an endodermal sinus tumor and is characterized by a reticular growth pattern (clear-cell endoblastic pattern) with glomerulus-like structures (Schiller-Duval bodies). The serum AFP levels are commonly high, and AFP is positive immunohistochemically within the tumor (Kim et al. 2009).

Carcinosarcoma consists of both carcinomatous and sarcomatous components. In the gastrointestinal tract, this tumor is most frequently seen in the esophagus and rarely in the stomach. Esophageal carcinosarcoma has also been referred to as sarcomatoid carcinoma, pseudosarcoma, pseudosarcomatous squamous cell carcinoma, spindle cell carcinoma, and polypoid carcinoma. Esophageal carcinosarcoma often presents as a large intraluminal polypoid mass and has a more favorable prognosis than other esophageal malignancies, probably because of its exophytic growth. It represents approximately 2% of all esophageal carcinomas. Histologically these carcinosarcomas are biphasic with a small epithelial component, while the bulk of the tumor has a pleomorphic sarcomatoid appearance. The epithelial component is usually squamous and ranges from focal areas with in situ carcinoma to infiltrating nests. The sarcomatous component is

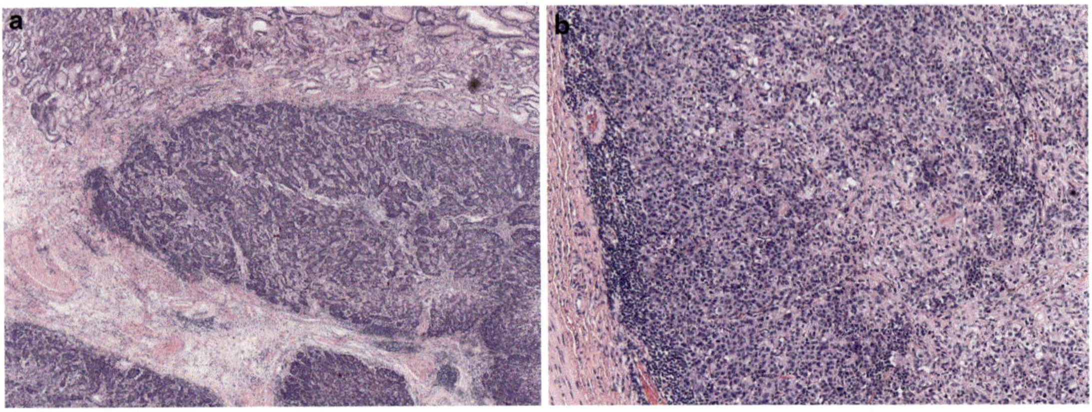

Adenocarcinoma, Upper Gastrointestinal Tract, Fig. 2 (**a**) Medullary gastric carcinoma with a submucosal growth pattern. (H&E, original magnification 25×); (**b**) Detail of a medullary gastric carcinoma. There is a pushing border with peri-tumoral lymphocytic infiltrate (H&E, original magnification 100×)

composed of undifferentiated, spindle-shaped cells arranged in a fascicular or storiform pattern. There can be differentiation with bizarre giant cells, osseous, cartilaginous, and rhabdomyoblastic cells (Raza and Mazzara 2011). In the stomach the epithelial component is composed of tubular or papillary adenocarcinoma with sometimes neuroendocrine carcinomatous differentiation. The mesenchymal sarcomatous component is variable and, as for the esophagus, may include leiomyosarcoma, rhabdomyosarcoma, osteosarcoma, or chondrosarcoma. Only approximately 50 cases have been reported of gastric carcinosarcoma, mainly in the Japanese literature. The epithelial component is cytokeratin, EMA, CEA positive, whereas the mesenchymal component shows strong immunoreactivity with vimentin, desmin, and α-smooth muscle actin (Cirocchi et al. 2012).

Extrarenal, primary malignant rhabdoid tumor of the stomach and the esophagus is rare with only a few case reports and associated with poor prognosis. These tumors share similar features with renal rhabdoid tumors with a typical rhabdoid morphology. The cells contain inclusion-like masses of densely acidophilic, homogeneous cytoplasmic material that displaces the nucleus toward the periphery of the cell. There are often giant multinuclear cells. The most consistent positive immunohistochemical marker is vimentin (Geramizadeh et al. 2010; Ng et al. 2003).

Gastric carcinoma with lymphoid stroma (lymphoepithelioma-like carcinoma or medullary carcinoma) is characterized by an organoid, solid, sheetlike, or trabecular pattern with a prominent lymphoid infiltration of the stroma. The etiology of gastric carcinomas with lymphoid stroma has been linked to microsatellite instability (and then called medullary carcinoma) or to Epstein-Barr virus (lymphoepithelioma-like cancer). In the stomach MSI and EBV are mutually exclusive, and it has been suggested that there are morphologic differences to distinguish lymphoepithelioma-like carcinoma from medullary carcinoma. Medullary carcinomas are organoid, syncytial, and sheetlike with a pushing non-infiltrative tumor front with a dense peri-tumoral lymphocytic infiltrate (Figs. 2a and 2b). Lymphoepithelioma-like carcinoma on the other hand is composed of single cells, small clusters of cells, and small glands with an infiltrative growth pattern and a dense intratumoral lymphoid infiltrate (Figs. 3a and 3b). These tumors frequently affect the proximal stomach or gastric stump and are more common in males, and >80% are associated with infection with Epstein-Barr virus (EBV). Both are associated with a more favorable prognosis than usual gastric adenocarcinoma (Chetty 2012).

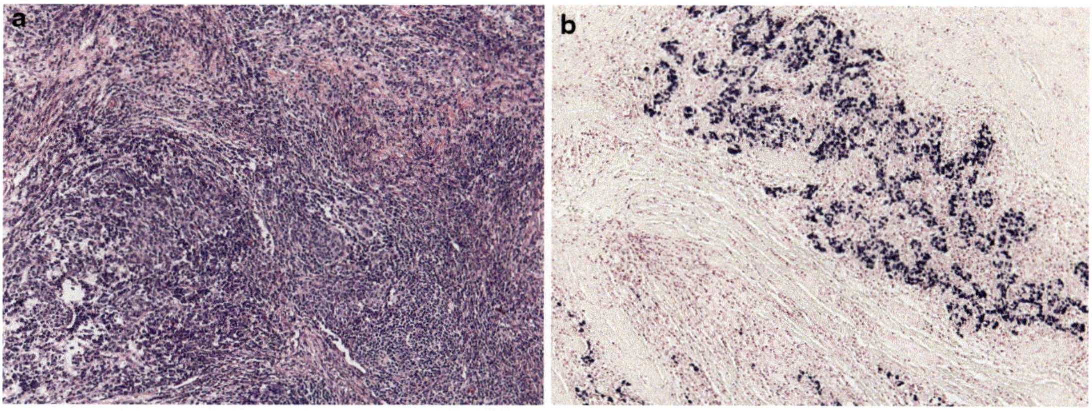

Adenocarcinoma, Upper Gastrointestinal Tract, Fig. 3 (**a**) Lymphoepithelioma-like carcinoma is composed of single cells, small clusters of cells and glands with an infiltrative growth pattern, and a dense intratumoral lymphoid infiltrate (H&E, original magnification 100×); (**b**) Lymphoepithelioma-like carcinoma is associated with Epstein-Barr virus (EBV) infection. (ISH EBER, original magnification 100×)

Immunophenotype

Gastric and esophageal adenocarcinomas are positive for pankeratin staining with varying degrees of CK7 and CK20 positivity. CK18 or CAM5.2 are most often negative. The majority of gastric carcinomas express Hep Par 1, heterogeneous CDX-2, MUC2, and MUC5AC.

See the description of relevant immunohistochemical markers of separate histological subtypes under "Microscopy."

Molecular Features

In the development and progression of adenocarcinoma there are multiple genetic alterations identified in tumor suppressor genes, oncogenes, growth factor receptors, signal transduction genes, or enzymes functioning in cell-cycle control, apoptosis, cell signaling or cell adhesion. The main genetic alterations in esophageal adenocarcinomas are found in the *TP53, CDKN2A, SMAD4, PIK3CA, CCND1, ERBB2/HER2-neu, EGFR, KRAS, PTGS2, AMACR* and *IMP3* genes. Recent exome studies also added mutations in chromatin modifying factors and candidate contributors: *SPG20, TLR4, ELMO1* and *DOCK2* (Dulak et al. 2013). Loss and gains of several chromosomal loci have been identified. The majority of studies demonstrate gains in the region of 8q, 6p, 10q and 20q, and losses at 3p, 4q, 5q and 18q. Considerable negative prognostic impact has been demonstrated for *ERBB2/HER2-neu* amplification or overexpression, *TP53* mutations, expression of *COX2, PRAP1/UPA* and *MMP1* and DNA ploidy. NFκB expression is also associated with negative clinical outcome. MicroRNAs are a class of small noncoding regulatory RNAs that play a major role in the pathogenesis of cancer. Dysregulation of micro-RNA expression has been identified to contribute to the development of cancer through altering processes as proliferation, apoptosis, invasion, and metastasis. In Barrett's esophagus, decreased expression of miR-31 and miR-375 is involved in progression to esophageal cancer (Leidner et al. 2012; WHO 2010).

Chromosomal instability also manifests in gastric cancer as gain or loss of whole chromosomes (aneuploidy) or parts of chromosomes (loss of heterozygosity, translocations and amplifications). Comparative genomic hybridization analysis has revealed many DNA copy number variations. In gastric cancer decreased levels of miR-451 and miR-485 have been described. The miR-200 family is important in the epithelial-mesenchymal transition in advanced gastric cancer (Thiel and Ristimaki 2012). Microsatellite instability is seen in 15–20% of intestinal-type gastric cancers, with a higher frequency in familial cases. Mutations in oncogenes include *KRAS* in intestinal-type gastric cancer and overexpression of *ERBB2/HER2-neu*, a cell surface receptor of the tyrosine kinase family. Tumor suppressor genes *TP53, PTEN, RUNX3* are frequently inactivated in gastric carcinomas. Studies applying exome sequencing identified frequent somatic mutations in the *ARID1A* gene which is involved in processes of DNA repair, differentiation, development and has a regulatory role in proliferation. Other identified mutated driver genes involved in gastric tumorigenesis are *PIK3CA, APC, STK11, CTNNB1, CDKN2A, ERBB2/HER2-neu, EGFR, FGFR2, MUC6, CTNNA2, GLI3, RNF43* (Zang et al. 2012; Wang et al. 2014). The most important described genetic pathway for diffuse gastric cancer is the loss of function of E-cadherin. Diffuse-type or signet ring cell carcinomas have been considered to start developing through the loss of function of the *CDH1* gene encoding for E-cadherin, a transmembrane glycoprotein involved in cell-cell adhesion. In recent next generation studies also *RHOA* mutations (normally functions in mediating anoikis) were frequently specifically found in diffuse-type tumors (Kakiuchi et al. 2014; Wang et al. 2014).

The *Cancer Genome Atlas* recently proposed a molecular classification dividing gastric adenocarcinomas into four molecular subtypes, namely:

- Epstein-Barr virus-infected tumors (10% of the subtypes), which contained recurrent *PIK3CA* mutations, DNA hypermethylation and amplification of *JAK2, ERBB2/HER2-neu, PD-L1* (*CD274*) and *PD-L2* (*PDCD1LG2*). These tumors were most frequently found in the gastric fundus or body;
- Microsatellite unstable tumors (20% of the subtypes), which had elevated mutation rates including the genes *PIK3CA, ERBB3, ERBB2/HER2-neu* and *EGFR*;
- Chromosomally unstable tumors (50% of the subtypes), which show frequent *TP53* mutations, marked aneuploidy and focal amplification of receptor tyrosine kinases. These tumors were of intestinal-type histology. Oesophageal adenocarcinomas strongly resembled the chromosomally unstable variant of gastric adenocarcinoma, suggesting that these cancers could be considered a single disease entity. However, some molecular features, including DNA hypermethylation, occurred disproportionally in oesophageal adenocarcinomas;
- Genomically stable tumors (20% of the subtypes), which are enriched for the diffuse-type histology and harbored mutations of *CDH1* and *RHO* family genes (including often *RHOA*)

Further integrated molecular and histological research may lead to a robust molecular classification that may serve as a valuable adjunct to histopathology (Cancer Genome Atlas Research).

Differential Diagnosis

An attempt should be made to distinguish the different subtypes of gastrointestinal carcinomas since they are often associated with important prognostic, therapeutic, or etiological factors. For example, medullary and lymphoepithelioma-like carcinomas of the gastrointestinal tract have slightly different morphological criteria and are associated with distinct molecular pathways.

The distinction between high-grade dysplasia and early-invasive adenocarcinoma can be sometimes very difficult.

In rare histological subtypes, the distinction between primary and metastatic disease should be made, for instance, for hepatocellular carcinoma and hepatoid adenocarcinoma and the same for primary gastric chorioadenocarcinoma and metastatic trophoblastic tumor, particularly gonadal or gestational primaries in women of reproductive age.

References and Further Reading

Allum, W. H., Blazeby, J. M., Griffin, S. M., Cunningham, D., Jankowski, J. A., & Wong, R. (2011). Guidelines for the management of oesophageal and gastric cancer. *Gut, 60*(11), 1449–1472.

Bosman, F. T., Carneiro, F., Hruban, R. H., & Theise, N. D. (2012). *WHO Classification of Tumours of the Digestive System* (4th ed.). IARC Science Publication.

Chen, S., Chen, Y., Yang, J., Yang, W., Weng, H., Li, H., et al. (2011). Primary mucoepidermoid carcinoma of the esophagus. *Journal of Thoracic Oncology, 6*(8), 1426–1431.

Chetty, R. (2012). Gastrointestinal cancers accompanied by a dense lymphoid component: An overview with special reference to gastric and colonic medullary and lymphoepithelioma-like carcinomas. *Journal of Clinical Pathology, 65*(12), 1062–1065.

Cirocchi, R., Trastulli, S., Desiderio, J., Grassi, V., Barillaro, I., Santoro, A., et al. (2012). Gastric carcinosarcoma: A case report and review of the literature. *Oncology Letters, 4*(1), 53–57.

Dye, D. W., Broadwater, R., & Lamps, L. W. (2005). Uncommon malignancies: Case 2. Gastric choriocarcinoma. *Journal of Clinical Oncology, 23*(25), 6251–6253.

Ferlay, J., Ervik, M., Dikshit, R., Eser, S., Mathers, C., Rebelo, M., et al. (2013). GLOBOCAN 2012 v1.0, cancer incidence and mortality worldwide: IARC CancerBase No. 11. from http://globocan.iarc.fr

Geramizadeh, B., Nikeghbalian, S., & Abolghasem-Hosseini, S. (2010). Primary malignant rhabdoid tumor of the stomach, a rare case report and review of literature. *Journal of Gastrointestinal Cancer, 41*(4), 269–271.

Kakiuchi, M., Nishizawa, T., Ueda, H., Gotoh, K., Tanaka, A., Hayashi, A., et al. (2014). Recurrent gain-of-function mutations of RHOA in diffuse-type gastric carcinoma. *Nat Genet, 46*(6), 583–587.

Kim, Y. S., Kim, S. H., Seong, J. K., Lee, B. S., Jeong, H. Y., & Song, K. S. (2009). Gastric yolk sac tumor: A case report and review of the literature. *The Korean Journal of Internal Medicine, 24*(2), 143–146.

Kobayashi, A., Hasebe, T., Endo, Y., Sasaki, S., Konishi, M., Sugito, M., et al. (2005). Primary gastric choriocarcinoma: Two case reports and a pooled analysis of 53 cases. *Gastric Cancer, 8*(3), 178–185.

Na, Y. J., Shim, K. N., Kang, M. J., Jung, J. M., Ha, C. Y., Jung, H. S., et al. (2007). Primary esophageal adenoid cystic carcinoma. *Gut and Liver, 1*(2), 178–181.

Ng, W. C., Leong, H. T., Ma, K. F., Yip, W. L., & Suen, W. M. (2003). Malignant rhabdoid tumour of the oesophagus: A case report. *Journal of Clinical Pathology, 56*(9), 713–714.

Parkin, D. M., Bray, F., Ferlay, J., & Pisani, P. (2005). Global cancer statistics, 2002. *CA: A Cancer Journal for Clinicians, 55*(2), 74–108.

Raza, M. A., & Mazzara, P. F. (2011). Sarcomatoid carcinoma of esophagus. *Archives of Pathology & Laboratory Medicine, 135*(7), 945–948.

Shastri, A., Daver, N. G., & Hayes, T. G. (2011). Primary gastric chorioadenocarcinoma: A needle in a haystack. *Rare Tumors, 3*(2), e19.

Stolte, M., & Dostler, I. (2012). Good handling and pathological examination of endoscopic resections of early Barrett's cancer. *Diagnostic Histopathology, 18*(21), 498–502.

Su, J. S., Chen, Y. T., Wang, R. C., Wu, C. Y., Lee, S. W., & Lee, T. Y. (2013). Clinicopathological characteristics in the differential diagnosis of hepatoid adenocarcinoma: A literature review. *World Journal of Gastroenterology, 19*(3), 321–327.

Takubo, K., Honma, N., Sawabe, M., Arai, T., Izumiyama-Shimomura, N., Kammori, M., et al. (2002). Oncocytic adenocarcinoma of the stomach: Parietal cell carcinoma. *The American Journal of Surgical Pathology, 26*(4), 458–465.

The Cancer Genome Atlas Research Network (2017). Integrated genomic characterization of oesophageal carcinoma. *Nature, 541*, 169–175.

Thiel, A., & Ristimaki, A. (2012). Gastric cancer: Basic aspects. *Helicobacter, 17*(Suppl 1), 26–29.

Wang, K., Yuen, S. T., Xu, J., Lee, S. P., Yan, H. H., Shi, S. T., et al. (2014). Whole-genome sequencing and comprehensive molecular profiling identify new driver mutations in gastric cancer. *Nat Genet, 46*(6), 573–582.

Yachida, S., Nakanishi, Y., Shimoda, T., Nimura, S., Igaki, H., Tachimori, Y., et al. (2004). Adenosquamous carcinoma of the esophagus. Clinicopathologic study of 18 cases. *Oncology, 66*(3), 218–225.

Zang, Z. J., Cutcutache, I., Poon, S. L., Zhang, S. L., McPherson, J. R., Tao, J., et al. (2012). Exome sequencing of gastric adenocarcinoma identifies recurrent somatic mutations in cell adhesion and chromatin remodeling genes. *Nature Genetics, 44*(5), 570–574.

Adenoid Cystic Carcinoma, Esophageal

Isabel Fonseca
Serviço de Anatomia Patológica, Instituto Português de Oncologia Francisco Gentil – Lisboa, Lisbon, Portugal
Faculdade de Medicina de Lisboa, Instituto de Anatomia Patológica, Lisbon, Portugal

Synonyms

Cylindroma

Definition

Adenoid cystic carcinoma is a basaloid tumor consisting of epithelial and myoepithelial cells (WHO) in variable architectural configurations, including tubular, cribriform, and solid patterns.

Clinical Features

- **Incidence**
  Adenoid cystic carcinoma is extremely rare in the esophagus, accounting for less than 0.1% of esophageal carcinomas.
- **Age**
  Most patients are in their seventh decade.
- **Sex**
  Males are more commonly affected with a reported M-F ratio of 3:1.
- **Site**
  More than half of the cases occur in the middle third of the esophagus. They rarely arise in the upper third.
- **Treatment**
  Surgery is the treatment of choice. In cases with positive margins, radiotherapy is warranted.
- **Outcome**
  The prognosis is poor, usually fatal. However, some cases have slow progression over large periods of time. Recurrence is found in regional lymph nodes as well as distant organs.

Macroscopy

The most common macroscopic presentation pattern is as an intraluminal, polypoid mass. Four cases of intramural, submucosal growth have also been reported. Ulceration of the overlying mucosa can be present.

Microscopy

Adenoid cystic carcinoma is formed by ductal, epithelial cells and myoepithelial cells that can be arranged in solid, cribriform, or tubular architectural patterns. The most common is the cribriform pattern, formed by nests of cells with microcystic spaces that contain hyaline, basal membrane-like material. The solid pattern presents sheets and nests of basaloid cells, without microcyst formation. The tubular pattern shows small duct lines by the two cell types with a central lumen containing hyaline material. Most cases show mixed architectural patterns. The stroma is usually hyalinized. Perineural invasion is almost invariably present. Mitoses are rarely seen in the cribriform and tubular types but they can occur in the solid variant. Necrosis is not a common feature except in the solid variant.

Immunophenotype

The ductal component of adenoid cystic carcinoma is stained by low molecular weight cytokeratins. The myoepithelial cells can be highlighted by muscle-specific actin, S100 protein, calponin, or p63. It has recently been shown that around 90% of salivary and breast adenoid cystic carcinomas express c-kit (CD117), at the ductal component. Basement membrane proteins, such as collagen IV, stain the hyaline material within the microcysts (Figs. 1 and 2).

Molecular Features

Adenoid cystic carcinoma has a recurrent translocation, the t(6:9)(q21-24:p13-23), and losses at 12q, 6q-23-qter, 13q21-q22, and 19q. The t(6:9) translocation fuses exon 14 of the *MYB* gene to the

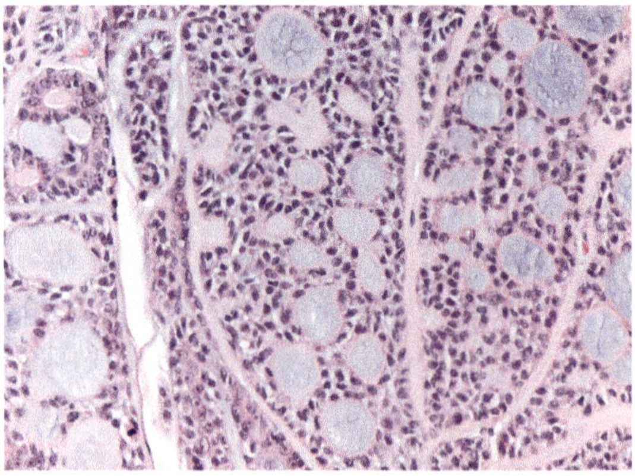

Adenoid Cystic Carcinoma, Esophageal, Fig. 1 Adenoid cystic carcinoma: in the cribriform variant there are nests of cells, both epithelial and myoepithelial, with microcyst formation. The microcysts contain hyaline material. The nests are surrounded by basement membrane-like material (H&E)

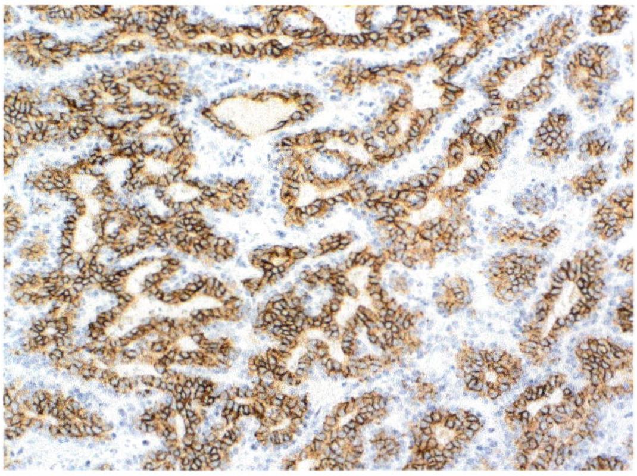

Adenoid Cystic Carcinoma, Esophageal, Fig. 2 Adenoid cystic carcinoma: staining with CD117 (c-kit) highlights the ductal cell component

last coding gene of the *NFIB* gene. None of these findings were reported in esophageal adenoid cystic carcinoma.

Differential Diagnosis

The main morphological differential diagnosis for esophageal adenoid cystic carcinoma is *basaloid squamous carcinoma*. The demonstration of squamous cell carcinoma (in situ or invasive) and the absence of myoepithelial markers in the latter allow the distinction. The role of novel specific biomarkers, namely, the *MYB-NFIB* fusion, in the differential diagnosis remains to be elucidated.

References and Further Reading

El-Naggar, A. K., & Huvos, A. G. (2005). Adenoid cystic carcinoma. In L. Barnes, J. W. Eveson, P. Reichart, & D. Sidransky (Eds.), *World Health Organization classification of tumours. Pathology and genetics of head and neck tumours* (pp. 221–222). Lyon: IARC Press.

Lieberman, M. D., Franceschi, D., Marsan, B., & Burt, M. (1994). Esophageal carcinoma. The unusual variants. *The Journal of Thoracic and Cardiovascular Surgery, 108*, 1138–1146.

Morisaki, Y., Yoshizumi, Y., Hiroyasu, S., Shibata, H., Terahata, S., Tamai, S., Sugiura, Y., Shima, S., & Tanaka, S. (1996). Adenoid cystic carcinoma of the esophagus: Report of a case and review of the Japanese literature. *Surgery Today: The Japanese Journal of Surgery, 26*, 1006–1009.

Persson, M., Andrén, Y., Mark, J., Horlings, H. M., Persson, F., & Stenman, G. (2009). Recurrent fusion of MYB and NFIB transcription factor genes in carcinomas of the breast and head and neck. *Proceedings of the National Academy of Sciences of the United States of America, 106*, 18740–18744.

Adenoma, Colorectal

Sibel Erdamar
Department of Pathology, Cerrahpasa Medical College, Istanbul, Turkey

Synonyms

Adenomatous polyp; Intraepithelial neoplasia

Definition

Adenomas, the precursor lesions of colorectal carcinomas, are dysplastic and noninvasive proliferations of colonic epithelium. Dysplastic epithelium is characterized by enlarged, hyperchromatic nuclei and nuclear stratification. Adenomas are well recognized histologically, with an abrupt transformation between dysplastic and nondysplastic epithelium. Adenomas are further classified as tubular, tubulovillous, and villous according to their architectural pattern.

Clinical Features

- **Incidence**
  Autopsy series reveal an incidence of approximately 30–35% in adults. Lifetime prevalence of an adenoma is 30–50% (Western countries) and increases with age. African-Americans have a lower prevalence than Caucasians.
- **Age**
  The frequency increases by age (20–30% by 50, 40–50% by 60). In the first two or three decades of life, adenomas are extremely uncommon unless the patient has some form of polyposis. By the fifth decade of life,

approximately 12% of individuals have adenomas, of which about 25% are high-risk lesions.

- **Sex**
  There is a slight male predominance.
- **Site**
  Sixty to 70% of adenomas are located distal to the splenic flexure. In some series, there is a tendency for a large proportion of adenomas to be in the rectum and sigmoid. On the other hand, one-fourth of patients have adenomas presenting only proximal to the splenic flexure.
- **Treatment**
  Complete removal (polypectomy) is indicated for all adenomas regardless of size, the presence of dysplasia, or villous component. Since the advent of fiber-optic scope, the indication is for any polypoid lesion anywhere in the large bowel to be removed as soon as it is detected, unless obvious contraindications exist.
- **Outcome**
  Most adenomas are asymptomatic, but they may cause bleeding due to twisting or vascular obstruction. If they are large, they may cause changes in bowel habits, intussusception, iron deficiency anemia, and stool incontinence. Almost 50% of adenomas increase in size with time. Five to 10% of them progress to CRC, in approximately 10 years. Size of an adenoma is the best predictor of carcinoma risk. Patients at initial examination with multiple adenomas, adenomas of size >0.5 cm, or with a family history of colorectal cancer should be followed after 3 years; those with a single tubular adenoma of size <0.5 cm and no family history should be followed up every 5 years.

Macroscopy

Most adenomas measure <1 cm in diameter. They may be sessile or pedunculated and single or multiple (Fig. 1). However intermediate forms between sessile and pedunculated forms may develop as well.

Tubular adenoma presents as a small, spherical pedunculated lesion. Larger lesions show a lobulated, bosselated, villous, raspberry-like, friable surface (Fig. 2).

Villous adenomas are seen in three macroscopic types: flat, carpet-like masses; lobulated bulky sessile masses; and pedunculated lesions with short, broad peduncles.

Adenomas can present also as superficial, flat (nonprotruding), or depressed lesions. Depressed (flat) adenomas are defined as dysplastic lesions without polypoid component, hardly detected in endoscopy.

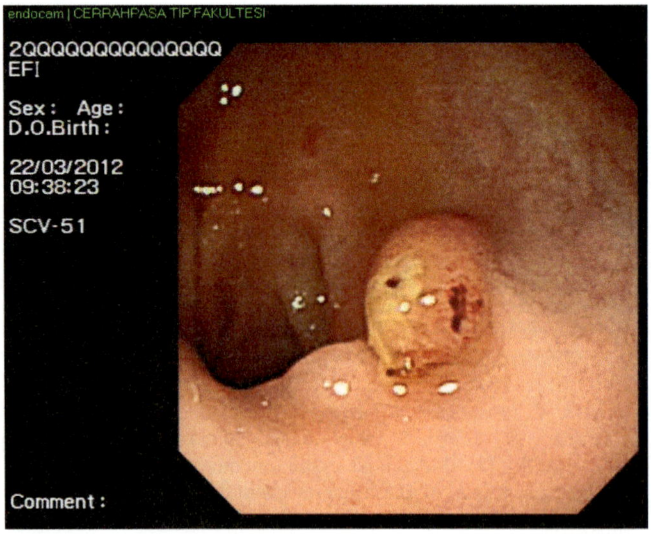

Adenoma, Colorectal, Fig. 1 Sessile tubular adenoma with a smooth surface in endoscopy

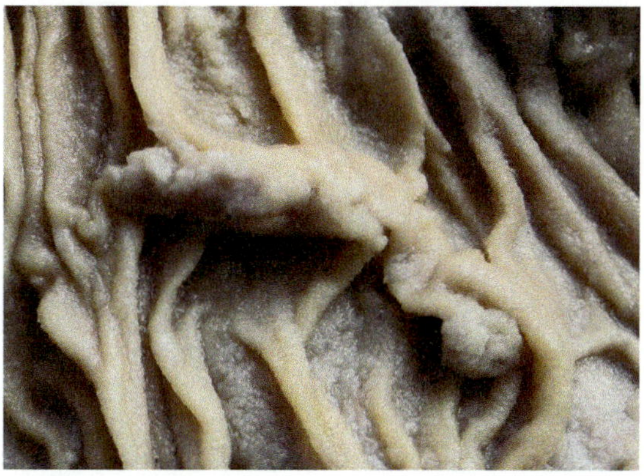

Adenoma, Colorectal, Fig. 2 Gross appearance of a sessile adenoma

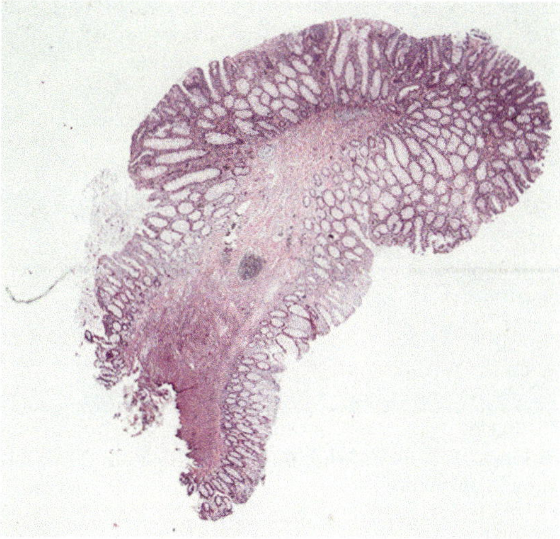

Adenoma, Colorectal, Fig. 3 Microscopic appearance of a tubular adenoma with a stalk

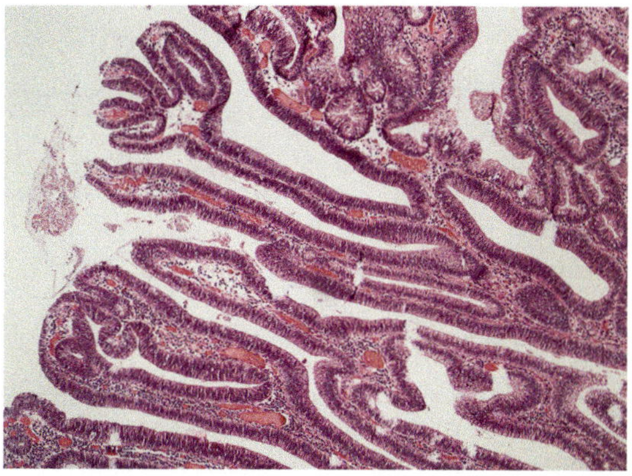

Adenoma, Colorectal, Fig. 4 Microscopic appearance of a villous adenoma

Microscopy

Adenomas (conventional) appear to arise in the upper parts of a single crypt. Dysregulation in proliferation and failure to full differentiation of colonic epithelium are basic features of neoplasia. Once the initial dysplastic event has occurred, adenomas grow by spreading along the basal lamina of the surface epithelium, into adjacent crypts. They replace the entire crypt and invaginate into the lamina propria; the new crypt formation tends to go up the mucosa to form a polyp. The lamina propria of adenomas may contain variable numbers of acute and chronic inflammatory cells including eosinophils. Paneth cell, neuroendocrine cell, and squamous cell aggregates can also be seen in adenomas.

Adenomas are traditionally categorized according to their architecture as *tubular adenoma*, if the villous component accounts for <25% of the lesion; *villous adenoma*, if >75%; and *tubulovillous adenoma*, if between 25% and 75% (Figs. 3 and 4). Villous component can be defined as elongated leaflike projections of dysplastic epithelium forming a height of more than twice the thickness of normal colonic mucosa.

Flat adenoma is a variant of adenoma that its height is less than twice the thickness of the adjacent mucosa.

Dysplasia can be low grade or high grade, depending on the degree of architectural complexity. By definition adenomas display at least low-grade dysplasia, characterized by nuclear stratification, enlargement, elongation, and hyperchromasia and mucin depletion (Fig. 5). The degree of dysplasia is related to increasing age, number of polyps, size of polyps, and the presence of villous changes. High-grade dysplasia (and carcinoma in situ) is defined by marked stratification, of neoplastic nuclei which extend toward the luminal part of the cells with significant pleomorphism, open chromatin, prominent nucleoli, increased mitotic activity, and loss of

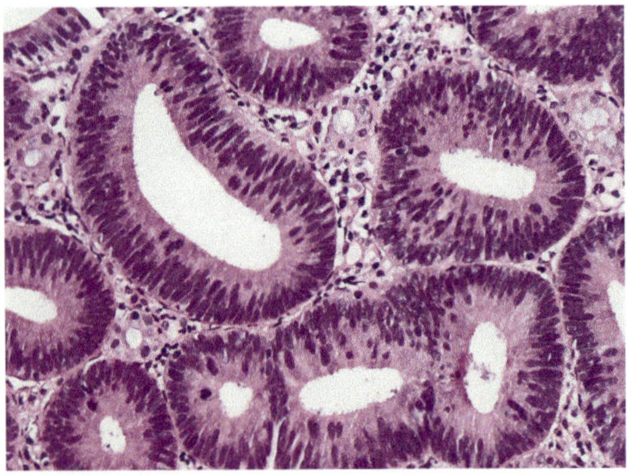

Adenoma, Colorectal, Fig. 5 Low-grade dysplasia and tubular adenoma

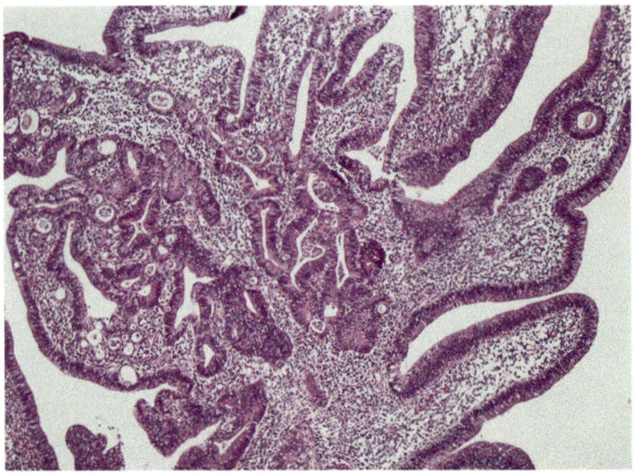

Adenoma, Colorectal, Fig. 7 Intramucosal carcinoma arising in villous adenoma: increased architectural complexity with irregular back-to-back glands

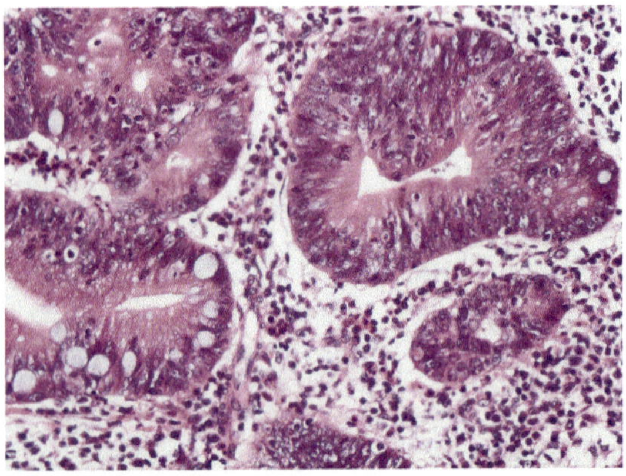

Adenoma, Colorectal, Fig. 6 High-grade dysplasia: note marked nuclear stratification and loss of polarity

polarity (Fig. 6). Architectural complexity such as back-to-back gland configuration and cribriform pattern can be seen as well. With neoplastic progression, the nucleus-to-cytoplasm ratio of the cells increases and loss of polarity becomes marked. Larger adenomas have a greater likelihood of harboring high-grade dysplasia.

Intramucosal carcinomas should be considered if the neoplastic cells show single-cell infiltration through the basement membrane into the surrounding lamina propria but not through muscularis mucosa (Fig. 7). They do not have metastatic risk since there is paucity of lymphatics in colorectal mucosa.

Pseudoinvasion is a misplaced (herniated) epithelium of adenoma in the submucosa. Pedunculated polyps can show pseudoinvasion that should be careful to misdiagnose as carcinoma.

In adenoma with invasive carcinoma, carcinoma invades through muscularis mucosa into the submucosa. Haggitt's levels are described as four levels of invasion of pedunculated polyps from the head to the submucosa of the underlying colonic wall. Sessile polyps do not have stalk, so they are all level 4. For the pedunculated polyps, evaluation of margin is very important. Cauterized margin is accepted as safe if there is >2 mm (or >1 mm according to some guidelines) distance from the neoplastic tissue to the margin. Poor differentiation of invasive component, the presence of lymphovascular invasion, tumor budding, and close proximity to the margin of stalk are poor prognostic features in adenomas with invasive carcinomas.

Immunophenotype

Immunohistochemical staining pattern of conventional adenomas is similar to that seen in colorectal adenocarcinomas. The upward shift in proliferative component of colonic epithelium can be highlighted by the use of proliferation markers such as antibody ki67 (MIB-1).

Molecular Features

Adenoma of the colon is a clonal disorder that is initiated and progresses by series of somatic and sometimes germline mutations. Initiation starts with inactivation of APC/β-catenin pathway. There are stepwise accumulations of genetic mutations. The earliest recognizable alteration is aberrant crypt foci (ACF).

There is more detailed information of colorectal carcinogenesis in *colorectal cancer* chapter; and brief information only is given here.

Homeostasis of the intestinal crypts of the colorectal mucosa depends on the balance between cell multiplication in the basal segment, upward cell migration, and surface apoptosis. An imbalance follows the increased cell multiplication and the progressive inhibition of surface apoptosis controlled by the Bcl-2 gene and the antiapoptosis protein survivin. There are two mechanisms suggested for the progression from a monocryptal event to a macroscopically visible lesion: (1) top-down theory proposes that abnormal cells born at the base of one crypt migrate to the surface, expand laterally, and fill adjacent crypts from top to bottom; (2) the bottom-up theory proposes that stem cells at the crypt base colonize in a second hit of the entire crypt and that lateral expansion occurs by crypt fission.

In 80% of conventional adenomas, a somatic mutation of adenomatous polyposis coli (APC) gene is the initial event. APC gene is located on chromosome 5. KRAS mutation is found in 50% of adenomas. TP53 gene (located on chromosome 17) mutation is also seen. General profile of conventional adenoma is CIN positive, MSS, CIMP negative, and negative for BRAF mutation. KRAS and APC mutations are found less frequently in nonpolypoid and depressed one.

For serrated adenomas BRAF mutation is the initial event, independent of CIMP or MSI status. Molecular features for *serrated polyps* are summarized elsewhere.

Differential Diagnosis

Reactive/regenerative changes in colonic mucosa sometimes can be misdiagnosed as dysplastic epithelium.

Traditional serrated adenomas are usually located in the left colon. They have serrated/sawtooth lumina contour with papillary infolding and surface nuclear tufting. The epithelium shows typically pseudostratification, nuclear elongation with hypereosinophilia in the cytoplasm.

References and Further Reading

Fenoglio-Preiser, C. M. (2008). Epithelial neoplasms of colon. In *Gastrointestinal Pathology an atlas and text* (pp. 899–1035). Philadelphia: Wolters Kluwer.

Giacosa, A., Frascio, F., & Munizzi, F. (2004). Epidemiology of colorectal polyps. *Techniques in Coloproctology, 8*, 243–247.

Lambert, R., & Triadafilopoulos, G. (2009). Pragmatic classification of superficial neoplastic colorectal lesions. *Gastrointestinal Endoscopy, 70*, 1182–1199.

Adenoma, Upper Gastrointestinal Tract

Chella R. S. van der Post[1] and Fátima Carneiro[2]
[1]Department of Pathology, Radboud University Medical Center, Nijmegen, The Netherlands
[2]Faculty of Medicine of Porto University, Centro Hospitalar São João and Ipatimup/i3S, Porto, Portugal

Synonyms

Intestinal-type adenoma; Polyps

Definition

An adenoma is defined by the World Health Organization as a "circumscribed benign neoplasm composed of tubular and/or villous structures lined by dysplastic epithelium." Gastric adenomas are depicted as raised, protruding, or polypoid lesions composed of dysplastic epithelium that project above the surrounding gastric mucosa and therefore distinct from flat mucosal dysplasia or intraepithelial dysplasia like formerly termed flat adenomas or depressed adenomas. The grade of the dysplastic epithelium that comprises the adenoma is classified as low grade or high grade. Gastric adenomas are histologically divided into intestinal- and gastric- types based on the type of glandular epithelium they display. In this entry, intestinal-type gastric adenoma is being discussed.

Sporadic gastric adenomas often occur in a background of chronic gastritis with atrophy and intestinal metaplasia. Adenomas may actually represent polypoid areas of dysplasia that develop as a result of underlying chronic gastritis, similar to polypoid dysplasia in ulcerative colitis. The exact pathogenesis of gastric adenomas is unresolved. Unlike colorectal adenomas, gastric adenomas do not appear to represent the major precursor lesion for gastric adenocarcinoma since gastric adenocarcinoma is almost never associated with an identifiable adenoma precursor lesion. However, gastric adenomas are a direct precursor to gastric carcinoma with much higher incidence of adenocarcinoma within the adenoma than seen in colonic adenomas. Next to this, they serve as markers for synchronous or metachronous adenocarcinoma in other areas of the stomach.

Gastric adenomas are frequently seen in patients with familial adenomatous polyposis (FAP) with an incidence of 1–15%. Gastric adenomas are much less frequent in FAP than fundic gland polyps, duodenal adenomas, and of course colonic adenomas. Gastric adenomatous polyposis is rarely seen. Among Asian patients with FAP, the risk of gastric carcinoma is increased by tenfold, this is not seen in Western patients with FAP and adenocarcinoma is almost never present in gastric adenoma. FAP-associated adenomas are most commonly of the gastric type.

Adenomas may also occur in the gastroesophageal junction in the setting of Barrett's esophagus. Polypoid dysplasia is however uncommon. Its precise frequency is unknown since most gastroesophageal adenomas have been described as individual case reports. As in the colon and stomach, the polyps are raised sessile or pedunculated lesions and histologically display a tubular, tubulovillous, or villous architecture; show varying degrees of dysplasia; and may contain areas of invasive carcinoma.

Clinical Features

- **Incidence**
  Gastric adenomas rank third in overall incidence of all gastric polyps after fundic gland and hyperplastic polyps. Adenomas account for 8–10% of gastric polyps in most large reported series. Their incidence increases progressively with patient age. There is considerable variation in the incidence of gastric adenomas, depending upon the geographic population analyzed that, generally, parallels the incidence of adenocarcinoma. For example, gastric adenomas are much more common in Japanese series (where the incidence of adenocarcinoma is higher and an active screening program has been ruled out) compared to series reported from Western countries.
- **Age**
  Incidence increases with age, with peak incidence in the sixth to seventh decade of life. FAP patients are considerably younger with mean age between the 30 and 40 year.
- **Sex**
  Males are more affected than females, with a male-to-female ratio of 3:1
- **Site**
  Gastric intestinal-type adenomas are predominantly located in the antrum; however, they can occur throughout the stomach.
- **Treatment**
  Adenomas should be removed completely when safe to do so, since they can progress to cancer. An examination of the entire gastric mucosa should be made for abnormalities. Endoscopic mucosal resection (EMR) and endoscopic submucosal dissection (ESD) are regarded as standard treatments for gastric adenoma. Large adenomas may sometimes require surgical resection. The patient needs endoscopic follow-up because of the increased risk of developing new adenomas and/or

carcinoma. Endoscopy should be repeated at 6 months for incomplete resection of polyps or those with high-grade dysplasia. Upper endoscopy can be repeated after 1 year for all other polyps.

- **Outcome**

  Gastric adenomas are true neoplasms and precursors of gastric adenocarcinoma. The risk of presence of carcinoma is strongly related to the presence of high-grade dysplasia and size of the lesion and is particularly high in high-grade adenomas with a size greater than 2 cm. Other risk factors include location, biopsy number, histological type (tubulovillous), redness, and ulceration. Therefore, evaluation of the entire polyp by resection is warranted, to obtain an accurate diagnosis and management plan. Malignant transformation may be present in 5–40% of gastric adenomas and seems to be more prevalent in villous adenomas compared to tubular adenomas.

Macroscopy

Adenomas are polypoid or protruding noninvasive neoplastic processes. More than 80% of adenomas are solitary. In patients with FAP, multiple adenomas can be present; however, more than 2 or 3 gastric adenomas is, also in the setting of FAP, rare. Grossly, adenomas are typically well-circumscribed sessile or pedunculated lesions measuring from a few millimeters to many centimeters in diameter. The average size is 1 cm. They are covered by an erythematous, velvety mucosa.

Microscopy

Gastric adenomas are histologically divided into intestinal- and gastric-types based on the type of glandular epithelium that they are composed of. Gastric-type adenomas are further divided into pyloric-gland adenoma and foveolar-type adenoma. Gastric foveolar-type adenomas are lined entirely by gastric mucin cells, while intestinal-type adenomas contain at least focal goblet cells and/or Paneth cells. Pyloric gland adenomas are rare and histologically characterized by pyloric-type glands with cuboidal epithelium with pale or eosinophilic cytoplasm. Intestinal-type adenomas are more prevalent than the gastric-type adenomas. The importance of the phenotype (intestinal versus gastric type) is debated, and there are also hybrid forms of adenomas with features of both phenotypes.

Intestinal-type adenomas are composed of intestinal-type columnar epithelium with absorptive cells, goblet cells, endocrine cells, and/or Paneth cells (Figs. 1 and 2). The glands show (pseudo-)stratification and elongated, hyperchromatic nuclei with increased mitotic activity. Often, a distinct brush border is detectable that confirms intestinal differentiation in the dysplastic epithelium. They can be classified into tubular, tubulovillous, and villous types, depending on their growth pattern.

Adenomas can be graded low or high grade. Adenomas with low-grade dysplasia show elongated, hyperchromatic, and crowded nuclei with mild pseudostratification. There is no complex architecture. Features of high-grade dysplasia are cribriform architecture, marked glandular crowding, full-thickness nuclear stratification, and severe cytonuclear atypia. Intramucosal carcinomas are defined by invasion into the lamina propria; it is difficult to distinguish cytonuclear features of intramucosal carcinomas from high-grade dysplasia. Features in favor of carcinoma

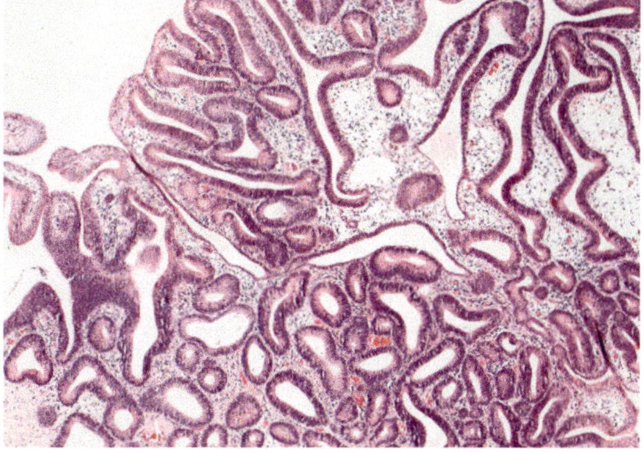

Adenoma, Upper Gastrointestinal Tract, Fig. 1 Intestinal-type tubular adenoma with low-grade dysplasia (H&E, Original magnification 25×)

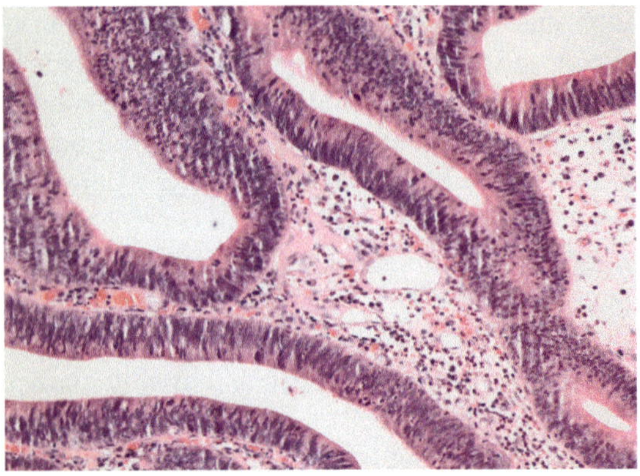

Adenoma, Upper Gastrointestinal Tract, Fig. 2 The glands show elongated, hyperchromatic, and crowded nuclei with pseudostratification (H&E, Original magnification 200×)

are syncytial growth pattern, effacement of normal architecture with back-to-back glands, and single cells within the lamina propria. Often there are cystic glands. The malignant potential of adenomas has been demonstrated in long-term follow-up studies, even in low-grade dysplasia; therefore, resection of adenomas is recommended.

Intestinal-type adenomas frequently arise on a background of atrophic gastritis and intestinal metaplasia but there is no proven association with *H. pylori* infection. Surrounding epithelium frequently shows features of intestinal metaplasia and atrophy. This is in contradiction to colonic adenomas that most often occur in a normal mucosal background.

Immunophenotype

Intestinal-type adenomas express variably the intestinal markers MUC2 and CD10. They are negative for gastric mucins MUC5AC and MUC6.

Molecular Features

The molecular features of gastric adenomas are not fully understood. Microsatellite instability is present in a minority of lesions, but its incidence increases in adenomas that contain carcinoma. Gastric adenomas show molecular alterations in the *APC*, *KRAS*, and *Tp53* genes.

Differential Diagnosis

- Hyperplastic polyps with dysplasia contain foveolar hyperplasia, cystic change, and inflammation in the underlying polyp. In addition, dysplasia is often focal or patchy in hyperplastic polyps.
- Fundic gland polyps with dysplasia are extremely uncommon, except in FAP patients or in the setting of GAPPS syndrome (gastric adenocarcinoma and proximal polyposis of the Stomach). The presence of cystically dilated fundic glands lined by parietal and chief cells beneath the area of dysplasia is helpful in diagnosing a dysplastic fundic gland polyp.
- Adenomas with high-grade dysplasia may be difficult to distinguish from intramucosal carcinomas. Features in favor of carcinoma are syncytial growth pattern, effacement of normal architecture with back-to-back glands, and single cells within the lamina propria.

References and Further Reading

Abraham, S. C., Mongomery, E. A., Singh, V. K., Yardley, J. H., & Wu, T. T. (2002). Gastric adenomas: Intestinal-type and gastric-type adenomas differ in the risk of adenocarcinoma and presence of background mucosal pathology. *The American Journal of Surgical Pathology, 26*(10), 1276–1285.

Abraham, S. C., Park, S. J., Lee, J. H., Mugartegui, L., & Wu, T. T. (2003). Genetic alterations in gastric adenomas of intestinal and foveolar phenotypes. *Modern Pathology, 16*(8), 786–795.

Choi, C. W., Kang, D. H., Kim, H. W., Park, S. B., Kim, S., & Cho, M. (2012). Endoscopic submucosal dissection as a treatment for gastric adenomatous polyps. *Scandinavian Journal of Gastroenterology, 47*(10), 1218–1225.

Goddard, A. F., Badreldin, R., Pritchard, D. M., Walker, M. M., Warren, B., & British Society of Gastroenterology. (2010). The management of gastric polyps. *Gut, 59*(9), 1270–1276.

Park do, Y., Srivastava, A., Kim, G. H., Mino-Kenudson, M., Deshpande, V., Zukerberg, L. R., et al. (2008). Adenomatous and foveolar gastric dysplasia: Distinct patterns of mucin expression and background intestinal metaplasia. *The American Journal of Surgical Pathology, 32*(4), 524–533.

Adenosquamous Carcinoma, Upper GI Tract

Maria Gabriela Gasparinho[1,2] and
Isabel Fonseca[3,4]
[1]Instituto Português de Oncologia de Lisboa Francisco Gentil, Lisboa, Portugal
[2]Instituto de Anatomia Patológica da Faculdade de Ciências da Saúde da Universidade da Beira Interior, Covilhã, Portugal
[3]Serviço de Anatomia Patológica, Instituto Português de Oncologia Francisco Gentil – Lisboa, Lisbon, Portugal
[4]Faculdade de Medicina de Lisboa, Instituto de Anatomia Patológica, Lisbon, Portugal

Synonyms

There are no current synonyms for this neoplasm. Historically, it has been often confounded with mucoepidermoid carcinoma.

Definition

A malignant epithelial neoplasm that has mixed elements of glandular and squamous cell differentiation, which remains clearly distinguishable within the tumor.

Clinical Features

- **Incidence**
  Adenosquamous carcinoma (ASC) is a rare disease. No worldwide incidence data is available. In the largest published series, it represented 1.0% of all esophageal cancers.
- **Age**
  In the largest published series, patients' age range from 51 to 85 years, with a mean age of 64 years.
- **Sex**
  The disease is more frequent in males.
- **Site**
  Adenosquamous carcinoma is somewhat more frequent in the middle and lower thirds of the esophagus.
- **Treatment**
  Surgery is the treatment of choice and can be followed by radiotherapy. This particular histological type does not change the usual treatment for esophageal carcinomas.
- **Outcome**
  ASC seems to have a better prognosis than conventional squamous cell carcinomas or adenocarcinomas. In the largest series, reporting 18 cases, the survival rate at 3, 5, and 10 years was, respectively, 71.5%, 63.6%, and 47.7%.

Macroscopy

ASC has similar macroscopic features similar to conventional squamous cell carcinoma. It can present as ulcerative and infiltrative masses, as well as protruding or flat tumors. No special macroscopic type has been reported.

Microscopy

ASC is characterized by the presence of definite squamous cell differentiation and glandular differentiation, clearly demarcated from each other (Figs. 1, 2, and 3). Squamous elements can be identified by keratin pearl formation or by differentiation into prickle cells in the tumor nests. Glandular elements are generally clearly tubular, with occasional mucus secretion visible in the lumina, which can be highlighted with PAS (Fig. 4). In the glandular component, ciliated cells were also reported. ASC has also been described in association with Barrett's metaplasia.

Immunophenotype

CD44 has been shown to be an effective marker of squamous elements in ASC of various locations. In head and neck ASCs, the glandular differentiated structures are mostly positive for CEA and

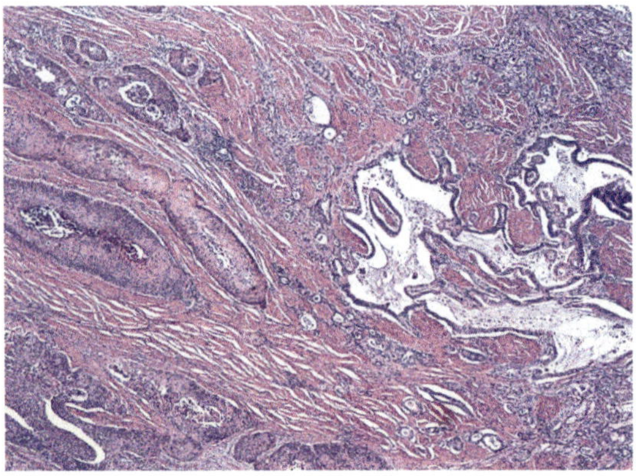

Adenosquamous Carcinoma, Upper GI Tract, Fig. 1 Adenosquamous carcinoma (hematoxylin-eosin, low power). The malignant squamous components can be seen on the *left* side of the image; the malignant glandular component can be identified on the *right*

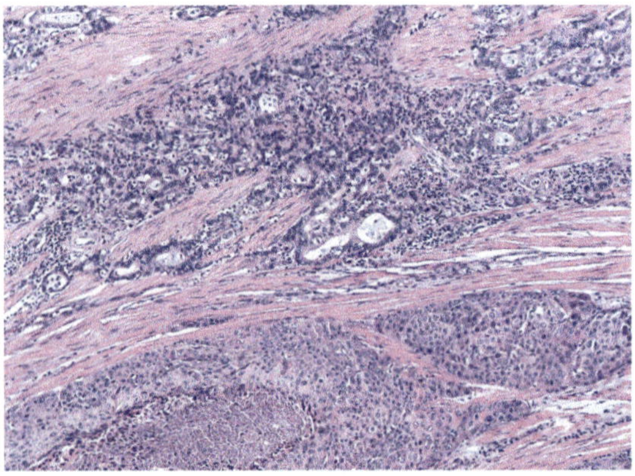

Adenosquamous Carcinoma, Upper GI Tract, Fig. 2 Adenosquamous carcinoma (hematoxylin-eosin, high power). The two malignant components can be clearly identified on the *top* and *bottom* of the image

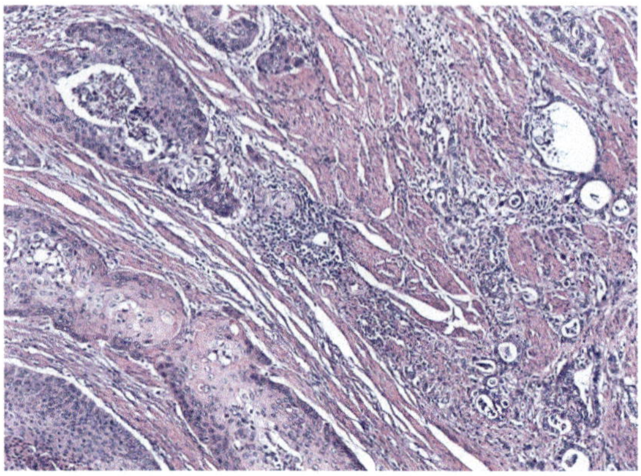

Adenosquamous Carcinoma, Upper GI Tract, Fig. 3 Adenosquamous carcinoma (hematoxylin-eosin, high power). Squamous elements display prickle cells in the center of the nests (*lower left*). The glandular component is poorly differentiated (*right*)

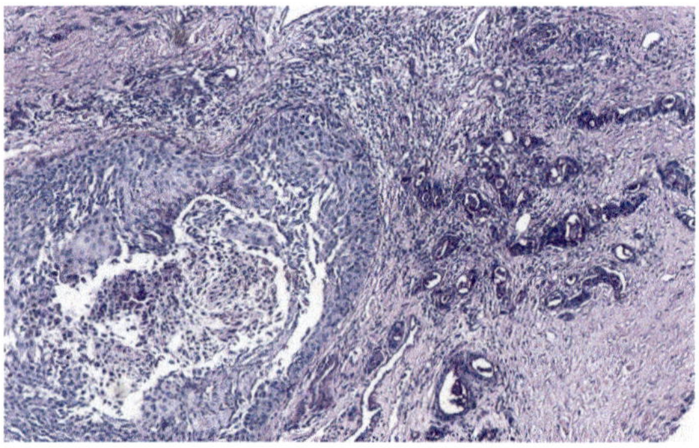

Adenosquamous Carcinoma, Upper GI Tract, Fig. 4 Adenosquamous carcinoma (periodic acid-Schiff (PAS), high power). PAS highlights the mucin produced by the glandular component of the tumor

CAM 5.2, while squamous elements are negative; nevertheless, both components have been shown to be reactive to 34βE12 antibody. In these series, cytokeratin 7 stains the glandular component more intensely than the squamous component, while cytokeratin 20 is negative in both elements. However, these findings were only described in the head and neck locations and they have not been validated in esophageal ASC.

Molecular Features

The only available information on molecular features of adenosquamous carcinoma stems from one case report, demonstrating the same clonal origin of both components of the tumors. Both displayed allelic losses at levels of 3p, 5q, 10q, 14q, and 18q, as well as the same missense mutation at p53 gene.

Differential Diagnosis

The main differential diagnosis is to be done with *mucoepidermoid carcinoma* and the acantholytic variant of *squamous cell carcinoma*. As major differences, mucoepidermoid carcinoma contains intermediate cells (which are absent from ASC), has an intimate admixture of squamous and glandular elements (which are clearly separated from each other in ASC), and generally does not display keratinization of the epidermoid component (which is frequent in ASC). Moreover, mucoepidermoid carcinoma has a characteristic lobular architecture, which is not found in ASC. The study of the CRTC1/3-MAML2 fusion gene, characteristic feature of mucoepidermoid carcinoma, can also be of use in the differential diagnosis. In the acantholytic variant of squamous cell carcinoma, tumor cells display pseudoglandular spaces due to acantholysis, but no mucin can be identified in these spaces, which are filled with dyskeratotic neoplastic cells. *Basaloid squamous cell carcinoma* can also be misinterpreted as ASC. Nevertheless, the absence of a true glandular element and the typical basaloid appearance of the cells is generally enough to disclose the diagnosis.

References and Further Reading

Alos, L., Castillo, M., Nadal, A., Caballero, M., Mallofre, C., Palacin, A., & Cardesa, A. (2004). Adenosquamous carcinoma of the head and neck: Criteria for diagnosis in a study of 12 cases. *Histopathology, 44*, 570–579.

Rees, B. P., Rouse, R. W., Wit, M., Noesel, C. J. M., Tytgat, G. N. J., Lanschot, J. B., & Offerhaus, G. J. A. (2002). Molecular evidence for the same clonal origin of both components of an adenosquamous Barrett carcinoma. *Gastroenterology, 122*, 784–788.

Yachida, S., Nakanishi, Y., Shimoda, T., Nimura, S., Igaki, H., Tachimori, Y., & Kato, H. (2004). Adenosquamous carcinoma of the esophagus, clinicopathologic study of 18 cases. *Oncology, 66*, 218–225.

Ylagan, L. R., Scholes, J., & Demopoulos, R. (2000). CD44, a marker of squamous differentiation in adenosquamous neoplasms. *Archives of Pathology and Laboratory Medicine, 124*, 212–215.

Adipose Tissue Tumors, Stomach

José Manuel Lopes
Faculty of Medicine of the University of Porto and Institute of Molecular Pathology and Immunology of the University of Porto, Porto, Portugal

Synonyms

Atypical lipomatous tumor/well differentiated liposarcoma; Dedifferentiated liposarcoma; Lipoma; Myxoid liposarcoma; Pleomorphic liposarcoma

Definition

Lipoma is a benign tumor consisting of mature adipocytes.

Atypical lipomatous tumor/well-differentiated liposarcoma is an intermediate malignant tumor consisting of pleomorphic adipocytes and stromal cells with at least focal nuclear atypia.

Dedifferentiated liposarcoma: tumor displaying transition from atypical lipomatous tumor/well-differentiated liposarcoma to other non-adipocytic type mesenchymal tumor with variable malignant grade (sarcoma).

Myxoid liposarcoma is a sarcoma containing variable number of signet-ring lipoblasts and round/oval mesenchymal primitive cells surrounded by a myxoid stroma with delicate arborizing vessels.

Pleomorphic liposarcoma: high-grade sarcoma consisting of variable number of pleomorphic lipoblasts in the absence of atypical lipomatous tumor/well-differentiated liposarcoma features.

Clinical Features

- **Incidence**
  Adipose tumors are unusual in the stomach (<1% of gastric mesenchymal tumors) including mostly lipomas (Thompson et al. 2003) and

other extremely rare histological subtypes (Seki et al. 1998).

- **Age**
  The peak incidence of gastric lipomas is by the seventh decade, but they can occur from the pediatric age to the elderly; the exceptionally rare gastric liposarcomas seem to occur by the fifth/seventh decade.
- **Sex**
  There are no consistent data regarding incidence of gastric adipose tumors by gender (male: female).
- **Site**
  Most gastric lipomas develop in the submucosa (~90%), and infrequently in the subserosa or muscular propria. The antrum is the most frequent location (~90%), but they can localize in the gastric body/fundus.
- **Treatment**
  Safe treatment decision of gastric adipocytic tumors should be based on a confirmed or highly suggestive pretreatment/intraoperative diagnosis. Despite remaining controversies, adequate surgical resection is a treatment that can be advised for large symptomatic gastric lipomas. Active observation, partial resection, tumor enucleation, and endoscopic and laparoscopic resection may be adequate options (Krasniqi et al. 2008) without major adverse events (e.g., hemorrhage, perforation), depending on the exact tumor location (e.g., submucosa tumors <3 cm) and on the attending doctor experience. The treatment of the atypical lipomatous tumor/well-differentiated liposarcoma and of other rare gastric liposarcomas should be decided on an individual base following strict oncologic principles.
- **Outcome**
  Gastric lipomas are always benign, but some may cause comorbidities and life-threatening settings if not diagnosed/treated adequately. There are few data regarding the other rare adipose tumor subtypes.

Macroscopy

Adipose tissue tumors may present as polypoid, mostly submucosa (Fig. 1) or rarely subserosa well-circumscribed ovoid soft yellowish solid masses; some may display central overlying mucosa ulceration/depression, areas of necrosis, or hemorrhage. Tumors may be <2 cm in largest dimension, reported average size is 6.5 cm, but they may attain larger dimensions.

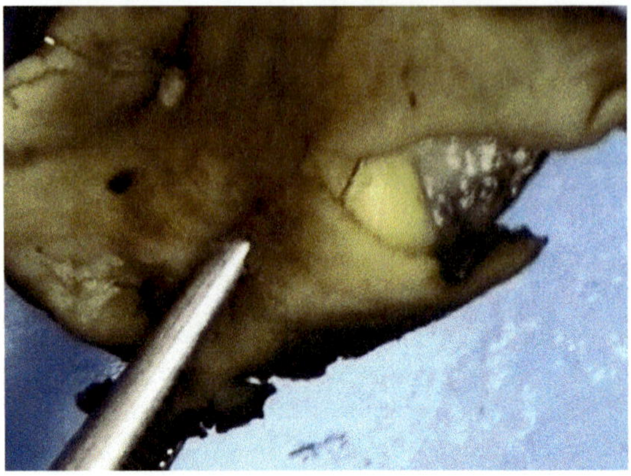

Adipose Tissue Tumors, Stomach, Fig. 1 Macroscopy of submucosal gastric lipoma

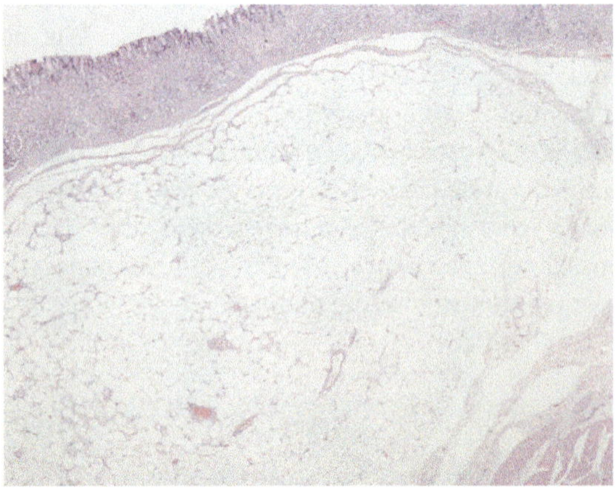

Adipose Tissue Tumors, Stomach, Fig. 2 Low power features of well-circumscribed submucosal gastric lipoma

Microscopy

See definition and the corresponding adipose tissue tumors of soft tissues (Fig. 2).

Immunophenotype

Most adipose tissue tumors express S100 protein in mature and atypical adipocytes as well as in round cells and lipoblasts. Vimentin and CD34 (cluster differentiation molecule 34) may be expressed in tumors with spindle cell component. Actin, desmin, myogenin, and MyoD1 (myogenic basic muscle-specific protein) may be useful to identify smooth and skeletal muscle tumor cell components. Nuclear expression of MDM2 (murine double minute 2) and CDK4 (cyclin-dependent kinase 4) in adipose and non-adipose components may be useful for the diagnosis of atypical lipomatous tumor/well-differentiated liposarcoma and of dedifferentiated liposarcoma.

Molecular Features

So far, there are no data on gastric lipomas to compare with the ordinary and special variants of soft tissue lipomas; FISH (fluorescence in situ hybridization) *MDM2* and *CDK4* gene amplification was reported in gastric atypical lipomatous tumor/well-differentiated liposarcoma (Kuhnen et al. 2010).

Differential Diagnosis

It may be difficult to distinguish whether well-differentiated fat is an adipose tumor or normal fat, particularly in fragmented or biopsy specimens. Adequate sampling is essential for the histological diagnosis, to evaluate nuclear atypia in adipocytes and non-adipocyte components, presence of round cells, lipoblasts, and other non-adipocyte components; immunohistochemistry, and genetic and molecular analyses may be useful to rule out other tumors that display microscopic features simulating adipose tissue tumors. See the corresponding adipose tissue tumors of soft tissues.

References and Further Reading

Krasniqi, A. S., Hoxha, F. T., Bicaj, B. X., Hashani, I. A., Hasimja, S. M., Kelmendi, S. M., & Gashi-Luci, L. H. (2008). Symptomatic subserosal gastric lipoma successfully treated with enucleation. *World Journal of Gastroenterology, 14*, 5930–5932.

Kuhnen, C., Mentzel, T., Haarmann, W., Schwegler, U., Sciot, R., Debiec-Rychter, M., et al. (2010). Atypical lipomatous tumors of the stomach. Clinical, morphological and molecular findings. *Pathologe, 31*, 199.

Seki, K., Hasegawa, T., Konegawa, R., Hizawa, K., & Sano, T. (1998). Primary liposarcorma of the stomach: A case report and a review of the literature. *Japanese Journal of Clinical Oncology, 28*, 284–288.

Thompson, W. M., Kende, A. I., & Levy, A. D. (2003). Imaging characteristics of gastric lipomas in 16 adult and pediatric patients. *American Journal of Radiology, 181*, 981–985.

Ampullary Carcinoma

Berna Savaş
Department of Pathology, Ankara University Medical School, Ankara, Turkey

Synonyms

Periampullary carcinoma

Definition

Ampullary carcinoma (AC) is an uncommon and heterogeneous neoplasm. AC can be broadly considered as tumors arising out of or within 1 cm of the papilla of Vater and include ampullary, pancreatic, bile duct, and duodenal carcinomas. Distinction may not be possible in advanced cases. There is a high incidence of these tumors in patients with FAP. AC can be broadly classified as primary, metastatic, or systemic. Primary cancers arise in the pancreas or other periampullary sites and can demonstrate either endocrine or nonendocrine differentiation. Ductal adenocarcinoma is by far the most common periampullary malignant tumor.

Clinical Features

- **Incidence**
  The incidence of AC was reported as 0.7 cases per 10,000 males and 0.4 cases for females between 1985 and 2005. AC represents 0.5% of all gastrointestinal malignancies.
- **Age**
  AC usually diagnosed in patients between the ages of 60 and 80 years (range 29–85 years).
- **Sex**
  ACs are more common in men than in women.
- **Site**
  Those tumors arising out of or within 1 cm of the papilla of Vater and include ampullary, pancreatic, bile duct, and duodenal carcinoma are considered as AC. AC can be centered on the ampulla, circumferentially involve it, or completely infiltrate the ampulla of Vater.
- **Treatment**
  Pancreaticoduodenectomy with or without (Whipple operation) pylorus preservation is the procedure of choice for AC. Local excision should only be attempted in patients with small adenocarcinoma of the ampulla of Vater who are unfit for or who refuse radical resection.
- **Outcome**
  Tumor stage, histological type, histological grade, and presence of preexisting adenoma are predictive factors. The best predictor of outcome is the stage of the disease. Cases with well-differentiated carcinomas have better prognosis than those with poorly differentiated carcinomas. Carcinomas that arise from the adenomas have better prognosis than the carcinomas not associated with preexisting adenomas. Size of the tumor, vascular and perineural invasion, and high level of microsatellite instability are other unfavorable prognostic factors. Overall ACs usually show aggressive behavior.

Macroscopy

Macroscopically tumors can be exophytic or mixed ulcerated and may involve the ampulla and periampullary duodenum. Large ampullary tumors usually involve multiple structures. Also tumors of the head of the pancreas, distal common bile duct, and duodenum may involve the ampullary region and may resemble primary AC.

Microscopy

The ampullary area represents different types of epithelium; hence, carcinomas that develop in this region may show an intestinal or pancreaticobiliary phenotype. Microscopic whole-mount sections that include the ampullary area are helpful to evaluate the relationship of these structures. Intestinal-type adenocarcinoma represents the most common histologic type (Figs. 1 and 2).

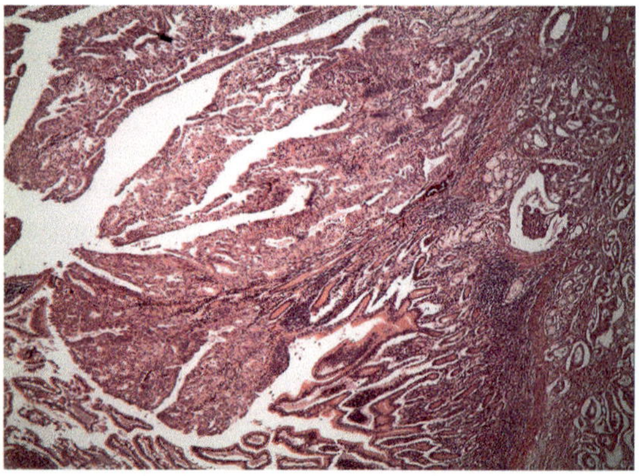

Ampullary Carcinoma, Fig. 1 Moderately differentiated adenocarcinoma of ampulla (H&E, ×25, respectively).

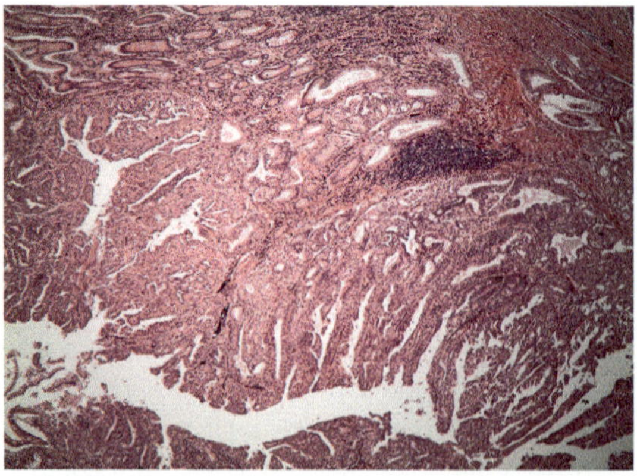

Ampullary Carcinoma, Fig. 2 Moderately differentiated adenocarcinoma of ampulla (H&E, ×100, respectively).

The intestinal-type ampullary adenocarcinomas are morphologically indistinguishable from adenocarcinomas that develop elsewhere in lower GI tractus. Pancreatobiliary-type carcinoma, the second more frequent subtype, is morphologically indistinguishable from the carcinoma of the pancreas and bile duct and usually shows a desmoplastic stromal reaction. AC usually shows tubular growth pattern. Tumors are classified according to the predominant component. Most of the ACs are adenocarcinomas with an intestinal phenotype (50–80%) or a pancreaticobiliary phenotype (15–20%). Adenosquamous carcinoma, clear cell carcinoma, hepatoid carcinoma, high grade neuroendocrine carcinoma and mixed carcinoma, mucinous adenocarcinomas, invasive papillary adenocarcinoma, signet ring adenocarcinoma, squamous carcinoma, and undifferentiated carcinoma are the rarely seen histological variants of ACs.

Immunophenotype

Pancreatobiliary-type carcinomas are usually negative for CK20, whereas most of the intestinal-type carcinomas of AC are positive for both CK7 and CK20. CDX2 and MUC2 as intestinal phenotype marker are usually negative in pancreatobiliary-type carcinomas which are positive for MUC1. CEA and CA19-9 expressions are also common.

Molecular Features

KRAS gene mutations (codon 12 and 13) have been recorded in 20–75% of ACs. Mutations in TP53 gene (exon 5, 6, and 7) have been shown in most of these tumors. Mutations in APC and beta-catenin genes, loss of SMAD4 gene, high level of microsatellite instability, and overexpression of EGF, ERBB2, and ERBB3 are other genetic abnormalities that have been reported in ACs.

Differential Diagnosis

Location of the ampulla makes identifying the origin of ACs very difficult. Pancreatic, bile duct, and duodenal carcinomas should be considered in the differential diagnosis. The size and the location of the tumor, determined both grossly and microscopically though not always, are considered as useful features. Similarly immunophenotype and molecular features of pancreatic and biliary carcinomas can overlap with those of pancreatobiliary-type ACs. However, evidence of a preexisting adenoma is a useful microscopic feature to determine the tumor origin.

References and Further Reading

Albores-Saavedra, J., Schwartz, A. M., Batich, K., & Henson, D. E. (2009). Cancers of the ampulla Vater; Demographics, morphology and survival based on 5628 cases from the SEER program. *Journal of Surgical Oncology, 100*, 598–605.

Albores-Saavedra, J., Hruban, R. H., Klimstra, D. S., & Zamboni, G. (2010). Invasive adenocarcinoma of the ampullary region. In F. T. Bosman, F. Carneiro, R. H. Hruban, & N. D. Theise (Eds.), *WHO classification of tumours of the digestive system* (pp. 87–91). Lyon-France: IARC.

Morini, S., Perrone, G., Borzomati, D., et al. (2012). Carcinoma of the ampulla Vater. Morphological and immunophynotypical classification predicts survival. *Pancreas, 42*, 60–66.

Ruemmele, P., Dietmaier, W., Terracciano, L., et al. (2009). Histopathologic features and microsatellite instability of cancers of the papilla of Vater and their precursor lesions. *The American Journal of Surgical Pathology, 33*, 691–704.

Amyloidosis, Gastrointestinal

Susana Rodrigues
Serviço de Gastrenterologia, Centro Hospitalar de São João, Alameda Professor Hernani Monteiro, Porto, Portugal

Synonyms

Gastrointestinal manifestations of amyloidosis; Systemic amyloidosis

Definition

Amyloidoses are a diverse group of diseases characterized by abnormal folding of proteins and the extracellular tissue deposition of fibrils of low molecular weight subunits of normal serum proteins which disrupt tissue structure and function. The conversion of peptides or proteins from their insoluble functional states into highly organized fibrillar aggregates showing a cross-beta supersecondary structure is termed as "amyloid." At least 28 different human proteins have been identified as amyloidogenic. Amyloidogenic deposition can be localized or systemic. Acquired causes of systemic amyloidoses include: (1) primary or AL amyloidosis in which the fibrils are composed of fragments of monoclonal light chains and affected patients may have amyloidosis alone or in association with other plasma cell dyscrasias, and (2) reactive (secondary) or AA amyloidosis in which the fibrils are composed of fragments of the acute phase reactant serum amyloid A, a structurally normal protein; or hereditary, as most commonly occurring by modulation of the transthyretin gene (mutant amyloid transthyretin, ATTR). Wild type transthyretin, TTR, can also form amyloid disease in older patients, in a process termed senile systemic amyloidosis (SSA). Both AL and ATTR amyloidoses are characterized by multi-system disease, involving more frequently the heart and kidneys, while ATTR preferentially affects the nervous system and heart. Among patients with systemic amyloidosis, histological involvement of the gastrointestinal (GI) tract is very common but is often subclinical. Localized amyloidosis of the GI tract is less frequent. GI involvement of the GI tract is defined as the presence of GI symptoms with direct biopsy verification. Patients with symptomatic gastrointestinal amyloidosis usually present in various forms. Among patients with amyloidosis and autonomic symptoms, the two most common presentations are orthostatic symptoms and gastrointestinal symptoms. The most common disease causes of reactive amyloidosis are chronic degenerative arthropathies, namely, rheumatoid arthritis. These include: gastrointestinal bleeding due to vascular friability and ulcers, chronic intestinal dysmotility resulting in dilatation of the intestine, malabsorption due to mucosal infiltration or bacterial overgrowth, and protein-losing gastroenteropathy.

Clinical Features

- **Incidence**
  The frequency of clinically apparent gastrointestinal involvement varies with the type of amyloidosis. Gastrointestinal disease is present in as many as 60% of patients with reactive amyloidosis (AA amyloidosis). It appears to be less common in AL amyloidosis, with biopsy diagnosed and clinically apparent disease occurring in around 7% of patients. In one case series from Japan, biopsies from senile systemic amyloidosis patients showed transthyretin amyloid deposits in 44% of patients.
- **Age**
  A retrospective review analyzing the 13-year experience of a single center showed a median age of 61 years.
- **Sex**
  There was a male predominance (62%) in a retrospective review of GI involvement of amyloidosis.
- **Site**
  Amyloidosis may involve the entire GI tract. The small bowel, in particular, the duodenum, is the most frequent organ affected, followed by the stomach, colon, and rectum and esophagus, in decreasing frequency. The oral cavity may also be affected manifesting as macroglossia which is very characteristic of systemic AL amyloidosis. It may lead to dysphagia, dysarthria, and, very infrequently, airway obstruction. Macroglossia is present in 10–23% of patients with systemic AL amyloidosis. Other oral manifestations may include bullous lesions, vesicles, and ulcers.
- **Treatment**
  Although the gastrointestinal complications can result in significant morbidity, they are

not usually the cause of death, which is most often due to renal failure, restrictive cardiomyopathy, or ischemic heart disease. Therapy is directed at symptomatic control of the gastrointestinal manifestations and is aimed at reducing the deposits of the amyloidogenic precursor protein, leading to the improvement of function of the organ involves. The treatment of AA amyloidosis relies on the control of inflammation of the underlying disease. The aim of therapy for patients with AA amyloidosis is to reduce the production of serum amyloid A (SAA) protein. Survival of the patient, amyloidotic organ survival, and change in amyloid load are directly influenced by SAA levels. The treatment of AL amyloidosis includes chemotherapy with melphalan and prednisolone and high-dose chemotherapy with hematopoietic stem cell transplantation. Dysmotility-related symptoms may be alleviated by prokinetic agents and total parenteral nutrition and antidiarrheal agents may also be beneficial. Severe diarrhea and protein loss due to gastrointestinal amyloidosis may respond to glucocorticoids and octreotide. Diarrhea may at least in part reflect the rapid intestinal transit that has been documented in patients with amyloidosis. Regarding novel therapies, there are case reports suggesting benefit of a humanized anti-IL6 receptor antibody. Surgical procedures should be contemplated only in an emergency setting because of the risk of decompensation of organs affected by amyloid deposition. Liver transplantation has been used most successfully for treatment of familial amyloid polyneuropathy.

- **Outcome**
  Gastrointestinal manifestations and malnutrition are common and multifactorial in etiology and have a negative impact on quality of life and survival. Nevertheless, the main determinant factor in survival is the extent of cardiac involvement. In a study carried out, an Italian center should have a median survival of 3.8 years in AL amyloidosis patients, with 27% dying within 1 year of diagnosis and a 10-cumulative proportion of 31% who survived.

Macroscopy

Amyloid deposition occurs predominantly, in AL amyloidosis, in the muscularis polypoid protrusions and thickening of the circular folds of the small bowel. In AA amyloidosis, fine, granular appearance, mucosal friability, and erosions are present. Consequently, AL amyloidosis usually presents with constipation, mechanical obstruction, or chronic intestinal pseudo-obstruction, while AA amyloidosis presents with diarrhea and malabsorption. In the colonic mucosa, some of the most common aspects include: submucosal hematomas, ulcers, hemorrhagic bullous colitis, and yellowish plaque-like infiltrative lesions. In familial amyloid polyneuropathy (FAP), a fine, granular appearance with smaller amount of amyloid deposition in the mucosa is more characteristic. Neuromuscular infiltration initially affects the intrinsic nervous system and results in a neuropathic process with uncoordinated contractions. At a later stage, tissue wall infiltration results in a myopathic process with low amplitude contractions associated with significantly prolonged transit.

No specific radiological features of gastrointestinal tract amyloidosis exist. The prevalence of radiological abnormalities in patients with systemic amyloidosis is highest in the small intestine.

Microscopy

Amyloid is defined as deposited fibrillar material detected by electron microscopy, amorphous eosinophilic appearance on hematoxylin and eosin staining (Fig. 1). Apple-green birefringence on Congo Red (Fig. 2) histological staining confirms the diagnosis. Immunohistochemistry should be routinely performed in biopsy samples from any patient with amyloidosis for precise identification of the amyloid fibril protein.

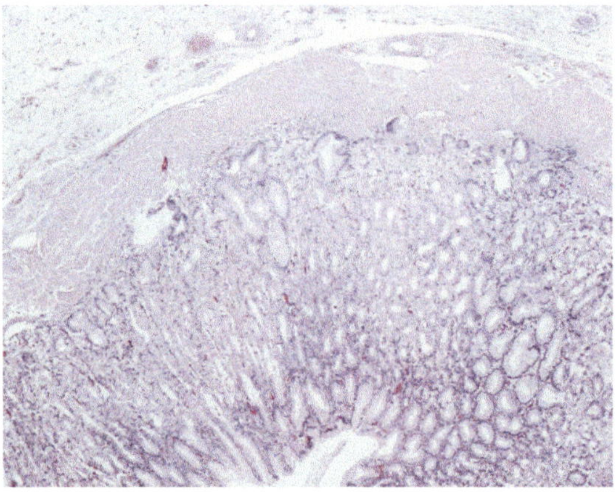

Amyloidosis, Gastrointestinal, Fig. 1 Gastric body biopsies, H&E stain showing amyloid substance deposits in the muscularis mucosa (original magnification, 40×)

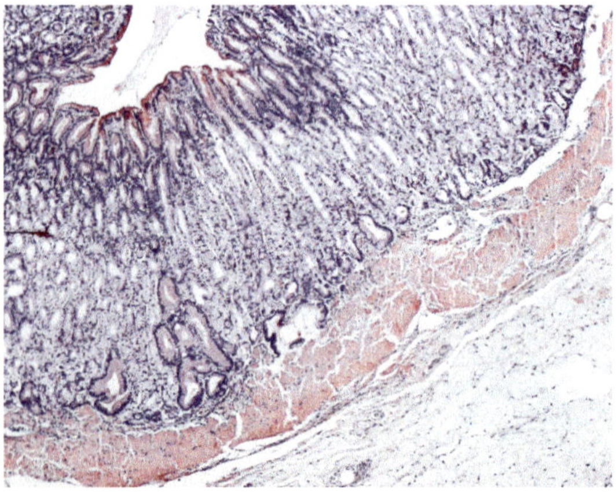

Amyloidosis, Gastrointestinal, Fig. 2 Gastric body biopsies, Congo Red stain showing amyloid substance deposits in the muscularis mucosa (original magnification, 40×)

Immunophenotype

Immunophenotyping may be used in the differential diagnosis between GI amyloidosis and malignant infiltrations, such as in the case of multiple myeloma. Markers such as CD38 (a surface protein that influences differentiation and proliferation of myeloma cells), CD45 (leukocyte common antigen), and CD19 and CD20 (B-cell associated antigens) may be used to differentiate between malignant involvement of the GI mucosa.

Differential Diagnosis

Symptoms related to GI amyloidosis may vary from bleeding to diarrhea and malabsorption syndromes to constipation and pseudo-obstruction. The relative rarity of amyloidoses, along with their variable clinical presentations and requirement for precise immunohistochemical staining of biopsy specimens, makes the diagnosis of amyloidosis challenging. The possibility of systemic amyloidosis is thus often overlooked, resulting in substantial delays in diagnosis. There should be a high index of suspicion in patients with disorders known to be associated with amyloidosis. These include multiple myeloma, a chronic inflammatory disease such as rheumatoid arthritis, and chronic renal failure treated with maintenance dialysis. Amyloidosis should also be suspected when there is involvement of other organs characteristic of systemic amyloid deposition such as the nephrotic syndrome, otherwise unexplained heart failure, or periarthritis. According to the organ affected, the differential diagnoses may diverge.

Esophagus: Cases of esophageal dysmotility may mimic achalasia on manometry studies.

Stomach: Bleeding related to amyloidosis may occur with Dieulafoy type ulcers and submucosal hematomas. Benign pyloric stenosis might be caused by amyloid-induced ulcers as opposed to peptic ulcers. Gastroparesis is common among patients with FAP and must be differentiated from other causes such as diabetic neuropathy.

Small bowel: Other causes of malabsorption syndromes such as infections (tuberculosis, *Giardia*), Crohn's disease, celiac disease, and lymphoma must be excluded.

Colon: Inflammatory bowel disease, Crohn's disease or ulcerative colitis, and irritable bowel syndrome are the most common differentials.

References and Further Reading

Cowan, A., Skinner, M., & Seldin, D. et al. (2012) Amyloidosis of the gastrointestinal tract: A 13-year single center referral experience. *Haematologica*, *97*. (epub ahead of print).

Madsen, L. G., Gimsing, P., & Schiødt, F. V. (2009). Primary (AL) amyloidosis with gastrointestinal involvement. *Scandinavian Journal of Gastroenterology, 44*, 708.
Merlini, G., Seldin, D., & Gertz, M. (2011). Amyloidosis: Pathogenesis and new therapeutic options. *Journal of Clinical Oncology, 14*, 1924–1933.
Sattianayagam, P. T., Hawkins, P. N., & Gillmore, J. D. (2009). Systemic amyloidosis and the gastrointestinal tract. *Nature Reviews. Gastroenterology & Hepatology, 6*, 608–617.
Tada, S., Iida, M., Yao, T., et al. (1994). Endoscopic features in amyloidosis of the small intestine: Clinical and morphologic differences between chemical types of amyloid protein. *Gastrointestinal Endoscopy, 40*, 45.

Anal Adenocarcinoma

Denis Chatelain[1] and Jean-François Fléjou[2]
[1]Service d'Anatomie Pathologique, Centre Hospitalier et Universitaire du Nord, Amiens, France
[2]Faculté de Médecine Pierre et Marie Curie, Service d'Anatomie et Cytologie Pathologiques, Hôpital Saint-Antoine, Paris, France

Synonyms

Glandular carcinoma

Definition

The most frequent type of anal cancer is squamous cell carcinoma, described in a specific chapter (see entry "► Squamous Cell Carcinoma, Anus"). Other types of anal carcinoma, i.e., adenocarcinoma, neuroendocrine carcinoma, Paget's disease, and basal cell carcinoma, can also be observed.

Adenocarcinoma of the anal canal is a malignant epithelial tumor arising from glandular cells lining the upper anorectal part of the anal canal, anal transitional zone (ATZ) mucosa, the anal glands, or the epithelium lining of fistulous tracts.

Most adenocarcinomas found in the anal canal represent downward spread from a rectal adenocarcinoma or arise from colorectal-type mucosa lining the ATZ above the dentate line. Rare cases, described as extramucosal perianal adenocarcinomas, develop in pre-existing congenital or acquired anal sinuses or fistulae (in patients with Crohn's disease). Some adenocarcinomas develop from anal glands or ducts that drain the anal glands (anal duct carcinoma). They differ from the former colorectal-type anal adenocarcinoma by the presence of an overlying nonneoplastic, non-dysplastic mucosa (which may sometimes be ulcerated by the tumor), while carcinomas arising in ATZ show dysplasia or intraepithelial neoplasia in the surface epithelium.

Clinical Features

Patients complain of similar symptoms to those of patients with anal squamous cell carcinoma: anal pain, rectal bleeding, and presence of a perianal mass. Some adenocarcinomas may develop from a chronic fissure or fistula that has been present for many years. Symptoms may also be nonspecific and this can contribute to delayed diagnosis.

- **Incidence**
  Adenocarcinoma of the anal canal accounts for approximately 10% (5–19%) of all anal canal cancers. The incidence of anal adenocarcinoma arising from an anal fistula is estimated to be 0.3–0.7% in patients with Crohn's disease. The mean interval between the onset of perianal Crohn's disease and the development of anal adenocarcinoma is 7 years.
- **Age**
  Extramucosal adenocarcinoma is usually diagnosed in patients aged from 50 to 70 years.
- **Sex**
  Extramucosal adenocarcinomas seem to be more frequent in males.
- **Site**
  Adenocarcinoma arises from anal glands of the anal mucosa or from glandular cells that line the ATZ mucosa.
- **Treatment**
  There is no consensus for the treatment of anal adenocarcinoma due to rarity of this tumor. Treatment modalities include abdominoperineal

resection, local excision, chemotherapy, and radiotherapy. Most patients are treated by abdominoperineal resection, in order to remove the entire lesion and diminish the risk of local recurrence. Half of the patients undergo adjuvant therapy with either radiotherapy alone or in combination with chemotherapy (with 5-FU, capecitabine, mitomycin, cisplatin, or oxaliplatin). The role of subsequent radiation therapy and or chemotherapy has not yet been defined.

- **Outcome**
  Anal adenocarcinoma often has an aggressive course. Prognosis is related to the stage at diagnosis and is graver than that of squamous cell carcinoma.
  The reported 5-year survival rate ranges from 5% to 93%, but the overall 5-year survival is generally accepted to be less than 20%. Metastases at time of presentation vary from 13.5% to 62%. Most common sites of metastases are the lymph nodes, liver, lung, and peritoneum. A possible explanation for the poor prognosis of anal adenocarcinoma is the delay in diagnosis due to symptomatic overlap between these tumors and benign conditions such as hemorrhoids.

Macroscopy

Anal adenocarcinomas present as ulcerated or polypoid indurate or friable mucinous or whitish masses. They measure from 1 to 5 cm in diameter and can induce obstruction of the anal canal. Metastases can be present in superficial inguinal, pelvic, and abdominal lymph nodes.

Microscopy

Adenocarcinomas arising in the anal canal are divided into three subcategories: colorectal-type adenocarcinoma, adenocarcinoma arising within anorectal fistula, and anal duct carcinoma.

Colorectal-type adenocarcinoma is the most common subtype of anal adenocarcinoma. It arises from the colorectal-type mucosa above the dentate line, from the glandular cells of the anal transitional zone, or sometimes from a previous dysplastic adenoma. It has the same microscopic features as a colorectal adenocarcinoma and consists of glands often with a cribriform pattern, lined by columnar cells with basophilic cytoplasm, and marked nuclear atypia with a high mitotic activity (Fig. 1). The lumen of the tumor glands often contains eosinophilic dirty necrosis with necrotic nuclear debris and neutrophils. These tumors carry a higher risk of inguinal and femoral metastatic lymph nodes than rectal adenocarcinoma.

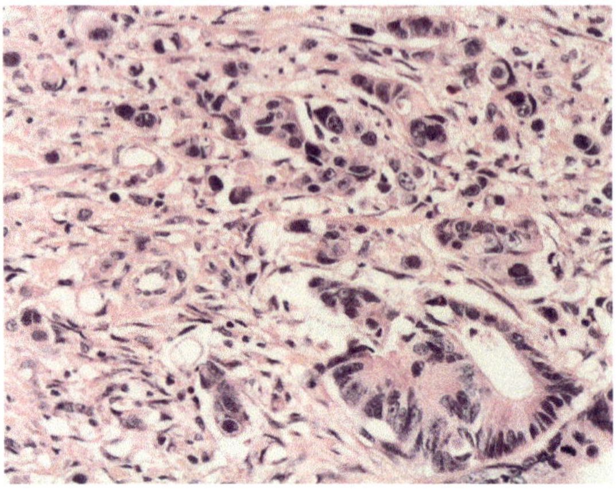

Anal Adenocarcinoma, Fig. 1 Moderately well-differentiated adenocarcinoma of the anus, with a similar morphology to a rectal adenocarcinoma

Adenocarcinoma within anorectal fistula is more frequently of the mucinous type, with atypical columnar cells, signet ring cells, or solid islands floating within mucin pools (Fig. 2).

Anal duct carcinoma arising from anal glands consists of small acini and tubules originating from ducts that open onto the mucosal surface. The acini are lined by cuboidal cells showing scanty mucin secretion. Nuclei are pleomorphic with a high nuclear-to-cytoplasmic ratio and prominent nucleoli. Tumors can have a papillary or cribriform architecture. Atypical ductular structures invade the surrounding tissues without necessarily causing ulceration of the overlying anal mucosa. Focal pagetoid spreading into the overlying squamous epithelium can be seen.

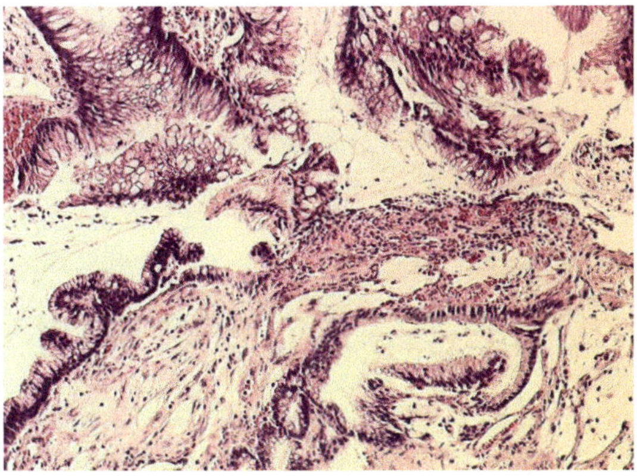

Anal Adenocarcinoma, Fig. 2 Mucinous adenocarcinoma arising within an anal fistula

Immunophenotype

Colorectal-type adenocarcinoma of the anal canal stains positive for cytokeratin 20 but may also have unexpected cytokeratin 7 expression. Adenocarcinoma of the anal glands expresses cytokeratin 7 as well as cytokeratin 19, cytokeratins 5/6, and MUC5AC. It does not show positivity for p63 protein, cytokeratin 20, and CDX2.

Molecular Features

Molecular features of anal adenocarcinoma are still unknown due to the rarity of this tumor.

Differential Diagnosis

A prostate carcinoma that invades the anal mucosa can mimic the growth pattern of an anal gland carcinoma. This tumor usually expresses prostate-specific antigen (PSA) on immunohistochemical study, and clinical evaluation for prostate carcinoma can help in the distinction between these two tumors. CK7 and CK20 can help distinguish anal gland carcinoma (CK7+ CK20−) from rectal-type adenocarcinoma (CK20+, CK7−). Histochemical strong PAS reactivity that is lost after periodate-borohydride/saponification indicates the absence of O-acylated sialic acids in tumor cells and could sign an origin from anal glands.

References and Further Reading

Meriden, Z., & Montgomery, E. A. (2012). Anal duct carcinoma: A report of 5 cases. *Human Pathology, 43*, 216–220.
Shia, J. (2010). An update on tumors of the anal canal. *Archives of Pathology and Laboratory Medicine, 134*, 1601–1611.

Angiodysplasia

Maria Sotiropoulou
Department of Pathology, Alexandra Hospital, Athens, Attica, Greece

Synonyms

Colonic angiomas; Colonic arteriovenous malformation; Vascular ectasia of the colon

Definition

Angiodysplasia is characterized by the presence of malformed dilated blood vessels in submucosa, extending into the overlying intestinal mucosa. It is the second most common colonic lesion (after diverticulosis) which may cause gastrointestinal bleeding, though it may be asymptomatic. Most cases are acquired degenerative lesions of the elderly people. Early in the nineteenth century (1839), Phillips described a vascular abnormality that caused gastrointestinal bleeding, but it was Margoulis and colleagues who first used the term angiodysplasia in 1960.

Angiodysplasia may present as multiple vascular lesions or as an isolated lesion. When there is GI bleeding without obvious reason, small bowel angiodysplasia may account for 30–40% of cases. Low-grade bleeding is characterized by melena or hematochezia in clinical presentation.

Rarely, (15% of cases) bleeding can be massive, and in 10–15%, iron deficiency anemia or positivity for occult blood can be the only manifestation. Although in a great percentage (≈90%) of cases bleeding stops spontaneously, it often reoccurs.

Chronic venous obstruction plays a role in the pathogenesis. Repeated episodes of colonic distention causing high lumen pressure slow down the submucosal venous outflow with subsequent local hypoxygenation. Over the years, which explains the higher incidence in aged people, this process causes gradual dilatation of venules, arterioles, or capillaries of the mucosa and submucosa. Ultimately the precapillary sphincter loses its capacity and small arteriovenous communications occur. This theory matches the clinical and pathologic features with the more common location in the cecum and proximal right colon where the tension is higher because of greater diameter. The presence of dilated submucosal veins, which is one of the most stable histologic features, supports this theory in pathogenesis. Angiodysplasia is not associated with angiomatous lesions of the skin and other viscera in contrast to other congenital or neoplastic vascular lesions. However, gastrointestinal angiodysplasias, including colon location, occur more frequently in individuals with scleroderma. A relative deficiency of collagen type IV in mucosal vessels and vascular immunoreactivity for angiogenic factors such as fibroblastic growth factor (VEGF) has been observed in patients with angiodysplasia. Characteristic is the fact that there are no pathologic changes in the arterioles in any of the mucosal lesions.

Diseases such as von Willebrand, aortic stenosis (as already mentioned) may have a link with angiodysplasia. Other factors including diverticula, portal hypertension colopathy, and vascular ectasia in patients receiving high-dose chemotherapy and stem cell transplantation have been correlated to the entire GI angiodysplasia.

Although colonoscopy is the principal method in the evaluation of gastrointestinal bleeding, angiograph plays an important complementary role. Colonoscopic signs, in incidentally found angiodysplasias, are pale in color, while those in patients with recent hemorrhage are bright with slight raised centers. In colonoscopy angiodysplastic lesions are described as small, frondlike, or scalloped edges. Colonoscopy's sensitivity exceeds 80% and has the advantage of obtaining biopsies from suspected lesions, especially when colonoscopic signs are not clear. Capsular endoscopy has shown that angiodysplasia is the most common reason (50%) for obscure gastrointestinal bleeding and can be used combined with magnetic resonance enterography (MRE) with better results in the small bowel disease. Only in rare cases (2,6%), angiodysplasia can be diagnosed by visual inception at laparotomy.

Clinical Features

- **Incidence**
  The real incidence of angiodysplasia is unknown. Study from Foutch et al. found that the prevalence in 964 asymptomatic individuals (mean age 60 years) at screening colonoscopy was 0,83%. However, in cases of lower gastrointestinal bleeding, the incidence is estimated at 6%, and angiodysplasia is the second leading cause after diverticulosis in patients older than 60 years.
- **Age**
  Angiodysplasia usually occurs in individuals older than 60 years, with mean age in the 70th year. In any case it can happen at any age even in young people.
- **Sex**
  Men and women have the same frequency of angiodysplasia.
- **Site**
  Angiodysplasia is usually located in the right colon and actually 77% in cecum and ascending colon and 15% in small intestine (jejunum and ileum).
- **Treatment**
  Conservative management is recommended in hemodynamically stable patients. Endoscopic techniques with obliteration of angiodysplastic lesions have beneficial results in 50% of patients. Heater probe and multipolar

electrocoagulation probe have been successful in colonic lesions. Selective embolization of visceral arterial branches achieves immediate cessation of bleeding in 97% of patients. Especially in right-side lesions, endoscopic laser photocoagulation has been successful with the disadvantage of complications (15%). Other methods such as emergency embolization with liquid polyvinyl alcohol copolymer or endoclips have been used.

Angiography and injection of dyes play an important role in preoperative localization of small bowel lesions before surgical procedures. Surgical resection such as right hemicolectomy is the second-line therapy after endoscopic ablation, with high mortality rate, because patients are aged with coexisting medical problems.

In refractory cases, somatostatin analogues, continuous octreotide administration, and thalidomide play a role in the management of bleeding from angiodysplasia.

- **Outcome (Prognosis)**
  Fifteen percent (15%) of individuals with colonic angiodysplasia never bleed. Hemorrhage ceases spontaneously in most patients (90%). Recurrence of hemorrhage is the major problem and occurs in 30% of patients. Predictive factors of recurrence are the earlier history of bleeding after treatment, over-anticoagulation, and multiple lesions. Individuals with more than 10 angiodysplastic lesions or a diameter of 10 mm or more have worse clinical impact.

Macroscopy (Gross)

Angiodysplasia is extremely difficult to detect in gross examination of the surgical resected specimen. If there is suspicion of angiodysplasia, the bowel needs to be received fresh and sometimes we can see small foci of vascular marking and erythema. These difficult to confine features are not visible after formalin fixation. Only few laboratories have the equipment to perform injection studies which facilitate the revelation of the lesions. The injected substance is a combination of Indian ink (which remains after fixation) and a radiopaque dye and then x-ray examination follows. In fixed specimens slicing at the site of suspected mucosal lesions with a sharp blade can detect the lesion. Grossly the lesions, which are more often multiple, consist of small (usually 1–2 mm or less, <5 mm) fan shaped with central vessel, cherry-red in color, and flat, while rarely may coexist with mucosal erosions. When angiodysplastic foci have been cauterized, the lesion will be a heaped-up ulcer.

Microscopy

Endoscopic biopsies have diagnostic histopathologic features of angiodysplasia in 31–60% of specimens. The characteristic lesion is the presence of irregularly shaped clusters of ectatic arterioles, venules, and their capillary connections (Fig. 1). Vessels are dilated (twice the normal diameter) with distorted thin wall with variable smooth muscle, usually composed only of endothelium. The lesion at first is identified in submucosa and later more advanced lesions involve the mucosa too (Fig. 2). Most endoscopically obtained biopsies have not submucosa, where the major and early portion of the lesion is present. Mucosal biopsies may show few ectatic capillaries which may collapse and be difficult to identify. In advanced cases the dilated vessels distort

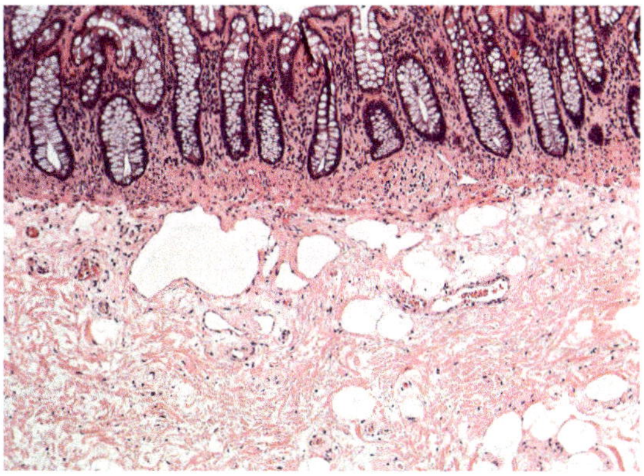

Angiodysplasia, Fig. 1 Large bowel specimen: in low power there are thin-walled submucosal veins and arteries with arteriovenous anastomoses

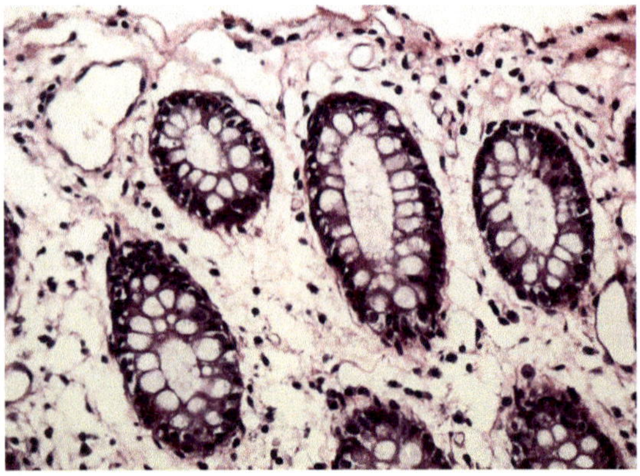

Angiodysplasia, Fig. 2 Colon biopsy in high power with clusters of dilated tortuous veins and capillaries

the normal mucosal architecture, displacing glands and separating crypts from each other, and sometimes there is only a layer of endothelial cells between the vascular channel and the intestinal lumen. Submucosal arteries may have mild to moderate sclerotic changes in some cases with atheromatous emboli, while arterialization of veins with hypertrophy of intima and smooth muscle may also happen. There are cases with full-thickness involvement from serosa to mucosa. Ultrastructural characteristics by electron microscopy are modified shape of endotheliocytes, impaired structure of the basal membrane, and reduced count of pericytes.

Immunophenotype

Study with collagen IV, which forms the basement membrane of the vascular endothelium, has demonstrated relative deficiency in mucosal vessels with angiodysplastic features. Vascular endothelial growth factor (VEGF) expression is higher in angiodysplasias than normal mucosal and submucosal vessels.

Molecular Features

There are no specific molecular studies concerning angiodysplasia.

Differential Diagnosis

Vascular tumors and lesions associated with congenital or systematic disease and radiation damage with similar histologic findings must be kept in mind in the differential diagnosis. Colonic arteriovenous malformation tends to be solitary and large in size in contrast to angiodysplasia which is isolated or diffuse and small.

References and Further Reading

Anne, H. (1988). Angiodysplasia: Current concepts. *Postgraduate Medical Journal, 64*, 259–263.

Fenoglio-Preiser, C., Noffsinger, A., Stemmermann, G., et al. (2008). *Gastrointestinal pathology. An atlas and text* (3rd ed., pp. 863–864). Philadelphia: Lippincott, Williams and Wilkins.

Kheterpal, S. (1991). Angiodysplasia: A review. *Journal of Royal Society of Medicine, 84*, 615–618.

Roskell, D. E., Biddolph, S. D., & Warren, P. F. (1998). Apparent deficiency of mucosal vascular collagen type IV associated with angiodysplasia of the colon. *Journal of Clinical Pathology, 51*, 18–20.

West, B., Mitchell, K. (2009). In R. Odze, J. Goldblum (Eds.), *Surgical pathology of the GI tract, liver, biliary tract and pancreas* (2nd ed., pp.196–199). Saunders Elsevier.

Antibiotic-Associated Colitis

Liesbeth Ferdinande
Department of Pathology, Ghent University Hospital, Ghent, Belgium

Definition

Antibiotic-associated diarrhea is defined as otherwise unexplained diarrhea that occurs in association with antibiotic use. The antibiotic types most often related to antibiotic-associated diarrhea are cephalosporins, clindamycin, broad-spectrum penicillins, and ampicillin/amoxicillin. The clinical manifestations range from mild complaints of frequent loose and watery stools to severe, fulminant colitis (pseudomembranous colitis) with possible fatal outcome.

The mechanisms behind this antibiotic-associated diarrhea are multiple.

First, antibiotics may have direct effects on the gastrointestinal tract that contribute to the development of diarrhea. Erythromycin, for example, has a motilin receptor stimulating activity, and this prokinetic action results in faster gastric emptying and a shorter oro-cecal transit time.

Secondly, the antibiotic-induced alterations in the composition of resident microflora in the intestinal tract may influence normal gut functioning. Anaerobes are involved in the breakdown of carbohydrates, and the use of antibiotics active on this anaerobic flora may result in osmotic diarrhea due to the impaired colonic carbohydrate fermentation. It was suggested that also a decrease in degradation of bile acids, which is dependent on bacterial enzymes, plays a role in antibiotic-associated diarrhea as bile acids are potent colonic secretory agents.

Thirdly, changes in the gut flora allow overgrowth of various infectious agents that were previously present in the resident flora or that were acquired from the environment. *Clostridium difficile* is described to be the major infectious agent in this context. *Clostridium difficile* is a Gram-positive, spore-forming, anaerobic bacillus. It may be part of the normal microflora of the gut, especially in children and young adults, but is found in only 0–3% of healthy adults. Colonization is significantly more frequent in hospitalized patients. The spores that are formed by *Clostridium difficile* may persist in the environment for years. Ingested spores are resistant to the acidic milieu of the stomach and germinate in the colon. Symptoms are generated by the action of two exotoxins: toxin A and toxin B. More than 60% of adults or older children have antibodies against these toxins, and the level and quality of this specific antibody response determines susceptibility to *Clostridium difficile* infection. Clinical manifestations may be variable ranging from mild diarrhea to pseudomembranous colitis. Cephalosporins, clindamycin, and broad-spectrum penicillins are the antibiotics that are most frequently associated with *Clostridium difficile* infection, but virtually any antibiotic may be implicated.

Antibiotic-associated hemorrhagic colitis is a distinct form of antibiotic-associated colitis in which *Clostridium difficile* is absent. *Klebsiella oxytoca* was identified as the causative agent. This type of colitis is characterized by the sudden onset of bloody diarrhea within 1 week of antibiotic therapy, often associated with severe abdominal cramps. Endoscopy shows mucosal hemorrhage, mucosal edema, and ulcers, predominantly localized in the right colon. *Klebsiella oxytoca* is a Gram-negative enterobacterium that expresses a β-lactamase, making it resistant to penicillins which may explain why this type of colitis is mainly seen during therapy with penicillin derivatives. Overgrowth of *Klebsiella oxytoca* in the colon due to penicillin treatment may lead to high cytotoxin concentrations and subsequent mucosal damage. Frequent use of nonsteroidal anti-inflammatory drugs (NSAID) was reported to aggravate colitis.

Other enteric pathogens described in the pathogenesis of antibiotic-associated colitis are *Clostridium perfringens*, *Staphylococcus aureus*, *Candida* species, and *Salmonella*.

Clinical Features

- **Incidence**
  The incidence of antibiotic-associated diarrhea ranges from 5% to 25% in literature, depending on the definition of diarrhea and the type of antibiotic used. Infection with *Clostridium difficile* accounts for 10–20% of cases of antibiotic-associated diarrhea, with significantly higher incidence in hospitalized patients than in outpatients. *Clostridium difficile* is responsible for almost all cases of antibiotic-associated pseudomembranous colitis. The incidence and mortality of *Clostridium difficile* infection is increasing worldwide. In most areas, this is believed to be due to the appearance and spread of a hypervirulent strain that has acquired resistance to many commonly used antibiotics. Next to antibiotic use, major risk factors associated with *Clostridium difficile* infection are advanced

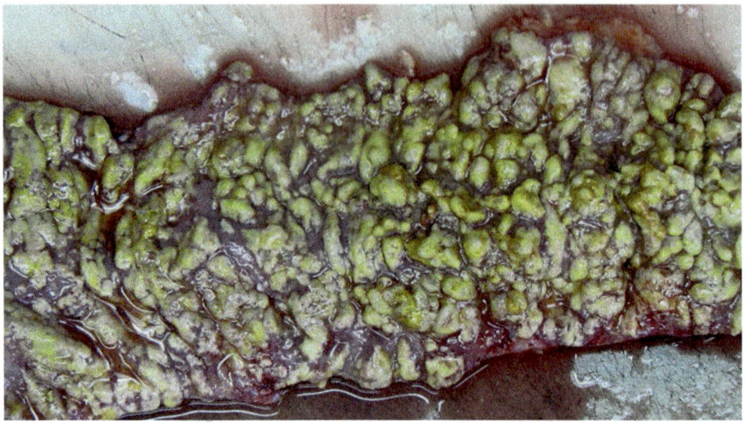

Antibiotic-Associated Colitis, Fig. 1 Gross appearance of pseudomembranous colitis: pseudomembranes present as yellow, adherent mucosal plaques

age, hospitalization, and contact with other infected patients. Recent evidence proposes the use of proton pump inhibitors as a risk factor in the development of *Clostridium difficile* infection owing to their effects on the intestinal microflora.

Klebsiella oxytoca-induced antibiotic-associated hemorrhagic colitis is rare, but its exact incidence is not known.

- **Treatment**

  In patients with *Clostridium difficile*-associated diarrhea, cessation of the inciting antibiotic therapy combined with supportive treatment if necessary results in resolution of diarrhea in 25% of patients. In patients with moderate or severe disease or significant underlying conditions, administration of oral metronidazole or vancomycin hydrochloride is indicated. Occasionally, surgery (subtotal colectomy) is required.

  To avoid the outbreak of *Clostridium difficile* infections, especially in hospitals and care facilities, preventive measures should be taken. These include restricted prescription and use of antibiotics, education of hospital personnel, isolation of patients, and disinfection of rooms of infected patients to remove the persistent spores.

  In patients with *Klebsiella oxytoca*-induced antibiotic-associated hemorrhagic colitis, discontinuation of the antibiotic and NSAID in combination with symptomatic therapy is usually sufficient.

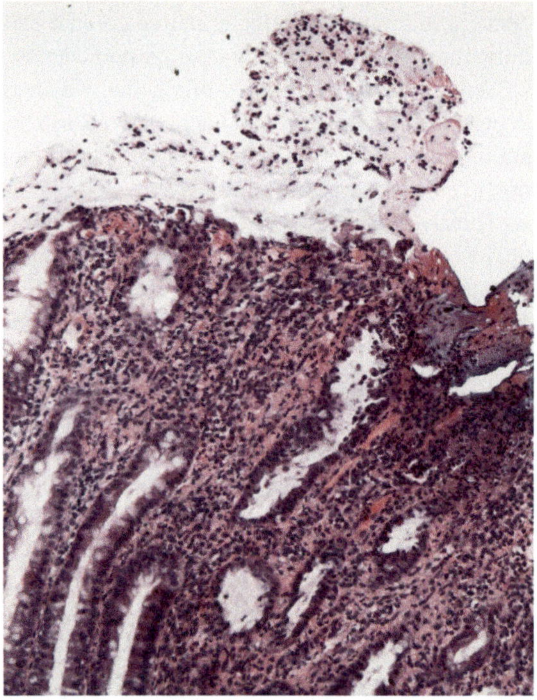

Antibiotic-Associated Colitis, Fig. 2 Early lesion in pseudomembranous colitis: accumulation of polymorphonuclear cells in the lamina propria and focal eruption with fibrin, polymorphonuclear cells, and debris spraying into the lumen

Macroscopy

Macroscopic findings of *Clostridium difficile* infection are rather unspecific in cases of colitis without pseudomembranes. Pseudomembranous

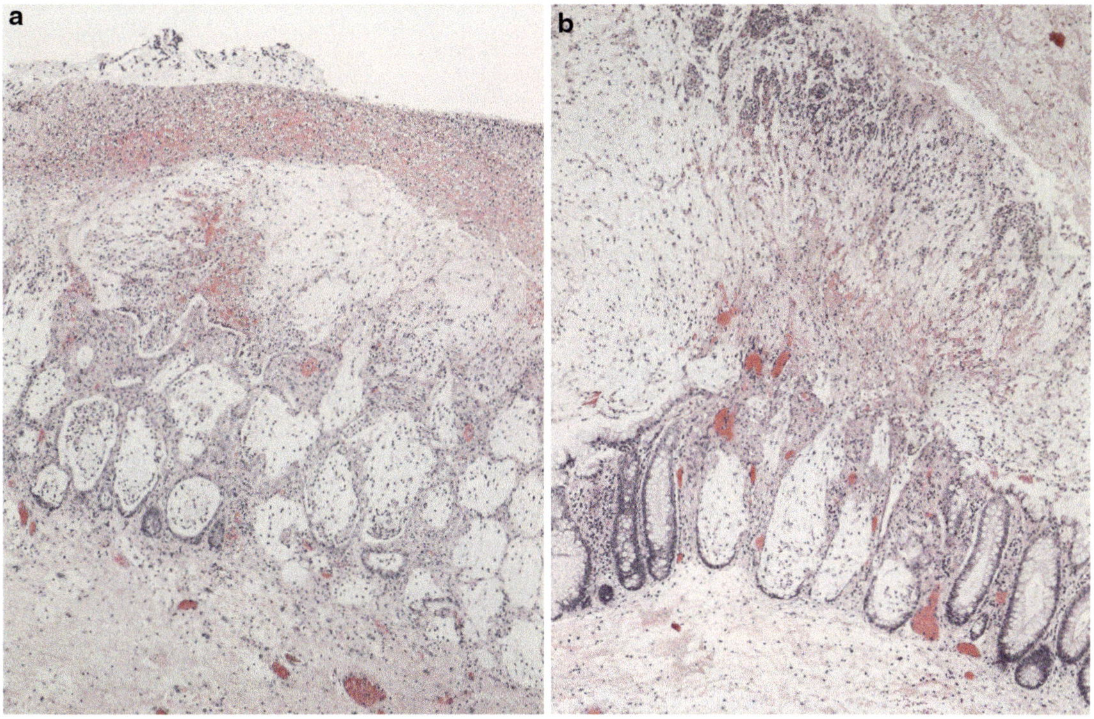

Antibiotic-Associated Colitis, Fig. 3 "Volcano" lesions in pseudomembranous colitis. (**a**) Dilated glands are filled with mucin and polymorphonuclear cells. The mucosa is covered by a laminated pseudomembrane. (**b**) Smaller lesion with normal adjacent mucosa

colitis, however, has a characteristic gross appearance (Fig. 1). Pseudomembranes can be recognized as yellow plaques adherent to the colonic mucosa. They are variable in size and occur most commonly in the left colon. In later stages, the plaques coalesce to form areas of complete mucosal necrosis.

Microscopy

The earliest recognizable mucosal abnormality in pseudomembranous colitis ("summit" lesion) shows subepithelial accumulation of polymorphonuclear cells, nuclear dust, and eosinophilic material with a focal, small eruptive focus spraying fibrin, polymorphonuclear cells, and debris into the lumen (Fig. 2). Typically, the surrounding mucosa is normal or shows minimal inflammatory changes. The more advanced lesions, the so-called "volcano" lesions, consist of a variable number of dilated glands that are partially disrupted (Fig. 3). The deeper epithelial cells are often preserved, but the more superficial epithelial cells are destroyed. This mucosal lesion is covered by a pseudomembrane composed of mucin, polymorphonuclear cells, nuclear debris, and fibrin. Again, these lesions are separated by normal or mildly inflamed mucosa. Progression and merging of these lesions result in complete mucosal necrosis.

Colon biopsies of patients with *Klebsiella oxytoca*-induced antibiotic-associated hemorrhagic colitis show mucosal hemorrhage as an accumulation of erythrocytes in the lamina propria. There is a mild inflammatory infiltrate in the lamina propria. Crypt abscesses are usually absent in contrast to other forms of infectious colitis. Epithelial alterations can be observed featuring goblet cell loss, anisonucleosis, increased rate of mitosis and apoptosis, or desquamation.

Differential Diagnosis

Pseudomembranous colitis is a descriptive entity, and although most cases are inflicted by *Clostridium difficile* infection, other causative factors should be excluded. Other infectious agents can cause pseudomembranous colitis. Also ischemic colitis can present with pseudomembranes, and differential diagnosis can be challenging, especially in older, hospitalized patients with comorbidity. A history of antibiotic use and detection of *Clostridium difficile* toxins in stool can aid in this differentiation. The diagnosis of ischemic colitis should be favored in colonic biopsies where hyalinization of the lamina propria, atrophic micro-crypts, and more diffuse involvement of the mucosal surface by pseudomembranes are found.

Signet-ring cell change (Fig. 4) was described in pseudomembranous colitis and should be recognized as a possible diagnostic pitfall, particularly in small biopsies or patients with an oncological history. These alterations should be differentiated from a neoplastic infiltrate, although both primary and metastatic signet-ring cell carcinomas of the colon are uncommon. The benign signet-ring cells show intracytoplasmic vacuoles and peripherally located nuclei without nuclear atypia or mitotic figures. The cells are present in the crypts of the mucosa or in the pseudomembrane, but not in the lamina propria outside the crypts. Some studies suggest that signet-ring cell morphology of crypt cells in pseudomembranous colitis is associated with a fulminant clinical course, but others could not confirm this.

In the stage of complete mucosal necrosis, macroscopy or microscopy is not diagnostic of pseudomembranous colitis anymore as this type of injury can occur in ischemic colitis or ► inflammatory bowel disease as well. Evaluation of adjacent vital mucosa can offer some clues to the diagnosis and etiology of the necrosis. In ► inflammatory bowel disease, inflammatory and architectural changes will be prominent. Ischemic colitis will show glandular atrophy and hyalinization of the lamina propria. In pseudomembranous colitis, transition from necrotic zones to relatively normal mucosa is quite abrupt. In areas with preserved mucosal structure, early summit and volcano lesions can be identified as part of the spectrum of lesions.

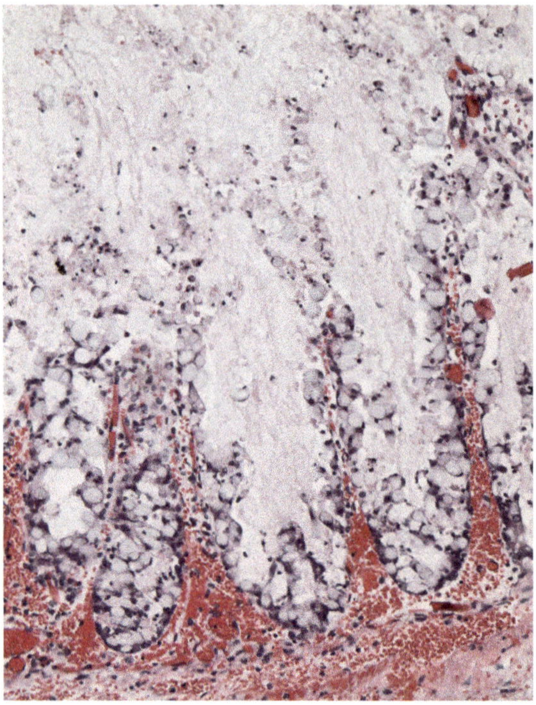

Antibiotic-Associated Colitis, Fig. 4 Pseudomembranous colitis with signet-ring cell change

Histology of biopsies from patients with *Klebsiella oxytoca*-induced antibiotic-associated hemorrhagic colitis is similar to that of other toxin-induced forms of colitis. This type of colitis may also resemble ischemic colitis. The diagnosis should therefore be confirmed by stool cultures.

References and Further Reading

Beaugerie, L., & Petit, J. (2004). Antibiotic-associated diarrhea. *Best Practice & Research Clinical Gastroenterology, 18*, 337–352.

Cameselle-Teijeiro, J., Abdulkader, I., & Forteza, J. (2004). Signet-ring cell change in pseudomembranous colitis versus signet-ring cell carcinoma. *The American Journal of Surgical Pathology, 28*, 1111.

Högenauer, C., Langner, C., Beubler, E., Lippe, I. T., Schicho, R., Gorkiewicz, G., Krause, R., Gerstgrasser, N., Krejs, G. J., & Hinterleitner, T. A. (2006). *Klebsiella oxytoca* as a causative organism of antibiotic-

associated hemorrhagic colitis. *The New England Journal of Medicine, 355*, 2418–2426.
Mylonakis, E., Ryan, E. T., & Calderwood, S. B. (2001). *Clostridium difficile*-associated diarrhea. A review. *Archives of Internal Medicine, 161*, 525–533.
Price, A. B., & Davies, D. R. (1977). Pseudomembranous colitis. *Journal of Clinical Pathology, 30*, 1–12.

Anus

Jean-François Fléjou[1] and Denis Chatelain[2]
[1]Faculté de Médecine Pierre et Marie Curie, Service d'Anatomie et Cytologie Pathologiques, Hôpital Saint-Antoine, Paris, France
[2]Service d'Anatomie Pathologique, Centre Hospitalier et Universitaire du Nord, Amiens, France

Synonyms

Anal canal

Anatomy

Classically, the generic term "anus" encompasses two parts: the anal canal and the anal margin or perianal skin. This terminology applies to the classification of anal tumors, which can be located either in the anal canal or in the anal margin. However, only the anal canal is precisely defined, and this term is often employed synonymously to the term anus.

The anus constitutes the distal 30–40 mm of the gastrointestinal tract. It extends from the rectum superiorly to the perianal skin inferiorly. The anal canal is defined surgically by the borders of the internal anal sphincter (Parks 1958). Anatomists use the levels of the anal valves and the anal orifice, respectively, to mark the upper and lower limits of the anus (Fenger 2007).

The mucosa comprises successive zones, with in the upper part vertical folds known as the anal columns, joined at their lower end by the anal valves marking the position of the dentate or pectinate line (see section "Microscopy").

Musculature

From the inside out, the anal musculature comprises the musculus submucosae ani, the internal anal sphincter, the intersphincteric longitudinal muscle, and the external sphincter. The internal sphincter is a continuation of the distal part of the internal circular layer of the rectal muscularis propria but is considerably thicker, measuring 5–8 mm in thickness. The internal sphincter is under autonomic control and is responsible for the major part of resting anal canal tone. The external sphincter is a surrounding sleeve of striated muscle that blends into the puborectalis muscle proximally and extends just below the internal sphincter margin distally. It is a voluntary muscle with innervation from the pudendal nerve. It can be divided into three parts: a deep part and a superficial part that surround the internal sphincter and a subcutaneous part.

Blood Supply and Vessels

The arterial supply to the anus comes from the superior, middle, and inferior rectal arteries, with large individual variation in anatomical details. The terminal branches of the arteries split up into small tortuous vessels, with some arteriovenous anastomoses with the submucosal venous plexus. This plexus is modified in three specialized vascular anal cushions, located in the left lateral, right anterior, and right posterior zones of the upper two-thirds of the anal canal. The plexuses consist of submucosal anastomosing networks of arterioles and venules showing similar features to erectile tissue. Hemorrhoids are defined as enlarged and prolapsed anal cushions. The superior, middle, and inferior rectal veins make the venous drainage of the anus.

Lymphatics

The lower part of the anal canal below the dentate line and the perianal skin are drained to the superficial inguinal nodes. The lymphatic drainage of the anal canal above the dentate line passes to the superior rectal group of lymph nodes.

Nerves

Ganglion cells present in submucous and myenteric plexuses in the rectum are absent or sparse in the first centimeter of the anal canal above the dentate line.

The sensory innervation of the lower part of the anal canal is accomplished by the inferior rectal nerves.

Function

The role of the anus is to control the expulsion of feces. Anal continence is maintained by the internal and external anal sphincters and the muscles of the pelvic floor.

Size

The anal canal measures 30–40 mm in length. It is a few millimeters shorter in females (Nivatvongs et al. 1981).

Macroscopy

The anal canal extends from the level of the pelvic floor to the anal opening. The lower border of the anal canal gradually merges to the perianal skin, at the level of the anal verge. This transition can be recognized by the presence of skin appendages. The anal lumen forms a triradiate slit, with the stem of the Y located posteriorly and the arms anteriorly. Three folds are present, named the anal cushions. The initial part of the mucosa shows a similar appearance to the mucosa of the rectum above. The mucosa of the upper half of the anal canal forms six to ten vertical folds designated as the anal columns (or columns of Morgagni), separated by the anal sinuses. The bases of the anal columns are connected by semilunar valves. Anal valves are usually more visible in children but may also become more prominent in elderly individuals. The line composed of anal valves and sinuses and the bases of the columns is designated by the term dentate line or pectinate line. Distal to the dentate line and sinuses, a smooth gray area is present, corresponding to the squamous epithelium. At the lower border of the anal canal, the perianal skin is easily recognized with hair follicles.

Microscopy

Mucosa

The mucosa of the anal canal contains four successive zones: the colorectal zone, immediately distal to the rectum; the anal transitional zone (often designated by its acronym ATZ); the uninterrupted nonkeratinizing squamous zone; and the distal zone made of keratinizing squamous epithelium (Fenger 1988) (Fig. 1).

- Colorectal zone: this zone succeeds to the rectal mucosa, and no line of demarcation marks the transition. Compared to the rectal mucosa, the crypts are shorter and more irregular.
- Anal transitional zone: this zone has irregular limits and varying locations and extents. It constitutes the only specific type of mucosa in the anal region. The ATZ epithelium consists of four to nine cell layers (Fig. 2). The basal cells are small with nuclei arranged perpendicularly to the basement membrane and correspond to the proliferative compartment. Intermediate cells have a shape between that of basal cells and surface cells. Surface cells can be columnar, cuboidal, or flattened; they resemble urothelial or immature metaplastic squamous epithelium

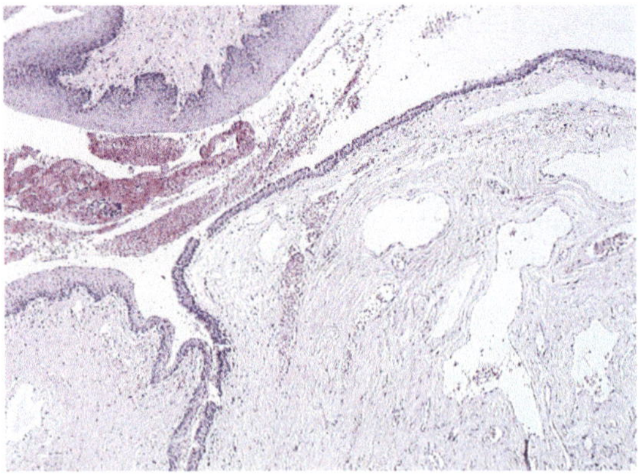

Anus, Fig. 1 Anal mucosa with areas of transitional epithelium (*lower part*) and unkeratinized squamous epithelium (*upper*)

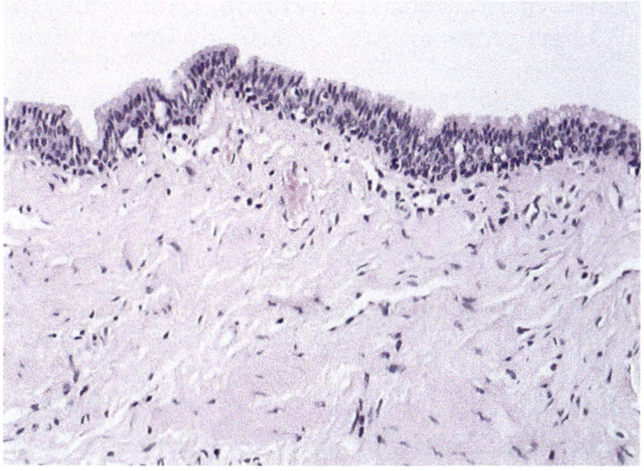

Anus, Fig. 2 Multilayered epithelium of the anal transitional zone (*ATZ*)

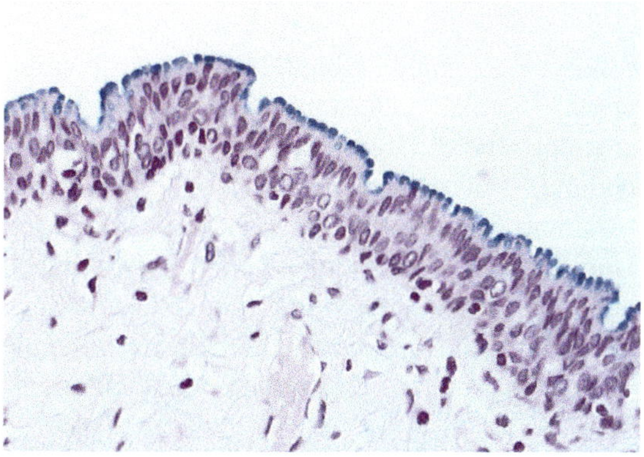

Anus, Fig. 3 Mucus secreting cells in the upper part of the anal transitional epithelium (*Alcian blue*)

and may contain sparse mucus (Fig. 3). Mature goblet cells may also be present, and occasional melanocytes can be seen. Mitoses are rare in the absence of mucosal injury.

The anal glands open in the ATZ. Their median number is six, with a range of three to ten. They are located in the submucosa, and some penetrate into the internal sphincter and even reach the intersphincteric space and the external sphincter (Fig. 4). The epithelial lining is similar to the ATZ surface epithelium. A characteristic feature is the presence of intraepithelial microcysts. These glands discharge into the anal crypts through long tubular anal ducts. Lymphoid nodules are often present around these ducts.

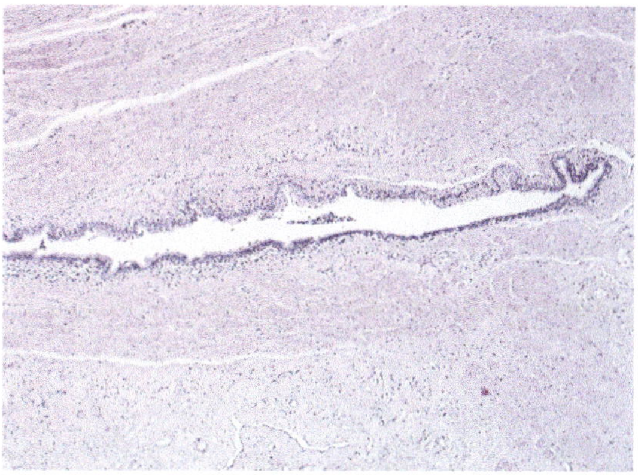

Anus, Fig. 4 Anal gland penetrating the internal sphincter

Endocrine cells are present in the colorectal mucosa, in the transitional mucosa, in anal glands and ducts, and in perianal sweat glands.

- Squamous zone: this zone begins at the level of the dentate line. The squamous epithelium is unkeratinized, with short or no papillae (Fig. 1). Melanocytes are more numerous as in the ATZ, and the epithelium contains dendritic cells, T lymphocytes, and Merkel cells. Glands and skin appendages are absent in this region.
- Perianal skin: keratinization appears at the lower end of the anal canal, and the squamous zone merges into the perianal skin, with sweat glands, hair follicles, sebaceous glands, and apocrine glands. The sweat glands are lined by columnar epithelium with characteristic cytoplasmic "snouts" protruding in the lumen and resting on flat myoepithelial cells. These glands are at the origin of papillary hidradenoma.

Lamina Propria and Submucosal Connective Tissue

The lamina propria is made of loose connective tissue with variable numbers of mast cells and CD34-positive cells of fibroblastic origin that may give rise to fibroepithelial polyps. The muscularis mucosa of the rectum extends to the colorectal zone of the anal canal and may still be present in the upper part of the ATZ. The submucosal connective tissue is loose in the upper anal canal, but it is denser in the lower part, anchoring the epithelium to the superficial part of the internal sphincter.

Immunophenotype

The colorectal epithelium in the upper part of the anal canal is CK20+/CK7-. The ATZ epithelium and anal glands are CK7+/CK20-. Androgen, estrogen, and, to a lesser degree, progesterone receptor are present in the squamous epithelium and in the underlying connective tissue of the anal canal. Endocrine cells express synaptophysin and chromogranin A, and the largest population expresses serotonin. Melanocytes express S100 protein, Melan A, and HMB-45.

Important Diseases

Name of the disease
Abscess
Adenocarcinoma, Anal
Atresia
Basal Cell Carcinoma, Anal Margin
Bowen Disease
Bowenoid Papulosis
► Condyloma, Anal
Fibroepithelial Polyp
► Hemorrhoid
► Inflammatory Cloacogenic Polyp
Melanoma
Neuroendocrine Neoplasms, Anal
Paget's Disease, Anal
► Squamous Cell Carcinoma, Anus
Verrucous Carcinoma, Anal

References and Further Reading

Fenger, C. (1988). Histology of the anal canal. *The American Journal of Surgical Pathology, 12*, 41–55.

Fenger, C. (2007). Anal canal. In S. E. Mills (Ed.), *Histology for pathologists* (3rd ed., pp. 663–683). Philadelphia: Lippincott Williams & Wilkins.

Nivatvongs, S., Stern, H. S., & Fryd, D. S. (1987). The length of the anal canal. *Diseases of the Colon and Rectum, 24*, 600–601.

Parks, A. G. (1958). Modern concepts of the anatomy of the anal canal. *Postgraduate Medical Journal, 34*, 360–366.

Appendiceal Tumors

Magali Svrcek
Hôpital Saint-Antoine, Service d'Anatomie Pathologique, AP-HP, Hôpitaux Universitaires de l'Est Parisien, Paris, France

Synonyms

Adenocarcinoma; Carcinoid; Crypt cell carcinoma; Goblet cell tumor; Goblet cell-type adenocarcinoid; High-grade neuroendocrine carcinoma; Microglandular carcinoma; Mucinous carcinoid tumor; Neuroendocrine neoplasm; Non-mucinous carcinoma; Poorly differentiated endocrine carcinoma; Signet ring cell carcinoma; Small cell and large cell endocrine carcinoma; Well-differentiated endocrine tumor/carcinoma

Definition

One of the particularities of the appendix is the higher incidence of neuroendocrine neoplasms than carcinomas. Neuroendocrine neoplasms (NENs) of the appendix correspond to neoplasms with neuroendocrine differentiation and include neuroendocrine tumors (NET), neuroendocrine carcinoma (NEC), and mixed adenoneuroendocrine carcinomas (MANEC). In the latter, both the endocrine and exocrine components exceed 30%.

Primary adenocarcinomas of the appendix are rare after one eliminates low-grade appendiceal mucinous neoplasms (LAMNs) and mucinous adenocarcinomas. In the current UICC/AJCC TNM staging (7th edition, 2010), appendiceal adenocarcinomas are separated into mucinous and non-mucinous types because of a significant 5-year survival difference (UICC/AJCC TNM staging 2010). Two entries of the present encyclopedia are specifically devoted to the description of these types of mucinous neoplasms (see "▶ Mucinous Cystadenoma, Appendix" entry, and "▶ Mucinous Cystadenocarcinoma, Appendix" entry).

Here, the different types of NENs of the appendix and, briefly, non-mucinous adenocarcinoma are described. A short paragraph will also be devoted to miscellaneous tumors.

Tumors of the appendix composed entirely or partially of neuroendocrine cells are divided into two distinct categories: classic carcinoid tumors (with a minor variant) and goblet cell carcinoid (GCC) tumors and their variants. GCCs have mixed phenotypes, with partial neuroendocrine differentiation and intestinal goblet cell morphology. They are considered to represent a separate clinicopathological entity, distinct from both appendiceal NETs and appendiceal adenocarcinomas.

The different types of appendiceal tumors are summarized in Table 1.

Appendiceal Tumors, Table 1 The World Health Organization (WHO) classification of appendiceal tumors (from WHO 2010)

Epithelial tumors:
Premalignant lesions
Adenoma
Dysplasia (or intraepithelial neoplasia)
Serrated lesions
Hyperplastic polyp
Sessile serrated adenoma/polyp
Traditional serrated adenoma
Carcinoma
Adenocarcinoma
Mucinous adenocarcinoma
Low-grade appendiceal mucinous neoplasm
Signet ring cell carcinoma
Undifferentiated carcinoma
Neuroendocrine neoplasms
Neuroendocrine tumor (NET)
NET G1 (carcinoid)
NET G2
Neuroendocrine carcinoma (NEC)
Large cell NEC
Small cell NEC
Mixed adenoneuroendocrine carcinoma (MANEC)
EC cell, serotonin-producing NET
Goblet cell carcinoid
L cell, Glucagon-like peptide and PP/PYY-producing NETs
Tubular carcinoid
Mesenchymal tumors
Leiomyoma
Lipoma
Neuroma
Kaposi sarcoma
Leiomyosarcoma
Lymphomas
Secondary tumors

Clinical Features

- **Incidence**

  Appendiceal tumors constitute <0.4% of all intestinal neoplasms. NENs have been reported with an incidence rate of approximately 0.15/100,000/year in the SEER databases (Yao et al. 2008). Similarly, recent data from European registries reported an incidence of 0.08/100,000. Appendiceal NENs comprise the largest subgroup of appendiceal neoplasms with 50–77% of all appendiceal neoplasms, including both benign and malignant neoplasms, and are the second most frequently occurring digestive NETs, with a relative frequency of 25–30%. They affect 0.3–0.9% of patients undergoing appendectomy. Because not all cases are reported, particularly when NETs are less than 1 cm, this rate might be however underestimated. NECs, on the other hand, are very rare.

  Because of its rarity, exact figures on incidences and percentage of GCCs among appendiceal neoplasms vary depending on the data source. The incidence of GCCs is estimated to be one-tenth of that for appendiceal NENs.

  Appendiceal NENs are sporadic tumors unrelated to familial tumor syndromes.

- **Age**

  Appendiceal NETs occur in all age groups, including childhood, but are most common in the third, fourth, and fifth decades of life. The age of presentation of appendiceal NETs is significantly younger than in patients with appendiceal adenocarcinomas (sixth or seventh decade of patients' life).

GCCs mostly occur during the fifth decade.

- **Sex**
Appendiceal NETs occur more frequently in females than males, although this increased incidence in females is probably exaggerated by the fact that incidental appendicectomy during laparotomy for unrelated conditions (notably gynecological conditions) is more frequent in females. NETs may also be more frequent in the Caucasian subpopulation than in the African-American and Asian subpopulations.

  In contrast to classic appendiceal NETs, roughly equal numbers of men and women develop GCCs. An ethnic preference for Caucasians is clearly described with more than 80% of GCCs reported in this population. An association of GCCs with schistosomiasis has recently been reported in a Chinese series.
- **Site**
Most appendiceal NETS are asymptomatic and are found incidentally in appendectomy specimens removed for some unrelated condition. Thus, the detection of these neoplasms requires a careful histological examination.

  Contrary to appendiceal carcinomas which develop at the base of the appendix, appendiceal carcinoid tumors usually develop near the tip (70% or more) (Fig. 1). Indeed, the cell of origin of appendiceal NET is the subepithelial Kultschitzky cells, which are more numerous toward the appendiceal tip. Tubular carcinoid tumors, which are a rare variant of appendiceal "classic" NETs, also tend to develop at the tip of the appendix. Some NETs are located in the mid-appendix (5–20%) and the smallest fraction (less than 10%) at the base of the appendix. In the case of a close localization to the base of the appendix (10% of cases), the neoplasm may obstruct the lumen and produce appendicitis. An extremely rare carcinoid syndrome, resulting from the systemic effects of vasoactive peptide secretion by the tumor and almost always related to widespread metastases, has been described in less than 1% of cases.

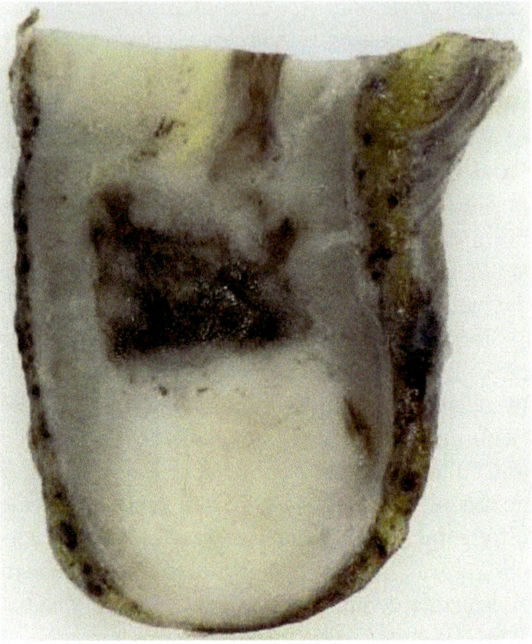

Appendiceal Tumors, Fig. 1 Gross appearance of a neuroendocrine tumor (NET) G1 (carcinoid) located at the tip of the appendix. The tumor has a typical *yellow* coloration

  GCCs are usually located in the middle third of the appendix and may cause appendicitis. They may be found in any portion of the appendix and appear as an area of whitish, sometimes mucoid induration without dilatation of the lumen. At diagnosis, approximately 10% of these tumors are already widespread with distant metastases to the liver, the ovaries, and the peritoneum.
- **Treatment**
Despite the fact that NETs are invasive neoplasms, often showing perineural spread or lymphatic invasion and extending through the wall of the appendix to the serosa or mesoappendix, simple appendectomy is adequate therapy for the vast majority of these neoplasms.

  For NETs, tumor size plays a major role when deciding upon type of surgery. The influence of several other parameters, such as lymphovascular invasion, subserosal invasion, extension to the mesoappendix, and the distance from the mesoappendiceal resection margin, remains to be defined.

Two surgical procedures can be applied to treat appendiceal NETs: simple appendicectomy and oncological right-sided hemicolectomy.

Most classic carcinoid neoplasms of the appendix being very indolent and any metastatic spread being usually restricted to tumors greater than 2 cm in diameter, most authors agree that simple appendectomy is adequate therapy for carcinoid neoplasms measuring less than 1 cm. These tumors ever hardly metastasize. Right hemicolectomy (including lymphadenectomy) is however indicated for tumors measuring more than 2 cm in diameter. The indications for further surgery are based on the location of neoplasms (at the base of the appendix with involvement of the surgical margin or the cecum) or a strong clinical evidence of metastases to regional lymph nodes.

The treatment of NETs measuring 1–2 cm remains controversial. Complementary surgery (right hemicolectomy) and/or follow-up is debated in case of a deep mesoappendiceal infiltration (beyond 3 mm), positive or unclear margins, higher proliferative rate (G2; see below), and/or angioinvasion (Deschamps and Couvelard 2010).

In summary, indications for right-sided hemicolectomy in patients with appendiceal NETs are:

- **Tumor located at the base of the appendix**
- **Tumor present in resection margin**
- **Tumor extending to mesoappendix**
- **Presence of angioinvasion**
- **Tumor measuring ≥2 cm**
- **Evidence of metastases**
- **High mitotic activity**

GCCs are considered as MANEC, a biological subtype of adenocarcinoma. They require a different therapeutic approach. Due to a higher metastatic risk, right-sided hemicolectomy, usually performed after initial appendectomy even when the appendiceal margin is negative for cancer cells, is considered the standard surgical treatment for the majority of GCCs. This right-sided hemicolectomy is recommended within 3 months of the appendectomy. In very rare cases (tumor measuring less than 1 cm, a localized tumor, without serosal, mesoappendiceal, or cecal invasion, and a low proliferative index), an appendectomy alone can be proposed. Cytoreductive surgery with adjuvant chemotherapy or intraperitoneal chemotherapy can be proposed in cases with advanced peritoneal dissemination. Treatment of liver metastases might follow the corresponding recommendations for colonic adenocarcinomas.

- **Outcome**

NETs

The prognosis is generally good, with a reported 5-year survival varying from 88% to 94% in patients with localized disease, 78–84% in patients with regional dissemination, and 25–31% in patients with distant metastasis (Yao et al. 2008).

Location at the base of the appendix does not modify the prognosis, but may change the therapeutic decision in case of involvement of the surgical margin.

The significance of several parameters other than tumor size, such as lymphovascular invasion, subserosal invasion, extension to the mesoappendix, and the distance from the mesoappendiceal resection margin, remains to be defined.

The evaluation of mitotic and proliferative index is now part of the WHO classification (7th edition) scheme of gastrointestinal NENs, but its relevance in appendiceal NENs is not as precisely defined as it is for other endocrine tumors. The proposed grading based on morphological criteria and proliferation has three tiers (G1, G2, G3) with the following definitions of mitotic count and Ki67 index (Rindi et al. 2010):

- G1: mitotic count <2 per 10 high-power fields (HPF) and/or ≤2% Ki67 index
- G2: mitotic count 2–20 per 10 HPF and/or 3–20% Ki67 index
- G3: mitotic count >20 per 10 HPF and/or >20% Ki67 index

Grading is combined with a site-specific staging system to improve prognostic strength. Two different staging systems exist, one proposed by the European Neuroendocrine Tumor Society (ENETS) in 2007 and the other recently proposed by the American Joint Committee on Cancer (AJCC) (7th edition, 2010). Tumors are classified according to their size and infiltration into the appendiceal wall. This classification has some differences with those used for appendiceal carcinomas. Moreover, this classification for NENs of the appendix has also differences with other well-differentiated gastrointestinal NENs. This is due to the fact that NETs of the appendix have no apparent in situ state and may arise in deep mucosa or submucosa, and that the tumor size, more than its depth, is considered as a major criterion of aggressiveness for a localized tumor. It is worthy to note that the 2 systems differ considerably in the cutoff values and classification rules.

An invasion of more than 3 mm in depth has been suggested to reflect the aggressiveness of the disease and is therefore used in the TNM classification by ENETS to distinguish T2 from T3 tumors, even in tumors <2 cm.

The most clinically relevant parameters for the pathologic characterization of appendiceal NENs remain to be defined. A recent Italian retrospective study of 138 appendiceal NENs was designed with the aim of testing the applicability and prognostic significance of the previous and current WHO classifications, different pathologic parameters, and TNM staging systems (2010 WHO/AJCC and ENETS 2007) (Volante et al. 2013). Interestingly, in the specific appendiceal location, at variance with midgut/hindgut NENs, mesoappendix invasion (and the 2000 WHO classification) performs better than the grading-based 2010 WHO scheme and, together with tumor stage, seems to be the most relevant parameter associated with clinical aggressiveness. It seemed that the ENETS system produced an overestimation, whereas the 2010 WHO/AJCC TNM system was more accurate and specific in selecting the very few aggressive and fatal cases.

Appendiceal Tumors, Table 2 Comparison of WHO 2010 classification of appendiceal NEN versus WHO 2000 classification

WHO 2000	WHO 2010
A. Well-differentiated endocrine tumor	A. NET G1 (carcinoid)
1. Benign behavior	
Nonfunctioning	
Confined to appendiceal wall	
≤2 cm	
Nonangioinvasive	
Ki67 index ≤2%	
Mitoses of ≤2 cells/HPF x40	
2. Uncertain behavior	
Nonfunctioning	
Confined to subserosa	
>2 cm	
Angioinvasive	
B. Well-differentiated endocrine carcinoma, low-grade, malignant	B. NET G2
Invading the mesoappendix or beyond	
With metastases	
With or without a functioning (carcinoid) syndrome	
C. Poorly differentiated endocrine carcinoma/ small cellcarcinoma	C. NEC (large cell and small cell type)
D. Mixed exocrine-endocrine carcinoma	D. Mixed adenoneuroendocrine carcinoma (MANEC)

The comparisons of WHO 2010 classification of appendiceal NEN versus WHO 2000 classification and of TNM classification of appendiceal NENs according to ENETS versus UICC/AJCC are shown, respectively, in Tables 2 and 3.

In summary, for well-differentiated tumors, diagnosed incidentally, with a maximum diameter of 1 cm and R0 resection, no follow-up is required when considered cured. For well-differentiated tumors of 1–2 cm and R0 resection, there is no sufficient data for a clear-cut decision. A follow-up is not necessarily required. However, in cases

Appendiceal Tumors, Table 3 Comparison of TNM classification of appendiceal NEN according to ENETS versus UICC/AJCC (TNM classification) (from Pape et al., 2012)

ENETS	UICC/AJCC
T: primary tumor	
x: primary tumor cannot be assessed	
0: no evidence of primary tumor	
1: tumor ≤ 1 cm invading submucosa and muscularis propria	
1a	Tumor <1 cm in greatest dimension
1b	Tumor >1 cm but ≤2 cm in greatest dimension
2: tumor ≤2 cm invading submucosa, muscularis propria, and/or minimally (up to 3 mm) invading subserosa/ mesoappendix	Tumor > 2 cm but ≤4 cm or with extension to the cecum
3: tumor > 2 cm and/or extensive (>3 mm) invasion of subserosa/ mesoappendix	Tumor > 4 cm or with extension to the ileum
4: tumor invades peritoneum/other organs	Tumor perforates peritoneum or invades other adjacent organs or structures, e.g., abdominal wall and skeletal muscle
N: regional lymph node metastasis	
x: regional lymph nodes cannot be assessed	
0: no regional lymph node metastasis	
1: regional lymph node metastasis	
M: distant metastasis	
X: distant metastasis cannot be assessed	
0: no distant metastasis	
1: distant metastasis	

with deep mesoappendiceal infiltration or angioinvasion, imaging may be performed to rule out any residual tumor. All other patients with either tumor size >2 cm, metastases, or additional risk factors (including R1 resection) should be followed initially after 6 and 12 months postoperatively and then annually (Pape et al. 2012).

GCCs

GCCs have a worse prognosis than appendiceal NENs. The 5-year survival of patients with GCCs is 86% for localized disease, 74% for regional disease, and 18% when distant metastases are present.

Serosal involvement, invasion of the mesoappendix, and extension into the peritoneum or adjacent organs are prognostic factors. The pattern of extension is predominantly limited to the pelvic organs with peritoneal spread.

GCCS are classified according to the TNM staging of adenocarcinomas because their behavior appears closer to them rather than to appendiceal carcinoids (see "▶ Mucinous Cystadenocarcinoma, Appendix" entry).

After curative surgical treatment, patients should be followed every 3–6 months, then yearly, mimicking the guidelines for colorectal adenocarcinoma. Gastrointestinal follow-up is recommended because of the high incidence (up to 48%) of gastrointestinal neoplasms in these patients.

Macroscopy

During macroscopic examination, margin of the appendix must be individualized, as well as the entire tip of the appendix. When an appendiceal NEN is found by histological analysis, the entire tumor and the totality of the appendix should be submitted in this examination in order to rule out size and invasion.

Grossly, appendiceal NETs are firm, grayish white (yellow after formalin fixation), well circumscribed, but not encapsulated. The size distribution is 60–80% for tumors smaller than 1 cm, 4–37% for those between 1 and 2 cm, and 2–17% for those larger than 2 cm.

GCCs range in size from 1 to 5 cm, with a mean of 2 cm. However, they usually lack a well-defined tumor mass structure, making somewhat difficult the accurate assessment of their size.

Microscopy

Histology is always necessary to establish the diagnosis. However, cytology may be helpful, particularly in the rare metastatic setting.

NETs

Appendiceal NETs display several distinct histological patterns: the large majority of classic appendiceal carcinoid tumors are enterochromaffin (EC) cell, serotonin-producing tumors. Only a minority are glucagon-like peptide, PP/PYY-producing, or L cell NETS.

In EC cell NET, tumor cells are arranged in rounded, solid nests ("insulae") (Fig. 2a), with some peripheral palisading infiltrating the appendiceal wall. A minority of tumors exhibit glandular formations or a mixture of the two. Tumor cells are uniform, with little or no pleomorphism. Mitoses are rare and Ki67 proliferative index is mostly <2% (G1 class) (Fig. 2b). A retraction of the tumor periphery from the stroma is usually evident and sometimes prominent. An acinar component can be present; in that case, the cells differentiate into solid rosettes containing small amounts of mucin. In that variant, some of the cells may appear clear, a pattern termed "clear cell" or "balloon cell carcinoid." Occasionally, cells may appear vacuolated, perhaps related to degeneration. Most EC cell NETs involve deeper layers of the appendiceal wall and display also lymphatic and perineural invasion. Spread to the peritoneal surface is not rare. Despite such aggressive growth patterns, the behavior of most classic appendiceal NETs is very indolent, and metastatic spread is uncommon. More aggressive NETs display nuclear pleomorphism and a higher mitotic rate.

A minority of classic carcinoid tumors are composed of L cells rather than EC cells. They produce glucagon-like peptides (GLP1, GLP2, and the enteroglucagons glicentin and oxyntomodulin) and PP/PYY. They tend to feature tubular or trabecular patterns rather than solid nests. These tumors are usually small, measuring only 2–3 mm in size. Tumor cells are regular and mitotic activity is little. Occasionally, mucin is present in the lumen of the tubules.

Tubular carcinoid tumors do not resemble the typical EC cell NETs: they show little contact with the mucosa and originate from the base of the glands. These tumors have a distinctive appearance with small, discrete tubules or linear structures in an abundant fibrosis. Solid nests are generally absent. The tumor cells have round or oval regular nuclei and contain variable amounts of eosinophilic cytoplasm. Inspissated mucin can be observed in their lumen.

D-cell tumors are extremely rare in the appendix.

Neuroendocrine Carcinomas

Neuroendocrine carcinomas (NECs) are exceedingly rare in the appendix. Both the histology and

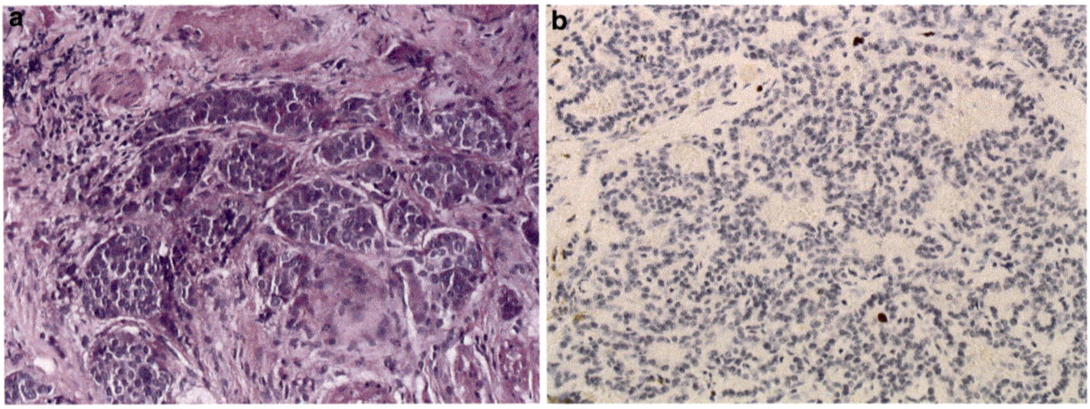

Appendiceal Tumors, Fig. 2 (**a**) Appendiceal neuroendocrine tumor (NET) of classic (insular) type (A) (×200 magnification); (**b**) Tumor cells scarcely (<1%) express Ki67 (×200 magnification)

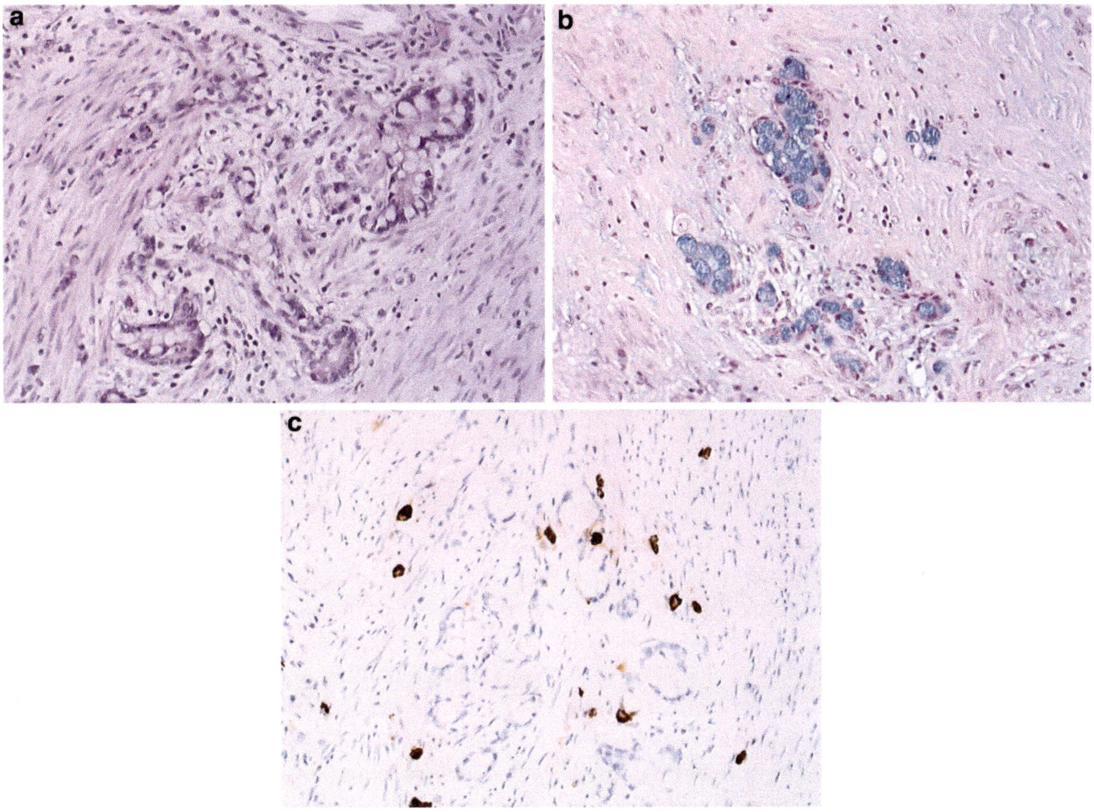

Appendiceal Tumors, Fig. 3 Appendiceal goblet cell carcinoid. (**a**): Typical clusters of goblet cells; (**b**): Goblet cells positive with alcian blue staining; (**c**): Focal positivity is detected with chromogranin antibody (×200 magnification)

the immunoprofile are similar to those reported at other sites of the gastrointestinal tract.

GCCs

GCC is the other major type of appendiceal tumor. Typical GCCs have a mixed phenotype, with partial neuroendocrine differentiation and predominant intestinal-type goblet cell morphology. Goblet cells are arranged in small uniform nests, often in a microglandular fashion, and are sometimes accompanied by extracellular mucus. The intestinal-type goblet cells exhibit minimal cytological atypia (Fig. 3a–c). Mitotic figures are rarely identified. Smaller numbers of endocrine cells with finely granular eosinophilic cytoplasm are also normally present. A component of lysozyme-positive cells with features similar to Paneth cells may also be observed, as well as foci resembling Brunner glands. GCCs are characterized by predominantly submucosal growth. They typically infiltrate the appendiceal wall in a concentric manner, with a common extension into the muscle and serosa, but the mucosa is characteristically spared, except where the tumor touches the bases of the crypts. These tumors often elicit a considerable desmoplastic response.

The proportion of each of the two components varies markedly within the tumors. Typically, the EC cell component is small. In some cases, GCCs resemble a signet ring cell carcinoma, and the neuroendocrine component is only detectable after the use of stains for neuroendocrine differentiation. That is why Fenoglio-Preiser et al. advocate that all appendiceal lesions that look like signet ring cell carcinomas be stained with neuroendocrine markers to exclude the presence of the biologically less aggressive GCCs.

GCCs are thought to be intermediate between classic carcinoid tumors and adenocarcinomas. Mixed GCC-adenocarcinomas are also reported. Adenocarcinoma (either a signet ring cell type or poorly differentiated adenocarcinoma type) appears to arise from a preexisting GCC.

As seen previously (see "Outcome" section), nomenclature and classification of neuroendocrine neoplasms of the digestive system have changed since 2010. Two complementary classification tools, including a grading classification and a site-specific staging system, are now used.

In summary, histological report should include:

- **An immunohistochemical staining (synaptophysin and chromogranin A, or CD56) to prove the neuroendocrine character of the tumor. Tumor subtyping by immunohistochemistry is not necessary on a routine basis.**
- **A mitotic count per 10 HPF (2 mm^2, at least 40 fields at ×40 magnification) evaluated in areas displaying the highest mitotic density. Histological grading is not carried out for carcinoid tumors, but a mitotic count of 2–10 per hpf and focal necrosis are features of atypical carcinoids (well-differentiated neuroendocrine carcinomas), a type seen much more commonly in lungs than in appendix.**
- **The Ki67 index (using the MIB1 antibody as a percentage of 500–2,000 cells counted in areas displaying the strongest nuclear labeling) to determine the proliferative capacity of the tumor. The Ki67 index allows the determination of tumor grading based on the current WHO classification.**
- **The presence or not of angioinvasion, perineural spread, or necrosis and the distance from the mesoappendiceal resection margin.**
- **ENETS-TNM classification in addition to the AJCC/UICC TNM staging.**
- **Surgical margin status (R0/R1) must be reported clearly.**

Immunophenotype

NETs

The tumor cells are argentaffin and argyrophilic and positive with the neuroendocrine cell markers (chromogranin A, synaptophysin, and CD56) and serotonin (Fig. 4). Occasional cells stain for somatostatin, glucagon, calcitonin, CCK, gastrin, ACTH, neurotensin, and PP. The tumor cells are also positive for keratins 8 and 19 and usually negative for keratins 7 and 20, CEA, and TTF1. Keratin staining tends to be weaker than in ileal carcinoids. The tumor cells characteristically express CDX2, a marker of midgut derivation, and are intimately associated with a population of S-100 protein-positive cells, forming subepithelial neuroendocrine complexes.

In contrast to carcinoid tumors made of EC cells, those composed of L cells tend to be negative for chromogranin A. The tumor cells are cytokeratin immunoreactive.

Tubular carcinoid tumors are positive for chromogranin A, synaptophysin, and serotonin. Contrary to other types of NETs, these tumors produce proglucagon mRNA and are frequently immunoreactive for glucagon. S-100-positive cells are absent.

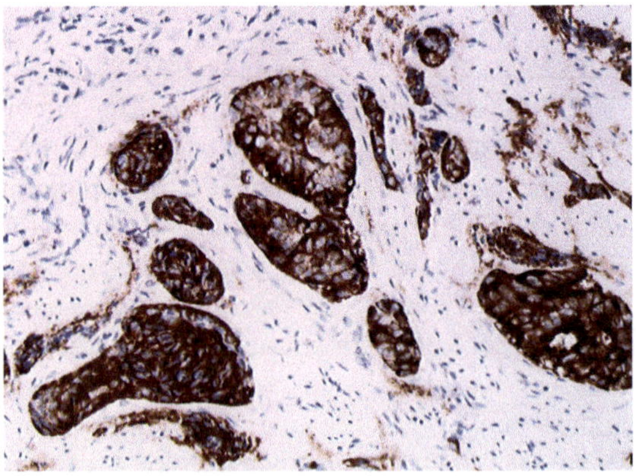

Appendiceal Tumors, Fig. 4 Chromogranin A immunostaining of the appendiceal NET illustrated in Fig. 2a (×200 magnification)

GCCs

Mucin stains (periodic acid-Schiff, periodic acid-Schiff diastase, Alcian blue) are strongly positive within goblet cells and may underline the presence of pools of extracellular mucin. Contrary to most classic NETs, immunohistochemistry performed in GCCs with neuroendocrine markers demonstrates focal positivity (in 5–25% of tumor cells) and not a diffuse staining. The goblet cells stain MUC2. CK20 is present in all cases and CK7 in about 70%. There is also frequent expression of CK18.

Molecular Features

KRAS mutations are rarely found in NETs and GCCs. Unlike other NETs of the gastrointestinal tract, loss of heterozygosity (LOH) at the MEN1 gene locus appears to be rare. Expression of additional immunohistochemical markers such as p53 is still unclear and remains to be investigated in larger series.

In GCCS, *TP53* mutations are present in about 25% of cases. These tumors classically lack *DPC4/SMAD4* mutations, as well as mutations of the gene coding for beta-catenin (*CTNNB1*).

Differential Diagnosis

NETs

Retraction artifacts mimic angioinvasion.

Tubular carcinoid tumors can mimic a primary or metastatic adenocarcinoma because tumoral cells show little contact with the overlying mucosa and cause an ill-defined thickening of the appendiceal wall. The lack of mitoses and atypia, orderly arrangement, and integrity of the overlying mucosa should lead to the correct diagnosis. It is also important to distinguish tubular carcinoid tumors from GCCs that have a worse prognosis and require more aggressive treatment. In tubular carcinoid tumors, all of the tumor cells are positive with neuroendocrine markers, the glandular lumens contain mucin but there is no intracytoplasmic mucin, and Paneth cells are generally absent.

GCCs

A conventional variant of lipid-rich well-differentiated appendiceal NENs is a morphological differential diagnosis to GCCs because of their clear appearance. A periodic acid-Schiff (PAS) staining of mucin (with or without Alcian blue) is helpful to differentiate these two different entities.

Another differential diagnosis of GCC includes signet ring cell carcinoma. Signet ring cell carcinomas show much more architectural and cytological atypia. A mucin stain may be used, in some cases, because signet ring cell carcinomas frequently produce pools of extracellular mucin. The expression of E-cadherin and B-catenin is preserved in goblet cell carcinoid and is lost in signet ring cell carcinoma.

Other Appendiceal Tumor: Non-mucinous Adenocarcinomas and Miscellaneous Tumors of the Appendix

One entry of this encyclopedia of pathology is specifically devoted to mucinous adenocarcinomas (see "▶ Mucinous Cystadenocarcinoma, Appendix" entry).

Non-mucinous Adenocarcinomas of the Appendix

Adenocarcinomas of the appendix occur in 0.1–0.2% of appendicectomies, corresponding to an estimated incidence of 0.2 per 100,000 per year, and are accounted for 60% of malignant appendiceal tumors in the US Surveillance, Epidemiology, and End Results (SEER 1981).

Outcome

The 5-year survival of appendiceal non-mucinous carcinomas with distant metastasis is around 10% (versus 40–50% for mucinous appendiceal carcinomas), which justifies the separation between mucinous and non-mucinous adenocarcinomas. Contrary to mucinous adenocarcinomas, non-mucinous carcinomas tend not to produce pseudomyxoma peritonei. Non-mucinous appendiceal carcinomas behave like colorectal adenocarcinomas, metastasizing to the regional lymph nodes or to the liver. Nodal metastases are present in approximately 25% of resection specimens.

The prognosis of patients with appendiceal signet ring cell carcinomas is poor, tumors being frequently detected at an advanced stage. Thus, many patients die of their disease within 1 year or two of their original diagnosis.

Right hemicolectomy and regional lymphadenectomy are the treatment of choice for adenocarcinoma.

Macroscopy

The appendix may be enlarged, deformed, or completely destroyed by a polypoid, ulcerating, or infiltrative mass usually present at the base contrasting with carcinoid tumors that classically develop on the tip of the appendix. Tumors may also cause appendiceal intussusception. A mucinous cystadenocarcinoma can display exuberant mucus secretion giving rise to the gross appearance of a mucocele.

Perforation or diverticula may be present. Perforations of appendiceal adenocarcinomas develop in 50–62% of tumors and are responsible for the dissemination into the peritoneum.

Cecum can be involved with advanced tumor stages, making it difficult to determine the exact site of origin. If the major part of the tumor lies in the appendix or if microscopic examination reveals a precursor lesion in the appendix, one can consider that the tumor is of appendiceal origin.

During macroscopic examination, margin of the appendix must be individualized. In right hemicolectomy specimens, the ileal and colonic margins are the proximal and distal margins, respectively. In right hemicolectomy specimens, pathologic assessment of the regional lymph node should be performed.

Differential Diagnosis

Adenocarcinomas of the cecum can secondarily involve the base of the appendix and thus are sometimes erroneously assumed to be of primary appendiceal origin. A signet ring cell carcinoma needs to be distinguished from a metastasis of a gastric or mammary origin and from a GCC.

Appendiceal tumors pathologically resemble their small and large intestinal counterparts. Non-mucinous adenocarcinomas of the appendix are graded using the criteria for colorectal cancers. Grading is based on the extent of glandular appearances and comprises well, moderately, and poorly differentiated carcinomas. Well-differentiated (grade 1) carcinomas exhibit glandular structures in >95% of the tumor, moderately differentiated (grade 2) adenocarcinomas show 50–95% gland formation, poorly differentiated (grade 3) adenocarcinomas show 5–50% gland formation, and finally, undifferentiated (grade 4) carcinomas have less than 5% gland formation. Non-mucinous appendiceal adenocarcinomas arise in preexisting adenomas.

Signet ring cell carcinoma is an adenocarcinoma in which the predominant component (more than 50%) is composed of isolated malignant cells containing intracytoplasmic mucin.

Miscellaneous Tumors of the Appendix

Miscellaneous tumors of the appendix include neural proliferations, lymphomas, and secondary tumors. Neural proliferations are common in the appendix. The most frequent is the neuroma, also called neurogenous hyperplasia. The normal mucosa and lymphoid tissue are replaced by a proliferation of spindle cells associated with nerve fibers, accompanied by neuroendocrine cells, and causing obliteration of the appendiceal lumen. However, there is considerable controversy over whether they represent true neoplasms or nonneoplastic neuronal proliferation, possibly resulting from previous episodes of inflammation.

Primary lymphomas of the appendix are rare and are usually part of a more general intestinal spread. Some are of Burkitt type. Secondary

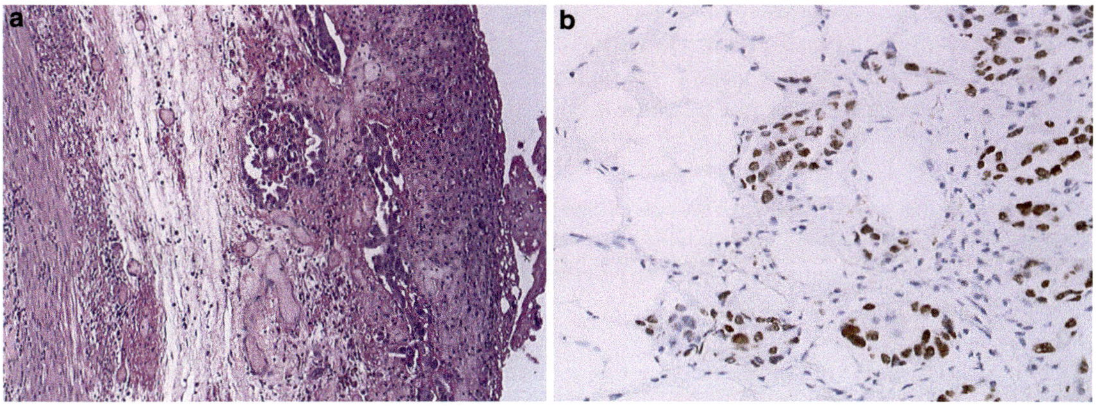

Appendiceal Tumors, Fig. 5 (**a**) Metastatic adenocarcinoma of lung involving the appendix (×100 magnification); (**b**) Tumor cells express TTF1 (×200 magnification)

tumors of the appendix are unusual and have been described from primary tumors of the breast, stomach, or bronchus (Fig. 5a, b).

References and Further Reading

Deschamps, L., & Couvelard, A. (2010). Endocrine tumors of the appendix. *Archives of Pathology & Laboratory Medicine, 134*, 871–875.

Edge, S. B., Byrd, D. R., Compton, C. C., Fritz, A. G., Greene, F. L., & Trotti, A. (2010). Appendix. In *AJCC cancer staging handbook, from the AJCC cancer staging manual* (7th ed., pp. 161–171). New York: Springer.

Komminoth, P., Arnold, R., Capella, C., Klimstra, D.S., Kloppel, G., Solcia, E., & Rindi, G. (2010). Neuroendocine neoplasms of the appendix. In F. T. Bosman, F. Carneiro, R. H. Hruban, & N. D. Theise (Eds.), *WHO classification of tumours of the digestive system* (pp. 126–128). Lyon: IARC Press.

Pape, U.-F., Perren, A., Niederle, B., et al. (2012). ENETS consensus guidelines for the management of patients with neuroendocrine neoplasms from the jejuno-ileum and the appendix including goblet cell carcinomas. *Neuroendocrinology, 95*, 135–156.

Rindi, G., Arnold, R., Bosman, F. T., & Capella, C. (2010). Nomenclature and classification of neuroendocrine neoplasms of the digestive system. In F. T. Bosman, F. Carneiro, R. H. Hruban, & N. D. Theise (Eds.), *WHO classification of tumours of the digestive system* (pp. 13–14). Lyon: IARC Press.

Volante, M., Daniele, L., & Asioli, S. (2013). Tumor staging but not grading is associated with adverse clinical outcome in neuroendocrine tumors of the appendix. A retrospective clinical pathologic analysis of 138 cases. *The American Journal of Surgical Pathology, 37*, 606–612.

Yao, J. C., Hassan, M., Phan, A., et al. (2008). One hundred years after "carcinoid": Epidemiology of and prognostic factors for neuroendocrine tumors in 35,825 cases in the United States. *Journal of Clinical Oncology, 26*, 3063–3072.

Appendicitis, Etiology, Macroscopy, and Histology of

Iva Brcic
Institute of Pathology, Medical University of Graz, Graz, Austria

Synonyms

Typhilitis; Typhlitis

Definition

Acute appendicitis is an acute emergency characterized by inflammation of the appendix. It is associated with lumen obstruction and infection. Obstruction is usually due to a fecalith; however, other causes have been described: food fragments, lymphoid hyperplasia (mostly in children), endometriosis, and primary and secondary tumors. Regarding infection, *Fusobacteria* (*F. nucleatum and F. necrophorum*) was identified in 62% of patients with acute appendicitis (Swidsinski et al. 2012). Other bacterias (*Salmonella, Shigella, C. difficile, Campylobacter*), viruses (*Adenovirus, CMV, measles, infectious mononucleosis*), and parasites (*Enterobius vermicularis, Schistosoma, Trichuris, Ascaris, Amoebae,* etc.) have been reported. Complications include perforation, peritonitis, periappendiceal abscesses and fibrosis, fistula formation, pylephlebitis with thrombosis of portal venous drainage, and liver abscess formation (Riddell 2014).

Clinical Features

- **Incidence**
  140 per 100,000 inhabitants (Søreide 1984).
- **Age**
  Usually found in children and young adults but can occur at any age.
- **Sex**
  There is slight male predominance over females as 1.4: 1 (Addiss et al. 1990).
- **Site**
  Appendix.
- **Treatment**
  Surgery (appendectomy).
- **Outcome**
  Good prognosis. In case of perforation, up to 2% mortality (higher rate in older population) (Peltokallio and Tykka 1981).

Macroscopy

Macroscopic appearance varies with the stage of the inflammation. Initially the appendix can look almost normal, with congested vessels on the serosal surface. With progression of the inflammation through the wall, appendix becomes enlarged and tan colored. Serosal surface can be covered with tan-yellow exudates. Eventually, appendix becomes gangrenous leading to perforation, leaving a well-circumscribed hole (Fig. 1). On the cut surface, yellowish-tan mucosal exudation with a hyperemic border can be found. After resolution of inflammation, luminal obliteration (also called obliterative fibrosis) is usually found.

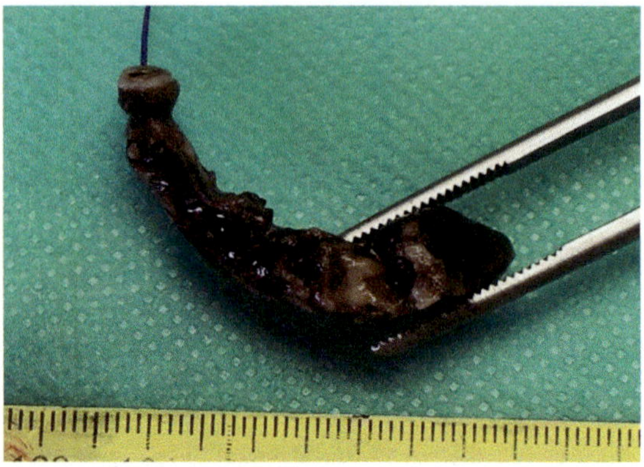

Appendicitis, Etiology, Macroscopy, and Histology of, Fig. 1 Acute appendicitis, macroscopic image. Appendix is enlarged and tan colored with visible perforation; serosal surface is covered by tan-yellow exudates

Microscopy

Earliest changes are neutrophils infiltrating lamina propria with migration into the surface epithelium causing erosions. Further on, they migrate to adjacent crypts and form crypt abscesses and ulcers. Neutrophils can also be found in lymphoid follicles where they cause deep suppuration. Later, full-thickness mucosal ulceration develops and crypt abscesses advance into submucosa and muscularis propria (Fig. 2). In the later stage, we can see acute inflammation of submucosa, visceral peritoneum, and mesoappendix. In advanced forms, the entire wall of the appendix is necrotic and filled with pus and perforation can occur. Rarely, due to perforation, appendix mucosa can be found growing along the external surface of the appendix. Resolution of inflammation can leave architectural distortion with focal dense submucosal fibrosis and duplicated muscularis mucosae. Eventually, obliteration of the appendix with neuronal hyperplasia develops.

Immunophenotype

There is no distinctive immunophenotypic feature for appendicitis.

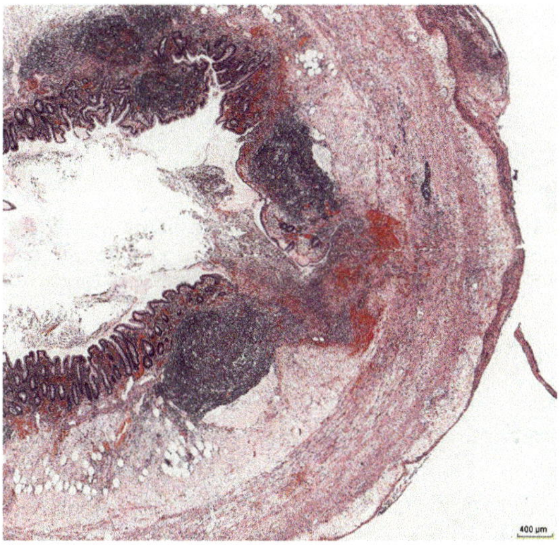

Appendicitis, Etiology, Macroscopy, and Histology of, Fig. 2 Acute appendicitis, microscopic images. On low-power image, mucosa ulceration with transmural inflammation is seen with preserved surface epithelium in the surrounding. On the serosal surface an extensive neutrophilic exudate is seen

Molecular Features

There is no distinctive molecular feature for appendicitis.

Differential Diagnosis

Differential diagnosis of appendicitis includes IBD (Crohn's disease and ulcerative colitis), infectious enterocolitis, and neutropenic (agranulocytic) enterocolitis.

References and Further Reading

Addiss, D. G., Shaffer, N., Flower, B. S., & Tauxe, R. V. (1990). The epidemiology of appendicitis and appendectomy in the United States. *American Journal of Epidemiology, 132*, 910–925.

Peltokallio, P., & Tykka, H. (1981). Evolution of the age distribution and mortality of acute appendicitis. *Archives of Surgery, 116*, 153–156.

Riddell, R. (2014). Appendix. In R. Riddell & D. Jain (Eds.), *Lewin, Weinstein, and Riddell's gastrointestinal pathology and its clinical implications* (pp. 806–824). Philadelphia: Lippincott Williams & Wilkins/Walter Kluwer.

Søreide, O. (1984). Appendicitis – A study of incidence, death rates and consumption of hospital resources. *Postgraduate Medical Journal, 60*, 341–345.

Swidsinski, A., Dörffel, Y., Loening-Baucke, V., Tertychnyy, A., Biche-Ool, S., Stonogin, S., Guo, Y., & Sun, N. D. (2012). Mucosal invasion by fusobacteria is a common feature of acute appendicitis in Germany, Russia and China. *Saudi Journal of Gastroenterology, 18*, 55–58.

Autoimmune Gastritis

Chella R. S. van der Post and
J. Han van Krieken
Department of Pathology, Radboud University Medical Center, Nijmegen, The Netherlands

Synonyms

Autoimmune chronic gastritis; Autoimmune metaplastic atrophic gastritis (AMAG); Autoimmune-associated gastritis; Type A gastritis

Definition

Autoimmune gastritis is an immune-mediated gastritis, and in its development, anti-parietal cell and anti-intrinsic factor antibodies are involved. There is typical loss of oxyntic cells in the gastric corpus and fundus. Autoimmune gastritis is characterized by hypochlorhydria or achlorhydria, hypergastrinemia, low pepsinogen I/pepsinogen II ratio, and vitamin B_{12} deficiency that can lead to pernicious anemia. The declining incidence of *Helicobacter pylori* gastritis parallels a growing clinical focus on autoimmune gastritis.

Hypochlorhydria results from loss of oxyntic mucosa and possibly from the disruption of normal parietal cell maturation. This can already occur in patients with a large number of preserved parietal cells, suggesting that there may be a role for anti-proton pump antibodies or inhibitory lymphokines released by inflammatory cells in the pathogenesis of this disease. Achlorhydria, which is a direct result of destruction of acid-producing parietal cells, typically occurs in the most advanced stage of disease. Normally, the gastric acidic pH has an inhibitory effect on gastrin production through release of somatostatin produced by D cells. Patients with atrophy of the corpus have a higher pH in the stomach because of less acid secretion. Loss of acid production leads to hypergastrinemia, the level of which tends to correlate with disease severity. Damage to chief cells leads to a reduction in pepsin activity within gastric juice and in the level of pepsinogens in serum. The finding of a low pepsinogen I level (<20 ng/mL) is both a sensitive and specific indicator for the presence of corpus atrophy.

A considerable proportion of patients develop either iron-deficiency anemia or pernicious anemia. Pernicious anemia is the end stage of atrophic corpus gastritis. Achlorhydria is a major contributor to the pathogenesis of anemia. Gastric acid is important for absorption of non-heme iron, which supplies at least two-third of the nutritional iron supply in most Western diets. Pernicious anemia, which results from loss of intrinsic factor production by parietal cells, is usually preceded by corpus-restricted chronic autoimmune gastritis and reduced acid secretion of at least 10 years duration.

The etiology of autoimmune gastritis is unknown. One theory suggests the disease may be initiated by *H. pylori* infection. A high prevalence of antibodies with specificity for gastric mucosal antigens has been reported among patients with *H. pylori*-associated gastritis. Furthermore, 20% of *H. pylori*- positive subjects have autoantibodies that react with canaliculi of parietal cells, which represent one of the main antibody targets in autoimmune gastritis. Recent studies using cloned T cells from both *H. pylori*-infected patients and patients with autoimmune atrophic gastritis have identified molecular mimicry between *H. pylori* and H^+, K^+, and ATPase, suggesting that infection may stimulate T cells that target parietal cells. These studies provide support for the concept that there is a cross-reactive mechanism between *H. pylori* organisms and gastric epithelial antigens that may be responsible for, or at least participate in, the pathogenesis of autoimmune gastritis.

Clinical Features

The clinical presentation is often insidious and progression is slow. Patients present with abdominal discomfort, weight loss, diarrhea, malabsorption, and sometimes neurologic complications in advanced stage, but nowadays that is almost never seen. Neurologic complications include peripheral neuropathy and subacute combined degeneration of spinal cord related to severe vitamin B_{12} deficiency. Unspecific symptoms related to anemia include weakness, asthenia, decreased mental concentration, headache, and cardiac symptoms such as palpitations and chest pain. Autoimmune gastritis does not cause specific clinical manifestations until a critical decrease has occurred in the parietal cell mass, beyond which anemia develops. Years before the onset of anemia, patients may show various degrees of hypochlorhydria, hypergastrinemia, and loss of pepsin and pepsinogen secretion.

Iron-deficiency anemia can be seen in 20–40% of patients, whereas pernicious anemia is seen in 15–25% of patients. Reduced gastric acid plays a role in iron deficiency, because gastric acid is necessary to release iron from bound protein, as well as reduce ferric iron to ferrous state necessary for absorption. Pernicious anemia is a macrocytic anemia due to cobalamin (vitamin B_{12}) deficiency. It is the result of deficiency of intrinsic factor, a protein that binds to dietary vitamin B_{12} and promotes its transport to the terminal ileum for absorption. The deficiency of intrinsic factor is a direct consequence of the gastritis and destruction of oxyntic mucosa with loss of parietal cells, which normally produce chlorhydric acid as well as intrinsic factor. Pernicious anemia is characterized by macrocytosis, megaloblasts, pancytopenia, atrophic glossitis, low serum vitamin B_{12} concentration, and normal folate level. Pernicious anemia is a late manifestation of autoimmune gastritis, taking 20–30 years to develop and is caused by progressive loss of parietal cell, which are necessary for intrinsic factor production, as well as autoantibody targeted at intrinsic factor preventing the formation of B_{12} intrinsic factor complex.

Laboratory findings include a low vitamin B_{12} level, and high gastrin levels. Serum analysis frequently demonstrates anti-parietal cell antibodies targeted against H+/K+ ATPase in 60–85% and intrinsic factor antibodies in 30–50% of patients.

- **Incidence**
  Autoimmune gastritis may be underdiagnosed, because most patients present with either microcytic or macrocytic anemia and are treated with iron, folate, and cobalamin without having undergone a thorough investigation for the underlying cause. However, targeted studies suggest an overall prevalence rate of 1–2%, with a peak of 4–5% among elderly women. Autoimmune gastritis is more common among individuals of Scandinavian, English, and Irish ancestry, while it is less commonly in Caucasians of Italian or Greek origin. The disease has sporadically been reported in African-American and Latin-American subjects.
- **Age**
  Autoimmune gastritis is a disease of adults around or above 50–60 years of age.
- **Sex**
  Male-to-female ratio is 1:1.7–3.
- **Site**
  Autoimmune gastritis affects primarily the gastric corpus and fundus.
- **Treatment**
  The clinical management of patients with autoimmune gastritis concerns different aspects. First, the treatment of cobalamin deficiency (by administration of vitamin B_{12}) and the monitoring of onset of iron deficiency. Second, the surveillance to early detection of long-term consequences of autoimmune gastritis such as gastric carcinoma and carcinoids needs attention.
- **Outcome**
  The early recognition of, especially neurological, symptoms is important, because neurological lesions may not be reversed after replacement therapy with vitamin B_{12}.

Autoimmune gastritis is a benign disorder; however, it is epidemiologically and biologically linked to the development of intestinal-type gastric adenocarcinoma and gastric carcinoid type I. Hypochlorhydria, developing as a consequence of atrophy of the oxyntic mucosa, has a crucial role in the development of gastric cancer. Hypochlorhydria leads to an overgrowth of nitrosamine-producing bacteria with potential carcinogen activity. In literature, annual incidence rates of gastric cancer in patients with pernicious anemia range from 0.1% to 0.5%. Due to the atrophic changes, autoimmune gastritis is listed among the gastric precancerous conditions.

Long-standing hypo/achlorhydria triggers enterochromaffin-like (ECL) cell hyperplasia, which may develop to gastric carcinoids. It has been reported that one in 25 patients with pernicious anemia develops gastric carcinoids. These carcinoid tumors are typically indolent. Removal of the antrum results in disappearance of these lesions.

Gastric polyps are detected in 20–40% of patients with pernicious anemia; they are mostly sessile, less than 2 cm in diameter, and often multiple in number. Most are hyperplastic, but up to 10% contain foci of dysplasia.

The disease may coexist with other autoimmune disorders, such as autoimmune thyroid disease (Hashimoto's thyroiditis, Graves' disease), type I diabetes mellitus, vitiligo, and myasthenia graves. HLA-DR genotypes suggest a role of genetic susceptibility in pernicious anemia.

Macroscopy

Endoscopic and gross features include a thinner corpus and fundic mucosa resulting from reduction or complete absence of rugal folds. The mucosa is shiny and red with a prominent submucosal vascular pattern becoming visible due to mucosal atrophy. Multiple pseudopolyps can be seen, representing preserved islands of oxyntic mucosa surrounded by flattened corpus mucosa.

Other associations that can be found in the surrounding mucosa are hyperplastic polyps, carcinoids, and adenocarcinoma.

Microscopy

The histology of autoimmune gastritis typically features a corpus mucosa restricted chronic atrophic gastritis with mild to moderate intestinal metaplasia. Findings vary depending on the stage of the disease. In the absence of synchronous *H. pylori* infection or bile reflux, the antrum is typically relatively spared. However, concomitant antral atrophic gastritis may be observed. Autoimmune gastritis is often easily recognized when changes are fully developed and adequately sampled, but earlier manifestations are more challenging to recognize (Fig. 1).

In the early (non-atrophic) stage, the oxyntic mucosa shows a diffuse or multifocal dense, full-thickness lymphocytic infiltrate. The prominent lymphoplasmacytic infiltration of the lamina propria is often mixed with eosinophils and mast cells and directed at the oxyntic glands. The chronic inflammation is often more prominent in the deeper mucosa, contrasting with *H. pylori* gastritis, which presents with prominent and active inflammation superficially. Focal lymphocytic infiltration and destruction of individual oxyntic glands may be seen. There may be patchy atrophy of oxyntic mucosa with pseudopyloric and/or intestinal metaplasia. The remaining parietal cells show pseudo-hypertrophic changes and luminal snouting similar to that seen in patients on proton-pump inhibitors. Hypertrophic changes are indicative of a high level of functional stimulation, possibly related to hypergastrinemia, and can be found in parietal cells of patients with autoimmune atrophic gastritis.

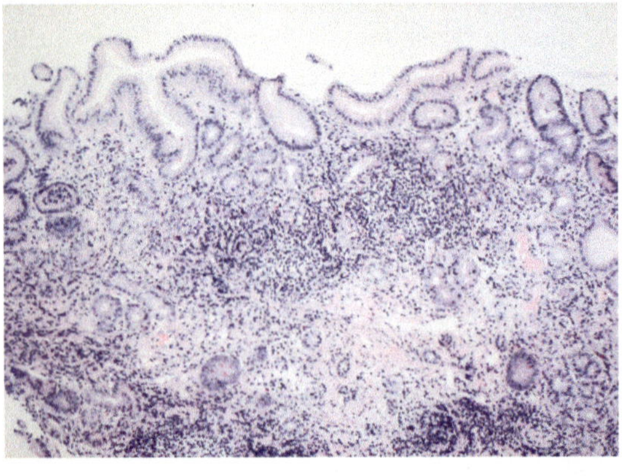

Autoimmune Gastritis, Fig. 1 Gastric corpus biopsy from a patient with autoimmune gastritis. There is loss of oxyntic cells and presence of antralized mucosa with focal intestinal metaplasia. There is a prominent lymphoplasmacytic infiltration of the lamina propria (H&E, original magnification 25×)

In a later (florid atrophic) stage, there is, next to diffuse lymphoplasmacytic infiltrate, atrophy of oxyntic glands and fibrosis of the lamina propria. These atrophic changes include the loss of glandular units, resulting in fibrosis of the lamina propria and the metaplastic replacement of native oxyntic glands. Metaplastic glands including two different phenotypes, which can coexist simultaneously, replace the chief and parietal cells. Pseudopyloric metaplasia (i.e., spasmolytic polypeptide-expressing metaplasia or SPEM) is first seen, consisting of glands that resemble mucous glands in the antrum, but the glands do not produce gastrin since they lack gastrin cells. This is followed by or coexists with intestinal metaplasia of the glands characterized by goblet and Paneth cells.

The end stage of disease is marked by further reduction in oxyntic glands, foveolar hyperplasia with elongation and microcystic change, hyperplastic polyp formation, and increasing degrees of pseudopyloric, pancreatic, and intestinal metaplasia. The muscularis mucosae may be thickened. Parietal cells are difficult to detect and the degree of inflammation is usually minimal or absent, although scattered lymphoid aggregates may persist.

Extensive gastric metaplastic atrophy is a risk factor for adenocarcinoma; that is why autoimmune gastritis is listed among the gastric precancerous conditions. *H. pylori* infection may coexist with autoimmune gastritis, and this condition is an additional factor for atrophic transformation and, as a consequence, for gastric carcinoma. During the florid and end stages, hypo- and achlorhydria cause physiologic increased production of gastrin from the antral G cells which stimulates ECL cells in the corpus, leading to ECL cell hyperplasia. A second mechanism that also contributes to ECL cell hyperplasia is the destruction and atrophy of oxyntic glands, which results in condensation and coalescence of the spared ECL cells. Morphologic patterns of gastrin-driven ECL cell hyperplasia include simple hyperplasia representing an increased (at least double) number of ECL cells in the corpus; linear hyperplasia, which represents a chain-forming proliferation of ECL cells within the glands; and (micro-)nodular hyperplasia marked by an organized collection of ECL cells that form nodules.

ECL proliferations may lead to carcinoid tumors; an intramucosal carcinoid tumor is defined as an expansive or infiltrative endocrine growth that measures >0.5 mm in diameter. Invasive carcinoids are those in which the tumor invades the submucosa. Although ECL cell carcinoids may arise during the florid phase, they are found most commonly in patients with end-stage disease. Carcinoid tumors associated with ECL cell hyperplasia occur in 5–8% of patients with autoimmune gastritis and account for 65% of all gastric carcinoid tumors. These tumors are relatively harmless with a >95% 5-year survival rate, which is in sharp contrast to the less common solitary, sporadic type of carcinoid tumors that are biologically more aggressive (<35% 5-year survival).

In the majority of patients, antral mucosa remains either completely normal or shows only focal mild chronic inflammation, either with or without intestinal metaplasia, similar to that observed in the age-matched general population. Hyperplasia of gastrin cells secondary to achlorhydria is often present in the antrum. Of course, concurrent *H. pylori* infection may involve the antrum and cause neutrophilic inflammation in addition to chronic antritis.

Immunophenotype

In autoimmune gastritis, the corpus mucosa loses oxyntic glands and looks like antrum ("antralized corpus"). Immunostaining for gastrin is useful in discriminating corpus, which lacks G cells, from antrum, which contains G cells (Fig. 2). A negative immunostain for gastrin indicates that the biopsy specimen is truly from the corpus and not from the antrum or antral-oxyntic transitional zone. This is especially useful to check the biopsy location since multiple gastric biopsies are often provided in a single box, without specifying the exact location. G-cell hyperplasia in the antrum can be observed in autoimmune gastritis. Seldom gastrin-positive cells may be seen in foci with intestinal metaplasia.

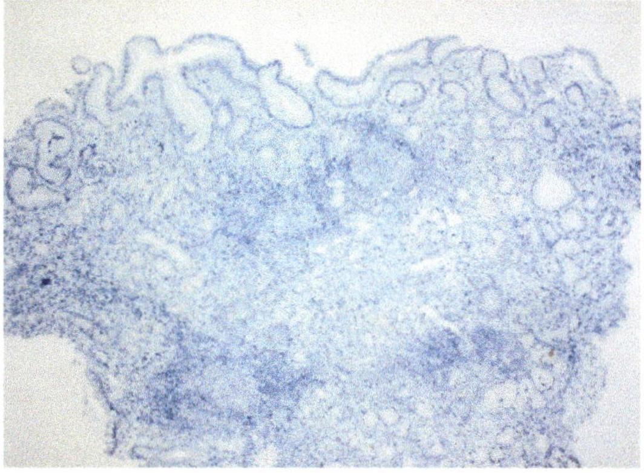

Autoimmune Gastritis, Fig. 2 A gastrin stain shows absence of G cells in the corpus mucosa (gastrin, original magnification 25×)

Gastrin stimulates the enterochromaffin-like (ECL) cells of the oxyntic compartment. This may result in linear and micronodular ECL cell hyperplasia, which can be stained with chromogranin A immunostaining (Fig. 3). A progression of the stimulation into gastric carcinoid is also highlighted with chromogranin A.

Molecular Features

Not applicable.

Differential Diagnosis

H. pylori-associated gastritis: *H. pylori* gastritis often shows a superficial band-like infiltrate with neutrophilic granulocytes, whereas autoimmune gastritis shows diffuse or patchy

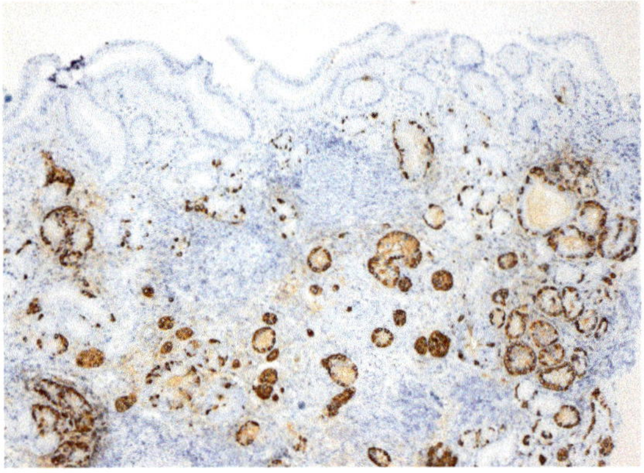

Autoimmune Gastritis, Fig. 3 Typical nodular and linear hyperplasia of endocrine cells in the corpus is highlighted with a chromogranin stain (chromogranin, original magnification 25×)

lymphoplasmacytic infiltration of lamina propria often with deep predominance. *H. pylori* gastritis predominantly affects the antrum and corpus, while autoimmune gastritis is restricted to the corpus.

MALT lymphoma: Lymphoma of the mucosal-associated lymphoid tissue (MALT) can occasionally be in the differential diagnosis and is differentiated by the dense, destructive nature of the neoplastic B-cell infiltrates in MALT lymphoma. Immunohistochemistry can be helpful in difficult cases.

Autoimmune polyglandular syndrome type 1: It presents in childhood and can resemble autoimmune gastritis. Antibodies against gastrointestinal endocrine cells cause this rare disorder. The destruction of gastrin cells results in low serum gastrin and leads to loss of parietal cells.

References and Further Reading

Annibale, B., Lahner, E., & Fave, G. D. (2011). Diagnosis and management of pernicious anemia. *Current Gastroenterology Reports, 13*(6), 518–524.

Odze, R. D., & Goldblum, J. R. (2009). *Surgical pathology of the GI tract, liver, biliary tract, and pancreas* (2nd ed.). Philadelphia: Saunders.

Rugge, M., Fassan, M., Pizzi, M., Zorzetto, V., Maddalo, G., Realdon, S., et al. (2012). Autoimmune gastritis: Histology phenotype and OLGA staging. *Alimentary Pharmacology & Therapeutics, 35*(12), 1460–1466.

Torbenson, M., Abraham, S. C., Boitnott, J., Yardley, J. H., & Wu, T. T. (2002). Autoimmune gastritis: Distinct histological and immunohistochemical findings before complete loss of oxyntic glands. *Modern Pathology, 15*(2), 102–109.

B

Bacterial Enterocolitis

Anne Jouret-Mourin
Department of Pathology, Cliniques Universitaires St. Luc, UCL, Brussels, Belgium

Synonyms

Dysentery

Definition

Bacterial colitis is an inflammatory-type diarrhea which can be caused by a variety of enteric pathogenic bacteria and affects both the small and large intestine or exclusively the large intestine (Table 1).

The diarrhea is the result of two major mechanisms: the production of toxins and the ability of the pathogens to survive in the intestine. Some toxins are either ingested in a preformed state (food intoxication by bacteria) or produced within the lumen of the intestine like enterotoxin produced by noninvasive *E. coli*. Some strains induce mainly intestinal secretion without tissue damage while others cause histological damage. Infections with *Vibrio cholerae*, *Klebsiella*, or noninvasive *E. coli* are examples of a severe pure secretory diarrhea. These organisms do not invade the mucosa. They induce minimal mucin depletion in the goblet cells and mucosal edema without acute inflammation. Other bacteria such as *Campylobacter*, *Shigella*, *Salmonella*, and *Yersinia* cause mucosal damage which results in bloody inflammatory diarrhea with fever.

Clinical Features

- **Incidence**
  Escherichia coli, *Salmonella*, *Campylobacter*, *Yersinia*, and *Shigella* represent the most common food- and waterborne pathogens worldwide. Their incidence differs depending on whether developing or industrialized countries are considered (a figure like ...%). Common modes of transmission include the fecal-oral pathway, animal host transmission, ingestion of contaminated food or water, and close human-to-human contact. The features specific for a variety of other pathogenic bacteria are discussed separately.
- **Age**
  Children, elderly persons, and immunocompromised individuals are especially susceptible to these infections.
- **Clinical Symptoms**
  Bacterial infections can be classified according to their clinical presentation. Some bacteria can induce either acute watery diarrhea or bloody diarrhea. Production of bloody stools means a mucosal break caused by enteroinvasive bacteria.

F. Carneiro et al. (eds.), *Pathology of the Gastrointestinal Tract*, Encyclopedia of Pathology,
DOI 10.1007/978-3-319-40560-5

Bacterial Enterocolitis, Table 1 Histologic patterns of bacterial colitis

	Mild or no histological changes	Acute self-limiting colitis	IBD-like		Ischemic pattern	Pseudomembranous pattern
			CD	UC		
Clostridium difficile			+ (early stage)		+ (later stage)	++
Salmonella typhimurium		+	++	+		
Non-typhoid		++		+		
(O1)*V. cholerae*	++	+				
Shigella		++	+	+		+
Campylobacter		++	+	+		
Aeromonas (sp.)		++	+	+	+	
Yersinia			++ (YP)			
E. coli						
EPEC	++					
EAEC	++					
EHEC	+	+			++	+

++: most often
+: rarely
EPEC enteropathogenic *E. coli*
EAEC enteroadherent *E. coli*
EHEC enterohemorrhagic *E. coli*
YP Yersinia pseudotuberculosis

- **Microscopic Findings**
  The morphological changes of bacterial infections are nonspecific or show a pattern of acute self-limited colitis (see description entry "► Infectious Colitis"). Some organisms produce characteristic histological features like a pseudomembranous or granulomatous pattern.
  Bacterial infections can also mimic chronic idiopathic inflammatory bowel disease (IBD) or ischemic colitis. These typical patterns and the differential diagnosis are detailed in the chapter dedicated to each bacterium.
- **Prognosis**
  Most bacterial infections resolve with antibiotics or supportive care, but in elderly, immunocompromised, or very young patients, the illness may be more severe causing septicemia and death.

Escherichia coli

Escherichia coli is one of the most common gram-negative human pathogens. It is found in the normal intestinal flora in human and animals but can act as pathogen. Five major subgroups based on serotyping cause enteric infections. Enterotoxigenic *E. coli* (ETEC), enteropathogenic *E. coli* (EPEC), and enteroadherent *E. coli* (EAEC) are noninvasive pathogens. ETEC is more frequently reported in travelers from tropical or subtropical areas as well as in children living in developing countries. EPEC is more common in young infants and neonates, and EAEC is more frequent in AIDS patients and pediatric patient.

The noninvasive *E. coli* (EPEC, EAEC, ETEC) cause profuse watery diarrhea, sometimes mucoid for EPEC, associated with fever, cramps, malaise, and vomiting. Diarrhea may be chronic in AIDS patients.

Enteroinvasive *E. coli* (EIEC) and enterohemorrhagic *E. coli* (EHEC) cause frequent watery or mucoid diarrhea which may be bloody when EHEC is responsible.

EIEC cause an illness similar to *Shigella* with direct invasion of the distal ileum and colonic mucosa. It occurs primarily in the tropics and is a cause of traveler's diarrhea.

EHEC (major strain O157:H7) is a virulent organism. It produces a cytotoxin without tissue invasion. This subtype is the focus of the following data.

- **Incidence**
  Contaminated meat (contaminated hamburger, unpasteurized milk, water or contact with swimming pool water, or sometimes person-to-person contact) is the most frequent mode of transmission requiring 10–100 organisms to produce illness. The bacteria are noninvasive and cause injury by attachment to epithelial cells and the production of toxins. These toxins are associated with the development of the hemolytic-uremic syndrome in children or the elderly at particular risk for severe illness and may cause encephalopathy.
- **Clinical Symptoms**
  Symptoms occur 3–4 days after infection and include severe abdominal pain, mild or no fever, and watery diarrhea followed in 1 or 2 days by bloody diarrhea and abdominal tenderness. Resolution of the diarrhea occurs after 4–10 days.
- **Age**
  Usually children or young patients.
- **Site**
  Lesions occur in the terminal ileum and right colon.

Macroscopic Data

Endoscopically, the right colon is most often involved. The mucosa is edematous with some erosions, ulcers, or hemorrhage. Transmural edema may be so important that it causes obstruction.

Microscopic Features

EHEC infection may show five major patterns:

(a) Marked edema and hemorrhage in the mucosa or submucosa with microthrombi even in areas away from ulcers and crypt withering causing an ischemic pattern of injury (Fig. 1)
(b) Pseudomembranous colitis-like
(c) Acute self-limited colitis characterized by cryptitis, less commonly crypt abscesses with or without neutrophil leukocytic infiltrate in the lamina propria
(d) Focal active colitis
(e) Normal aspect or mild focal increase in mononuclear cells

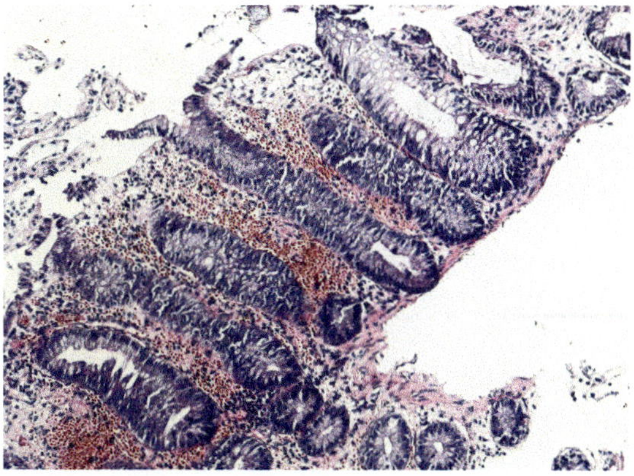

Bacterial Enterocolitis, Fig. 1 Enterohemorrhagic *E. coli* infection showing mucosal hemorrhage, reactive epithelial changes, and lamina propria fibrosis

Differential Diagnosis

The differential diagnosis includes *Clostridium difficile*-related colitis and ischemic colitis from which EHEC may be microscopically indistinguishable. Knowledge of clinical history, type of onset, age, history of antibiotic use, and endoscopic findings may help to distinguish these two entities. Ischemia rarely involves the right colon.

Useful Tests

The *Clostridium difficile* antigen test may be very helpful for the differential diagnosis.

Routine stool culture is useless because it cannot distinguish 0157:H7 from normal intestinal flora. Specific culture as early as possible and serotyping are the mainstay for diagnosing the pathogen.

Specific immune histochemical staining is available.

Yersinia

Yersinia pseudotuberculosis (YP) and *Yersinia enterocolitica* (YE), both gram-negative bacilli, are the species that cause human enteritis and mesenteric lymphadenitis.

- **Incidence**
  They are frequently diagnosed in Europe and the USA and are one of the most common causes of bacterial enteritis with a worldwide distribution. The genus *Yersinia* is responsible for 60–80% of cases of terminal ileitis and mesenteric lymphadenitis. The incidence is rising in Europe and the USA.
- **Epidemiology**
  The main source is food contamination (chicken, fish, and pork meat), water, and milk. Transmission from domestic animals is less common. Epidemiologic studies have revealed clustering of infections during fall and winter.
- **Pathogenesis**
  The pathogenic mechanism is invasion of the intestinal mucosa. After ingestion, *Yersinia* sp. penetrates through M cells and multiplies in underlying tissues.
- **Site**
  The primary infected site is the terminal ileum, the cecum, the ascending colon, and the appendix.
- **Age**
  Infants, children, and young adults are most commonly infected.
- **Clinical Symptoms**
  Yersinia may mimic acute appendicitis. Symptoms of ileitis or colitis may also be observed. Abdominal pain, diarrhea, nausea, and vomiting are commonly present. Although yersiniosis is usually a self-limited disease, chronic infection may be observed.
- **Prognosis**
  Most infections are self-limited. Immunocompromised or debilitated patients are at risk of more severe disease with sepsis and intestinal perforation. Chronic colitis is possible but uncommon. Symptoms may be present for months misleadingly suggesting IBD.

Macroscopic Features

Yersinia enterocolitica involves the ileum, right colon, and appendix and may be segmental and patchy.

It can infect any part of the bowel. Endoscopically mucosal ulceration or scattered punctate aphthous ulcers with mucosal hyperemia may be present.

Involved segment looks edematous and congested causing a thickened wall with nodularities around Peyer's patches. Sometimes mesenteric lymph nodes are enlarged and show central foci of necrosis.

Microscopic Findings

Microscopy shows mucosal ulceration surrounded by edematous and actively inflamed mucosa. Common features include lymphoid hyperplasia with active germinal centers both in the intestinal wall and the mesenteric lymph node, formation of epithelioid granulomas with central coagulative necrosis and microabscess formation (especially in YP infection), and transmural lymphoid aggregates.

YE is more characterized by mucosal ulceration with hyperplastic Peyer's patches associated with acute inflammation and diffuse increase of histiocytes.

An overlap between YE and YP has been described.

Differential Diagnosis

The major differential diagnosis includes other types of infectious colitis particularly by mycobacteria and *Salmonella*. Acid-fast staining and culture may help to distinguish mycobacteria infections. Microabscesses and granulomas may help to distinguish yersiniosis from salmonellosis.

Crohn's disease and yersiniosis may be difficult to distinguish from one another on histologic grounds alone. The transmural inflammation, epithelioid granulomas, fissuring lesions, and skip lesions may closely mimic Crohn's disease. Fat wrapping and prominent neural hyperplasia are in favor of Crohn's disease.

Useful Tests

Cultures, serologic studies, and PCR assays may be of help to confirm the diagnosis.

Shigella

Shigella species are virulent, gram-negative, non-motile bacilli causing dysentery. *Shigella dysenteriae* is the most common and most virulent, but *Shigella sonnei*, *Shigella flexneri*, and *Shigella boydii* are also reported.

- **Incidence**
  Shigella infection is a major cause of infectious colitis worldwide and more frequent and endemic in subtropical and tropical climates. The infective dose is as low as 10–100 species in *Shigella dysenteriae*.
- **Pathogenesis**
  The basic pathogenetic mechanism is the ability of the bacterium to penetrate the intestinal mucosa. The bacilli invade enterocytes by a bacterium directed macropinocytotic process, multiply within the epithelium and then enter the lamina propria. They may produce apoptosis.
- **Age**
  Infants, debilitated patients, and homosexuals are most commonly affected in developed countries.
- **Site**
  Lesions are usually concentrated in the left colon; the ileum may also be involved.
- **Clinical Symptoms**
  Symptoms are usually watery diarrhea, abdominal pain, fever followed by rectal tenesmus, and bloody diarrhea. Chronic disease is rare. The onset of the symptoms is usually within 12–50 h after contamination.

Macroscopic Findings
The colonic mucosa is edematous and hemorrhagic with pseudomembranes as well as ulceration.

Mucosal defects start with a superficial necrosis of the colonic mucosa, beginning as a focal process on the surface and in severe cases becoming confluent. Distribution is often continuous.

Microscopic Features
Early shigellosis is characterized by cryptitis and ulceration. Pseudomembranes as well as aphthoid ulcers may be observed. The lesion appears as a small defect in the epithelium subjacent to which is a mucosal damage in which only the deeper parts of the crypts persist.

Later, the mucosal defect increases; architectural distortion and an important mixed inflammatory infiltrate will appear.

Differential Diagnosis
In the early stage, *Shigella* may mimic pseudomembranous colitis caused by *C. difficile* and *E. coli*. Later, the differential diagnosis is needed with ulcerative colitis or Crohn's disease. Marked architectural distortion is commonly leading to a misdiagnosis of IBD.

Useful Test
Stool culture may be of help for diagnosis. PCR and serological studies are also available.

- **Treatment**
  Most often supportive care but selected antibiotics may be useful.

Clostridium
Clostridia are potent toxigenic bacteria responsible for severe gastrointestinal diseases including pseudomembranous colitis (*Clostridium difficile*), necrotizing enterocolitis (NEC) (*Clostridium perfringens*), neutropenic enterocolitis (*Clostridium septicum*), and botulism (*C. botulinum*).

The colon is affected essentially by *C. difficile* and *C. septicum*.

- **Site**
  Anywhere in the colon and the disease may be patchy or segmental. In pseudomembranous colitis, the distal left colon is most commonly involved. In 10% of cases, only the proximal colon is involved.
  For NEC, the right colon (cecum) is preferentially involved.
- **Age**
  Infants as well as adults may suffer from *C. difficile* infections, but the majority of patients are elderly.
- **Incidence**
  C. difficile is the most common nosocomial pathogen producing two toxins: toxin A which leads to fluid secretion and mucosal permeability and toxin B with an enterotoxic activity. *Clostridium difficile* infections

account for 10–25% of all cases of antibiotic-associated diarrhea (postoral antibiotic treatment) and virtually all cases of antibiotic-associated pseudomembranous colitis. Other risk factors are comorbid conditions as well as underlying illness, intensive care unit stay, and prolonged hospitalization. The incidence is also increased in patients with IBD, although in these patients the presentation is usually atypical. *C. septicum* is usually observed in the context of previous chemotherapy corresponding to a complication of neutropenia.

Clinical Features

Watery diarrhea is the first symptom of pseudomembranous colitis accompanied by abdominal pain, cramping, and fever. Bloody diarrhea may be seen. Symptoms can occur up to several weeks after antibiotic therapy. Toxic megacolon and perforation are possible complications.

Necrotizing enterocolitis (NEC) is more frequently associated with *C. septicum* especially in adults. GI hemorrhage, diarrhea, fever, abdominal pain, and distension are the most common symptoms.

Macroscopic Features

In pseudomembranous colitis, round, yellow-white adherent false membranes either isolated or confluent are observed, most often in the left colon sparing sometimes the rectum. Between the false membranes, the mucosa appears normal or erythematous. Small lesions like aphthoid ulcers are also seen.

The right colon is the most common localization of NEC with diffuse dilatation, marked edema, hemorrhage, and ulceration. Pseudomembranes can also be seen in NEC.

Microscopic Features

Three grades of histological lesions are described for pseudomembranous colitis.

Type I is the earliest lesion and consists of a superficial inflammatory reaction with neutrophilic subepithelial exudates, focal areas of epithelial necrosis, and widening of the crypt opening. The early lesions reflect local epithelial damage occurring on the luminal surface.

Type II lesion consists of a well-demarcated group of disrupted and distended crypts containing mucous with neutrophils at their bases. The overlying epithelial cells become flattened and necrotic and are progressively lost. Occasional thrombi are found in superficial mucosal capillaries. Mucous, fibrin, and cellular debris are projected into the intestinal lumen forming a pseudomembrane like a mushroom or volcanic eruptions overlying the necrotic mucosa (Figs. 2 and 3).

Type III lesion is rare and occurs late in the evolution. This lesion consists of complete necrosis with a few surviving glands covered by a membrane of fibrin, mucous, and cellular inflammatory debris.

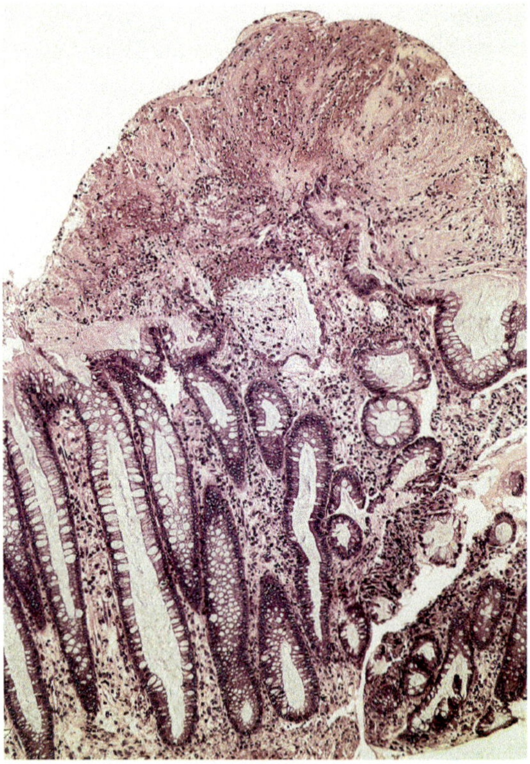

Bacterial Enterocolitis, Fig. 2 *C. difficile* infection. Mushroom- or volcano-like pseudomembrane overlying the mucosa is the classical feature of pseudomembranous colitis

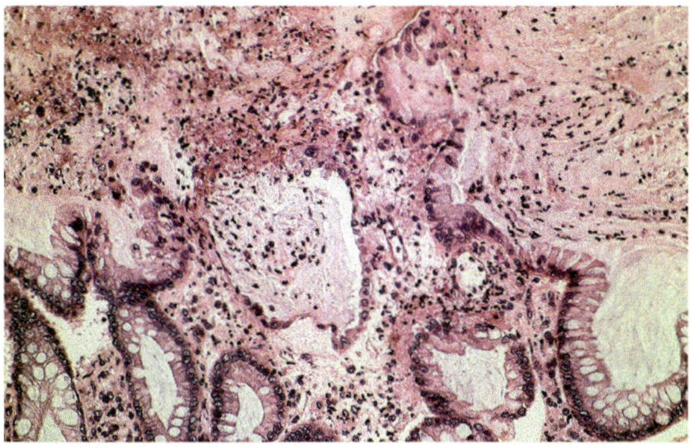

Bacterial Enterocolitis, Fig. 3 *C. difficile* infection. Dilated and ballooned crypts with necrosis giving rise to the membrane

Less characteristic lesions such as focal active colitis with some crypt abscesses have also been described.

In the resolving phase, residual glandular irregularity or regenerative changes with pseudopolypoid features may be seen.

In NEC, mild hemorrhage to prominent submucosal edema with mucosal ulceration and focal hemorrhagic necrosis can be seen. Lack of neutrophils is common. Perforation is a frequent complication.

- **Prognosis**
  Recurrent disease is common and seen in up to 5% of cases.

Differential Diagnosis

In the earliest stage, the differential diagnosis involves other infections. Pseudomembranes can be seen with other infectious entities such as *E. coli*, *Shigella*, and *Salmonella*. More rarely, in the earliest stage, *Clostridium difficile* can mimic Crohn's disease with identical mucosal changes and inflammation extending into the submucosa.

In the latest stage (type III), ischemic colitis is the most important differential diagnosis because this may also produce pseudomembranes. Areas of focal fibrosis and hyalinization of the lamina propria are more likely associated with ischemia.

The differential diagnosis for NEC includes ischemic colitis.

Useful Test

The bacterial diagnosis is based on the isolation or detection of components of the organism. Stool anaerobic cultures and assays for *C. difficile* toxin are positive in 95% of contaminated patients. The cytotoxin assay is the gold standard for the diagnosis (sensitivity, 94–100%; specificity, 99%) for the *C. difficile*. *Clostridium difficile* toxin can be also identified by PCR.

Stool culture is the most helpful technique for diagnosing *C. septicum*.

B

References and Further Reading

Aslam, S. (2006). An update on diagnosis, treatment and prevention of Clostridium difficile-associated disease. *Gastroenterology Clinics of North America, 35*, 315–335.

Gleason, T. H., et al. (1982). The pathology of Yersinia enterocolitica ileocolitis. *American Journal of Surgical Pathology, 6*, 347–355.

Gomez, L., et al. (1998). Necrotizing enterocolitis: Spectrum of the disease and comparison of definite and possible cases. *Clinical Infectious Diseases, 27*, 695–699.

Griffin, P. M., et al. (1990). Escherichia coli 0157: H7-associated colitis: A clinical and histological study of 11 cases. *Gastroenterology, 99*, 142–149.

Islam, M. M. (1994). Pathology of shigellosis and its complications. *Histopathology, 24*, 65–71.

Kelly, J., et al. (1987). The histopathology of rectosigmoid biopsies from adults with bloody diarrhea due to verotoxin-producing *Escherichia coli. American Journal of Clinical Pathology, 88*, 78–82.

Lamps, L. W. (2007). Infective disorders of the gastrointestinal tract. *Histopathology, 50*, 55–63.

Naktin, J., et al. (1999). Yersinia enterocolitica and Yersinia pseudotuberculosis. *Clinics in Laboratory Medicine, 19*, 523–536.

Otaibi, A., et al. (2002). Neutropenic enterocolitis after pediatric bone marrow transplant. *Journal of Pediatric Surgery, 37*, 770–772.

Price, A. B., et al. (1977). Pseudomembranous colitis. *Journal of Clinical Pathology, 30*, 1–12.

Speelman, P., et al. (1984). Distribution and spread of colonic lesions in shigellosis: A colonoscopic study. *Journal of Infectious Diseases, 150*, 899–903.

Surawicz, C. M. (1999). Pseudomembranous colitis. Causes and cures. *Digestion, 60*, 91–100.

Welinder-Olsson, C., et al. (2005). Enterohemorrhagic Escherichia coli (EHEC). *Scandinavian Journal of Infectious Diseases, 37*, 405–416.

Bacterial Overgrowth Syndrome

Arzu Ensari
Department of Pathology, Ankara University Medical School, Sihhiye, Ankara, Turkey

Synonyms

Blind loop syndrome; Small bowel bacterial overgrowth (SIBO) syndrome; Stasis syndrome

Definition

SIBO occurs when small bowel motility is altered under conditions causing luminal stasis and colonization of the normal microfloral bacteria in the lumen resulting in mucosal damage and malabsorption. Regardless of the underlying cause, SIBO is a very heterogeneous syndrome characterized by the presence of an increased number and/or abnormal type of bacteria normally confined to the colon, within the small intestine. Normally, small intestinal lumen is colonized by facultative anaerobe or obligate bacteria, particularly bacteroides species, which are predominantly found in the distal ileum, while proximal small intestinal mucosa is usually colonized by bacteria ingested with food. Bacteria in SIBO might significantly interfere with enzymatic, absorptive, and metabolic actions of the small intestinal mucosa. Any condition causing disruption of intestinal luminal flow including motor and neural disorders such as scleroderma, diabetes, pseudo-obstruction and amyloidosis, structural defects such as diverticulosis and strictures, and surgery leading to isolated bowel segments like Billroth II anastomosis may all lead to SIBO and resultant malabsorption. In addition irritable bowel syndrome, immunodeficiencies, and long-term treatment with proton pump inhibitors may also cause predisposition to SIBO. The diagnosis relies on the presence of increased intestinal volume and bacterial concentrations, hydrogen breath tests, and response to antibiotics. Small bowel aspirate and quantitative cultures with more than 10^5 bacteria CFU/mL of proximal jejunal aspiration are the diagnostic procedures.

Clinical Features

- **Incidence**
  The overall prevalence of SIBO in the general public is unknown. SIBO is generally left undiagnosed. According to different studies, the incidence of SIBO was found between 2.5% and 22%. However, the prevalence varies depending on the population studied and the diagnostic methods used.
- **Age**
  Bacterial overgrowth syndrome is more prevalent in elderly population because of diminished gastric acid secretion and consumption of medications that can cause hypomotility.
- **Sex**
  No known predilection for either sex is present.
- **Site**
  The entire small intestine may be involved.
- **Treatment**
  Bacterial overgrowth is treated with antibiotics and nutritional support which help to restore the normal microflora. However, underlying causes should also be treated when possible.
- **Outcome**
  The outcome is usually good if diagnosed early and antibiotic therapy is started before severe malabsorption is developed. The prognosis largely depends on the underlying disease leading to bacterial overgrowth. Ultimately, SIBO might result in intestinal failure as it has a high relapse rate.

Macroscopy

Macroscopic changes may be visible in some patients in the form of small intestinal mucosal breaks (erosions or ulcers) on capsule endoscopy.

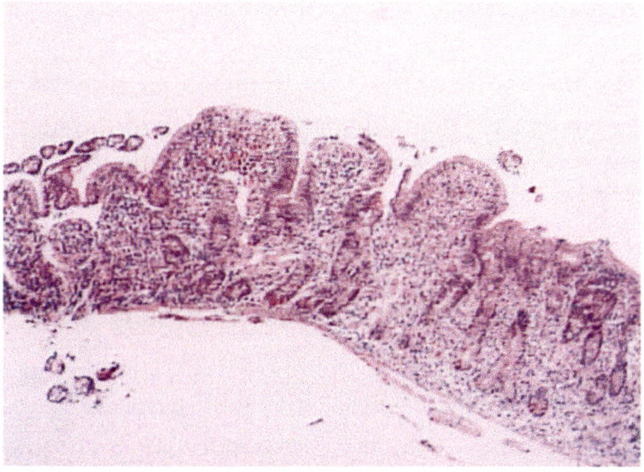

Bacterial Overgrowth Syndrome, Fig. 1 Villous blunting and crypt hyperplasia with mixed cellular inflammatory infiltration of the lamina propria (H&E; ×100)

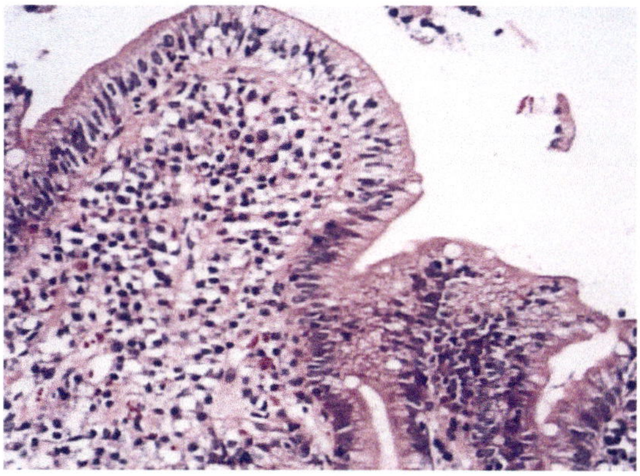

Bacterial Overgrowth Syndrome, Fig. 2 IELs and neutrophils in the surface epithelium showing lipid vacuolization (H&E; ×200)

Microscopy

The mucosal biopsy may be normal but histopathologic picture may vary between mild to moderate villous shortening and blunting with increased chronic inflammatory cells in the lamina propria (Fig. 1). There may be intraepithelial lymphocytosis and neutrophilic infiltration of the surface epithelium. Enterocyte vacuolization due to lipid accumulation may also be seen (Fig. 2). However, these features are usually patchy in nature and multiple biopsies are necessary for diagnosis in the right clinical setting. Histology does not correlate with clinical severity.

Immunophenotype

No immunophenotypic feature has been reported.

Molecular Features

No molecular feature has been reported.

Differential Diagnosis

Differential diagnosis of SIBO is difficult if it is not considered. It is necessary to distinguish functional disorders (e.g., flatulence, abdominal bloating and distension, and malabsorption of mono- or disaccharides) and chronic gastrointestinal infections (e.g., giardiasis). Moreover, the differential diagnosis must focus on the underlying cause including irritable bowel syndrome, Crohn's disease, chronic pancreatitis, scleroderma, or coeliac disease nonresponding to adequate gluten-free diet. Under these clinical settings, unexplained deterioration of the clinical status of the patient is an indication to search for SIBO.

References and Further Reading

Bohm, M., Siwiec, R. M., & Wo, J. M. (2013). Diagnosis and management of small intestinal bacterial overgrowth. *Nutrition in Clinical Practice, 28*, 289–299.

Bures, J., Cyrany, J., Kohoutova, D., Förstl, M., Rejchrt, S., Kvetina, J., Vorisek, V., & Kopacova, M. (2010). Small intestinal bacterial overgrowth syndrome. *World Journal of Gastroenterology, 16*(24), 2978–2990.

Petrone, P., Sarkisyan, G., Fernández, M., Coloma, E., Akopian, G., Ortega, A., & Kaufman, H. S. (2011). Small intestinal bacterial overgrowth in patients with lower gastrointestinal symptoms and a history of previous abdominal surgery. *Archives of Surgery, 146*(4), 444–447.

Rana, S. V., & Bhardwaj, S. B. (2008). Small intestinal bacterial overgrowth. *Scandinavian Journal of Gastroenterology, 43*(9), 1030–1037.

Sachdeva, S., Rawat, A. K., Reddy, R. S., & Puri, A. S. (2011). Small intestinal bacterial overgrowth (SIBO) in irritable bowel syndrome: Frequency and predictors. *Journal of Gastroenterology and Hepatology, 26* (Suppl 3), 135–138.

Barium Sulfate, Esophageal Inclusions

Mário Ferraz de Oliveira
Serviço Anatomia Patológica, Centro Hospitalar Lisboa Central EPE, Lisbon, Portugal

Synonyms

Barium granuloma

Definition

Barium sulfate is an inorganic compound ($BaSO_4$) used since the early 1900s in colloidal suspension as a contrast medium in the gastrointestinal tract. Extravasation of barium into the wall of the esophagus through an injury in the mucosa (whatever the cause) provokes a reaction against it, as a granulation tissue or more commonly as a granulomatous reaction.

Clinical Features

It is a very rare complication and usually an incidental finding in biopsies or resection specimens for other reasons, but can present as a polypoid or ulcerative lesion.

Macroscopy

Barium granulomas, when large enough, produce brownish-green masses associated with fibrosis.

Microscopy

Barium sulfate can be seen in histological sections in two ways, depending on the method the commercial suspensions are prepared:

- Fine gray/greenish non-refringent granules (PAS negative)
- Larger birefringent rhomboid crystals

Barium is located in the cytoplasm of macrophages and extracellular tissues (sometimes associated with foreign giant cells granulomas) and can be stained by the rhodizonate method or demonstrated by paraffin block radiographic study. We can identify barium in the mucosa and submucosa.

References and Further Reading

Levison, D. A., Crocker, P. R., Smith, A., Blackshaw, A. J., & Bartram, C. I. (1984). Varied light and scanning electron microscopic appearances of barium sulphate in smears and histological sections. *Journal of Clinical Pathology, 37*(5), 481–487.
Morson, B. C., & Dawson, I. M. P. (2003). *Gastrointestinal pathology* (4th ed., p. 86). Malden: Blackwell.
Womack, C. (1984). Unusual histological appearances of barium sulphate – A case report with scanning electron microscopy and energy dispersive X ray analysis. *Journal of Clinical Pathology, 37*(5), 488–493.

Barrett's Esophagus

Paula Chaves[1,2] and António Dias Pereira[3]
[1]Serviço de Anatomia Patológica, Instituto Português de Oncologia de Lisboa de Francisco Gentil, Lisbon, Portugal
[2]Faculdade de Ciências da Saúde, Universidade da Beira Interior, Covilhã, Portugal
[3]Instituto Português de Oncologia de Lisboa Francisco Gentil, E.P.E., Lisbon, Portugal

Synonyms

Barrett's metaplasia; Esophageal columnar metaplasia

Definition

Barrett's esophagus (BE) results from the metaplastic replacement of the normal squamous esophageal lining by a columnar epithelium. Currently, there are two distinct definitions of BE stating two different proposals of patient's management. The American Gastroenterological Association (AGA) defines BE as "the condition in which any extent of metaplastic columnar epithelium that predisposes to cancer development replaces the stratified squamous epithelium that normally lines the distal esophagus." Currently, the AGA understanding is that "intestinal metaplasia is required for the diagnosis of Barrett's esophagus because intestinal metaplasia is the only type of esophageal columnar epithelium that clearly predisposes to malignancy" (The AGA Institute Medical Position Panel 2011). The British Society of Gastroenterology (BSG), on the other hand, defines BE as "an endoscopically apparent area above the esophagogastric junction that is suggestive of Barrett esophagus (salmon-colored mucosa) which is supported by the finding of columnar-lined esophagus on histology" (Playford 2006).

These two different statements are based on the recognition of BE as the premalignant condition that predispose to esophageal adenocarcinoma. Both the BSG and the AGA recognize BE as the gastroesophageal reflux (GER)-induced replacement of the normal squamous esophageal lining by a columnar metaplastic epithelium that is endoscopically recognized and that exhibits gastric and intestinal features. Nevertheless, as intestinal metaplasia (IM) is the sole feature unequivocally associated to malignancy, the AGA requires its presence for the diagnosis of BE.

Since its first reference on the medical literature by Tileston in 1906 as a peptic ulcer of the esophagus, and the first description of a columnar lining in the distal esophagus by Lyall in 1937, the BE entity, described in the early 1950s simultaneously in France by Lortat-Jacob and in England by Norman Barrett, has suffered a lot of misunderstandings and had multiple definitions. These definitions, established by researchers to characterize study populations and used by clinicians to manage patients, express the absence of consensus in the different biopathogenic aspects of BE.

In the 1980s BE was restricted to the columnar-lined segments longer than 3 cm. This definition is mostly due to Hayward who stated in the early 1960s that the distal 2 cm of the normal esophagus was lined by the columnar epithelium, thus sustaining that the use of the 3 cm rule would avoid over diagnosis. The recognition by Haggitt in the early 1990s of IM as the sole columnar esophageal metaplastic epithelium clearly associated with cancer supported the recognition of goblet cells as the hallmark for BE diagnosis.

Today, it is recognized that BE is a multistep process in which IM is a late event (Dias Pereira and Chaves 2012), but the sole type of columnar esophageal epithelium undoubtedly associated to malignancy is IM (The AGA Institute Medical Position Panel 2011).

Clinical Features

- **Incidence**
  There is no data on the incidence of BE. The prevalence of BE in symptomatic reflux disease patients has been described to be up to 12%. Its prevalence in the general population still remains a matter of discussion. The two largest and well-designed studies, from Sweden and the United States, have produced widely ranging results, 1.6% and 6.8%, respectively. Despite the extensive discussion on the reasons for this difference, it is not clear if we are facing a true difference or a methodological bias.
- **Age**
  Our knowledge about the natural history of BE is limited. As a rule, BE is generally diagnosed in the first endoscopy; the diagnosis is uncommon in pediatric age. Most of the cases of columnar-lined esophagus diagnosed at this age do not fulfill the criteria of intestinal metaplasia required by some authors for the diagnosis of BE. Generally, this condition is diagnosed after the fifth decade of life. BE is an uncommon diagnosis under the age of 40.

Although this data may be biased by the higher utilization of endoscopy in the elderly, there is evidence that the likelihood of finding BE increases with age.

- **Sex**
  BE affects mainly men. Among individuals with GER symptoms, BE risk is higher in males than in females. Cohort studies of Barrett's patients also show predominance of men, with a pooled relationship of 2:1. The reasons for this male preponderance in BE are not yet fully understood. Besides this gender difference in BE prevalence, there is also evidence that it is far more common in non-Hispanics white subjects than in blacks.
- **Site**
  BE is located at the distal portion of the esophagus, as circumferential, tongue, or isle-like metaplastic segments.
- **Treatment**
  Treatment of reflux disease in patients with BE does not differ from treatment of reflux in subjects without Barrett's. Medical proton pump inhibitors (PPIs)-based treatment has been associated with a slight, although not significant, decrease in Barrett's length. The impact of reflux control in the cancer risk associated to BE has not yet been established. Though it has been claimed that surgical anti-reflux procedures have benefits over medical treatment in the reduction of cancer incidence, there is no definite data on this question. From available published data, there is some evidence that proton pump inhibitors, nonsteroidal anti-inflammatory drugs, and statins are associated with a low risk of cancer in BE. There are some prospective trials ongoing in this field. Recently, a prospective study on a cohort of BE patients showed that the use of PPIs was associated with a reduced risk of neoplastic progression.

  Until recently, surgery (esophagectomy) was the option for patients that progressed to cancer. Moreover, due to the relatively high proportion of patients whose surgical specimen showed invasive cancer despite a preoperative diagnosis of high-grade dysplasia, many centers considered this diagnosis, after confirmation by two independent pathologists, as an indication for surgery.

  In the last two decades, several endoscopic ablative techniques (laser, argon plasma, photodynamic therapy, radiofrequency ablation, mucosectomy, submucosal dissection) that proved to be efficient in the elimination of neoplastic lesions and in the eradication of BE have been developed. Importantly, it has also been shown that when reepithelialization of the esophagus occurs in a nonacidic environment, squamous rather than columnar lining is observed. Today, it is consensual that the endoscopic management of dysplastic BE should include resection of visible lesions (either by mucosectomy or by submucosal resection) and ablation of residual metaplastic mucosa, being radiofrequency the preferred method. Indeed, radiofrequency has been shown to be highly effective and safe in the eradication of BE with high-grade dysplasia not associated to visible lesions. Outcomes of endoscopic and surgical management of BE with high-grade dysplasia and/or cancer are not substantially different. Whereas endoscopic approach is associated with a higher rate of local recurrence of the neoplasia, surgery is associated with a higher post-procedural mortality and morbidity. Nevertheless, the quality of life seems to be superior after endoscopic ablation than after esophagectomy.
- **Outcome**
  BE is associated to esophageal adenocarcinoma (EA), the malignancy with the highest increasing incidence in the past four decades in the western world. The risk of cancer in BE is not completely established yet. Given the association between BE and EA, the risk of cancer in BE was initially thought to be very high, and until the new millennium, the pooled risk of cancer in BE was established as 1% per year. However, it was later shown that this 1% risk was an overestimation due to bias publication and a 0.5% risk per year was judged as a reasonable estimation. Recent population-based studies showed an incidence of cancer

as low as 0.12% per year and four recent meta-analyses reported annual incidences of adenocarcinoma in Barrett's from 0.33% to 0.63%. The magnitude of cancer risk in BE is an important issue since there is evidence from cost-effectiveness studies of surveillance that if cancer risk is too low, surveillance may be not justified.

Macroscopy

BE is macroscopically recognized at endoscopy as a red gastric-type or salmon-colored mucosa of any length in the distal esophagus, just above the gastroesophageal junction (GEJ) (Fig. 1). For the diagnosis of BE, the endoscopist must recognize two landmarks: the GEJ, the imaginary line where the esophagus ends and the stomach begins, generally accepted as the most proximal extent of the gastric folds, and the squamous columnar junction (SCJ), the line where the squamous epithelium meets the columnar lining. Normally, the GEJ and the SCJ or Z-line coincides. BE is suspected when a proximal displacement of the SCJ in relation to the GEJ is observed. According to the length of this proximal displacement, BE is traditionally classified as short (<3 cm) or long ($\geq$3 cm) segments. For a better estimation of the metaplastic segments extent, a new classification based on both, the circular and maximal extents, was proposed (the Prague C&M classification) and is now widely accepted.

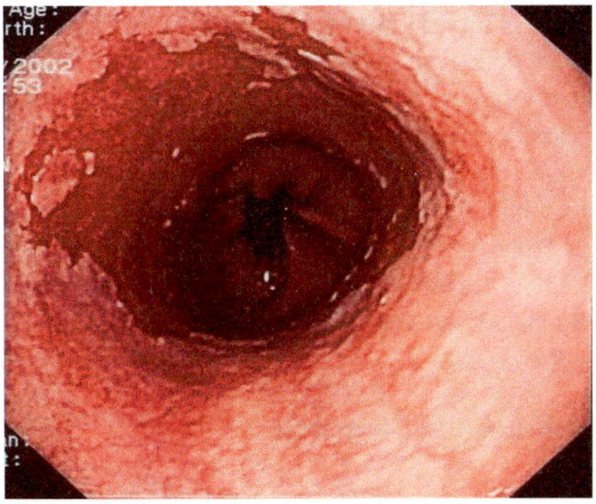

Barrett's Esophagus, Fig. 1 Barrett segment

Microscopy

BE is histologically characterized by a columnar-lined mucosa that displays a spectrum of histological features which combines an assortment of columnar epithelia with gastric and intestinal characteristics. In 1976, Paul described two gastric-type epithelia, the *junctional* and the *atrophic fundic*, and one intestinal type, the *specialized columnar epithelium*, which in 2000 were nominated by Chandrasoma as *oxynto-cardiac* (Fig. 2), *cardiac* (Fig. 3), and *intestinal metaplasia (IM)* (Fig. 4), respectively.

For the microscopic confirmation of BE in the biopsy material from a suspected esophageal segment, the AGA requires the recognition of IM (The AGA Institute Medical Position Panel 2011), while the BSG (Playford 2006) do not

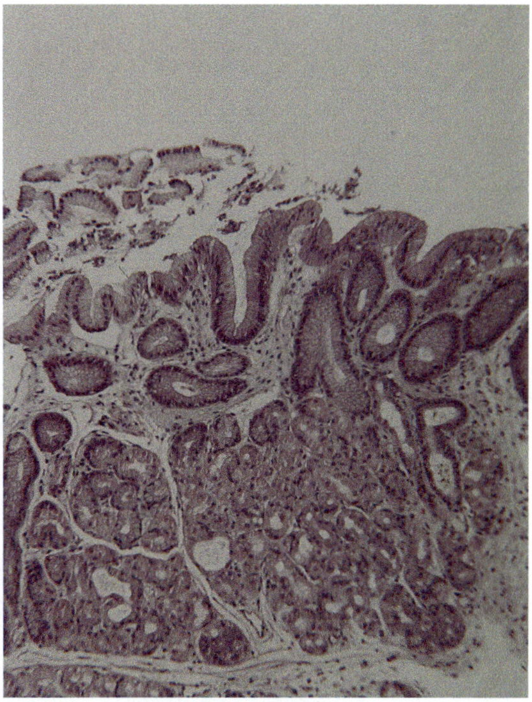

Barrett's Esophagus, Fig. 2 BE Oxyntico-cardiac mucosa

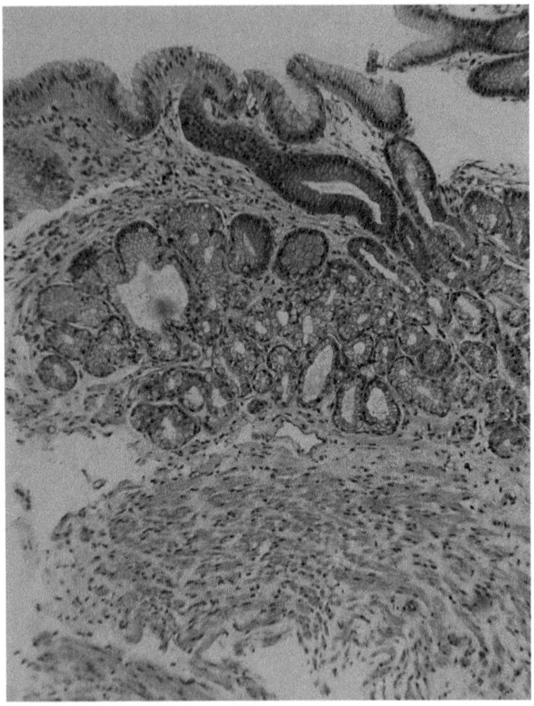

Barrett's Esophagus, Fig. 3 BE Cardiac mucosa

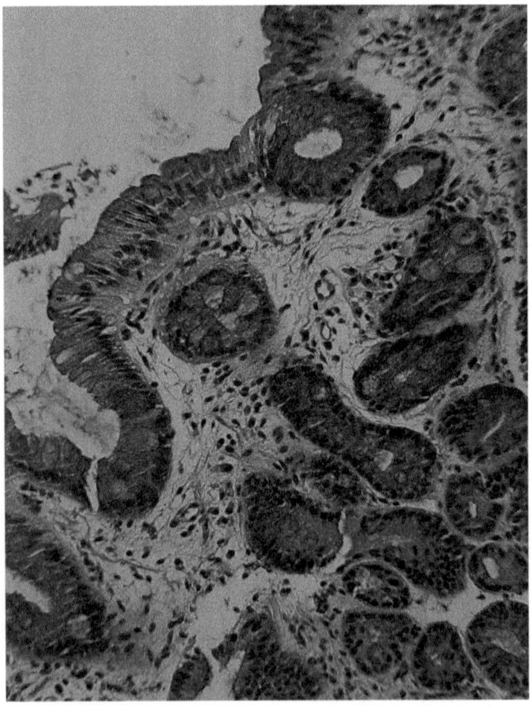

Barrett's Esophagus, Fig. 4 BE Intestinal metaplasia

require the demonstration of goblet cells being the finding of a columnar-lined mucosa the only prerequisite.

Immunophenotype

BE has a mixed, gastric and intestinal, phenotype expressed by the presence of gastric and intestinal markers in columnar as well as in goblet cells (Hahn et al. 2009). The intestinal phenotype is associated with an increased risk for adenocarcinoma, and it is recognized that the expression of gastric features are early changes in BE pathogenesis, while the late metaplastic steps lead to an epithelium with assorted gastric and intestinal characteristics (Dias Pereira and Chaves 2012; Hahn et al. 2009). Cytokeratins 7 and 20 in BE exhibit a characteristic, but not specific, pattern of expression (Nurgalieva et al. 2007) that does not allow the differential diagnosis between IM of the stomach and IM of the distal esophagus.

Molecular Features

BE progresses through the morphological sequence metaplasia-dysplasia-carcinoma corollary of a successive accumulation of molecular genetic alterations (Goldblum 2003). Some of the well-recognized abnormalities, such as abnormal expression of growth factors and p16 hypermethylation or mutation, are consistently related to the earliest steps of progression, whereas others, namely, p53 alteration and inhibition of apoptosis, appear as late events. Some of them, like telomerase upregulation, are detected in early dysplastic as well as in non-dysplastic BE. Nevertheless a magic marker to select patients that will progress for cancer has not yet been identified.

Differential Diagnosis

BE is distinguished from IM at the junction by the recognition of a normal junction or of a metaplastic segment, long or short, at endoscopy.

References and Further Reading

Dias Pereira, A., & Chaves, P. (2012). Columnar-lined oesophagus without intestinal metaplasia: Results from a cohort with a mean follow-up of 7 years. *Alimentary Pharmacology & Therapeutics, 36*, 282–289.
Goldblum, J. R. (2003). Barrett's esophagus and Barrett's-related dysplasia. *Modern Pathology, 16*, 316–324.
Hahn, H. P., Blount, P. L., Ayub, K., Das, K. M., Souza, R., Spechler, J. S., & Odze, R. D. (2009). Intestinal differentiation in metaplastic, nongoblet columnar epithelium in the esophagus. *The American Journal of Surgical Pathology, 33*, 1006–1015.
Nurgalieva, Z., Lowrey, A., & El-Serag, H. B. (2007). The use of cytokeratin stain to distinguish Barrett's esophagus from contiguous tissues: A systematic review. *Digestive Diseases and Sciences, 52*, 1345–1354.
Playford, R. J. (2006). New British Society of Gastroenterology (BSG) guidelines for the diagnosis and management of Barrett's oesophagus. *Gut, 55*, 442–443.
The AGA Institute Medical Position Panel. (2011). American gastroenterological association medical position statement on the management of Barrett's esophagus. *Gastroenterology, 140*, 1084–1091.

Basal Cell Carcinoma of the Anal Margin

Denis Chatelain[1] and Jean-François Fléjou[2]
[1]Service d'Anatomie Pathologique,
Centre Hospitalier et Universitaire du Nord,
Amiens, France
[2]Faculté de Médecine Pierre et Marie Curie,
Service d'Anatomie et Cytologie Pathologiques,
Hôpital Saint-Antoine, Paris, France

Definition

Basal cell carcinoma of the anal margin is a malignant epithelial neoplasm. It consists of basaloid cells, and on microscopic examination, it is similar to conventional basal cell carcinoma of the skin (Gibson and Ahmed 2001).

The etiology of this tumor is unknown, but there is neither an evidence for a role of infection by HPV nor a role of ultraviolet radiation, unlike other basal cell carcinoma occurring in the sun-exposed skin. Some patients have a history of radiotherapy in the pelvic area. For some authors, the occurrence of this tumor could be favored by chronic skin irritation or a local trauma.

B

Clinical Features

Patients present with a perianal ulcerated tumor and complain of itching or local irritation. Some physicians sometimes initially misdiagnose these cancers as inflammatory or infectious skin lesions. Some patients have multiple basal cell carcinomas at other anatomic sites and the diagnosis of basal cell carcinoma of the anal margin should prompt an examination of the whole cutaneous surface.

- **Incidence**
  The incidence of this rare tumor is difficult to assess. It represents less than 0.5% of all basal cell carcinomas.
- **Age**
  Basal cell carcinoma of the perianal margin is diagnosed in middle aged and elderly patients (generally aged between 60 and 70).
- **Sex**
  This tumor is more frequently diagnosed in males.
- **Site**
  Basal cell carcinoma originates from the skin of the anal margin.
- **Treatment**
  Basal cell carcinoma of the anal margin is treated by local excision. Recurrences are rare if the surgical excision is complete.
- **Outcome**
  Basal cell carcinoma seems to be a purely locally aggressive tumor. No metastatic site has been described.

Macroscopy

Perianal basal cell carcinoma presents as erythematous papules, patches or nodules, plaques or ulcers. A polypoid appearance has also been described. The average size of the tumor is 2 cm (0.5–5 cm). Some tumors occasionally involve the squamous zone below the dentate line.

Microscopy

Histologically perianal basal cell carcinoma shows the same variability morphologic patterns as conventional basal cell carcinoma of the skin with nodular, superficial, infiltrative, basosquamous, or fibroepithelioma patterns. The tumors consist of small- or medium-sized round or cylindrical cells with basophilic cytoplasm and round or oval uniform nuclei (Fig. 1). Peripheral cell layers of the tumor masses can show a palisade arrangement of the nuclei, and there is sometimes retraction of the stroma from tumor islands, resulting in peritumoral lacunae. Cystic spaces may be present in the center of nodules, horn cysts and pseudoglands can be seen.

Immunophenotype

Perianal basal cell carcinoma is positive for Ber EP4 and negative for keratins 13, 19, 22, CEA, and Ulex Europaeus A1, while the basaloid variant of squamous cell carcinoma usually shows the opposite pattern.

Molecular Features

Molecular features of perianal basal cell carcinoma have not been described specifically.

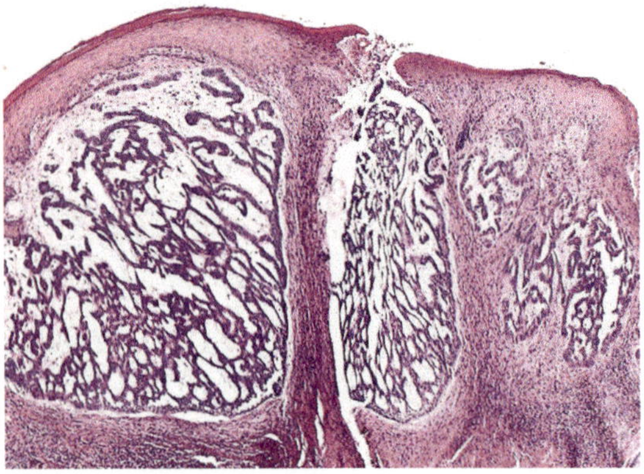

Basal Cell Carcinoma of the Anal Margin, Fig. 1 Anal basal cell carcinoma

Differential Diagnosis

It is important to distinguish basal cell carcinoma from squamous cell carcinoma because treatments are different. The differential diagnosis may be difficult on small biopsies. However, the basaloid variant of squamous cell carcinoma usually shows less conspicuous peripheral palisading, more cellular pleomorphism, and often shows larger eosinophilic necrotic areas.

Cross-References

- ▶ Basal Cell Carcinoma of the Anal Margin
- ▶ Paget's Disease of the Anus
- ▶ Squamous Cell Carcinoma, Anus

References and Further Reading

Gibson, G. E., & Ahmed, I. (2001). Perianal and genital basal cell carcinoma: A clinicopathologic review of 51 cases. *Journal of the American Academy of Dermatology, 45*, 68–71.

Shia, J. (2010). An update on tumors of the anal canal. *Archives of Pathology & Laboratory Medicine, 134*, 1601–1611.

Basaloid Squamous Cell Carcinoma, Esophageal

Maria Gabriela Gasparinho[1,2] and
Isabel Fonseca[3,4]
[1]Instituto Português de Oncologia de Lisboa Francisco Gentil, Lisboa, Portugal
[2]Instituto de Anatomia Patológica da Faculdade de Ciências da Saúde da Universidade da Beira Interior, Covilhã, Portugal
[3]Serviço de Anatomia Patológica, Instituto Português de Oncologia Francisco Gentil – Lisboa, Lisbon, Portugal
[4]Faculdade de Medicina de Lisboa, Instituto de Anatomia Patológica, Lisbon, Portugal

Synonyms

There are no current synonyms for this neoplasm. Historically, it has been confused with another neoplastic entity, namely *adenoid cystic carcinoma*.

Definition

A malignant epithelial neoplasm composed of closely packed cells with hyperchromatic nuclei and scant cytoplasm, with a solid growth pattern, small cystic spaces, and foci of necrosis. The diagnosis depends on the demonstration of squamous cell dysplasia/carcinoma in situ in the overlying mucosa.

Clinical Features

- **Incidence**
  Basaloid squamous cell carcinoma (BSCC) is a rare entity and there are no global worldwide incidence data available. In most published series, the incidence ranges from 0.07% to 11.3% of all esophageal carcinomas.
- **Age**
  In the published series, the mean age at the time of diagnosis is around 60 years.
- **Sex**
  There is a slight predominance in males.
- **Site**
  This type of neoplasm has been classically described in the upper aerodigestive tract, namely at the larynx and the esophagus, but it can also be encountered in other organs, such as the uterine cervix or the anal canal.
- **Treatment**
  Surgical resection is the treatment of choice. Depending on the stage of the disease, chemotherapy and radiotherapy may be added. This particular histological type does not change the usual treatment for esophageal carcinomas.
- **Outcome**
  Basaloid squamous cell carcinoma has been considered to harbor a dim prognosis. Nevertheless, recent series have failed to demonstrate that point, suggesting it might have a similar prognosis to moderate/poorly differentiated squamous cell carcinoma. In the most recent series, the mean 5-year survival rate was 36.6%. Lymph node metastases are seen at presentation in 20–67% of cases, depending on the series.

Macroscopy

Basaloid squamous cell carcinoma can present as a polypoid mass or an ulcerated/infiltrative tumor. In the latest series, it was more frequently encountered in the middle and inferior thirds of the esophagus.

Microscopy

Basaloid squamous cell carcinoma is composed of cells with hyperchromatic nuclei, inconspicuous nucleoli and scant cytoplasm, and has a high nuclear-cytoplasmic ratio. The cells are arranged in solid, nesting, sharply demarcated lobules, surrounded by a fibrous stroma. Often, necrotic foci are seen in the center of the lobules (comedo-like necrosis; Fig. 1). The tumor may also assume a trabecular pattern, displaying anastomosing trabeculae, or show microcystic/pseudoglandular structures (Fig. 2). A cribriform pattern and ductal differentiation were also reported. The

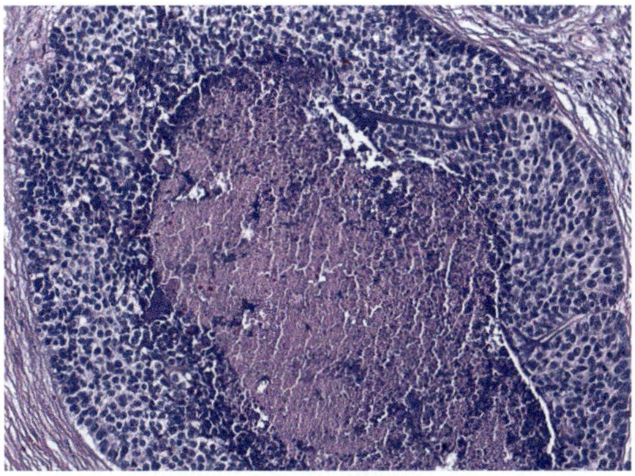

Basaloid Squamous Cell Carcinoma, Esophageal, Fig. 1 Basaloid squamous cell carcinoma (hematoxylin–eosin, medium-power). Comedo-type necrosis in the center of a lobule. This is composed of basaloid cells, with hyperchromatic nuclei and a high nuclear–cytoplasmic ratio. There is slight palisading at the periphery of the lobule

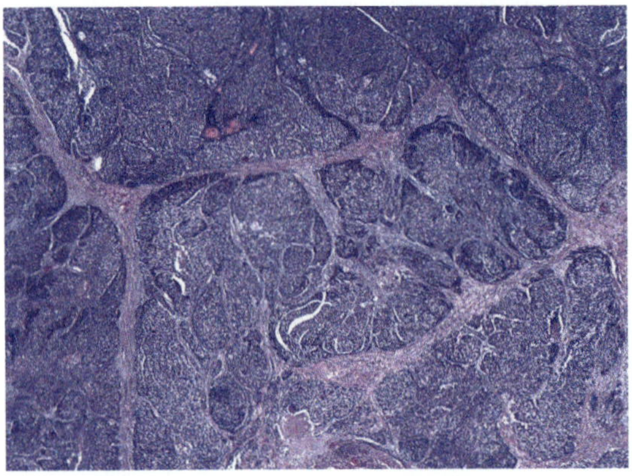

Basaloid Squamous Cell Carcinoma, Esophageal, Fig. 2 Basaloid squamous cell carcinoma (hematoxylin–eosin, low power). The tumor grows as lobules and anastomosing trabeculae

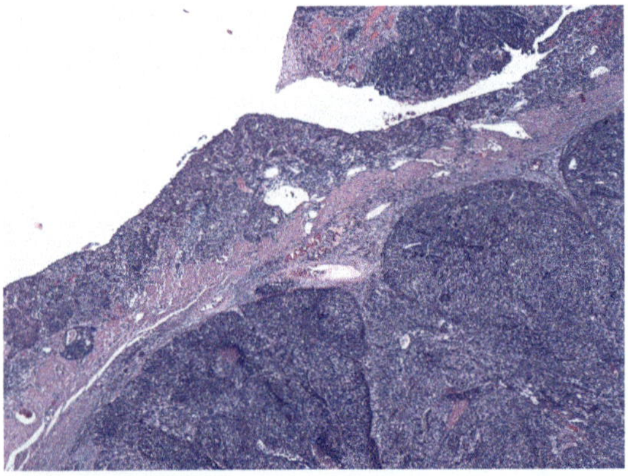

Basaloid Squamous Cell Carcinoma, Esophageal, Fig. 3 Basaloid squamous cell carcinoma (hematoxylin–eosin, medium power). The squamous cell dysplasia of the overlying epithelium is evident

interlobular stroma and microcysts demonstrate hyaline basement membrane-like material deposits, which are PAS positive. This neoplasm is typically associated with squamous dysplasia/squamous cell carcinoma in situ or even invasive squamous cell carcinoma, by definition in less than 50% of the tumor (Fig. 3). The transition between the two components is generally abrupt. Nevertheless, focal squamous cell differentiation within basaloid nests can also be seen.

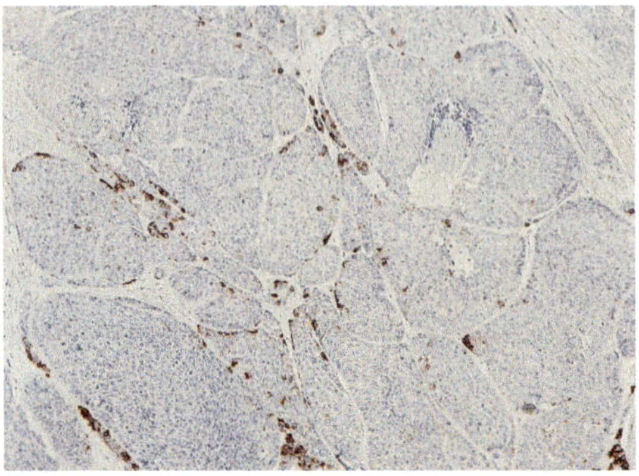

Basaloid Squamous Cell Carcinoma, Esophageal, Fig. 4 Basaloid squamous cell carcinoma (immunohistochemistry anti-cytokeratin 14, medium power). Cytokeratin 14 decorates cells of the basal layer, leaving the more luminal cells unstained

Immunophenotype

There is no specific immunophenotype for BSCC. The neoplasm displays epithelial membrane antigen (EMA) and cytokeratins expression (e.g., MNF116); cytokeratins 14 and 19 generally stain the basal layer of the tumor (Fig. 4), while cytokeratin 13 decorates the other layers. P53, EGFR, and BCL2 overexpression, as well as nuclear expression of beta-catenin, are often seen. Occasional positivity with smooth muscle actin and S100 protein has been reported. Neuroendocrine markers are largely negative.

Molecular Features

There are no characteristic molecular features. A low incidence of EGFR amplifications and mutations (exons 18–21) has been reported. Several mutations of the *p53* gene have also been described. Despite the presence of the nuclear expression of beta-catenin, no CTNNB1 mutations have been identified so far.

Differential Diagnosis

The differential diagnosis of BSCC includes *adenoid cystic carcinoma*, *small cell carcinoma*, poorly differentiated conventional *squamous cell carcinoma* and *adenosquamous carcinoma*. The neoplasm can be distinguished at a light microscopy level on architectural and cytological grounds. The association between the tumor and squamous cell dysplasia/in situ squamous carcinoma, which is typical for BSCC, as well as the lobular and cribriform patterns, often dominant in BSCC, are not seen in the small cell carcinoma. The absence of neuroendocrine markers helps to support the diagnosis (nevertheless, positivity for one neuroendocrine marker can be seen in BSCC). Despite the fact that BSCC and the solid variant of adenoid cystic carcinoma can be very similar, mitoses, nuclear pleomorphism, and necrosis are much more prominent in BSCC. The existence of two cell types, as seen in adenoid cystic carcinoma, is not encountered in BSCC. Immunohistochemical stains are of limited importance, since smooth muscle actin and S100 protein may be encountered in BSCC. The role of the determination of *MYB-NFIB* fusion, recently described in adenoid cystic carcinoma, remains to be validated.

References and Further Reading

Chen, S.-B., Weng, H.-R., Wang, G., Yang, W.-P., Li, H., Liu, D.-T., & Chen, Y.-P. (2012). Basaloid squamous cell carcinoma of the esophagus. *Journal of Cancer Research and Clinical Oncology, 138*(7), 1165–1171.

Imamhasan, A., Mitomi, H., Saito, T., Hayashi, T., Takahashi, M., Kajiyama, Y., & Yao, T. (2012). Immunohistochemical and oncogenetic analyses of the esophageal basaloid squamous cell carcinoma in comparison with conventional squamous cell carcinomas. *Human Pathology, 43*(11), 2012–2023.

Sarbia, M., Verreet, P., Bittinger, F., Dutkowski, P., Heep, H., Willers, R., & Gabbert, H. E. (1997). Basaloid squamous cell carcinoma of the esophagus – Diagnosis and prognosis. *Cancer, 79*(10), 1871–1878.

Zhang, X.-H., Sun, G.-Q., Zhou, X.-J., Guo, H.-F., & Zhang, T.-H. (1998). Basaloid squamous carcinoma of esophagus: A clinicopathological, immunohistochemical and electron microscopic study of sixteen cases. *World Journal of Gastroenterology, 4*(5), 397–403.

C

Cameron's Ulcer

Pedro Pimentel-Nunes[1,3], Ricardo Marcos-Pinto[1,2] and Mário Dinis-Ribeiro[1,3]
[1]Serviço de Gastrenterologia, Portuguese Oncology Institute, Porto, Portugal
[2]Centro Hospitalar do Porto, Instituto de Ciências Biomédicas Abel Salazar (ICBAS-UP), Cintesis (FMUP-UP), Porto, Portugal
[3]Instituto Português de Oncologia (IPO - Porto), Cintesis (FMUP-UP), Porto, Portugal

Synonyms

Cameron erosions; Cameron lesions

Definition

Cameron lesions are benign, superficial, and linear erosions or ulcers associated with gastroesophageal hiatal hernia, generally large hernias. They are named in tribute of Adrian J Cameron who in 1986 first described these lesions as a cause of anemia in patients with hiatal hernias. The lesions are located in the proximal body of the stomach at the end of the hernia, near the diaphragmatic impression. They are thought to be caused primarily by mechanical trauma and local ischemia caused by the repeated movements of the diaphragm against the hernia. Secondarily, acid and pepsin may perpetuate the lesions. They are a rare cause of overt gastric bleeding; however, they are a common cause of obscure gastrointestinal bleeding and of ferropenic anemia in patients with hiatal hernias.

Clinical Features

- **Incidence**
  Cameron lesions are uncommon, with an estimated incidence of 5% in patients with hiatal hernia. The risk is around 10–20% when the hernia size is >5 cm.
- **Age**
  They are more common in older patients (>60 years); however, they may affect any age, particularly if patients have large hiatal hernias (>5 cm).
- **Sex**
  They affect equally men and women.
- **Site**
  They are found on the mucosal folds near the diaphragmatic impression, generally on the lesser curvature of proximal gastric body.
- **Treatment**
  Medical therapy includes iron supplementation (to control anemia) and acid suppression (to heal the lesions). Some patients with refractory, transfusion-dependent anemia due to Cameron erosions may respond to surgical repair of the hernia.

F. Carneiro et al. (eds.), *Pathology of the Gastrointestinal Tract*, Encyclopedia of Pathology,
DOI 10.1007/978-3-319-40560-5

- **Outcome**
  Medical therapy is very effective for the treatment of these lesions. Acid suppressive therapy may heal these lesions in more than 65% of the patients after 6 weeks. Nevertheless, 20% of the patients may have complications such as recurrence of bleeding or persistent anemia. After surgery the recurrence of these lesions is extremely rare.

Macroscopy

At endoscopy Cameron lesions appear as linear and longitudinal erosions or ulcers at the end of the hernia, near the diaphragmatic impression. If small or if the endoscopist is not looking for it, they may go unnoticed.

Microscopy

It is not usual to take biopsy samples from these lesions and so histology is rarely described. When biopsied they present the same characteristics of other benign ulcerations with a mucosal defect with some inflammatory exudate and granulation tissue without atypical cells. However, many of these lesions also present focal ischemic changes consisting of coagulation necrosis supporting the role of ischemia as a possible cause of these lesions.

Immunophenotype

Not applied

Molecular Features

Not applied

Differential Diagnosis

Peptic ulcer/erosion (different location, microscopy can be exactly the same), reflux esophagitis (different location, near the esophagogastric junction and extending into the esophagus), malignant ulcer (e.g., lymphoma or adenocarcinoma, different endoscopic appearance with irregularity, rarely localized in a hiatal hernia; histology confirms the diagnosis).

References and Further Reading

Byron, C., & Stuart, J. S. (2010). Peptic ulcer disease. *Sleisenger & Fordtran's gastrointestinal and liver disease*. (9th ed.). Saunders: Elsevier.
Cameron, A. J., & Higgins, J. A. (1986). Linear gastric erosion. A lesion associated with large diaphragmatic hernia and chronic blood loss anemia. *Gastroenterology, 91*, 338–342.
Maganty, K., & Smith, R. L. (2008). Cameron lesions: Unusual cause of gastrointestinal bleeding and anemia. *Digestion, 77*, 214–217.
Moskovitz, M., Fadden, R., Min, T., Jansma, D., & Gavaler, J. (1992). Large hiatal hernias, anemia, and linear gastric erosion: Studies of etiology and medical therapy. *The American Journal of Gastroenterology, 87*, 622–626.

Campylobacter Enterocolitis

Anne Jouret-Mourin
Department of Pathology, Cliniques Universitaires St. Luc, UCL, Brussels, Belgium

Definition

Campylobacter enterocolitis is an inflammation of the colon caused by *Campylobacter* species which is a curved or spiral gram-negative rod. *Campylobacter* species is part of the natural flora in many wild and domestic animals including household pets.

Campylobacter enterocolitis is one of the most common causes of acute bacterial gastroenteritis. Numerous *Campylobacter* species exist within the genus *Campylobacter* including *Campylobacter jejuni*, *Campylobacter coli*, *Campylobacter laridis*, *Campylobacter fetus*, *Campylobacter upsaliensis*, *Campylobacter sputorum*, *Campylobacter concisus*.

Epidemiology

The vast majority of food-borne enterocolitis is caused by *Campylobacter jejuni* along with *C coli* and *C laridis*. *C fetus* is most often seen in immune-suppressed patients and homosexual men. There is a higher incidence in HIV-positive patients.

Transmission occurs most commonly through consumption of raw milk, contaminated meat, untreated water, or undercooked poultry. It is a common animal pathogen. Person-to person transmission by oro-fecal contamination can also occur. The infective dose is low, and as few as 500 organisms can cause symptomatic disease.

Pathogenesis

Regarding the pathophysiology, *Campylobacter* organisms produce diarrhea after adhesion and bacterial invasion into the enterocytes. Such invasion leads to the loss of function and erosion of the surface epithelial cells. The organisms are able to invade and replicate in infected epithelia via TLR-2 and TLR-4 receptors and may also produce both an enterotoxin and a cytotoxin, damaging the cells. *C jejuni* organisms seem more enterotoxigenic and probably more virulent than *C coli* and *C laridis*.

Clinical Features

- **Incidence**
  Campylobacter species is one of the most frequently isolated enteric stool pathogens encountered in man and accounts for up to 14% of all cases of infectious diarrheas worldwide. *Campylobacter jejuni* is a common cause of traveler's diarrhea. Its incidence differs from one country to another.
- **Age**
  Campylobacter infections affect persons of all ages, with a peak of incidence in children (highest under 1 year) and young adults (between 15 and 30 years of age).
- **Site**
  Campylobacter infections are thought to involve the small bowel especially the terminal ileum as well as the colon especially the cecum.

Clinical Symptoms

The incubation period ranges from 1 to 7 days. Approximately 20% of the infected patients remain asymptomatic. The clinical symptoms classically result in a self-limited gastroenteritis including fever, malaise, abdominal pain, and watery and sometimes bloody diarrhea. Abdominal pain, often cramping, diarrhea and fever are the most common symptoms. Other symptoms such as nausea, headache, vomiting, and myalgia can be present. As *Campylobacter* infections involve the terminal ileum or the cecum, the infection can suggest a clinical picture of acute appendicitis.

Campylobacter enterocolitis lasts for 1–2 weeks but can occasionally be longer.

Immune-compromised patients, the elderly, and very young children are at particular risk for prolonged infection. In these cases, *Campylobacter*, most frequently *Campylobacter fetus*, may present as severe, diffuse, or pancolitis with bloody diarrhea in an acute or even fulminant manifestation or toxic megacolon. It has been suggested that such cases may be clinically, endoscopically, and histologically difficult to distinguish from acute noninfectious inflammatory bowel disease. These severe forms must be distinguished for the proper early management of patients because corticosteroids or immunosuppressive therapies required for the treatment of severe ulcerative colitis may exacerbate infectious enterocolitis.

- **Treatment**
  Symptoms generally resolve spontaneously within 1–2 weeks. Sometimes, antibiotics may be required especially in the severe form or in the immune-compromised patients.
- **Prognosis**
  Most of the *Campylobacter* infections are self-limited infections particularly in healthy patients. The disease usually lasts about 1 week. Immune-compromised patients have more frequently a severe infection with sometimes systemic illnesses that are often fatal. Relapse is common as many as in 25% of patients. There are rare but significant systemic complications including Reiter syndrome and Guillain-Barre syndrome.

Macroscopic Features

Campylobacter causes both small and large intestinal disease, most often nonspecific at endoscopy. The colonoscopy may reveal different features from normal mucosa or mild mucosal erythema to friable colonic mucosa with a segmental or diffuse distribution and often with hemorrhage.

In the early stage of the illness (within 4 days after the onset of clinical disease), the mucosa is typically hyperaemic and edematous with sometimes aphthoid erosions or superficial ulcers. Contact bleeding is not frequently present.

Later in the course of the illness, granularity and hyperemia without edema or ulceration may be observed.

More frequently, the lesions are segmental but severe diffuse pancolitis mimicking IBD can occasionally be observed.

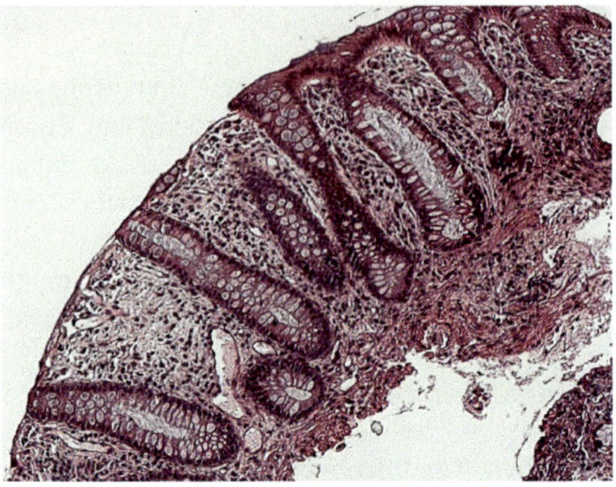

***Campylobacter* Enterocolitis, Fig. 1** *Campylobacter colitis*: Mild colitis with edema, hemorrhagic, and a few lympho-plasmocytic cells in the lamina propria

Microscopic Findings

Pathological examination usually shows acute infectious type self-limited colitis including preservation of crypt architecture with cryptitis, surface epithelial damage, and a superficial cellular infiltrate in the lamina propria with neutrophils often invading the upper crypts. Mild chronic nonspecific colitis with edema and a few lympho-plasmocytic cells in the lamina propria can also be observed (Fig. 1) as well as marked mucosal hemorrhage and superficial mucosal erosions.

In some cases of *Campylobacter* infections, biopsy findings are those of focal active colitis characterized only by focal neutrophilic crypt injury such as cryptitis in the absence of features of chronicity.

In the small intestine, mucosal edema, inflammation, architectural villous distortion, atrophy or flattening with goblet cell depletion, and cryptitis as well as some erosions can be observed.

In rare cases, more severe colitis with crypt abscesses and crypt distortion mimicking chronic idiopathic inflammatory bowel disease can be seen (Figs. 2 and 3).

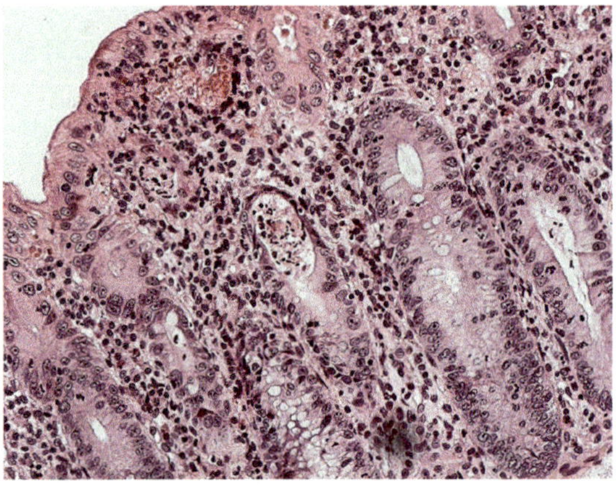

***Campylobacter* Enterocolitis, Fig. 2** *Campylobacter colitis*: colitis with neutrophils aggregates in the lamina propria and surrounding epithelium forming cryptitis and crypt abscesses

The timing of the biopsy does not appear to influence the specificity of the histopathological findings. Early microscopic changes include mucosal edema, superficial ulcers, neutrophilic surface exudates, and cryptitis. In the following days of the first week, active crypt lesions become focal and neutrophils in the lamina propria appear less prominent. In the later part of the second week of the infection, active crypt lesions have resolved while features of epithelial regeneration persist together with a slight increase of the cellularity in the lamina propria.

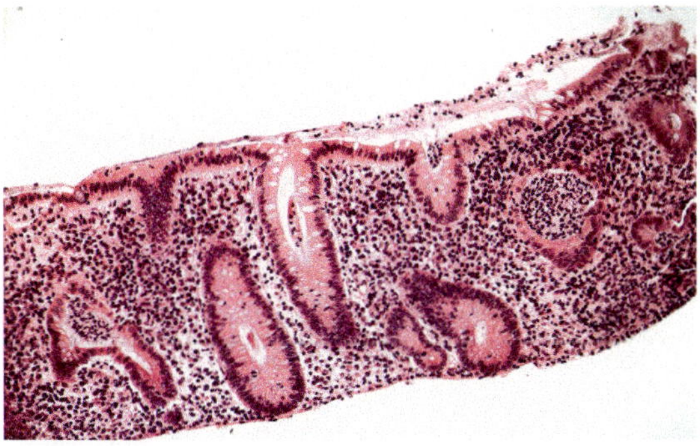

***Campylobacter* Enterocolitis, Fig. 3** *Campylobacter colitis*: distorted crypt may be present mimicking ulcerous colitis

Differential Diagnosis

The differential diagnosis predominantly includes other infections that provoke an acute self-limited pattern such as *Shighella*, *Salmonella*, *Yersinia enterocolitica*, and *Aeromonas*.

Sometimes, when *Campylobacter* infections persist for a longer time and are more severe, they can mimic inflammatory bowel disease, most often ulcerative colitis, especially when crypt distortion appears. Poorly formed mucosal granulomas are occasionally present and may suggest a diagnosis of Crohn's disease. Therefore, the differential diagnosis can be challenging and is very important. This problem can be solved by studying the plasma cells in the infiltrate. An increase of plasma cells can occur 7–10 days after the initial onset of the infection. In *Campylobacter colitis*, increased numbers of IgA and IgM containing plasma cells are found in the mucosa. In contrast, active IBD shows an increase of IgA and IgG for ulcerative colitis and of IgA, IgM, and IgG in Crohn's disease. Moreover, plasma cells are not usually located in a basal position in *Campylobacter colitis*, while this location is a frequent finding in IBD and a positive diagnostic predictive factor for both ulcerative colitis and Crohn's disease.

Numerous authors have tried to establish criteria to distinguish an infectious colitis from an IBD at the time of the first biopsies. One of the most important studies was by Schumacher in 1994 who carried out a prospective study showing significant features of IBD (see ► Infectious Colitis). Pointers to an infective cause were edema of the lamina propria and the presence of a cellular infiltrate mainly composed of neutrophils. The aggregates of neutrophils were usually conspicuous in the lamina propria and surrounded or infiltrated the upper crypt epithelium. However, more frequently, the histological features are not specific. A control repeat biopsy can help as it usually shows an improvement of the lesions. The absence of IBD criteria can also help to diagnose infectious colitis.

Useful Tests

Culture is the best test to aid in *Campylobacter* infection diagnosis. The yield of *C jejuni* is higher from colonic tissue culture than stool culture.

Serologic studies have been reported using a variety of techniques including agglutination, complement fixation, and ELISA technique. Serological evidence of a specific antibody response to *Campylobacter* permits confirmation of the diagnosis but positive serologies may persist for more than a year after an acute infection has resolved.

PCR analysis performed on fixed biopsies may be a diagnostic method for detection of this organism as well as Immunohistochemistry with a specific antibody. Identification of the organism from the stool by dark-field microscopy or DNA hybridization is also possible.

References and Further Reading

Lamps, L. W. (2007). Infective disorders of the gastrointestinal tract. *Histopathology, 50*, 55–63.

Mee, A. S., et al. (1985). *Campylobacter colitis*: Differentiation from acute IBD. *Journal of the Royal Society of Medicine, 78*, 217–223.

Quomdarcarlo, C., et al. (2003). *Capylobacter jejuni* enterocolitis presenting as IBD. *Techniques in Coloproctology, 7*, 173–177.

Schneider, E. S., et al. (2006). Molecular diagnosis of *C jejuni* infection in cases of focal active colitis. *American Journal of Surgical Pathology, 30*, 782–785.

Schumacher, G., et al. (1994). A prospective study of first attacks of IBD and infectious colitis. *Scandinavian Journal of Gastroenterology, 29*, 318–332.

Siegal, D., et al. (2005). *Campylobacter jejuni* pancolitis mimicking idiopathic ulcerative colitis. *Heart & Lung, 34*, 288–290.
Van Spreeuwel, J. P., et al. (1985). *Campylobacter colitis*: Histological, immunohistochemical and ultrastructural finding. *Gut, 26*, 945–951.

Carcinoma, Colorectal

Sibel Erdamar
Department of Pathology, Cerrahpasa Medical College, Istanbul, Turkey

Synonyms

Colorectal carcinomas, Malignant epithelial tumors of the large intestine

Definition

Colorectal carcinoma is a malignant tumor arising from colonic epithelium. More than 90% of colorectal carcinomas (CRC) are adenocarcinomas.

The cause and pathogenesis of CRC are related to both environmental and genetic factors. Environmental factors contain diet rich in meat, high fat, carbohydrate, low fiber; lifestyle risk factors like cigarette smoking and alcohol consumption; and those which have effect on the intestinal microflora and chemical composition of the intraluminal content. Bile acids and their metabolites derived from bacterial action could also be potential carcinogen. Some vitamin deficiencies (vitamins B2, B6, B12, C, D, folate, etc.) have risk for CRC. The repeated colonic mucosal injury and repair as occurs in chronic idiopathic inflammatory bowel disease are important in the development of CRC. Various genetic factors are as follows: there is high predisposition for CRC in patients with FAP, other forms of polyposis (MUTYH polyposis, juvenile polyposis, etc.), Lynch syndrome, and Peutz-Jeghers syndrome.

It is generally accepted that most colorectal carcinomas arise from adenomas. Residual adenoma is identified in about 10–30% of colorectal cancers.

Clinical Features

- **Incidence**
  An estimated 1.23 million new cases of CRC occurred worldwide in 2008, 9.7% of all new cancers. CRC is the fourth most common cancer in men, third in women. There is big difference in incidence in different locations in the world. For example, the incidence is high in industrialized, high-resource countries of Europe, North America, Australia, New Zealand, and Japan and low in countries like India, Asia, and Africa.
- **Age**
  Incidence increases with age. The risk for CRC rises significantly after age 40 in both men and women and doubles in each succeeding decade until age 75. Most patients are middle aged and elderly. Median age at diagnosis for cancer of colon and rectum is 71. The age of onset is younger, and tumors are more aggressive in low-risk countries.
- **Sex**
  Rates of rectal cancer are about 50% higher and colon cancer rates about 20% higher in men than in women. Women have higher rates of right-sided neoplasms and develop their cancers at earlier age than men.
- **Site**
  In low-risk countries, carcinomas of cecum and ascending colon occur more frequently than carcinomas of the left colon, whereas in high-risk countries, CRC more commonly arises in the rectosigmoid region. Generally, 50% of all carcinomas occur in the rectosigmoid area. CRCs like adenomas could be multiple. Multiple neoplasms may be synchronous or metachronous. Synchronous cancers often remain confined to some regions of the bowel.
- **Treatment**
  Surgical resection is typically the first line of treatment for CRCs. The type of surgery depends on the site of the tumor. Patients with advanced stage tumors (especially rectum tumors) may have chemoradiation prior to surgery. To date, fluorouracil (5-FU)-based chemotherapy is standard. Irinotecan or

oxaliplatin can be used in the advanced stage of the disease. As a second line treatment, anti-EGFR antibodies (panitumumab and cetuximab) may be used if the tumor has no KRAS mutation. Microsatellite instability status is important since MSI-H cancers do not benefit from 5-FU chemotherapy. Radiation therapy is often used in combination with chemotherapy in advanced disease and used preoperatively in rectal cancer to downstage of tumor. Hepatic arterial infusions are used to treat metastatic disease in liver.

- **Outcome**

  CRC may present with rectal bleeding, changes in bowel habits, anemia, and abdominal pain.

  The cancers located in the left colon may cause intestinal obstruction. Some cecal carcinomas can present symptoms of appendicitis.

  Differences in the death rates from colorectal cancer relate to differences in socioeconomic factors, diet, population longevity, genetic factors, and quality of available medical care. The overall 5-year relative survival rate is 64%. Only about 40% of patients present with localized disease, although remaining 40% of patients with regional metastases and 20% with distant metastases.

  Many factors influence the prognosis of patients with colorectal cancer, including the presence of preexisting diseases such as familial polyposis, ulcerative colitis, and Lynch syndrome and tumor growth characteristics. Prognosis largely depends on depth of invasion of large bowel wall and presence of lymph node involvement and of course stage. Other strong prognostic factors are extramural venous invasion, preoperative CEA level, residual tumor in surgical margin, and radial margin in rectum tumors. Histologic grading, microsatellite instability, tumor margins and inflammatory reaction, age, perineural invasion, and microscopic tumor type are considered also as poor prognostic markers. Currently, mucinous histology is not considered as an independent prognostic factor.

  Medical oncologists currently use MMR status to guide adjuvant 5-FU therapy decisions for new CRC patients with deep primary tumors without nodal or distant metastases (AJCC stage II).

Macroscopy

CRCs are often sharply circumscribed and grossly resemble adenomas. Some are elevated only a few millimeters, whereas others are almost hemispherical in shape. As carcinoma replaces the adenoma, the tumor becomes firmer and paler.

The gross appearance of colorectal carcinomas may be polypoid, fungating (exophytic) (Fig. 1), ulcerating (Fig. 2), stenosing, or diffusely infiltrating. Polypoid type of carcinoma forms an exophytic intraluminal mass usually with little surface ulceration. The diffusely infiltrative

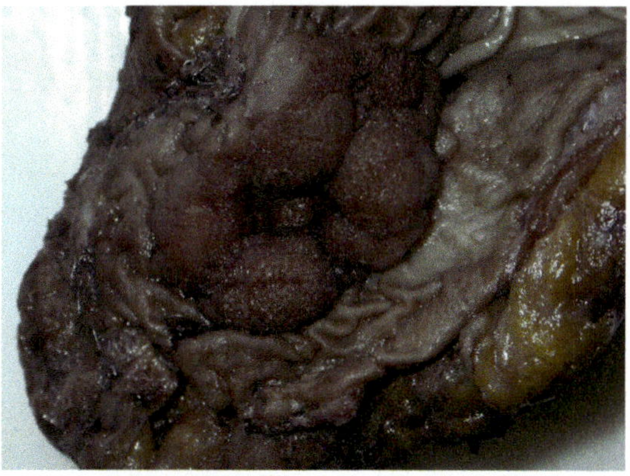

Carcinoma, Colorectal, Fig. 1 Fungating adenocarcinoma

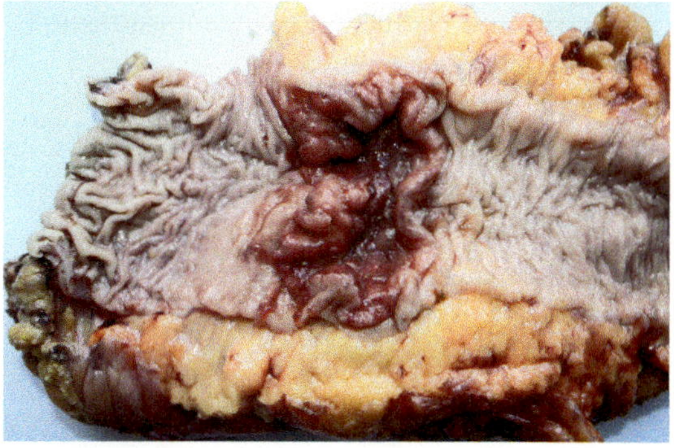

Carcinoma, Colorectal, Fig. 2 Ulcerating and infinltrating type carcinoma of colon

carcinoma infiltrates a segment of the intestinal wall, often in a circumferential fashion, without forming nodular mass.

Majority of carcinomas are centrally located and have raised everted edge. Carcinomas located in the cecum frequently protrude to the lumen; others may present as excavated ulcerating tumors with flat margins. Carcinomas arising in the transverse and descending colon usually become infiltrative and ulcerating, producing annular and constricting tumors. These tend to present with obstructive symptoms.

Approximately two thirds of all tumors are ulcerating; one third appear fungating. Ulcerating carcinomas deeply invade into the colonic wall. Most of them have solid white or yellowish white tissue in their cut surface. In contrast, approximately 10% of CRC have mucinous component display mucin/or gelatinous material on the cut surface. Least commonly, diffuse infiltrative/linitis plastica pattern can be seen. Overlaps among different macroscopic types and ulceration are common.

Infiltration through the intestinal wall ultimately may reach the serosa and contiguous structures and pericolic tissues.

Microscopy

More than 90% of CRC are adenocarcinomas. This is the list of microscopic types of CRC according to the WHO (2010):

Adenocarcinoma:
- Cribriform comedo-type adenocarcinoma
- Medullary carcinoma
- Micropapillary carcinoma
- Mucinous adenocarcinoma
- Serrated adenocarcinoma
- Signet ring cell carcinoma

Adenosquamous carcinoma
Spindle cell carcinoma
Squamous cell carcinoma
Undifferentiated carcinoma

Colorectal adenocarcinomas are histologically characterized by well-recognized gland formation with mostly well differantiated or moderate differantiated. These glands usually contain variable amount of musin secretion. Mostly these glands line by tall, columnar, malignant epithelium with high mitotic rate. Residual adenomatous mucosa may be seen at the edge of a malignancy, especially in smaller tumors. The majority of small carcinomas associated with residual carcinomas are well differentiated.

Grade (degree of differentiation) applies only to adenocarcinomas and is mainly based on gland formation and architectural features of tumors. Well-formed glands are present in >75% of the tumors that are well differentiated (simple tubules with little complex architectural complexity, maintained polarity), in 25–75% of moderately differentiated tumors (considerable architectural complexity, nuclei modestly enlarged, polarity largely maintained), and in <25% of poorly differentiated carcinomas (if glands present, nuclei have often prominent nucleoli and lost polarity).

Apart from 3 degrees of differantiation, two-tier grading system is also used: In this system, CRCs are classified as either low grade (well and moderately differentiated; >50% gland formation) or high grade (poorly differentiated; <50% gland formation) (Figs. 3, 4, and 5). Other microscopic types carry their own prognostic significance, and grading does not apply.

Mucinous carcinomas are defined as the tumors composed of >50% mucin secretion and are about 10% of all CRCs (Fig. 6). Mucinous

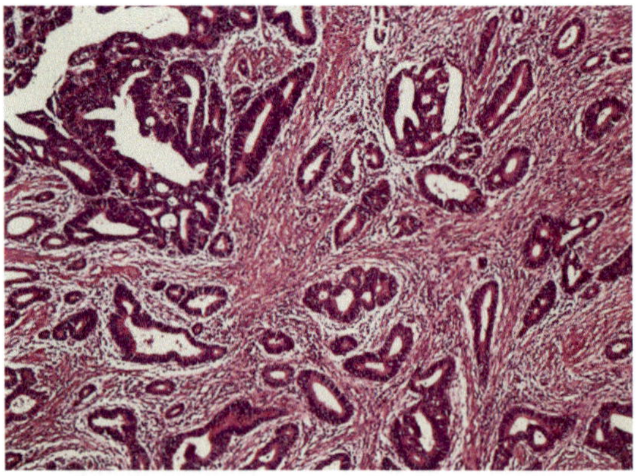

Carcinoma, Colorectal, Fig. 3 Well differantiated adenocarcinoma

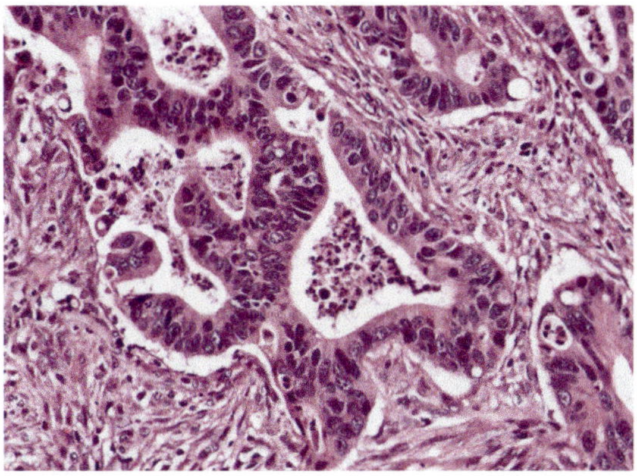

Carcinoma, Colorectal, Fig. 4 Typical colorectal adenocarcinoma with complex glandular structures and "dirty necrosis"

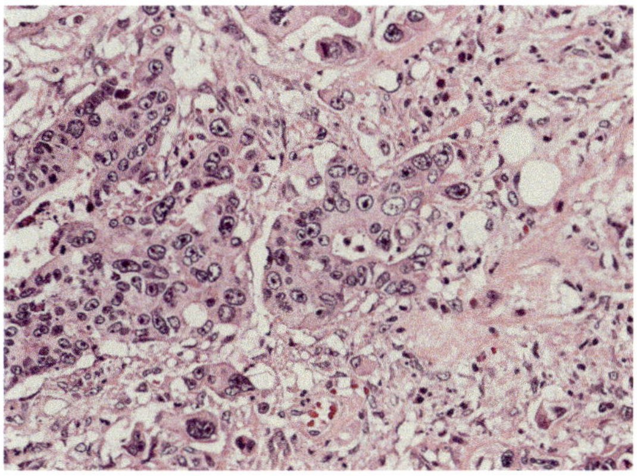

Carcinoma, Colorectal, Fig. 5 Poorly differantiated adenocarcinoma

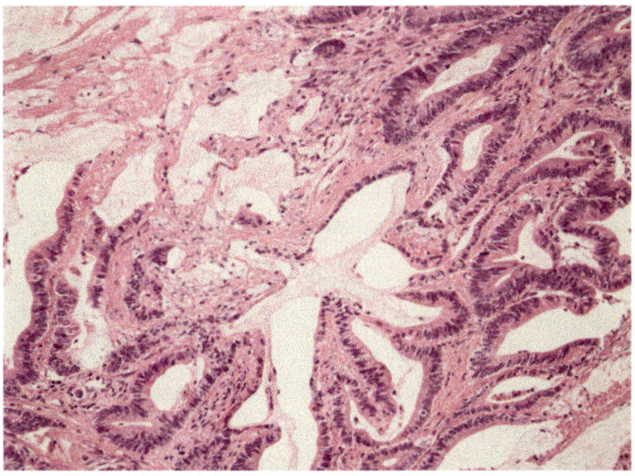

Carcinoma, Colorectal, Fig. 6 Mucinous adenocarcinoma with abundance of mucin pools

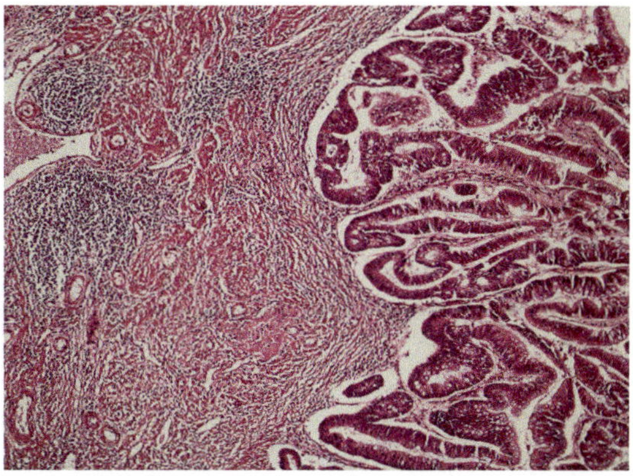

Carcinoma, Colorectal, Fig. 7 Adecarcinoma with peritumoral crohn-like lymphocytic reaction

material is an acid mucopolysaccharide that stains with periodic acid- schiff (PAS), mucicarmine, and acidic aniline blue stains.

Signet ring cell adenocarcinomas represent about 0.5–1.0% of all CRCs and are defined as a tumor composed of at least 50% signet ring cells.

Medullary carcinoma is a rare variant characterized by sheets of malignant cells with vesicular nuclei, prominent nucleoli, and abundant eosinophilic cytoplasm containing intraepithelial lymphocytes.

Serrated carcinomas have glandular serration with mucinous cribriform, lacy and trabecular areas, and low nucleus-to-cytoplasm ratio. Necrosis is not seen.

Inflammatory and lymphoid cell infiltration is one of the prominent features of many CRCs. Lymphoid aggregates can be seen at the advancing edge of the tumor and in the pericolic fat tissue which is called Crohn's disease-like lymphoid reaction in some CRC cases (Fig. 7). CRCs usually show development of desmoplastic stromal fibrous reaction.

According to infiltration at advancing margin of tumor in the bowel wall, CRCs have two distinct patterns: expanding pattern and infiltrating pattern (Figs. 8 and 9). Invasive front of some CRCs reveals isolated clusters of tumor cells, the so-called tumor budding, which are defined as less than four or five cells in one group (Fig. 10). They are more frequently seen in flat tumors.

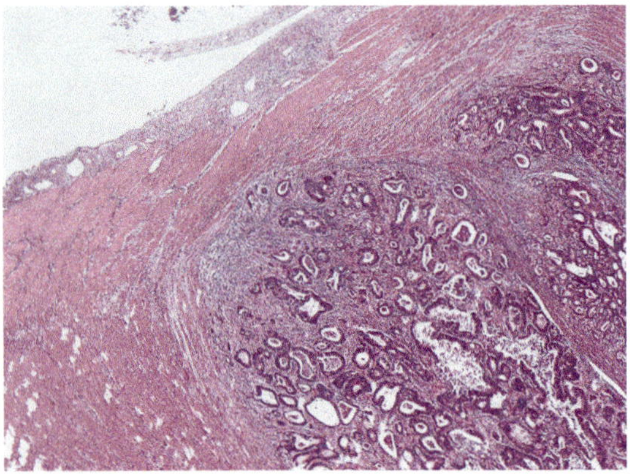

Carcinoma, Colorectal, Fig. 8 Expanding growth pattern

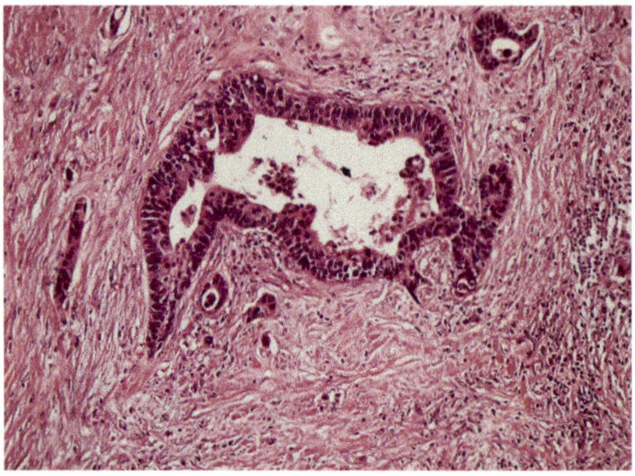

Carcinoma, Colorectal, Fig. 10 tumor budding with desmoplastic stroma

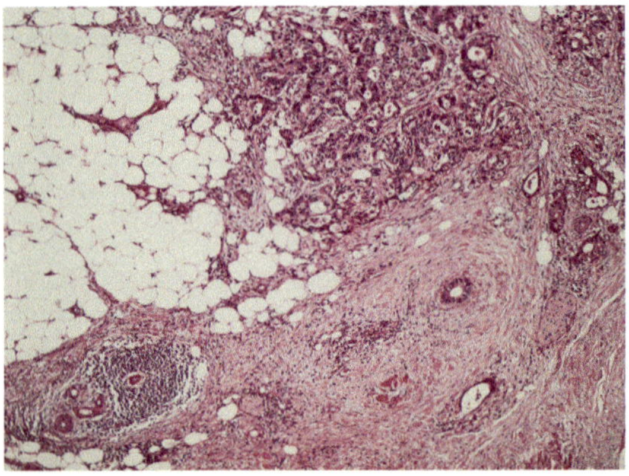

Carcinoma, Colorectal, Fig. 9 CRC showing infiltrating pattern

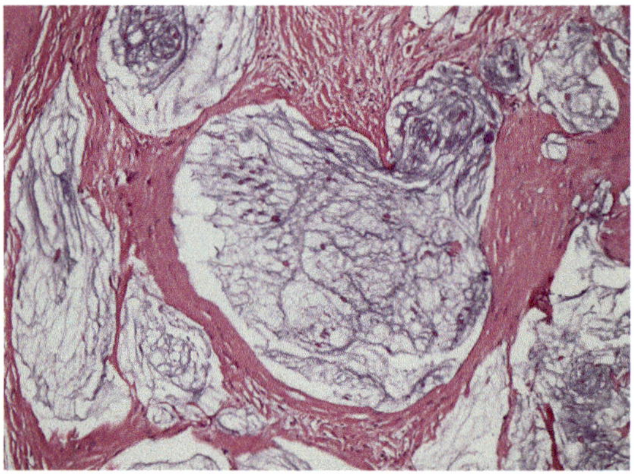

Carcinoma, Colorectal, Fig. 11 Acellular mucinous changes in tumor after CRT

Microscopic Features Suggesting Microsatellite Instability

The tumor that shows mucinous differentiation, poor differentiation with solid pattern, circumscribed growth pattern (or pushing margin), peritumoral Crohn's-like lymphoid aggregates, tumor infiltrating lymphocytes (>2/HPF), lack of dirty necrosis, preexisting serrated lesion, and right colon location should be analyzed for microsatellite instability.

Posttreatment Changes: Neoadjuvant (preoperative) chemoradiotherapy is increasingly used in tumors located in rectum. Posttreatment effects can be seen as acellular mucin lakes in the wall of rectum (Fig. 11). These should not be revealed as tumor infiltration. Residual tumors show radiation effects and its stroma is usually desmoplastic (Fig. 12).

Spreading of Colorectal Cancer

CRCs can spread by direct local invasion, lymphatic invasion (LI), blood vessel invasion (BVI), and perineural invasion (PNI) like other cancer types. Staging of CRCs according to TNM classification is shown in Table 1.

The tumor extends through the various intestinal wall layers or extends through the area of the penetrating vessels. Mural penetration results in direct involvement of serosa, adjacent organs or tissues, and peritoneal seeding (Figs. 13 and 14).

CRCs frequently metastasize to the regional lymph nodes. The incidence of LI ranges from

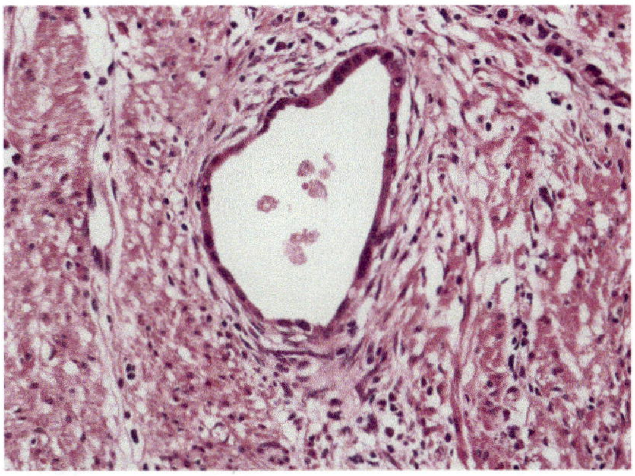

Carcinoma, Colorectal, Fig. 12 Post treatment changes in tumoral gland

8% to 73% and increases with tumor stage and grade (Fig. 15). Metastases usually progress from the closest one to the next lymph node in a fairly orderly fashion. The number of both total and metastatic lymph nodes affects the prognosis, so the lymph nodes should be carefully examined grossly and microscopically.

Spread of tumor through the veins draining ultimately to the portal vein and liver is important for distant organ metastases. Detection of intramural and extramural BVI is very important for prognosis (Fig. 16). The tumor located in the lower rectum can metastasize directly the lung via the middle and inferior hemorrhoidal veins.

PNI is an indicator of high risk of local recurrence and poor outcome (Fig. 17).

Carcinoma, Colorectal, Table 1 TNM staging for colorectal carcinomas (the original source of this material is AJCC cancer staging manual seventh edition)

Classification	Definition
T-primary tumor	
TX	Primary tumor cannot be assessed
T0	No evidence of primary tumor
Tis	Carcinoma in situ: intraepithelial or invasion of lamina propria
T1	Tumor invades submucosa
T2	Tumor invades muscularis propria
T3	Tumor invades subserosa or into non-peritonealized pericolic or perirectal tissues
T4	Tumor perforates visceral peritoneum and/or directly invades other organs or structures
T4a	Tumor perforates visceral peritoneum
T4b	Tumor directly invades other organ or structures
N- regional lymph node	
NX	Regional lymph nodes cannot be assessed
N0	No regional lymph node metastasis
N1	
N1a	Metastasis in 1–3 regional lymph nodes
N1b	Metastasis in 1 regional lymph node metastasis in 2–3 regional lymph node
N1c	Tumor deposits/satellites, in the subserosa, or in non-peritonealized pericolic or perirectal soft tissue without regional lymph node metastasis
N2	Metastasis in 4 or more lymph nodes
N2a	Metastasis in 4–6 regional lymph node
N2b	Metastasis in 7 or more regional lymph node
M-distant metastasis	
M0	No lymph node metastasis
M1	Distant metastasis
M1a	Metastasis confined to one organ
M1b	Metastasis in more than one organ or the peritoneum

Immunophenotype

The most common immunostaining pattern is cytokeratin (CK) 20 positivity and CK7 negativity. CK20 is an acidic cytokeratin that is generally expressed in colonic mucosa and CRC (Fig. 18). CDX2 is a caudal-type homeobox gene which encodes a transcription factor that plays an important role in the proliferation and differentiation of intestinal epithelial cells. Most of CRCs express nuclear CDX2 positivity (Fig. 19). MUC1 is not usually expressed in colonic epithelium but can be expressed by some CRC which has adverse prognosis. MUC2 is the most characteristic intestinal mucin (Fig. 20). MUC5AC and MUC6 can rarely express in some CRCs. CEA is expressed in the great majority of CRCs. *MMR proteins* (MLH1, MSH2, MSH6, and PMS2) normally show nuclear expression with immunostaining.

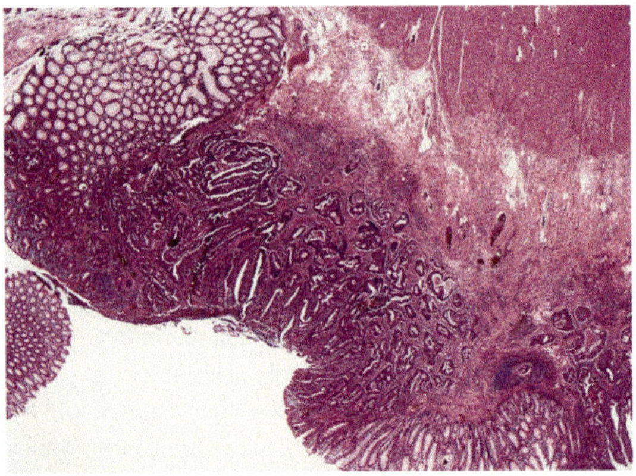

Carcinoma, Colorectal, Fig. 13 Submucosal invasion is seen in flat carcinoma

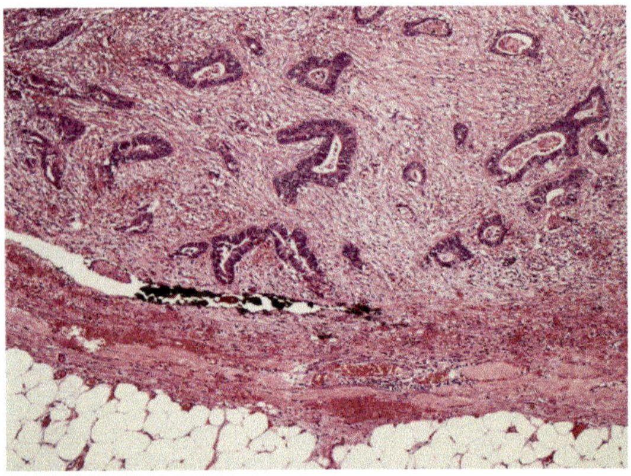

Carcinoma, Colorectal, Fig. 14 Tumor infiltrates serosa

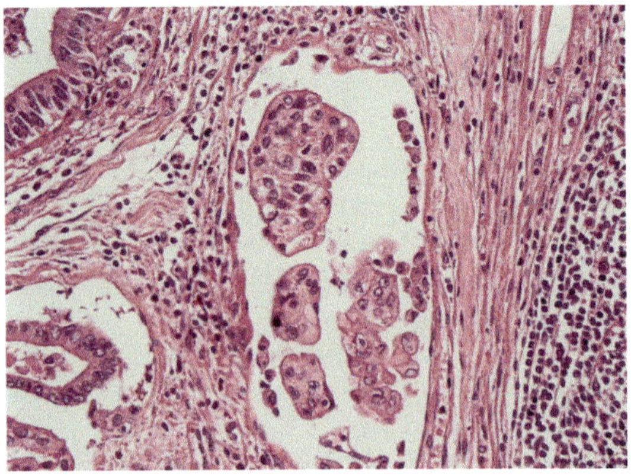

Carcinoma, Colorectal, Fig. 15 Lymphatic invasion is seen in submucosal lymphatic vessel

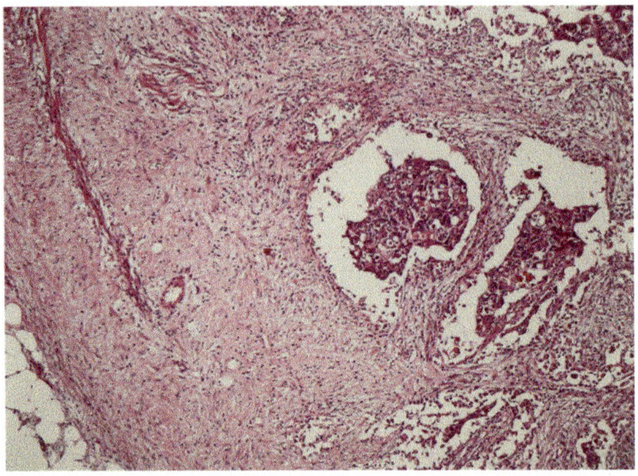

Carcinoma, Colorectal, Fig. 16 Extramural blood veesel invasion

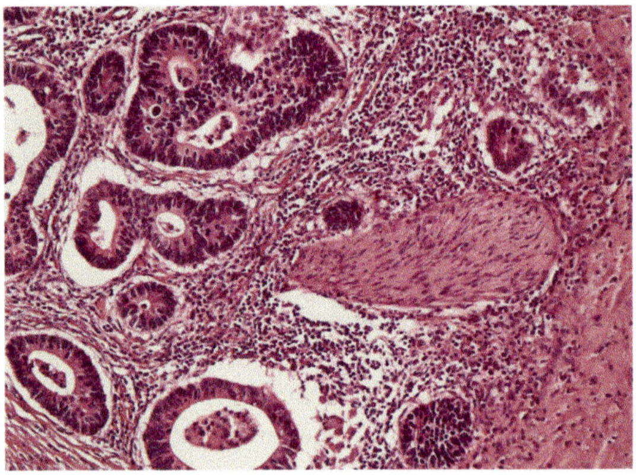

Carcinoma, Colorectal, Fig. 17 Perineural invasion

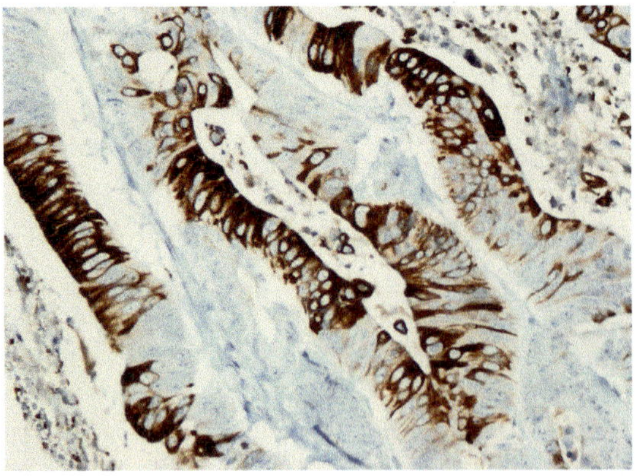

Carcinoma, Colorectal, Fig. 18 CK20 positivity in CRC cells

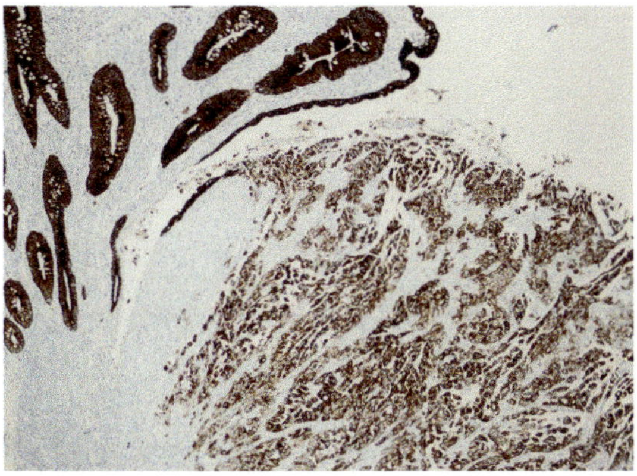

Carcinoma, Colorectal, Fig. 19 Diffuse and strong CK19 positivity in both normal colonic mucosa and carcinoma

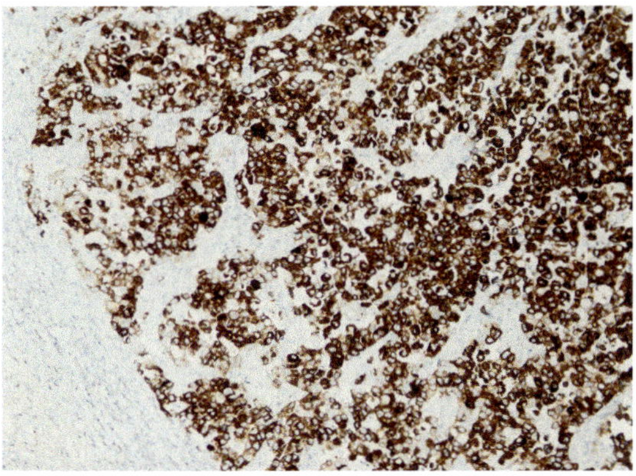

Carcinoma, Colorectal, Fig. 20 Strong MUC2 positivity

Molecular Features

Molecular features of CRCs are getting more complex compared to the past. Several broad clinicopathological pathways in the development of CRC are defined. It is understood that every colorectal carcinoma is genetically unique. Generally, the pathways lead to CRC: inherited pathways (FAP, Lynch syndrome (LS), MYH-associated polyposis, serrated polyposis, juvenile polyposis), sporadic pathways (conventional adenoma, serrated adenoma), and inflammatory bowel disease-associated pathway.

There are at least two general forms of genome instability important to the development of colorectal neoplasia. Approximately 85% of sporadic CRCs develop chromosomal instability (CIN) which is characterized by gross chromosomal abnormalities, aneuploid karyotype, large chromosome segment deletion and duplications, and increased DNA content. CRC with CIN also reveals abnormalities in DNA methylation, particularly hypermethylation of CpG dinucleotides in the promoter regions of genes. Microsatellite instability (MSI) is present in about 10–15% of CRC and is characterized by widespread alterations in the size of repetitive DNA sequences.

The development of most colorectal carcinomas is thought to be initiated by inactivation of the APC/ß-catenin/Wnt signaling pathway, usually by mutation of one copy of the APC gene followed by a second event that inactivates the other allele. The second inactivating event is usually described as allelic deletion or mutation but can be epigenetic methylation of cytosines in CpG islands of the promoter region of APC that results in transcriptional silencing. Altered APC has wide-ranging downstream effects on cell-cell adhesion, transcriptional regulation, chromosomal instability, cell migration, proliferation and cell cycle control, differentiation, and apoptosis. Somatic APC mutation is associated with the development of intraepithelial neoplasia (dysplasia) in aberrant crypt foci and early adenomas and is present in as many as 80% of sporadic colorectal adenomas and carcinomas. Mutations of the KRAS or BRAF gene in the RAS/RAF/MAPK pathway typically occur early in ACF or small adenomas and result in constitutive activation of the gene. Epigenetic silencing of MGMT by promoter methylation in normal colonic mucosa may be predisposing factor for cancer as a field effect and an early event colorectal carcinogenesis. Mutation and inactivation of the P53 gene are later genetic events in colorectal tumorigenesis. The deleted in colorectal carcinoma (DCC) gene is located in 18q. CRCs show 60–70% loss of heterozygosity (LOH) of 18q. DCC mutation is seen almost 50% of larger size of adenomas. SMAD2 and SMAD4 are also located on the same locus of 18q. SMAD4 mutations increase in frequency with the advancing stage of adenoma-carcinoma sequence.

The most frequent cause of sporadic MSI is tumor-acquired promoter hypermethylation of MLH1, which often occurs in the context of global hypermethylation of gene promoters known as CpG island methylator phenotype. When CpG sites in the promoter regions of both copies of MLH1 are hypermethylated, MLH1 expression is lost and genomic instability in the form of MSI ensues. In contrast to *LS*, in which a monoallelic mutation of one of the MMR genes is inherited germline, sporadic MSI is associated with acquired epimutation of both copies of MLH1. The V600E hotspot mutation (c. 1799 > A) in the BRAF oncogene occurs in 40–50% of sporadic MSI colorectal cancers and is highly associated with MLH1 promoter methylation. The mutational profile of sporadic MSI-H tumors includes APC and BRAF (approximately 50%) mutations. These cases have very rare KRAS mutation. *SSA/P* with dysplasia is considered the precursor for sporadic MSI-H CRC and shows unique molecular features, including BRAF V600E mutation, generalized increased in CpG island methylation (the CpG island methylator phenotype-CIMP), MLH1-promoter methylation (PHM), and MSI-H. Approximately 70% CIMP-H CRCs are sporadic MSI-H CRC. 85% of sporadic MSI-H CRCs are associated CIMP-H. A total of 5–10% of MSS sporadic CRC have BRAF mutation.

According to CIMP status, MLH1 status, MSI status, and chromosomal instability status, colorectal carcinomas are subdivided into five main groups (Table 2). Jass et al. suggested that groups 1 and 2 arise from serrated adenomas, groups 4 and 5 from conventional adenomas, and group 3 which is KRAS positive arises from either serrated or conventional adenomas.

Differential Diagnosis

Adenoma with pseudoinvasion can be described in the presence of lamina-propria-like inflammation surrounding dysplastic glands within polyp stalk.

Metastatic adenocarcinoma in the colon should be differentiated from primary CRC by the lack of adenoma at the edge of the tumor. However this feature is not always helpful if the tumor overgrowth of the preexisting adenoma.

Carcinoma, Colorectal, Table 2 Molecular classification of colorectal carcinomas

Group 1	CIMP-H, MLH1 methylation, BRAF mutation, CIN(−), MSI-H, serrated precursor
Group 2	CIMP-H, BRAF mutation, CIN(−), MSS or MSI-L, serrated precursor
Group 3	CIMP-L, KRAS mutation, MSS or MSI-L, CIN(+), serrated or conventional adenoma
Group 4	CIMP negative, MSS, CIN(+), APC mutation (conventional, FAP)
Group 5	CIMP negative, BRAF negative, CIN (−), MSI-H, Lynch syndrome

References and Further Reading

Bosmann, F. T., Carnerio, F., Hruban, R. H., & Theise, N. D. (2010). *WHO classification of tumours of the digestive system*. Lyon: IARC.

Funkhouser, W., Lubin, I. M., Monzon, F. A., Zehnbauer, B. A., Evans, J. P., Ogino, S., & Nowak, J. A. (2011). Relevance Pathogenesis and testing algorithm for mismatch repair-defective colorectal carcinomas (a report of association for molecular pathology). *Journal of molecular diagnostics, 14*, 91–103.

Jass, J. R. (2007). Classification of colorectal cancer based on correlation of clinical, morphological and molecular features. *Histopathology, 50*, 113–130.

Pritchard, C. C., & Grady, W. M. (2011). Colorectal cancer molecular biology moves into clinical practice. *Gut, 60*, 116–129.

Rosai, J. (2011). Gastrointestinal tract large bowel. In *Rosai and Ackerman's surgical pathology* (10th ed., pp. 731–802). Edinburgh: Mosby Elsevier.

Carcinoma, Small Intestine

Berna Savaş
Department of Pathology, Ankara University Medical School, Ankara, Turkey

Synonyms

Adenocarcinoma; Small Intestine

Definition

Briefly, small intestinal carcinoma is the malignant epithelial tumor of the small intestine. Though the small intestine has a larger surface area and higher rate of epithelial cell turnover, epithelial neoplasms develop less frequently than the other parts of the GI tract. Small intestinal carcinomas are most commonly located in duodenum, usually around the ampulla of Vater. Although adenocarcinomas are the most common primary tumors, small intestine is the most common part of the gastrointestinal tract for involvement by secondary tumors, which are more than twice as common as the primary neoplasm. Like colorectal carcinomas, most of the small intestine carcinomas are sporadic and develop from adenomas. Risk factors for sporadic carcinoma include smoking, alcohol consumption, and fat in diet. Chronic inflammation is an important predisposing condition, including long-standing ► Crohn's disease and gluten-sensitive enteropathy (GSE). Familial adenomatous polyposis (FAP) carries the greatest increase risk for small intestinal adenocarcinoma. Other polyposis syndromes with increased risk include ► Peutz-Jeghers syndrome, juvenile polyposis syndrome, and hereditary nonpolyposis colon cancer syndrome (HNPCCC). Carcinoma can also develop in ileostomies, and ileal reservoirs. The most common presenting symptoms of small intestinal carcinoma are abdominal pain, obstruction, and occult gastrointestinal bleeding. Duodenal and ampullary tumors may obstruct the bile duct and cause jaundice. Most cases with distal small intestinal carcinomas present with advanced disease.

Clinical Features

- **Incidence**
  6.8 per million (Data from United States Surveillance, Epidemiology and End Results (SEER), 1973–2005). Overall small intestine carcinomas are rare tumors, making up 2% of GI tumors and 1% of GI cancer deaths.
- **Age**
  Median age is approximately 67 years.
- **Sex**
  Men are affected slightly more often than woman.
- **Site**
  Duodenum is the main site of occurrence of carcinomas. In duodenum, carcinomas are most common around the ampulla of Vater (approximately 65% of the tumors). The incidence decreases progressively through the rest of the small intestine. Crohn's disease–associated tumors are found in the ileum, in the main site of the inflammatory pathology.
- **Treatment**
  Pancreaticoduodenectomy or endoscopic mucosectomy/polypectomy (for polypoid and superficial tumors) can be applied for proximally located tumors, while more distal tumors require segmental resection with accompanying mesentery. Chemotherapy and radiotherapy appear to have little proven effect on survival.
- **Outcome**
  Outcome of the patients is poor in all locations. In the SEER database for 1988–2001, the overall 5-year survival of small intestinal adenocarcinoma was 27% and median survival was 13.9 months. For the cases with localized tumors, the 5-year survival rate was 57%, regional disease was 34%, and metastatic disease was 3%.

Macroscopy

The macroscopic findings depend on the site of the carcinoma. Tumors may have flat, stenotic, ulcerative, infiltrative, or polypoid macroscopic appearance. Ampullary and duodenal tumors usually have small, exophytic appearance, whereas distal tumors tend to be large, constricting, and annular lesions. Stage of the tumor also affects the macroscopic appearance. Another determinant is the presence or absence of a predisposing factor, such as accompanying adenoma, GSE, Crohn's disease, polyposis syndromes, etc. Most of the tumors have already penetrated the muscularis layer or serosal surface at the time of diagnosis.

Duodenal carcinoma requires additional sampling to evaluate the involvement of the pancreas and depth of the retroperitoneal invasion.

Microscopy

Histologically, small intestine carcinomas resemble their colonic counterparts (Fig. 1). Most of the small intestine carcinomas are adenocarcinomas, while mucinous adenocarcinoma and signet ring cell carcinomas can also be seen. Carcinomas that develop in ampulla of Vater may show an intestinal or pancreaticobiliary phenotype. Differentiation of these phenotypes is important for treatment and also the prognosis of the intestinal type is better. Adenosquamous carcinoma, medullary carcinoma, squamous cell carcinoma, carcinomas with neuroendocrine cell component, and undifferentiated carcinomas are rarer types of small intestinal carcinomas.

Immunophenotype

Small intestinal carcinomas show a different keratin 7/keratin 20 profiles; nearly half of the cases are positive for keratin 7 and keratin 20. This feature can be useful in differential diagnosis of metastatic spread of colonic carcinoma. AMACR/P504S immunostaining can be helpful as this antibody is usually positive in colon cancer, but not in primary small intestinal carcinoma. Expression of CDX2 is observed in more than half of the cases and the staining pattern is usually diffuse, similar to colorectal carcinomas.

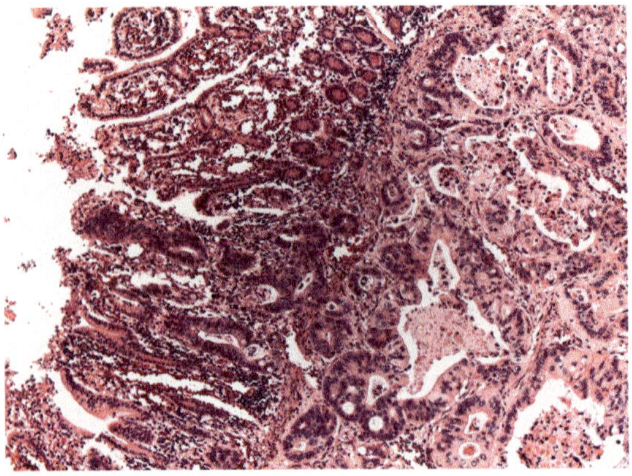

Carcinoma, Small Intestine, Fig. 1 Moderately differentiated adenocarcinoma of the duodenum (H&E, ×100)

Molecular Features

Molecular pathology is not very clear because of the relative rarity of these tumors. APC gene mutations are infrequent; however, overexpression of p53 is common. Loss of E-cadherin expression, mutation in beta-catenin, SMAD4, and KRAS genes, and activation of RAS-RAF-MAPK pathway are other genetic abnormalities that have been reported.

Differential Diagnosis

The main differential diagnostic consideration is metastatic tumor. Colorectal, breast, and lung adenocarcinoma and melanoma are among the most common secondary tumors involving the small intestine. Pancreatic and gastric cancer may directly involve the small intestine. Features favoring metastasis include the presence of multiple lesions and absence of a predisposing lesion. Immunohistochemistry is primarily used to exclude metastatic disease. Pancreaticobiliary neoplasms arising in the ampulla of Vater and periampullary area should be considered in the differential diagnosis of duodenal carcinomas. The size and the location of the tumor, determined both grossly and microscopically, are considered as useful features.

References and Further Reading

Lee, M. J., Lee, H. S., Choi, Y., & Yang, M. (2003). Expression of mucins and cytokeratins in primary carcinomas of the digestive system. *Modern Pathology, 16*, 403–410.

Scelo, G., Boffetta, P., Hemminki, K., Pukkala, E., Olsen, J. H., Andersen, A., et al. (2006). Associations between small intestinal cancer and the other primary cancers:

An international population-based study. *International Journal of Cancer, 118*, 189–196.
Schoftenfeld, D., Beebe-Diemmer, J. L., & Vigneau, F. D. (2009). The epidemiology and pathogenesis of neoplasia in small intestine. *Annals of Epidemiology, 19*, 58–69.
Shepherd, N. A., Carr, N. J., Howe, J. R., Noffsinger, A. E., & Warren, B. F. (2010). Carcinoma of small intestine. In F. T. Bosman, F. Carneiro, R. H. Hruban, & N. D. Theise (Eds.), *WHO classification of tumours of the digestive system* (pp. 98–101). Lyon, France: IARC.

Chagas Disease, Gastrointestinal Aspects

Rafaela L. Rego[1], Ivanir Martins[2], Janice Mary Chicarino Coelho[3] and Wilhermo Torres[4]
[1]Departamento de Diagnóstico Laboratorial – Serviço de Anatomia Patológica, Instituto Português de Oncologia Lisboa Francisco Gentil, IPOLFG, E.P.E, Lisbon, Portugal
[2]Serviço de Anatomia Patológica, Instituto Nacional do Cancer Rio de Janeiro, Rio de Janeiro, RJ, Brasil
[3]Fundação Oswaldo Cruz (Fiocruz) Instituto de Pesquisa Clínica Evandro Chagas, Rio de Janeiro, Brasil
[4]Departamento de Patologia, Universidade Federal Fluminense, Rio de Janeiro, Brasil

Synonyms

American trypanosomiasis

Definition

Chagas disease is an important parasitic disease resulting from the infection with *Trypanosoma cruzi* (*T. cruzi*), a hemoflagellate protozoa whose vectors are triatomine insects, a type of reduviid bug known as the "barber bug." It is one of the most serious public health problems in South America. The name was a tribute to its discoverer, the Brazilian medical doctor, scientist, and researcher Carlos Chagas (1879–1934). The achievement of Chagas, considered unique in the history of medicine, is a milestone in the history of Brazilian science and health (www.fiocruz.br/chagas).

In 1909, Carlos Chagas, from The Oswaldo Cruz Institute, announced the discovery of a new human disease. Chagas was the only researcher so far to completely describe a new infectious disease: its pathogen, vector (Triatominae), host, clinical manifestations, and epidemiology. The discovery brought immediate prestige and projection to the young scientist, who received several academic honors in Brazil and abroad, having been nominated for the Nobel Prize twice. Bringing an innovative contribution to the emerging field of tropical medicine and to the studies on parasitic diseases transmitted by insect vectors, Chagas also brought attention to the health and social reality of the countryside of Brazil, devastated by rural endemies.

Under natural conditions, *T. cruzi* exists in different populations of vertebrate hosts, sylvan, and domestic animals. It can also be found in invertebrates, such as in vector insects. During its phase in the invertebrate host, *T. cruzi* becomes epimastigotes and then, in the posterior intestine, these differentiate into trypomastigotes, which, after being eliminated with the feces and urine of the vector insect, are capable of infecting the vertebrate host.

The most important form of transmission of Chagas disease is either through skin break, resulting from the insect prick, or through mucous membranes, including conjunctive or oral/digestive mucosa. However, transfusional and congenital transmissions also have epidemiological importance. The determinants of Chagas disease result from the number of parasites in the initial infection, the infecting forms in the initial inoculum (number of trypomastigotes), the lineage of *T. cruzi* inoculated (I, II, Z3, or hybrid Z1/Z3), reinfection, the quality of the strains and clones (biodema), the specific clonal-histotrophic receptors of the host, and the patient's initial and late immune response (Andrade et al. 2006; Teixeira et al. 2006).

The parasites deposited on skin wounds or mucosa stimulate a local inflammatory reaction (inoculation chagoma or Romaña's sign) with a lymphoreticular response. The circulating trypomastigotes enveloped by macrophages can reach the liver, spleen, lymph nodes, skeletal, and cardiac muscles to form pseudocysts of amastigotes. With the rupture of the pseudocysts in the myocardium or myenteric plexuses, acute inflammatory reaction (mediated by CD4+ and CD8+ cells and interleukins, mainly IL-2 and IL-4) leads to muscle and neuron cell destruction, which is maintained by the presence of *T. cruzi* or its fragments and by the parasite's DNA. There is a late hypersensitivity reaction with dilated chronic myocardiopathy, arrhythmia, dysperistalsis, mega-esophagus, and megacolon (Coura 2007). There is evidence that the persistence of the parasite in the tissues, associated with unbalanced homeostatic mechanisms (oxidant/antioxidant and pro-inflammatory/anti-inflammatory processes), is critical for the pathogenesis and progression of Chagas disease (Higuchi et al. 2003; Lannes-Vieira 2003). The progression of the infection, as well as its resulting clinical picture, is dependent upon a complex parasite-host relationship, which involves environmental and genetic factors stemming either from the host or from the parasite. However, the specific pathophysiological factors influencing the clinical course remain unclear.

Chagas disease presents an initial or acute phase with evident parasitemia seen in direct blood examination. In most cases there are no symptoms, but in symptomatic cases there are entry point signs (inoculation chagoma or Romaña's sign), fever, generalized adenopathy, edema, hepatosplenomegaly, myocarditis, and meningoencephalitis in severe cases. This is followed by a chronic phase that in most cases presents as an indeterminate form (asymptomatic, with normal results from electrocardiogram and chest x-ray, no abnormalities in esophagus or colon), which may evolve to the cardiac and/or digestive form (megaesophagus and megacolon). The so-called congenital form may also occur, by means of transmission across the placenta or through the birth canal during delivery, and this may give rise to abortion, prematurity, or organic lesions in the fetus (Koberle 1961; Andrade 2000, 2005).

Acute Form

In the acute form, intracellular parasites are found in several organs, mainly inside the myocardium. Immunohistochemical tests are found to be helpful in the identification of *T. cruzi* and also the parasitism intensity. The myocardium inflammation is usually very intense, diffuse, and disproportional to the number of parasitic cells. There are morphological evidences indicative of the immune system's participation in the augmentation of this inflammatory response, such as the discovery of lymphocytes and adhered macrophages, membrane fusion in myocardial necrotic focuses, morphological data revealing cytoadherence and cytotoxicity, and also the presence of microangiopathy. The presence of non-parasitic myocardiocyte necrosis is also a usual finding. In other organs, the inflammation is focal or multifocal, always preserving a direct relationship with the parasited cells. These cells may be macrophages, flat muscular and grooved cells, and even gray fat adipocytes, as well as glial cells of the central nervous system and the corresponding satellite cells of the autonomic nervous system. In relation to the presence of parasitism and inflammation in their immediate neighborhoods, neurons of the myenteric plexus can exhibit regressive lesions at several levels or even necrosis and lyse. In the acute and chronic forms of Chagas disease, the etiological diagnosis can be accomplished by the detection of the parasite through the direct or indirect parasitological method and by the presence of antibodies in the serum through serological tests. The most used techniques are immunofluorescence, hemaglutination, and *enzyme-linked immunosorbent assay* (ELISA). Tests of greater complexity, such as the molecular test, using *polymerase chain reaction* (PCR) coupled with the hybridization with molecular probes and the *Western blot* (WB) have been showing promising results (www.fiocruz.br/chagas).

Indetermined Form

Most individuals infected with *T. cruzi*, having or not previously presented an evident acute form of infection, usually evolve into an apparent parasite-host state of equilibrium without clinical manifestations. This state of silent infection is denominated indetermined form. For a more precise diagnosis, it is necessary to identify this form not only by serological and/or parasitological evidences of the infection but also by normal results from radiology and electrocardiogram, confirming the digestive and circulatory systems normality. The inflammatory infiltrate is interstitial, does not hinder myocardiocytes, and is accompanied by a light, focal, and interstitial fibrosis, as well as by matrix expansion. After a certain time, the inflammatory infiltrate disappears, inflammatory cells exhibit apoptosis, while the excess of interstitial tissue is reabsorbed and degraded.

Chronic Cardiac Form

The chronic cardiac form is the most expressive manifestation of Chagas disease, both because of its frequency and because of its severity (Fig. 1). It generally appears between the second and fourth decades of life, 5–15 years after the initial infection. The signs and symptoms of chronic Chagas cardiopathy result from arrhythmia, cardiac insufficiency, auricular-ventricular and branch blockages, and thromboembolism.

This form presents an inflammatory fibrous essentially arrhythmic myocardiopathy that leads to a progressive lethal cardiac insufficiency. *T. cruzi* is not always demonstrated histologically; however, pathology findings are much more pronounced. Many times, a highly characteristic, if not pathognomonic, lesion occurs at the left ventricular end level, and it is usually called end lesion or aneurysm. It is a nonfibrous thinning, with myocardial fiber atrophy and protrusion of the left ventricular end. This lesion has an intimate connection with the peculiar involvement of the heart in this chronic form of Chagas disease. There is a delay in the arrival of electric impulses to the left ventricular end area. At each systole, the dorsal column blood pressure on a nonactivated region provokes herniation of the left ventricular apex. Histologically, it also has peculiarities and exhibits fibrous inflammation with several age-related alterations that reveal a dynamic, progressive process. This process involves the tissues that generate and transport electric impulses in a most varied pattern, with fibrosis, ectasis, and variable degrees of vascular sclerosis in several areas, which explains why this disease presents almost all the isolated or combined classified arrhythmias, like any other cardiopathy. With the dilation of the heart chambers and propagation of the inflammation to the endocardium, intracardiac thrombus frequently occur, especially in the terminal phases, generating embolus and infarctions in several organs, among which the most important is the central nervous system.

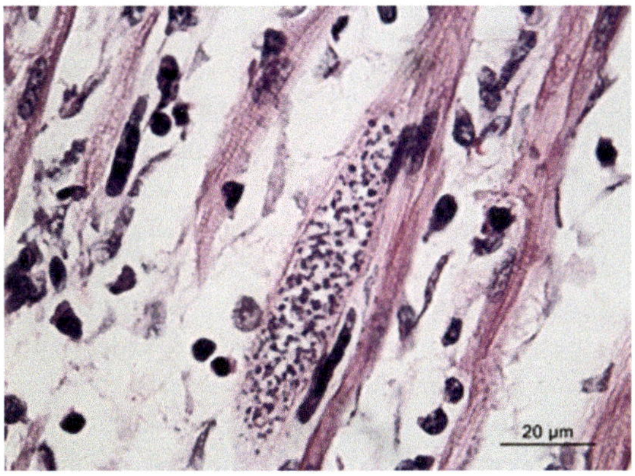

Chagas Disease, Gastrointestinal Aspects, Fig. 1 *T. cruzi*-infected heart muscle cells. Hematoxylin and eosin. Magnification: 1000×

Chronic Digestive Form

In the chronic digestive form of the disease, the clinical manifestations result from dysperistalsis of the esophagus and colon caused by destruction of the myenteric plexuses, which consequently leads to megaesophagus and megacolon. Complications include esophageal cancer, obstruction with twisting, and colon necrosis.

Congenital Form

The congenital form of Chagas disease seems to occur solely in pregnant women who have a lesion in the placenta that favors penetration by *T. cruzi* through the chorionic villi, where amastigote forms multiply (probably in Hofbauer cells) and subsequently invade the fetal circulation (Bittencourt 1963; Carlier and Torrico 2005).

Clinical Features

- **Incidence**
  A century after its discovery, Chagas disease remains a neglected tropical disease, and approximately 15 million people are infected in Latin America (Coura and Dias 2009).
- **Age and Sex**
  Chagas disease can infect anyone, but is diagnosed most often in children. There is no sex predilection.
- **Site**
  Since its discovery in 1909, Chagas disease started to be considered as one of the possible causes of an endemic condition in Brazil, known as choking disease ("mal de engasgo"), in which the symptoms are the same as those of achalasia of the esophagus (www.fiocruz.br/chagas). Choking disease is characterized by the loss of esophageal peristalsis and lack of lower esophageal sphincter relaxation in response to deglutition, with a consequent difficulty in the ingestion of food, being most of which retained in the esophagus, causing a progressive dilatation of the organ. The similarity between the two conditions led many authors to believe that this was a single morbid entity. What distinguished them was the unusual frequency of choking disease in certain regions of Brazil, in contrast to the rarity of achalasia in all parts of the world.

  About 10% of infected individuals develop the gastrointestinal form of the illness, which can result in megaesophagus and/or megacolon. This is frequently associated with cardiac disease, constituting the mixed chronic form. Although isolated cases of autonomic disorders of the esophagus have been described in the acute phase of the disease, these occur mostly in the chronic phase, when the dysperistalsis and spasms are accompanied by enlargement of the esophagus. The salivary glands, especially the parotid glands, are hypertrophied in patients with megaesophagus, a fact commonly occurring in any obstructive esophageal disease as a consequence of the esophagosalivary reflex, which produces hypersalivation. In Chagasic patients, however, the salivary glands are more sensitive to the mechanical stimulus of mastication and to the pharmacological stimulation by pilocarpine. In addition, hypersalivation and parotid hypertrophy persist in esophagectomized patients, demonstrating that this is not simply a situation regarding the esophagosalivary complex, but, instead, an impairment of the innervation of these glands in Chagas disease.

  Heart disease occurs in 30–40% of the infected individuals having manifestations such as myocarditis, fibrosis, cardiomyopathy, and heart dysfunction. The nervous form of Chagas disease has been observed in human immunodeficiency virus (HIV) positive patients, as well as in transplanted and cancer patients. In these cases, the specific anti-parasite treatment is effective in parasitemia control and leads to clinical improvement.
- **Treatment**
  Treatment for Chagas disease focuses on killing the parasite and managing signs and symptoms. During the acute phase of Chagas disease, the prescription medications benznidazole and nifurtimox may be of benefit. Once Chagas disease reaches the chronic phase, medications are not effective for curing the disease. Instead, treatment depends on the specific signs and symptoms and can include surgery/transplant.
- **Vaccine: Current Experience**
  Aiming at developing a recombinant vaccine against Chagas disease, researchers of both Oswaldo Cruz Institute and the Interdisciplinary Center of Gene Therapy at the Federal University of São Paulo developed a synergic work to generate recombinant adenoviruses expressing *T. cruzi* antigens [*trans*-sialidase (TS) and Amastigote Surface Protein 2 (ASP-2)] (www.fiocruz.br/chagas). Genes referring to these antigens were inserted into adenovirus type 5 genome, which is replication deficient. This vector is being used for the development of several commercial recombinant vaccines.
- **Outcome**
  The prognosis depends on the clinical form and the complications during its evolution. Many

cases may be asymptomatic and remain in the indeterminate form. In the acute phase, it depends on the patient's age and the severity and location of the lesions. In general, the acute phase is very severe among children that are less than 2 years old, and it is almost always fatal in those with myocarditis, cardiac insufficiency, and meningoencephalitis.

The prognosis for the digestive and indeterminate forms is generally good, except in cases of the digestive form with complications (esophageal cancer, obstruction with twisting, and colon necrosis).

In the chronic cardiac form, the prognosis varies considerably from one case to another. Patients with minimal lesions such as blockage of the right branch alone or unifocal ventricular or auricular extrasystole tend to remain stable and most of them survive for long periods and often end up dying for other reasons. Patients with complex arrhythmia, multifocal extrasystole, paroxystic tachycardia, auricular fibrillation, third-degree A-V blockage, or cardiac insufficiency have a very poor prognosis. A third group of patients with slightly increased heart area and changeable electrocardiographic findings and clinical manifestations have an uncertain prognosis.

The prognosis may also be very poor in the congenital form, which may lead not only to abortion and prematurity but also to organic lesions in the liver, spleen, heart, and central nervous system, with neurological sequelae and mental deficiency.

Macroscopy

The most important expression of the chronic digestive form is the endemic megaesophagus, encountered in Central Brazil, followed by the megacolon. Although neuronal lesions affect the myenteric plexus in several parts of the alimentary canal, the largest repercussions happen in the esophagus and colon. In those anatomic places, the content is usually solid and, therefore, more dependent on peristaltic forces. The presence of sphincters, either anatomic or physiological, contributes to dysperistalsis augmentation. Dysperistalsis then stimulates peristaltism, which is followed by hypertrophy of the muscular layers and, finally, by dilation or ectasis of the organs involved. In mega digestives, there is a narrowed cylindrical-fusiform area in the most distal portion that transitions between the normal part and the dilated one. The mucous membrane can present metaplastic areas that can be detected as whitish areas in the esophagus (squamous metaplasia). These may seem ulcerated areas, most usually found in the colon (stercoraceous ulcers). These features are seen in the chronic phase of the disease, and by the time symptoms are noted, the organisms can no longer be demonstrated in the myenteric plexus. The emergence of malignancy can be a complication of both conditions (megaesophagus and megacolon).

Microscopy

Parasitic involvement of the enteric nervous system is common in this disease, and an achalasia-like megaesophagus and megacolon are the most frequent manifestations. Microscopically, myenteric plexus appear destroyed, both in the narrowed and in the dilated areas, and histologically, Chagas disease cannot be distinguished from other causes of visceral neuropathy. There is inflammatory destruction of the myenteric plexus, with loss of up to 90% of neurons. However, the parasite is rarely visible in myenteric plexuses.

Immunophenotype

Immunohistochemical studies with polyclonal antibody for *T. cruzi* antigens can be used to identify the parasite and establish the diagnosis of Chagas disease (Carvalho et al. 2012) (Fig. 2).

Molecular Features

The diagnosis of Chagas disease can be accomplished through an array of strategies, depending

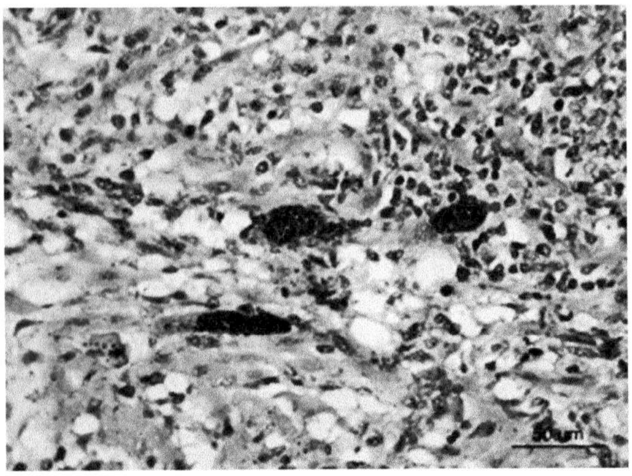

Chagas Disease, Gastrointestinal Aspects, Fig. 2 Amastigote nests of *T. cruzi* detected by immunohistochemistry. Magnification: 400×

upon the current phase of the disease (www.fiocruz.br/chagas). In the initial phase of *T. cruzi* infection, a large number of parasites circulate in the blood stream, and the diagnosis can be done by direct microscopic examination of peripheral blood. In contrast, during the chronic phase, parasitemia levels are quite below the threshold detection through microscopy, and, thus, diagnosis is mainly based on the host's serological response or on the in vitro amplification of the parasite population, especially by using methodologies such as xenodiagnosis or hemoculture. Despite its high specificity, xenodiagnosis presents a limited sensitivity, yielding parasite detection in only 20–60% of seropositive chronic patients, depending on the endemic area studied. Moreover, both biological amplification assays may select subpopulations of parasites, leading to distortions in the results of typing the etiological agent and in the epidemiological data obtained. The specificity of the conventional serological assays has been uncertain due to the frequency of infections by other trypanosomatids that cohabit in the same geographical region of *T. cruzi* (*Leishmania* spp. and *T. rangeli*), which are responsible for cross-antigenicity and false-positive results. In this sense, serological results need to be further confirmed by a parasitological test. Another problem related to serological diagnosis refers to the clinical profile of a patient, which may not be in accordance to the humoral response (during the first weeks of the infection, when no serological response is observed, or after a specific treatment, when the immune response may last for years, even in cases of successful treatment).

To date, the main technique tested for the identification of *T. cruzi* directly in the blood of chronic patients is the molecular assay using PCR. However, 20 years after the first reports of the use of PCR for the detection of *T. cruzi* infection, such test has not been made commercially available yet and has been used just in scientific research.

PCR strategy using kDNA as an amplification target employs oligonucleotides (primers) designed for the conserved minicircle regions, thus amplifying a specific 120 base pair (bp) (minicircle conserved region) or a 330 bp fragment (minicircle variable region). This approach has proven to be highly specific, as it allows the successful detection of distinct *T. cruzi* strains and does not recognize other protozoa kinetoplastids. The presence of an excess of human DNA does not interfere with the selective parasite DNA amplification process either. In the countries affected by Chagas disease, collecting clinical samples in rural areas, far from the laboratory that will perform the diagnosis, is a common practice, and this routine may interfere in the integrity of the sample to be analyzed. Nowadays, PCR can be considered a gold standard technique for the detection of circulating parasites in Chagas disease.

The use of Real-Time PCR, a quantitative automated approach based on the use of fluorescent probes ("TaqMan") or fluorescent dyes that have affinity to DNA molecules ("SYBR green"), has also been employed. Such procedure is able to measure the amplification rate of the reaction in real time. The implementation of a quantitative assay capable to estimate the parasite load in Chagasic patients in a highly accurate way and also to monitor parasitemia during specific therapy will certainly be particularly useful as an indicator of therapeutic efficacy. Some authors argue that chronic or asymptomatic patients that present extremely low or even undetectable circulating parasite levels should present a better response to treatment than those with patent parasitemia. This observation underlines the urgent need to join efforts for a standardization of both conventional and Real-Time PCR protocols, which will probably be the basis for the future establishment of more reliable cure criteria for patients submitted to Chagas disease therapy.

Differential Diagnosis

The differential diagnosis includes idiopathic primary achalasia as well as other visceral neuropathies. However, many of these latter disorders lack inflammation of the myenteric plexus. Unlike primary achalasia, Chagas disease usually involves other organ systems (especially the heart) or other areas of the GI tract. Nevertheless, often the differential is resolved only clinically.

References and Further Reading

Andrade, Z. (2000). Patologia da doença de Chagas. In Z. Brener, Z. Andrade, & M. Barral-Netto (Eds.), *Trypanosoma cruzi e doença de Chagas* (2nd ed., pp. 201–230). Rio de Janeiro: Guanabara-Koogan.

Andrade, S. G. (2005). Biodemas, zimodemas e esquisodemas: sua relação com a patologia da doença de Chagas. In J. R. Coura (Ed.), *Dinâmica das Doenças Infecciosas e Parasitárias* (pp. 621–637). Rio de Janeiro: Guanabara-Koogan.

Andrade, S. G., Campos, R. F., Sobral, S. C., Magalhães, J. B., Guedes, R. S. P., & Guerreiro, M. L. (2006). Reinfections with strains of Trypanosoma cruzi, of different biodemes as a factor of aggravation of myocarditis and myositis in mice. *Revista da Sociedade Brasileira de Medicina Tropical, 39*, 1–8.

Bittencourt, A. L. (1963). Placenta chagásica e transmissão da doença de Chagas. *Revista do Instituto de Medicina Tropical de São Paulo, 5*, 62–67.

Carlier, V., & Torrico, F. (organizers). (2005). Colóquio Internacional Infección Congênita por Trypanosoma cruzi: desde los mecanismos de transmissión hasta una estratégia de diagnóstico y control. *Revista da Sociedade Brasileira de Medicina Tropical, 38* (Suppl. II), 1–128.

Carvalho, C. M., Silverio, J. C., da Silva, A. A. et al. (2012). Inducible nitric oxide synthase in heart tissue and nitric oxide in serum of Trypanosoma cruzi-infected rhesus monkeys: Association with heart injury. *PLoS Neglected Tropical Diseases, 6*(5), e1644. doi:10.1371/journal.pntd.0001644. Epub 2012 May 8

Coura, J. R. (2007). Chagas disease: what is known and what is needed – A background article. *Memórias do Instituto Oswaldo Cruz, 102*(Suppl. I), 113–122.

Coura, J. R., & Dias, J. C. P. (2009). Epidemiology, control and surveillance of Chagas disease: 100 years after its discovery. *Memórias do Instituto Oswaldo Cruz, 104*, 31–40.

Higuchi, M. L., Benvenuti, L. A., Martins, R. M., & Metzger, M. (2003). Pathophysiology of the heart in Chagas' disease: Current status and new developments. *Cardiovascular Research, 60*, 96–107.

Koberle, F. (1961). Patologia y anatomia patológica de la enfermedadde Chagas. *Bol Ofic Sanit Panamer, 51*, 404–428.

Lannes-Vieira, J. (2003). Trypanosoma cruzi-elicited CD8 + T cell-mediated myocarditis: Chemokine receptors and adhesion molecules as potential therapeutic targets to control chronic inflammation? *Memórias do Instituto Oswaldo Cruz, 98*, 299–304.

Teixeira, A. R. L., Nascimento, R. J., & Sturm, N. R. (2006). Evolution and pathology in Chagas disease – A review. *Memórias do Instituto Oswaldo Cruz, 101*, 463–491.

www.fiocruz.br/chagas

CHARGE Syndrome, Esophagus

Ana Berta Sousa[1] and Ana Isabel Lopes[2]
[1]Departamento de Pediatria, Faculdade de Medicina de Lisboa, Serviço de Genética Médica, Hospital Universitário de Santa Maria/CHLN, Lisbon, Portugal
[2]Unidade de Gastrenterologia Pediátrica, Departamento de Pediatria, Faculdade de Medicina de Lisboa, Hospital Universitário de Santa Maria/CHLN, Lisbon, Portugal

Synonyms

Hall-Hittner syndrome

Definition

CHARGE is an acronym coined by Pagon et al. in 1981 to describe the nonrandom association of ocular *C*oloboma, *H*eart defects, choanal *A*tresia, *R*etardation of growth and/or development, *G*enital anomalies and *E*ar anomalies

CHARGE Syndrome, Esophagus, Table 1 Clinical criteria for the diagnosis of CHARGE syndrome

Diagnostic criteria		
Pagon et al. (1981)[a]	Blake et al. (1998)[b]	Verloes (2005)[c]
Coloboma[d]	Coloboma[d]	Coloboma[d]
Choanal Atresia	Choanal Atresia	Choanal Atresia
Ear anomalies and/or deafness	Characteristic ear anomalies[e]	Abnormal semicircular canals
Ear anomalies and/or deafness	Characteristic ear anomalies[e]	Abnormal ear
	Cranial nerve dysfunction[f]	Rhombencephalic dysfunction[g]
Heart defects	Heart defects	Malformation of mediastinal organs
	Traqueoesofageal defects	Malformation of mediastinal organs
Genital hypoplasia	Genital hypoplasia	Hypothalamo-hypophyseal dysfunction[h]
Retarded growth and/or development	Growth deficiency	Hypothalamo-hypophyseal dysfunction[h]
Retarded growth and/or development	Developmental Delay	Developmental Delay
	Orofacial cleft	
	Gestalt face[i]	
2 + 2 or 1 + 3	4 or 3 + 3	Typical = 3 or 2 + 2 Partial = 2 + 1 Atypical = 2 or 1 + 3

Explanations:
[a]Pagon, R. A., Graham, J. M. Jr., & Zonana J., et al. (1981). Coloboma, congenital heart disease, and choanal atresia with multiple anomalies: CHARGE association. *The Journal of Pediatrics*, *99*(2), 223–227
[b]Blake, K. D., et al. (1998). CHARGE association: An update and review for the primary pediatrician. *Clinical Pediatrics (Phila)*, *37*(3):159–173
[c]Verloes, A. (2005). Updated diagnostic criteria for CHARGE syndrome: A proposal. *American Jouranal of Medical Genetics. Part A*, *133A*(3), 306–308
[d]Coloboma of the iris, choroid, retina, and/or optic disk that may only be visible on fundoscopy
[e]Cup-shaped ear, wide with reduced vertical height, with a triangular concha and small/absent lobes; may include middle or inner ear malformations
[f]Anosmia (I), oculomotor dysfunction (VI), facial palsy (VII), sensorineural hearing loss and vestibular problems (VIII), swallowing difficulties (IX/X)
[g]Brainstem and cranial nerve dysfunction
[h]Hypogonadotropic hypogonadism, growth hormone deficiency
[i]Broad forehead, square face, facial asymmetry

(Table 1) (reviewed in Bergman et al. 2011; Zentner et al. 2010). These criteria were updated by Blake et al. in 1998 to include cranial nerve dysfunction and visceral malformations (Table 1). A few years later, in 2001, Amiel et al. stressed the specificity of inner ear anomalies in CHARGE patients, and suggested these should be included as major diagnostic criteria. Finally, in 2005,

Verloes proposed diagnosis should be based on the 3C-triad comprising *C*oloboma, *C*hoanal atresia, and abnormal semicircular *C*anals, and gave a formal definition of typical, partial, and atypical CHARGE (Table 1).

The condition was believed to be an association until recent years, when loss-of-function mutations in the *CHD7* gene were identified as causative in over two-thirds of patients with this clinical diagnosis (reviewed in Janssen et al. 2012).

CHD7 is a *C*hromodomain *H*elicase *D*NA-binding gene, located on chromosome 8q12. CHD proteins act by modifying chromatin structure to alter access of the transcriptional apparatus to its genomic template, thus interfering with gene expression. This class of proteins is thought to have pivotal roles in early embryonic development, in keeping with the large spectrum of abnormalities described in CHARGE patients.

Over 500 different mutations affecting *CHD7* have been described in CHARGE patients (a locus-specific database is accessible at www.CHD7.org). The mutation detection rate rises above 90% if only CHARGE patients meeting the diagnostic criteria of Blake et al. and/or Verloes et al. are taken into account, indicating *CHD7* mutations are the major cause of CHARGE syndrome. There are no mutational hotspots and recurrent mutations are rare. The mutations are equally distributed along the coding region of *CHD7*, and are mostly nonsense or frameshift. No clear genotype/phenotype correlation has been established, which is best demonstrated by intrafamilial variability as observed in sib pairs, including monozygotic twin pairs, and two generation families portraying dominant transmission from a very mildly affected parent. Germ-line and somatic mosaicism have been demonstrated; thus, the recurrence risk for parents of the novo patients is 2–3%.

Clinical Features

- **Incidence**
  CHARGE syndrome has been estimated to occur in 1:10,000 births. Incidence of tracheo-esophageal anomalies varies from 19% to 29% in different series (Bergman et al. 2011; Zentner et al. 2010).
- **Age**
  CHARGE syndrome presents at birth.
- **Sex**
  CHARGE syndrome affects both sexes equally.
- **Site**
  CHARGE is a highly variable multiple congenital anomalies syndrome (see above).

  Esophageal involvement in CHARGE syndrome may include a range of anomalies, most frequently esophageal atresia (EA) with or without tracheo-esophageal fistula (TEF).

  EA is a relatively common malformation, clinically and etiologically heterogeneous, occurring in approximately 1 in 3,500 births (Scott 2009). EA can be an isolated finding. However, in over half the cases, there are other anomalies, more commonly cardiac malformations. Complex cardiac malformations are often associated with multiple other anatomic defects and have a poorer outcome. EA with additional anomalies can be classified as either syndromic or non-isolated, depending on whether a specific genetic diagnosis can be made. A significant proportion of non-syndromic non-isolated cases of EA/TEF can be said to have VACTERL association (*v*ertebral, *a*nal, *c*ardiac, *t*racheo-*e*sophageal fistula, *r*enal, *l*imb defects). Besides CHARGE syndrome, examples of other syndromes featuring tracheo-esophageal anomalies are Feingold, Pallister-Hall, and Anophthalmia-Esophageal-Genital syndrome.

  More rarely, laryngo-tracheo-esophageal cleft (LC) may also occur in CHARGE syndrome (Leboulanger and Garabédian 2011). LC is also a feature of Opitz/BBB and Pallister-Hall syndromes and can be part of the VACTERL association.
- **Treatment**
  Treatment is supportive and site specific.

  An early multidisciplinary medical and surgical approach is required in the care of children born with multiple congenital anomalies. In fact, the increased survival of CHARGE children with EA and TEF is due not only to improved care for these particular defects, but also to a more aggressive approach to the treatment of serious associated anomalies. When appropriate, surgical repair of the EA/TEF may be postponed by gastrostomy, upper pouch suction, and parenteral nutrition until concomitant problems are treated.

Concerning LC, once the cleft is diagnosed, it is essential to determine its length to orient the management and treatment approach. Management involves maintenance of satisfactory ventilation, prevention of secondary pulmonary complications resulting from repeated aspirations, and adequate feeding. Endotracheal intubation may be required for respiratory distress in severe cases. Treatment requires endoscopic or external surgery to close the cleft (usually performed as early as possible to avoid complications related to aspiration and gastric reflux).

- **Outcome (Prognosis)**
  Life expectancy in CHARGE syndrome varies widely and is most influenced by the combined presence of choanal atresia and heart defects or TEF. Feeding and swallowing difficulties as well as gastroesophageal reflux (GER) resulting in aspiration of secretions also contribute to the mortality rate.

  As such, frequent feeding and gastrointestinal assessments, including combinations of barium swallow, reflux scan, and pH monitoring, should be conducted to diagnose swallowing dysfunction, esophageal dysmotility, GER, and tracheal aspiration.

  Regarding EA, over the past 50 years, refinements in neonatal surgical technique, preoperative support, anesthesia, and neonatal intensive care have considerably improved the outcome. It is also recognized that prompt diagnosis with appropriate clinical management and expeditious referral to a tertiary care center has had a dramatic impact on the improved survival of these infants.

  Concerning LC, the prognosis is variable depending on the severity of the LC and associated malformations. Early diagnosis and appropriate treatment and management help to reduce mortality and morbidity.

Macroscopy (Gross)

EA is characterized by incomplete formation of the esophagus. It is often associated with a fistula between the trachea and the esophagus. Many anatomic variations of EA with or without TEF have been described. The most common variant of this anomaly (about 80% of the cases) consists of a blind esophageal pouch with a fistula between the trachea and the distal esophagus, the fistula often entering the trachea close to the carina. The proximal esophageal pouch is often hypertrophied and dilated secondary to the fetus' efforts to swallow amniotic fluid. The muscular pouch may also compress the trachea, and this compression has been implicated in the development of the tracheomalacia that is sometimes reported in these infants. The second most common anomaly is pure atresia without TEF. This condition is usually associated with an underdeveloped distal esophageal remnant, making surgical repair more cumbersome. The third most common variation is the H-type fistula, which consists of a TEF without EA. This aberration is more difficult to diagnose clinically. If the fistula is long and oblique, the symptoms may be minimal, and the condition may remain unidentified for many years (Shaw-Smith et al. 2005).

LC is a congenital malformation characterized by an abnormal, posterior, sagittal communication between the larynx and the pharynx, possibly extending downward between the trachea and the esophagus. It results from failure of fusion of the posterior cricoid lamina and abnormal development of the tracheo-esophageal septum. Five types of laryngo-tracheo-esophageal cleft have been described based on the downward extension of the cleft, which typically correlates with the severity of symptoms.

Microscopy

Does not apply

Immunophenotype

Does not apply

Molecular Features

No mutation in *CHD7* is specifically or more frequently associated with tracheo-esophageal anomalies (see above).

Differential Diagnosis

Phenocopies of CHARGE syndrome can be due to chromosomal aberrations (namely 22q11.2 deletion) and teratogen exposure (e.g., retinoic acid, maternal diabetes). In particular, 22q11.2 deletion syndrome has a number of overlapping clinical features. However, TEF is more frequently found in patients with CHARGE syndrome. Conversely, feeding and swallowing difficulties are not clinically useful for differentiating the two syndromes, because of the clinical overlap between the dysfunction of cranial nerves IX, X, and XI in CHARGE syndrome and the dysphagia and velopharyngeal insufficiency seen in the 22q11.2 deletion.

Interestingly, a few patients with Kallmann syndrome (KS, characterized by the combination of anosmia and hypogonadotropic hypogonadism) have been found to harbor a *CHD7* mutation, suggesting KS might be seen as a mild presentation of CHARGE syndrome.

References and Further Reading

Bergman, J. E., Janssen, N., Hoefsloot, L. H., et al. (2011). CHD7 mutations and CHARGE syndrome: The clinical implications of an expanding phenotype. *Journal of Medical Genetics, 48*(5), 334–342.

Janssen, N., Bergman, J. E., Swertz, M. A., et al. (2012). Mutation update on the CHD7 gene involved in CHARGE syndrome. *Human Mutation, 33*(8), 1149–1160.

Leboulanger, N., & Garabédian, E. N. (2011). Laryngo-tracheo-oesophageal clefts. *Orphanet Journal of Rare Diseases, 6*, 81.

Scott, D. A. (2009). Esophageal atresia/tracheoesophageal fistula overview. In R. A. Pagon, T. D. Bird, & C. R. Dolan, et al., (Eds.), *GeneReviews™* [Internet]. Seattle: University of Washington; 1993. http://www.ncbi.nlm.nih.gov/books/NBK5192/

Shaw-Smith, C., Willatt, L., & Thalange, N. (2005). *Clinical Dysmorphology, 14*(3), 155–158.

Zentner, G. E., Layman, W. S., Martin, D. M., et al. (2010). Molecular and phenotypic aspects of CHD7 mutation in CHARGE syndrome. *American Journal of Medical Genetics. Part A, 152A*(3), 674–686.

C

Cholera

Xavier Sagaert
Department of Pathology, University Hospitals KU Leuven, Leuven, Belgium

Definition

Cholera is an infectious, often fatal bacterial disease of the intestine, caused by the Gram-negative bacterium *Vibrio cholera*. Infection with *V. cholerae* occurs after ingestion of contaminated food or water. In the developed world, shellfish is the usual cause, while in the developing world, it is mostly water. Direct person-to-person spread is rare but has been implicated in hospital outbreaks and during burial ceremonies requiring handling of intestinal contents. *V. cholerae* also colonizes arthropods, and flies have been postulated as potential hosts and possible disease vectors.

Most ingested *V. cholerae* bacteria are sensitive to the gastric acid barrier, and are rapidly killed. However, some bacteria may survive transit through the stomach by virtue of low gastric acidity of a compromised host, protection within food, rapid gastric emptying, or a large inoculum size. Following colonization of the small intestinal epithelium with the aid of flagella, *V. cholerae* start producing cholera toxin, a heterodimeric protein composed of one catalytic A subunit and five B subunits. The A subunit is cleaved to produce A1 and A2 fragments linked by a disulfide bond. The B subunit pentamer binds holotoxin to the enterocyte surface receptor, the ganglioside GM1. Following binding of holotoxin to GM1 and internalization, A1 catalyzes the adenosine diphosphate (ADP)-ribosylation of a guanosine triphosphate (GTP)-binding protein, leading to persistent activation of adenylate cyclase. This increase of cyclic adenosine monophosphate (cAMP) in the intestinal mucosa leads to increased chloride secretion and decreased sodium absorption, producing the massive fluid and electrolyte loss characteristic of the disease. Indeed, an untreated person with cholera may produce 10–20 l of diarrhea a day, leading to significant dehydration, electrolyte imbalance, and death within hours.

Clinical Features

- **Incidence**
  Globally, cholera incidence has increased steadily since the year 2005, with outbreaks persisting in Sub-Saharan Africa, Asia, and more recently in Hispaniola. Cholera continues to pose a public health problem among developing world populations without access to adequate water and sanitation resources. In 2011, a total of 58 countries from all continents reported 589 854 cases of cholera to the World Healt Organisation (WHO), of which 32% were reported from Africa and 61.2% from the Americas (where a large outbreak that started in Haiti at the end of October 2010 also affected the Dominican Republic). Globally, however, the true number of cholera cases is known to be much higher (probably a tenfold). Cases of cholera officially reported to WHO do not account for the estimated 500,000–700,000 cases labeled as acute watery diarrhea. These cases occur in vast areas of Central and South-East Asia, and in some African countries, leading to great underestimation of the global burden of this disease. Although United Nations members are required to report cholera to the WHO, member states generally underreport outbreaks of the diarrheal disease because of the potential effect on tourism and trade. Also contributing to underreporting is the inability of poor countries to initiate systematic surveillance. Another factor is that many cholera-associated deaths in developing countries probably occur before patients reach the hospital, so statistics are likely to be underestimated.
- **Age**
  Children younger than 5 years of age are the most vulnerable to infection, with nearly half of all cholera cases occurring in that age group. The estimated cholera incidence rate for children younger than 1 years is 7.3 cases per 1,000 in endemic areas, and for children aged 1–4 years, it is 7.0 per 1,000. Children in the next age group, 5–14 years, have an incidence rate less than one third of the youngest group, at 2.2 per 1,000.
- **Sex**
  Both sexes are equally affected by cholera.
- **Site**
  The effects of cholera are initially limited to the small intestine, where the bacteria starts producing toxic proteins which can cause (extreme) loss of fluids, thereby having a prominent cardiovascular impact.
- **Treatment**
  In most cases, cholera can be successfully treated with oral rehydration therapy, which is highly effective, safe, and simple to administer. Rice-based solutions are preferred to glucose-based ones due to greater efficiency. If commercially produced oral rehydration solutions are too expensive or difficult to obtain, solutions can be made. One such recipe is composed of 1 l of boiled water, 1/2 teaspoon of salt, and 6 teaspoons of sugar; mashed banana is added for potassium and to improve taste.

  In severe cases with significant dehydration, intravenous rehydration may be necessary, in addition to replacement of electrolytes such as potassium. Ringer's lactate is the preferred solution, often with added potassium. Large volumes and continued replacement until diarrhea has subsided may be needed. Ten percent of a person's body weight in fluid may need to be given in the first 2–4 h.

  People will recover without need for antibiotic treatment, on condition that sufficient hydration is maintained. Nevertheless, antibiotic treatment for 1 to 3 days not only shortens the course of the disease and reduce the severity of the symptoms, but also reduces fluid requirements. Doxycycline is typically used first line, although some strains of *V. cholerae* have shown resistance.

- **Outcome**
  If people with cholera are treated quickly and properly, the mortality rate is less than 1%. However, with untreated cholera, the mortality rate rises to 50–60%. For certain genetic strains of cholera, such as the one present during the 2010 epidemic in Haiti, death can occur within 2 h of becoming ill.

Macroscopy

Stools resemble "rice water" and contain mucus, although the macroscopic aspect of the intestines is mostly unaltered and cannot be distinguished from the intestine of a healthy individual.

Microscopy

Although direct microscopy of the stools is not recommended, dark field microscopic examination of stool sample will often show rapidly motile *V. cholerae* bacteria. Epithelial cells are also present in the stool sample.

Despite the severity of the disease, *V. Cholerae* is a noninvasive organism that causes minimal or no histological changes in the gut. Rare, nonspecific findings such as small bowel mucin depletion, degenerative surface epithelium changes, and a mild increase in lamina propria mononuclear cells have been described. Autopsy studies after severe cholera disease revealed that a spectrum of histologic changes was observed in the gut. The most consistent finding was vascular dilatation and congestion of the viscera. Specifically, when autopsies were cases performed 2–3 h post-mortem, the small intestine was essentially intact but edema and transudate between the epithelium and the stroma of the lamina propria were noted. The lamina propria contained increased numbers of cells associated with striking congestion of submucosal blood vessels. When the time between death and autopsy was increased, epithelial denudation and extensive sloughing were present. Variable degrees of smooth muscle degeneration were also observed in the musculature of the small intestine, characterized by patchy hypereosinophilia, muscle bundle disarray, and individual myofiber fusion with loss of cell borders. Nuclei were pale and vesicular; occasional others small and pyknotic. Small blood vessel walls were thickened and hyalinised with occasional exfoliation of cellular elements hyalinization into the lumens.

Immunophenotype

A rapid dip-stick test is available to determine the presence of *V. cholerae*. As such, stool and swab samples collected in the acute stage of the disease, before antibiotics have been administered, are the most useful specimens for laboratory diagnosis. If an epidemic of cholera is suspected, the most common causative agent is *V. cholerae* O1. If *V. cholerae* serogroup O1 is not isolated, the laboratory should test for *V. cholerae* O139. However, if neither of these organisms is isolated, it is necessary to send stool specimens to a reference laboratory. Infection with *V. cholerae* O139 should be reported and handled in the same manner as that caused by *V. cholerae* O1.

Differential Diagnosis

The clinical picture of severe cholera is so spectacular that differential diagnosis does not present many difficulties. Milder cholera may be similar to other forms of gastro-enteritis (but not to dysentery). A child above the age of 5 years who develops acute dehydration, or dies as the result of acute diarrhea, is always suggestive for cholera.

References and Further Reading

Gill, D. M. (1976). Arrangement of subunits in cholera toxin. *Biochemistry, 15*, 1242–1248.

Harris, J. B., LaRocque, R. C., Charles, R. C., Mazumder, R. N., Khan, A. I., & Bardhan, P. K. (2010). Cholera's western front. *Lancet, 376*, 1961–1965.

Harris, J. B., LaRocque, R. C., Qadri, F., Ryan, E. T., & Calderwood, S. B. (2012). Cholera. *Lancet, 379*, 2466–2476.

Nelson, E. J., Chowdhury, A., Harris, J. B., et al. (2007). Complexity of rice-water stool from patients with *Vibrio cholerae* plays a role in the transmission of infectious diarrhea. *Proceedings of the National Academy of Sciences of the United States of America, 104*, 19091–19096.
Norris, H. T. (1973). Changing pattern of autopsy findings in patients dying of cholera after 1960. *American Journal of Tropical Medicine and Hygiene, 22*, 215–222.

Choriocarcinoma, Gastrointestinal

Helena Baldaia
Serviço de Anatomia Patológica, Centro Hospitalar de São João, Porto, Portugal

Synonyms

Cytotrophoblast; Germ cell tumor; Nongestational choriocarcinoma; Syncytiotrophoblast

Definition

Choriocarcinoma is an aggressive germ cell tumor that can rarely occur in extragonadal location (Iyomasa et al. 2003). In the gastrointestinal tract, the occurrence of pure choriocarcinoma is very rare, being more frequently diagnosed in association with adenocarcinoma (Fenoglio-Preiser et al. 2008a). In the esophagus, a few of the reported cases were coexistent with squamous cell carcinoma (Glickman and Odze 2009).

This type of tumor presents itself commonly as massive gastrointestinal (GI) bleeding, liver hemorrhage from metastatic disease, or abdominal pain (Kobayashi et al. 2005).

Choriocarcinoma is frequently associated with markedly elevated serum human chorionic gonadotropin (hCG) levels (Fenoglio-Preiser et al. 2008b).

Given the rarity of this type of tumor, before a diagnosis of primary GI choriocarcinoma can be made, it is important to exclude the possibility of an ectopic pregnancy, a teratoma, or metastatic disease from an occult primary (Noffsinger 2009).

Although several hypotheses have arisen, the exact pathogenesis of this tumor is still unknown. The most commonly accepted mechanism is the dedifferentiation of malignant adenocarcinoma tissue to the level of embryonal ectoderm, retaining the ability to form trophoblast (Kobayashi et al. 2005). An argument favoring this hypothesis is the frequent occurrence of choriocarcinoma in association with adenocarcinoma.

Clinical Features

- **Incidence**
  The occurrence of GI choriocarcinoma is very rare. In the stomach, the most common GI location, it is reported to account for approximately 0.08% of all gastric cancers (Kobayashi et al. 2005). In the esophagus and small intestine, it is very rare. Presently, in the colon, there are fewer than 10 cases reported in the literature (Harada et al. 2012).
- **Age**
  GI choriocarcinoma occurs in adults of all ages. In a study on 53 cases of gastric choriocarcinoma, the mean age was 60.9 years (age range 26–83 years). Patients with choriocarcinoma of the colon tend to be younger than those with gastric choriocarcinoma (mean age 51.6 years; age range 29–74 years) (Harada et al. 2012). The age range of the cases of choriocarcinoma of the jejunum reported was 16–49 years (Iyomasa et al. 2003).
- **Sex**
  Choriocarcinoma occurs in both sexes. In gastric choriocarcinoma, there appears to be a slight male predominance (M/F ratio, 2.3:1) (Kobayashi et al. 2005), while in the colon there is a female predominance (Fenoglio-Preiser et al. 2008c).
- **Site**
  The stomach is the most commonly reported site of occurrence of GI choriocarcinoma. The lower third is the most common location (41% of cases in one study)(Kobayashi et al. 2005). Cases have also been reported in the esophagus, small intestine, and colorectal area. In the

latter, the left colon seems to be more frequently affected (Fenoglio-Preiser et al. 2008c).

- **Treatment**
  Surgery and multiple chemotherapy regimens have been used as the mainstay of therapy for choriocarcinoma. Chemotherapy is reported to be an important part of treatment because radiation and local treatment are thought to be ineffective against choriocarcinoma, which is characterized by rapid proliferation with generalized metastasis (Harada et al. 2012).
- **Outcome**
  The prognosis of choriocarcinoma is very poor. The mean reported survivals for patients with gastric and colic choriocarcinomas are 200 and 108 days, respectively (Harada et al. 2012). The majority of patients have metastatic disease at presentation. Choriocarcinoma metastasizes early to the lymph nodes, liver, lung, and spleen (Fenoglio-Preiser et al. 2008a). In a study on gastric choriocarcinomas, curative resection, appropriate chemotherapy, and the absence of synchronous liver metastasis were independent favorable prognostic factors (Kobayashi et al. 2005). The immunohistologic detection of hCG in colorectal choriocarcinomas has also been reported as a putative biologic marker of prognostic significance (Fenoglio-Preiser et al. 2008c).

Macroscopy

Choriocarcinomas are usually large masses (2–18 cm with a mean size of 7 cm in a study on gastric choriocarcinomas) with prominent necrosis and hemorrhage (Kobayashi et al. 2005).

C

Microscopy

Histology usually reveals variably differentiated adenocarcinoma admixed with cytotrophoblastic and syncytiotrophoblastic cells (Fig. 1). The former forms solid sheets of clear or pale mononuclear cells containing PAS-positive cytoplasmic granules (Fenoglio-Preiser et al. 2008a). Syncytiotrophoblastic giant multinucleated cells are easily encountered. Vascular invasion is common (Fenoglio-Preiser et al. 2008a).

Immunophenotype

Choriocarcinomas are typically positive for hCG in the syncytiotrophoblastic component (Fig. 1). The cytotrophoblastic cells can be positive for human placental lactogen (hPL). The adenocarcinomatous cells can also show immunoreactivity with hCG. In fact, it has been shown that 43% of

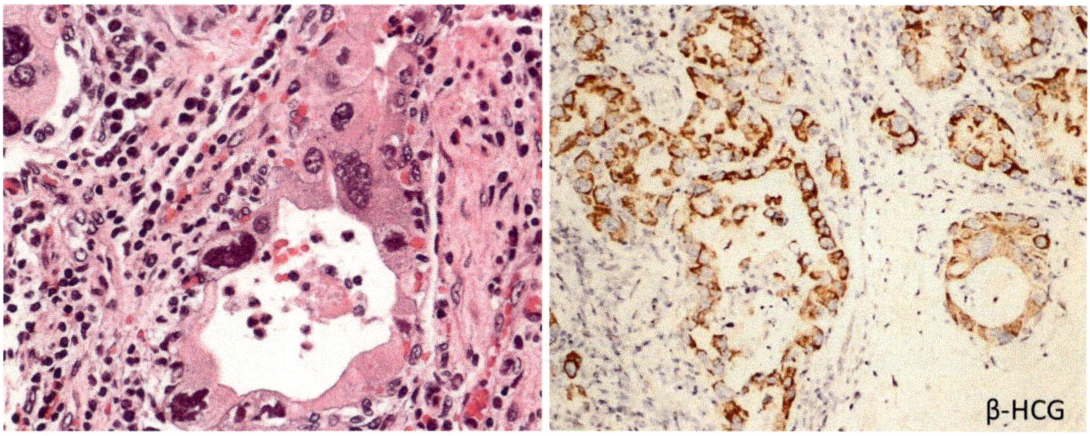

Choriocarcinoma, Gastrointestinal, Fig. 1 Gastric choriocarcinoma. This area of the tumor shows poorly differentiated adenocarcinoma admixed with atypical syncytiotrophoblastic cells, which stain for β-hCG

typical colic adenocarcinomas contain hCG-positive cells (Fenoglio-Preiser et al. 2008c) so that the presence of hCG immunoreactivity is insufficient to diagnose a choriocarcinoma (Fenoglio-Preiser et al. 2008c).

Molecular Features

At the present, there are no typical diagnostically or prognostically important molecular alterations reported in GI choriocarcinomas.

Differential Diagnosis

As was mentioned earlier, the diagnosis of GI choriocarcinoma implies exclusion of a primary elsewhere. The presence of adenocarcinoma in the vicinity of the choriocarcinomatous component is in favor of a primary choriocarcinoma, but a *metastasis* cannot be ruled out solely on morphologic grounds. Large *anaplastic cells* can be identified in the setting of an aggressive adenocarcinoma. However, even if it is possible, hCG-positivity is not a feature of anaplastic carcinoma cells. The positivity for hPL and the presence of the cytotrophoblastic component allow a differential diagnosis in this case (Fenoglio-Preiser et al. 2008a).

References and Further Reading

Fenoglio-Preiser, C. M., Noffsinger, A. E., Stemmermann, G. N., Lantz, P. E., & Isaacson, P. G. (2008a). The noplastic stomach. In J. McGouh & J. Pine (Eds.), *Gastrointestinal pathology an atlas and text* (p. 268). Philadelphia: Lippincott Williams & Wilkins.

Fenoglio-Preiser, C. M., Noffsinger, A. E., Stemmermann, G. N., Lantz, P. E., & Isaacson, P. G. (2008b). Epithelial tumors of the small intestine. In J. McGouh & J. Pine (Eds.), *Gastrointestinal pathology an atlas and text* (pp. 486–487). Philadelphia: Lippincott Williams & Wilkins.

Fenoglio-Preiser, C. M., Noffsinger, A. E., Stemmermann, G. N., Lantz, P. E., & Isaacson, P. G. (2008c). Epithelial neoplasms of the colon. In J. McGouh & J. Pine (Eds.), *Gastrointestinal pathology an atlas and text* (pp. 982–983). Philadelphia: Lippincott Williams & Wilkins.

Glickman, J. N., & Odze, R. D. (2009). Epithelial neoplasms of the esophagus. In R. Odze & J. Goldblum (Eds.), *Surgical pathology of the GI tract, liver, biliary tract and pancreas*. Philadelphia: Saunders.

Harada, M., Inoue, T., & Hamano, K. (2012). Choriocarcinoma of the sigmoid colon: Report of a case. *Surgery Today, 42*(1), 93–96.

Iyomasa, S., Senda, Y., Mizuno, K., et al. (2003). Primary choriocarcinoma of the jejunum: Report of a case. *Surgery Today, 33*(12), 948–951.

Kobayashi, A., Hasebe, T., Endo, Y., et al. (2005). Primary gastric choriocarcinoma: Two case reports and a pooled analysis of 53 cases. *Gastric Cancer, 8*(3), 178–185.

Noffsinger, A. (2009). Epithelial neoplasms of the small intestine. In R. Odze & J. Goldblum (Eds.), *Surgical pathology of the GI tract, liver, biliary tract and pancreas*. Philadelphia: Saunders.

Chronic Gastritis

Chella R. S. van der Post[1] and Fátima Carneiro[2]
[1]Department of Pathology, Radboud University Medical Center, Nijmegen, The Netherlands
[2]Faculty of Medicine of Porto University, Centro Hospitalar São João and Ipatimup/i3S, Porto, Portugal

Synonyms

Campylobacter pylori gastritis; Chronic antral gastritis; Diffuse antral gastritis; Helicobacter pylori gastritis; Multifocal gastritis; Superficial gastritis; Type B gastritis

Definition

Chronic gastritis refers to chronic inflammatory diseases of the stomach, which range from mild superficial involvement of the gastric mucosa to severe atrophy. Generally, chronic atrophic gastritis is divided into Autoimmune Metaplastic Atrophic Gastritis (AMAG) or type A gastritis and Environmental Metaplastic Atrophic Gastritis (EMAG) or type B gastritis mostly caused by *Helicobacter pylori* infection. This entry discusses especially EMAG/chronic *H. pylori* associated gastritis; for AMAG, the reader is referred to the entry ▶ "autoimmune gastritis." ▶ *H. pylori* gastritis is a chronic infectious form of gastritis caused by spiral, flagellated gram-negative rods and characterized by superficial chronic active gastritis.

Clinical Features

H. pylori infection is probably the most common cause of chronic environmental gastritis; most people acquire *H. pylori* infection during childhood. Symptoms of chronic *H. pylori* gastritis include abdominal pain, nausea, vomiting, dyspepsia, weight loss, iron deficiency anemia, and ulcer-related bleeding (melena).

Transmission of infection is human to human, with poor sanitary conditions and overcrowding being risk factors. Infection leads to a 15–20% lifetime risk of developing peptic ulcer disease. Other risks of *H. pylori* infection include gastric cancer and gastric mucosa–associated lymphoid tissue (MALT) lymphoma. Various dietary factors such as excessive salt, smoked food, lack of green vegetables and fruits, and nitrites and nitrosamines may also cause environmental metaplastic atrophic gastritis.

- **Incidence**
  The incidence is variable and more prevalent in areas endemic for *H. pylori* infection. *H. pylori* gastritis is an universal infection which is estimated to affect half up to two-thirds of the world's population. In many developing countries, the prevalence of *H. pylori* infection in adults approaches 90%. The prevalence of *H. pylori* infection and subsequently gastric ulcer disease and gastric cancer has been steadily declining in Western countries. In the East, however, large proportions of the population still acquire *H. pylori* infection in early childhood. Despite declining rates of *H. pylori* infection in general, the prevalence rate of *H. pylori* in patients who undergo endoscopy remains significant. The incidence rate of chronic atrophic gastritis is up to 10.9%, depending on the patient groups investigated. The highest incidence rate of chronic atrophic gastritis was observed in patients with ulcer disease and/or *H. pylori* infection.
- **Age**
  There is a high prevalence rate of infection in children, indicating that exposure to the bacterium probably occurs relatively early in life. The early phase of *H. pylori* infection causes an acute inflammatory response that is usually asymptomatic. Chronic atrophic gastritis and intestinal metaplasia are more often observed above 45 years. In Japan, atrophy appears already in patients aged 30–40 years. Atrophic gastritis develops approximately 20 years after the *H. pylori* acquisition and prevalence increases with age.
- **Sex**
  No sex predilection
- **Site**
  Predominantly, the antrum is affected with extension to the corpus; inflammation, atrophy, and intestinal metaplasia can be multifocal. Infrequently, some *H. pylori*–infected individuals show a corpus-predominant pattern that overlaps with autoimmune gastritis and lymphocytic gastritis.
- **Treatment**
  The best treatment option of *H. pylori* infection is proton-pump inhibitor–based triple therapy combining a proton-pump inhibitor combined with two antibiotics: clarithromycin (or another macrolide), a nitroimidazole (metronidazole or tinidazole), or amoxycillin. One-week triple therapy cures 85–95% of infected patients.
- **Outcome**
  H. pylori gastritis can lead to ulcer-related bleeding in the stomach, and is associated with gastric lymphoma and carcinoma. Chronic atrophic gastritis is considered a precursor condition of gastric carcinoma. *H. pylori*–related gastritis in the antrum is also a risk factor for duodenal ulcer.

Macroscopy

Endoscopic findings are variable and depend on the stage and type of gastritis. The antrum is predominantly affected, while the body is relatively spared. Multiple foci first appear in the incisura angularis, the transition zone between antrum and body. Various endoscopic findings include gastric mucosal erythema or hyperemia, erosions, atrophy, and hypertrophy with granularity and nodularity. The endoscopic appearance may even be normal, placing emphasis on the value of histological examination for *H. pylori* gastritis or by detection of urease in mucosal specimens by the CLO test or urea breath test.

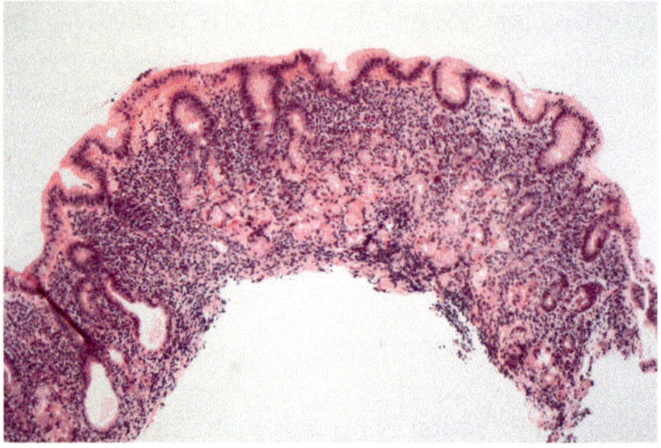

Chronic Gastritis, Fig. 1 Chronic active gastritis in a patient with *H. pylori* infection. There is a dense plasma lymphocytic infiltrate admixed with neutrophilic inflammation and gradual loss of glands

Microscopy

H. pylori gastritis is a chronic infectious form of gastritis caused by spiral, flagellated gram-negative rods and classically characterized by superficial chronic active gastritis. *H. pylori* organisms can be found especially in the mucous layer covering the gastric mucosa in both the corpus and antrum. Sporadically, the organisms can be present in biopsies of the cardia. Often, surface erosions and ulcers are present. Epithelial changes include irregularity and degeneration of epithelial cells with a reduction in the mucin content of the cytoplasm, an increase in nuclear size, and presence of one or more prominent nucleoli. Bacterial toxins, such as Vac A and Cag A, urease, ammonia, acetaldehyde, and phospholipases that have a direct effect on epithelial cells, cause these changes. At the base of the foveolae, there is an increased mitotic activity, reflecting a more rapid cell turnover. Features of epithelial damage and regeneration are not specific; they appear in biopsies of all forms of gastritis and reactive chemical gastropathy.

H. pylori gastritis is characterized by an infiltrate of neutrophils and mononuclear cells in the superficial portion of the mucosa. In all cases of active *H. pylori* gastritis, neutrophilic activity is present; however, sometimes, multiple biopsies have to be examined to detect focal infiltration (Fig. 1). The neutrophils can be observed in the lamina propria, with prominent infiltration in the surface epithelium and pits with formation of crypt abscesses. The amount and density of intraepithelial neutrophils is correlated with the extent of mucosal damage and *H. pylori* infection. Neutrophilic infiltrate will dissolve after successful treatment of *H. pylori*. Eosinophils are often observed in biopsies, but their pathogenetic role is unknown. In *H. pylori* gastritis, the chronic cellular infiltrate contains an increase in CD4+ and CD8+ T-lymphocytes, B-lymphocytes, plasma cells, monocytes, and mast cells. The superficial gastric stroma normally contains some chronic inflammatory cells, and it may be difficult to assess whether the amount of inflammatory cells are normal or increased; there is no simple satisfactory method of objective measurement though a maximum has been defined of 2–5 lymphocytes, plasma cells, and macrophages per high power field. Especially the presence of plasma cells is an important indicator of an inflammatory response, since plasma cells are sparse or absent in the gastric mucosa of healthy persons. Chronic inflammation disappears slowly after eradication therapy of *H. pylori*, and it may take over a year to see a marked decrease in the chronic inflammatory infiltrate (Fig. 2). In a later stage of chronic gastritis, the inflammation spreads deeply to involve the whole thickness of the mucosa with the formation of prominent lymphoid follicles especially in the region of the angulus. These lymphoid aggregates with germinal centers are characteristic of chronic *H. pylori* gastritis. The presence of a dense population of lymphocytes with infiltration in the epithelium should raise

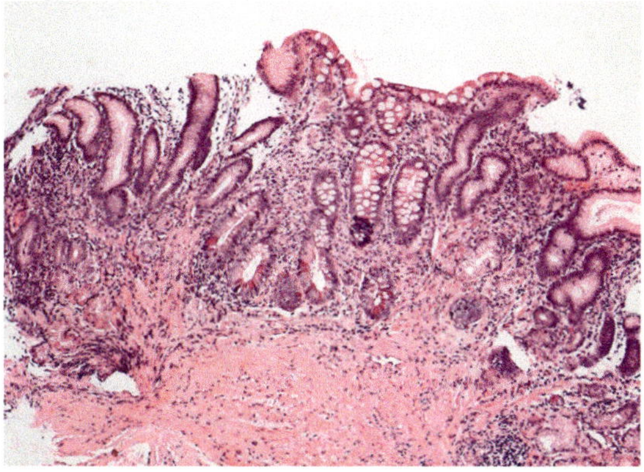

Chronic Gastritis, Fig. 2 Biopsy shows chronic gastritis with plasma cells and lymphocytes. There is intestinal metaplasia and atrophy of the corpus typical for environmental atrophic metaplastic gastritis

the suspicion of a mucosa-associated lymphoid tissue (MALT) lymphoma.

Other features of chronic gastritis include atrophy, defined as loss of glandular tissue with thinning of the mucosa and intestinal metaplasia. The loss of glands may follow erosion or ulceration of the mucosa or may result from prolonged inflammation where individual glands undergo destruction. Normally, three to four antral gland cross sections are observed; in the case of atrophy, this is reduced to two or fewer cross sections. Glands with a pyloric appearance, indicated as fundic antralization or spasmolytic polypeptide expressing metaplasia (SPEM), replace the native glands in the corpus. Discriminating between pseudopyloric and true antropyloric glands can be difficult. Pseudopyloric glands differ from true pyloric glands in that pseudopyloric glands do not possess G cells, which can be confirmed using an immunostain for gastrin. Furthermore, pseudopyloric glands contain both pepsinogens I and II whereas true antral glands show only pepsinogen II. Atrophy is often accompanied by intestinal metaplasia, characterized by the presence of goblet cells and absorptive cells. Intestinal metaplasia has been categorized into complete and incomplete forms. With the use of histochemistry for mucin, intestinal metaplasia has been divided into three main types according to morphology and glycoprotein content with variable risk for development of gastric cancer. In 1–2% of gastric biopsies, pancreatic metaplasia is detected; pancreatic acinar-like cells are characterized by abundant cytoplasm, acidophilic and finely granular in the apical and middle portions and basophilic in the basal compartment, arranged in nests or lobules among gastric glands. The presence of pancreatic metaplasia is associated with intestinal metaplasia and chronic gastritis; its significance remains unclear.

Chronic non-*H. pylori*–related gastritis can be caused by long-term use of proton-pump inhibitors and antibiotics. Both can reduce or suppress inflammation or infection, resulting in the absence of *H. pylori* organisms. The organisms may be focal and sparse and not easily identified in biopsies.

The updated Sydney-Houston System guidelines can be used to generate systematic, uniform diagnostic reports when a full set of biopsy specimens is available of patients with gastritis. A grading system for the morphological variables is useful in the evaluation to translate the histological observation into well-defined topographic patterns or for comparison purposes. The features, graded into mild, moderate, and marked, include the amount of *H. pylori* organisms, neutrophils, mononuclear cells, atrophy in the antrum and corpus, and intestinal metaplasia. Diagnoses related to chronic gastritis generated according to the recommendations of the updated Sydney System include chronic active antrum-predominant *H. pylori* gastritis, chronic active corpus-predominant *H. pylori* gastritis, chronic active *H. pylori* nonatrophic pangastritis, and chronic active *H. pylori* multifocal atrophic gastritis. However, in routine practice, only one or two gastric biopsies are provided and the Sydney system cannot be applied.

Although updated Sydney-Houston System guidelines brought some uniformity, they do not provide information about gastric cancer risk. The recently established OLGA staging system (Operative Link for Gastritis Assessment) aims to translate the histopathological data into a standardized report with information on the gastric condition (topography and extent of the atrophic changes) and sub-grouping of patients by cancer risk

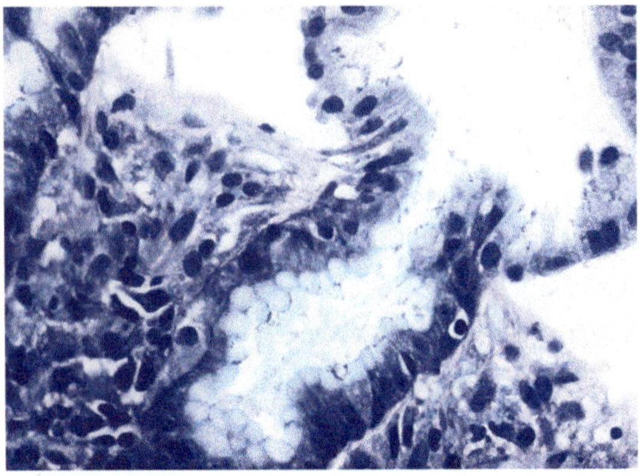

Chronic Gastritis, Fig. 3 Modified Giemsa highlights the slightly curved wing-shaped *H. pylori* organisms in the gastric pits and lining the foveolar epithelium

using the Sydney-Houston five biopsy protocol. The gastritis stage results from the combinations of the atrophy score (at the single biopsy level) with the atrophy topography (as obtained by gastric mapping). Another proposed classification system used intestinal metaplasia as a phenotypic marker of atrophy (OLGIM – Operative Link on Gastric Intestinal Metaplasia Assessment).

Immunophenotype

H. pylori organisms may be identified on hematoxylin and eosin (H&E); however, often additional stains are used to identify or confirm their presence, such as a modified Giemsa or an immunostain for *H. pylori* (Fig. 3). Special stains are particularly useful in detecting coccoid forms of *H. pylori*. Alcian-blue and periodic acid Schiff stain can be useful to demonstrate (focal) intestinal metaplasia. For the suspicion of atrophy in the corpus, gastrin stains can be used.

Molecular Features

Molecular tests to discover *H. pylori* organisms include a polymerase chain reaction (PCR)-based detection of *H. pylori* using various genetic targets such as 23S ribosome, Vac A, urea, and Cag A gene.

Differential Diagnosis

– Focally enhanced gastritis is seen in patients with Crohn's disease.
– Autoimmune gastritis: The antrum is normal in autoimmune gastritis, which is not the case in EMAG. The corpus shows atrophy with a marked reduction of oxyntic glands, intestinal metaplasia, and enterochromaffin-like (ECL) cell hyperplasia. Unlike in autoimmune gastritis, the gastrin level in chronic *H. pylori* associated gastritis is low or normal.
– Organisms that cause *Helicobacter heilmanii*-gastritis are longer, spiraled, and less tightly adherent to surface foveolar cells than *H. pylori*. It is responsible for circa 0.3% of cases and treatment is equal to *H. pylori* gastritis.
– The lymphoid hyperplasia in *H. pylori* gastritis can raise suspicion for low-grade MALT lymphoma. The infiltrate in MALT lymphoma extends below the muscularis mucosae, while *H. pylori* gastritis causes predominantly superficial inflammation. Immunostains for CD20 and CD3 demonstrate a reactive pattern in *H. pylori* gastritis consisting of mixed T- and B-lymphocytes.

References and Further Reading

Capelle, L. G., de Vries, A. C., Haringsma, J., Ter Borg, F., de Vries, R. A., Bruno, M. J., et al. (2010). The staging of gastritis with the OLGA system by using intestinal metaplasia as an accurate alternative for atrophic gastritis. *Gastrointestinal Endoscopy, 71*, 1150–1158.

Dixon, M. F., Genta, R. M., Yardley, J. H., & Correa, P. (1996). Classification and grading of gastritis. The updated Sydney System. International Workshop on the Histopathology of Gastritis, Houston 1994. *The American Journal of Surgical Pathology, 20*(10), 1161–1181.

Odze, R. D., & Goldblum, J. R. (2009). *Surgical pathology of the GI tract, liver, biliary tract, and pancreas* (2nd ed.). Philadelphia: Saunders/Elsevier.

Rocha, G. A., Queiroz, D. M., Mendes, E. N., Barbosa, A. J., Lima Junior, G. F., & Oliveira, C. A. (1991). *Helicobacter pylori* acute gastritis: Histological, endoscopical, clinical, and therapeutic features. *The American Journal of Gastroenterology, 86*(11), 1592–1595.

Rugge, M., & Genta, R. M. (2005). Staging and grading of chronic gastritis. *Human Pathology, 36*(3), 228–233.

Rugge, M., Correa, P., Di Mario, F., El-Omar, E., Fiocca, R., Geboes, K., et al. (2008). OLGA staging for gastritis: A tutorial. *Digestive and Liver Disease, 40*, 650–658.

Sipponen, P. (2001). Update on the pathologic approach to the diagnosis of gastritis, gastric atrophy, and Helicobacter pylori and its sequelae. *Journal of Clinical Gastroenterology, 32*(3), 196–202.

C-Kit (CD117), Gastrointestinal Stromal Tumors (GISTs)

José Manuel Lopes
Faculty of Medicine of the University of Porto and Institute of Molecular Pathology and Immunology of the University of Porto, Porto, Portugal

Synonyms

CD117; C-Kit synonyms include C-Kit; Mast/stem cell growth factor receptor Kit; p145 c-kit; PBT; Piebald trait protein; Proto-oncogene c-Kit; Proto-oncogene tyrosine-protein kinase Kit; SCFR; Soluble KIT variant 1; Tyrosine-protein kinase Kit; v-kit Hardy-Zuckerman 4 feline sarcoma viral oncogene-like protein

Definition

C-Kit (CD117) is an antibody that identifies the C-Kit protein.

Molecule Type and Chemical Structure

C-Kit belongs to the type III receptor tyrosine kinase (RTK) subfamily, whose members include platelet-derived growth factor receptors α and β (PDGFRα and PDGFRβ) (Roskoski 2005). All type III RTKs contain five immunoglobulin-like domains in their extracellular ligand-binding region followed by a single transmembrane domain and a cytoplasmic tyrosine kinase domain interrupted by a large kinase insert. The ligand of KIT is known as stem cell factor. *C-Kit* (the gene) is transcribed and ultimately translated into the KIT protein, a transmembrane receptor tyrosine kinase. CD117 is an antigenic marker of the KIT protein. As for other RTKs, stem cell factor induces dimerization of KIT followed by transautophosphorylation of the cytoplasmic tyrosine kinase domain, leading to activation of multiple signaling pathways, such as the PI3K (phosphoinositide 3-kinase)/AKT (serine-/threonine-specific protein kinase B) and mitogen-activated protein kinase pathways but seemingly not c-Jun N-terminal kinase or STAT (signal transducer and activator of transcription) pathways.

Physiological Relevance and Function

C-Kit belongs to the PDGF (platelet-derived growth factor)/C-Kit receptor tyrosine kinase family. C-Kit is a transmembrane tyrosine kinase normally expressed by Cajal interstitial cells (Fig. 1), melanocytes, mast cells, and germ cells. Intact signal transduction by C-Kit is crucial for the development and survival of germ cells, hematopoietic stem cells, melanocytes, mast cells, and interstitial cells of Cajal. In normal physiology the C-Kit ligand (also known as stem cell factor) binds to the extracellular domain of the C-Kit protein, resulting in receptor homodimerization and phosphorylation of critical tyrosine residues

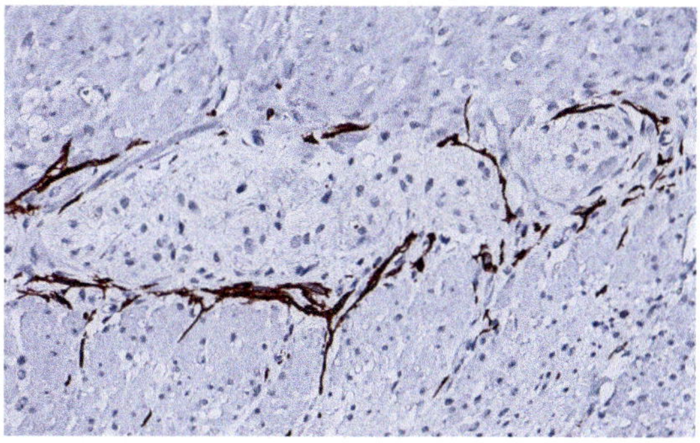

C-Kit (CD117), Gastrointestinal Stromal Tumors (GISTs), Fig. 1 Expression of CD117 in Cajal interstitial cells

in the intracellular portion of C-Kit, thus leading to downstream phosphorylation of intracellular substrates that results in activation of the Janus-associated tyrosine kinase/signal transducers and activators of transcription (JAK/STAT), phosphoinositide 3-kinase (PI3K), and mitogen-activated protein kinase (MAPK) pathways important in cell growth and differentiation.

Relevance for Pathology

A critical understanding of the molecular pathogenesis of GIST (gastrointestinal stromal tumor) came from a study (Hirota et al. 1998) which first reported activating mutations of the *C-Kit* proto-oncogene in GISTs. The classification and diagnosis of GISTs radically changed with the recognition of the *C-Kit* proto-oncogene mutation as the key molecular event in GISTs.

CD117 (cluster differentiation molecule 117) stains approximately 95% of GISTs and the expression is ligand independent. CD117 immunoreactivity in GISTs is typically strong and uniformly positive in a cytoplasmic pattern (Fig. 2), although a membranous pattern of staining can be seen (Fig. 3). Additionally, approximately 50% of GISTs can show a dot-like pattern of expression (Fig. 4); these tumors are more likely to be extra-intestinal in location and may show an epithelioid pattern of growth. The absence of CD117 staining in GISTs occurs in approximately 5% of the cases and may associate with a mutated platelet-derived growth receptor-alpha (*PDGFR-A*) gene. These CD117-negative GISTs typically have an epithelioid morphology and occur in the omentum or peritoneum. The markers for PDGFR-A and DOG1 (discovered in GIST 1) were reported to have high sensitivity and specificity in the diagnosis of C-Kit-negative GISTs (Wong 2011).

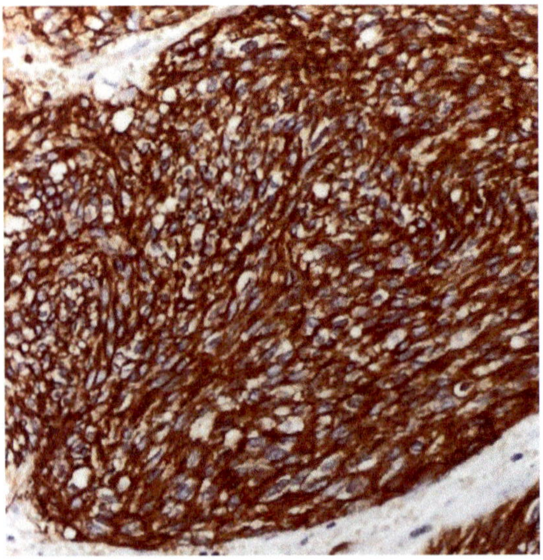

C-Kit (CD117), Gastrointestinal Stromal Tumors (GISTs), Fig. 2 CD117 cytoplasm expression in GIST tumor cells

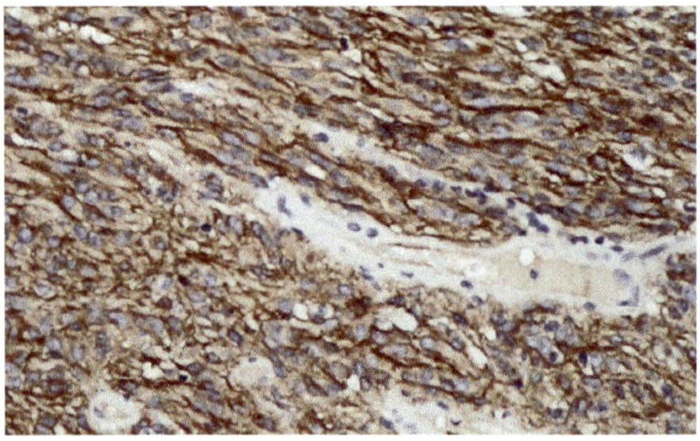

C-Kit (CD117), Gastrointestinal Stromal Tumors (GISTs), Fig. 3 CD117 membrane and cytoplasm expression in GIST tumor cells

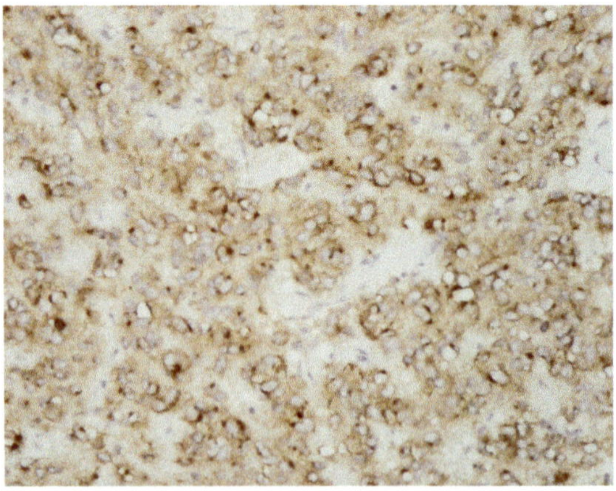

C-Kit (CD117), Gastrointestinal Stromal Tumors (GISTs), Fig. 4 Dot-like expression of CD117 in tumor paranuclear GIST cells

CD117 immunoreactivity is not restricted to GISTs and has been reported in a number of other neoplasms including melanoma, mastocytosis, renal cell carcinoma, and germ cell tumors. Sarcomas that have been reported to stain with C-Kit include angiosarcoma, clear cell sarcoma, Ewing sarcoma/primitive neuroectodermal tumor, neuroblastoma, and Kaposi sarcoma; very focal CD117 staining can be seen in retroperitoneal leiomyosarcomas and liposarcomas. Intra-abdominal desmoid-type fibromatosis may display minimal cytoplasmic staining in up to 5% of the cases.

The vast majority of GISTs are characterized by gain-of-function mutations in *C-Kit*, which lead to constitutive, uncontrolled activation of the receptor signaling cascade and resultant unchecked cell growth. Gain-of-function *C-Kit* mutations have been identified in several different "hot spots" in the gene, most in exon 11 (coding the justamembranar intracellular regulatory region) and then in exon 9 (coding the extracellular ligand-binding region) and exon 13 (coding an intracellular tyrosine kinase region), which results in constitutive activation of the C-Kit receptor and is thought to promote proliferation and/or decrease apoptosis. Approximately 5% of GISTs harbor mutations in the gene encoding the homologous receptor tyrosine kinase PDGF receptor-α (PDGFRA), most in exon 18. Most of GISTs display C-Kit or platelet-derived growth factor alpha (PDGFR-A) mutations. Approximately 5–10% of GISTs have no identifiable mutation in either the *C-Kit* or *PDGFRA* gene and are classified as "wild-type" GISTs; nearly all pediatric GISTs are wild type.

Although *C-Kit* gene mutations almost always result in CD117 immunoreactivity, CD117-positive lesions do not invariably indicate a *C-Kit* mutation. For example, approximately 25% of neurofibromatosis type I (NF1) patients develop GISTs that stain with CD117 and CD34 (cluster differentiation molecule 34) but lack *C-Kit* gene mutations. Instead, these lesions have the typical NF1 (17q11.2) gene mutations that are found in NF1-associated neurofibromas.

C-Kit is a transmembrane glycoprotein receptor tyrosine kinase with homologies to the platelet-derived growth factor (PDGF) and granulocyte-macrophage colony-stimulating factor (GM-CSF) receptors, making it a recent favorite target of molecular therapy with the, so far, approved small molecules (imatinib and sunitinib) that are tyrosine kinase inhibitors (Lennartsson and Rönnstrand 2006; Corless et al. 2011). Imatinib inhibits phosphorylation of the C-Kit in GIST and analogous molecules in other conditions, the bcr (breakpoint cluster region protein)/abl (named for a researcher whose last name was Abelson) gene kinase product of the t (9; 22) transformation in chronic myeloid leukemia and of *PDGFRβ* mutation in dermatofibrosarcoma protuberans. Response of GISTs to imatinib may be predicted based on the presence of exon-specific mutations in the *C-Kit* gene. Patients with tumors harboring exon 11 *C-Kit* mutations have better response rate compared with response rates of those with exon 9 mutations. Patients with no detectable *C-Kit* or *PDGFRα* mutation usually demonstrate no response to imatinib and may respond to sunitinib treatment. Patients with exon 11 mutations pursue longer progression-free survival times than other patients. The mechanisms of acquired resistance to imatinib include secondary mutations in exon 17 of *C-Kit* and may predict outcome in response to sunitinib, a second-line treatment approved for patients with intolerance or (primary/secondary) resistance to imatinib treatment of GISTs.

References and Further Reading

Corless, C. L., Barnett, C. M., & Heinrich, M. C. (2011). Gastrointestinal stromal tumours: Origin and molecular oncology. *Nature Reviews Cancer*, doi:10.1038/nr3143.

Hirota, S., Isozaki, K., Moriyama, Y., Hashimoto, K., Nishida, T., Ishiguro, S., Kawano, K., Hanada, M., Kurata, A., Takeda, M., Muhammad, T. G., Matsuzawa, Y., Kanakura, Y., Shinomura, Y., & Kitamura, Y. (1998). Gain-of-function mutations of c-kit in human gastrointestinal stromal tumors. *Science, 279*, 577–580.

Lennartsson, J., & Rönnstrand, L. (2006). The stem cell factor receptor/c-Kit as a drug target in cancer. *Current Cancer Drug Targets, 6*, 561–571.

Roskoski, R. (2005). Structure and regulation of Kit protein-tyrosine kinase – The stem cell factor receptor. *Biochemical and Biophysical Research Communications, 338*, 1307–1315.
Wong, N. A. C. S. (2011). Gastrointestinal stromal tumours – An update for histopathologists. *Histopathology, 59*, 807–821.

Coeliac Disease

Arzu Ensari
Department of Pathology, Ankara University Medical School, Sihhiye, Ankara, Turkey

Synonyms

Coeliac sprue; Gluten-induced enteropathy or gluten-sensitive enteropathy (GSE); Nontropical sprue

Definition

Coeliac disease (CD) is a chronic inflammatory disorder of the small intestine characterized by malabsorption after ingestion of wheat gluten or related proteins in rye (secalins) and barley (hordeins) in individuals with a certain genetic background. The pathogenesis involves a T cell-mediated immune response and autoreactive B lymphocytes that produce autoantibodies directed against gliadin, endomysium, or tissue transglutaminase in individuals with a genetic susceptibility related to HLA-DQ2 and HLA-DQ8. The diagnostic scheme of GSE consists of clinical history and symptomatology, HLA subtyping, serologic testing (tTG, EMA, and AGA), histological findings in proximal small intestinal biopsy, and clinical and serological (optionally histological) response to a GFD.

Clinical Features

- **Incidence**
  Current estimates show that the incidence is at 0.5–1% in wheat-eating populations such as Western Europe and North America, while the incidence continues to rise in Eastern societies, possibly, as a result of "western-style" eating habits.
- **Age**
  The mean age of diagnosis is in middle adulthood.
- **Sex**
  Coeliac disease is diagnosed in women more often than in men. The estimated male to female ratio is 1:3.2.
- **Site**
  The damage to the small intestinal mucosa classically involves the proximal small intestine including duodenum and upper jejunum and extends distally for a variable length into the ileum. Currently, many investigators believe that CD can exhibit a patchy distribution; that is, areas with villous flattening may occur in proximity to areas with mild villous shortening and also areas with normal histology, particularly, in pediatric patients.
- **Treatment**
  The treatment of CD involves the exclusion of the antigen from the diet. Lifelong gluten-free diet is the only way to treat these patients. Following treatment, clinical remission can be restored within few months, while healing of the small bowel mucosa may take at least 6 months and may even prolong up to 24 months after treatment with GFD.
- **Outcome**
  Patients with incomplete or no response to GFD are considered within the context of refractory sprue. Diagnosis of refractory sprue is rarely made and should be strictly limited to patients with clinical features of CD not responding to GFD for at least 6 months. It can be either primary, as lack of initial response to diet, or secondary, as unresponsiveness to diet in the form of a relapse. Primary refractory sprue can include many different pathologic conditions mimicking CD, comprising collagenous sprue, ulcerative jejunitis, lymphocytic colitis, collagenous colitis, and EITCL. Patients with long-standing malabsorption can develop EITCL as the most frequent fearsome complication of CD. They usually suffer from severe malabsorption refractory to GFD,

causing weight loss and complications such as perforations, bleeding due to ulcerative lesions. Histopathologically, the mucosa is flat with ulcerations. An atypical population of neoplastic lymphocytes infiltrate the mucosa. Lymphoma cells are pleomorphic large cells that are double-negative (CD8− and CD4−) with cell surface markers but almost always positive with CD30 which is also associated with poor prognosis. Patients with CD have a more than 30-fold increased risk of developing adenocarcinoma of the small bowel compared to general population.

Macroscopy (Endoscopy)

In most patients with flat mucosa, the duodenum shows typical endoscopic features described as mosaic appearance, scalloping, or reduction of duodenal folds.

Microscopy

Histologic evidence of CD depends on abnormalities in either architecture (villous shortening and crypt hyperplasia) or the number of IELs or both. In its classical form, CD results in shortened, widened villi or even totally flat mucosa with hyperplastic crypts. Overall thickness of the mucosa remains relatively unchanged, but villous/crypt ratio (normally, 3:1 in distal duodenum and 2:1 in bulbus) decreases as the villi become shortened. These architectural changes are preceded by an increase in the number of IELs over the normal numbers, corresponding to the cell-mediated immune nature of the disorder. The normal upper limit of IELs is accepted as 20 lymphocytes/100 enterocytes (a ratio of 1 IEL per 5 enterocytes) in H&E sections, whereas 25 IELs/100 enterocytes (or a ratio of 1:4) in CD3 immunostained slides are considered as the upper limit of normal. There is a heterogenous population of inflammatory cells in the lamina propria comprising plasma cells which locally produce AGA and EMA antibodies, T cells which include predominantly helper T cells, as well as few cytotoxic cells, neutrophils, eosinophils, and mast cells found in varying numbers. However, none of these changes is specific to CD, and IELosis with architectural changes effecting villous to crypt ratio remains as the main diagnostic parameters.

Marsh classification is being used to grade mucosal damage in CD comprising (i) infiltrative lesion (Figs. 1 and 2), increased IELs in the villus epithelium in an otherwise normal mucosa with normal villous/crypt ratio (Marsh type 1); (ii) hyperplastic lesion, crypt hyperplasia with normal villi showing increased IELs (Marsh type 2); (iii) destructive lesion (Figs. 3 and 4), flat mucosa with crypt hyperplasia and increased IEL (Marsh type 3); and (iv) atrophic lesion, flat mucosa with crypt

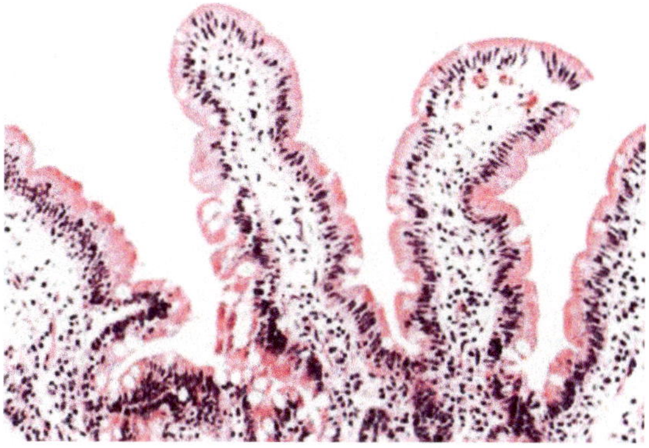

Coeliac Disease, Fig. 1 Duodenal mucosa with normal villi showing IELosis (H&E; ×100)

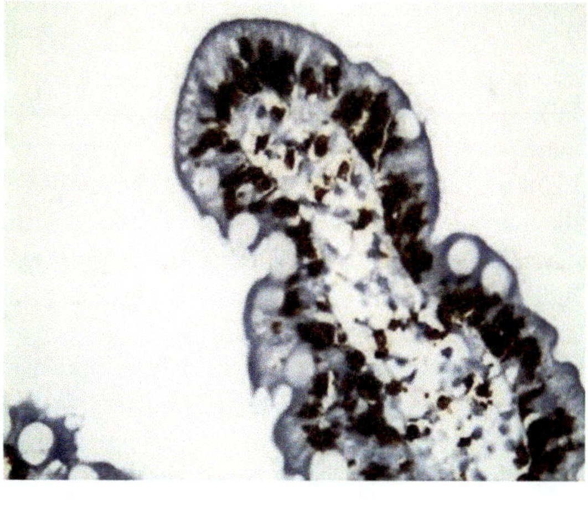

Coeliac Disease, Fig. 2 Normal villus with T lymphocytic infiltration in the epithelium (anti-CD3 IHC; ×200)

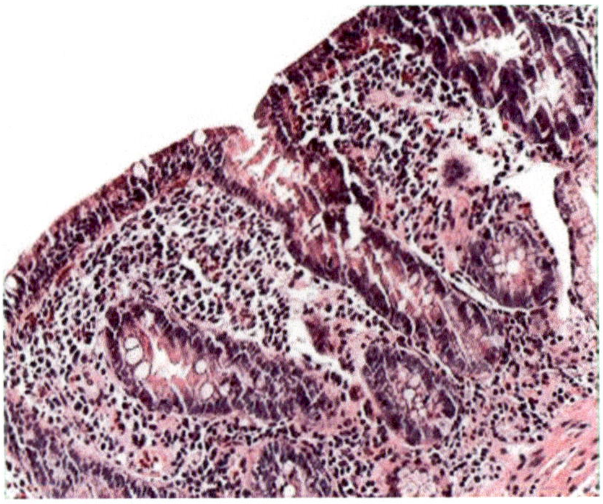

Coeliac Disease, Fig. 3 Flat mucosa with IELosis (H&E; ×200)

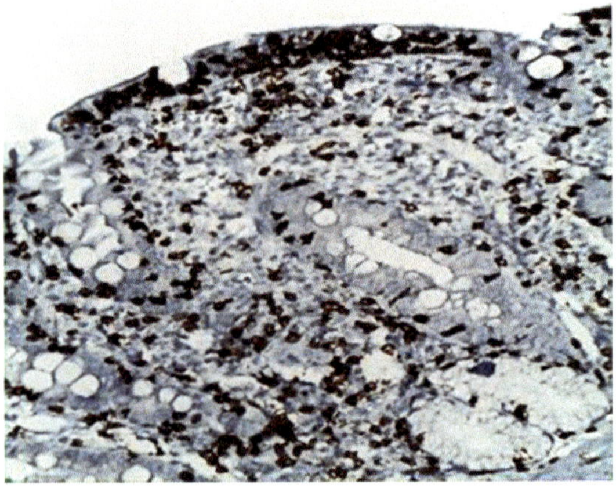

Coeliac Disease, Fig. 4 T lymphocytic infiltration of surface epithelium in flat mucosa (anti-CD3 IHC; ×200)

hypoplasia and mild inflammation (Marsh type IV). It is usually observed in refractory sprue patients or patients who develop enteropathy-induced T cell lymphoma (EITCL). The cutoff for the number of IELs has not been defined in Marsh classification. The updated classification proposed by Oberhuber et al. has indicated that 40 IELs/100 enterocytes should be the cutoff point for normal, a figure possibly derived from jejunal mucosal biopsies which used to be taken previously for the diagnosis of CD. They have also subgrouped type 3 flat mucosa into three grades (grades 3A, 3B, and 3C) with regard to the severity of villous atrophy. This classification has the potential to cause significant reproducibility problems leading to increased intra- and interobserver variations due to the greater number of diagnostic categories. Later, a new and relatively simpler classification was proposed by Corazza and Villanaci, in which lesions characterizing CD should be classified as non-atrophic (grade A) and atrophic (grade B) and that grade B lesions should be split into grade B1, characterized by a villous/crypt ratio <3/1, while B2 is characterized by completely flat mucosa with no detectable villi. Table 1 summarizes the classification schemes of CD. In 2010 Ensari proposed a simpler classification scheme based on the original Marsh classification in which types 1 and 3 were identical to original Marsh, namely intraepithelial lymphocytosis and flat mucosa, respectively, while type 2 was redefined as mucosa with (any degree of) villous shortening and crypt hyperplasia as well as intraepithelial lymphocytosis.

There is a group of patients with evidence of gluten sensitivity but without full-blown symptoms of sprue. Terms that have been applied to such cases include latent, subclinical, silent, or occult CD, gluten-sensitive disease with mild enteropathy, low-grade enteropathy, minimally symptomatic enteropathy, and potential CD. This form of CD is characterized by the presence of no or only mild changes in the proximal small intestinal mucosa, but in recent years, mucosal expression of tTG-specific IgA molecules as a subepithelial band has been demonstrated in such cases by immunofluorescence microscopy on fresh frozen tissue.

Immunophenotype

The vast majority of IELs are T lymphocytes, which are mostly cytotoxic T cells expressing $\alpha\beta$ TCR on their surface. The population specifically expanded in GSE is the CD3+/CD4−/CD8−, $\gamma\delta$ TCR-bearing IELs, which is only 5% of the total in normal mucosa.

Molecular Features

No molecular feature is reported.

Coeliac Disease, Table 1 Classification of CD

Marsh 1992	Oberhuber et al. 1999	Corazza & Villanaci 2005	Ensari 2010
Type 0	-	-	
Type 1 →	Type 1	Grade A →	Type 1
Type 2 →	Type 2		
Type 3 →	Type 3a	Grade B1	Type 2
	Type 3b		
	Type 3c →	Grade B2 →	Type 3
Type 4 →	Type 4	-	

Differential Diagnosis

Differential diagnosis of CD involves a great variety of disorders with architectural abnormalities and/or IELosis (see Table 2). Complete villous flattening usually indicates coeliac disease when coexisting crypt hyperplasia is present. However, there are some other entities which may cause villous flattening and crypt hyperplasia other than coeliac disease. The majority of disorders causing malabsorption, on the other hand, produce mild to moderate villus blunting and crypt hyperplasia without any specific diagnostic feature. Moreover, the recognition of mild villous blunting is a difficult task due to biopsy artifacts such as improper orientation of the biopsy, shallow biopsies which lack muscularis mucosae. The accompanying lamina propria inflammation and/or intraepithelial lymphocytosis should always be searched for before making a diagnosis. Pathologists can also be faced with a patient with malabsorption or chronic diarrhea and a biopsy that appears normal or near-normal architecturally on microscopy. In the presence of IEL increase, there are some disorders that can be diagnosed on light microscopy with very careful examination. In the absence of an appropriate clinical history, a number of additional entities can enter in the differential diagnosis of coeliac disease based on the histologic features, including tropical sprue, bacterial overgrowth syndrome, and various drug toxicities such as colchicine. In tropical sprue, the characteristic histology results from a postinfectious enteritis. A travel history and serologic studies for infectious microorganisms may help determine the possibility. In bacterial overgrowth in addition to villous atrophy, the degree of active inflammation of the villi and

Coeliac Disease, Table 2 Conditions that are included in the differential diagnosis of GSE

IELosis	Villous shortening/ flattening
HP-associated gastroduodenitis	Microvillus inclusion disease (MID)
Non-gluten food hypersensitivity	Autoimmune enteropathy
Infections	Tropical sprue
Bacterial overgrowth	Refractory sprue
Drugs (primarily NSAIDs)	Collagenous sprue
IgA deficiency	Radiochemotherapy
Common variable immunodeficiency	Graft versus host disease (GVHD)
Crohn's disease	Nutritional deficiencies
Small bowel allograft rejection	EITCL

crypts is more severe than coeliac disease. A prior history of surgery may be found in these patients. In some patients receiving colchicine treatment, features simulating coeliac disease can be seen. The histologic features comprise of ring mitoses and loss of goblet cell polarity.

References and Further Reading

Corazza, G. R., & Villanaci, V. (2005). Coeliac disease. *Journal of Clinical Pathology, 58*, 573–574.

Dickson, B. C., Streutker, C. J., & Chetty, R. (2006). Coeliac disease: An update for pathologists. *Journal of Clinical Pathology, 59*, 1008–1016.

Ensari, A. (2010). Gluten-sensitive enteropathy (celiac disease): Controversies in diagnosis and classification. *Archives of Pathology & Laboratory Medicine, 134*, 826–836.

Kurppa, K., Ashorn, M., Iltanen, S., Koskinen, L. L. E., Saavalainen, P., Koskinen, O., Maki, M., & Kaukinen, K. (2010). Celiac disease without villous atrophy in children: a prospective study. *The Journal of Pediatrics, 157*, 373–380.

Marsh, M. N. (1992). Gluten, major histocompatibility complex and the small intestine: A molecular and immunobiologic approach to the spectrum of gluten sensitivity ("coeliac sprue"). *Gastroenterology, 102*, 330–354.

Marsh, M. N., & Crowe, P. T. (1995). Morphology of the mucosal lesion in gluten sensitivity. *Baillière's Clinical Gastroenterology, 9*, 273–293.

Oberhuber, G., Granditsch, G., & Vogelsang, H. (1999). The histopathology of coeliac disease: Time for a standardized report scheme for pathologists. *European Journal of Gastroenterology and Hepatology, 11*, 1185–1194.

Özakıncı H, Kırmızı A, Savaş B, Kalkan Ç, Soykan İ, Çetinkaya H, Kuloğlu Z, Kansu A, Gürkan ÖE, Dalgıç B, Şentürk Z, Ensari A. (2016). Classification Chaos in coeliac disease: does it really matter? *Pathol Res Pract. 212*(12), 1174–1178.

Collagen Vascular Disorders, Esophagus

J. Alberto Pereira da Silva
Serviço de Reumatologia, Hospital de S. Maria, Lisbon, Portugal

Synonyms

Collagen diseases, esophagus; Connective tissue diseases, esophagus

Definition

Collagen vascular disorders include some multisystem diseases of unknown etiology associated with autoimmunity.

In Collagen vascular disorders, the involvement of the esophagus varies widely accordingly to the particular disease.

In these diseases the esophagus involvement is more important in scleroderma (see Scleroderma, esophageal), dermatomyositis/polymyositis (DM/PM), mixed connective tissue disease (MCTD), and Sjogren syndrome (SS).

In rheumatoid arthritis (RA) esophagus disease (esophagitis, ulcers, candidal esophagitis) may occur in consequence of the use of drugs like nonsteroidal anti-inflammatory drugs, steroids, and immunosuppressors. Esophagus involvement is not frequent in SLE (less than 5%), but some patients complain of dysphagia as a result of dysmotility; many of these patients also present Raynaud's phenomenon. In SLE dysphagia may also be caused by gastroesophageal reflux disease and esophageal candidiasis.

In dermatomyositis/polymyositis the involvement of the esophagus is characterized by myositis of the striated muscles in its superior third and of pharynges and may result in dysphonia, dysphagia, and aspiration pneumonitis which may lead to life-threatening bacterial pneumonia. In 15–50% of patients, there is smooth muscle involvement which results in dysmotility and reflux; in this case the clinical problems are similar to those observed in scleroderma (see ► Scleroderma, Esophageal).

In MCTD esophagus dysmotility is observed in 60–80% of patients which present the overlap with scleroderma; these patients often complain of heartburn or dysphagia. In those patients where the clinical features of myositis are predominant, dysphonia and aspiration pneumonia may be important features of the disease.

Dysmotility was found in 33% of patients with SS, using manometry. About 75% of patients with SS present dysphagia caused and aggravated by xerostomia. Strictures were reported in 10% of SS patients.

Clinical Features

- **Incidence**
  In rheumatoid arthritis, it is believed that disorders of the esophagus are those caused by drugs or are unrelated to RA. The prevalence of RA ranges from 0.3% to 1.5%, and the incidence was estimated to be 32 per 100,000 population.
  In SLE the esophagus is involved in less than 5%. Prevalence of SLE is 15–50 per 100,000 and the incidence 2–8 per 100,000 per year.
  Dysphagia occurs in 60% of patients with PM/DM; this may be due to striated muscle involvement of pharynges and upper esophagus and/or due to involvement of the smooth muscles of the two inferior thirds of the esophagus. The incidence of PM/DM is less than 10 per million per year. Juvenile-onset DM has an incidence of two to three cases per million per year.
  MCTD prevalence is 2.7–3.8 per million.
  The estimated prevalence of SS is 0.5–5% depending on the diagnostic criteria; about 50% of SS is secondary to RA, SLE, or scleroderma.
- **Age**
  RA is most commonly present in women ranging from 40 to 50 years.
  SLE has its main incidence between 15 and 45 years.
  Polymyositis/dermatomyositis most often begins between 40 and 60 years; the mean age of onset is 10 years in juvenile DM/PM.
  MCTD is usually diagnosed in the fourth decade of life.
  SS may appear after the menarche, but most of the patients are affected after the age of 55 years.
- **Sex**
  Collagen vascular disorders are more common in females.
  RA occurs in two to four females for each male.
  In SLE and SS there is a wider difference of genders (9:1).
  DM has a female preponderance of 2:1. When in association with other connective tissue diseases, the female-to-male ratio increases to 10:1. In contrast there is the same frequency in both genders in malignancy-associated DM.
  In MCTD the female-to-male ratio ranges from 3:3 to 9:1.
- **Site**
  In collagen vascular disorders esophageal involvement has two different patterns according to the site:
  Myositis concerns the striated muscles of the superior third of esophagus and pharynges in dermatomyositis/polymyositis and MCTD.
  Dysmotility of the two inferior thirds with or without gastroesophageal reflux may occur in scleroderma, MCTD, SS, and SLE.
- **Treatment**
  Treatment of myositis of striated muscle needs aggressive use of pulse steroids and intravenous gamma-globulin.
  Treatment of dysmotility and gastroesophageal reflux is similar to the treatment used in scleroderma for these conditions (see Scleroderma, esophageal).
- **Outcome**
  Esophageal and pharyngeal myositis is of particular concern in PM/DM and MCTD and may be a life-threatening situation when resulting in bronchial aspiration and bacterial pneumonia. Dysmotility and gastroesophageal reflux may interfere with the outcome in the individual patient when complications such as ulcers, hemorrhage, strictures, or candidal esophagitis appear.

Macroscopy

In collagen vascular disorders the macroscopic involvement of the esophagus results from dysmotility and gastroesophageal reflux (strictures, esophagitis) or the use of drugs (esophagitis, ulcers, and candidal esophagitis).

Microscopy

Biopsy of the esophagus is not used for the diagnosis of these diseases but may be important when ulcers or Barrett's metaplasia are present or suspected.

Immunophenotype

Collagen vascular diseases are characterized by the presence of autoantibodies.

Antinuclear antibodies are present in the serum of patients with collagen vascular disorders in particular in SLE (95%) and SS (75%), but its specificity is low. They may be found in other conditions such as autoimmune thyroiditis, autoimmune liver disease, neoplasms, and infections; moreover, they may be caused by several drugs, and its presence may be found in healthy people (up to 35% over 65 years of age).

Anticitrullinated peptide antibodies are found in 80–90% of patients with RA, are more specific for this disease than rheumatoid factors (RF), and are in association with patients presenting more cartilage and bone lesions. RF are present in the serum of 60–80% of RA patients but may be found as well in 50% of SLE and 75% of SS patients.

Autoantibodies against double-stranded DNA are specific for SLE and are present in 60% of patients. Anti-Sm antibodies (from "Smith") are also highly specific for SLE, are associated with renal involvement, and are present in 5–25% of patients.

Anti-SSA (Ro) antibodies are detected in 60% of primary SS, and antibodies to SSB (La) are present in 40% of patients with SS; both may be found in RA, SLE (35%), and PM/DM. In SLE the presence of anti-SSA in pregnant patients is associated with neonatal lupus and fetal heart block (risk: 1 in 15 to 20 patients).

Anti-ribonuclear protein (U1 RNP) antibodies and in particular antibodies to the 70 kDa antigen are associated with MCTD.

Anti-Jo-I (anti-histidyl-tRNA synthetase) antibodies are present in 20–40% of patients with PM/DM and anti-Mi-2 with DM.

Differential Diagnosis

In collagen vascular disorders impaired motility and the use of antacids, antibiotics, and immunosuppressors predispose to candidal esophagitis.

Inclusion body myositis should always be considered in the differential diagnosis of PM. It is more frequent in men older than 50 years.

References and Further Reading

Carsons, S. (2009). Sjogren's syndrome. In G. S. Firestein, R. C. Budd, E. D. Harris, I. B. McInnes, S. Ruddy, & J. S. Sergent (Eds.), *Kelley's textbook of rheumatology* (pp. 1149–1168). Philadelphia: Saunders Elsevier.

Doma, S., Wo, J. M., & Parkman, H. P. (2012). Esophageal Involvement in Systemic diseases. In J. E. Richter & D. O. Castell (Eds.), *The esophagus* (pp. 367–382). Chichester: Wiley-Blackwell.

Merieux, P., Verity, A., Clements, P. J., & Paulus, H. E. (1983). Esophageal abnormalities and dysphagia in Polymyositis and Dermatomyositis. *Arthritis and Rheumatism, 26*, 961–968.

Nagaraju, K., & Lundberg, I. E. (2009). Inflammatory diseases of muscle and other myopathies. In G. S. Firestein, R. C. Budd, E. D. Harris, I. B. McInnes, S. Ruddy, & J. S. Sergent (Eds.), *Kelley's textbook of rheumatology* (pp. 1149–1168). Philadelphia: Saunders Elsevier.

Sheldon, J. (2004). Laboratory testing in autoimmune rheumatic diseases. *Best Practice & Research. Clinical Rheumatology, 18*(3), 249–269.

Collagenous Colitis

Arzu Ensari
Department of Pathology, Ankara University Medical School, Sihhiye, Ankara, Turkey

Synonyms

Chronic watery diarrhea; Microscopic colitis

Definition

Collagenous colitis (CC) is defined as a chronic nondistorting colitis with the deposition of characteristic thick collagen band immediately beneath the surface epithelium. This layer has an irregular, jagged lower edge and consists of collagen fibers, inflammatory cells, and capillaries. The average collagen width has been reported as 10–20 μm, compared with the normal basement membrane width of up to 3 μm. Patients with CC generally suffer from chronic watery diarrhea. Colonoscopy is usually normal or near normal.

Clinical Features

- **Incidence**
  The reported incidence is between 1 and 2 in 100,000.
- **Age**
  Primarily affects middle-aged or older adults.
- **Sex**
  There is slight female predominance over males as 1.8:1.
- **Site**
  CC involves the entire colon in a patchy fashion. In some cases there may be rectal or left colonic sparing.
- **Treatment**
  Most patients with CC require anti-inflammatory therapy with either steroids or 5-ASA compounds.
- **Outcome**
  Spontaneous remission may occur in CC. Rarely, a diverting ileostomy may be necessary in refractory patients. There are normal periods in between diarrheal periods.

Macroscopy

The endoscopy is normal in the majority of patients. A few may show erosions, linear ulcers, or pseudomembranes.

Microscopy

Low power reveals an eosinophilic amorphous subepithelial band with an intact crypt architecture and an increase in lamina propria inflammatory cells superficially (Fig. 1). Higher magnification shows increased plasma cells and eosinophils in the lamina propria and patchy IELosis with surface epithelial damage. The surface epithelium may be stripped off from the underlying collagen band. Though there is no real consensus how thick the collagenous band should be, the average collagen width is usually greater than 10 μm, compared with the normal basement membrane width of 2–5 μm. However, measurements as thick as 70 μm for collagen deposition have been reported. The lower edge of the collagen layer usually shows an irregular contour; capillaries and inflammatory cells are entrapped within the collagen layer (Fig. 2). The collagen deposition can be patchy in distribution and thickness can be variable along the length of the colon, hence requiring multiple biopsies for diagnosis. A common pitfall for the diagnosis is the misinterpretation of the basement membrane as collagen deposition in poorly oriented, tangentially sectioned biopsies. A trichrome stain is a useful ancillary technique because it allows the identification of the presence of collagen. The density of the inflammatory cells in the epithelium and lamina propria is increased in CC. The composition of the infiltrate is also changed. Eosinophils may be markedly increased and are sometimes seen infiltrating crypt and surface epithelium together with lymphocytes. The number of mast cells and lymphocytes may also be increased. Neutrophils

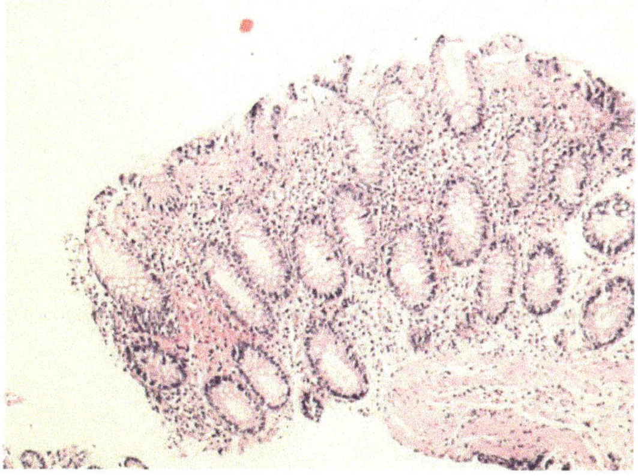

Collagenous Colitis, Fig. 1 A thick subepithelial band with jagged lower edge in a mildly inflamed colonic mucosa (H&E; ×100)

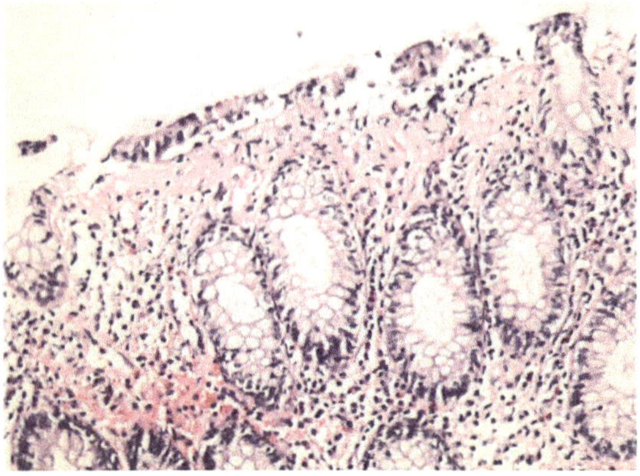

Collagenous Colitis, Fig. 2 Epithelial detachment with IELs and subepithelial collagen band containing blood vessels and inflammatory cells (H&E; ×200)

are often present and may induce occasional crypt abscesses.

Immunophenotype

The collagen band consists predominantly of type VI collagen and tenascin, with lesser amounts of collagen types I and III.

Molecular Features

There is no known molecular feature attributed to CC.

Differential Diagnosis

Thickening of the collagen band can be seen in other conditions such as lymphocytic colitis, IBD, enema effect, radiation colitis, ischemia, diverticular disease, mucosal prolapse, diabetes, and hyperplastic polyps. In these conditions however the inflammatory changes necessary for the diagnosis of CC are not present. Amyloid colitis can also show thickened eosinophilic material underneath the surface epithelium. This can be identified with specific stains such as Congo red. Drug damage is a category that can be much more difficult to distinguish from CC. There are many drugs that have diarrhea as a side effect. A relatively small subset of these medications are associated with histologic abnormalities in mucosal biopsies. Among these medications, NSAID substances are most commonly associated with gastrointestinal symptoms. Among their many toxic effects, several NSAIDs have been associated with endoscopic and histologic changes identical to CC. Whether the association is coincidental or causal is not clear. In some reports, patients respond entirely to withdrawal of NSAIDs, while in others, symptoms and histologic changes persist despite withdrawal of NSAIDs. In practice, a history of NSAID use should be sought in patients with a new diagnosis of CC. If possible, these medications should be discontinued prior to labeling the patient with a chronic colitic condition. Other medications that have been reported to result in CC include carbamazepine and lansoprazole. Pseudomembrane formation has been reported in association with CC by several groups. None of these reported cases showed C. difficile-positive stools. Overall, the clinical outcome of these patients in this retrospective series is similar to that of patients with classic CC without pseudomembrane formation. Histologically, the pseudomembrane seen in collagenous colitis consists of neutrophils, necrotic debris, fibrin, and, occasionally, detached epithelium. Collagenous colitis should therefore be added to the list of differential diagnoses for patients with pseudomembranous colitis. The presence of associated pseudomembranes supports the hypothesis that collagenous colitis may be caused by a toxic and/or ischemic mechanism. The coexistence of CC with IBD and autoimmune disorders such as celiac disease, thyroid disease, enteropathic arthritis, rheumatoid arthritis, myasthenia gravis, Sjogren's syndrome, scleroderma, pernicious anemia, and sarcoidosis has also been reported.

References and Further Reading

Fernández-Bañares, F., Salas, A., Esteve, M., et al. (2003). Collagenous and lympho-cytic colitis: Evaluation of clinical and histological features, response to treatment,

and long-term follow-up. *The American Journal of Gastroenterology, 98*, 340–347.
Lazenby, A. J., Yardley, J. H., Giardiello, F. M., et al. (1990). Pitfalls in the diagnosis of collagenous colitis: Experience with 75 cases from a registry of collagenous colitis at the Johns Hopkins Hospital. *Human Pathology, 21*, 905–910.
Lindstrom, C. G. (1976). 'Collagenous colitis' with watery diarrhoea: A new entity? *Pathologia Europaea, 11*, 87–89.
Widgren, S., Jlidi, R., & Cox, J. N. (1988). Collagenous colitis: Histologic morphometric immunohistochemical and ultrastructural studies. Report of 21 cases. *VirchowsArchiv Anatomy, 413*, 287–296.
Yuan, S., Reyes, V., & Bronner, M. P. (2003). Pseudomembranous collagenous colitis. *The American Journal of Surgical Pathology, 27*, 1375–1379.
Langner C, Aust D, Ensari A, Villanacci V, Becheanu G, Miehlke S, Geboes K, Münch A. (2015). Working Group of Digestive Diseases of the European Society of Pathology (ESP) and the European Microscopic Colitis Group (EMCG). Histology of microscopic colitis-review with a practical approach for pathologists. *Histopathology, 66*(5), 613–626.

Collagenous Gastritis

Helena Baldaia
Serviço de Anatomia Patológica, Centro Hospitalar de São João, Porto, Portugal

Synonyms

Microscopic gastritis

Definition

Collagenous gastritis is a rare entity characterized by the presence of an irregular and discontinuous subepithelial band of collagen of more than 10 μm in thickness in the gastric mucosa (Ravikumara et al. 2007).

The pathogenesis of this disease is still unknown. The most commonly accepted hypothesis is that the striking collagen deposition represents a reparative process subsequent to mucosal damage from chronic inflammation, an infectious agent, or toxic injury. This is supported by the fact that Type I and Type III collagen are associated with repair and have been demonstrated in the subepithelial collagen band present in this condition. An abnormality of the pericryptal fibroblast sheath or leakage of plasma protein with replacement with collagen has also been proposed to explain the collagen deposition (Ravikumara et al. 2007).

Clinical Features

- **Incidence**
  Collagenous gastritis is a rare disorder with scarce reports in the literature since its first description in 1989 (Ravikumara et al. 2007).
- **Age**
  This entity has been reported in a wide age range (1–77 years) (Jain and Chetty 2010). Clinical aspects have allowed segregation into two separate age groups, a pediatric-onset (children and young adults) and an adult-onset form, which is the most frequent.

  Pediatric collagenous gastritis is associated with severe anemia, sometimes with upper GI bleeding, and a nodular mucosa on endoscopy and is typically limited to the stomach.

  Adult-onset collagenous gastritis is, on the contrary, frequently associated with collagenous colitis, presenting with chronic watery diarrhea. There have been reports of association with immune-based disorders such as celiac disease, ulcerative colitis, Sjogren's syndrome, and autoimmune hemolytic anemia (Ravikumara et al. 2007).
- **Sex**
  The rarity of the condition has not allowed setting a difference in gender distribution. However, in pediatric cases of collagenous gastritis, there seems to be a slight female predominance (Jain and Chetty 2010).
- **Site**
  Gastric involvement is more often found in the body and fundus. However, involvement of the antrum and diffuse gastric involvement have also been reported.

  In the pediatric-onset collagenous gastritis, the disease is characteristically confined to the stomach. In the adult-onset form, there is often association with collagenous colitis (Suskind et al. 2009).

- **Treatment**
  Specific therapy has not been established. A number of therapies have been used (corticosteroids, ranitidine, omeprazole, 5-ASA, and hypoallergenic diets) with unreliable results (Ravikumara et al. 2007).
- **Outcome**
  The natural history of the disease is still unknown. There have been reports of symptomatic relief with persistence of the histological and endoscopic findings (Jain and Chetty 2010).

  In adults, the disease is characterized by a chronic intermittent course (Suskind et al. 2009).

  One report on pediatric collagenous gastritis found that a child developed psoriasis and achalasia and another child developed diabetes mellitus (Ravikumara et al. 2007). In the 12-year follow-up of the first case reported in 1989(a 15-year old girl), study of subsequent biopsies showed a lower number of antral gastrin cells and a significant corpus endocrine cell hyperplasia, suggesting, to the authors, an increased risk of endocrine neoplasia. Furthermore, the same study showed chronic atrophic gastritis, intestinal metaplasia, and epithelial changes indeterminate for dysplasia in these biopsies (Winslow et al. 2001).

Macroscopy

The most common endoscopic findings are nodularity and erythema of the gastric mucosa, particularly in the fundus and corpus. Mucosal erosions and diffuse thickening have also been described (Suskind et al. 2009).

Microscopy

Collagenous gastritis is a histological diagnosis. Gastric biopsies reveal a thickened, irregular band of collagen in subepithelial location which is more than 10 μm thick (usually between 10 and 25 μm) and frequently has entrapped inflammatory cells and dilated capillaries (Fenoglio-Preiser et al. 2008). It is believed that the anemia that characterizes the pediatric form stems from chronic bleeding from these dilated capillaries (Ravikumara et al. 2007). The inflammatory infiltrate is mainly composed of mononuclear cells with a number of neutrophils and eosinophils. The collagen band is irregular, showing a ragged transition to the lamina propria. There is frequently intraepithelial lymphocytosis (often exceeding 20 per 100 epithelial cells) and some degree of epithelial damage (Suskind et al.. 2009).

Histochemistry

The collagen band may be highlighted with the Masson trichrome stain.

Differential Diagnosis

The typical subepithelial collagen deposition allows a differential diagnosis with other fibrosis-associated lesions, such as scleroderma or changes associated with autoimmune gastritis or radiation therapy, in which the fibrosis is usually interstitial (Fenoglio-Preiser et al. 2008).

References and Further Reading

Fenoglio-Preiser, C. M., Noffsinger, A. E., Stemmermann, G. N., Lantz, P. E., & Isaacson, P. G. (2008). Inflammatory disorders of the stomach. In J. McGouh & J. Pine (Eds.), *Gastrointestinal pathology an atlas and text*. Philadelphia: Lippincott Williams & Wilkins.

Jain, R., & Chetty, R. (2010). Collagenous gastritis. *International Journal of Surgical Pathology, 18*(6), 534–536.

Ravikumara, M., Ramani, P., & Spray, C. H. (2007). Collagenous gastritis: A case report and review. *European Journal of Pediatrics, 166*, 769–773.

Suskind, D., Wahbeh, G., Murray, K. et al. (2009). Collagenous gastritis, a new spectrum of disease in pediatric patients: two case reports. *Cases Journal, 2*, 7511.

Winslow, J. L., Trainer, T. D., & Colletti, R. B. (2001). Collagenous gastritis: A long-term follow-up with the development of endocrine cell hyperplasia, intestinal metaplasia, and epithelial changes indeterminate for dysplasia. *American Journal of clinical pathology, 116*(5), 753–758.

Colon, Anatomy and Histology

Sibel Erdamar
Department of Pathology, Cerrahpasa Medical College, Istanbul, Turkey

Synonyms

Large bowel; Large intestine

Anatomy

The colon extends distally from the ileocecal valve to the anus and is subdivided into cecum, ascending, transverse, descending colon, sigmoid and rectum (Fig. 1).

The cecum, appendix, ascending and proximal portion of the transverse colon (right colon) are derived from midgut, while the distal transverse, descending, sigmoid colon and rectum (left colon) are derived from hindgut. The colon comes to lie in its final position in the abdominal cavity through a complex series of rotations.

The large intestines have omental appendices which are small, fatty, omentum-like projections.

The teniae coli are thickened bands of smooth muscle representing most of the longitudinal coat and begin at the base of appendix as the thick longitudinal layer of the appendix splits to form three bands: T.mesocolica, T.omentalis, and T.libera. Mesocolon attach to T.mesocolica on cecum and transverse colon, and omental appendices attach to T.omentalis. Since the teniae are shorter than intestine, the colon becomes sacculated between the teniae, forming haustra.

The right colon receives its blood supply from the superior mesenteric artery, parasympathetic nervous innervation from vagus nerve, and sympathetic innervation from the superior mesenteric ganglia. The left colon receives its blood supply from the inferior mesenteric artery, parasympathetic innervation from sacral nerves S2, S3, and S4 through the nervi erigentes; and sympathetic innervation from the inferior mesenteric ganglia. Venous drainage is predominantly portal. Veins from entire colon and that part of the

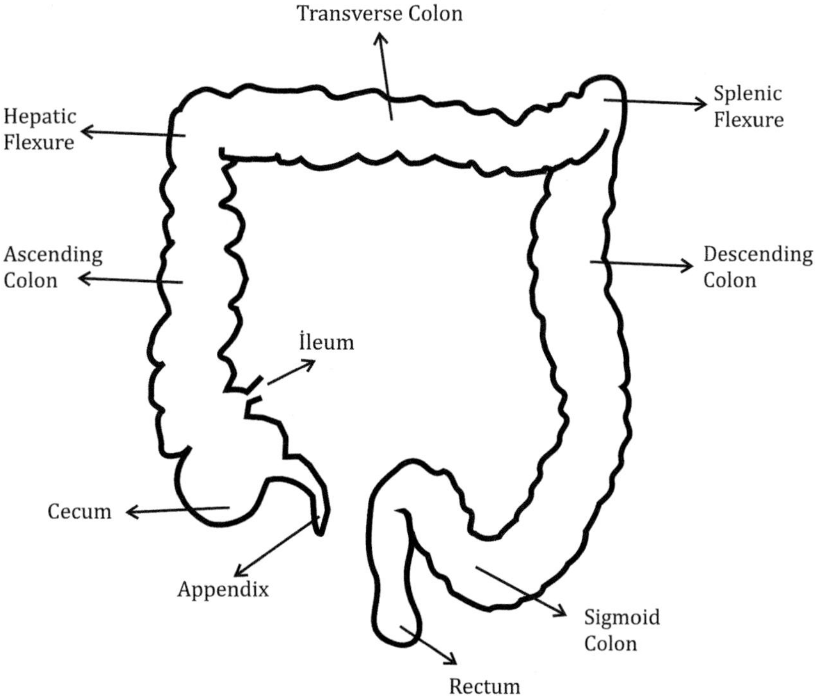

Colon, Anatomy and Histology, Fig. 1 Anatomic parts of colon

rectum served by the superior rectal artery drain into the portal system, but veins from the remainder of the rectum drain into systemic circulation. Portal-systemic anastomoses occur by communication of the superior rectal with the middle and inferior rectal veins.

Interaction between colon and peritoneal membrane varies according to anatomic subdivision.

The cecum is defined as the saccular part of colon and the first part of the large intestine that is continuous with the ascending colon. Cecum has no mesentery and is completely intraperitoneal, so it is mobile within right iliac fossa. The ileocecal valve is a combination valve and weak sphincter, actively opening periodically to allow entry of ileal contents and forming a largely passive one-way valve between the ileum and the cecum, preventing reflux.

The ascending colon is the second part of the large intestine. It passes superiorly on the right side of the abdominal cavity from the cecum to the right lobe of liver, where it turns to the left at the right colic flexure (hepatic flexure). It is covered by peritoneum anteriorly and separated from the anterolateral abdominal wall by the greater omentum.

The transverse colon is the third longest and most mobile part of the large intestine. It extends in abdomen from right colic flexura to the left colic flexure. The transverse colon is suspended by transverse mesocolon and its descending level various according to body type. The root of the transverse mesocolon lies along the inferior border of the pancreas and is continuous with the parietal peritoneum.

The descending colon locates a secondarily retroperitoneal position between the left colic flexure and the left iliac fossa. The peritoneum covers the colon anteriorly and laterally and binds it to the posterior abdominal wall. As it descends, the colon passes anterior to the lateral border of the left kidney.

The sigmoid colon is typically S-shaped, suspended by sigmoid mesocolon. It is highly variable in length and disposition and ends in rectosigmoid junction.

The rectum is the distal 8–15 cm of extra-peritoneal large bowel which is placed between pelvis and end part of anal canal. Its upper third is covered by peritoneum both anteriorly and laterally; more distally it becomes progressively devoid of serosal covering. Retroperitoneally and subperitoneally, the rectum is surrounded by a fatty mesorectum, which contains lymph nodes and is enveloped by an embryologic plane of cleavage that is called the mesorectal fascia. This whole mesorectal fatty tissue is removed during mesorectal excision for carcinoma of the rectum, and it is vital for the pathologist to examine its entire circumferential margin.

Function

The colon is the site where water is absorbed from the indigestible residues of the liquid chyme, converting it into semisolid stool or feces that is stored temporarily and allowed to accumulate until defecations occurs. The colon is an absorptive organ for electrolytes, bile salts, and other substances produced by bacterial degradation. On a daily basis, about 1 L of fluid enters the colon from ileocecal valve, and this is reduced to about 100 ml that is eliminated. The histologic organization of he colon reflects its functions (resorption of water and elimination of undigested material, feces). Elimination is provided by the secretion of mucus that lubricates and protects the mucosa from the luminal contents. Large intestine has immune and endocrine functions, like the small intestine. Lymphoid follicles and immune cells play important roles in this immune function. Heterogeneous population of endocrine cells provides its endocrine function.

Size

In normal adults, the length of the colon is variable and ranges 0.8–1.5 m. The cecum is a blind intestinal pouch, approximately 7.5 cm in both length and breadth. The ascending colon is 15–20 cm in length and extends up to the hepatic flexure. Transverse colon is somewhat u shaped mobile segment, 30–60 cm in length. The length of the sigmoid colon and its mesentery is very variable measuring 20–85 cm, with average length of about 40 cm. The rectum continues for 10–15 cm to the dentate line. The rectum is longer in men than in women.

Macroscopy

The large bowel is hollow muscular organ which begins at ileocecal valve and at the anus. The cecum has the largest diameter and is nestled in the right iliac fossa. The diameter of the colon decreases as it proceeds distally so that lumen of sigmoids is considerably smaller than that of cecum.

Externally, the presence a complete mesentery suggests the transverse or sigmoid colon, while the flaring of teniae and gradual loss of peritoneum denotes the rectum. The greater and lesser omentum are attached to the transverse colon in the immediate vicinity of an adjacent teniae.

Internally, the surface of the large intestine has typically series of haustra. Numerous, fine innominate grooves which run mainly transversely across the mucosa can be seen in every milimeter. Those grooves are actually crypt opennings. Mucosal lymphoid nodules can occasionally be seen as tiny dimples. They increase progressively in frequency from cecum to rectum.

Lymph nodes draining the large intestine can be divided into two major groups: those that lie immediately adjacent to the bowel wall (paracolic and pararectal nodes), and those that follow the course of the blood supply.

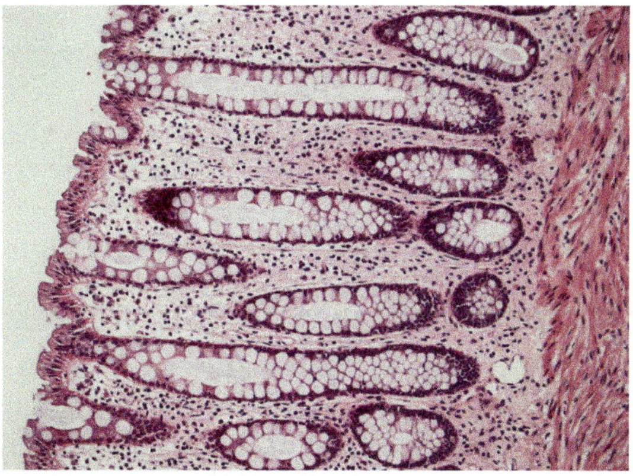

Colon, Anatomy and Histology, Fig. 2 Normal colonic mucosa

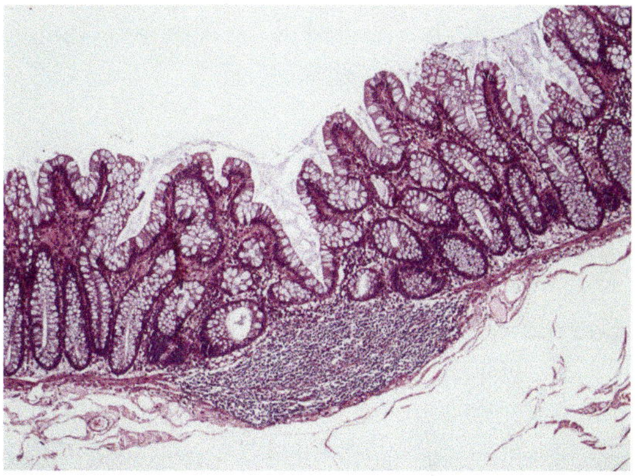

Colon, Anatomy and Histology, Fig. 3 Disorientation of crypts due to colonic lymphoid agregate

Microscopy

The colon wall is composed of mucosa, submucosa, muscularis propria, subserosa, and serosa. The mucosa contains epithelium, lamina propria, and muscularis mucosae. Function of the colon is to reclaim luminal water and electrolytes. The surface epithelium is composed of single layer of columnar to cuboidal absorptive cells, which have shorter and less abundant microvilli than those in the small intestine and goblet cells. The crypts have a tubular, test tube-like shape, and are rearranged parallel to each other (Fig. 2). Occasional branching crypts or slight architectural distortion may be seen in rectum and sigmoid colon and in areas adjacent to lymphoid aggregates (Fig. 3). The epithelial cells that reach the mucosal surface undergo apoptosis, and apoptotic bodies may be seen on either side of the basement membrane. Apoptosis is infrequent within crypts. The crypt epithelium contains mature absorptive cells and goblet cells, but in addition, it has immature and undifferentiated precursor cells, endocrine cells, and Paneth cells. Goblet cells show positivity with diastase-PAS, alcian-blue, and high iron-diamine reaction. Precursor and endocrine cells are seen mostly at the base of the crypts. Paneth cells are normally present only in the cecum and proximal right colon. Endocrine cells are found throughout the length of the large intestine but tend to increase in frequency distally. Serotonin-containing enterochromaffin cells and neurotensin-containing N cells are most numerous in the proximal colon; L cells are predominant distally.

Lamina propria of large intestine has a highly organized, loose connective tissue which provides a supporting scaffold for the epithelium and pericryptal sheath of myofibroblasts. Macrophages, plasma cells, histiocytes, eosinophils, lymphocytes, and sometimes mast cells are seen in lamina propria. The plasma cells, mostly IgA containing with occasional IgM and IgG varieties, are mostly located in upper zones of mucosa. The density of eosinophils varies depend on different geographic areas.

Intraepithelial lymphocytes can be prominent in epithelium overlying lymphoid aggregates.

In the lamina propria of the large bowel, the lymph vessels are limited to the area immediately above the muscularis mucosa.

Immunophenotype

Colonic epithelium shows immunoactivity with *CK20, pCEA, mCEA, villin, CDX2, AE1/AE3* and negative staining with *CK7*. Immunostaining for mucin profile shows positive immunoactivity in surface and crypt goblet cells with *MUC1, MUC2. MUC3* shows positivity in surface cells but not in crypt cells. Intraepithelial cells are positive with CD3, *CD45RO*. Plasma cells in lamina propria show positivity with *CD79a, CD138*.

References and Further Reading

Dahl, J., & Greenson, J. K. (2012). Colon. In S. E. Mills (Ed.), *Histology for pathologist* (pp. 673–695). Philadelphia: Wolter Kluwer/Lippincott Wiliams & Wilkins.

Moore, K. L., & Dalley, A. F. (2006). *Clinically oriented anatomy* (pp. 241–289). Philadelphia: Lippincott Williams & Wilkins.

Netter, F. H. (1989). Abdomen. In F. H. Netter, & S. Colacino (Eds.), *Atlas of human anatomy* (pp. 251–256, 264–268). Summit: Ciba-Geigy.

Condyloma, Anal

Denis Chatelain[1] and Jean-François Fléjou[2]
[1]Service d'Anatomie Pathologique, Centre Hospitalier et Universitaire du Nord, Amiens, France
[2]Faculté de Médecine Pierre et Marie Curie, Service d'Anatomie et Cytologie Pathologiques, Hôpital Saint-Antoine, Paris, France

Synonyms

Anal wart

Definition

Anal condyloma is a benign squamous epithelial lesion caused by Human Papilloma Virus (HPV) infection.

Several pathways can transmit HPV: sexual contact, autoinoculation, or contact with infected materials. The incubation period usually lasts 2–3 months before the development of condyloma. HPV 6 and 11 are the cause of over 90% of the exophytic anal warts (anal condyloma acuminatum), and they tend to be associated with low-grade dysplastic cellular changes (or anal intraepithelial neoplasia – AIN), and with other low-risk HPV subtypes such as 16 and 39. HPV 16 and 18 are responsible for most of the chronic infections that cause flat squamous lesions, often with high-grade dysplasia, favoring the development of squamous cell carcinoma (with other high-risk subtypes of HPV such as 31, 33, 35, 39, 45, 51, 52, 56, 58, 59, 66, 69).

Risk factors for the development of anal or perianal warts are: immunosuppression (iatrogenic on long-term steroids for connective tissue diseases or autoimmune disorders, transplant recipients, or HIV-induced), concurrent genital HPV-related diseases, anal intercourse, number of sexual partners, history or presence of other sexually transmitted infections, chronic irritation, and poor personal hygiene.

Clinical Features

Anal condyloma presents as exophytic lesion of the perianal zone (anal margin) or the anal canal (Fig. 1). Most patients are asymptomatic and can be diagnosed incidentally in the management of another anal or colorectal disease or found through screening with anal cytology in selected patients. Some patients may experience pruritus, mild burning, anal discharge bleeding, or irritation. The diagnosis is made primarily on visual inspection. Clinical impression may be confirmed by a biopsy in special circumstances, when the diagnosis is uncertain or when the lesions fail to respond to treatment.

- **Incidence**
  Anal condylomas are diagnosed in 20–30% of homosexual men. The prevalence among sexually abused children varies widely from 5% to 33%.

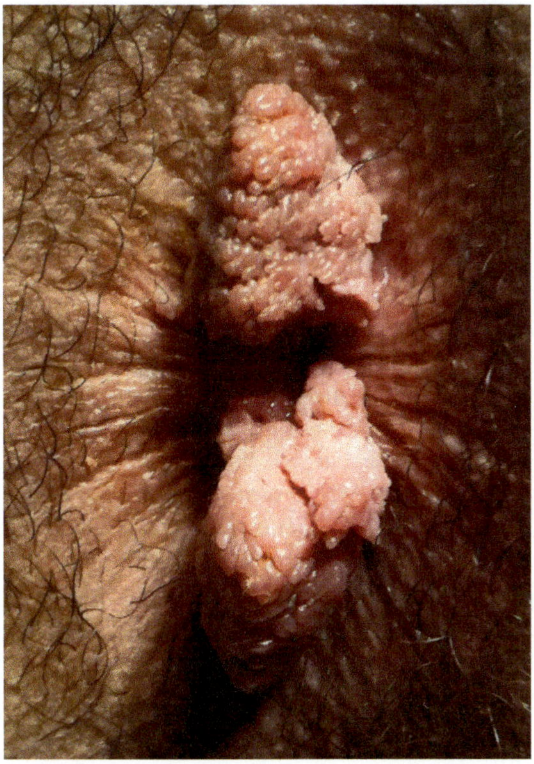

Condyloma, Anal, Fig. 1 Anal condylomas of the anal margin, with multiple exophytic verrucous lesions

The exact prevalence of AIN in the general population is unknown although the incidence is probably rising. The prevalence of AIN ranges from less than 1% to 5% in non-immunosuppressed patients to 3–5% in renal allograft recipients, 30% in women with HPV disease, and 26–89% in HIV patients.

- **Age**
  Anal condyloma is usually diagnosed in young sexually active women and men. The prevalence of AIN decreases in older women. In men having sex with men, anal condyloma can be diagnosed in older patients, and the prevalence of AIN in HIV-negative men who have sex with men does not change with age.

  The significance of anal warts in children has been debated, because they may suggest sexual abuse, but other ways of transmission cannot be excluded (hetero-inoculation by caregivers or self-inoculation with cutaneous types of HPV).
- **Sex**
  Anal condylomas occur regardless of gender but are specially frequent in HIV-infected homosexual men.
- **Site**
  Anal condyloma occurs in the skin of the perianal region or in the squamous epithelium lining the anal canal or the anal transitional zone.
- **Treatment**
  Anal condyloma and AIN can be treated by cryotherapy, CO_2 laser, or topical application of podophyllin, imiquimod, or trichloroacetic acid. AIN can also be treated by dynamic phototherapy. Larger lesions can be treated by local surgical excision.
- **Outcome**
  Most perianal condylomas harbor low-risk HPV (HPV 6 and 11) and have a minimal risk of progression to cancer. Those of the anal canal are more often associated with high-risk HPV (HPV 16 and 18) and may develop malignancy, particularly in immunocompromised patients. The reported incidence of squamous cell carcinoma of the anus in patients with anal condyloma is 3–4%.

  The natural history of AIN is uncertain. Low-grade AIN may spontaneously regress but high-grade AIN rarely regresses. AIN seems to pursue a more aggressive course in HIV-positive patients. Progression from low-to high-grade AIN is seen in 62% of HIV-positive and 36% of HIV-negative men having sex with men in a 2-year follow-up. The risk of progression of AIN to invasive anal cancer approximates 10% at 5 years. Patients most at risk of invasive cancer are those with multifocal disease and immunosuppression. At least, regular 6-month surveillance is recommended for immunocompromised patients and yearly for immunocompetent patients. Follow-up should be closer for patients with high-grade AIN, every 3 months. The recurrence rate of anal condyloma is high after treatment, ranging from 20% to 60%.

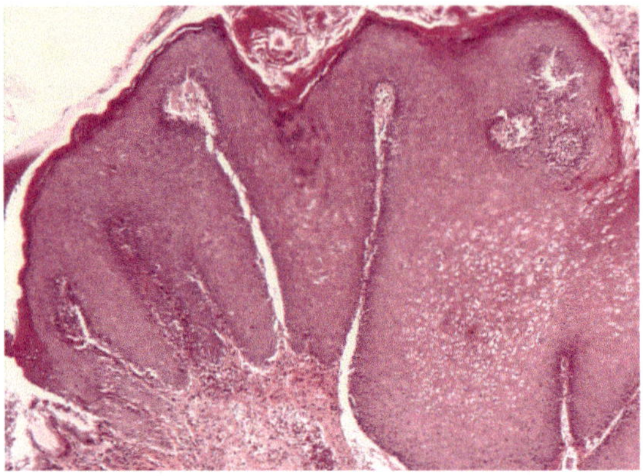

Condyloma, Anal, Fig. 2 Anal condyloma, with hyperpapillomatous and hyperkeratotic squamous epithelium

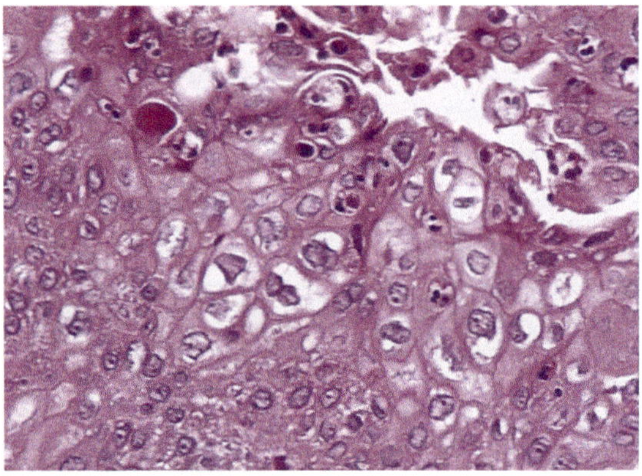

Condyloma, Anal, Fig. 3 Cytopathic effect of HPV in an anal condyloma

Macroscopy

Anal condylomas can be single or multiple. They usually measure from 2 to 5 mm, but they may grow to form large confluent masses. They present as papular lesions or acuminate cauliflower-like masses, with a slightly verrucous surface, and harbor a pinkish to salmon red or more grayish or whitish color (Fig. 1). Flat non-exophytic condylomas are more difficult to diagnose and may require high resolution anoscopy (HRA) and acetic acid test for identification.

Microscopy

Anal condyloma is a polypoid and verrucous squamous lesion. It is composed of papillary excrescences lined by hyperkeratotic and hyperplastic squamous epithelium (Fig. 2). The cytopathic effect due to HPV is characterized by the presence of cytoplasmic keratohyaline granules of different sizes, shapes, and stainability within vacuolized granular cells in the upper layers of the epidermis. It is also characterized by the presence of koilocytic changes with cells in the upper epidermis showing vacuolated cytoplasm with perinuclear cavitation and an enlarged and hyperchromatic nucleus with irregular nuclear membranes, with sometimes binucleation (Fig. 3). Some condylomas show evidence of low-grade AIN, with architectural disorganization, nuclear atypia, and mitoses in the lower half of the epithelium (low-grade squamous intraepithelial lesion – LSIL) (Fig. 4).

High-grade AIN is characterized by architectural disorganization, encompasses the upper half of the epithelium, and consists of round squamous cells, smaller than those of normal epithelium. These cells have a basophilic cytoplasm and a high nuclear cytoplasmic ratio, with an enlarged atypical nucleus, and with sometimes atypical mitoses, reaching the upper half of the epithelium (Fig. 5).

Anal cytology screening, as a diagnostic tool, can be used in patients with high-risk factors of

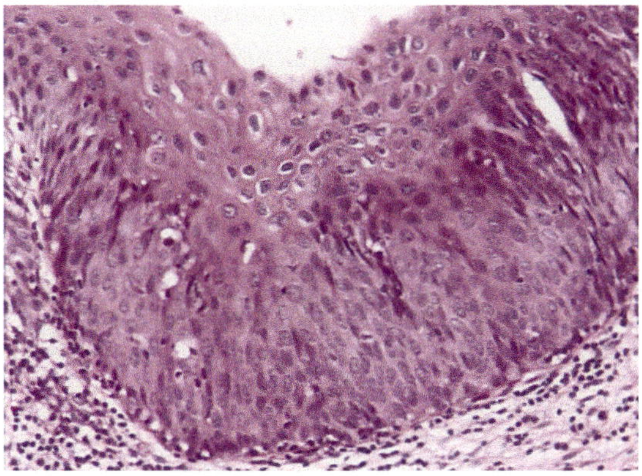

Condyloma, Anal, Fig. 4 Anal condyloma with low-grade AIN

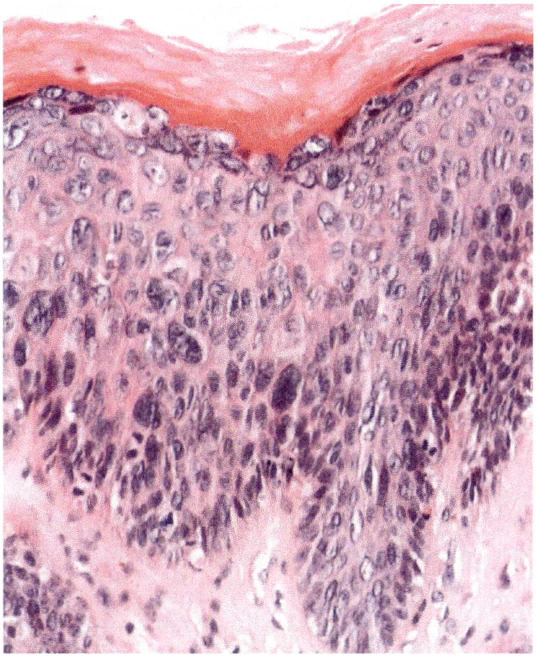

Condyloma, Anal, Fig. 5 Anal condyloma with high-grade AIN

AIN, such as men having sex with men, immunosuppressed patients, and patients with a concurrent HPV infection in another site. Anal screening has a sensitivity that ranges from 47% to 90% and a specificity that ranges from 16% to 92%. There is a moderate interobserver agreement for cytology specimens. Detection of DNA of HPV by hybrid capture testing and p16 immunoreactivity in anal cytology specimens can be useful to enhance the diagnostic performances of anal cytology. However, patients with abnormal cytology should be evaluated by HRA and AIN has to be confirmed by histopathological examination of anal biopsies.

C

Immunophenotype

Some commercially available HPV immunohistochemical stains and in situ hybridization tests can be used to confirm the presence of HPV subtypes in epithelial lesions suspicious of condyloma acuminatum. However, these tests are generally insensitive and HPV detection in formalin-fixed paraffin-embedded tissue is best accomplished using polymerase chain reaction (PCR)-based assays. But HPV PCR is not routinely performed due to the high cost of this labor-intensive technique. p16 and Ki-67 immunohistochemical staining can be useful to confirm a diagnosis of high-grade AIN. High-grade AIN tends to show diffuse p16 staining with a band-like strong cytoplasmic and nuclear staining of the basal and intermediate cell layers of the squamous epithelium, with or without staining of the cells of the superficial layers (Fig. 6). Ki67 shows an increased number of nuclear positivity in the middle or upper third of the epithelium (Fig. 7).

Molecular Features

Molecular features of anal condyloma are still unclear, but principally linked to HPV infection.

Differential Diagnoses

The fibroepithelial anal polyp can mimic condyloma acuminatum on microscopic examination. It differs from the former by the lack of typical koilocytic changes, and by the absence of Ki67 positive cells in the intermediate and superficial layers of the squamous epithelium.

Reactive inflammatory changes in immature squamous epithelium of the anal transitional

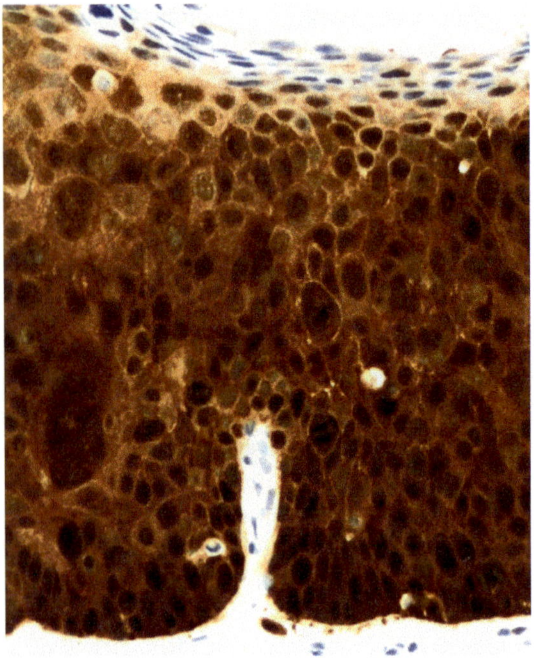

Condyloma, Anal, Fig. 6 Strong p16 staining in high-grade AIN

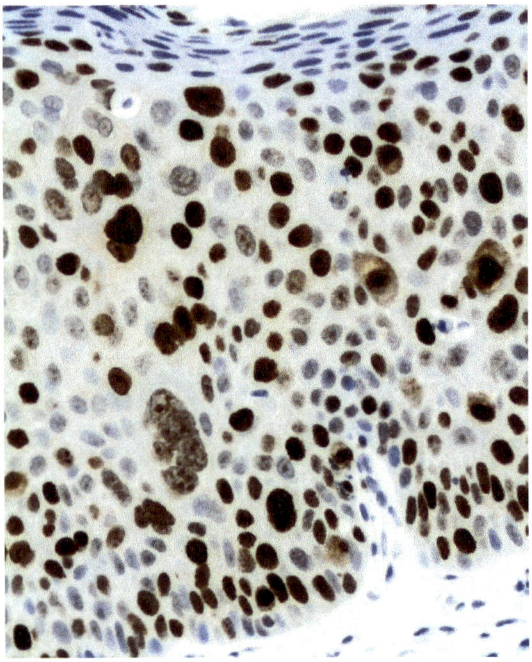

Condyloma, Anal, Fig. 7 Strong Ki67 positivity in high-grade AIN

zone can simulate the appearance of high-grade AIN. However, contrary to high-grade AIN, metaplastic epithelium does not show strong band-like positivity of the basal and intermediate layers of the epithelium with p16 immunohistochemical stain.

Bowen's disease has the same microscopic appearance as high-grade AIN on microscopic examination. Bowen's disease shows a marked epidermal hyperplasia with thickening of the rete ridges. The entire thickness of the squamous epithelium is disorganized with large squamous cells with marked nuclear atypia, abnormal mitosis, and a few small round eosinophilic dyskeratotic cells extending from the base to the surface of the epithelium. The horny layer is thickened and consists of parakeratotic cells with atypical nuclei. The lesion sometimes extends to follicular infundibula. However, Bowen's disease is a distinct entity that can be differentiated from AIN by its epidemiological and clinical features. Bowen's disease can be defined as a nonkeratinizing intraepithelial squamous cell carcinoma of the perianal skin. It is more common in females aged over 50 and presents as a solitary nummular, reddish, slowly enlarging erythemato-squamous scaling and oozing plaque. It is associated with HPV types 16 and 18. The natural history of Bowen's disease is relatively benign and progression to invasive squamous cell carcinoma is observed in only 2–5% of the cases.

Bowenoid papulosis has the same microscopic appearance as Bowen's disease and high-grade AIN. It is induced by HPV 16 but is never transformed into invasive squamous cell carcinoma. This distinctive entity differs from Bowen's disease by its epidemiological and clinical features. Bowenoid papulosis occurs in young sexually active adults or adolescents. It presents as multiple maculo-papular lesions, 2–10 mm in diameter, erythematous, reddish or violaceous brown with a smooth velvety surface. The lesions have a typically bilateral distribution in the genital, perianal, and inguinocrural folds. Whereas some lesions spontaneously regress, others may appear that in turn may also regress.

References and Further Reading

Chin-Hong, P. V., & Palefsky, J. M. (2002). Natural history and clinical management of anal human papillomavirus disease in men and women infected with human immunodeficiency virus. *Clinical Infectious Diseases, 35*, 1127–1134.

Longacre, T. A., Kong, C. S., & Welton, M. L. (2008). Diagnostic problems in anal pathology. *Advances in Anatomic Pathology, 15*, 263–278.

Rock, B., Shah, K. V., & Farmer, E. R. (1992). A morphologic, pathologic, and virologic study of anogenital warts in men. *Archives of Dermatology, 128*, 495–500.

Scholefield, J. H., Harris, D., & Radcliffe, A. (2011). Guidelines for management of anal intraepithelial neoplasia. *Colorectal Disease, 13*, 3–10.

Cowden's Syndrome

Özgür Ekinci
Department of Pathology, Gazi University, Ankara, Turkey

Synonyms

Multiple hamartoma syndrome; PTEN hamartoma syndrome

Definition

This is an autosomal dominant condition with hamartomatous lesions in various organs, including the GI tract, with an increased risk of malignancy in extraintestinal organs such as the breast and thyroid. There does not seem to be sufficient evidence to render a causal relationship between Cowden's syndrome (CS) and GI cancer. It is part of the PTEN hamartoma tumor syndrome also including Bannayan–Riley–Ruvalcaba, Proteus, and Proteus-like syndromes.

This syndrome can be characterized by hamartomatous lesions of the skin (trichilemmoma is the classical lesion), benign breast lesions, uterine leiomyomas, macrocephaly, mental retardation, and Lhermitte–Duclos disease of the cerebellum, each being present in varying rates.

The World Health Organization has put forth the following diagnostic criteria based on the International Cowden Consortium:

Pathognomonic criteria:

- Mucocutaneous lesions:
  - Trichilemmomas, facial
  - Acral keratoses
  - Papillomatous papules
  - Mucosal lesions

Major criteria:

- Breast carcinoma
- Thyroid carcinoma (nonmedullary), especially follicular thyroid carcinoma
- Macrocephaly (megalencephaly) (more than 97%)
- Lhermitte–Duclos disease

Minor criteria:

- Other thyroid lesions (e.g., adenoma or multinodular goiter)
- Mental retardation (IQ $\leq$ 75)
- Gastrointestinal hamartomas
- Fibrocystic disease of the breast
- Lipomas
- Fibromas
- Genitourinary tumors (e.g., uterine fibroids) or malformation

Operational diagnosis in an individual:

1. Mucocutaneous lesions alone if:
   (a) There are six or more facial papules, of which three or more must be trichilemmoma.
   (b) Cutaneous facial papules and oral mucosal papillomatosis.
   (c) Oral mucosal papillomatosis and acral keratoses.
   (d) Palmoplantar keratoses, six or more.
2. Two major criteria, but one must include macrocephaly or Lhermitte–Duclos disease
3. One major and three minor criteria
4. Four minor criteria

Operational diagnosis in a family where one individual is diagnostic for Cowden:

1. One or more pathognomonic criterion

2. Any one major criterion with or without minor criteria
3. Two minor criteria

Clinical Features

- **Incidence**
  CS is estimated to be present in one individual per million. There are, however, reports of an incidence of 1 in 200,000.
- **Age**
  There are no confident findings as to the age of inflicted individuals. However, the associated cancers present at an early age.
- **Sex**
  As with age, the predilection for sex remains undetermined.
- **Site**
  CS is a multisystemic condition comprising hamartomatous and various lesions in organ systems deriving from all of the three germ layers. The skin, mucosae, breast, GI tract, uterus, and the central nervous system are at the front.
- **Treatment**
  The primal problem in managing these patients is in diagnosing them correctly and – because of the multisystemic involvement – approaching them accordingly, relevant to the related site and the lesion, and the subsequent follow-up by a specialist knowledgeable of the condition.
- **Outcome**
  The prognosis depends largely on the correct diagnosis and requisite management. As the primary concern is on the breast (in female patients, though males are not spared) and thyroid, a specialist in the area would be needed. The breast cancers mostly are ductal carcinomas, and the thyroid tumors are follicular or papillary carcinomas.

Macroscopy

CS affects multiple sites. For tricholemmomas, breast lesions such as fibrocystic disease and cancer, and thyroid carcinomas, the reader is referred to the relevant chapters.

The GI polyps can look on gross examination quite indifferent to adenomas or hamartomatous polyps.

Microscopy

The polyps show a nonspecific morphology consistent with a hamartomatous polyp of the GI tract. The general appearance includes an inflamed lamina propria on which are dispersed glandular structures with roundish outlines. The epithelial cells in these glands are columnar enterocyte-type cells and goblet-type cells. Dysplasia is not seen, but as with the hyperplastic polyps, the basally located glands may have cellular features of the "proliferative" type: larger and more crowded nuclei, darker cytoplasm, and a less-differentiated appearance, which should not be considered as dysplasia.

In some Cowden polyps, a lamina propria containing spindly cells as would be seen in a neural sheath tumor (e.g., neurofibroma) can occur. Other polyps may contain adipocytic cells or ganglionic cells with associated Schwann-like cells. Fibrous-type spindle cells can also be encountered.

Immunophenotype

There is no specific immunohistochemical profile to a Cowden polyp. As these are deriving from certain parts of the GI tract, they are expected to exhibit the epithelial profile of the relevant site, such as a gastric polyp would be positive for cytokeratin 7 and MUC5AC or an intestinal one can be positive for cdx2, cytokeratin 20, etc.

Molecular Features

PTEN gene mutation is the mainstay of CS. This gene is expressed in virtually every tissue in the human body, especially the skin, thyroid, and central nervous system (CNS). The PTEN protein normally acts as a tumor suppressor. It acts as an inhibitor of the AKT–mTOR pathway, which leads to cellular proliferation and survival among other effects.

Differential Diagnosis

The main issue in distinguishing a Cowden's polyp from that of other hamartomatous polyposis syndromes lies not in the morphology but the involved organs, extraintestinal findings, family history, and molecular features. Still, in a patient with multiple hamartomatous polyps throughout the GI tract, there can be a number of syndromes in the differential diagnosis at hand, as follows.

Distinction from Peutz–Jeghers' polyps would necessitate the absence of tree-like musculature, more crowded glandular proliferation, and lack of molecular features of the latter syndrome. Peutz-Jeghers' polyps may lack this classical morphology in several sites of the GI tract, especially the stomach, where in a proven case of Peutz–Jeghers syndrome, the polyps may appear like an inflammatory, hyperplastic, or juvenile polyp.

Differentiation has to be done – quite expectedly – also from juvenile polyposis syndrome, which can be impossible in a single polyp examined by microscopy. Nevertheless, juvenile polyps – either sporadic or syndromic – tend to have an ulcerated surface, fewer, more irregular, and larger glandular elements, and a lobulated overall structure. They can have foci of dysplastic change and even carcinomatous transformation. The so-called atypical juvenile polyp is multilobated, larger (i.e., more than a few centimeters), and believed to be unique to the syndromic cases.

Bannayan–Riley–Ruvalcaba polyps are believed to be identical to the Cowden polyps, so molecular and/or clinical aspects should be taken into consideration.

Hyperplastic polyps, as the state-of-the-art recommendations propose, can be divided into three types: goblet cell, microvesicular, and the rare mucin-poor types. Because an hyperplastic polyp can be viewed as a "hyperplasia" of the normal colorectal mucosal components, there is a regularity in the pattern of distribution of the glandular structures that resemble the normal mucosa. Besides, especially in the microvesicular type, serration may be found, which is not expected in a Cowden's polyp. For that matter, serrated polyps are not in the differential diagnosis.

In an hamartomatous-looking, non-dysplastic polyp from the GI tract, if there are adipocytic or ganglioneuromatous components, the diagnosis of CS should be entertained and the suspicion put in the pathology report.

For cutaneous, mammary, and thyroid tumors, the reader is kindly referred to the relevant chapters, as there is are morphological differences than these latter in a CS patient.

References and Further Reading

Nelen, M. R., Padberg, G. W., Peeters, E. A., Lin, A. Y., van den Helm, B., Frants, R. R., Coulon, V., Goldstein, A. M., van Reen, M. M., Easton, D. F., Eeles, R. A., Hodgsen, S., Mulvihill, J. J., Murday, V. A., Tucker, M. A., Mariman, E. C., Starink, T. M., Ponder, B. A., Ropers, H. H., Kremer, H., Longy, M., & Eng, C. (1996). Localization of the gene for Cowden disease to chromosome 10q22-23. *Nature Genetics, 13*, 114–116.

Zbuk, K. M., & Eng, C. (2007). Cancer phenomics: RET and PTEN as illustrative models. *Nature Reviews Cancer, 7*, 35–45.

Crohn's Disease

Karel Geboes
Department of Pathology, N. Goormaghtig Institute, University Gent, Gent, Belgium
Department of Pathology, KU Leuven, Leuven, Belgium

Synonyms

Regional enteritis, ileitis terminalis (the first name used in the original paper by Dr. Burrill Crohn and colleagues)

Definition

Crohn's disease is a life-long relapsing inflammatory disease of unknown aetiology, mainly affecting the gastrointestinal tract with extraintestinal manifestations and associated immune disorders. The disease can involve different segments of the gastrointestinal tract. Various theories have been proposed for the pathogenesis of Crohn's disease with implications for specific therapies. Genome-wide association studies identified susceptibility loci that, triggered by environmental factors, may result in a disturbed innate and adaptive immune response. Dysfunction of innate immunity includes a disturbed intestinal barrier, Paneth cell dysfunction, endoplasmic reticulum stress, defective unfolded protein response and autophagy, impaired recognition of microbes by pattern recognition receptors, such as nucleotide-binding domain and Toll-like receptors on dendritic cells and macrophages. Because of the similarities between infectious colitis and Crohn's disease, infections have repeatedly been proposed as a potential responsible factor. Thus far, however, no single pathogenetic agent has been identified. The prevailing concept today is either an abnormal interaction between the intestinal flora and the immune system or an abnormal composition of the intestinal flora. Cigarette smoking is another important harmful factor. The hypothesis implying a role for microorganisms in the pathogenesis is strengthened by the increased familial occurrence of the disease as well as by the observations obtained with genetic studies. Epidemiological studies in monozygotic and dizygotic twins, as well as family studies, indicate that genetic factors may have a dominant role in Crohn's disease. The search for susceptibility genes had its first success in 1996, when the first susceptibility locus was identified in the pericentromeric region of chromosome 16, which was called IBD1. In 2001, a caspase recruitment domain-containing protein, CARD15/NOD2, was found to be mutated in 20–30% of Crohn's disease patients, establishing a proof of principle for the genetic concept. Multiple mutations in the CARD15/NOD2 gene have since been identified.

The major differences between Crohn's disease and ulcerative colitis are the distribution of the lesions, presence or absence of transmural inflammation, and the ability of Crohn's disease to form fistulas. Crohn's disease is a segmental disease with skip areas that is more prevalent in the proximal colon and ileum, but can involve the entire GI tract. A diagnosis of Crohn's disease is therefore often not based on histology alone but confirmed by clinical evaluation and a combination of endoscopic, histological, radiological, and biochemical investigations.

Clinical Features

- **Incidence**
  Crohn's disease affects individuals in many parts of the world. The incidence differs depending on the region studied. Studies assessing the incidence (the number of new cases per year per 10^5 inhabitants in a given place) show that the United Kingdom, North America, and the northern part of Europe are the areas with the highest incidence. A north–south axis has been found in both Europe and in the United States, with higher incidence and prevalence in the northern regions. Incidence rates have increased after the Second World War and especially since the mid-1970s. The incidence rate in Olmsted County, Minnesota, United States, was 1.0 in 1940–1943, while the rate in 1984–1993 was 6.9. The incidence seems to level off around 6.0 per 100,000. A plateau in incidence has been found in five studies but a continuous increase in incidence is demonstrated in four other studies involving populations from Derby, Florence, Iceland, and Copenhagen. A Danish study found a peak incidence among 15–29-year olds, with an incidence rate among men and women of 5.3 and 9.1, respectively. The increase in incidence occurred in all disease locations but was relatively more common in colonic Crohn's disease. The prevalence rate in Europe varies from less than 10 to about 150 per 100,000

inhabitants. One study from South Korea indicated a prevalence of 11.2.

- **Age**
  Crohn's disease tends to present initially in the teens and 20s, with another peak incidence in the 50s to 70s, although the disease can occur at any age. From a population-based cohort from Copenhagen county, it appears that approximately 6% of the patients had an onset before 15 years of age, but overall the age at diagnosis is approximately 30.
- **Sex**
  The sexes are affected approximately evenly, although there is a mild female predominance with female-to-male ratios being 1.3–1.89 to 1.0. In Japan, there is a male predominance. The incidence is 0.51 per 100,000 (male: 0.71; female: 0.32).
- **Site**
  The terminal ileum and proximal colon are the commonest sites involved, followed by the anorectum and colon. The terminal ileum is involved in approximately 2/3 cases. Perianal disease is also common. The frequency varies between 14% and 76%. The rectum may appear unaffected in a large number of cases. Involvement of the upper gastrointestinal tract is uncommon, and usually associated with disease of the terminal ileum. The ileocolonic lesions may however take time to develop, and occasionally, Crohn's disease can start as isolated gastric or gastroduodenal disease.
- **Treatment**
  CD is a chronic disorder that is not yet curable. The induction and maintenance of symptom improvement and, at best, the induction and maintenance of mucosal healing are the goals of both medical and surgical treatment. Corticosteroids have a favorable effect on the symptoms intestine but will not achieve a significant reduction in endoscopically observed inflammation. Active colonic disease may be treated with sulfasalazine if only mildly active. Both azathioprin and 6-mercaptopurine have a positive effect on maintaining remission. The introduction of antitumor necrosis factor (TNF) agents has changed the treatment of refractory CD. Anti-TNF agents have shown the ability to induce mucosal healing and to reduce the need for surgery in randomized, placebo-controlled studies. It is not known, however, if they can reduce the risk of recurrence after surgery. Complications such as stenoses, fistulas, and abscesses are the main reasons for bowel resection in patients with CD.
- **Outcome**
  The majority of patients experience progression from inflammatory disease to the development of strictures and fistulas. Within the first 5 years of the disease, at least one third of the patients have had intestinal surgery, where ileocecal resection is the most commonly performed procedure. The overall mortality in most studies is comparable to the background population, although subgroups of CD patients seem to have slightly increased mortality. There are only few reports on sick leave and unemployment, but overall, it is concluded that having CD is correlated to an increased unemployment rate.

Macroscopy

The macroscopic lesions of Crohn's disease are apparent both on the mucosal and serosal side of the bowel wall. The length of the segments involved is variable. The mucosal appearance is heterogeneous. Lesions of different size (and probably of variable duration) are simultaneously present and found in the same surgical specimen or seen during endoscopy. The mucosa may appear normal or may show small, punctiform, rounded superficial erosions, often in the proximity of the section margin. These ulcers are called "aphthoid or aphthous ulcers." Over a period of time, the erosions become confluent and give rise to larger longitudinal ulcers, which are known as serpiginous ulcers, separated by normal-appearing mucosa. The combination of longitudinal and transverse ulceration in an edematous mucosa is responsible for a characteristic cobble stone aspect. More severe ulcerations with complete circumferential loss of the mucosa are seen in stenosing areas. These can be fissural ulcers

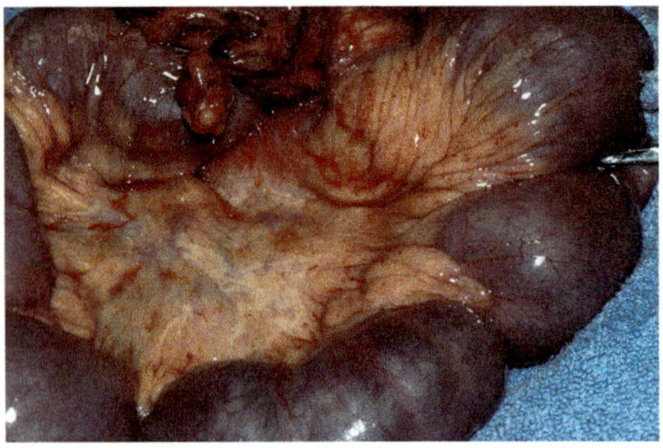

Crohn's Disease, Fig. 1 Surgical specimen of small intestine showing fat wrapping

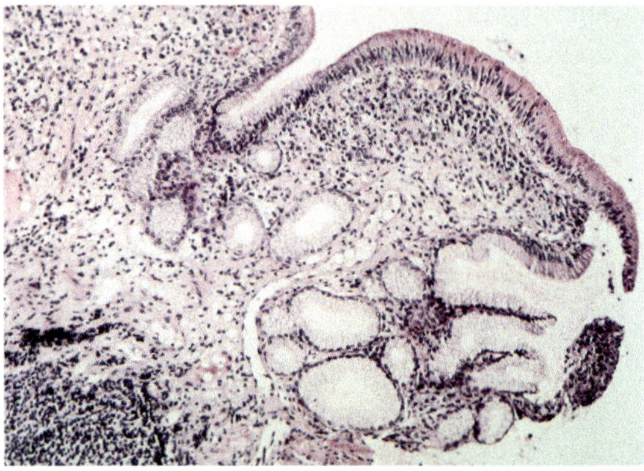

Crohn's Disease, Fig. 2 Microphotograph of ileal biopsy showing disturbed villous architecture and pseudopyloric gland metaplasia

reaching the muscularis propria. Fistulas are often associated with strictures Strictures are characterized by luminal narrowing, often circular, and bowel wall thickening with or without prestenotic dilatation. Inflammatory pseudopolyps of the colon and even small intestine (in approximately 20% of the cases) can be found. Usually the bowel wall is thickened with involvement of the submucosa, the muscularis propria, the subserosa, and mesenteric fat. The serosal surface reveals distended blood vessels and may be covered by a fibrinous exudate, with or without adhesions to adjacent loops. Mesenteric fat partially surrounds the intestine, extending from the mesenteric attachment anteriorly and posteriorly, corresponding to the involved segment. This phenomenon, known as fat wrapping or creeping fat, is specific for Crohn's disease (Fig. 1).

Microscopy

The histological diagnosis of Crohn's disease in the colon is based on the analysis of a full colonoscopic biopsy series. Rectal biopsies are necessary to either confirm or reject rectal involvement and may additionally be helpful in differentiating Crohn's disease from other inflammatory lesions. Ileoscopy with biopsy is recommended as additional step, the diagnostic value of terminal ileum biopsies being highest in patients with known or suspected Crohn's disease

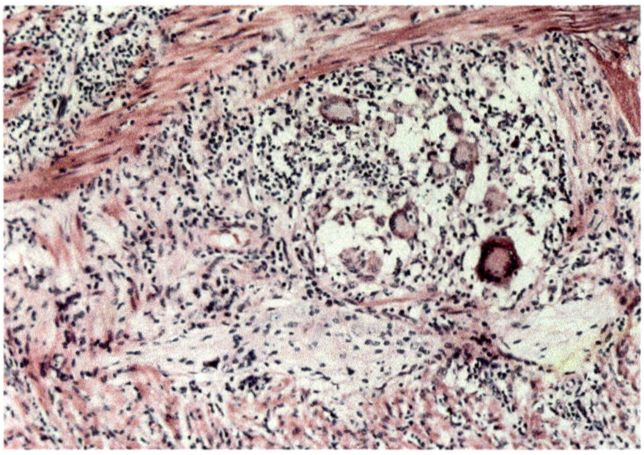

Crohn's Disease, Fig. 3 Loosely arranged granuloma with multinucleated giant cell in the vicinity of the myenteric plexus

(Fig. 2). Focal (discontinuous) chronic inflammation, focal crypt irregularity (discontinuous crypt distortion), and granulomas (not related to crypt injury) are the generally accepted microscopic features (on endoscopic biopsies). The same features and, in addition, an irregular villous architecture can be used for samples from the ileum. The granuloma is defined as a collection of epithelioid histiocytes (monocyte/macrophage cells), the outlines of which are often vaguely defined (Fig. 3). Multinucleated giant cells are not characteristic, and necrosis is usually not apparent. Yet noncaseating granulomas or isolated giant cells can be observed in other conditions such as

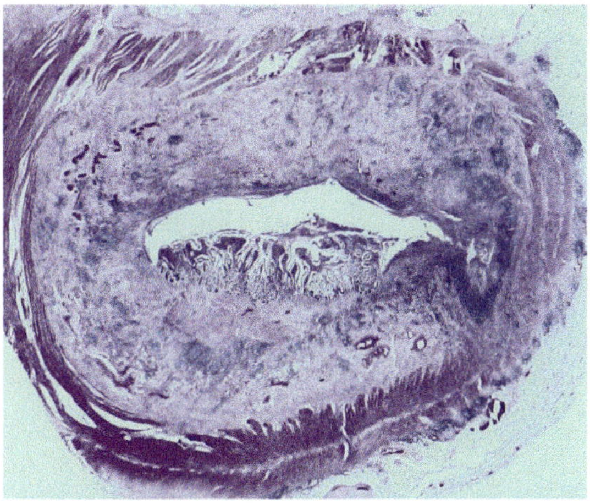

Crohn's Disease, Fig. 4 Transmural lymphoid hyperplasia

infectious colitis (Tuberculosis) and should therefore not simply be regarded as diagnostic for Crohn's disease. Indeed, the presence of one single feature is not regarded as sufficient for a reliable diagnosis of Crohn's disease. For surgical material, it has been suggested that a diagnosis of Crohn's disease should be made when three features are present in the absence of granulomas, or when an epithelioid granuloma is present with one other feature provided that specific infections are excluded. In young children, the diagnosis may be more difficult although granulomas are more common. Surgical specimens allow also the evaluation of the transmural nature of the disease. The presence of lymphoid aggregates in the submucosa, the muscularis propria, in the vicinity of the myenteric plexus, and in the subserosa is a specific indicator of Crohn's disease (Fig. 4). They may be numerous and their presence in the muscularis propria and subserosa together may form an appearance resembling two or three rows of beads (rosary-bead effect). Widening of the submucosa by edema and fibromuscular obliteration is also very common. Lymphangiectasias and abnormalities of the enteric nervous system in the submucosa are other common findings. The major structural abnormalities of the nervous system are irregular hypertrophy and hyperplasia of nerve fibers.

Immunophenotype

The prevailing view was that Crohn's disease is a primary T cell autoimmune disorder. One theory is that the inflammation of Crohn's was caused by an overactive Th1 cytokine response. More recent studies argue that Th17 is more important. A newer view is that Crohn's disease results from an impaired innate immunity.

Molecular Features

Several susceptibility genes have been identified. These include CARD15/NOD2, the organic cation transporters OCTN1 and 2 on chromosome 5q31, the Drosophila disc large homologue 5 (DLG5) on chromosome 10, and the receptor for interleukin-23 (IL23R) on chromosome 1p31, among others. A defective secretion or production of local antibiotic peptides such as defensins seems to be another defect.

Differential Diagnosis

The main differential diagnostic entities to be considered are infectious enterocolitis, drug-induced colitis, diverticular-disease-associated colitis, and diversion colitis. Infectious colitis is usually a transient disorder presenting with sudden onset of bloody diarrhea. The distinction between Crohn's disease and infective type colitis relies mainly on the absence of features which direct toward a diagnosis of chronic idiopathic inflammatory bowel disease (mainly architectural distortion and basal plasmocytosis). In patients presenting with persistent or long-standing diarrhea, in immigrants or in travelers, the problem may be more difficult. Tuberculosis is a granulomatous inflammation that also presents as a segmental disease. It involves most commonly the ileocecal region, but it can also be localized in the remainder of the colon and rectum. Unlike the longitudinal serpiginous ulcers of Crohn's disease, tuberculous ulcers tend to be circumferential or transverse. The diagnosis relies upon the presence of necrotizing granuloma with giant cells, of confluent granulomas and/or multiple granulomas (>10 per biopsy field). Overall however, less than 5% of the mucosal biopsies are positive. Drug-induced colitis must be considered in middle aged patients. The main drugs implicated are antibiotics and nonsteroidal anti-inflammatory drugs. Diverticular-disease-associated colitis is also more common in elderly patients. Diversion colitis is an inflammatory process that occurs in the bypassed colonic segment after surgical diversion of the fecal stream. Microscopic lesions similar to Crohn's disease have been reported in ileal and colonic biopsies from patients with reactive arthritis and ankylosing spondylitis. However, only a minority of these patients developed genuine Crohn's disease.

References and Further Reading

Baumgart, D. C., & Sandborn, W. J. (2012). Crohn's disease. *Lancet, 380*, 1590–1605.

Geboes, K., Ectors, N., D'Haens, G., & Rutgeerts, P. (1998). Is ileoscopy with biopsy worthwhile in patients presenting with symptoms of IBD. *The American Journal of Gastroenterology, 93*, 201–206.

Gledhill, A., & Dixon, M. F. (1998). Crohn's-like reaction in diverticular disease. *Gut, 42*, 392–395.

Harpaz, N., & Sachar, D. B. (2006). Segmental colitis associated with diverticular disease and other IBD look-alikes. *Journal of Clinical Gastroenterology, 40* (Suppl 3), S132–S135.

Hovde, O., & Moum, B. A. (2012). Epidemiology and clinical course of Crohn's disease: Results from observational studies. *World Journal of Gastroenterology, 18*, 1723–1731.

Stange, E. F., Travis, S. P., Vermeire, S., Beglinger, C., Kupcinkas, L., Geboes, K., Barakauskiene, A., Villanacci, V., Von Herbay, A., Warren, B. F., Gasche, C., Tilg, H., Schreiber, S. W., Scholmerich, J., & Reinisch, W. (2006). European evidence based consensus on the diagnosis and management of Crohn's disease: Definitions and diagnosis. *Gut, 55* (Suppl 1), i1–i15.

Van Assche, G., Dignass, A., Panes, J., Beaugerie, L., Karagiannis, J., Allez, M., Ochsenkühn, T., Orchard, T., Rogler, G., Louis, E., Kupcinskas, L., Mantzaris, G., Travis, S., & Stange, E. (2010). The second European evidence-based Consensus on the diagnosis and management of Crohn's disease: Definitions and diagnosis. *Journal of Crohn's & Colitis, 4*, 7–27.

Cronkhite–Canada Syndrome

Andreia Albuquerque
Serviço de Gastrenterologia, Centro Hospitalar de São João, Porto, Portugal

Synonyms

CCS

Definition

Cronkhite–Canada syndrome (CCS) was first described in 1955 by Leonard W. Cronkhite and Wilma Jeanne Canada as a new distinct clinical entity, occurring in two patients with generalized gastrointestinal polyposis, pigmentation of the skin, alopecia, and atrophy of the fingernails and toenails.

Is a rare, non-inherited gastrointestinal polyposis syndrome characterized by diffuse distribution of hamartomatous or juvenile-type polyps throughout the gastrointestinal tract, except for the characteristic sparing of the esophagus and specific ectodermal abnormalities, including alopecia, onychodystrophy, and skin hyperpigmentation.

CCS is a chronic disorder of unknown etiology. An autoimmune origin has been suggested but not proved. Other proposal theories included an infectious cause, nutritional deficiency, altered intestinal mucin production, and mast cell dysfunction.

Diarrhea is the most prominent feature, and patients also can have weight loss, abdominal pain, nausea and vomiting, hypogeusia, and anorexia. The nails can have several degrees of dystrophy, such as thinning and splitting, and partial separation from the nail bed, onycholysis. Hair loss usually occurs rapidly over a period of a few weeks. In most patients, hair loss is simultaneous from the scalp, eyebrows, face, axillae, pubic areas, and extremities, but in some patients, only loss of the scalp is described. Hyperpigmentation areas are "lentigolike," light to dark brownish macules, ranging from a few mm to 10 cm in diameter, and can be seen in the buccal mucosa, retina, and abdomen. Laboratory analyzes can reveal anemia, electrolyte disturbances, or hypoalbuminemia. Paresthesias, seizures, and tetany, apparently related to electrolyte abnormalities, have also been reported.

Clinical Features

- **Incidence**
  CCS has a worldwide distribution, and 75% of case reports come from Japan. Is a rare disorder, until 2002, only 467 cases have been reported in the literature, 354 of which were reported by Japanese groups.
- **Age**
  The typical onset is during middle or old age; mean age is 59 years, with a range of 31–86 years. At the time of presentation, 80% of the patients were over 50 years of age.
- **Sex**
  There is slight male predominance, male-to-female ratio is approximately 1.3–1.5:1.
- **Site**
  CCS is a gastrointestinal polyposis syndrome characterized by diffuse distribution of polyps throughout the gastrointestinal tract, except for the characteristic sparing of the esophagus and specific ectodermal abnormalities, involving the skin and nails.
- **Treatment**
  Several therapies have been used in patients with CCS. Due to the rarity of the disease, controlled therapeutics trials have not been possible. Nutritional support, antibiotics, corticosteroids, anabolic steroids, histamine receptor, and surgical treatment have all been used with varying degrees of success.

The majority of patients require nutritional support, and this should be used in patients with weight loss, malnourishment, or electrolyte abnormalities but in addition to other medical therapies, namely, corticosteroids. Aggressive nutritional support, including electrolyte replacement and parenteral nutrition when necessary, is often utilized, and there have been reports of patients achieving remission for more than 5 years with complete symptomatic improvement and resolution of ectodermal changes.

Corticosteroids have been used in a large number of cases and are related with resolution of the symptoms and ectodermal abnormalities. Steroids such as prednisone 40 mg/day or the equivalent should be considered the mainstay of medical treatment. In some patients, corticosteroids were used for induction and as a bridge to allow time for the immunomodulatory agent, azathioprine, to take effect.

Anabolic steroids are not recommended for CCS treatment due to the limited data concerning effectiveness and adverse effects. There is no definitive evidence for an infectious etiology for CCS, but coexisting infections, including septicemia, have occurred. There are no firm recommendations for the use of antibiotics in the absence of infection. A combination regimen using histamine-receptor antagonist, cromolyn sodium, prednisone, and suppressive antibiotics has also been described. Surgical treatment should be reserved for complications, namely, uncontrolled gastrointestinal bleeding, intussusception, and perforation. Routinely endoscopic exams are important to remove large polyps (>10 mm), allowing the early detection of adenomas and presumably prevention of colorectal cancer.

The symptoms and ectodermal changes are partial or completely reversible with specific treatment, and a diminution in the size and density of polyps has also been reported, but total disappearance of all polyps has not been documented.

- **Outcome**
  Complications as gastrointestinal bleeding, infection, and malnutrition commonly occur, and the mortality rate has been estimated to be 60%.

The malignant potential of CCS polyps is controversial, several reports documented gastrointestinal malignancy in patients with CCS. There are case reports to suggest that both typical adenomatous and serrated polyp pathways may be involved, and the overall risk of colorectal cancer has been suggested to be as high as 20–25%, whether the duration and/or extent of polyp formation accelerate the risk for neoplasia in CCS is unknown [3]. Large polyps (> 10 mm) need to be removed, with histological examination.

Macroscopy

Multiple sessile or semipedunculated polyps ranging from 0.5 to 2 cm in diameter located principally in the colon but also in the stomach ("carpetlike" polyposis) and small intestine. The number of polyps appeared to be greater in the duodenum and in the terminal ileum and less in the jejunum and proximal ileum. Other common feature includes superficial erosion of polyps and gross thickening of the polyp-bearing mucosa which may contain ulcers. The mucosa thickening is attributed to the severe edema, glandular ectasia, and inflammation found in the lamina propria and submucosa. In the stomach, this thickening often occurs in the greater curvature and may appear as giant rugal folds. In the small bowel, edema and inflammation of the transverse folds produce prominent valvulae conniventes. In the large bowel, the edema and inflammation of transverse folds may result in a thickening bowel wall with normal haustrations.

Microscopy

In CCS, polyps are hamartomatous or juvenile-type polyps. Mucosa is characterized by an intact epithelium, proliferated tortuous glands, some of which were cystically dilated and filled with proteinaceous fluid or mucus, and edematous chronically inflamed lamina propria. The mucosa often contains engorged vascular channels, surface erosions, and prominent eosinophilic infiltration. The mucosa between the polyps showed edema, congestion, and inflammation of the lamina propria and focal glandular ectasia.

Morphologically, the gastric mucosa in CCS resembles that seen in Ménétrier's disease.

The polyps of juvenile polyposis coli may also be indistinguishable from those of CCS but differ from the latter in that the intervening mucosa is histologically normal.

Single or multiple carcinomas, often near the polyps, have been documented. Almost 40 cases of colorectal cancer have been reported in association with CCS.

Hyperpigmentation in CCS is due to an increase of melanin in the basal layer and not to proliferation in the number of melanocytes.

Scalp biopsy shows a marked non-inflammatory loss of follicular units, miniaturization of the hair shafts, markedly dilated follicles, and a heavy deposition of glycosaminoglycans in the reticular dermis.

Immunophenotype

A study including cases of CCS seen at Mayo Clinic showed that immunostaining for the autoimmune-related IgG4 antibody is significantly increased in CCS polyps compared to juvenile polyposis syndrome hamartomas and normal control tissue. Immunostaining for IgG4 was performed on 42 polyps from CCS cases and on control tissues, including 46 histologically similar hamartomas (from juvenile polyposis syndrome) and 20 normal mucosae. More studies concerning this issue are needed.

Molecular Features

Not described.

Differential Diagnosis

The main differential diagnosis is sporadic juvenile polyps or juvenile polyposis syndrome (JPS). Both JPS and CCS have nonneoplastic hamartomas with cystic dilation and typical glandular. Although, JPS is an inherited condition associated with mutations in the *SMAD4 (MADH4)* and *BMPR1A* genes, does not have the ectodermal changes typical of CCS, and polyps do not regress with steroid treatment. CCS polyps tend to be less pedunculated, and the nonpolypoid mucosa of CCS is histologically abnormal (edema, dilated crypts), while the mucosa between JPS polyps is normal. Despite these differences, CCS and JPS can occasionally be confused both clinically and histologically.

A relationship between CCS and Ménétrier's disease has been reported by some authors, the gastric mucosa is similar and both are associated with protein-losing enteropathy and symptomatic remissions, although, Ménétrier's disease is confined to the stomach and not associated with ectodermal changes.

References and Further Reading

Cronkhite, L. W., Jr., & Canada, W. J. (1955). Generalized gastrointestinal polyposis; an unusual syndrome of polyposis, pigmentation, alopecia and onychotrophia. *The New England Journal of Medicine, 252*, 1011–1015.

Daniel, E. S., Ludwig, S. L., Lewin, K. J., Ruprecht, R. M., Rajacich, G. M., & Schwabe, A. D. (1982). The Cronkhite-Canada Syndrome. An analysis of clinical and pathologic features and therapy in 55 patients. *Medicine (Baltimore), 61*, 293–309.

Sweetser, S., Ahlquist, D. A., Osborn, N. K., et al. (2012). Clinicopathologic features and treatment outcomes in Cronkhite-Canada syndrome: support for autoimmunity. *Digestive Diseases and Sciences, 57*(2), 496–502.

Ward, E. M., & Wolfsen, H. C. (2003). Pharmacological management of Cronkhite-Canada syndrome. *Expert Opinion on Pharmacotherapy, 4*, 385–389.

Ward, E. M., & Wolfsen, H. C. (2002). Review article: The non-inherited gastrointestinal polyposis syndromes. *Alimentary Pharmacology & Therapeutics, 16*, 333–342.

Cushing's and Curling's Ulcer

Ricardo Marcos-Pinto[1,2], Pedro Pimentel-Nunes[1,3] and Mário Dinis-Ribeiro[1,3]

[1]Serviço de Gastrenterologia, Portuguese Oncology Institute, Porto, Portugal

[2]Centro Hospitalar do Porto, Instituto de Ciências Biomédicas Abel Salazar (ICBAS-UP), Cintesis (FMUP-UP), Porto, Portugal

[3]Instituto Português de Oncologia (IPO - Porto), Cintesis (FMUP-UP), Porto, Portugal

Synonyms

Stress-related mucosal disease; Stress ulcer

Definition

Cushing's ulcer is considered a stress ulcer, a condition that results from an imbalance between gastric protection and gastric acid production in response to a major insult (traumatic brain injury in the case of Cushing's ulcer). Harvey Cushing published in 1932 a paper with the description of patients who postoperatively and unexpectedly died of perforated peptic ulcers. It was one of the first descriptions of a stress ulcer and a treatise on the brain-stomach connection. The lesions arise from the action of the parasympathetic centers of the hypothalamus and their connections to vagal nuclei in the medulla increasing gastric acid production. The pathogenesis includes the disequilibrium between major destructive factors like acid and pepsin and the protective factors like mucosal blood flow, mucous bicarbonate layer, epithelial renewal, and prostaglandin production. On the other side, in 1842, Curling reported 12 cases of duodenal ulceration in burn patients establishing the relationship of stress secondary to burns leading to peptic ulceration. Harvey Cushing published his theories on stress ulceration related to hypothalamic lesions in 1932; these are similar lesions, but with a different cause. The relationship between extent of burn and frequency of ulceration has not been precisely determined, but the majority occurs in patients with significant burns covering 30–60% of body surface. The pathogenesis includes the disequilibrium between major destructive factors like acid and pepsin and the protective factors like mucosal blood flow (postburn hemoconcentration), mucous bicarbonate layer, epithelial renewal, and prostaglandin production. Other risk factors for stress ulcer, validated in prospective multicenter cohorts, include burns, respiratory failure, severe coagulopathy, and renal and hepatic failure.

Clinical Features

- **Incidence**
  Nowadays acute gastric lesions associated with burn injury are not commonly seen, this may

C

be due to prophylactic use of gastric protective agents, first used in burn patients and later in similarly critically ill patients. Old studies described 86% of patients with gastric erosions following large burns and 22% with the development of gastric ulcer. Actual incidence of gastrointestinal bleeding estimates a prevalence of 8.5% among intensive care unit patients (who do not receive stress ulcer prophylaxis).

- **Age**
  The typical traumatic brain injury patient is a male between 15 and 24 years of age.
- **Sex**
  The typical traumatic brain injury patient is a male between 15 and 24 years of age.
- **Site**
  Stress ulcerations usually occur in the fundus and body of the stomach, but sometimes develop in the antrum or duodenum.
- **Treatment**
  Medical therapy includes treatment of the established stress ulcer that parallels that of traditional peptic ulcer, including medical therapy with proton pump inhibitors (PPI) and endoscopic therapy in the presence of high-risk stigmata. Nowadays prophylactic therapy is assuming a relevant role. Clinical trials have demonstrated that H2 blockers, PPI, and anti-acid reduce the frequency of GI bleeding related to stress ulceration compared to placebo or no prophylaxis. Current guidelines suggested the use of prophylactic agents in intensive care unit setting in the presence of major risk factors like coagulopathy (defined as platelet count < 50,000/ml or an international normalized ratio (INR) > 1.5), mechanical ventilation for more than 48 h, or traumatic brain injury/burn injury. On the other hand, some randomized trials suggested that increasing gastric pH with those prophylactic agents may increase the frequency of nosocomial pneumonia and *Clostridium difficile* infection.
- **Outcome**
  Cushing's ulcer is one of the severe complications of traumatic brain injury with a substantial mortality rate. Overt gastrointestinal bleeding due to stress ulceration is associated with increased mortality (OR 1.8–4.9). Curling's ulcer is one of the severe complications of severe burns with a substantial mortality rate.

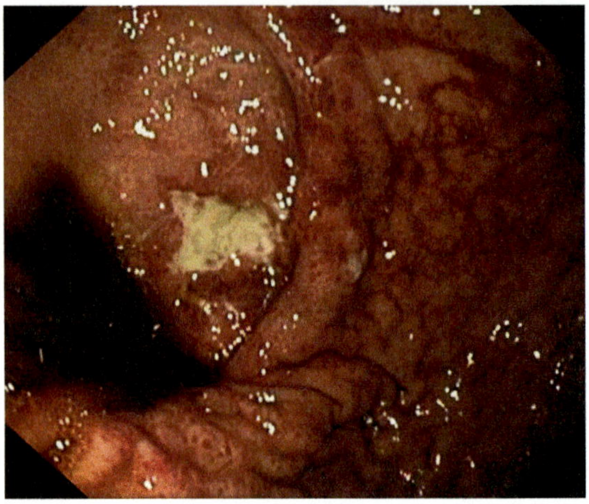

Cushing's and Curling's Ulcer, Fig. 1 Fundic stress ulcer

Macroscopy

At endoscopy, stress ulcers tend to be shallow and cause oozing of blood from superficial capillary beds. Deeper lesions may also occur, which can erode into the submucosa and cause significant hemorrhage or perforation. Figure 1 shows a fundic stress ulcer with multiple erosions in the surrounding mucosa; the patient presented with a significant upper GI bleeding.

Microscopy

It is not usual to take biopsy samples from these lesions and so histology is rarely described. When biopsied, they present as acute with minimal reactive fibrosis (manifesting their acute nature) which is the principal feature distinguishing stress ulcers from common peptic ulcer of the stomach.

Immunophenotype

Not applied

Molecular Features

Not applied

Differential Diagnosis

- Peptic ulcer/erosion (different location and microscopy)
- Malignant ulcer (e.g., lymphoma or adenocarcinoma, different endoscopic appearance with irregularity)
- Ischemic ulcer

References and Further Reading

Alain, B. B., & Wang, Y. J. (2008). Cushing's ulcer in traumatic brain injury. *Chinese Journal of Traumatology, 11*(2), 114–119.

Marik, P. E., Vasu, T., Hirani, A., & Pachinburavan, M. (2010). Stress ulcer prophylaxis in the new millennium: A systematic review and meta-analysis. *Critical Care Medicine, 38*(11), 2222–2228.

Wijdicks, E. F. (2011). Cushing's ulcer: The eponym and his own. *Neurosurgery, 68*(6), 1695–1698.

D

Diaphragmatic Hernia

Miguel Serrano and Susana Mão de Ferro
Department of Gastroenterology, IPOLFG, E.P.E., Lisbon, Portugal

Synonyms

Acquired diaphragmatic hernia; Congenital diaphragmatic hernia

Definition

A hernia is a protrusion of the abdominal cavity beyond its fascial or muscular walls through fascial or muscular openings or defects. Diaphragmatic hernias (DH) include acquired hernias through the esophageal hiatus and hernias through post-traumatic or congenital (such as the foramina of Bochdalek or Morgagni) defects in the diaphragm. The majority of DH are sliding hernias of the stomach through the esophageal hiatus.

Congenital and post-traumatic DH will be reviewed here. Hiatal hernias are discussed elsewhere (see entry on "▸ Diaphragmatic Hernia").

Congenital Diaphragmatic Hernia

Congenital diaphragmatic hernia (CDH) is a developmental defect in the diaphragm that allows abdominal viscera to herniate into the chest, thereby interfering with normal lung development.

The ventral part of the diaphragm is derived from the septum transversum, which in the early embryo separates the heart from the abdominal contents. Normally it fuses with rib cage and sternum, but small canals, the foramina of Morgagni, remain lateral to the sternum on either side. The dorsal part forms from the dorsal mesentery, but posterolateral communications, known as the canals of Bochdalek, persist on either side between the pleural and peritoneal cavities. At first, only the pleural and peritoneal membranes fuse. Latter, muscle grows into them from the body wall.

CDH results from failure of fusion of the multiple developmental components of the diaphragm. Morgagni hernias form anteriorly at the sternocostal junctions of the diaphragm and Bochdalek hernias posterolaterally at the lumbocostal junctions of the diaphragm.

The pathophysiology of CDH involves compression of the developing lung by the herniated abdominal contents which decrease bronchial and pulmonary arterial branching resulting in lung hypoplasia and pulmonary arterial muscle hyperplasia. Pulmonary hypertension resulting from these arterial anomalies leads to right-to-left shunting at atrial and ductal levels. This persistent fetal circulation leads to right-sided heart strain or failure and to the vicious cycle of progressive hypoxemia, hypercarbia, acidosis, and pulmonary hypertension observed in the neonatal period.

F. Carneiro et al. (eds.), *Pathology of the Gastrointestinal Tract*, Encyclopedia of Pathology,
DOI 10.1007/978-3-319-40560-5

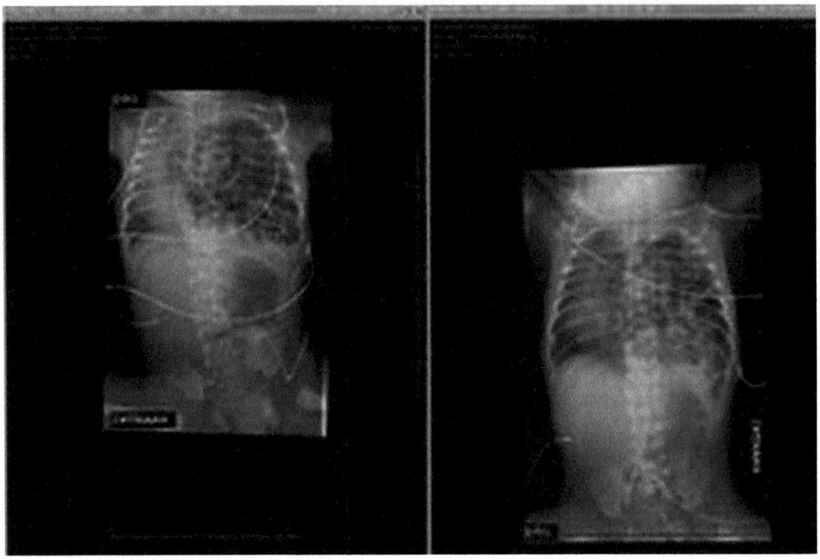

Diaphragmatic Hernia, Fig. 1 Chest radiography showing herniation of abdominal contents into the left hemithorax (Courtesy of Dr. João Paulo Conceição e Silva, Department of Radiology, IPOLFG, EPE, Lisbon Portugal)

Biochemical analysis also indicates potential deficiencies in the surfactant and antioxidant enzyme system.

The most common CDHs are posterolateral hernias through the foramen of Bochdalek, more frequently left-sided and unilateral, while Morgagni hernias occur in only 5–10% of cases.

The presentation of CDHs varies greatly, from death in the neonatal period to an asymptomatic finding in adults.

Newborns with Bochdalek hernia most often develop respiratory distress in the first few hours or days of life, and examination will reveal scaphoid abdomen and absence of breath sounds on the ipsilateral side. Associated anomalies are seen in approximately 50% of CDH cases and include chromosomal abnormalities (trisomy 13, 18, and 21), congenital heart disease, renal anomalies, genital anomalies, and neural tube defects. Intestinal malrotation is commonly observed in children with CDH (30–62%). Volvulus is a complication in a small minority of these cases. The kidneys are often enlarged and hyperplastic. CDH can also occur as a part of De Lange syndrome (an autosomal dominant disorder with microbrachycephaly and limb and digital anomalies) and as a part of Fryns syndrome (an autosomal recessive disorder with variable features that include DH, cleft lip and palate, and distal digital hypoplasia).

Associated anomalies confer a twofold relative risk of mortality when compared with patients with isolated CDH. In stillborn infants, associated anomalies are more common.

With the routine use of prenatal ultrasound, the diagnosis of CDH is frequently made prenatally. Ultrasonography reveals polyhydramnios, an absent intra-abdominal gastric air bubble, mediastinal shift, and hydrops fetalis. In those where CDH was not diagnosed in utero, the diagnosis is made by chest radiography showing herniation of abdominal contents into the hemithorax (Fig. 1).

In older children and adults, a Bochdalek hernia may manifest as an asymptomatic chest mass. About one half of adult patients present with acute emergencies due to incarceration. Gastric volvulus is common. The diagnosis may be suspected on chest radiograph, particularly a lateral view, because Bochdalek hernias occur in the posterior chest.

Morgagni hernias are most likely to manifest in adult life. They may contain omentum, stomach, colon, or liver. The diagnosis is often made by chest radiograph, particularly the lateral view because Morgagni hernias are anterior.

Post-traumatic Diaphragmatic Hernia

Post-traumatic diaphragmatic hernias (PTDH) are due to blunt trauma (such as motor vehicle accidents) in about 80% of cases and to penetrating trauma (such as gunshot or stab wounds) in the remainder. Other rare causes of traumatic rupture include labor in women with prior DH repair and barotrauma during underwater dives in patients with history of Nissen fundoplications. Blunt diaphragm rupture usually causes large radial tears of the diaphragm, while penetrating injury leads to smaller rents that approximate the size of the penetrating impalement. As such, penetrating injuries are more likely to be missed. Blunt trauma is more likely than penetrating trauma to lead to herniation of abdominal contents into the chest because the defect is usually larger.

PTDH require a high level of suspicion to detect. Patients can be asymptomatic in up to 53% of hernias from blunt trauma and 44% from penetrating trauma. After serious trauma, rupture of the diaphragm is often masked by other injuries. Respiratory or abdominal symptoms manifesting several days to weeks after injury should suggest the possibility of diaphragmatic injury. At least 50% of patients with diaphragmatic injury also suffer associated injuries. Routine chest radiograph is diagnostic in only one half of the cases. The use of rapid helical CT, especially with sagittal reconstruction, has facilitated the diagnosis. Symptoms may also manifest long after injury.

Clinical Features

- **Incidence**
  CDH is estimated to occur in 1 out of 2,000–10,000 births, with Bochdalek hernia making up the majority of cases.
  The incidence of PTDH is uncertain since many cases likely go undiagnosed. It is estimated that 3–5% of patients admitted to the hospital for multiple traumatic injuries have a DH.
- **Age**
  As many as 90% of patients with CDH present in the neonatal period or within the first year of life (most often Bochdalek hernias). History and clinical findings vary with the presence of associated anomalies and the degree of pulmonary hypoplasia and visceral herniation. In neonates, variable respiratory distress and cyanosis, feeding intolerance, and tachycardia are noted. Older children or adults present with obstructive symptoms from protrusion of the colon, chest pain, tightness or fullness in the chest, sepsis following strangulation or perforation, or respiratory symptoms.
  Morgagni hernias are most likely to manifest in adulthood. The symptoms are usually those of intestinal obstruction and may affect one or more of the following: stomach, small intestine, and colon.
  Most of patients with PTDH present in the third decade of life.
- **Sex**
  CDH seem to be slightly more frequent in males and less frequent in blacks.
  The male-to-female ratio is 4:1 in patients with PTDH.
- **Site**
  In CDH the defect is usually posterolateral (Bochdalek hernia) but may be anterior retrosternal or parasternal (Morgagni hernia) or rarely central. Herniation usually occurs on the left (80–85%); right-sided DH occur in only 10–15% of cases. Bilateral herniation is rare.
  In patients presenting with PTDH, 69% of hernias are left-sided, 24% are right-sided, and 15% are bilateral. This difference is probably related to hepatic protection and increased strength of the right hemidiaphragm. Children have equal rates of rupture per side, likely due to laxity of liver attachments.
- **Treatment**
  Congenital Diaphragmatic Hernia
  Since the mid-1980s, when it was recognized that the major determinants of mortality were pulmonary hypoplasia and pulmonary hypertension, the treatment paradigm of CDH has shifted from early surgical intervention to preoperative care directed towards optimal management of pulmonary hypoplasia and pulmonary hypertension, followed by surgical repair.
  Preoperative care is directed towards stabilizing the infant's oxygenation, blood pressure, and acid–base status. Aggressive medical management consists of

decompression of the lung tissue, cardiovascular support, and ventilatory support including high-frequency oscillatory ventilation and extracorporeal membrane oxygenation that minimize lung injury.

Once the child has stabilized from a pulmonary standpoint, the hernia will then be repaired through reduction of the abdominal viscera and primary closure of the diaphragmatic defect, using sutures alone or large mesh prosthesis.

Post-traumatic Diaphragmatic Hernia

Traumatic rupture of the diaphragm requires surgical intervention whether the patient presents immediately or sometime after the trauma. The high incidence of concomitant intra-abdominal injuries dictates the need for emergency abdominal exploration in the acute trauma setting after initial resuscitation is accomplished. Patients who present in the latent phase or long after the trauma require repair because the hernia contents may become incarcerated and strangulated.

If the diaphragmatic injury is discovered during the acute phase of trauma, the standard surgical approach is laparotomy. For long-standing hernias, a transthoracic or thoracoabdominal approach should be used, because the herniated intra-abdominal contents tend to be firmly attached to intrathoracic structures, making a trans-abdominal approach difficult.

- **Outcome**

The degree of pulmonary dysfunction determines the child's prognosis with CDH. Mortality and morbidity are due to the amount of pulmonary hypoplasia, the response on artificial ventilation, and the presence of therapy-resistant pulmonary hypertension. Thirty nine to 77% of infants survive the neonatal period after repair, but a significant number have long-term neurologic and musculoskeletal problems and as many as 50% experience gastroesophageal reflux.

In PTDH, the outcome is generally related to the trauma mechanism and presence of associated injuries. Reported mortality ranges from 5.5% to 51%. People with isolated diaphragmatic injuries tend to recover without long-term disability.

Macroscopy

When the defect is located on the left side, the thorax may contain small and large bowel, the spleen, the stomach, the left lobe of the liver, and, occasionally, the kidney (Fig. 2). Right-sided CDHs usually contain part of the right lobe of the liver and sometimes the bowel and/or the kidney. A sac may cover the herniated abdominal

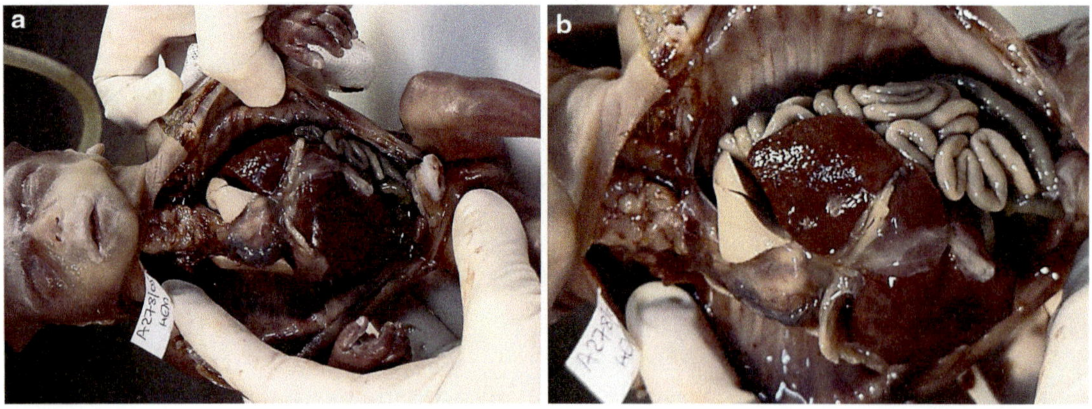

Diaphragmatic Hernia, Fig. 2 Gross pathology of left sided Bochdalek hernia containing small and large bowel. The ipsilateral lung is hypoplastic, but the contralateral one is also affected (Courtesy of Drª. Lucília Monteiro, Fetopathology Unit, CHLO, EPE, Lisbon Portugal)

contents. DH tend to be smaller than diaphragmatic eventrations.

The lung is hypoplastic on the ipsilateral side, but the contralateral one is also affected to a variable extent. Lung weight is decreased and the number of alveoli is reduced due to insufficient branching. In addition, hypoplasia of the left ventricle with a left-sided hernia or pleural effusions caused by right-sided involvement is frequently observed. The size of the pulmonary vascular bed is decreased in the hypoplastic lungs, and the adventitia and media of the pulmonary arterial walls are thickened.

Microscopy

The histology of the herniated bowel is normal unless a complication such as ulceration or incarceration with obstruction and/or ischemia has occurred. Then, the histology reflects the complication.

Microscopic examination of the hypoplastic lung shows a reduced number of alveoli due to insufficient branching. Respiratory epithelial maturity is delayed with hyaline membrane disease patterns similar to those found in prematures, and the distal bronchiolar arteries have muscularized walls and the wall thickness is increased particularly at the expense of the media and adventitial layers.

Immunophenotype

Not applicable.

Molecular Features

Experimental models have shown a link between CDH and defects in the retinoid signaling pathway, a key regulator of embryonic morphogenesis.

Differential Diagnosis

Thoracic lesions that should also be considered when the diagnosis of CDH is made prenatally by ultrasound include diaphragmatic eventration, congenital cystic adenomatoid malformation, bronchopulmonary sequestration, bronchogenic cysts, bronchial atresia, enteric cysts, and teratomas. In the full-term neonate with severe respiratory distress, the differential diagnosis includes other causes of pulmonary hypoplasia either primary or secondary (e.g., oligohydramnios from chronic amniotic fluid leak or renal hypoplasia/dysplasia) and persistent pulmonary hypertension.

References and Further Reading

Blitz, M., & Louie, B. E. (2009). Chronic traumatic diaphragmatic hernia. *Thoracic Surgery Clinics, 19*, 491–500.

Gaxiola, A., Varon, J., & Valladolid, G. (2009). Congenital diaphragmatic hernia: An overview of the etiology and current management. *Acta Paediatrica, 98*, 621–627.

Hanna, W. C., & Ferri, L. E. (2009). Acute traumatic diaphragmatic injury. *Thoracic Surgery Clinics, 19*, 485–489.

Tovar, J. A. (2012). Congenital diaphragmatic hernia. *Orphanet Journal of Rare Diseases, 7*, 1.

Waag, K. L., Loff, S., Zahn, K., et al. (2008). Congenital diaphragmatic hernia: A modern day approach. *Seminars in Pediatric Surgery, 17*, 244–254.

Dieulafoy's Lesion

Francisco Ferro de Beça and
Elisabete Rios
Department of Pathology, Centro Hospitalar de São João, Porto, Portugal
Faculty of Medicine of the University of Porto, Porto, Portugal
IPATIMUP – Institute of Pathology and Molecular Immunology of the University of Porto, Porto, Portugal

Synonyms

Caliber-persistent artery; Exulceratio simplex; Gastric atherosclerotic aneurysm

Definition

Named after Paul Georges Dieulafoy (1839–1911), a French surgeon and professor of pathology, Dieulafoy's lesion is a cause of acute GI bleeding. This is a potentially life-threatening lesion due to the presence of an enlarged artery in the submucosa that protrudes through small (2–5 mm) mucosal defects with exposure of the vessel wall in the lumen causing intraluminal hemorrhage. Dieulafoy's lesion is often recurrent and causes obscure massive GI hemorrhage, manifested by hematemesis and/or melena (Ding et al. 2010). Patients usually have no prior history of GI pathology or symptoms and typically have no significant NSAIDs or alcohol use. Although this lesion presents more commonly in a population with comorbidities, such as cardiopulmonary dysfunction or renal failure, which has led some researchers to propose causal links with these diseases, etiology for Dieulafoy's lesion remains largely unknown.

Clinical Features

- **Incidence**
  Approximately 1–5% of acute GI bleeding.
- **Age**
  The mean age of presentation is within the sixth decade of life, having most patients at presentation between 50 and 70 years old. Nevertheless recent series have described several cases in pediatric populations (Senger and Kanthan 2012).
- **Sex**
  More common in men than women, at a 2:1 ratio.
- **Site**
  The stomach is the most common site (approx. 70%), with 80–95% occurring in the lesser curvature within 6 cm of the gastroesophageal junction (Montgomery and Voltagio 2012). Extragastric lesions occur most frequently in the duodenum, followed by the colon. Other uncommon sites include the esophagus, rectum, and anus.
- **Treatment**
  Endoscopic hemostatic procedures are the treatment of choice in most cases. Angiography with embolization and surgery are also treatment options, especially when the lesion is beyond reach of the endoscope or when there are difficulties controlling recurrent bleeding (Baxter and Aly 2010).
- **Outcome**
  The risk of re-bleeding is between 9% and 40%. Mortality risk decreased from 80% to 8.6% due to endoscopic therapeutic modalities currently used.

Macroscopy

Although sometimes visualization of these lesions is difficult due to large amounts of blood, hematin, and its location, the majority can be identified on endoscopic examination of the GI tract. The macroscopic appearance on endoscopic examination is of a 2–5 mm mucosal defect, sometimes with visible a protruding vessel, surrounded by normal-appearing mucosa (Montgomery and Voltagio 2012).

Microscopy

Due to the straightforward endoscopic diagnosis when this lesion is identified, microscopic evaluation is usually limited to cases of resection and autopsy specimens. Still, the usual microscopic appearance of this lesion is of an artery, primary located in the superficial submucosa, which extends through the mucosa (Fig. 1). The vessel typically presents with focal disruption covered by a fibrin clot, without evidence of atherosclerotic or aneurysmal dilatations. The mucosa adjacent may be obliterated with fibrin and show some degree of chronic inflammation, without any other specific pathological findings (Montgomery and Voltagio 2012).

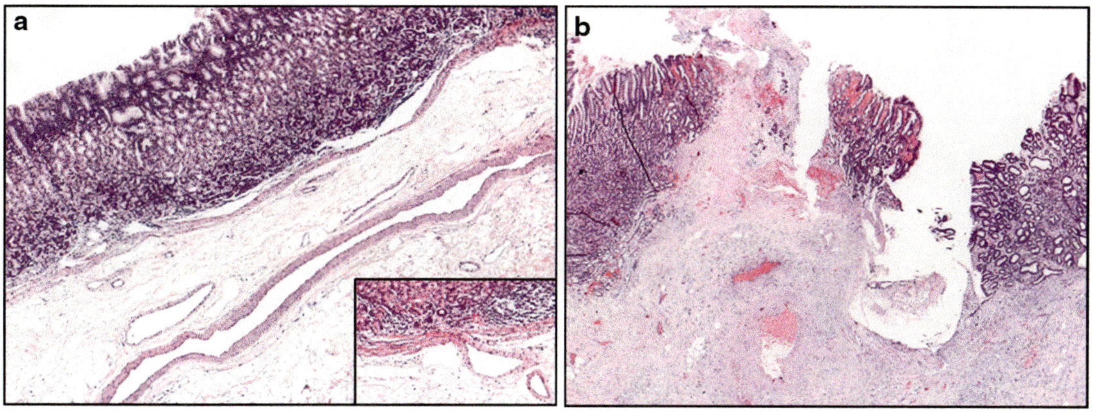

Dieulafoy's Lesion, Fig. 1 Histopathological findings. (**a**) – Large caliber-persistent artery running on superficial submucosa of the gastric wall, lacking atherosclerotic or aneurysmal dilatations (H&E; objective lens x10). Inset: higher amplification (objective lens x40) showing a focal protrusion into the gastric mucosa of an artery running of superficial submucosa. (**b**) – Gastric ulceration with underlying tortuous and dilated arteries in the submucosa with hemorrhagic infiltrate (H&E; objective lens x4)

Differential Diagnosis

The histological differential diagnosis is usually made with other vascular lesions causing obscure GI bleeding. In the stomach, common differential diagnosis should consider both GAVE (gastric antral vascular ectasia or "watermelon stomach") and portal gastropathy. In other GI tract sites, as the colon, lesions such as angiodysplasia, diverticular disease, telangiectasias, vascular neoplasms, and disorder of connective tissue-affecting blood vessels should be considered as possible differential diagnosis (Jain and Chetty 2009).

References and Further Reading

Baxter, M., & Aly, E. H. (2010). Dieulafoy's Lesion: Current trends in diagnosis and management. *Annals of the Royal College of Surgeons of England, 92*, 548–554.

Ding, Y., Zhao, L., Liu, J., & Luo, H. S. (2010). Clinical and endoscopic analysis of gastric Dieulafoy's lesion. *World Journal of Gastroenterology, 16*(5), 631–635.

Montgomery, E. A., & Voltagio, L. (2012). Chapter 2, Stomach. In: *Biopsy interpretation of the gastrointestinal tract mucosa. Vol 1: Non-neoplastic*. 2nd ed, (pp. 89–91). Philadelphia: Lippincott Williams & Wilkins.

Jain, R., & Chetty, R. (2009). Dieulafoy disease of the colon. *Archives of Pathology & Laboratory Medicine, 133*(11), 1865–1867.

Senger, J. L., & Kanthan, R. (2012). The evolution of Dieulafoy's Lesion since 1897: Then and now-a journey through the lens of a pediatric lesion with literature review. *Gastroenterology Research and Practice*. 2012: 432517.

Disaccharidase Deficiency

Arzu Ensari
Department of Pathology, Ankara University Medical School, Sihhiye, Ankara, Turkey

Synonyms

Lactase, sucrose, and maltase deficiencies

Definition

The deficiency of disaccharidases is defined as the absence of the enzymes which are located in the brush border of the small intestinal mucosa and that break down dietary carbohydrates into simple sugars so that the intestine can absorb the nutrients. The major dietary disaccharides are lactose, maltose, and sucrose. These are broken down by lactase, maltase, and the sucrase-isomaltase

Disaccharidase Deficiency, Table 1 Causes of disaccharidase deficiency

Primary	Secondary
Hereditary	Acquired
Very rare[a]	Relatively common
Usually affects one disaccharidase only	Affects all disaccharidases
Presents at birth	Presents at any age
Small intestinal mucosa is normal	Associated with small intestinal mucosal abnormality
Irreversible	May be reversed if the mucosa heals
Managed by dietary control	Treatment of the underlying disorder

[a]Except adult-onset lactase deficiency

Disaccharidase Deficiency, Table 2 Causes of secondary disaccharidase deficiency

Pancreatic insufficiency
Loss/damage of intestinal brush border
Celiac disease
Infectious gastroenteritis
Crohn's disease
Ulcerative colitis
Lymphoma
Antibiotics
Chemotherapy
Alcoholism
Short gut syndrome

complex in the duodenum. A deficiency of these enzymes in the duodenum results in a range of gastrointestinal symptoms including diarrhea, abdominal pain, and bloating. Disaccharidase deficiency may be congenital or acquired (Table 1). With the exception of adult-onset lactase deficiency, hereditary disorders are rare and present at birth. They usually only affect one disaccharide and are irreversible. They include congenital sucrase-isomaltase deficiency, an autosomal-recessive disease caused by a mutation in the SI gene, glucose-galactose malabsorption, due to a glucose transporter deficiency, and starch malabsorption due to glucoamylase deficiency. Acquired disaccharidase deficiency is relatively common, affects all disaccharides, and is associated with intestinal mucosal injury – damage to the small intestinal brush border. The injury can be due to a genetic abnormality; or autoimmune disorders such as celiac disease or Crohn's disease; or some other malabsorption syndrome (Table 2). It may also be transient. It can be due to extended use of drugs including antibiotics and other drugs and toxins, including alcohol and chemotherapeutic agents. Diagnostic laboratory tests include stool analysis to identify the presence of reducing sugars in feces, a sucrose hydrogen breath test to detect an abnormally high level of hydrogen in the breath of an affected individual after sucrose ingestion, and a sugar tolerance test in which a flat blood serum curve will indicate an abnormality. Intermittent distribution of lactase on the brush border revealed by immunohistochemistry, hydrogen breath tests, and response to an exclusion diet are the diagnostic procedures for lactase deficiency. However, gold-standard to achieve a definitive diagnosis is a small bowel biopsy and small bowel enzyme test which is performed on the crushed piece of tissue by radioimmunoassay.

Clinical Features

- **Incidence**
  The incidences of disaccharidase deficiencies are largely underestimated. By far the most common form of disaccharidase disorder is adult-onset lactase deficiency. This is present in 70% of the world's population, though not all are symptomatic. Congenital form on the other hand is extremely rare. Isosucrase-maltase deficiency has a prevalence of 2% among Caucasian populations. Lactase activity declines with age, and by adulthood, the loss of the enzyme leads to lactose intolerance. This is highly prevalent among Asian, African, Native-American, and Mediterranean populations.
- **Age**
  Congenital forms present soon after the introduction of carbohydrates in the diet of the infant, while secondary forms can occur at any age.

- **Sex**
  Males and females are affected with equal frequency.
- **Site**
  Small intestinal mucosa is involved in the secondary form.
- **Treatment**
  After the diagnosis of disaccharidase deficiency, treatment is by dietary modification. This may include the removal of offending sugars or the use of enzymes to aid digestion.
- **Outcome**
  An accurate diagnosis of disaccharidase deficiency is particularly important in children, given the potentially serious consequences of prolonged symptoms. The consequences include low levels of body fluids, malnutrition, and a failure to thrive. In a child with gastrointestinal symptoms, the first step in diagnosis is typically diet modification. Foods containing the suspected offending substance are withheld and then reintroduced to assess whether symptoms resolve and then recur.

Macroscopy

In the secondary form, the intestinal mucosa may show a range of abnormalities depending on the underlying disorder, whereas the congenital form causes no such change in the mucosa.

Microscopy

A normal histology in small intestinal biopsy may suggest primary deficiency, while the preceding disorder such as celiac disease may also be diagnosed by histology.

Immunophenotype

Immunohistochemistry performed using brush border hydrolases may aid in the diagnosis when there is lack of staining.

Molecular Features

Primary deficiencies show a range of genetic abnormalities.

Differential Diagnosis

The differential diagnosis comprises of all other causes of malabsorption.

References and Further Reading

Mones, R. L., Yankah, A., Duelfer, D., Bustami, R., & Mercer, G. (2011). Disaccharidase deficiency in pediatric patients with celiac disease and intact villi. *Scandinavian Journal of Gastroenterology, 46*(12), 1429–1434.

Murray, I. A., Smith, J. A., Coupland, K., Ansell, I. D., & Long, R. G. (2001). Intestinal disaccharidase deficiency without villous atrophy may represent early celiac disease. *Scandinavian Journal of Gastroenterology, 36*(2), 163–168.

Nichols, B. L., Avery, S. E., Karnsakul, W., Jahoor, F., Sen, P., Swallow, D. M., Luginbuehl, U., Hahn, D., & Sterchi, E. E. (2002). Congenital maltase-glucoamylase deficiency associated with lactase and sucrase deficiencies. *Journal of Pediatrics Gastroenterology and Nutrition, 35*(4), 573–579.

Nichols, B. L., Jr., Adams, B., Roach, C. M., Ma, C. X., & Baker, S. S. (2012). Frequency of sucrase deficiency in mucosal biopsies. *Journal of Pediatrics Gastroenterology and Nutrition, 55*(Suppl 2), S28–S30.

Volonaki, E., Sebire, N. J., Borrelli, O., Lindley, K. J., Elawad, M., Thapar, N., & Shah, N. (2012). Gastrointestinal endoscopy and mucosal biopsy in the first year of life: Indications and outcome. *Journal of Pediatrics Gastroenterology and Nutrition, 55*(1), 62–65.

Diversion Colitis

Gert De Hertogh
Department of Pathology, Pathologische Ontleedkunde, UZ Leuven, Leuven, Belgium

Synonyms

Nonspecific colitis of the excluded colonic segment

Definition

Diversion colitis is an inflammatory process occurring in an empty colon or rectum after surgical diversion of the fecal stream. It was first recognized in patients with chronic inflammatory bowel disease (IBD). It is still more common in these patients, although it has been reported with other, non-inflammatory conditions. Most patients have mild to moderate symptoms, typically tenesmus and diarrhea which may be mucous or bloody. Rare cases present with fulminant colitis. It is commonly believed that diversion colitis starts in the mucosa, with damage to the colonic epithelium. The colonocytes use mainly luminal short-chain fatty acids (SCFAs) as nutrients. SCFAs are metabolites of carbohydrate and peptide fermentation by obligate anaerobic bacteria. The number of these bacteria is reduced in an excluded colon.

Clinical Features

- **Incidence**
  The incidence and prevalence of this disease are difficult to estimate since many cases with histologic changes in the bowel wall remain asymptomatic. Numbers of up to 91% of adults following diversion have been cited, with the highest rates in IBD.
- **Age, Sex, Site**
  There is no age, sex, or site predilection.
- **Treatment**
  The preferred treatment for diversion colitis of relatively short duration is surgery to restore bowel continuity. This is usually curative and quickly reverses both the symptoms and the lesions. With long-standing diversion, surgery is less successful as the excluded bowel segment may have become completely atrophic. In such cases, patients may be treated with SCFA enemas or sometimes with anti-inflammatory agents (5-aminosalicylate or hydrocortisone enemas). Also irrigation with enemas containing soybean fibers has been applied with some success.
- **Outcome**
  The outcome is generally good after restoration of the fecal stream.

Macroscopy

Lesions may develop in the excluded colon segment within months of surgical diversion. In a typical case, the bowel is overall narrow with a stiff wall. The endoscopist may see mucosal edema, erythema, friability, nodularity, and ulcers, which are typically aphtous. In long-standing disease, inflammatory pseudopolyps and strictures may develop. The presence of linear ulcers and segmental strictures should alert one to the possibility of recurrent IBD in a patient who was already known with Crohn's disease.

Microscopy

The diagnosis rests on clinical grounds, endoscopic evaluation, and histology of mucosal biopsies. The clinician should alert the pathologist that the tissue fragments were taken in an excluded bowel segment. The reason for exclusion, particularly prior IBD, should be mentioned in the pathology request form.

Microscopically, one may see a spectrum of changes, both of the architecture and the cellular composition of the mucosa. Crypts can have an irregular course and may show branching or atrophy. The crypt epithelium can contain metaplastic Paneth cells. The lamina propria is filled with an increased, irregularly distributed mononuclear cell infiltrate. Prominent lymphoid follicles are a typical finding and may explain the endoscopically observed nodularity (Fig. 1). These follicles are commonly larger than what is expected for Crohn's disease. The muscularis mucosae is usually thickened. With active diversion colitis, neutrophils are present in the lamina propria and in the crypts. One may see cryptitis, crypt abscesses, signs of crypt rupture with mucin granulomas, and aphtous or larger ulcerations (Fig. 2). Some of these findings may also be recognized with confocal laser endomicroscopy.

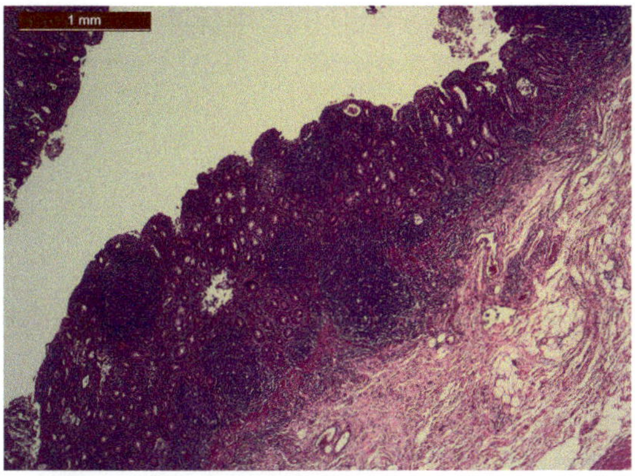

Diversion Colitis, Fig. 1 Low power H&E stain shows colon mucosa with a nodular surface due to the presence of prominent lymphoid aggregates

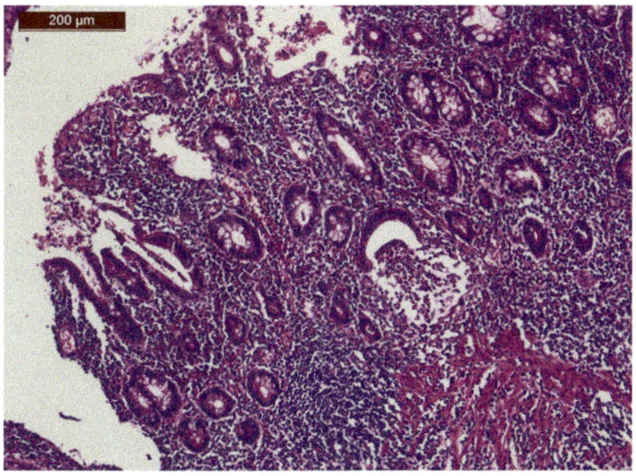

Diversion Colitis, Fig. 2 In this medium power H&E stain, one can discern a disturbed mucosal architecture (irregular branching crypts), an increased mixed inflammatory cell infiltrate in the lamina propria (with cryptitis, crypt abscesses, and surface erosions), and a thickened muscularis mucosae

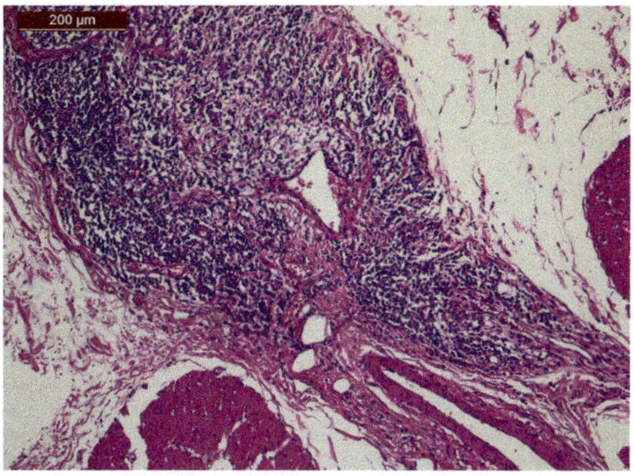

Diversion Colitis, Fig. 3 Low power H&E. Enterocolic lymphocytic phlebitis. The mesocolic vein wall in the center of the image is infiltrated by numerous lymphocytes, while the corresponding artery in the lower half of the picture is spared

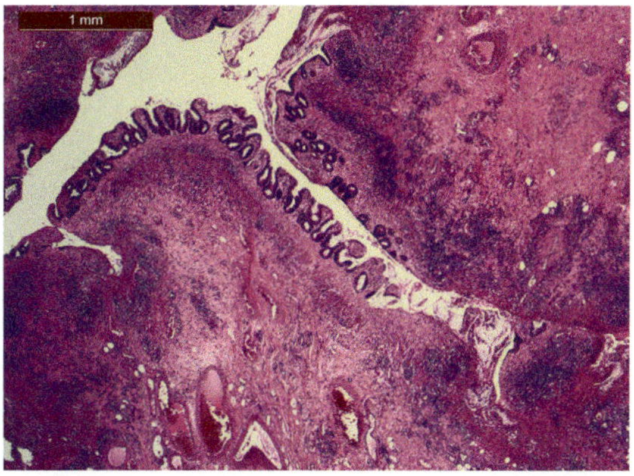

Diversion Colitis, Fig. 4 Low power view of longstanding diversion colitis, H&E stain. The mucosa is atrophic, there are large superficial ulcers, and the submucosa shows fibrosis and some lymphoid aggregates. The bowel caliber was severely reduced

The diagnosis is usually straightforward in a patient without preexisting IBD. The investigations can be supplemented with examination of stools for ova, parasites, *Clostridium difficile* toxin, and bacterial cultures when needed.

Occasionally, the diverted bowel segment is completely excised when the disease is difficult to treat. In such a case, penetrating ulcers, localized strictures, transmural lymphoid hyperplasia, and classical epithelioid granulomas point to a diagnosis of recurrent Crohn's disease in a patient known with this diagnosis. Rarely, similar changes may be seen after diversion for rectal ulcerative colitis. Diversion colitis in a patient with preexisting IBD may also be complicated by the development of enterocolic lymphocytic phlebitis (artery-sparing, venulocentric lymphoid inflammation which in the long term leads to vascular compromise) (Figs. 3 and 4). Another rare finding in surgical specimens is osseous metaplasia, presumably due to secretion of bone morphogenic proteins and increased alkaline phosphatase activity in epithelial and stromal cells. Also the presence of hyperplasia of neuroendocrine cells and microcarcinoids has been described.

Immunophenotype, Molecular Features

These techniques are not usually employed for the diagnosis. In one study, the effect of diversion on the cellular composition and function of the small bowel mucosa was investigated. The authors described a significant decrease of the number of spontaneously interferon-gamma-secreting CD3 lymphocytes both in the epithelium and in the lamina propria, and similar results for interleukin-4, especially in the lamina propria T-cells.

Differential Diagnosis

The main differential diagnosis is recurrent IBD as described earlier. One should also exclude infections, e.g., reactivation of CMV-infection or pseudomembranous colitis due to *Clostridium difficile* toxin.

References and Further Reading

Cook, S. I., & Sellin, J. H. (1998). Review article: Short chain fatty acids in health and disease. *Alimentary Pharmacology and Therapeutics, 12*, 499–507.
Edwards, C. M., George, B., & Warren, B. (1999). Diversion colitis – New light through old windows. *Histopathology, 1999*(34), 1–5.
Haas, P. A., Fox, T. A., Jr., & Szilagy, E. J. (1990). Endoscopic examination of the colon and rectum distal to a colostomy. *The American Journal of Gastroenterology, 85*, 850–854.
Ma, C. K., Gottlieb, C., & Haas, P. A. (1990). Diversion colitis: A clinicopathologic study of 21 cases. *Human Pathology, 21*, 429–436.
Schmit, A., Van Gossum, A., Carol, M., et al. (2000). Diversion of intestinal flow decreases the numbers of interleukin 4 secreting and interferon gamma secreting T lymphocytes in small bowel mucosa. *Gut, 46*, 40–45.

Diverticular Colitis

Gert De Hertogh
Department of Pathology, Pathologische Ontleedkunde, UZ Leuven, Leuven, Belgium

Synonyms

Crescentic fold disease; Diverticular disease-associated chronic colitis; Isolated sigmoiditis; Segmental colitis associated with diverticulosis (SCAD)

Definition

Diverticular colitis can be defined operationally as mucosal inflammation within a colon segment containing diverticula. It primarily affects the sigmoid colon. It is however distinct from diverticulitis, which is inflammation of one or more diverticula and the surrounding connective and muscle tissues. Diverticular colitis is noteworthy for mimicking chronic inflammatory bowel disease (IBD), both endoscopically and histologically.

Clinical Features

- **Incidence**
  Only a subset of patients with diverticulosis coli also develops diverticular colitis. Estimates vary between less than 1% and 4%. The true incidence and prevalence are probably underestimated as many patients do not develop worrisome symptoms. The most common presenting complaints are cramping left lower quadrant pain or tenesmus, constipation or diarrhea which may be mucous, and rectal bleeding. The classic radiologic exam shows only diverticular disease. The preferred diagnostic technique is endoscopy with biopsies.
- **Age, Sex**
  Similar to diverticulosis, diverticular colitis is mainly a disease of elderly persons.

- **Site**
  The inflammation is limited to the diverticular segment of the bowel. Diverticular colitis typically involves the mucosa between the diverticular ostia and only occasionally spreads to the diverticula proper (although without erosions or large numbers of neutrophils). In contrast, diverticulitis always involves the diverticula and their ostia, and may spread to the surrounding mucosa, but only when severe.
- **Treatment and Outcome**
  Diverticular colitis may be treated conservatively with the same measures as for diverticular disease (e.g., a high-fiber diet and antibiotics when needed). It also responds to treatment with 5-aminosalicylic acid (5-ASA) compounds, with over half of the patients achieving clinical remission. In most cases, the clinical course is benign and self-limited, although some patients may require sigmoid colectomy for bleeding or stricture complications. An increased risk for diverticulitis or colon cancer seems to be remote.

Macroscopy

At endoscopy, the lesions are typically situated in the sigmoid. In addition to diverticula, one sees mucosal erythema, friability, and erosions. This pattern can be very similar to the one observed with ulcerative colitis (UC). Also linear ulcerations in a longitudinal pattern and a cobblestone appearance may be present, causing confusion with Crohn's disease (CD). Clues to the correct diagnosis are that the inflammation is limited to the diverticular colon segment, and that the rectum is characteristically spared.

Microscopy

The pathogenesis of the mucosal inflammation has been ascribed to abnormal prominence of mucosal folds with chronic or recurrent mucosal prolapse, ischemia, and inflammation. Abnormal exposure to luminal antigens and toxins in a context of altered bowel flora due to stasis has also been implicated. Finally, the mass effect of peridiverticulitis and serosal abscesses may play a role (although it has been observed that diverticular colitis can develop even before the diverticula themselves are well formed).

Biopsies should be taken from the most inflamed-looking mucosa, preferably at some distance from the diverticular ostia. The endoscopist should warn the pathologist that the biopsies are taken from a diverticular colon segment. Preferably, rectal biopsies should be taken for microscopic examination to rule out inactive or previously treated UC. When mucosal biopsies are taken from areas between the diverticular openings, the histological aspect may mimic IBD to perfection. There are two patterns, one with diffuse and the other with patchy mucosal disease, potentially causing confusion with UC or CD, respectively.

In the first form, there is widespread architectural disturbance with crypt branching and shortening, together with the presence of an evenly spread, dense mononuclear cell infiltrate admixed with eosinophils. Basal lymphoid aggregates may be present, as basal plasmocytosis which may be focal or diffuse. With active disease, one may see neutrophils in the lamina propria, cryptitis, multiple crypt abscesses, erosions, and granulation tissue. Paneth cell metaplasia may be present (Figs. 1 and 2). More than 80% of the patients with this pattern respond to medical or surgical treatment, although a few develop classical UC.

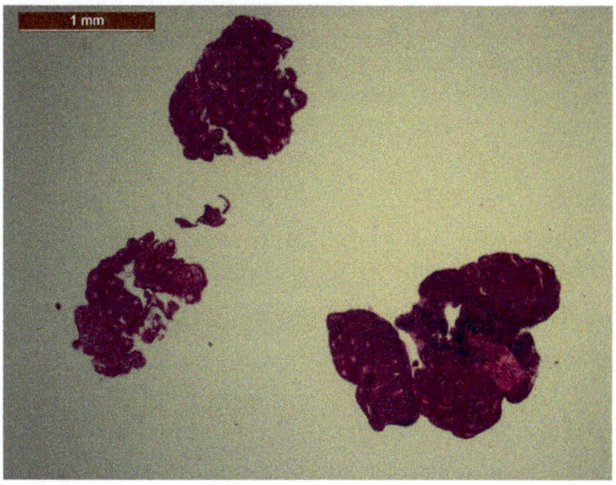

Diverticular Colitis, Fig. 1 Low power H&E stain shows colon mucosa with crypt distortion and an overall increased inflammatory infiltrate

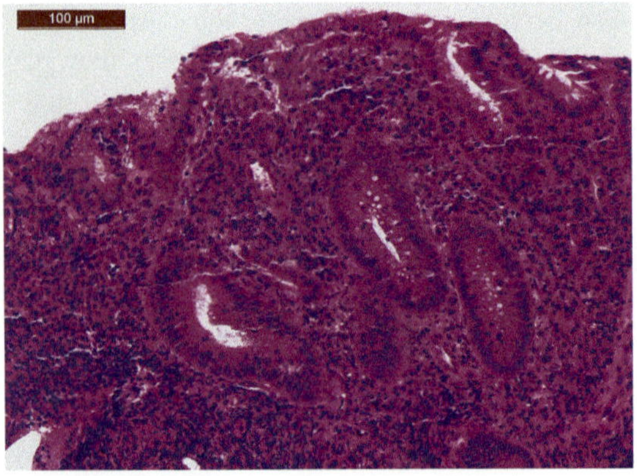

Diverticular Colitis, Fig. 2 (Detail of Fig. 1). Basal lymphoid aggregates, dense mixed inflammatory infiltrate with cryptitis. These changes were limited to the mucosa of a diverticular sigmoid and descending colon. The patient has not developed ulcerative colitis over a follow-up period of 4 years

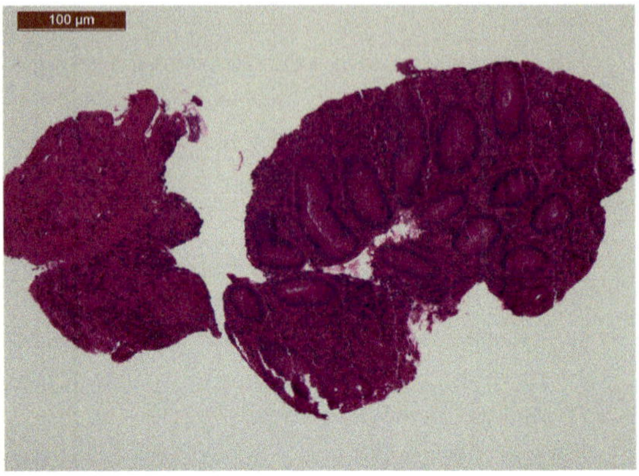

Diverticular Colitis, Fig. 4 (Detail of Fig. 3). Presence of giant cells and an epithelioid granuloma. The changes were limited to a diverticular sigmoid. The patient had no changes suggestive of Crohn's disease elsewhere at the time of biopsy 3 years ago, and has not developed them since

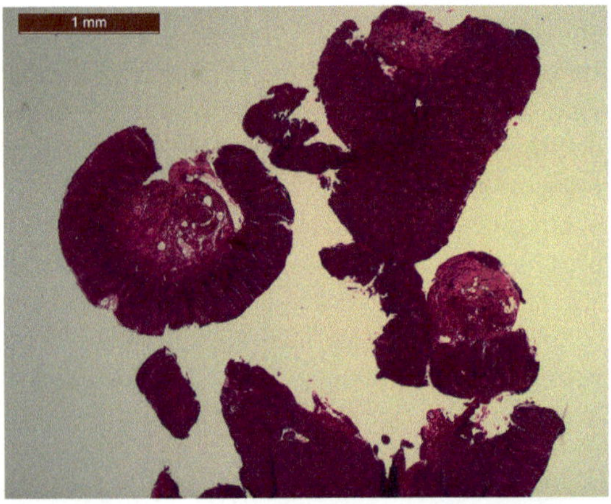

Diverticular Colitis, Fig. 3 Low power H&E. Colon mucosa. Irregularly distributed crypt distortion and patchy infiltrate

Such a disease course is unlikely when the rectal mucosa is completely normal, although one should recall that rectal histology may normalize in UC patients treated topically with enemas or suppositories.

In the second form, mucosal disease is more patchy with an irregularly distributed architectural distortion and a variably dense inflammatory cell infiltrate. Granulomas, both due to crypt rupture or classical epithelioid forms, may be present (Figs. 3 and 4). This may cause confusion with Crohn's disease, a problem which may be aggravated in colectomy specimens as other hallmarks of CD (such as thin deep ulcers, transmural lymphoid aggregates, serositis and creeping fat, and mural or lymph node granulomas) can then also be observed. The pathologist should be reluctant to offer a diagnosis of CD when these changes are limited to a diverticular sigmoid in an elderly person. In fact, the only strong argument for CD in such cases is the presence of histologically documented classical lesions elsewhere in the gastrointestinal tract.

Immunophenotype, Molecular Features

These techniques are not used for diagnosis or stratification.

Differential Diagnosis

As indicated above, a small subset of patients with diverticular colitis, when followed endoscopically over time, evolves into a picture typical for ulcerative proctosigmoiditis or Crohn's colitis. Therefore, a patient with presumed diverticular colitis should be re-evaluated clinically and endoscopically when symptoms persist or are progressive.

References and Further Reading

Burroughs, S. H., Bowrey, D. J., Morris-Stiff, G. J., et al. (1998). Granulomatous inflammation in sigmoid diverticulitis: Two diseases or one? *Histopathology, 33*, 349–353.

Goldstein, N. S., Leon-Armin, C., & Mani, A. (2000). Crohn's colitis-like changes in sigmoid diverticulitis specimens is usually an idiosyncratic inflammatory response to the diverticulosis rather than Crohn's colitis. *The American Journal of Surgical Pathology, 24*, 668–675.

Lamps, L. W., & Knapple, W. L. (2007). Diverticular disease-associated segmental colitis. *Clinical Gastroenterology and Hepatology, 5*, 27–31.

Makapugay, L. M., & Dean, P. J. (1996). Diverticular disease-associated chronic colitis. *The American Journal of Surgical Pathology, 20*, 94–102.

Tursi, A. (2011). Segmental colitis associated with diverticulosis: Complication of diverticular disease or autonomous entity? *Digestive Diseases and Sciences, 56*, 27–34.

Diverticular Disease, Colon

Iva Brcic
Institute of Pathology, Medical University of Graz, Graz, Austria

Synonyms

Outpouchings, herniations, or protrusions of the colon; Pseudodiverticulosis

Definition

Diverticulosis of the colon is characterized by diverticula in the colon. They represent herniations of the colonic mucosa and submucosa through thickened muscularis mucosae into the pericolic fatty tissue (Riddell et al. 2014). This happens in individuals who eat low-fiber diets when intraluminal pressure is increased and muscle layers of the colon wall are weak (West and Losada 2004). Uncomplicated diverticular disease (*diverticulosis*) may be asymptomatic or may present with left lower abdominal pain, fever, and diarrhea alternating with constipation. The symptoms are more prominent when inflammation of diverticula occurs (refer to as *diverticulitis*). This can lead to perforation with abscess or fistula formation. Gastrointestinal hemorrhage can also occur, usually arteriolar, causing bright red blood on the stool. Further complications are strictures of the colon and segmental colitis associated with diverticulosis (SCAD), also known as diverticular colitis. Prolapse-associated polyps may form at the diverticular orifices.

Clinical Features

- **Incidence**
  Diverticular disease is among the most common acquired disorder of the colon, especially in Western society (Weizman and Nguyen 2011).
- **Age**
  Usually found in patients over 60 years.
- **Sex**
  No sex predilection.
- **Site**
  Two forms of diverticular disease have been described: left-sided and right-sided. More common left-sided disease is predominantly found in the sigmoid and descending colon but can be distributed throughout the colon. Right-sided form is more commonly found in non-Western communities and involves cecum and proximal colon (Golder et al. 2011).
- **Treatment**
  Appropriate antibiotic therapy with high-fiber diet in uncomplicated disease. Surgery in case of complications.
- **Outcome**
  Generally good prognosis. In case of perforation, up to 5% mortality (Floch et al. 2004).

Macroscopy

External inspection of the surgical specimen reveals diverticula, around 1 cm in diameter, situated between the mesenteric and antimesenteric teniae, sometimes forming two rows on either side of the colon. Bowel can appear shortened. Open

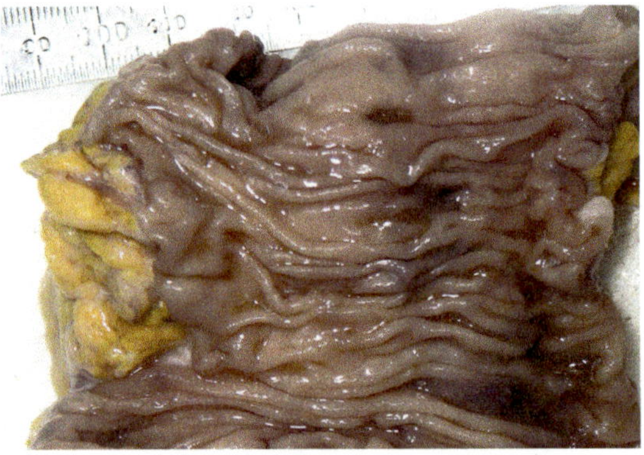

Diverticular Disease, Colon, Fig. 1 Macroscopic image of colon resection showing opening of a diverticulum filled with fecolith

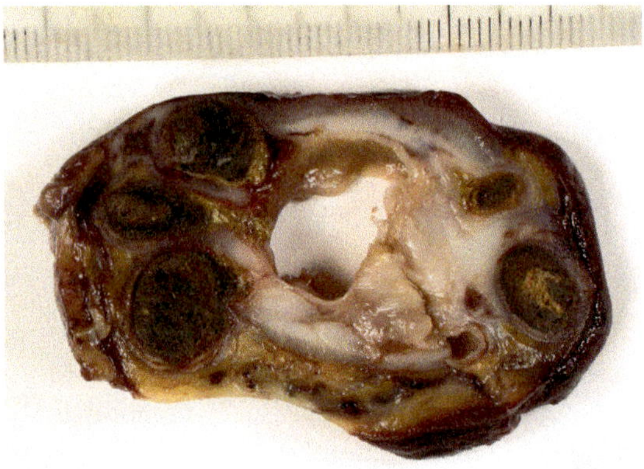

Diverticular Disease, Colon, Fig. 2 Cross section of the colon showing the thickened muscularis propria and multiple outpouchings of mucosa and submucosa through muscularis propria (diverticula) filled with fecolith

specimen shows prominent mucosal ridges and saccular dilatations where orifices of diverticula are apparent (Fig. 1). On the cut surface, thickened muscularis propria is present with visible herniations of the mucosa and submucosa (Fig. 2).

Microscopy

Upon histology, we see herniation of the colonic mucosa and submucosa between thickened muscularis mucosae into the subserosal adipose tissue (Fig. 3). In case of diverticulitis, mucosa changes can be found, namely architectural

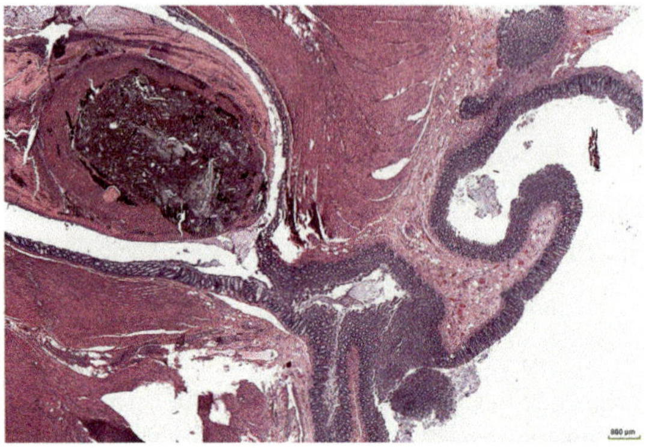

Diverticular Disease, Colon, Fig. 3 Microscopic image showing intact colon mucosa lining the bowel wall and the mucosa/submucosa invagination into the muscularis propria (diverticulum)

distortion, mucin depletion, mild cryptitis, increased lamina propria cellularity by lymphocytes and plasma cells, Paneth cell metaplasia, lymphoid aggregates, and erosions/ulcerations. Inflammation usually starts at the apical part of the diverticulum. When perforation occurs, localized abscess formation with occasional foreign-body giant cells can be found. In SCAD, the mucosal changes are located in the area of diverticulosis. In majority of cases, mucosa proximal and distal to the diverticula shows no inflammation (which can be helpful in the differential diagnosis). In later stages, with resolution of the inflammation, fibrosis leads to thickened and stenotic large bowel wall.

Immunophenotype

There is no distinctive immunophenotypic feature for diverticular disease.

Molecular Features

There is no distinctive molecular feature for diverticular disease.

Differential Diagnosis

Differential diagnosis of diverticular disease includes IBD (Crohn's disease and ulcerative colitis), diversion disease, and infection.

References and Further Reading

Golder, M., Ster, I. C., Babu, P., Sharma, A., Bayat, M., & Farah, A. (2011). Demographic determinants of risk, colon distribution and density scores of diverticular disease. *World Journal of Gastroenterology, 17*, 1009–1017.

Maconi, G., Barbara, G., Bosetti, C., Cuomo, R., & Annibale, B. (2011). Treatment of diverticular disease of the colon and prevention of acute diverticulitis: A systematic review. *Diseases of the Colon and Rectum, 54*, 1326–1338.

Riddell, R., El-Zamaity, H., & Jain, D. (2014). Motility disorders. In R. Riddell & D. Jain (Eds.), *Lewin, Weinstein, and Riddell's gastrointestinal pathology and its clinical implications* (pp. 227–238). Philadelphia: Lippincot Williams & Wilkins/Walter Kluwer.

Weizman, A. V., & Nguyen, G. C. (2011). Diverticular disease: Epidemiology and management. *Canadian Journal of Gastroenterology, 25*, 385–389.

West, A. B., & Losada, M. (2004). The pathology of diverticulosis coli. *Journal of Clinical Gastroenterology, 38*, S11–S16.

Diverticulum Epiphrenic

Bruno Pereira[1,2] and António Dias Pereira[1]
[1]Instituto Português de Oncologia de Lisboa Francisco Gentil, E.P.E., Lisbon, Portugal
[2]Servico de Gastrenterologia, Hospital Amato Lusitano, ULS de Castelo Branco, Castelo Branco, Portugal

Synonyms

Lower esophageal diverticulum; Supra-diaphragmatic diverticulum

Definition

A diverticulum is an outpouching of a hollow organ. Diverticula arising from the esophagus and hypopharynx are usually classified into three types according to anatomical location and pathogenesis. Zenker's diverticulum (pharyngoesophageal diverticulum) arises from the posterior hypopharynx, just above the upper esophageal sphincter, as a result of increased pressure during swallowing. Middle esophageal diverticula are usually secondary to an inflammatory process in the carinal lymph nodes (e.g., tuberculosis) which exert a traction force over the esophageal wall. Diverticula arising from the distal esophagus, usually within 10 cm of the cardia, are called epiphrenic diverticula.

In terms of pathogenesis, epiphrenic diverticula are generally classified as pulsion diverticula, although there have been reports of cases where a traction form seems to occur. The diverticula are thought to be the result of increased intraluminal pressure secondary to neuromuscular dysfunction. Most are associated with an underlying esophageal motility disorder, including distal esophageal spasm, achalasia, and hypertensive lower esophageal sphincter. Esophageal contractions against a closed lower sphincter seem to play an important role. Strictures, most often peptic in nature, may also act as an obstacle to esophageal peristalsis, thus contributing to diverticula formation. Protrusion of the diverticulum usually develops through a muscular defect in the esophageal wall. Conditions in which there is an increased weakness of the esophageal wall, like iatrogenic surgical injury or Ehlers-Danlos syndrome, have also been associated with epiphrenic diverticula.

Most epiphrenic diverticula are false diverticula (pseudodiverticula) since they only contain the mucosa and submucosa layers which protrude into the circular and longitudinal muscle of the esophagus. In a series by Bruggeman et al., all 11 resected epiphrenic diverticula lacked a muscularis propria. However, there have been several reports of surgically excised diverticula containing all layers of the esophagus, including a thin muscularis propria. Congenital epiphrenic diverticula, which are extremely rare, have a normally developed muscular layer. It is believed that they result from esophageal duplication which eventually develops a connection with the esophageal lumen.

Epiphrenic diverticula may present with a wide spectrum of symptoms, which are mostly related to underlying esophageal motility disorders. In the absence of associated esophageal disease, small diverticula are usually asymptomatic. Large diverticula (over 5 cm) are more frequently associated with esophageal abnormalities and more likely to be symptomatic. The accumulation of significant amounts of undigested food can lead to regurgitation in the recumbent position, particularly during the night, or when bending over. Dysphagia and chest pain are also common complaints. Some patients may present with cough or recurrent pneumonia due to aspiration of esophageal contents. Least common symptoms include heartburn, epigastric pain, halitosis, hematemesis, melena, and weight loss. There are no remarkable findings on physical examination. Halitosis and signs of pneumonia may be present in some patients.

Asymptomatic epiphrenic diverticula are usually found incidentally on radiographic or endoscopic studies performed for unrelated reasons. Even when symptomatic, the diagnosis can be often delayed due to attribution of the symptoms to other more common conditions. Chest radiographs may demonstrate a mediastinal air-fluid level within the diverticulum. Upper gastrointestinal endoscopy can not only detect the diverticulum but also play an important role in the exclusion of associated disorders like strictures. Barium esophagogram is the diagnostic gold standard for epiphrenic diverticula. It provides a precise definition of the location, number, and diverticulum structure, particularly the length and direction of protrusion of the neck, important parameters in the presurgical evaluation. Barium studies can also raise suspicion to an underlying esophageal motility disorder. An esophageal manometry should be performed if a motility disorder is suspected or if a surgical approach is being considered.

Clinical Features

- **Incidence**
  Epidemiologic data of esophageal diverticula are scarce. Epiphrenic diverticula constitute less than 10% of all esophageal diverticula. Contrast esophagograms performed in patients undergoing evaluation for dysphagia revealed epiphrenic diverticula in around 0.015% of the exams in the United States, 0.77% in Japan, and 2% in Europe. While the true prevalence in the general population remains unknown, epiphrenic diverticula appear to be significantly less common than Zenker's diverticulum, which has an estimated prevalence between 0.01% and 0.11%. The estimated annual incidence of epiphrenic diverticula is approximately 1:500.000.
- **Age**
  Esophageal diverticula are usually diagnosed in middle-aged adults and in the elderly. Age of diagnosis has been described to range from 18 to 88 years, with 75% of patients in the fifth, sixth, or seventh decades of life (Bruggeman and Seaman 1973).
- **Sex**
  A male to female ratio of 2:3 has been reported (Bruggeman and Seaman 1973). Several other series have not shown a significant male or female preponderance. This seems to be in accordance with epidemiologic data of esophageal motility disorders, frequently associated with epiphrenic diverticula. Achalasia is estimated to affect both sexes in equal numbers.
- **Site**
  Epiphrenic diverticula are located in the distal third of the esophagus, usually within 10 cm of the cardia.
- **Treatment**
  Due to its rarity, the appropriate treatment of esophageal diverticular disease remains somewhat controversial. Most literature on the management of epiphrenic diverticula consists of case series. Controlled clinical trials are lacking and unlikely to be performed considering the extremely low incidence and prevalence of the condition.

  A barium esophagogram should be performed to obtain the precise location, number, and structure of the diverticula. Upper gastrointestinal endoscopy is useful to rule out associated conditions like peptic or malignant strictures which might play a role in the pathogenesis of the diverticulum and alter the approach. Due to the strong association between epiphrenic diverticula and esophageal dysmotility, a manometry should be performed and treatment eventually directed to specific esophageal motility disorders, which are responsible for the symptoms in most cases. The management options for achalasia include endoscopic intrasphincteric injection of botulinum toxin, endoscopic pneumatic dilatation, and laparoscopic Heller myotomy. Symptoms related to esophageal spasm can sometimes improve with calcium channel blockers or nitrates.

All patients with epiphrenic diverticula and moderate to severe esophageal symptoms should be considered for surgical treatment. Asymptomatic or minimally symptomatic patients do not warrant treatment and should be followed. Most diverticula seem to have reached a stable size when diagnosed. Among 25 cases of epiphrenic diverticula followed for 1–12 years, an increase in size occurred in only 4 (Bruggeman and Seaman 1973). Worsening of an underlying motility disorder is believed to be the cause of size increase.

If surgical treatment is indicated, the traditional approach is a diverticulectomy through open transthoracic surgery (Hudspeth et al. 1993; Varghese et al. 2007). Underlying esophageal motility disorders should also be addressed at the time of surgery. By resolving the distal obstruction, an esophagomyotomy not only relieves dysmotility related symptoms but also decreases diverticular recurrence and postsurgical suture dehiscence. The myotomy should be performed opposite the location of the diverticulum. In order to minimize acid reflux caused by the disruption of the gastroesophageal junction, an antireflux procedure should be added to the myotomy.

Surgery for diverticular disease of the esophagus has been associated with high rates of morbidity and mortality. Various series, including 16–35 patients, have been published regarding the results of epiphrenic diverticula managed through open transthoracic surgery. Reported mortality rates ranged from 0% to 11% and postoperative leakages from 0% to 21%. The largest series (Varghese et al. 2007) achieved excellent results with no residual symptoms in 76% of patients, with an additional 21% only reporting relatively mild dysphagia. Median hospital stay was only 7 days.

Recent advances in minimally invasive techniques have led to thoracoscopic and laparoscopic management of epiphrenic diverticula in some centers. A recent meta-analysis (Kilic et al. 2009) included 10 studies reporting the outcome of 85 patients undergoing minimally invasive surgery for epiphrenic diverticula, 86% of them through laparoscopy. Conversion to an open procedure was necessary in only one patient. Mortality rates ranged from 0% to 7.7% and postoperative leakages from 0% to 33%. A positive surgical outcome, defined by symptom resolution or minimal symptoms, was reported in 83–100% of patients after a follow-up period ranging from 5 to 58 months. In the hands of experienced surgeons, a laparoscopic approach can be considered a viable alternative to open transthoracic surgery.

- **Outcome**

Diverticulum recurrence following surgery is rare. Asymptomatic epiphrenic diverticula can grow in size, usually in parallel with the worsening of an underlying esophageal dysmotility. When significant symptoms develop, a surgical approach should be considered. Delayed diagnosis and surgical referral can result in more severe and potentially life-threatening complications. Large symptomatic diverticula have been associated with recurrent aspiration pneumonia, ulceration, upper gastrointestinal bleeding, and perforation. The most serious complication arising from epiphrenic diverticula is carcinoma, which has an estimated incidence between 0.3% and 3%. There have been around 100 case reports in the medical literature. The pathogenesis is not completely understood but is thought to be related to chronic inflammation and injury due to food stasis. Carcinoma arising from epiphrenic diverticula is usually diagnosed in advanced stages and has a poor prognosis. If confirmed preoperatively, an esophagogastrectomy should be attempted instead of a diverticulectomy.

Macroscopy

Epiphrenic diverticula are usually single but can be multiple in up to 10% of patients. Size may vary from less than a cm to over 15 cm. One of the largest published series included 88 diverticula with 59% measuring 3 cm or less and 25% over 5 cm. Diverticula seem to arise more commonly on the right side comparing to the left side of the esophagus. They rarely protrude through the anterior or posterior wall. The right side preponderance is mostly attributed to large diverticula. The aforementioned series included 21 large diverticula (greater than 5 cm) with 71% located on the right side as opposed to only 19% on the left. However, taking into account only 67 small diverticula, the distribution was practically even (45% on the right side versus 46% on the left). One possible explanation is that the heart and aorta might prevent significant enlargement on the left side. The diverticulum orifice on the esophageal wall can be infracentimetric or measure up to 7 cm. Shapes can vary, with some diverticula being relatively flat with a poorly defined neck, while others have the more typical rounded sac form.

Microscopy

Most epiphrenic diverticula are false diverticula, and therefore, resected specimens usually contain the mucosa and submucosa layers and lack a muscularis propria. Diverticula containing all layers of the esophagus, including a thin muscularis propria, have also been reported. Chronic inflammation can be found in nearly all resected epiphrenic diverticula. Erosions and ulcerations can also occur. Dysplasia and carcinoma must be ruled out in view of the apparently increased cancer risk.

Differential Diagnosis

The clinical presentation of epiphrenic diverticula is diverse. Many potential diseases should be considered during the initial approach. Common conditions like gastroesophageal reflux disease can sometimes mimic the clinical features of diverticular disease. Obstructive disorders, including esophageal cancer, strictures, rings, and webs, should be ruled out in any patient presenting with dysphagia. Achalasia, distal esophageal spasm, and other motility disorders are frequently associated with epiphrenic diverticula. Symptoms are mostly related to the underlying esophageal motility disorder rather than the diverticulum itself. Other diverticula arising from the esophagus and hypopharynx, including mid-thoracic or Zenker's diverticulum, should also be considered. The finding of an air-fluid level on chest radiograph can raise suspicion of hiatal hernia, achalasia, and epiphrenic diverticulum. Upper gastrointestinal endoscopy and contrast esophagogram wield a high diagnostic accuracy and can usually differentiate between all of the aforementioned conditions.

References and Further Reading

Bruggeman, L. L., & Seaman, W. B. (1973). Epiphrenic diverticula. An analysis of 80 cases. *The American Journal of Roentgenology, Radium Therapy, and Nuclear Medicine, 119*(2), 266–276.

Fasano, N. C., Levine, M. S., Rubsein, S. E., et al. (2003). Epiphrenic diverticulum: Clinical and radiographic findings in 27 patients. *Dysphagia, 18*, 9–15.

Hudspeth, D. A., Thorne, M. T., Conroy, R., et al. (1993). Management of epiphrenic esophageal diverticula. A fifteen-year experience. *The American Surgeon, 59*(1), 40–42.

Kilic, A., Schuchert, M. J., Awais, O., et al. (2009). Surgical management of epiphrenic diverticula in the minimally invasive era. *Journal of the Society of Laparoendoscopic Surgeons, 13*(2), 160–164.

Varghese, T. K., Marshall, B., Chang, A. C., et al. (2007). Surgical treatment of epiphrenic diverticula: A 30-year experience. *The Annals of Thoracic Surgery, 84*(6), 1801–1809.

Drug-Induced Esophagitis

Mário Ferraz de Oliveira
Serviço Anatomia Patológica, Centro Hospitalar Lisboa Central EPE, Lisbon, Portugal

Synonyms

Drug; Iatrogenic; Medication-induced esophagitis; Pill

Definition

First described in 1970 by Pemberton, drug-induced esophagitis is an underdiagnosed entity, which affects all ages but is more frequent in the elderly (specially women).

It is caused by attached and prolonged mucosal contact of the ingested tablets/capsules with posterior damage to the mucosa due to the following mechanisms: production of a caustic solution (acidic or alkaline), creation of a hyperosmolar solution, or direct drug toxicity.

The patients normally have no previous esophageal pathology, although some cases are related with decreased salivary flow, esophageal motility abnormalities, or extrinsic compression. The more common causes are ingested pills with either very little fluid or without, before night time sleep, or other recumbent positions.

The common symptoms are odynophagia, retrosternal pain, and dysphagia, which start a few hours or days after the ingestion of the pill, sometimes with hematemesis and melena.

There is a growing list of more than one hundred drugs related with pill esophagitis, but the more frequent are nonsteroidal anti-inflammatory drugs (NSAIDs), antibiotics (specially doxycycline and tetracycline), emepronium bromide, potassium chloride, ferrous sulfate, quinidine, and alendronate. Almost 50% are due to antibiotics, but the more complicated cases are from NSAIDs and specially from biphosphatases (alendronate), with formation of strictures.

Clinical Features

- **Incidence**
  The incidence reported varies between 3,9/100,000 per year (Wright 1991) and 4/100,000 per year (Sweden study 1978) but is probably higher today.
- **Age**
  It affects patients of all age groups (reports from 3 to 98 years) but is more frequent in the elderly.
- **Sex**
  Females are more affected (around 70% of reported cases).
- **Site**
  Lesions are usually located at the junction of proximal and middle third of the esophagus (where the aortic arch compresses the esophagus and the peristaltic amplitude is low), but can appear above or below this zone.
- **Treatment**
  Discontinuation of the drug, sometimes with anti-reflux therapy and topical anesthetics.
- **Outcome**
  After discontinuation of the drug, the most uncomplicated cases may heal spontaneously, with resolution of symptoms in a few days.

Macroscopy

Injury occurs due to the direct irritant effects of the medications on the mucosa, with formation of erosions or discrete ovoid ulcers with normal or only mildly inflamed adjacent esophageal mucosa. Ulcers can be superficial or deep, sometimes with perforation, depending on the composition of the pill.

Microscopy

Histologic appearance is of an acute nonspecific inflammation, with desquamation, spongiosis, and necrosis of the squamous epithelium (Figs. 1 and 2), sometimes associated with prominent eosinophilic infiltration.

In cases of ferrous sulfate-induced disease, there is crystalline stainable iron, and in

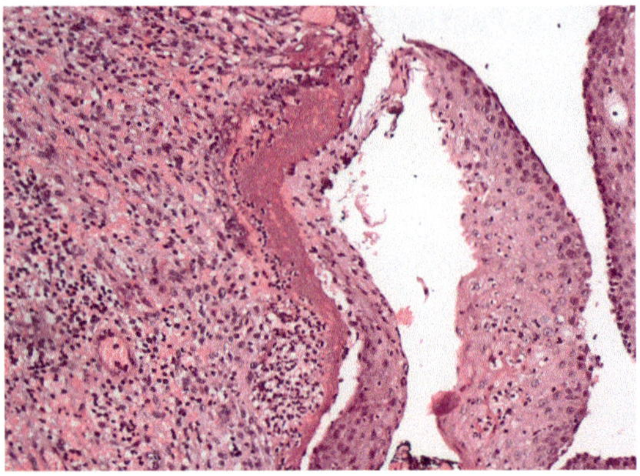

Drug-Induced Esophagitis, Fig. 1 Esophageal mucosa with ulceration and nonspecific inflammation (hematoxylin–eosin, ×100)

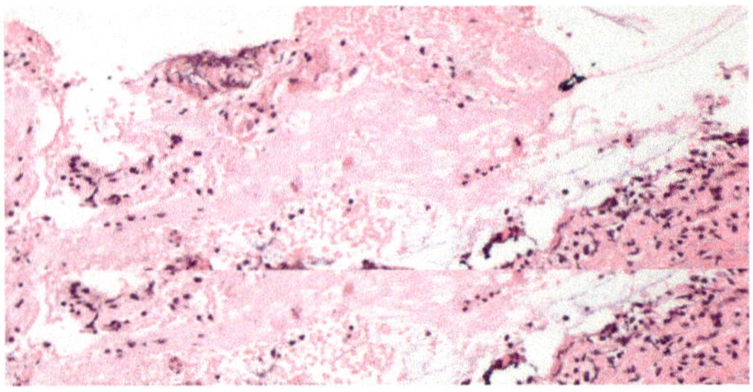

Drug-Induced Esophagitis, Fig. 2 Erosion with fibrin and necrotic cells (hematoxylin–eosin, ×100)

alendronate-induced injury, we can observe polarizable crystalline foreign material (sometimes with multinucleated giant cells).

Immunophenotype

Noncontributory

Molecular Features

Noncontributory

Differential Diagnosis

Infectious esophagitis (CMV, herpes, and *Candida*).

Gastroesophageal reflux disease

Neoplastic lesions

References and Further Reading

Arora, A. S., & Murray, J. A. (2000). Iatrogenic esophagitis. *Current Gastroenterology Report, 2*(3), 224–229.

Jaspersen, D. (2000). Drug-induced oesophageal disorders: Pathogenesis, incidence, prevention and management. *Drug Safety, 22*(3), 237–249.

Kikendall, J. W. (1999). Pill esophagitis. *Journal of Clinical Gastroenterology, 28*(4), 298–305.

Noffsinger, A. E. (2009). Update on esophagitis-controversial and underdiagnosed causes. *Archives of Pathology and Laboratory Medicine, 133*, 1087–1095.

Young, P. E., & Kikendall, J. W. (2012). Pill-induced esophageal injury. In J. E. Richter & D. O. Castell (Eds.), *The esophagus* (pp. 707–724; 5th ed.). Wiley-Blackwell.

Drug-Induced Gastritis

Wen-Yih Liang[1] and Gregory Y. Lauwers[2]
[1]Department of Pathology, Taipei Veterans General Hospital, Taipei, Taiwan
[2]Department of Pathology, Massachusetts General Hospital, Harvard Medical School, Boston, MA, USA

Synonyms

Iatrogenic gastritis

Definition

Drug-induced gastritis refers to gastric mucosal injury related to the adverse effects of therapeutic/pharmacological agents.

Clinical Features

- **Incidence**
  The incidence varies significantly between agents, but over the last 10 years, there has been greater recognition of iatrogenic-related gastric mucosal alteration.
- **Presentation**
  Drug-induced gastritis is characterized by the diversity and the nonspecific nature of the

presentation. Some patients are asymptomatic, but common clinical manifestations include upper abdominal discomfort or pain, loss of appetite, nausea, and vomiting. More severe presentations may include hematochezia, melena, hemorrhagic shock, and even gastric perforation.

- **Age**
  Drug-induced gastritis is more frequently diagnosed in adults and seniors. This is likely directly related to the increased use of therapeutic agents in older age-groups, such as anti-inflammatory or antioncologic therapy. However, younger patients are also affected if treated with the same medications.
- **Sex**
  There is no sex-related predilection.
- **Site**
  Body fundus and antrum can be equally affected by most drugs.
- **Treatment/Outcome**
  In most cases, the symptoms will subside after withdrawal of the causative agent.

Macroscopy

In many cases, the endoscopic appearance may be normal. In others, nonspecific alterations can be detected, such as erosion, ulceration, stenosis, mucosal erythema, or polyp.

Microscopy

The gastric mucosa can be affected differently by various drugs. Erosion and ulceration, acute hemorrhagic gastritis, reactive gastropathy, parietal cell hyperplasia, fundic gland polyp, epithelial atypia and apoptosis, and crystal deposition can be detected. (See discussions in subsections below.) Given the ever-growing number of drugs associated with noxious mucosal effects, an exhaustive review cannot be offered here, but several of the most recently highlighted iatrogenic effects will be described.

Nonsteroidal Anti-inflammatory Drugs (NSAIDs)

NSAIDs are widely used, and about 30–40% of individuals taking them may show gastric mucosal changes. Topically, NSAIDs, which are weak organic acids, can insult mucosal cells directly. NSAIDs also inhibit cyclooxygenase enzymes required for conversion of arachidonic acid to protective prostaglandins. Alteration of cellular proliferation and repair, blood flow, and growth factor expression occur as well. Finally, inhibition of cyclooxygenase also leads to diminished bicarbonate and mucus secretion with decrease in hydrophobicity of the mucus.

Several patterns of mucosal damage can be seen: acute hemorrhagic gastritis, erosions, ulcers, and chemical gastritis. Acute hemorrhagic gastritis is an early lesion, characterized by damaged surface epithelium, edema, hemorrhage of the lamina propria, and little inflammation (Fig. 1). Stromal eosinophilia can be seen as well. This alteration usually develops within the first hour after ingestion. Reactive gastropathy is the second most common histological diagnosis made on gastric biopsies and is noted in 35–45% of chronic NSAID users. The diagnostic hallmarks include foveolar hyperplasia lined by tall columnar cells with variable mucin depletion with hyperchromatic nuclei (Fig. 2). Other features include ectatic capillaries, minimal edema, and

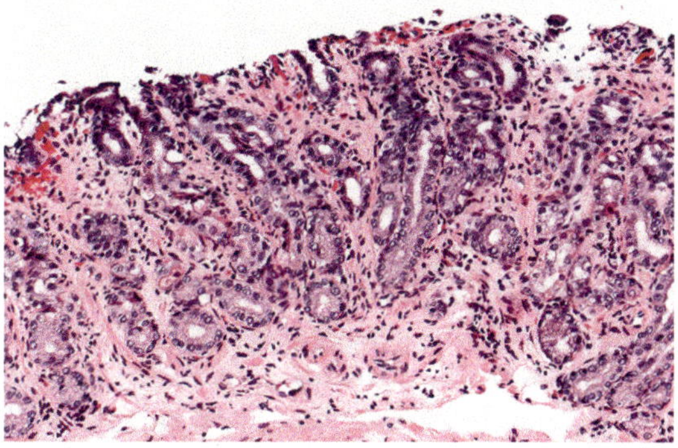

Drug-Induced Gastritis, Fig. 1 Example of erosive acute gastritis. The surface epithelium has been sloughed off, while the lamina propria demonstrates evidence of hemorrhage and hyalinization. The epithelium is regenerative and should not be mistaken for dysplasia

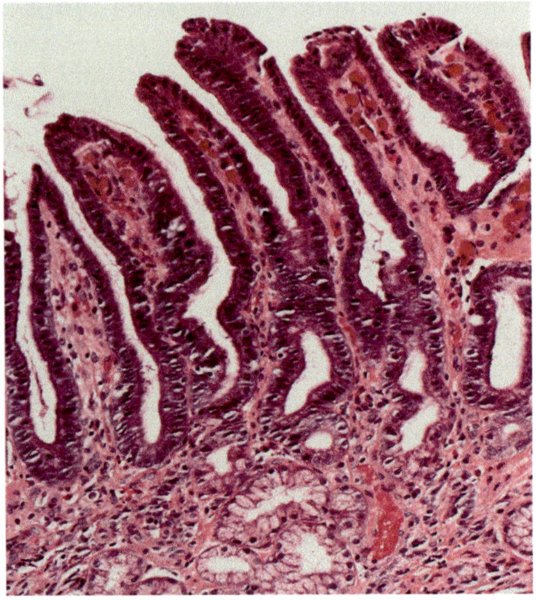

Drug-Induced Gastritis, Fig. 2 Example of reactive gastropathy. In this patient known to take NSAIDs, the foveolar epithelium shows mucin depletion, while the pit regions have mild serration

prominence of smooth muscle with minimal inflammation of the lamina propria.

Chronic NSAID use also can lead to the development of ulcers that are often large and multiple, and often painless.

Proton Pump Inhibitors

Proton pump inhibitors (PPIs) block gastric acid production by binding the H^+, K^+ -ATPase on the canalicular surface of the parietal cell membrane. Most patients also develop parietal cell hyperplasia of the corpus characterized by enlarged and more numerous parietal cells that protrude into the gland and confer a serrated appearance to the gland lumen. This change is reported in 90% of patients using PPI daily after 1 year. A few deep glandular cysts may be present and are attributed to obstruction of acid flow out of the gland due to the protruding parietal cells. Fundic gland polyps may develop in 17% and 35% of patients receiving PPI after 3 and 12 months of treatment, respectively (Fig. 3).

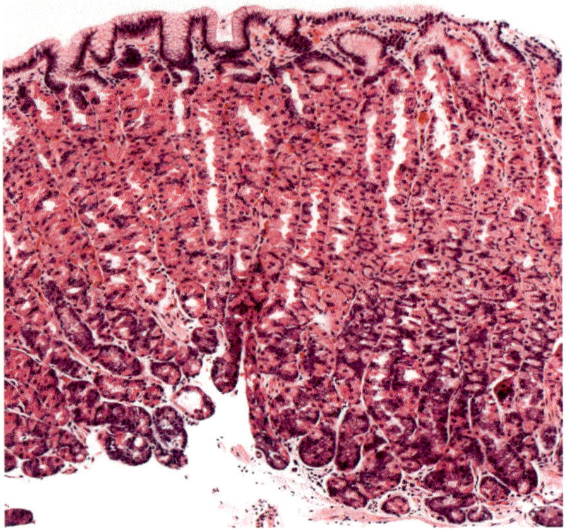

Drug-Induced Gastritis, Fig. 3 Example of parietal cell hyperplasia in a patient taking a proton pump inhibitor

Iron

Iron supplements (ferrous sulfate) is locally corrosive and is associated with erosions, ulcers, and in some cases infarct-like necrosis of the mucosa. The golden-brown pigment of iron is easily visible on H&E stains, embedded in granulation tissue, crusting the top of damaged epithelium, or detected in the lamina propria. Prussian blue stain may be helpful in confirming the diagnosis (Figs. 4a, b).

Gastric Mucosal Calcinosis

This refers to small, deeply eosinophilic crystals typically found beneath the surface epithelium of the mucosa, and more often in the antrum than in the body. The crystals may stain deeply pink or be only partially calcified refractile material. Usually, the mucosa is otherwise unremarkable or shows some degree of foveolar hyperplasia and edema. This condition has been associated with hypercalcemia, but also antacids, isotretinoin, and citrate-containing blood products.

Doxycycline

Recently, an example of doxycycline-associated erosive gastritis has been reported. The

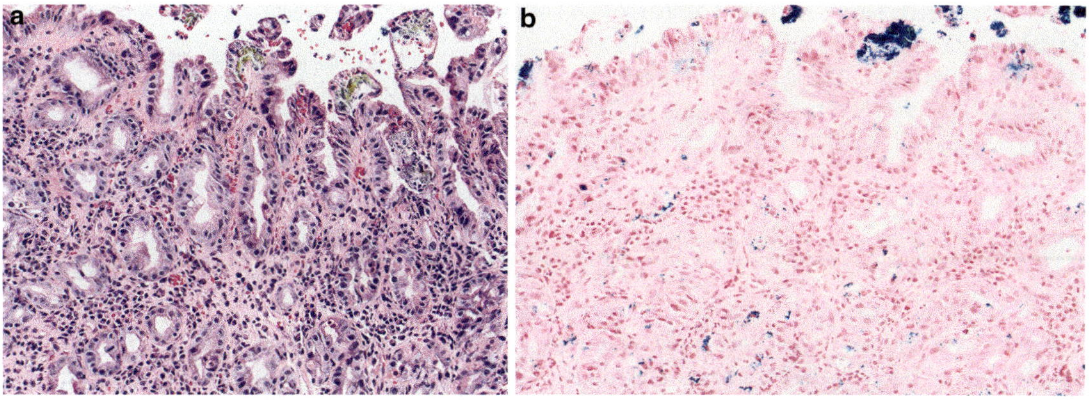

Drug-Induced Gastritis, Fig. 4 (**a**) Iron pill gastritis. Moderate chronic inflammation is noted, along with regenerative epithelium. Note the presence of golden brown pigment encrusted in the superficial lamina propria. (**b**) Prussian blue stain highlights the presence of iron within the lamina propria and also in a few epithelial and stromal cells

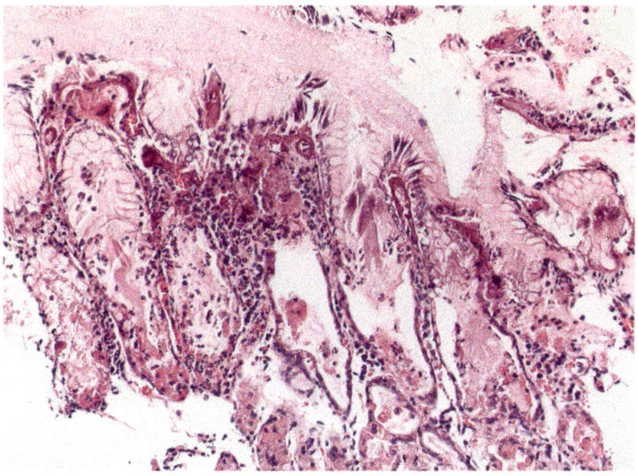

Drug-Induced Gastritis, Fig. 5 Example of doxycycline associated erosive gastritis. Vascular degeneration and microthrombi in the superficial lamina propria are easily observed

histological characteristics include superficial erosion with dense exudate associated with vascular degeneration and microthrombi (Fig. 5).

Colchicine

This alkaloid binds to tubulin and inhibits its polymerization into microtubules. The most characteristic finding is the presence of numerous epithelial mitotic figures arrested in metaphase, with the chromosomes often arranged as "ring" mitoses. Epithelial pseudostratification and loss of polarity are common as well and should be distinguished from dysplasia. Apoptoses can be prominent, typically located in the proliferative region of the crypt or gland neck.

Chemotherapy

Many therapeutic agents (e.g., 5-FU, mitomycin C) delivered either orally or systemically or via arterial infusion (e.g., hepatic arterial infusion) can be associated with significant epithelial damage. The damage can be observed at the architectural and cellular level, and variation is noted between different agents. However, most descriptions include regenerative foveolar changes with cellular and nuclear atypia particularly associated with the proliferative zone, eosinophilic transformation of the epithelium and vacuolization, few or no mitotic figures, and bizarre cellular atypia accompanied by stromal and architectural cellular atypia.

Biological Agents

Over the last decades, novel biological agents with either an immune modulatory role or an antineoplastic effect have been developed, with the expectation of biological specificity with fewer side effects. However, many of these novel agents have been associated over time with various mucosal injuries. The lesions that have been related to use of the CTLA-4 molecule antibody and mycophenolate mofetil will be described.

Alpha CTLA-4 Monoclonal Antibody

This antibody, directed against cytotoxic T lymphocyte antigen 4, has been used as adjuvant therapy to tumor in the treatment of renal cell carcinoma, malignant melanoma, and ovarian cancer. In the stomach, the immune-mediated toxicity is characterized by increased basal apoptosis, expansion of the lamina propria, and increased intraepithelial lymphocytes.

Mycophenolate Mofetil (MMF)

MMF inhibits the enzyme inosine monophosphate dehydrogenase and arrests the cell cycle, and affects the production of T and B cell lymphocytes. It is used to prevent rejection in individuals who have undergone solid organ transplantation.

Increased apoptosis, glandular withering, and elevation of the number of eosinophils in the lamina propria are the characteristic features.

Olmesartan

This recently developed angiotensin II receptor antagonist used in the treatment of hypertension has been associated with the development of severe sprue-like enteropathy. Gastric side effects have also been reported, including lymphocytic gastritis and collagenous gastritis.

References and Further Reading

Haig, A., et al. (2006). Iron-induced mucosal injury to the upper gastrointestinal tract. *Histopathology, 48*(7), 808–12.

Lauwers, G. Y., Fujita, H., Nagata, K., & Shimizu, M. (2010). Pathology of non-Helicobacter pylori gastritis: Extending the histopathologic horizons. *Journal of Gastroenterology, 45*(2), 131–45. Review.

Oble, D. A., Mino-Kenudson, M., Goldsmith, J., Hodi, F. S., Seliem, R. M., Dranoff, G., Mihm, M., Hasserjian, R., & Lauwers, G. Y. (2008). Alpha-CTLA-4 mAb-associated panenteritis: A histologic and immunohistochemical analysis. *The American Journal of Surgical Pathology, 32*, 1130–7.

Xiao, S. Y., Zhao, L., Hart, J., & Semrad, C. E. (2013). Gastric mucosal necrosis with vascular degeneration induced by doxycycline. *The American Journal of Surgical Pathology, 37*, 259–63.

Drug-Induced Intestinal Injury

Liesbeth Ferdinande
Department of Pathology, Ghent University Hospital, Ghent, Belgium

Definition

A large number of drugs can cause intestinal side effects with clinical symptoms ranging from diarrhea or constipation to ulceration, bleeding, or perforation. One drug can be responsible for different clinical presentations and variable pathological findings. As these microscopic injury patterns are often not specific or pathognomonic, making a correct diagnosis of drug-induced pathology can be very difficult. Moreover, pathologists are usually not informed about the drugs that a patient has been taking, although this information together with the clinical history is essential in establishing the diagnosis. The possibility of a drug-related etiology should be considered, especially in cases of unusual pathology without apparent explanation. Drug-induced damage is mostly a reversible condition if drug intake is stopped, emphasizing the importance of recognizing this pathology.

Demonstrating that the drug is the cause of the pathological findings is difficult. A correlation can be suggested if there is a temporal relationship between the start of the drug and the onset of the clinical symptoms and pathological changes and if these features regress when the drug is withdrawn. A subsequent challenge with the drug and re-appearance of the symptoms can prove a causal relationship, but is often not applied in daily clinical practice.

Clinical Features

- **Incidence**
  The precise incidence of drug-induced intestinal damage is not known. Reports in literature are usually limited to cases or small series. However, diarrhea accounts for about 7% of all drug-related adverse effects in which more than 700 drugs are implicated, indicating that drug-induced intestinal injury is probably not uncommon.
- **Treatment**
  In most cases, drug-induced intestinal injury will heal after cessation of drug intake. The interval between drug discontinuation and resolution of clinical symptoms and microscopic findings is variable. For mycophenolate mofetil, for example, persistent microscopic changes were found up to 12 months after administration of this agent was stopped. When severe complications occur, additional active treatment may be required.

Macroscopy

The pathognomonic macroscopic finding of diaphragm disease is discussed elsewhere (▶ Diaphragm Disease/▶ Nonsteroidal Anti-inflammatory Drug Injury).

Microscopy

Table 1 gives an overview of the different injury patterns that were reported in literature to be associated with specific drugs (▶ Nonsteroidal Anti-inflammatory Drug Injury and ▶ Antibiotic-Associated Colitis are reviewed elsewhere). The major injury patterns of drug-induced intestinal disease include ulceration, stricture formation, variable inflammatory processes, and ischemia. These nonspecific microscopic patterns can display certain clues, indicating that a drug-induced etiology should be considered: apoptotic epithelial cells, increased intra-epithelial lymphocytes, or eosinophils (Fig. 1).

Drug-Induced Intestinal Injury, Table 1 Drugs causing various types of gastrointestinal injury

Erosion and ulceration
NSAID, KCl, iron, kayexalate, colchicine, ergot alkaloids, local analgesics (e.g., in suppositories)
Strictures and diaphragms
NSAID, KCl, pancreatic enzyme replacement
Perforation
Corticosteroids, contrast media
Acute colitis
NSAID, antibiotics, carbamazepine, oral contraceptive steroids, laxatives, $NaPO_4$, glutaraldehyde, mycophenolate mofetil
Focal active colitis
NSAID, $NaPO_4$
Pseudomembranous colitis
Antibiotics, PPI, chemotherapy
Neutropenic enterocolitis
Cytosine arabinoside, cisplatin, vincristine, adriamycin, 5-FU, mercaptopurine
Opportunistic infections
Immunosuppressive agents, corticosteroids
Malakoplakia
Corticosteroids
Ischemic-type colitis
Cardiovascular drugs (digoxin, α-adrenergic blockers, antihypertensive drugs, diuretics), oral contraceptive steroids, cocaine, ergot alkaloids, vasopressin and other vasoconstrictors, neuroleptics, NSAID, sumatriptan, alosetron hydrochloride, glutaraldehyde, flutamide, α-interferon, mycophenolate mofetil
Microscopic colitis
PPI, NSAID, H2 receptor antagonists (ranitidine, cimetidine), ticlopidine, simvastatin, flutamide, carbamazepine, paroxetine, sertraline, penicillin V, veinotonics (Cyclo 3 Fort), vinbumine, ferrous sulfate, levodopabenserazide
Inflammatory bowel disease-like colitis
Gold salts, NSAID, aminogluthemide, mycophenolate mofetil
Graft-versus-host-like disease
Mycophenolate mofetil
Epithelial apoptosis
NSAID, $NaPO_4$, anthraquinones, 5-FU, irinotecan
Pseudodysplastic changes
Cyclosporin

D

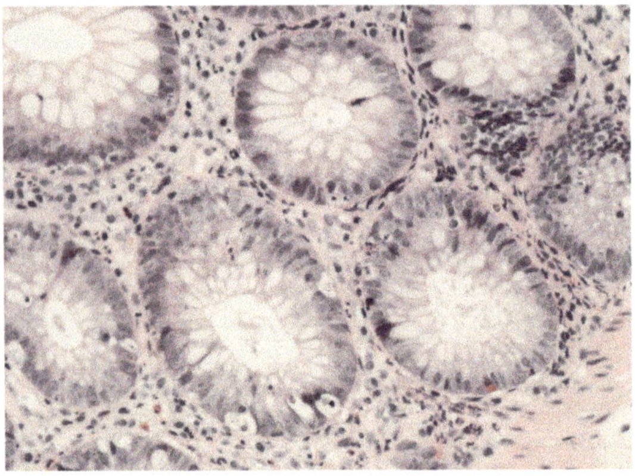

Drug-Induced Intestinal Injury, Fig. 1 Prominent epithelial apoptosis in a colon biopsy of a patient treated with capecitabine, a prodrug of 5-FU

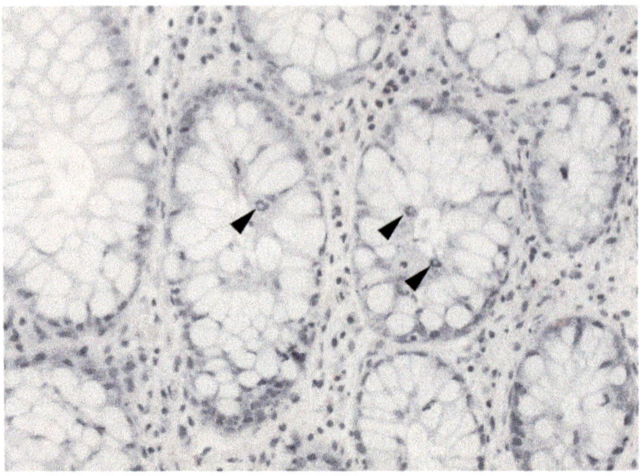

Drug-Induced Intestinal Injury, Fig. 2 Epithelial ring mitoses (*arrowheads*) in a colon biopsy of a patient with metastatic breast cancer treated with paclitaxel 2 days prior to colonoscopy

Specific hallmark features that lead to the diagnosis of a certain drug-induced pathology are rare, but if present, they can be a helpful tool in establishing the diagnosis. These features include specific histological patterns (as seen in treatment with colchicine, taxanes, mycophenolate mofetil, or in melanosis coli) or crystal deposition in the tissue (as seen in treatment with kayexalate or cholestyramine) as morphological evidence of drug-induced injury.

Colchicine and Taxanes

Colchicine is an alkaloid with antimitotic activity used in the treatment of gout and other medical conditions. It binds tubulin and inhibits its polymerization into microtubules, thereby causing mitotic arrest. Patients with renal or hepatic failure are at risk to develop colchicine toxicity, leading to a cholera-like syndrome associated with dehydration and shock that, if left untreated, can progress to multiorgan failure and death. Colchicine toxicity affects rapidly proliferating tissue like the gastrointestinal mucosa. Mainly the stomach and duodenum are involved, but also the colon can be affected. The most discriminating histologic feature is the presence of abundant epithelial mitotic figures arrested in metaphase. Metaphase mitoses can be identified as enlarged epithelial cells with condensed chromatin in ring formation within the center of the cell ("ring" mitoses). Epithelial pseudostratification and loss of epithelial polarity can be seen as well, mimicking epithelial dysplasia. The lack of nuclear hyperchromasia or atypia, general preservation of mucosal architecture, and the presence of surface maturation can distinguish these cases of colchicine toxicity from true dysplasia. Remarkably, none of these characteristic morphologic features were seen in gastrointestinal biopsies from patients under colchicine therapy without clinical evidence of colchicine toxicity.

Taxanes are a class of chemotherapeutic agents commonly used in the treatment of malignancies like breast cancer. These alkaloids bind to microtubules, thus promoting polymerization and forming extremely stable and nonfunctional microtubules. Gastrointestinal biopsies from patients under taxane therapy show similar epithelial changes as described for colchicine toxicity, most prominent in the first 3 days after taxane administration (Fig. 2). As in cases of colchicine toxicity, the greatest number of ring mitoses and accompanying apoptosis is found within the proliferative region of the mucosa. These findings are not specific for taxane toxicity, but may also reflect taxane effect.

Mycophenolate Mofetil

Mycophenolate mofetil (MMF) is an immunosuppressive agent used in the setting of solid organ transplantation. MMF is an inactive prodrug that is converted into mycophenolic acid (MPA) by intestinal esterases. MPA inhibits inosine monophosphate dehydrogenase (IMPDH), an enzyme in the de novo pathway of purine synthesis. As B- and T-lymphocytes lack a salvage pathway for this purine synthesis, MMF prevents proliferation of these cells and formation of antibodies from B cells. In addition, it may inhibit recruitment of leukocytes to inflammatory sites. Side effects of this drug mainly affect the lower gastrointestinal tract. Up to 40% of patients under MMF therapy develop persistent diarrhea. Maes et al. studied this population in 2003 and identified an infectious etiology in about 60% of the patients. Antibacterial or antiviral therapy was effective here. In another subgroup of patients, no clinical explanation was found for the diarrhea. The endoscopic biopsies, however, showed an inflammatory bowel disease-like injury pattern featuring patchy architectural changes with slight to moderate distortion of the crypt architecture, difference in diameter between individual crypts and preserved or slightly increased mucus secretion. The mucosal infiltrate, composed of lymphocytes, plasma cells, and some neutrophils, was slightly increased, but usually milder than in real ► Inflammatory Bowel Disease. Focally, crypts can be dilated and lined by flattened epithelium, infiltrated by macrophages and neutrophils. Beside this inflammatory bowel disease-like pattern, which is the most frequent, other histologic patterns are described under MMF therapy. Changes are considered graft-versus-host-disease-like when increased enterocyte apoptosis is observed without lamina propria inflammation or distortion of crypt architecture. The differential diagnosis with true ► Graft-Versus-Host Disease is clinically important, but may be nearly impossible based on the histologic findings. Other causes of increased apoptosis, such as intake of other types of drugs (e.g., NSAID), bowel preparation, or cytomegalovirus infection, should be kept in mind. Additional patterns that are described in the context of MMF use mimic self-limited colitis or ischemia.

Melanosis Coli

Melanosis coli or pseudolipofuscinosis coli is defined as the presence of lipofuscin-type pigment in macrophages of the lamina propria of the colon (Fig. 3). This can occur after long-term use or abuse of anthraquinone-containing laxatives. These drugs belong to the class of contact laxatives. The active compound is released in the caecum by bacteria, which means that melanosis will never affect the small intestine, it starts in the right colon and gradually involves the more distal parts of the colon. The active drug binds to surface epithelial cells and promotes apoptosis of these cells. Cell remnants together with the drug metabolites are then engulfed by the macrophages, resulting in the typical color. The epithelial cell damage is usually associated with mild mucosal inflammation.

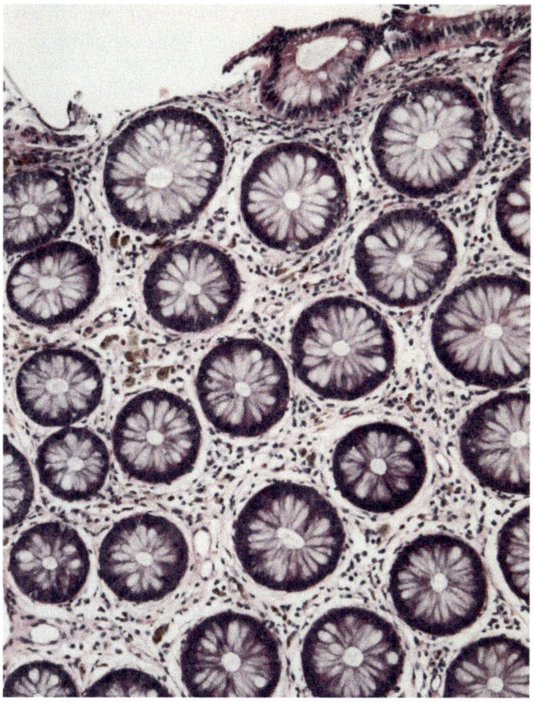

Drug-Induced Intestinal Injury, Fig. 3 Melanosis coli with pigmented macrophages in the lamina propria of a colon biopsy

Kayexalate and Cholestyramine

Kayexalate or sodium polystyrene sulphonate, a cation exchange resin, is used in the treatment of hyperkalemia. Kayexalate can be administered as an enema, orally or by nasogastric tube. When administered into the upper gastrointestinal tract, sodium cations are released from the resin and

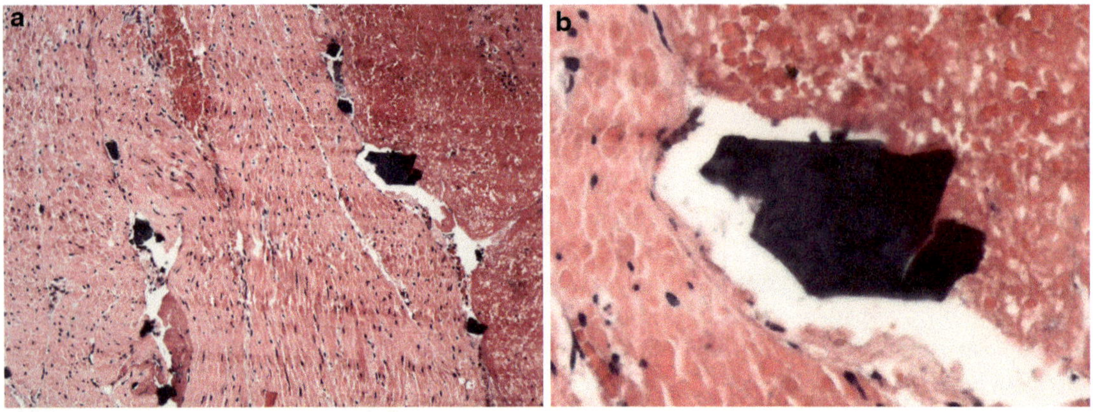

Drug-Induced Intestinal Injury, Fig. 4 (**a**) Kayexalate crystals in the muscular layer of the large bowel wall in a resection of a patient with colonic perforation due to kayexalate treatment. (**b**) Higher power view of **a** shows the characteristic features of kayexalate crystals: polygonal basophilic crystals with fish-scale appearance

exchanged for hydrogen ions in the acidic milieu of the stomach. As the resin passes through the intestine, hydrogen is exchanged for potassium, which is subsequently eliminated in the feces along with the remainder of the altered resin, thereby lowering serum potassium over a period of hours to days. Initially, kayexalate was administered as a suspension in water. Some patients however developed crystalline resin concretions. Later, the resin was mixed with a hypertonic solution of sorbitol, an osmotic laxative, to improve efficacy and to avoid complications of constipation and fecal impaction. The sorbitol is believed to be the component that leads to the intestinal damage that presents as mucosal ulcerations and necrosis, particularly in uremic patients. The erosive and ulcerative injuries can also occur in the upper gastrointestinal tract, but these lesions are less common and usually less severe (Gastric Injury from Kayexalate). Kayexalate can be recognized by the presence of rhomboid or triangular basophilic crystals, showing a mosaic pattern resembling fish scales and staining red with a PAS stain and maroon with an acid fast stain (Fig. 4). These crystals can be observed as an incidental finding in normal mucosa or adjacent to ulcerations. In the absence of injury, the crystals are located at the mucosal surface of small or large intestine. Kayexalate crystals can be recognized adherent to a mucosal ulceration or on the serosal surface in case of a perforation.

Kayexalate crystals should be differentiated from cholestyramine, a bile acid–binding resin. These crystals are more intensely basophilic and opaque and do not show the typical mosaic pattern of kayexalate. Cholestyramine crystals stain red with a PAS stain and pink with an acid fast stain.

References and Further Reading

Daniels, J. A., Gibson, M. K., Xu, L., Sun, S., Canto, M. I., Heath, E., Wang, J., Brock, M., & Montgomery, E. (2008). Gastrointestinal tract epithelial changes associated with taxanes: marker of drug toxicity versus effect. *The American Journal of Surgical Pathology, 32*, 473–477.

Geboes, K., De Hertogh, G., & Ectors, N. (2006). Drug-induced pathology in the large intestine. *Current Diagnostic Pathology, 12*, 239–247.

Iacobuzio-Donahue, C. A., Lee, E. L., Abraham, S. C., Yardley, J. H., & Wu, T. (2001). Colchicine toxicity. Distinct morphological findings in gastrointestinal biopsies. *The American Journal of Surgical Pathology, 25*, 1067–1073.

Parfitt, J. R., & Driman, D. K. (2007). Pathological effects of drugs on the gastrointestinal tract: a review. *Human Pathology, 38*, 527–536.

Rashid, A., & Hamilton, S. R. (1997). Necrosis of the gastrointestinal tract in uremic patients as a result of sodium polystyrene sulfonate (kayexalate) in sorbitol: an underrecognized condition. *The American Journal of Surgical Pathology, 21*, 60–69.

Selbst, M. K., Ahrens, W. A., Robert, M. E., Friedman, A., Proctor, D. D., & Jain, D. (2009). Spectrum of histologic changes in colonic biopsies in patients treated with mycophenolate mofetil. *Modern Pathology, 22*, 737–743.

Duplication, Esophagus

Susana Mão de Ferro and Miguel Serrano
Department of Gastroenterology, IPOLFG, E.P.E., Lisbon, Portugal

Synonyms

Congenital duplications; Gastrointestinal duplication cyst

Definition

Gastrointestinal duplication (GD) is a rare congenital anomaly that arises during early embryonic development and may occur anywhere along the gastrointestinal tract, from the mouth to the anus.

The cause of GD remains unclear. The most popular theory is the abnormal recanalization hypothesis. During the sixth week of fetal development, a proliferation of epithelium completely occludes the lumen of the gut, and vacuoles develop within the occluded lumen. Vacuoles coalesce until the lumen of the gut tube is fully recanalized. Duplication may occur due to an abnormal persistence of vacuoles. Other hypotheses include persistent embryologic diverticulum, bronchopulmonary foregut malformations, or intrauterine vascular accidents.

There are two general types of GD. Cystic duplications account for approximately 80% of cases, are spherical in shape, and have no communication with the bowel lumen. Tubular duplications account for 20% of GD, are tubular in shape, and communicate directly with the bowel lumen.

GD is usually asymptomatic and found accidentally during endoscopic or imaging exams. Symptoms may be vague and diverse as they vary with the location of the GD and are caused by compression or displacement of the surrounding structures. Complications are rare but include obstruction by volvulus or intussusception, bleeding, infection, and perforation. Bleeding usually occurs due to the presence of gastric ectopic mucosa in the GD. Malignant tumors may develop from the mucosa, but this complication is rare.

Unlike GD in other parts of the gastrointestinal tract, esophageal duplications frequently cause symptoms as dysphagia, retrosternal pain, cough, or respiratory distress due to esophageal or respiratory tract compression.

GD present at endoscopy as a submucosal lesion or as a diverticulum that can vary in size from several millimeters to over 5 cm. They have a smooth and regular appearance without mucosal irregularities.

At endosonography GD are usually anechoic homogeneous lesions, with regular margins, arising from the submucosa (third layer) or extrinsic to the gastrointestinal wall. Their walls can be characterized by three- or five-layer structures. They also can contain septae, fluid levels, or echogenic material consisting of layering debris or mucin.

At CT GD presents as a fluid-filled cystic mass with a thick, slightly enhancing wall that either arises from or is extrinsic to the gastrointestinal wall. An area of high attenuation within the cyst may be seen, a finding due to protein-rich material or hemorrhage. Occasionally, a cyst appears as a solid lesion on CT scan due to the higher density elicited from debris particles within a cyst. Enhancing solid foci within the cyst are suggestive of malignant change.

Clinical Features

- **Incidence**
  GD are rare conditions. Their true incidence is unknown as many cases are asymptomatic and remain undetected.
  Congenital duplications of esophagus are estimated to occur in 1 in 8,000 live births.
- **Age**
  More than 60% of symptomatic GD manifest during the first year of life. However, some GD may not be symptomatic until school age or adulthood. As GD is seldom symptomatic, it is usually found incidentally at endoscopy or imaging studies.

- **Sex**
  GD occurs both in females and males.
- **Site**
  GD is most common in the distal ileum, followed by the esophagus, colon, jejunum, stomach, and duodenum. Most esophageal duplications occur distally and on the right due to elongation and dextrorotation of the foregut.
- **Treatment**
  Surgical excision via an open or laparoscopic approach is the treatment of choice in symptomatic or complicated GD. The main considerations in the management of GD are the age and the condition of the patient and the location and type of GD (cystic or tubular). Generally total excision is preferred. Sometimes a segment of normal gastrointestinal tract must be excised due to the intimate contact to the GD or due to complications such as infection or ischemia. Long segment resections should be avoided as they may result in short bowel syndrome.

  Endoscopic management of tubular duplication of the esophagus has been described in few case reports using fine needle aspiration, needle knife cystostomy, and, when small, snare excision.

  The management of asymptomatic GD is usually expectant. However, some authors believe that surgery should be offered to asymptomatic patients due to the risk of complications, including malignancy, and to the impossibility to achieve the diagnosis.
- **Outcome**
  Prospective studies evaluating the outcome of GD are lacking. Cases described in the literature are mainly those of symptomatic or complicated GD. Even in these cases, the outcome is generally good. Mortality did not exceed 20% in any published series.

Macroscopy

GD is usually attached to the gastrointestinal tract. Cystic duplications are spherical in shape and have no communication with the bowel lumen. Tubular duplications are tubular in shape and communicate directly with the bowel lumen. Cysts contain a mucoid fluid.

Microscopy

GD has smooth muscle in its wall and is lined with gastrointestinal epithelium with a mucosal pattern of the adjacent gut and contains a mucoid fluid. Heterotopic gastric mucosa may be present in up to one third of cases. Ectopic pancreatic mucosa may also be present. Epithelial malignant transformation is rare.

Immunophenotype

Not applicable.

Molecular Features

Not applicable.

Differential Diagnosis

The differential diagnoses of GD include gastrointestinal submucosal lesions and other cystic lesions adjacent to the gastrointestinal tract.

References and Further Reading

Banner, K., Helft, S., Kadam, J., Miah, A., & Kaushik, N. (2008). An unusual cause of dysphagia in a young woman: Esophageal duplication cyst. *Gastrointestinal Endoscopy, 68*(4), 793.

Lee, K. N., Kim, S., Jeon, T. Y., Sung, H., Kim, H. S., Kim, D. H., Seo, H. I., Park, D. Y., Jang, H. J., et al. (2010). Complications of congenital and development abnormalities of the gastrointestinal tract in adolescents and adults: Evaluation with multimodality imaging. *Radiographics, 30*, 1489–1507.

Long, J., Orlando, R. Esophageal duplication. In Sleisenger and Fordtran's gastrointestinal and liver disease (9th edn, p. 671). Saunders Elsevier.

Olajide, A. R., Yisau, A., Abdulraseed, N., Kashim, I., Olaniyi, A., & Morohunfade, A. (2010).

Gastrointestinal duplications: Experience in seven children and review of the literature. *Saudi Journal of Gastroenterology, 16*(2), 105–109.
Tahri, N. (2012). Complete endoscopic management of tubular esophageal duplication in a young woman. *Endoscopy, 44*, E261–E262.

Duplication, Intestinal

Maria Sotiropoulou
Department of Pathology, Alexandra Hospital, Athens, Attica, Greece

Synonyms

Diverticula; Dorsal enteric cysts; Dorsal enteric remnants; Enterocysts; Enterogenous cysts; Giant diverticula; Neurenteric cysts; Persistent neurenteric canal; Posterior mediastinal cysts; Thoracic duplications of the intestine

Definition

Gastrointestinal duplications (GIDs) are rare congenital malformations that consist of cystic or tubular replicas involving any segment of the gastrointestinal tract from the mouth to the anus and containing all three layers. The histologic criteria applied for the diagnosis of GIDs include (1) attachment to a segment of the GI tract, the mesenteric site of which is typically involved and with which they share a common blood supply; (2) a well developed smooth muscle envelope mimicking the normal muscularis propria; and (3) an epithelial lining derived from the alimentary or respiratory tract.

Among the validated theories to define the embryogenesis of GIDs are the fusion of embryological longitudinal folds; persistence of the normal transient diverticula, applying especially in the formation of the ileal Ds; abortive partial twinning; aberrant luminal recanalization, applying mainly to the Ds in these portions of the GI tract that develop through a "solid" stage such as the esophagus, small bowel, and colon; intrauterine intestinal ischemia; and developmental abnormalities of the notochord, neurenteric canal, and related midline structures (split notochord).

GIDs present with a wide spectrum of symptoms and unspecific signs, frequently simulating other diseases, and their varied clinical appearance depends largely on the site, size, location, mucosal lining of D, and the age of the patients. Infants and children may present with high level GI obstruction, vomiting, abdominal pain, poor feeding and a palpable mass in case of a gastric or small intestinal D, or respiratory distress due to airway compression in case of esophageal and thoracoabdominal Ds. Likewise, the presence of gastric mucosa can lead to melena or hematemesis and perforation. Small cystic Ds predispose to intussusception or volvulus, whereas long tubular ones with proximal opening result in cystic dilatation and obstruction. Colonic Ds are usually asymptomatic, but can manifest with abdominal mass, abdominal pain, bleeding, or acute intestinal obstruction, especially in newborns, while constipation, hematochezia, rectal prolapse, and perirectal abscess are some of the main presenting signs and symptoms of rectal Ds. Adults present with symptoms including anemia, abdominal pain, nausea, relapsing pancreatitis, hematemesis or melena, ulceration, bowel obstruction, infection, and neoplastic transformation.

Although the diagnosis of a D cyst is difficult to make clinically or based upon conventional radiologic study (including barium examinations), gastrointestinal series may demonstrate extrinsic pressure produced by the cyst to the neighboring gut. Ultrasonography may reveal a characteristic double wall or "muscular rim" sign with an inner hyperechoic rim representing the mucosa-submucosa and an outer surrounding hypoechoic layer reflecting muscularis propria. Technetium 99 m pertechnetate could be useful in demonstrating the bleeding mucosa from the ectopic tissue as in Meckel's diverticulum. CT is useful especially in the diagnosis of duodenal Ds due to clear and unequivocal resolution without overshadowing, and MRI allows an accurate assessment of the topography and close relations of the cysts to each other, the diaphragm, and the alimentary tract as well as evaluating synchronous spinal cord anomalies and defining complications such as intra-abdominal hemorrhage.

Clinical Features

- **Incidence**
  GIDs are observed in 1/4,500 autopsies (appendix duplication is extremely rare, 0.004–0.009% of appendectomies).
- **Age**
  Eighty percent of GIDs become symptomatic within the first 2 years of life with approximately half of them occurring during the neonatal period. The colonic lesions usually remain asymptomatic and undiagnosed. GIDs are rare in adults.
- **Sex**
  There is a white male predominance with the exception of gastric Ds which are more common in females without any distinct geographical or racial distribution.
- **Site**
  GIDs occur more frequently in the small intestine with the ileum being involved in nearly one third of cases, whereas gastric, duodenal, rectal, and thoracoabdominal involvement is relatively rare and the occurrence within the liver substance exceptional. Synchronous GIDs occur in as many as 15% of the patients (Fig. 1).
- **Treatment**
  The treatment is surgical and, generally, total excision is preferred, except in cases of thoracic and thoracoabdominal duplications where staged approaches are more appropriate, colonic Ds with a free flow of intestinal contents through both lumens; where stool softeners and enemas can improve symptoms and gastric Ds; and where resection is not required. The age and condition of the patient, the location, regarding the presence or not of a common blood supply, the multiplicity and the cystic or tubular nature of the lumen, the presence of heterotopic gastric mucosa, the proximity to the biliary or pancreatic ducts, and the possible association with other abnormalities, like the genitourinary ones in colonic tubular Ds, are the main considerations in the management of intestinal Ds.

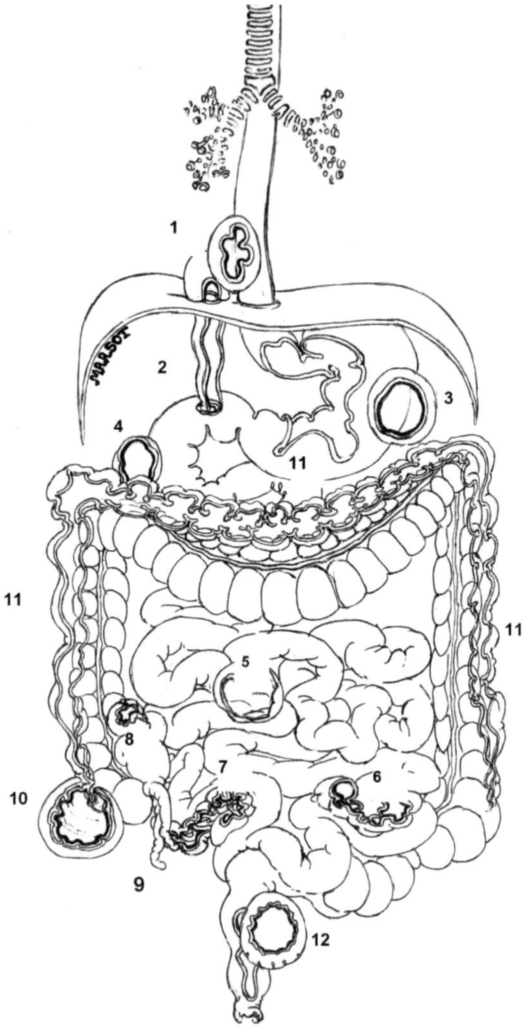

Duplication, Intestinal, Fig. 1 Distribution of duplications along the gastrointestinal tract: *1:* esophageal, *2:* thoracoabdominal, *3:* gastric, *4:* duodenal, *5:* jejunal, *6–7:* ileal, *8:* involving the ileocecal valve, *9:* appendiceal, *10:* cecal, *11:* involving the whole large bowel, *12:* rectal

Drainage procedures should be discouraged owing to the high incidence of heterotopic gastric mucosa and the lack of autonomy of the duplication's blood supply and such managements are acceptable only, provided that the presence of gastric mucosa has been ruled out, in selected cases such as in duodenal Ds, where excision is not feasible due to potential injury to the biliary or pancreatic duct and rectal Ds and where rectal cysts can be drained through the posterior rectal mucosa, the stripping of the cyst wall mucosa following.

Localized cystic Ds of the small intestine and colon can be excised with safety, but longer tubular ones, where a long segment resection resulting in a short bowel syndrome should be avoided, can be managed by lengthening procedures, the Wrenn method of mucosal stripping through multiple incisions, or excising part of the common rectal wall.

- **Outcome**
  Despite the occurrence of certain complications including injury to the pancreatobiliary tree and secondary pancreatitis, following the excision of gastric or duodenal Ds, recurrent bleeding after mucosal stripping, and the need for regular clinical evaluation and continence studies for patients with cystic colonic Ds undergoing medical therapy with stool softeners and patients treated for rectal Ds, respectively, the outcome of surgical or medical management is favorable and excision is generally curative with not more than 20% mortality in any reported series and morbidity and mortality rate depending significantly on the presence of bowel necrosis, the length of the resected segment, the type and extent of the associated malformations, and the rare, but possible, neoplastic development.

Macroscopy

In general, GIDs involve the mesenteric side and share a common blood supply with the native intestine. Most are attached along the dorsal or mesenteric border, but some are attached to the lateral border forming parallel side-by-side segments referred to as double-barrel Ds. Rarely the duplication has a separate mesentery and blood supply and is called loop duplication. According to the shape and length of the intestinal segment involved, Ds can morphologically be divided to *spherical-cystic* and *tubular*, according to the sort of attachment to the bowel wall and sharing a common muscular wall with the normal segment to *complete* and *incomplete* and depending on the presence of an opening to the normal intestinal lumen to *communicating* and *noncommunicating*. The communicating ones are further differentiated according to the location of the opening, meaning proximally, distally, or at both ends, which results in different clinical presentation, severity of symptoms, complications, and type of therapy.

GIDs are usually single (multiple GIDs occur in as many as 15% of patients), noncommunicating, and spherical-cystic with a size ranging from a few millimeters to over 10 cm. Foregut Ds are associated with anomalies of the thoracic spine ranging from spina bifida and hemivertebra to vertebral fusion defects, an association that is not noted with more distal cysts; midgut cystic Ds coexist with intestinal atresias and hindgut Ds with complex genital and urinary abnormalities (Table 1).

Microscopy

From the three criteria used to define a lesion as duplication, meaning the intimate anatomic relation to a segment of the GI tract, the epithelial lining, and the presence of an organized smooth muscle coat, only the latter is absolutely necessary. As a rule, the epithelium lining a duplicated segment mimics the native one, meaning that esophageal Ds are usually lined by stratified

Duplication, Intestinal, Table 1 A useful topographical categorization of GIDs

Cervical	Usually cystic in the lower third of esophagus
Thoracic and thoracoabdominal	Large tubular of the posterior mediastinum
Gastric	Non communicating intramural of the great curvature
Duodenal	Mixed in second portion
Small intestinal	Cystic, 35% in the ileum
Colonic and rectal	Isolated cysts (fistula to skin, urinary tract, or normal colon), tubular (duplication of the entire colon)

squamous mucosa and gastric Ds usually contain gastric mucosa, but heterotopic tissues, including thyroid stroma, gastric mucosa, pancreatic rests, lymphoid aggregates resembling Peyer patches, ciliated bronchial epithelium, lung tissue, and cartilage can be present as well. Beneath the epithelium, a normal submucosa and submucosal plexus and an inner circular muscle layer and myenteric plexus are also present, although as some lesions become cystic, both the epithelial lining and the muscle component become atrophic and may appear incomplete.

Different types of epithelium have different clinical implications, and the main clinically significant heterotopia, the ectopic gastric mucosa, which is also the most prevalent (with an incidence ranging from 15% to 40–50%) usually in esophageal and small intestinal Ds, predisposes to peptic ulceration, painless gastrointestinal hemorrhage, and perforation. Otherwise, secondary inflammatory changes may supervene, as is the case with communicating Ds having a blind distal end, where the accumulation of intestinal contents and secretions cause cystic dilatation, inflammation, necrosis, and fistula formation.

Finally several cases of neoplastic transformation, mainly adenocarcinomas, developing within the duplicated bowel, have been reported.

Differential Diagnosis

Esophageal duplication cysts may be difficult to differentiate from bronchogenic cysts. Adding to the diagnostic confusion is the rare occurrence of cartilaginous heterotopias within the wall of the esophageal cyst, but the presence of a close attachment to the esophagus than to the bronchial tree and of an extensive stratified squamous, gastric, or intestinal lining mucosa (than a respiratory one) with a muscularis propria and submucosal and myenteric plexuses aids in the distinction.

Other diagnostic considerations include diverticula, retention cysts originating from cystic dilation of the submucosal esophageal wall, any posterior or middle mediastinal mass such as meningocele, pulmonary sequestration, neoplasms of the sympathetic chain, and, especially, neurenteric cysts, which bear a close resemblance to duplication cysts and contain various intestinal epithelia, present in the posterior mediastinum much more frequently associated with spinal defects, but are not attached to the esophageal wall and are thought to have a different embryological origin.

Midgut intestinal Ds must be differentiated from enteric cysts and congenital diverticula, which are more localized lesions with a less organized smooth muscle and usually associated with vertebral body abnormalities, acquired diverticula, mesenteric cysts, Meckel's diverticulum, choledochal cysts, pancreatic abscesses, and cystic necrotic tumors.

Finally, rectal duplication cysts should be distinguished from epidermoid-dermoid cysts (both unilocular, but the latter have squamous epithelium and lack an organized muscular wall) and retrorectal cystic hamartomas (tailgut) cysts, which are multilocular with a varying presence of solid areas; a squamous, transitional, or glandular epithelium; a disorganized smooth muscle wall; and occasional foreign body giant cell granulomatous inflammation.

Immunohistochemistry

Immunohistochemistry is noncontributory in intestinal duplication.

Molecular Studies

There are not molecular studies concerning intestinal duplication.

References and Further Reading

Fenoglio-Preiser, C., Noffsinger, A., Stemmermann, G., et al. (2008). *Gastrointestinal pathology* (3rd ed., pp. 746–747). Lippincott: Williams and Wilkins.

Macpherson, R. I. (1993). Gastrointestinal tract duplications: clinical, pathologic, etiologic and radiologic considerations. *Radiographics, 13*(5), 1063–1080.

Plummer, J. M. (2009). Intestinal duplication presenting with recurrent abdominal pain. *Canadian Journal of Surgery, 52*(4), 103–104.
Puligandla, P. S., Ngugen, L. T., St Vil, D., et al. (2003). Gastrointestinal duplication. *Journal of Pediatric Surgery, 38*(5), 740–744.
Stern, L. E., & Warner, B. W. (2000). Gastrointestinal duplications. *Seminars in Pediatric Surgery, 9*(3), 135–140.

Dysentery, Bacillary

Xavier Sagaert
Department of Pathology, University Hospitals KU Leuven, Leuven, Belgium

Synonyms

Shigellosis

Definition

Dysentery is an infection of the digestive tract, characterized by inflammation of the colon wall, frequent loose stools, cramping abdominal pain, appearance of mucus, blood and pus in the feces.

Bacillary dysentery is a type of dysentery that is caused by bacteria of the genus *Shigella*, although sometimes *Campylobacter, Salmonella*, and other related bacteria may cause clinically similar diseases. In the Western world, bacillary dysentery is most commonly transmitted through fecal-oral route, e.g., during care for a sick person or through a variety of household items contaminated with secretions of the patient. It is highly contagious as symptoms may result from ingestion of only 10–100 organisms. As such, *Shigella* outbreaks are often associated with crowded living conditions and less than optimal hygiene conditions, e.g., military troops deployed in camps, nursing homes, day-care centers, and prions. *Shigella* contamination can also occur during sexual intercourse.

Shigellae are virulent, invasive gram-negative bacilli that include four species: *S. dysenteriae, S. flexneri, S. boydii*, and S. *sonnei*. *Shigella dysenteriae* is the most virulent and the most common species isolated, although *S. sonnei* and *S. flexneri* are increasingly reported in the western world. All four *Shigella* species produce a toxin that damages the endothelial cells in the microvasculature of the colon. As a consequence, intestinal epithelial cells begin to exude that leads to diarrhea, liquid stools containing mucus, pus, and often blood, similar to the secretions in cholera. Later the toxin-damaged cells die, and their death is accompanied by inflammation, ulceration of the intestinal wall, and other symptoms of dysentery.

Bacillary dysentery symptoms begin within 2–10 days of consumption of contaminated food or water. The illness often starts with fever, nausea, vomiting, abdominal cramps, and diarrhea. Episodes of diarrhea may increase to as much as once an hour, with mucus, pus, and blood in the stool. Vomiting and diarrhea may result in rapid and severe dehydration, which may lead to shock and death if not treated. Signs of dehydration include an extremely dry mouth, sunken eyes, and poor skin tone. In children and older patients, general intoxication can be accompanied by neurological symptoms, as they can be restless, irritable, and possibly lethargic. Children may also have sunken eyes and may not be able to produce tears or urine, the latter appearing very dark and concentrated. Unlike amoebic dysentery, the bacillary dysentery is characterized by the rapid growth of symptoms, fever, and dehydration. Also, the bacillary dysentery is usually less lasting and does not have a chronic form.

Clinical Features

- **Incidence**
  Shigellosis is endemic throughout the world, where it is held responsible for some 120 million cases of severe dysentery (with blood and mucus in the stools). Recent estimates fix the Shigella disease burden at 90 million episodes and 108,000 deaths per year, the overwhelming majority of which occur in developing countries and involve children less than 5 years. In addition, about 500,000 cases of

shigellosis are reported each year among military personnel and travelers from industrialized countries.

- **Age**
  Young children (ages 1–4) living in poverty, travelers to tropical regions, and adults living in crowded environments with poor hygiene are most likely to contact bacillary dysentery.
- **Sex**
  There is no gender predilection for bacillary dysentery.
- **Site**
  In most cases, the effects of the Shigella toxin are limited to the large intestines, with a predilection for the rectum.
- **Treatment**
  The main component in the treatment of the bacterial dysentery treatment is to hydrate the patient by drinking plenty of liquids, containing sugar and mineral salts. This oral replacement is satisfactory for most people, but some may need to receive fluids intravenously. In most cases, the disease resolves within 4–8 days without antibiotics. Severe infections may last 3–6 weeks.

  Antibiotics (e.g., trimethoprim- norfloxacin, ciprofloxacin, sulfamethoxazole, or furazolidone) may be given when the disease is severe, when the person is very young or very old, or when there is a high risk of the infection spreading to other people. Additionally, ampicillin (but not amoxicillin) is effective in treating this disease. Antibiotics accelerate recovery, but may develop antibiotic-resistant forms of the disease, and therefore, their use is discouraged.
- **Outcome**
  Bacillary dysentery is usually curable in 7 days with treatment. Most Shigella infections are mild and do not require drastic treatment. In a severe attack, excessive dehydration can be fatal if treatment is unsuccessful (especially in infants and young children). Also, during the recovery period or even in the acute phase, exudative arthritis may occur. In pregnant, critically ill patients, the *Shigella* toxin can cause miscarriage or premature birth. When poorly treated, bacillary dysentery can also lead to sepsis, perforation, toxic megacolon, rectal prolapse, Reiter's syndrome, a leukemoid reaction, otitis media, angular stomatitis, or hemolytic uremic syndrome.

Macroscopy

Grossly, the large bowel is typically affected (the distal left side usually more severely), but the ileum may be involved as well. Initially, distribution is often continuous and can mimic ulcerative colitis; patchy involvement is more common as the disease resolves. The mucosa is edematous and hemorrhagic, with exudates that may form from pseudomembranes. Ulcerations are variably present.

Microscopy

Morphologic changes are usually most severe in the rectum. Early changes are generally those of acute infectious-type colitis, including a superficial neutrophilic infiltrate, edema, mucin depletion, cryptitis, crypt abscesses, and ulceration. Apthoid ulcers similar to Crohn's disease are variably present. Pseudomembranes similar to *Clostridium difficile* infection are fairly common, and microtrombi can even be seen. As the disease continues, there is increased mucosal destruction with many neutrophils and mononuclear inflammatory cells in the lamina propria. Architectural changes mimicking idiopathic inflammatory disease are well described in shigellosis, including crypt branching, crypt disorganization, crypt dilatation, and marked crypt distortion.

Differential Diagnosis

The differential diagnosis of early shigellosis is primarily that of other infections, particularly enteroinvasive *Escherichia coli* and non-typhoid *Salmonella*. Pseudomembranous shigellosis may closely resemble the colitis caused by *Clostridium difficile*, and the *Clostridium difficile* antigen test may be very helpful in this instance. Later in the course of the disease, it may be extremely difficult to distinguish shigellosis from Crohn's disease or ulcerative colitis, both endoscopically and histologically. Clinical presentation (e.g., rapid onset of symptoms) may be very helpful in resolving the differential diagnosis. Stool cultures are essential, and specimens should be rapidly inoculated onto appropriate culture plates, since *Shigella* is fastidious and dies quickly. Multiple cultures may be necessary. Molecular essays for the diagnosis of shigellosis are also available.

References and Further Reading

Edwards, B. H. (1999). *Salmonella* and *Shigella* species. *Clinics in Laboratory Medicine, 19*, 469.

Niyogi, S. K. (2005). Shigellosis. *Journal of Microbiology, 43*, 133–143.

Pfeiffer, M. L., Dupont, H. L., & Ochoa, T. J. (2012). The patient presenting with acute dysentery–A systematic review. *Journal of Infection, 64*, 374–386.

Phalipon, A., & Sansonetti, P. J. (2003). Shigellosis: Innate mechanisms of inflammatory destruction of the intestinal epithelium, adaptive immune response, and vaccine development. *Critical Reviews in Immunology, 23*, 371–401.

Walker, C. L. F., Applegate, J. A., & Black, R. E. (2012). Haemolytic-uraemic syndrome as a sequela of diarrhoeal disease. *Journal of Health, Population and Nutrition, 30*, 257–261.

E

E-Cadherin, Hereditary Diffuse Gastric Cancer

Chella R. S. van der Post[1] and Fátima Carneiro[2]
[1]Department of Pathology, Radboud University Medical Center, Nijmegen, The Netherlands
[2]Faculty of Medicine of Porto University, Centro Hospitalar São João and Ipatimup/i3S, Porto, Portugal

Synonyms

HDGC; Hereditary diffuse gastric carcinoma

Definition

E-cadherin gastric carcinoma or hereditary diffuse gastric carcinoma (HDGC) is a form of gastric cancer in patients with germline alterations in the *CDH1* gene. HDGC is an autosomal-dominant cancer-susceptibility syndrome and is characterized by diffuse gastric cancer and lobular breast cancer. In 1998, Guildford et al. identified germline mutations in the *CDH1* gene to be the cause of HDGC by linkage analysis and mutation screening in three Maori kindreds with multi-generational gastric cancer in New Zealand.

CDH1 encodes the protein E-cadherin, which plays an important role in cell polarity and the maintenance of epithelial integrity. Due to mutations in *CDH1*, the cell-cell adhesion mediated by E-cadherin is lost, which causes disruption of the correct spatial organization of the cells. This interferes with processes that regulate cell division, such as the orientation of the mitotic spindle. Abrogated cell polarity may also lead to the disruption of cell fate determination, which can result in the displacement of cells with self-renewal capacity into the lamina propria. This may lead to formation of multiple small signet ring cell (diffuse) carcinomas with the potential to progress into widely invasive carcinoma.

Genetic counseling is essential in the evaluation and management of HDGC. The genetic evaluation should include a careful three-generation family pedigree and histopathological confirmation of gastric (pre-)malignancies. Genetic testing should be initiated in an affected proband. The revised international criteria as established by the International Gastric Cancer Linkage Consortium (IGCLC) to identify patients eligible for *CDH1* genetic testing include:

(1) Two or more documented cases of gastric cancer at any age in first- or second-degree relatives, with at least one confirmed diffuse-type;
(2) Personal history of diffuse-type gastric cancer before the age of 40 years;
(3) Personal or family history (first- or second-degree relatives) of diffuse-type gastric cancer and lobular breast cancer, one diagnosed before the age of 50 years.

F. Carneiro et al. (eds.), *Pathology of the Gastrointestinal Tract*, Encyclopedia of Pathology,
DOI 10.1007/978-3-319-40560-5

In addition, genetic testing can be considered in families with bilateral or multiple cases of lobular breast cancer before the age of 50 years; families with clustering of diffuse-type gastric cancer and cleft lip/cleft palate and; any patient that is diagnosed with *in-situ* or pagetoid spread of signet ring cells.

Clinical Features

- **Incidence**
  Familial clustering is observed in approximately 10% of gastric cancer cases; 1.4% (1–3%) of all gastric cancers are caused by heterozygous inactivating germline mutations in *CDH1*. These mutations are found in about 45% of families fulfilling the diagnostic criteria for HDGC mentioned above. Germline *CDH1* mutations are found in all ethnic groups but are rare in countries with high rates of sporadic gastric cancer, including Japan and Korea. The reason for this uneven distribution is not known.
- **Age**
  The overall risk of HDGC before the age of 20 is very low but is increasing with reported cumulative risks of developing advanced gastric carcinoma of 60–70% by age 80. The mean age at diagnosis is 40 years (range 14–85 years). Besides the high risk of developing gastric cancer, female *CDH1* mutation carriers have an additional high lifetime risk of developing lobular breast cancer (around 40% in women by age 80).
- **Sex**
  No clear predominance of gender. Women have next to the gastric cancer risk a high risk of developing breast cancer.
- **Site**
  In Maori families in New Zealand, a predilection was observed for gastric cancer to occur in the body-antral transitional zone. This was not confirmed in North American and European families, where carcinomas were observed from the cardiac to prepyloric region, being more frequently identified in the corpus/fundus. Since all topographic regions in the stomach are at risk and new gastric cancer can develop in any remaining gastric mucosa, histological confirmation of resection margins after surgery is important.
- **Treatment**
  Endoscopic surveillance is not standard recommended, since this is ineffective to detect small *foci* of signet ring cell (diffuse) carcinoma, which are often <1 mm and located in a normal mucosa. Multiple endoscopic biopsies carried out before prophylactic gastrectomy in these patients failed to detect small *foci* of mucosal signet ring cell carcinomas. Further research using chromoendoscopy or other techniques is under way. Endoscopic surveillance is now recommended for proven *CDH1* mutation carriers under 20 years, for carriers above 20 years who are willing to postpone surgery, or for whom prophylactic gastrectomy (biopsy-negative) is unacceptable but gastrectomy with curative intent (biopsy-positive) is acceptable and those with mutations of undetermined significance (e.g., missense). Total prophylactic gastrectomy is recommended in proven *CDH1* mutation carriers above 20 years. A curative total gastrectomy is advised in patients with positive biopsies at any age.
- **Outcome**
  The outcome of advanced diffuse gastric cancer is poor and depends on the stage of cancer. Prophylactic gastrectomy has an estimated mortality rate of up to 2%. Morbidity after prophylactic surgery includes abdominal pain, dumping syndrome, lactose intolerance, fat malabsorption, steatorrhea, bacterial overgrowth, and postprandial fullness. All patients lose weight and require lifelong vitamin B12 injections and follow-up for conditions such as anemia and trace element deficiencies. However, most patients undergoing prophylactic gastrectomy are young, and negative consequences of surgery seem to improve in the first year after surgery. Small tumor *foci* found in the prophylactic gastrectomy specimens do not influence outcome, since there are no nodal metastases or spread of tumor below the muscularis mucosa.

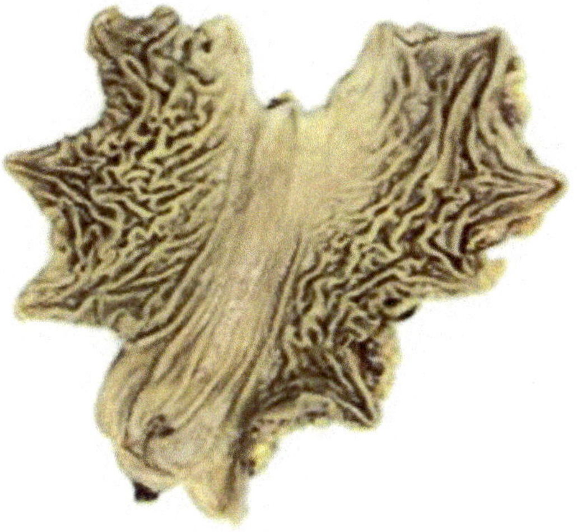

E-Cadherin, Hereditary Diffuse Gastric Cancer, Fig. 1 Gross image of macroscopically "normal" gastrectomy specimen, opened along the greater curvature without macroscopically visible abnormalities in preventive setting but with microscopically numerous small pT1a signet ring cell carcinomas

Macroscopy

Advanced HDGC presents as sporadic diffuse cancers with grossly either a more localized tumor or a diffuse linitis plastica appearance. This contrasts with prophylactic gastrectomy samples, where there are generally no abnormalities visible macroscopically (Fig. 1). These specimens are best included in total to find small invasive tumors. The "Swiss roll" technique can be used for including the complete mucosa.

Microscopy

Pathological mapping of complete prophylactic gastrectomy specimens has shown that early-stage HDGC is characterized by the presence of a few up to hundred *foci* of stage T1a signet ring cell (diffuse) carcinoma restricted to the superficial lamina propria. The majority of these *foci* appear relatively indolent and are composed of mitotically inactive neoplastic cells. In the mucosa, these cells are small at the neck-zone level and usually enlarge towards the surface of the gastric mucosa. Signet ring cells are typically found in

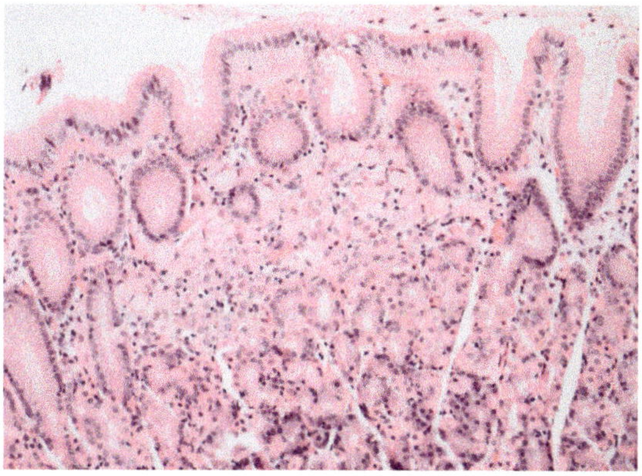

E-Cadherin, Hereditary Diffuse Gastric Cancer, Fig. 2 Signet ring cell lesion confined to the mucosa, exhibiting typical signet ring cell morphology with little architectural distortion

these lesions, characterized by a large, mucus-filled vacuole in the cytoplasm and an eccentric displaced nucleus. HDGC development is thought to start with signet ring cell carcinoma *in situ* (Tis), corresponding to the presence of signet ring cells within the basal membrane. This is followed by a pagetoid spread pattern of signet ring cells below the preserved epithelium of glands and foveolae still within the basal membrane. Increased proliferation of signet ring cells eventually will lead to invasive carcinoma. Striking is the discrepancy between the numerous T1a carcinomas and most often absence of carcinoma *in situ* (Tis) lesions, indicating that invasion usually occurs without morphologically detectable carcinoma *in situ* (Figs. 2 and 3).

In almost all prophylactic total gastrectomy specimens, multiple small T1a mucosal signet ring cell (diffuse) carcinomas are identified. The presence of *in situ* lesions and pagetoid spread of signet ring cells are distinct features in the stomach and highly indicative for the presence of germline *CDH1* mutations, since these features are not reported in the gastric mucosa of patients with sporadic diffuse gastric cancer (Figs. 4 and 5). These features should always be brought to the attention of clinicians, and referral of the patient to a geneticist is indicated. Background changes in the gastric mucosa of prophylactic gastrectomy specimens consist of foveolar hyperplasia, tufting of surface epithelium, vacuolization

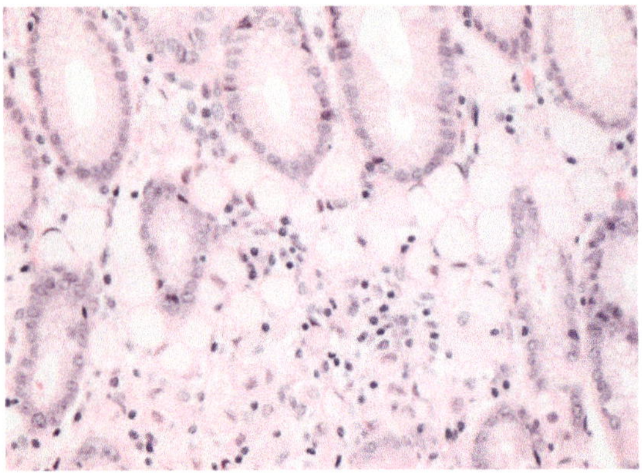

E-Cadherin, Hereditary Diffuse Gastric Cancer, Fig. 3 Detail of signet ring cells between glands

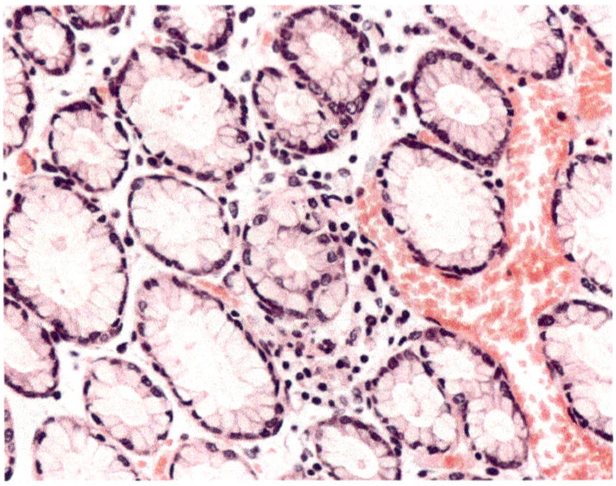

E-Cadherin, Hereditary Diffuse Gastric Cancer, Fig. 5 Pagetoid spread of signet ring cells below the epithelium

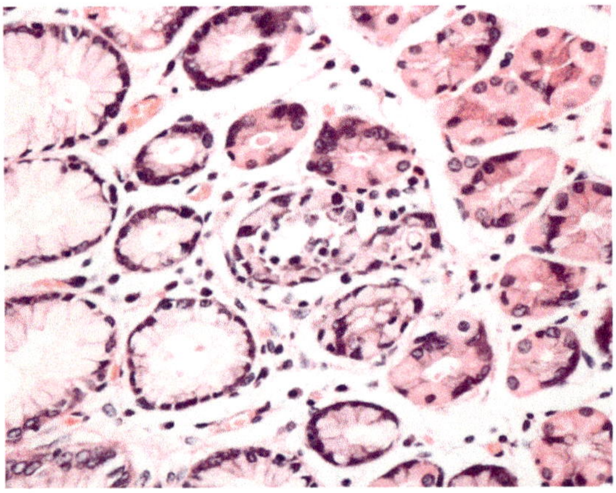

E-Cadherin, Hereditary Diffuse Gastric Cancer, Fig. 4 *In situ* signet ring cell carcinoma

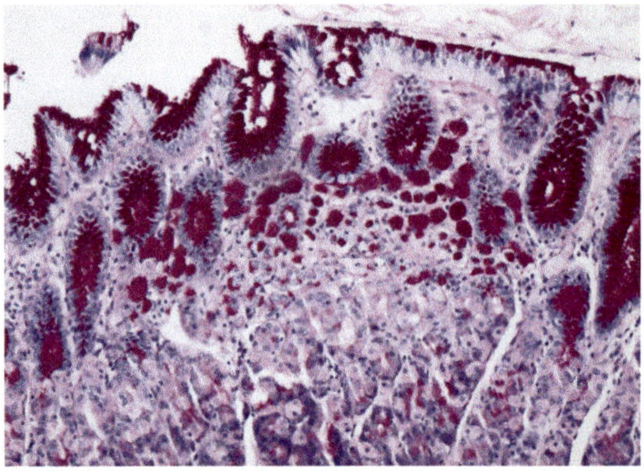

E-Cadherin, Hereditary Diffuse Gastric Cancer, Fig. 6 PAS staining outshining the signet ring cells

of surface epithelium, and mild chronic lymphocytic gastritis, generally without *H. pylori* infection or intestinal metaplasia.

Pathological analysis of the entire gastrectomy sample includes a thorough assessment microscopically with hematoxylin and eosin (H&E) and a histochemical mucin stain, such as periodic acid-Schiff (PAS) or Alcian Blue. PAS staining has proven to be helpful as a primary stain, increasing the detection rate of small invasive signet ring cell *foci* and reducing screening time (Fig. 6). The pathology report should mention all gastric abnormalities and localizations in the stomach, as well as (pre-)malignant lesions, intestinal metaplasia, dysplasia, inflammation, and signs of *H. pylori* gastritis. Histological confirmation of resection margins consisting of proximal squamous esophageal and distal duodenal mucosa is essential, since new gastric cancer can develop in any gastric mucosa left in the patient.

Advanced HDGC presents as signet ring cell carcinomas or poorly differentiated diffuse carcinomas (linitis plastica), in which sometimes only a few signet ring cells can be identified. Mixed carcinomas and mucinous differentiation can be observed. These advanced gastric carcinomas of *CDH1* mutation carriers normally do not show any distinct

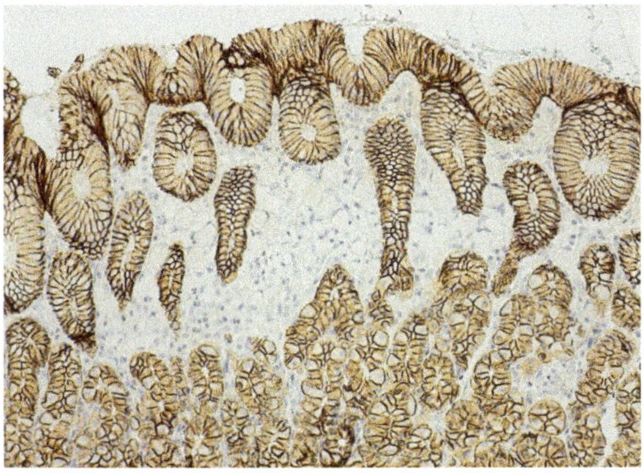

E-Cadherin, Hereditary Diffuse Gastric Cancer, Fig. 7 Loss of E-cadherin expression in signet ring cells, with positive surrounding mucosa

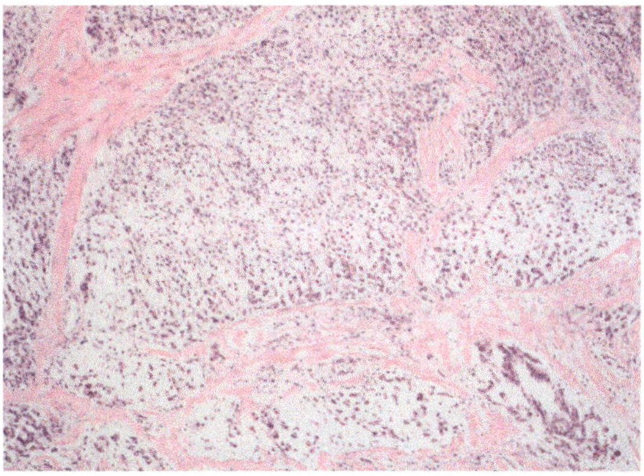

E-Cadherin, Hereditary Diffuse Gastric Cancer, Fig. 8 Advanced gastric carcinoma presenting as a poorly differentiated diffuse carcinoma

characteristics and are therefore indistinguishable from sporadic diffuse gastric cancer at advanced stage.

Immunophenotype

Immunohistochemical expression using E-cadherin staining has been shown to be often reduced or absent in HDGC and precursor lesions such as pagetoid spread lesions and *in situ* carcinomas. In routine pathology practice, staining is of little value since E-cadherin expression is not always reduced or absent, depending on the mutation localization and specific mechanisms of inactivation of the wild-type allele. Furthermore, it has been shown that E-cadherin expression is often reduced or absent in sporadic diffuse gastric cancer, due to somatic mutation in the tumor. A cytokeratin stain can be helpful to confirm the epithelial nature of a small invasive tumor, sometimes clear glassy changes, inflammatory infiltrate, and small capillaries can mimic small *foci* of signet ring cell carcinoma (Fig. 7).

Molecular Features

More than 100 germline alterations in the *CDH1* gene have been published to date. The mutation detection rate is approximately 45% of all families fulfilling the strict HDGC criteria. These alterations are small frameshifts (28%), splice-site mutations (27%), nonsense (20%), and 3′-end large deletions (1.6%). "Nonexpressing" mutations (predicted to lead to complete ablation of mRNA expression) account for 4.1% of the cases. A single family has been reported to carry promoter methylation (0.8%) and four families (3.3%) to carry 5′-end deletions that impair transcription initiation. Missense mutations affect 18.0% of all HDGC families, and a single family has been reported to carry an in-frame deletion (0.8%).

Examination of the genetic and epigenetic second hits that occur in HDGC revealed somatic alterations in 75% of signet ring cell carcinomas. The most frequent second hit was promoter hypermethylation (32%) followed by loss of heterozygosity (LOH) (25%) and a combination of both promoter hypermethylation and LOH (18%).

Differential Diagnosis

- Advanced gastric carcinomas of *CDH1* mutation carriers present as diffuse carcinomas that are indistinguishable from diffuse sporadic gastric cancers (Fig. 8). Patient and family characteristics are important to suspect a genetic cause.

- An increased risk of developing diffuse gastric cancer has been shown in several well-known hereditary cancer syndromes, which include Lynch syndrome, Peutz-Jeghers syndrome, Li-Fraumeni syndrome, hereditary breast and ovarian cancer, familial adenomatous polyposis (FAP), *MUTYH*-associated adenomatous polyposis (MAP), juvenile polyposis syndrome, and Cowden syndrome. In these syndromes gastric cancer is more often of the intestinal type. The typical pagetoid spread of signet ring cells and *in situ* lesions have only been observed in patients with germline *CDH1* mutations. In many families (50–60%) fulfilling the strict HDGC criteria, no *CDH1* mutation is identified and remains genetically unexplained. It is likely that most of these families carry mutations in other gastric cancer-susceptibility genes. Very recently, a mutation in *CTNNA1* gene has been identified in a family.

References and Further Reading

Carneiro, F., Huntsman, D. G., Smyrk, T. C., Owen, D. A., Seruca, R., Pharoah, P., et al. (2004). Model of the early development of diffuse gastric cancer in E-cadherin mutation carriers and its implications for patient screening. *The Journal of Pathology, 203*(2), 681–687.

Guilford, P., Hopkins, J., Harraway, J., McLeod, M., McLeod, N., Harawira, P., et al. (1998). E-cadherin germline mutations in familial gastric cancer. *Nature, 392*(6674), 402–405.

Guilford, P., Humar, B., & Blair, V. (2010). Hereditary diffuse gastric cancer: Translation of CDH1 germline mutations into clinical practice. *Gastric Cancer, 13*(1), 1–10.

Hansford, S., Kaurah, P., Li-Chang, H., et al. (2015). Hereditary Diffuse Gastric Cancer Syndrome: CDH1 Mutations and Beyond. *JAMA Oncology.*

Majewski, I. J., Kluijt, I., Cats, A., Scerri, T. S., de Jong, D., Kluin, R. J., et al. (2013). An α-E-catenin (CTNNA1) mutation in hereditary diffuse gastric cancer. *The Journal of Pathology, 229*(4), 621–629.

Oliveira, C., Sousa, S., Pinheiro, H., Karam, R., Bordeira-Carrico, R., Senz, J., et al. (2009). Quantification of epigenetic and genetic 2nd hits in CDH1 during hereditary diffuse gastric cancer syndrome progression. *Gastroenterology, 136*(7), 2137–2148.

van der Post, R. S., Vogelaar, I. P., Carneiro, F., et al. (2015). Hereditary diffuse gastric cancer: updated clinical guidelines with an emphasis on germline CDH1 mutation carriers. *Journal of medical genetics. 52*(6), 361–374.

Enteropathy, AIDS

Xavier Sagaert
Department of Pathology, University Hospitals KU Leuven, Leuven, Belgium

Definition

AIDS enteropathy is a syndrome in an HIV-positive individual characterized by chronic, well-established diarrhea (greater than 1 month in duration) without an identified infectious cause after thorough evaluation (Zeitz et al. 1998). As such, AIDS enteropathy is a diagnosis of exclusion and can only be made after other forms of diarrheal illness have been ruled out. Indeed, reported evidence suggests that HIV itself may be an indirect diarrheal pathogen because viral proteins have been found in the gut. *In situ* hybridization of biopsies specimens obtained from the rectum and duodenum revealed HIV-infected cells in both the base of the crypts and within the lamina propria in up to 40% of patients; but while the virus was confined to lamina propria macrophages and enterochromaffin cells, it was found in epithelial cells (Nelson et al. 1988). Intestinal HIV infection may also affect local humoral immunity (with presence of high levels of interleukins IL-6, IL-10 and interferon in the lamina propria) and cause motility disturbances via effects on autonomic nerves. While the exact working mechanisms of HIV-induced diarrhea remains unclear, there are currently two hypotheses: (1) mucosal HIV infection disrupts tight junctions or epithelial apoptotic activity (or both), thereby affecting intestinal permeability; and (2) coupled with a coreceptor, the HIV protein gp120 causes calcium-mediated loss of microtubuli, with subsequent cellular instability (Kotler 2005).

Clinical Features

- **Incidence**
  Diarrhea is the most common gastrointestinal symptom in patients with HIV. In outpatient

studies, the prevalence of diarrhea without identifiable pathogen ranged from 0.9% to 14%. Prevalence was increased in homosexual men (as compared to the heterosexual population) and individuals with lower CD4-positive T-cell counts. In hospitalized individuals with advanced HIV, 50–80% of all patients suffered from mild to severe diarrhea. Furthermore, there is considerable geographic variation in the frequency of diarrhea and the spectrum of enteric pathogens.

- **Age**
  HIV patients of all ages can be affected by AIDS enteropathy.
- **Sex**
  HIV patients of both sexes can be affected by AIDS enteropathy.
- **Site**
  AIDS enteropathy is a disease entity limited to the intestines.
- **Treatment**
  HIV-infected patients with complaints of chronic diarrhea should be treated symptomatically. Antidiarrheals, including Lomotil, Imodium, or tincture of opium drops, are often required and should be titrated individually. Bulk-forming agents may be helpful. While nutritional repletion will increase the patient's sense of well-being, it has not been linked to an overall survival benefit. In cases of severe diarrhea, short- or long-term intravenous fluid repletion may be indicated.

  Importantly, one should always investigate whether an enteric pathogen is present when confronted with diarrhea in AIDS patients, and if one is found, a specific therapy should be administered. Chronic administration of alternating antibiotics may be necessary for recurrent *Salmonella*, *Shigella*, *Campylobacter*, *Cryptosporidia*, or *Isospora* infections. An empiric trial of oral antibiotics or antiparasite therapy for the possibility of small bowel overgrowth, undetected *Campylobacter*, *Isospora* enteritis, or undetected protozoa can be considered. Ciprofloxacin, tetracyclines, sulfonamides, ciprofloxacin, or metronidazole may be appropriate in this setting (Cello and Day 2009).

  Numerous agents have been tested in patients with HIV-associated diarrhea, and controlled studies have failed to define a definitive treatment for cryptosporidiosis, microsporidiosis, or pathogen-negative diarrhea. Especially cryptosporidiosis has been a challenge to treat, because of its intracellular location within enterocytes and innate resistance. However, promising new data indicate that cryptosporidiosis infection may be cleared in patients receiving highly effective antiretroviral therapy. Also, the somatostatin analogue octreotide (administered subcutaneously) appears to be particularly effective in patients with diarrhea who lack a specific infection and thus fulfill the criteria of AIDS enteropathy. This drug inhibits a broad array of gastrointestinal hormones that regulate intestinal fluid and electrolyte secretion, resulting in a decrease of the diarrhea complaints. As a result of its inhibition of cholecystokinin, gallbladder ileus with stone formation and increased fat malabsorption may occur.
- **Outcome**
  Outcome will largely depend on effectiveness of antiretroviral therapy, nutritional supplementation, electrolyte replacements, targeted therapy for infection if indicated, and medications for symptom control.

Macroscopy

HIV enteropathy has no specific macroscopic features.

Microscopy

Histologically, the affected bowel will display atypical features, such as villus atrophy, crypt hyperplasia, or villous blunting in the small bowel, and colitis resembling ulcerative colitis in the large bowel. Some authors have described in small bowel and colon biopsies of patients suffering from AIDS enteropathy a decrease in immunoglobulin IgA-producing plasma cells, and a relative increase in IgM-producing plasma

E

cells (Kotler et al. 1987). Furthermore, enteric HIV infection may lead to mucosal atrophy, which in turn impairs small-bowel absorption, causing diarrhea and weight loss. Importantly, one can only establish a diagnosis of HIV colitis when other possible infectious organisms have been ruled out, and the pathologist should keep an eye out for these opportunistic microorganisms, such as *cryptosoridia* and *Mycobacterium avium, which* can be seen under the microscope.

Differential Diagnosis

It is very important in HIV/AIDS patient suffering from diarrhea to rule out an infectious origin of the complaints. Indeed, a wide variety of protozoal, viral, and bacterial organisms have been implicated as diarrheal pathogens in HIV/AIDS patients, and these should be ruled out before establishing the diagnosis of AIDS enteropathy. Some pathogens, like *Mycobacterium avium*, are quite unique to HIV disease. Others, like *Cryptosporidium*, cause self-limited diarrheal illness in healthy hosts but chronic diarrhea in immunosuppressed patients. The degree of immunodeficiency as reflected by the CD4 cell count is an important determinant of enteric pathogens : *Mycobacterium avium* and CMV infections are not observed in patients with CD4 cell count $>100/\text{mm}^3$.

In earlier studies, pathogens were identified in over half of patients with advanced HIV disease and diarrhea. However, in larger, more recent series, a changing clinical spectrum of diarrhea was revealed, with pathogen-negative diarrhea now representing the majority of patients. In all series, simultaneous infections were common, emphasizing the need to exclude all pathogens thoroughly when evaluating diarrheal symptoms.

Also, pathogens are not always to blame in AIDS patients suffering from diarrhea. In patients with "early" HIV disease, medications are the most common cause of diarrhea, especially protease inhibitors such as Nelfinavir and Saquinavir. This drug-induced type diarrhea is often self-limited, lasting no more than 4 weeks from initiation of medication use. Chronic/uncontrollable diarrhea, however, does occur in spite of improved CD4 cell count and decreased viral load. Other etiologies of diarrhea include enteropathogenic *Escherichia coli*, idiopathic colitis, and small bowel bacterial overgrowth.

References and Further Reading

Cello, J. P., & Day, L. W. (2009). Idiopathic AIDS enteropathy and treatment of gastrointestinal opportunistic pathogens (Vol.136, p. 1952, 2009). *Gastroenterology, 137*, 393.

Kotler, D. P. (2005). HIV infection and the gastrointestinal tract. *Aids, 19*, 107–117.

Kotler, D. P., Scholes, J. V., & Tierney, A. R. (1987). Intestinal plasma-cell alterations in acquired-immunodeficiency-syndrome. *Digestive Diseases and Sciences, 32*, 129–138.

Nelson, J. A., Reynoldskohler, C., Margaretten, W., Wiley, C. A., Reese, C. E., & Levy, J. A. (1988). Human immunodeficiency virus detected in bowel epithelium from patients with gastrointestinal symptoms. *Lancet, 1*, 259–262.

Zeitz, M., Ullrich, R., Schneider, T., Kewenig, S., Hohlock, K., & Riecken, E. O. (1998). HIV/SIV enteropathy. *Intestinal Plasticity in Health and Disease, 859*, 139–148.

Enteropathy, Neonatal (Congenital)

Arzu Ensari
Department of Pathology, Ankara University Medical School, Sihhiye, Ankara, Turkey

Synonyms

Childhood enteropathy; Congenital enteropathy; Primary enteropathies; Severe (primary) enteropathies of infancy

Definition

Primary enteropathies of infancy comprise of epithelial defects including microvillus inclusion disease, tufting enteropathy, and enteroendocrine cell dysgenesis and autoimmune enteropathies. The diseases in this group cause severe chronic (>2–3 weeks) diarrhea starting in the first weeks of life and resulting in failure to thrive in the infant. The diarrhea is either "intractable," that is, chronic, unexplained diarrhea, or "protracted" describing infants with loose and frequent stools which resolves despite initial severity. Both forms are usually associated with malabsorption. Causes of intractable or protracted diarrhea in infancy can be classified as entities showing a normal villus/crypt axis and those associated with villous atrophy. Congenital enteropathies are presented in Table 1. Congenital defects in the transport of sodium, chloride, glucose/galactose and bile acids, and congenital enterokinase deficiency can cause prolonged diarrhea in the neonates, while enterocyte defects many of which have been recently described may also cause similar symptoms. Microvillus inclusion disease (MID) and epithelial dysplasia (ED) or tufting enteropathy (TE) is the most frequent cause of intractable diarrhea with persistent villous atrophy and indefinite dependence on total parenteral nutrition (PN) from early infancy. Since these are intractable diseases, they have been proposed to be elective indication for early bowel transplantation in order to avoid complications, such as PN-related liver disease, that would require a combined small bowel-liver transplant.

Enteropathy, Neonatal (Congenital), Table 1 Classification of neonatal enteropathies

Normal V/C axis	Villus atrophy
Transport defects	Microvillus inclusion disease
Cl-losing diarrhea	Tufting enteropathy
Congenital Na diarr.	Autoimmune enteropathy
Glucose-galactose malabsorption	IPEX syndrome
Micronutrient deficiency	Infectious enteropathy
Acrodermatitis enteropathica	Postinfectious enteropathy
	Allergic enteropathy
	Idiopathic enteropathy
Enzyme deficiencies	
Enterokinase deficiency	
Congenital short bowel	

Clinical Features

- **Incidence**
  A rare group of disorders affecting less than 1: 100,000 infants annually.
- **Age**
  Primary enteropathies of infancy affect infants in the first 6 months of life.
- **Sex**
  There is no known sex predilection.
- **Site**
  In the majority of disorders included in primary enteropathies, the small bowel is affected, although some may also affect the colon (e.g., tufting enteropathy).
- **Treatment**
  Primary enteropathies cause intractable diarrhea which requires long-term TPN, immunosuppression, and/or intestinal transplantation.
- **Outcome**
  Severe intractable diarrhea of infancy has a poor prognosis. The reported mortality rates for primary enteropathies range between 5% and 47%. However, recent developments promise better outcomes after successful intestinal transplantations.

Macroscopy

Endoscopy may be normal in those with a normal villous/crypt axis, while entities causing villous atrophy show flat mucosa with mosaic pattern.

Microscopy

Duodenal mucosa is usually normal in primary enteropathies related to congenital transport or enzyme deficiencies, while biopsy reveals a wide range of abnormalities varying between normal villous morphology to villous atrophy and/or inflammation and specific features including

Enteropathy, Neonatal (Congenital), Table 2 Histopathologic spectrum of neonatal enteropathies

Normal villus morphology
Congenital chloride diarrhea
Carbohydrate malabsorption
Sucrose isomaltase deficiency
Villus atrophy/inflammation
Autoimmune enteropathy and IPEX
Microvillus inclusion disease
Tufting enteropathy
Gluten-sensitive enteropathy
Eosinophilic gastroenteritis
Congenital immunodeficiency disorders
Specific or characteristic features
Fat-filled enterocytes (abetalipoproteinemia, chylomicron retention disease)
Infectious agents
Absence of plasma cells (immunodeficiency)
Lymphangiectasia
Metabolic storage disorders

enterocyte abnormalities. The spectrum of histopathologic features of neonatal enteropathies is summarized in Table 2.

Immunophenotype

No specific immunophenotypic feature has been reported for primary enteropathies.

Molecular Features

Molecular/genetic abnormalities have been described for primary enteropathies depending on the underlying disorder.

Differential Diagnosis

Neonatal early-onset severe diarrhea may be caused by ion transport defects. However, congenital chloride diarrhea (CLD) or congenital sodium diarrhea (CSD) can be easily distinguished from the absence of hydramnios and by blood and stool electrolyte assessment. CLD is a rare autosomal recessive disorder of intestinal Cl/HCO_3 exchange caused by mutations in the *SLC26A3* gene and characterized by persistent Cl-rich diarrhea from birth. Chloride is low in urine and very high in stools. CSD is caused by defective sodium/proton exchange with only few sporadic cases reported. The genetics of the disease have not yet been established. Patients have acidosis and hyponatremia, and stools show high concentrations of HCO_3 and sodium.

Glucose-galactose malabsorption (GGM) is an autosomal recessive disease that presents in newborn infants as a life-threatening diarrhea. The diarrhea ceases after removing the oral intake of lactose, glucose, and galactose.

MID is a congenital disorder of the intestinal epithelial cells that presents with persistent life-threatening watery diarrhea and is characterized by morphological enterocyte abnormalities. MID is a very rare disorder transmitted as an autosomal recessive trait. Recently, mutations in MYO5B gene located on 18q21 which encodes myosin Vb responsible for actin-dependent organelle transport and regulation of endosome distribution were identified. Light microscopy shows accumulation of PAS-positive granules at the apical pole of immature enterocytes, together with atrophic band indicating microvillus atrophy and, in parallel, an intracellular PAS or CD10 positive line. Ultrastructural analysis reveals a partial to total atrophy of microvilli on mature enterocytes with apical accumulation of numerous secretory granules in immature enterocytes.

TE should be suspected in neonates with early-onset intractable diarrhea persisting at bowel rest. In patients with neonatal diarrhea and villous atrophy in which MID has been ruled out, the evidence of a punctuated keratitis is very relevant for the diagnosis of TE, since more than 60% of the cases have this association. The diagnosis of TE is especially problematic when the tufts are missing or hard to find and often leads to treat the disease as an immune enteropathy.

References and Further Reading

Cuenod, B., Brousse, N., Goulet, O., De Potter, S., Mougenot, J. F., Ricour, C., Guy-Grand, D., &

Cerf-Bensussan, N. (1990). Classification of intractable diarrhea in infancy using clinical and immunohistological criteria. *Gastroenterology, 99*(4), 1037–1043.
Gambarara, M., Diamanti, A., Ferretti, F., Papadatou, B., Knafelz, D., Pietrobattista, A., & Castro, M. (2003). Intractable diarrhea of infancy with congenital intestinal mucosa abnormalities: Outcome of four cases. *Transplantation Proceedings, 35*(8), 3052–3053.
Girault, D., Goulet, O., Le Deist, F., Brousse, N., Colomb, V., Césarini, J. P., de Potter, S., Canioni, D., Griscelli, C., Fischer, A., et al. (1994). Intractable infant diarrhea associated with phenotypic abnormalities and immunodeficiency. *The Journal of Pediatrics, 125*(1), 36–42.
Goulet, O., Kedinger, M., Brousse, N., Cuenod, B., Colomb, V., Patey, N., de Potter, S., Mougenot, J. F., Canioni, D., Cerf-Bensussan, N., et al. (1995). Intractable diarrhea of infancy with epithelial and basement membrane abnormalities. *The Journal of Pediatrics, 127*(2), 212–219.
Sherman, P. M., Mitchell, D. J., & Cutz, E. (2004). Neonatal enteropathies: Defining the causes of protracted diarrhea of infancy. *Journal of Pediatric Gastroenterology and Nutrition, 38*, 16–26.

Eosinophilic Colitis

Karel Geboes
Department of Pathology, N. Goormaghtig Institute, University Gent, Gent, Belgium
Department of Pathology, KU Leuven, Leuven, Belgium

Synonyms

Allergic colitis (proctitis or proctocolitis); Milk-protein proctocolitis

Definition

Eosinophilic colitis is a heterogeneous disorder characterized by the presence of a dense eosinophilic infiltration in the colon that can be segmental or diffuse (Fig. 1). It may affect children as well as adults. Three different types must be distinguished: primary eosinophilic colitis, which belongs to the family of primary eosinophilic gastrointestinal disorders (EGID), secondary eosinophilic colitis, and colitis in the framework of the hypereosinophilic syndrome (HES). Secondary eosinophilic colitis is observed in a variety of diseases such as idiopathic inflammatory bowel disease (IBD), parasitic and helminthic infections with *Strongyloides stercoralis*, *Enterobius vermicularis*, and drug-associated colitis. Drugs involved include clozapine, carbamazepine, gold salts, rifampicin, antiplatelet agents, tacrolimus, and naproxen. Other associations include vasculitis (Churg-Strauss), autoimmune connective tissue disease (scleroderma, dermatomyositis, polymyositis), systemic mastocytosis as well as allogenic bone marrow transplantation and the rare Tolosa-Hunt syndrome characterized by headache, ophthalmoplegia, and cranial nerve palsies. Classically, the HES exhibits markedly increased levels of blood eosinophilia (>1,500 μl) persistent for at least 6 months, clonal eosinophilia, and involvement of multiple organs. Two distinct subcategories of clonal eosinophilia are however recognized: chronic eosinophilic leukemia-NOS (not otherwise specified) and myeloid/lymphoid neoplasms involving platelet-derived growth factor A &B (PDGFRA, PDGFRB) or fibroblast growth factor receptor 1 (FGFR1). The gut is rather an innocent bystander with eosinophils infiltrating various sites.

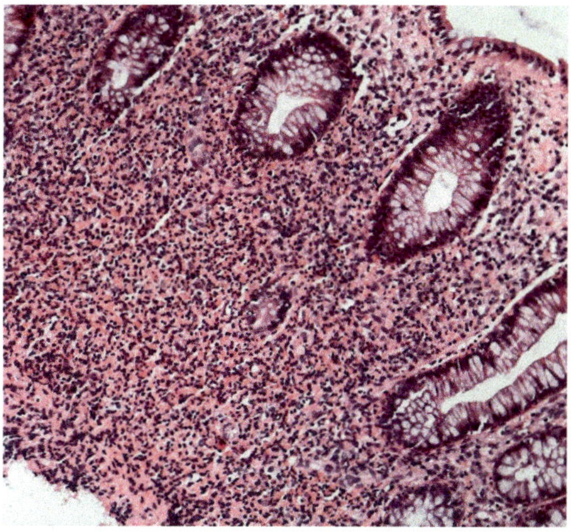

Eosinophilic Colitis, Fig. 1 Microphotograph showing a diffuse infiltrate of eosinophils in the lamina propria (Courtesy of Dr A. Jouret-Mourin)

Primary eosinophilic colitis may present with the classical hallmarks of EGID including peripheral eosinophilia (in the range of 5–35%), segmental eosinophilic infiltration, and functional abnormalities. Symptoms are usually nonspecific and depend on the affected segment. The disease may affect primarily the mucosa or the serosa or may be transmural. Clinical complaints include abdominal pain, nausea, vomiting, diarrhea, bleeding, weight loss, and ascites. Mucosa-predominant disease results in diarrhea, while transmural disease may be associated with obstruction, volvulus, intussusceptions, and even perforation.

No single test is the gold standard for diagnosis. The final diagnosis of primary eosinophilic colitis is based on endoscopic biopsies demonstrating colonic tissue hypereosinophilia and the absence of any other primary disorder that may cause secondary eosinophilic infiltrates. Peripheral eosinophilia is present in 20–90% of the patients. Eosinophils in the stools are also suggestive of eosinophilic colitis.

The precise etiology of primary eosinophilic colitis is unclear. There is an interaction between genetic and environmental factors. Approximately 75% of affected young patients have a history of allergy or atopy. Cow's milk and soy proteins are the foods most frequently implicated in the infantile form, although the condition has been reported in infants exclusively breast-fed or given protein-hydrolyzed formulas. The disease is due to the exposure to food allergens, causing a mixed IgE and non-IgE allergic reaction. Mast cell accumulation and degranulation in colonic tissue has been reported which supports the role of IgE in eosinophilic colitis. Furthermore, the reaction may induce a Th2-related immune response. The Th2 lymphocytes release cytokines such as IL-3, IL-4, IL-5, which function as chemo-attractants of inflammatory cells (mast cells, eosinophils). Besides these cytokines other chemokines, such as eotaxin-1, eotaxin-2, eotaxin-3, are involved in the recruitment and tissue infiltration of eosinophils. Less is known about the potential causes of the adult form. Food-related anaphylaxis is uncommon.

Clinical Features

- **Incidence**
  EGID, originally described by Kaijser in 1937, is a rare spectrum of gastrointestinal disorders. It affects the pediatric population although it has been reported also in patients up to 68 years of age. While eosinophilic esophagitis is diagnosed in about 1% of the population, primary eosinophilic colitis is the least frequent manifestation of EGID and exceptionally rare. Five cases were observed between 2003 and 2010 at the University of Minnesota. In contrast to increased trends seen in primary eosinophilic esophagitis, the prevalence of eosinophilic colitis does not appear to be increasing.
- **Age**
  Primary eosinophilic colitis appears to have a bimodal distribution that affects neonates (presenting at approximately 60 days) with a relatively high prevalence and a separate group presenting during adolescence and early adulthood.
- **Sex**
  No gender preference has been noted.
- **Site**
  Eosinophilic colitis is limited to the colon, but primary and secondary eosinophilic infiltration of the colon may also occur as part of a larger condition which is then called enterocolitis or gastro-enterocolitis.
- **Treatment**
  To date, there are no prospective controlled randomized trials on medical treatment for primary eosinophilic colitis. Corticosteroid therapy is the most common commonly used initial treatment and most effective for symptom control. Up to 90% of patients will respond within 2 weeks but relapse is frequent. A role for budesonide has been demonstrated particularly in the right colon. The beneficial effect of elimination and elemental diets is limited to cases with specific food allergies, especially in neonates. Expertise with other medical treatments such as antihistamine therapy, mast cell stabilizers, and leukotriene inhibitors in eosinophilic colitis is limited. More recently, the

role of biologics is considered. Chemokines such as eotaxin are involved in eosinophil recruitment. This provides a rationale for blocking this agent, either by immunomodulatory agents such as azathioprine or by biologicals. Other biologic drugs target the binding of IgE to the high-affinity receptor, Fc epsilon RI, or IL-5, involved in maturation and proliferation, survival of eosinophils. Clinical studies are however needed to validate these approaches.

The treatment for secondary eosinophilic colitis is essentially the treatment of the primary disease. In ulcerative colitis, the persistence of tissue eosinophilia in the colon may be a marker of possible relapse.

- **Outcome**

  Eosinophilic colitis of infancy is usually a benign disease. On withdrawal of the offending protein, gross blood in the stools usually resolves within 72 h. The vast majority of patients are able to tolerate the culprit food by 1–3 years of age. The prognosis for eosinophilic colitis at later age is good.

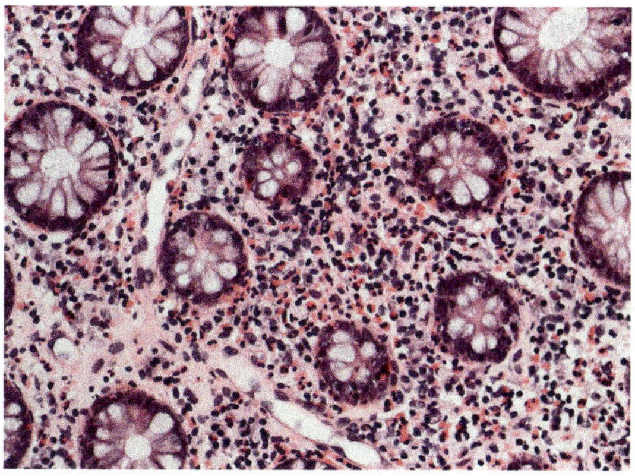

Eosinophilic Colitis, Fig. 2 Diffuse increase of eosinophils in the lamina propria exceeding 20 per high-power field (Courtesy of Dr A. Jouret-Mourin)

Macroscopy

The gross aspect of the colon is nonspecific. Endoscopy may be normal, limited to lymphonodular hyperplasia which is not uncommon in young patients, or reveal edematous mucosa with a loss of the normal vascular pattern, punctate erythematous changes, and even superficial ulcerations. Changes can occur throughout the colon but tend to be more prominent in the ascending colon and rectum.

Microscopy

No clear consensus exists with regard to the degree of tissue eosinophilia or the presence of distinct pathologic findings necessary for the diagnosis of eosinophilic colitis. With exception of the esophagus, eosinophils are normal constituents of the whole gastrointestinal tract, be it that their number varies in function of the segment of the gut. For the colon, most authors propose a diagnostic threshold of 20 eosinophils per high-power field present as focal aggregates or more diffuse in the lamina propria and muscularis mucosae (Fig. 2). However, normal values for tissue eosinophils in the colon vary widely. Location of the biopsy is an important variable. Lamina propria eosinophils are, on average, 3 times more numerous in the ascending compared with the descending colon. The normal value may range from <10 per high-power field in the rectum to >30 in the cecum, where the highest normal number can be found. The number of eosinophils may also vary in function of the season and the geography. Mucosal eosinophils are slightly more numerous in samples obtained in April and May, corresponding to periods of high pollen counts. A 35-fold difference between the mean eosinophil numbers was found when patients from New Orleans and Boston were compared. Eosinophils are not normally present in Peyer's patches or intraepithelial locations.

Diagnostic criteria for primary eosinophilic colitis therefore include certainly the presence of focal aggregates of eosinophils in the (crypt) epithelium (Fig. 3). The lesions can be associated with epithelial damage such as erosions and crypt abscesses.

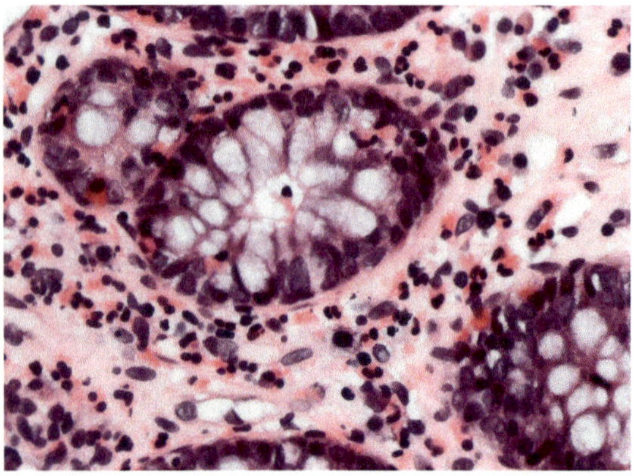

Eosinophilic Colitis, Fig. 3 Eosinophils in the lamina propria and in an intraepithelial position (Courtesy of Dr A. Jouret-Mourin)

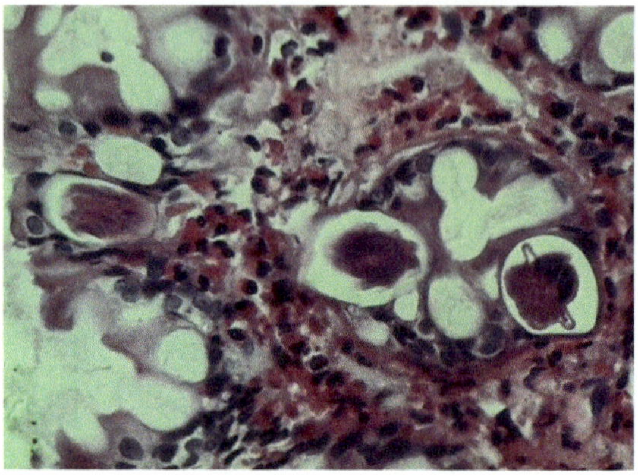

Eosinophilic Colitis, Fig. 4 Presence of numerous eosinophils in association with parasitosis (Courtesy of Dr Sihosptp)

Immunophenotype

There are no specific studies for primary eosinophilic colitis. In eosinophilic esophagitis, it was reported that levels of surface CD66b as well as levels of intracellular phospho-STAT1 and phospho-STAT6, (STAT: Signal Transducers and Activators of transcription), both transcription factors involved in inflammatory processes, were significantly higher in peripheral blood eosinophils for untreated subjects compared with healthy controls. These findings need however confirmation, and their meaning is not yet clear.

Molecular Features

Eosinophils are formed in the bone marrow. Maturation is regulated by transcription factors GATA-1, GATA-2, and c/EBP (GATA: transcription factor family related by a high degree of amino acid sequence identity; zinc finger family member; EBP: enhancer-binding protein). They cooperate with "permissive" eosinophil growth factors IL-3, IL-5, and GM-CSF. IL-5 is responsible for the release of eosinophils into the peripheral circulation. Finally, eosinophils relocate into specific tissues. They are normally present in the lamina propria of the stomach, small intestine, and colon. Homing occurs in the prenatal period independent of indigenous flora. The function of eosinophils in the digestive tract is not well known. They might have a role in tissue or organ development and mucosal defense. They can release preformed granule constituents including four cytotoxic cationic proteins: eosinophilic peroxidase (EPO), major basic protein (MBP), eosinophilic cationic protein (ECP) and eosinophil-derived neurotoxin (EDN), and a variety of cytokines, neuromediators, and lipid mediators. They are also involved in propagating immune responses by presenting antigens to T cells.

Differential Diagnosis

It is essential to differentiate between primary eosinophilic colitis and secondary forms such as parasitosis (Fig. 4), because the treatment is different. A complete workup of the patient is therefore needed. The finding of an increased eosinophil count in the left colon could be an indication of drug-related disease.

References and Further Reading

Casella, B., Villanaci, V., Fisogni, S., Cambareri, A. E., Di Bellas, C., Corazzi, N., Gorlas, S., Baldini, V., & Bassotti, G. (2009). Colonic left-side increase of eosinophils: A clue to drug-related colitis in adults. *Alimentary Pharmacology & Therapeutics, 29*, 535–541.

Gaertner, W. B., MacDonald, J. E., Kwaan, M. R., Shepela, C., Madoff, R., Jessurun, J., & Melton, G. B. (2011). Eosinophilic colitis: University of Minnesota experience and literature review. *Gastroenterology Research and Practice, 2011*, 857508.

Nguyen, T., Gernez, Y., Fuentebella, J., Patel, A., Tirouvanziam, R., Reshamwala, N., Bass, D., Berquist, W. E., Cox, K. L., Kerner, J. A., & Nadeau, K. C. (2011). Immunophenotyping of peripheral eosinophils demonstrates activation in eosinophilic esophagitis. *Journal of Pediatric Gastroenterology and Nutrition, 53*, 40–47.

Pascal, R. R., Gramlich, T. L., Parker, K. M., & Gansler, T. S. (1997). Geographic variations in eosinophil concentration in normal colonic mucosa. *Modern Pathology, 10*, 363–365.

Polydorides, A. D., Banner, B. F., Hannaway, P. J., & Yantiss, R. K. (2008). Evaluation of site-specific and seasonal variation in colonic mucosal eosinophils. *Human Pathology, 39*, 832–836.

Powell, N., Walker, M. M., & Talley, N. J. (2010). Gastrointestinal eosinophils in health, disease and functional disorders. *Nature Reviews. Gastroenterology & Hepatology, 7*, 146–156.

Rothenberg, M. (2004). Eosinophilic gastrointestinal disorders (EGID). *The Journal of Allergy and Clinical Immunology, 113*, 11–28.

Eosinophilic Esophagitis

Rafaela L. Rego[1] and Jason T. Lewis[2]
[1]Departamento de Diagnóstico Laboratorial – Serviço de Anatomia Patológica, Instituto Portugues de Oncologia Lisboa Francisco Gentil, IPOLFG, E.P.E, Lisbon, Portugal
[2]Division of Anatomic Pathology, Department of Laboratory Medicine and Pathology, Mayo Clinic, Jacksonville, FL, USA

Synonyms

Eosinophilic (allergic, idiopathic) esophagitis; Primary eosinophilic esophagitis

Definition

Eosinophilic esophagitis has been described as a variant of the family of presumably allergic eosinophilic disorders that can involve any portion of the gastrointestinal tract (Antonioli and Furuta 2005). The favored interpretation is that it is the result from local hypersensitivity to food- or blood-borne allergens and that antigen-presenting cells play an important role in its pathogenesis (Lucendo et al. 2007). It is a recently recognized disorder that has some features that may mimic gastroesophageal reflux disease (GERD) clinically, endoscopically, and histologically. By definition, patients have normal pH monitoring levels and fail to respond to antireflux therapy. Eosinophilic esophagitis tends to occur in children or young adults, with a strong male predominance, and its pathogenesis is not fully understood. Many affected patients reveal an allergic history and have peripheral eosinophilia [$>0.45 \times 10^9$/L (450/μl)]. Symptoms manifest differently according to the age groups: infants and young children often present with feeding difficulties, whereas older children and adults usually complain of dysphagia and food impaction. If not recognized early, it can progress to odynophagia and stenosis. Most authorities believe that this disorder is caused by a combination of allergic and immunologic factors (Liacouras and Ruchelli 2004). Affected patients often reveal other forms of atopy, such as atopic dermatitis, allergic rhinitis, and bronchial asthma (about 60–75%), and some patients show symptomatic improvement when a particular type of food allergen is identified and eliminated from their diet (Markowitz et al. 2003), for example, cow's milk and soy products. Some authors also believe that injury to the squamous epithelium secondary to GERD increases epithelial permeability and facilitates penetration by large-sized allergic peptides that could potentially trigger a local type of allergic response (Genta et al. 2007).

Clinical Features

- **Incidence**
  The incidence of eosinophilic esophagitis is increasing markedly (Furuta et al. 2007), and it is not an uncommon entity seen in pediatric gastroenterology services.

- **Age**
  Eosinophilic esophagitis occurs in all ages, but it is more common in the pediatric age group.
- **Sex**
  Strong male predominance.
- **Site**
  Along the length of the esophagus.
- **Treatment**
  Therapy includes dietary elimination of offending food and swallowing of topical steroids.
- **Outcome (prognosis)**
  The prognosis is excellent when treatment is given promptly. Progression of the disease is seen when an incorrect diagnosis of reflux is rendered. Improvements are sometimes dramatic.

Macroscopy (Gross)

Endoscopically, patients with eosinophilic esophagitis often exhibit characteristic concentric mucosal rings, also referred to as "trachealization" of the esophagus, or "ringed" esophagus (Gonsalves 2007; Spechler et al. 2007). Other endoscopic findings include small, punctate mucosal whitish plaques/exudates, narrow-caliber esophagus, and mucosal tears (Siafakas et al. 2000). Occasionally, the esophagus in patients with eosinophilic esophagitis may appear entirely normal. However, more than 90% of affected patients display one or more of the endoscopic abnormalities listed above (Potter et al. 2004).

Microscopy

Histologically, the features of eosinophilic esophagitis overlap with those of GERD (Fig. 1), particularly in distal esophageal biopsies, and in both of these conditions, intraepithelial eosinophils may be patchy in distribution (Fig. 2). Thus, sampling error may also affect one's ability to establish a correct diagnosis. Although biopsies of patients with eosinophilic esophagitis tend to reveal more prominent intraepithelial eosinophilia, typically in the range of 15–20 or more eosinophils per high-power field (400× – Fig. 3), severe GERD also may produce pronounced intraepithelial eosinophilia in this range in a minority of cases. Histologic features that favor eosinophilic esophagitis include the presence of aggregates or microabscesses of eosinophils (defined as an organized collection of eosinophils associated with cell necrosis), a predominance of eosinophils located within the superficial layers of the squamous epithelium, and abundant eosinophils mixed with superficial desquamated luminal debris (Fig. 4) (Gonsalves, 2007; Spechler et al. 2007). The American Gastroenterological Association (AGA)-sponsored

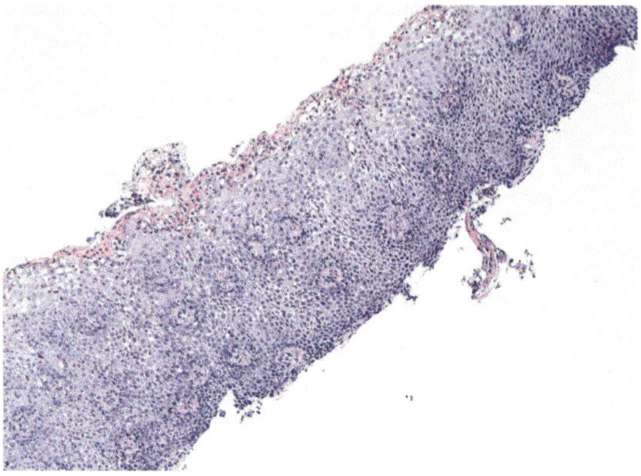

Eosinophilic Esophagitis, Fig. 1 Eosinophilic esophagitis with marked reactive squamous hyperplasia (H&E, 100×)

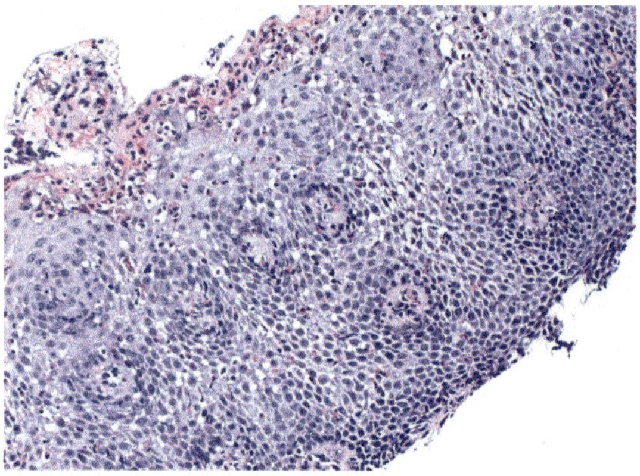

Eosinophilic Esophagitis, Fig. 2 Intraepithelial eosinophils may be patchy in distribution; consequently, multiple biopsies and multiple levels of each biopsy are recommended in suspected cases (H&E, 200×)

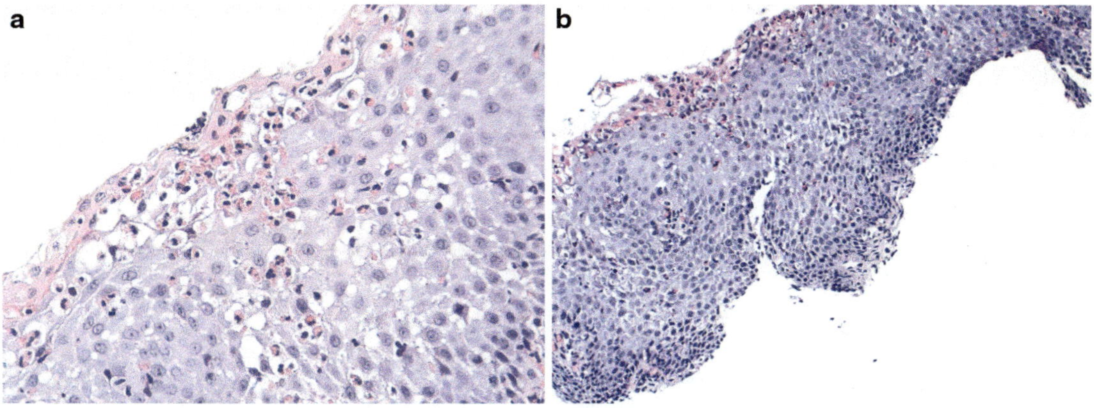

Eosinophilic Esophagitis, Fig. 3 Increased number of intraepithelial eosinophils (>20 per high-power field) (H&E, 400× – **a**), predominantly in the superficial portions of the epithelium (H&E, 200× – **b**)

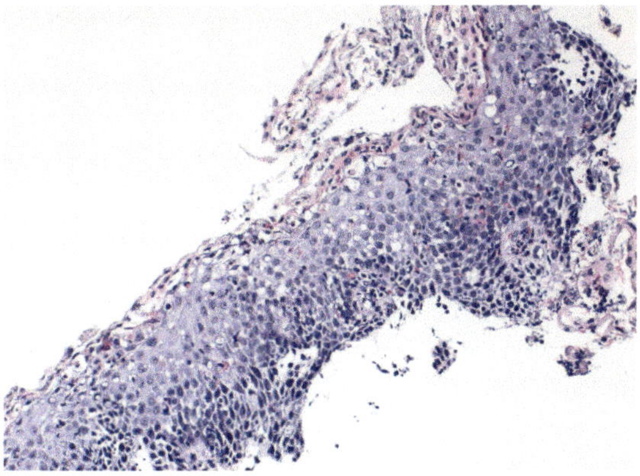

Eosinophilic Esophagitis, Fig. 4 Accumulation of eosinophils within the superficial necroinflammatory debris (H&E, 200×)

review on eosinophilic esophagitis, published in 2007, defines this condition as one in which more than 15 eosinophils per high-power field are identified in esophageal mucosal biopsies from patients who lack a positive response to proton pump inhibitor therapy, have normal pH monitoring values, or both (Furuta et al. 2007). Other histologic features of eosinophilic esophagitis include the presence of prominent eosinophilic degranulation and marked basal zone hyperplasia and lengthening of the lamina propria papillae. These histologic features, although helpful, are not considered perfect for discriminating eosinophilic esophagitis from GERD, particularly in biopsies from the distal esophagus. However, biopsy-proven involvement of the mid or upper regions of the esophageal mucosa has greater diagnostic significance for eosinophilic esophagitis, because GERD only rarely extends to the more proximal aspects of the esophagus.

Molecular Features

Eotaxin-3, a gene that encodes a component of the immunologic cascade, has been shown to be highly induced in patients with eosinophilic esophagitis compared with normal controls, a finding that suggests a component of genetic susceptibility (Mishra and Rothenberg 2003).

Differential Diagnosis

The differential diagnosis of eosinophilic esophagitis includes GERD, eosinophilic gastroenteritis, Crohn's disease, collagen-vascular diseases, infectious esophagitis (secondary to herpes, Candida, or parasites), drug-associated esophagitis, and hypereosinophilic syndrome. As previously discussed, given the overlap of histologic features of GERD and eosinophilic esophagitis, biopsy evaluations from the mid and proximal esophagus are the most diagnostically useful. Careful examination of histologic sections to exclude parasitic and fungal infection is also important. The types of plaques observed in patients with eosinophilic esophagitis may suggest Candida esophagitis endoscopically, but upon microscopy, the plaques in the former condition consist of sloughed squamous cells admixed with eosinophils, which are easily distinguished from the fungal elements characteristic of Candida esophagitis. Distinguishing eosinophilic esophagitis from eosinophilic gastroenteritis can be a challenge, particularly if the stomach and duodenum have not been biopsied. Most cases of eosinophilic gastroenteritis reveal gastric antral involvement, and a smaller proportion shows duodenal involvement as well. Nevertheless, mucosal biopsies in patients with eosinophilic gastroenteritis often show numerous eosinophils, frequently degranulated, infiltrating both the lamina propria and epithelium, and usually involve one or more of the esophagus, stomach, and duodenal regions. In addition, correlation with clinical symptoms of generalized mucosal involvement, such as nausea, vomiting, and diarrhea, is also helpful in establishing a correct diagnosis. Because the eosinophilic infiltrate in eosinophilic esophagitis is often focal, multiple biopsies and multiple levels of each biopsy should be evaluated in suspected cases. Finally, the diagnosis of eosinophilic esophagitis is best rendered in biopsies obtained after anti-GERD therapy.

References and Further Reading

Antonioli, D. A., & Furuta, G. T. (2005). Allergic eosinophilic esophagitis: A primer for pathologists. *Seminars in Diagnostic Pathology, 22*, 266–272.

Furuta, G. T., Liacouras, C. A., Collins, M. H., et al. (2007). Eosinophilic esophagitis in children and adults: A systematic review and consensus recommendations for diagnosis and treatment. *Gastroenterology, 133*(4), 1342–1363.

Genta, R. M., Spechler, S. J., & Souza, R. F. (2007). The twentieth eosinophil. *Advances in Anatomic Pathology, 14*, 340–343.

Gonsalves, N. (2007). Food allergies and eosinophilic gastrointestinal illness. *Gastroenterology Clinics of North America, 36*, 75–91.

Liacouras, C. A., & Ruchelli, E. (2004). Eosinophilic esophagitis. *Current Opinion in Pediatrics, 16*, 560–566.

Lucendo, A. J., Navarro, M., Comas, C., Pascual, J. M., Burgos, E., Santamaría, L., & Larrauri, J. (2007). Immunophenotypic characterization and quantification of the epithelial inflammatory infiltrate in eosinophilic esophagitis through stereology: an analysis of the cellular mechanisms of the disease and the immunologic capacity of the esophagus. *The American Journal of Surgical Pathology, 31*, 598–606.

Markowitz, J. E., Spergel, J. M., Ruchelli, E., & Liacouras, C. A. (2003). Elemental diet is an effective treatment for eosinophilic esophagitis in children and adolescents. *The American Journal of Gastroenterology, 98*, 777–782.

Mishra, A., & Rothenberg, M. E. (2003). Intratracheal IL-13 induces eosinophilic esophagitis by an IL-5, eotaxin-1, and STAT6-dependent mechanism. *Gastroenterology, 125*, 1419–1427.

Potter, J. W., Saeian, K., Staff, D., et al. (2004). Eosinophilic esophagitis in adults: An emerging problem with unique esophageal features. *Gastrointestinal Endoscopy, 59*, 355–361.

Siafakas, C. G., Ryan, C. K., Brown, M. R., & Miller, T. L. (2000). Multiple esophageal rings: An association with eosinophilic esophagitis: Case report and review of the literature. *The American Journal of Gastroenterology, 95*, 1572–1575.

Spechler, S. J., Genta, R. M., & Souza, R. F. (2007). Thoughts on the complex relationship between gastroesophageal reflux disease and eosinophilic esophagitis. *The American Journal of Gastroenterology, 102*, 1301–1306.

Eosinophilic Gastritis

Helena Baldaia
Serviço de Anatomia Patológica, Centro Hospitalar de São João, Porto, Portugal

Synonyms

"Allergic" gastroenteritis; Eosinophilic gastroenteritis

Definition

Eosinophilic gastritis is characterized by a prominent eosinophil-rich inflammation in the gastric wall (Lash et al. 2009) without known cause. Isolated gastric eosinophilia is very rare and it is usually associated with involvement of the duodenum, esophagus, or other gastrointestinal

(GI) segments, which is also referred as eosinophilic gastroenteritis (Lash et al. 2009).

As the gastric mucosa has a variable number of eosinophils, the diagnosis, especially in biopsy material, can be difficult. One study addressed the number of eosinophil counts in the normal gastric mucosa and other eosinophil-rich entities in the stomach and the authors proposed working diagnostic criteria: (1) patients who have gastric biopsies that show an average density of >127 eosinophils/mm^2 (or ≥ 30 eosinophils per HPF in microscopes equipped with wide-lens oculars) and (2) patients that have no known associated causes of eosinophilia. These criteria were proposed in an attempt to homogenize the diagnosis of this entity and for further characterization of the disease (Lwin et al. 2011).

Eosinophilic gastroenteritis can be classified on the basis of the GI segments involved but also the layers of the GI tract involved (mucosal, mural, and serosal types). Previous studies have shown that, in the stomach mucosal, involvement is the commonest type (approximately 60%), with muscular and serosal involvement seen in approximately 30% and 10% of the cases, respectively (Holroyd et al. 2010). Clinical manifestations are related to the latter classification. Mucosal involvement of eosinophilic gastroenteritis is associated with hemorrhage, nausea, vomiting, and malabsorption, while muscular (mural) involvement is frequently associated with wall thickening and obstructive symptoms. Serosal involvement can result in eosinophil-rich ascites (Lash et al. 2009).

The pathogenesis of eosinophilic gastroenteritis is still unknown but an allergic etiology, probably with the involvement of eotaxin-1, is supported by the fact that 75% of patients are atopic. Also a reduction of the severity of the disease is sometimes seen when certain foods are eliminated from the diet and mast cell degranulation is usually found in tissue specimens (Lash et al. 2009). In some patients there is IgE elevation (Robert 2009) and blood eosinophilia (Lash et al. 2009). Approximately 10% of patients with this condition have an immediate family member with a similar affliction (Lash et al. 2009).

Clinical Features

- **Incidence**
  Eosinophilic gastroenteritis is an uncommon condition (Fenoglio-Preiser et al. 2008). Isolated gastric involvement is very rare (Lash et al. 2009).
- **Age**
  Eosinophilic gastroenteritis usually presents between the second and fifth decades of life (Fenoglio-Preiser et al. 2008). Children are more frequently affected than adults (Lash et al. 2009).
- **Sex**
  There is no gender predilection reported.
- **Site**
  The stomach is the most common site of involvement in eosinophilic gastroenteritis, frequently associated with small bowel disease (Robert 2009).
- **Treatment**
  Treatment modalities include dietary eviction of certain allergenic foods and steroid therapy (Robert 2009). There have also been reports on the use of leukotriene inhibitors. Even if gastroesophageal reflux is not present, neutralization of gastric acidity may improve symptoms. In severe, refractory cases immunosuppressive antimetabolite therapy has been advocated as an alternative (Rothenberg 2004). Sometimes, in obstructive disease, resection may be necessary before a diagnosis can be established (Robert 2009).
- **Outcome**
  The natural history of this condition has not been well documented. Although there have been reports of good results with steroid therapy, these diseases are often chronic with a waxing and waning course.

  When the disease presents in infancy, and specific food sensitization can be identified, there is a high likelihood of disease remission by late childhood (Rothenberg 2004).

Macroscopy

In one case series, the most common endoscopic findings were a normal stomach or erythema and gastritis, with or without erosions (Lwin et al. 2011).

Microscopy

One important aspect of eosinophilic gastroenteritis is the frequent patchy aspect of the lesions that may hamper the diagnosis. Multiple biopsies should be evaluated, including deeper biopsies (Fenoglio-Preiser et al. 2008). The histological hallmark is the presence of a variably dense eosinophilic infiltrate in the gastric wall, frequently with numerous eosinophils in the lamina propria and foveolar surface (Lash et al. 2009) (Fig. 1). Some biopsies may show eosinophilic crypt abscesses, surface erosion, or ulceration (Robert 2009). Of note is that the absence of mucosal alterations in a patient suspected of having eosinophilic gastroenteritis does not exclude the diagnosis, since the disease can be very patchy in distribution and the involvement may be predominantly mural or serosal. In the former, the muscular layer may be thickened and infiltrated by eosinophils, with marked submucosal edema. In the serosal form, edema and eosinophils are limited to the subserosal layers. In this case a cytological diagnosis can usually be made (Robert 2009).

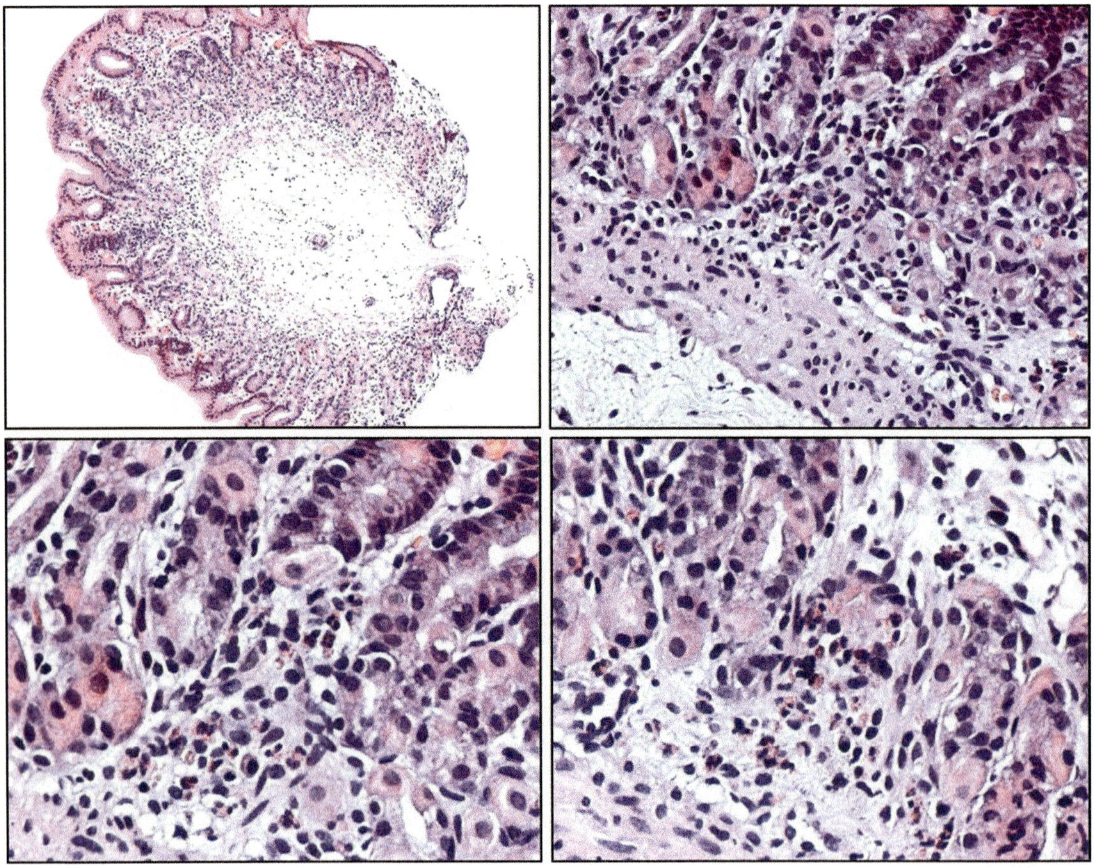

Eosinophilic Gastritis, Fig. 1 Eosinophilic gastritis. Gastric corpus mucosa with numerous eosinophils in the lamina propria

Immunophenotype

There are no immunophenotypical aspects characteristic to this disease.

Molecular Features

At the present there are no reports of molecular aspects characteristic of this disease.

Differential Diagnosis

The differential diagnosis is with other eosinophil-rich gastritis. *Parasitic infections* must be thoroughly excluded by histological, clinical, and microbiological methods. *Crohn's disease* may be difficult to distinguish from eosinophilic gastroenteritis. However, granulomas are not a feature of the latter (Robert 2009). *Drug reactions* usually are not associated with such a massive eosinophil infiltration. In this case clinical information can be helpful determining the correct diagnosis (Lash et al. 2009).

References and Further Reading

Fenoglio-Preiser, C. M., Noffsinger, A. E., Stemmermann, G. N., Lantz, P. E., & Isaacson, P. G. (2008). The non-neoplastic stomach. In J. McGouh & J. Pine (Eds.), *Gastrointestinal pathology an atlas and text* (pp. 196–197). Philadelphia: Lippincott Williams & Wilkins.

Holroyd, D. J., Banerjee, S., Chaudhary, K. S., et al. (2010). Transmural eosinophilic gastritis with gastric outlet obstruction: Case report and review of the literature. *Annals of the Royal College of Surgeons of England, 92*(4), W18–W20.

Lash, R. H., Lawuers, G. Y., Odze, R. D., & Genta, R. M. (2009). Inflammatory disorders of the stomach. In R. Odze & J. Goldblum (Eds.), *Surgical pathology of the GI tract, liver, biliary tract and pancreas*. Philadelphia: Saunders.

Lwin, T., Melton, S. D., & Genta, R. M. (2011). Eosinophilic gastritis: Histopathological characterization and quantification of the normal gastric eosinophil content. *Modern Pathology, 24*, 4,556–563.

Robert, M. E. (2009). Inflammatory disorders of the small intestine. In R. Odze & J. Goldblum (Eds.), *Surgical pathology of the GI tract, liver, biliary tract and pancreas*. Philadelphia: Saunders.

Rothenberg, M. E. (2004). Eosinophilic gastrointestinal disorders (EGID). *The Journal of Allergy and Clinical Immunology, 113*(1), 11–28.

Epstein-Barr Virus (EBV), Esophagitis

Paula Borralho Nunes
Hospital Cuf Descobertas and Escola Superior de Tecnologia da Saúde de Lisboa and Instituto de Anatomia Patológica, Faculdade de Medicina da, Universidade de Lisboa, Lisboa, Portugal

Synonyms

Human herpesvirus four esophagitis

Definition

Epstein-Barr virus (EBV) esophagitis is a form of esophagitis caused by herpesvirus in immunocompetent or immunocompromised patients.

EBV is a ubiquitous virus that infects and establishes a persistent infection in the host. Clinically, it causes two types of infection: the primary infection, which ranges from a mild self-limited illness in children to infectious mononucleosis in adolescents and adults, and the reactivation of latent infection in immunocompromised patients (Gesser 1997). EBV replicates and is shed periodically from epithelial cells in the oropharynx or from salivary glands and persists through interactions with two different host cell types: epithelial cells at the surface of the body that are fully permissive for the production of infectious virus and serve to transmit the virus from person to person and cells situated deeper in the body that generally are non-permissive and function as a reservoir of latent virus.

At least in theory, virus infecting epithelial cells in the oropharynx could potentially infect esophageal epithelial cells as well, causing esophagitis in predisposed patients. In fact, evidence has emerged to show that the prime target EBV is the epithelial cell (Pattengale et al. 1973), rendering esophageal squamous stratified epithelium a potential candidate for infection. The pathogenesis of Epstein-Barr virus (EBV) esophagitis is not well known. However, in immunocompromised patients infected with human immunodeficiency virus (HIV) infection, in oral hairy leukoplakia, Epstein-Barr virus (EBV) has been shown to replicate in the squamous epithelium of the oral mucosa, with Langerhans cell depletion showing to play an important part in the pathogenesis of these lesions.

Although EBV is undoubtedly important in many human benign and malignant conditions, its exact role in esophageal pathology remains unclear.

Clinical Features

- **Incidence**
  EBV infects and establishes latency in virtually everyone. More than 90% of the adult population carries this virus in a latent form, usually acquired asymptomatically during early childhood. The exact prevalence of EBV esophagitis, however, remains undefined in both immunodeficient and immunocompetent individuals, only sporadically reported (Pape et al. 2009). It might be a condition underdiagnosed, probably more frequent in immunocompromised patients.
- **Age and Sex**
  As the prevalence of EBV esophagitis, the age and sex of affected patients are unknown.
- **Site**
  The effects of EBV esophagitis are limited to the esophagus.
- **Treatment**
  In general, although a number of antiviral drugs can inhibit EBV replication, none of them have been licensed for the treatment of EBV infection. Regimens that have been used empirically and in clinical trials have been largely ineffective. Measures aimed at reconstituting specific host cellular immunity are more likely to clear and prevent the pathological changes associated with this disorder in immunocompromised patients.
- **Outcome**
  Although not very well documented, EBV esophagitis is probably a self-limiting illness in immunocompetent patients. In immunocompromised patients, the severity of diminished cellular immunity will probably determine the outcome of the disease. Local cellular immunity has previously been shown in association with oral hairy leukoplakia, and remission of both oral and esophageal lesions may be related to spontaneous improvement in local cellular immunity and Langerhans cell function or number.

Macroscopy

The macroscopic description is limited to endoscopic examination. In fact, the few reports describe multiple, well-circumscribed ulcerations identified in the upper and middle section of the esophagus. The ulcers are characterized as either shallow or of intermediate depth. A few deep ulcers were also seen (Pape et al. 2009). In the immunocompromised patients the ulcers are described as different from those usually associated with cytomegalovirus or herpes simplex virus infections, being deeper, often linear, and found in the mid-esophagus (Kitchen et al. 1990).

Microscopy

In the few reports, biopsy specimens show nonspecific features of active esophagitis, including ulceration or erosion, neutrophilic and eosinophilic inflammation, and basal cell hyperplasia. No viral inclusions, hyperchromicity, or atypical mitoses were described in the immunocompetent patient. In contrast, Kitchen et al. report a series of Epstein-Barr virus-associated esophageal ulcers in AIDS patients that also showed epithelial hyperplasia and koilocytes with multinucleated cells and individual cell keratinization (Kitchen et al. 1990). As all these features are nonspecific, histopathologic examination alone may lead to incorrect diagnosis.

Immunophenotype

Immunohistochemistry with anti-EBV antibodies is achievable in paraffin-embedded sections and is the single most informative protein-based assay for latent and lytic viral factors. It permits localization of protein in the context of histopathology, facilitating assessment of the medical significance of the infection.

Molecular Features

In biopsy tissues, molecular detection of EBV-encoded RNA transcripts by *in situ* hybridization remains important for proving that a histopathologic lesion is EBV related, as there are no specific histopathologic features. EBV DNA can also be detected in tissue samples by real-time polymerase chain reaction, with some benefits. Advantages over EBV-encoded RNA *in situ* hybridization are PCR's relatively low cost, its applicability to specimens with poor quality RNA, and its ability to detect infection lacking EBV-encoded RNA transcripts. It is important that the PCR assay be quantitative and that parallel Q-PCR of an endogenous human gene be used to normalize the number of nucleated cells represented in the reaction (Gulley 2001).

Differential Diagnosis

EBV infection should be considered in all symptomatic patients, immunocompetent or not, in whom esophageal ulceration is identified endoscopically and in the absence of any other demonstrable causes such as drug-induced esophagitis.

References and Further Reading

Gesser, R. M. (1997). The role of latency in herpesvirus infections. *Seminars in Pediatric Infectious Diseases, 8*(3), 128–135.

Gulley, M. L. (2001). Molecular diagnosis of Epstein-Barr virus-related diseases. *The Journal of Molecular Diagnostics, 3*(1), 1–10.

Kitchen, V. S., Helbert, M., Francis, N. D., Logan, R. P. H., et al. (1990). Epstein-Barr virus associated oesophageal ulcers in AIDS. *Gut, 31*, 1223–1225.

Pape, M., Mandraveli, K., Sidiropoulos, I., et al. (2009). Unusual Epstein-Barr esophageal infection in an immunocompetent patient: A case report. *Journal of Medical Case Reports, 3*, 7314.

Pattengale, P. K., Smith, R. W., & Gerber, P. (1973). Selective transformation of B lymphocytes by EB virus. *Lancet, ii*, 93–94.

Esophageal Atresia

Tiago Henriques-Coelho[1] and
Fátima Carneiro[2]
[1]Department of Paediatrics, University of Porto, Porto, Portugal
[2]Faculty of Medicine of Porto University, Centro Hospitalar São João and Ipatimup/i3S, Porto, Portugal

Synonyms

Atresia, upper GI; Congenital anomaly of the esophagus

Definition

Esophageal atresia (EA) is a congenital anomaly of the esophagus caused by an interruption of primitive foregut resulting in a proximal and a distal esophageal pouch. Usually, there is a tracheoesophageal fistula (TEF). The diagnosis is normally made in the first hours after birth by the impossibility to pass a feeding cannula into the stomach.

Symptoms: excessive salivation; regurgitation, choking, and coughing after the first feeding

Clinical Features

- **Incidence**
  The reported incidence is 1:3,500 live-born infants, with some geographic variability. There is a higher prevalence in white mothers, first pregnancy, and increased maternal age.
- **Age**
  Present at birth. Usually, without prenatal diagnosis but polyhydramnios and absence of stomach bubble can be present in the fetal ultrasound.
- **Sex**
  Slight male predominance. Male-to-female ratios varied among types of EA.

E

- **Site**
  Posterior mediastinum.
- **Treatment**
  Treatment of EA is surgical. In most infants, the division of tracheoesophageal fistula and primary anastomosis between two esophageal pouches are possible. The approach can be performed by open thoracotomy or, more recently, by thoracoscopy (Fig. 1).
- **Outcome**
  The survival is mainly related to the presence of major cardiac anomalies and the birth weight (Okamoto et al. 2009). The overall survival is 85–95%. Long-term symptoms include dysphagia, esophageal foreign body obstruction, gastroesophageal reflux disease, and recurrent respiratory problems. Thoracic deformities can be a problem after an open thoracotomy.

Macroscopy

Five types are described based on the location of the EA and the type of fistula between the trachea and esophagus (Harmon and Coran 2012):

1. EA with a distal TEF (84%)
2. EA without TEF (6%)
3. TEF without EA (4%)
4. EA with a fistula to both pouches (1%)
5. EA with a proximal TEF (5%)

Microscopy

Esophageal dysmotility can be present after a successful surgical repair of EA. The etiology of this motility disorder is still unknown. Histological studies of the upper pouch, fistulous portion, and lower pouch of the esophagus revealed some clues regarding abnormal innervation and neuromuscular defects. There is a high incidence of gastric-type mucosa in the upper esophageal pouches. Esophageal fistula can have several tracheobronchial remnants, namely, abnormal mucous glands and ducts, abnormal mucin secretion, presence of cartilage, and a disorganized muscle coat. Dilated epithelial clusters of seromucous glands and cartilage and irregularity of the smooth muscle fibers were described in the lower esophageal pouch. Regarding innervation pattern, there is a delay in neuronal differentiation and myenteric plexus organization. In both the upper and lower esophageal pouches, there is a reduction of neurocells (more notorious in the distal pouch), an increase of Schwann cells, the presence of immature neural cells, and a granin deficit with subsequent altered activity of

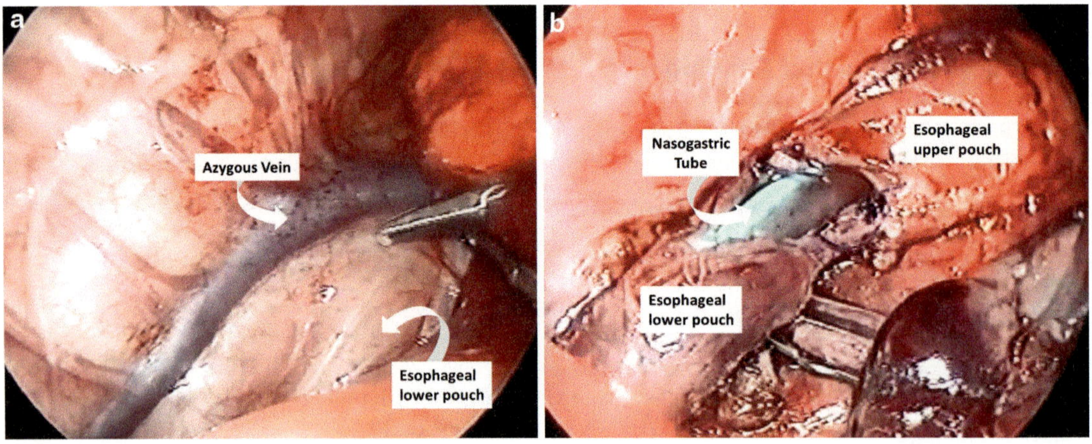

Esophageal Atresia, Fig. 1 Thoracoscopic view of an EA with TEF. (**a**) View of the lower esophageal pouch and the azygous vein before the surgical dissection. (**b**) Anastomosis of the posterior wall of the esophagus with a nasogastric tube in place

neurotransmitter release (Dutta et al. 2000; Zuccarello et al. 2009).

Molecular Features

EA is a multifactorial disease with genetic and environmental contributing factors. In only 10% of infants, a defined genetic syndrome can be diagnosed. In Table 1, there is a summary of the genetic mutations and chromosomal abnormalities described for EA (de Jong et al. 2010).

Differential Diagnosis

Tracheoesophageal fistula
Congenital stenosis of the esophagus
Laryngotracheoesophageal cleft
Disorders of esophageal function
Gastroesophageal reflux

Esophageal Atresia, Table 1 Genetic and chromosomal abnormalities in esophageal atresia

	Gene	Locus
Single-gene mutations		
Feingold syndrome	MYCN	2p24.1
CHARGE syndrome	CHD7	8q12
AEG syndrome	SOX2	3q26.3-q27
Pallister-Hall syndrome	GLI3	7p13
Opitz G syndrome	MID1	Xp22
Fanconi anemia	FANCA	16q24.3
Associations		
VACTERL association	FOXF1 MTHFSD FOXC2	16q24 cluster
	FOXL1	
Chromosomal abnormalities		
Full trisomies		21, 13, and 18
Di George and Opitz syndromes	TBX1	22q11.2
13d deletions	ZIC2	13q22-qter
17q deletions	RARa	17q21.3-q24.2
	NOG	
	TBX4	

References and Further Reading

de Jong, E. M., Felix, J. F., de Klein, A., & Tibboel, D. (2010). Etiology of esophageal atresia and tracheoesophageal fistula: "mind the gap". *Current Gastroenterology Reports, 12*, 215–222.

Dutta, H. K., Mathur, M., & Bhatnagar, V. (2000). A histopathological study of esophageal atresia and tracheoesophageal fistula. *Journal of Pediatric Surgery, 35*(3), 438–441.

Harmon, C. M., & Coran, A. G. (2012). Chapter 69: Congenital anomalies of the esophagus. In A. G. Coran (Ed.), *Pediatric surgery*. Philadelphia: Elsevier/Saunders.

Okamoto, T., Takamizawa, S., Arai, H., Bitoh, Y., Nakao, M., Yokoi, A., & Nishijima, E. (2009). Esophageal atresia: Prognostic classification revisited. *Surgery, 145*, 675–681.

Zuccarello, B., Spada, A., Turiaco, N., Villari, D., Parisi, S., Francica, I., Fazzari, C., Pederiva, F., & Tovar, J. A. (2009). Intramural ganglion structures in esophageal atresia: A morphologic and immunohistochemical study. *International Journal of Pediatrics, 2009*, 695837.

Esophageal Squamous Cell Carcinoma

Wen-Yih Liang[1] and Gregory Y. Lauwers[2]
[1]Department of Pathology, Taipei Veterans General Hospital, Taipei, Taiwan
[2]Department of Pathology, Massachusetts General Hospital, Harvard Medical School, Boston, MA, USA

Definition

Esophageal squamous cell carcinomas are neoplasms that develop from the mucosal squamous lining.

Clinical Features

- **Incidence**
  Esophageal squamous cell carcinoma (SCC) is the predominant subtype of esophageal cancer, with approximately 400,000 new cases diagnosed worldwide each year. An "esophageal

cancer belt" has been described where most cases are detected. It extends from northern Iran through central Asia to northern and central parts of China. In comparison, esophageal SCC is now relatively rare in the USA and most Western European countries. Instead, an increasing number of adenocarcinomas arising in Barrett's esophagus, particularly among white men in the west, has been noted since the turn of the century. However, squamous cell carcinoma still represents 38% of all esophageal malignancies.

- **Etiologic factors**
The role of alcohol and tobacco consumption (particularly in combination) is well known and associated with an increased risk of aerodigestive malignancies. Of interest, genetic factors such as *1/*2 heterozygous polymorphism of the *ALDH2* gene (involved in alcohol metabolism) is believed to confer an increased risk. Chewing betel quid, areca nut, or gutka also has been postulated to have a synergistic effect with alcohol and tobacco in increasing the risk.

A diet rich in pickled vegetables (with N-nitroso compounds) and also beverages at very high temperatures (e.g., tea, maté) is important in increased risk, as is human papillomavirus, particularly types 16 and 18.

Achalasia and caustic injury, conditions leading to the stasis of food or saliva and to chronic mucosal irritation, are associated with an increased occurrence of esophageal SCC as well.

Finally, Paterson-Kelly or Plummer-Vinson syndrome (iron deficiency anemia, dysphagia, and upper esophageal webs) and tylosis (a rare autosomal-dominant disorder characterized by hyperkeratosis of the squamous epithelium of the palmar and plantar surfaces) are associated with a higher-risk of esophageal SCC.

- **Clinical presentation**
Patients with squamous intraepithelial neoplasia and over half of patients with superficial esophageal SCC are asymptomatic when diagnosed. Symptoms are present only when the

Esophageal Squamous Cell Carcinoma, Table 1 Classification of superficial SCC

	Nomenclature	Level of invasion	TNM classification
Early SCC	M1	Epithelium	pTis
	M2	Lamina propria	pT1a
	M3	Muscularis mucosa	
	SM1	Upper third of submucosa	pT1b
	SM2	Middle third of submucosa	
	SM3	Lower third of submucosa	

tumors are large enough to interfere with esophageal function or have spread. At that point, the most common symptom is intermittent dysphagia occurring only with large food boluses.

- **Age**
Esophageal SCC is predominantly diagnosed in adults. The risk increases with age, particularly beyond the age of 60.
- **Sex**
Esophageal squamous cell carcinoma has a distinct male predominance.
- **Site**
Squamous cell carcinoma can develop along the entire length of the esophagus, but is more frequently diagnosed in the middle third of the esophagus.
- **Treatment**
Early esophageal cancer, that is, limited to the mucosa (pT1a, M1, and M2), can be treated successfully by either endoscopic mucosal resection (EMR) or endoscopic submucosal dissection (ESD), since there is little or no risk of lymph node metastasis (Table 1).

When superficial esophageal SCCs extend more deeply into the mucosa (M3) or the submucosal layer, the probability of lymph nodes harboring metastases is between 17% and 55%. Consequently, these esophageal SCCs are indications for esophagectomy with lymphadenectomy, either by transhiatal esophagectomy or transthoracic esophagectomy. Neoadjuvant therapy (chemotherapy alone or radiochemotherapy) is also the standard in the care of patients with advanced SCC.

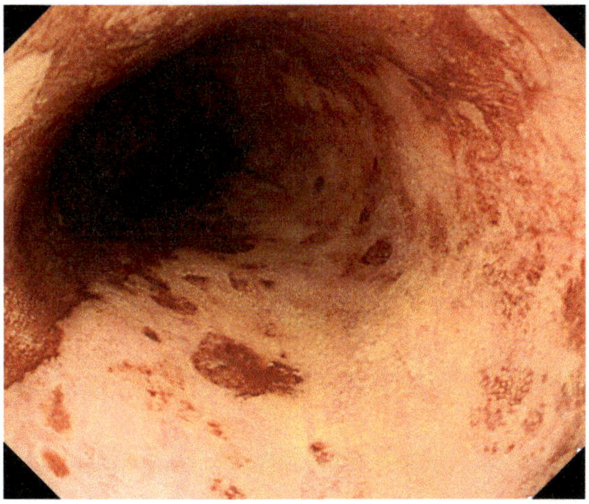

Esophageal Squamous Cell Carcinoma, Fig. 1 Endoscopic view of esophageal squamous cell carcinoma, superficial type. Lugol's iodine solution facilitates the detection of the carcinoma, which remains unstained

Macroscopy

Superficial squamous cell carcinomas are often subtle, and their detection demands an attentive examination. The visualization of the tumors is enhanced by chromoendoscopy (using Lugol's iodine solution or methylene blue) or narrow band imaging (Fig. 1). An advanced tumor can present as a friable, fungating, ulcerated mass variably extending into and partially occluding the esophageal lumen (Fig. 2).

E

Microscopy

Squamous intraepithelial neoplasia (or dysplasia) is defined by both architectural and cytological features that vary in extent and severity (see Table 2). A sharp demarcation commonly delineates the neoplastic epithelium from the surrounding normal epithelium. The diagnostic characteristics are confined to the basal layer in low-grade intraepithelial neoplasia (Fig. 3) and involve the full thickness of the epithelium in high-grade intraepithelial neoplasia (which encompasses the former carcinoma *in situ* and severe dysplasia) (Fig. 4). A diagnosis of invasive SCC is warranted when extension into the lamina propria is detected (Fig. 5).

Esophageal Squamous Cell Carcinoma, Fig. 2 Macroscopic appearance of advanced esophageal squamous cell carcinoma, protruding type

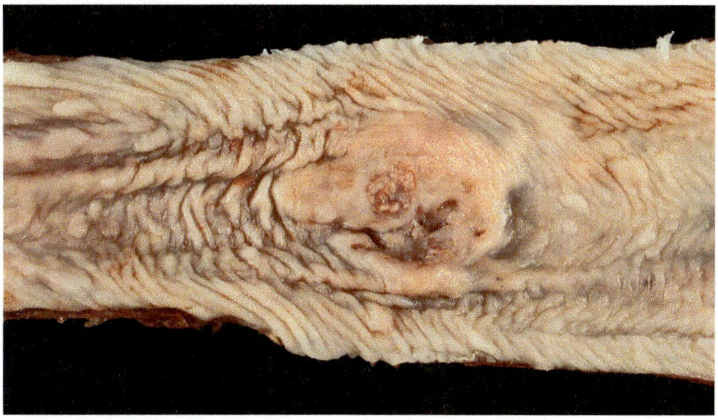

Advanced SCC can display a wide spectrum of histologic patterns. It can range from well differentiated with recognizable keratinization and defined intercellular bridges to poorly differentiated and composed of cells with no apparent squamous differentiation (Figs. 6, 7). Various subtypes of SCC have been recognized (see Table 3) (Fig. 8).

Esophageal Squamous Cell Carcinoma, Table 2 Cytologic and architectural characteristics of squamous intraepithelial neoplasia

Architectural characteristics	Cytologic characteristics
Loss of cell polarity	Pleomorphic and hyperchromatic nuclei
Overlapping nuclei	Increased nuclear to cytoplasmic ratio
Lack of surface maturation	Increased mitotic activity

Differential Diagnosis

Severe reactive and hyperplastic changes can develop in the setting of severe esophagitis or at the edge of an ulcer. These may be diagnostically challenging, particularly when pseudoepitheliomatous hyperplasia is present. Mucosal inflammation, spongiosis, vascular congestion, and surface maturation are helpful in confirming a benign diagnosis. Homogenous and fine nuclear chromatins, as well as prominent nucleoli, are also characteristically observed in benign reactive epi-

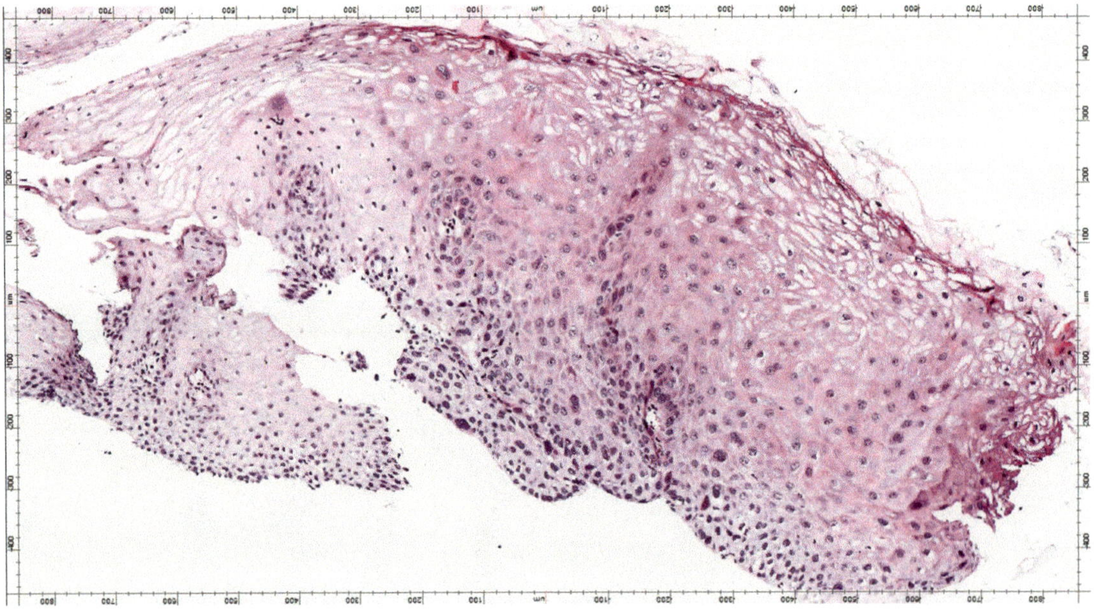

Esophageal Squamous Cell Carcinoma, Fig. 3 Intraepithelial neoplasia, low grade. Note the mild cytologic atypia, including nuclear irregularity and increased nuclear to cytoplasmic ratio. Note also the sharp oblique demarcation with the normal epithelium on the left

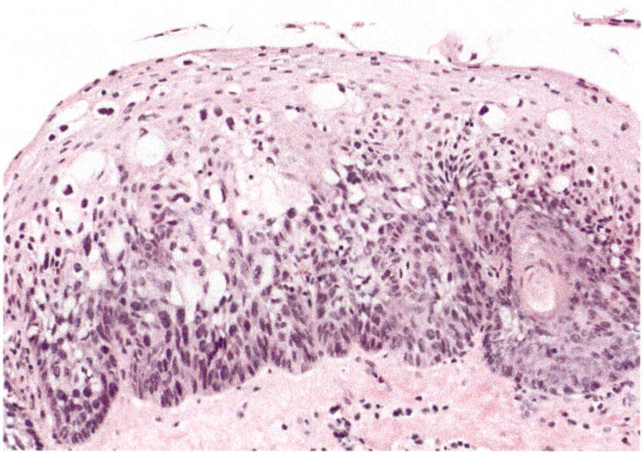

Esophageal Squamous Cell Carcinoma, Fig. 4 Intraepithelial neoplasia, high grade, characterized by marked architectural disarray with loss of polarity and cellular atypia

thelium. A series of negative findings are also noted, including the absence of irregular nuclear membranes, nuclear hyperchromasia and pleomorphism, and nuclear overlapping. Increased nuclear to cytoplasmic ratio, eosinophilic nucleoli, increased mitotic activity, and abnormal mitoses are also absent in reactive hyperplastic processes. Finally, highly atypical and keratinizing cells are also features of neoplastic lesions.

Esophageal Squamous Cell Carcinoma, Fig. 5 Early esophageal squamous cell carcinoma. Most of the neoplasm is limited to the epithelium, but focal extension into the lamina propria (pT1a) is seen

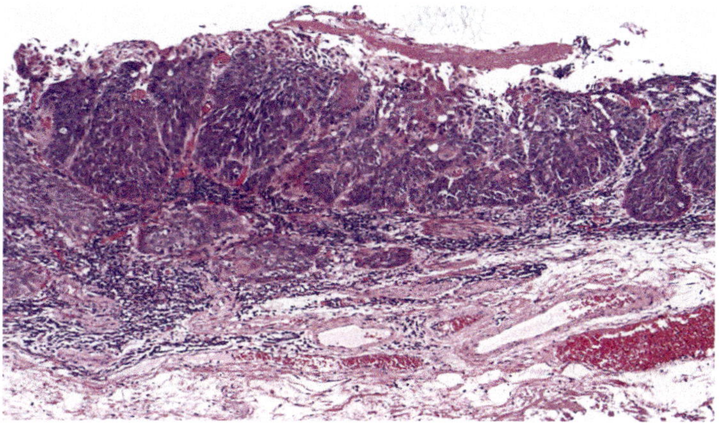

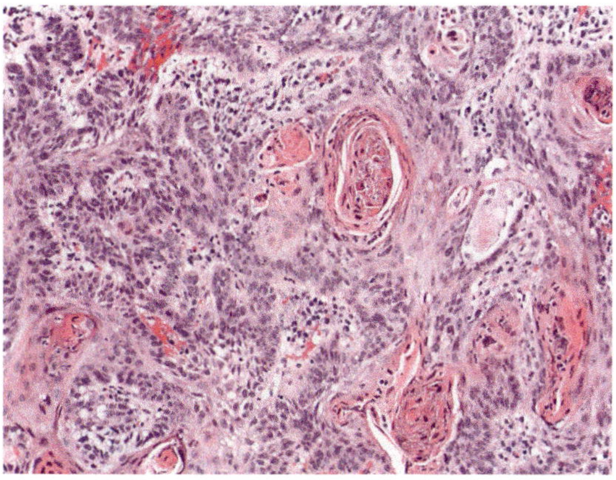

Esophageal Squamous Cell Carcinoma, Fig. 6 Invasive well-differentiated esophageal squamous cell carcinoma with keratin pearls

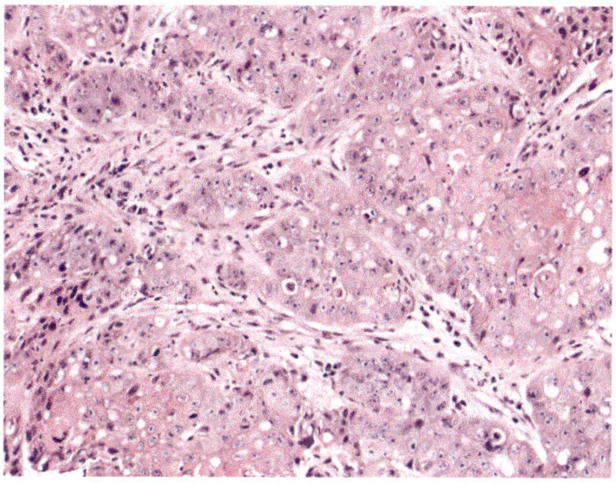

Esophageal Squamous Cell Carcinoma, Fig. 7 Invasive moderately differentiated esophageal squamous cell carcinoma

Esophageal Squamous Cell Carcinoma, Table 3 Histologic variants of esophageal squamous cell carcinoma

Histologic variants	Characteristics
Verrucous variant	Well-differentiated neoplasm characterized by broad papillae of keratinizing squamous epithelium with minimal atypia
	Broad epithelial tongues invade the underlying tissues
Basaloid carcinoma variant	Solid neoplasm characterized by discrete nests of small cells with hyperchromatic nuclei. Mitoses are numerous
	Microcystic spaces with basophilic material can be seen
Spindle cell variant	Biphasic neoplasm composed of malignant spindle component and an *in situ* or invasive squamous carcinoma. Heterologous components can be seen. This variant characteristically presents as an exophytic polypoid neoplasm with superficial invasion

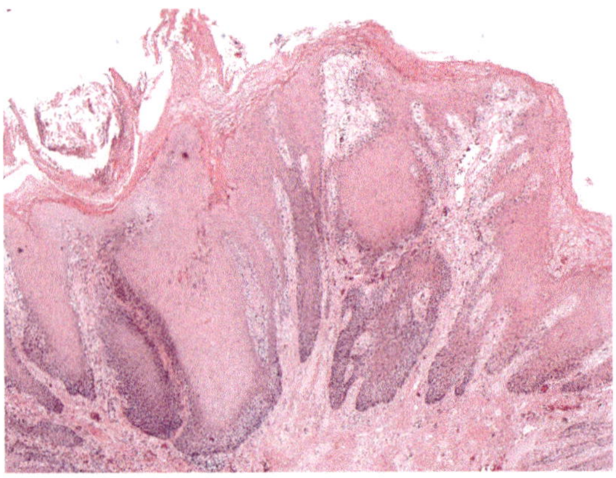

Esophageal Squamous Cell Carcinoma, Fig. 8 Verrucous squamous carcinoma. Note invasive pushing broad fronds at the base of the tumor

References and Further Reading

Campbell, F., & Lauwers, G. Y. (2013). Tumors of the esophagus and stomach. In C. D. M. Fletcher (Ed.), *Diagnostic histopathology of tumors* (4th ed., pp. 378–433). Philadelphia: Elsevier Saunders.

Montgomery, E., Field, J. K., Boffetta, P., Daigo, Y., Shimizu, M., & Shimoda, T. (2010). Squamous cell carcinoma of the esophagus. In F. T. Bosman, F. Carneiro, R. H. Hruban, & N. D. Theise (Eds.), *WHO classification of tumours of the digestive system* (pp. 18–24). Lyon: IARC.

Shimizu, M., Zaninotto, G., Nagata, K., Graham, D. Y., & Lauwers, G. Y. (2013). Esophageal squamous cell carcinoma with special reference to its early stage. *Best Practice and Research Clinical Gastroenterology, 27*, 171–186.

Srivastava, A., & Odze, R. D. (2013). Tumours of the oesophagus. In N. A. Shepherd, B. F. Warren, G. T. Williams, J. K. Greenson, G. Y. Lauwers, & M. R. Novelli (Eds.), *Morson and Dawson's gastrointestinal pathology* (5th ed., pp. 56–82). Hoboken: Wiley-Blackwell.

Takubo, K. (2007). Squamous epithelial dysplasia and squamous cell carcinoma. In *Pathology of the esophagus. An atlas and textbook* (pp. 145–190). Tokyo: Springer.

Esophageal Squamous Columnar Junction

Paula Chaves[1,2] and António Dias Pereira[3]
[1]Serviço de Anatomia Patológica, Instituto Português de Oncologia de Lisboa de Francisco Gentil, Lisbon, Portugal
[2]Faculdade de Ciências da Saúde, Universidade da Beira Interior, Covilhã, Portugal
[3]Instituto Português de Oncologia de Lisboa Francisco Gentil, E.P.E., Lisbon, Portugal

Synonyms

Esophageal squamous-columnar junction

Definition

The Z-line or squamous-columnar junction (SCJ) is the point of the esophagus where the stratified squamous esophageal lining meets the columnar epithelium (Spechler 2004). The esophagus is normally lined by a stratified squamous epithelium, whereas the gastric body and fundus exhibit a columnar lining with abundant mucous cells at the foveolar surface and numerous parietal and chief cells at the deep glands. These two types of epithelia normally meet together in an abrupt transition that is endoscopically and histologically recognized. Though the Z-line or SCJ is a very well-defined anatomical structure, its precise anatomical location and histological features are still disputed.

Clinical Features

- **Incidence**
  Not applicable.
- **Age**
  Not applicable.
- **Sex**
  Not applicable.
- **Site**
  The Z-line is located at the body of the esophagus.
- **Treatment**
  Not applicable.
- **Outcome**
  Not applicable.

Macroscopy

The Z-line or SCJ may or may not be coincident with the gastroesophageal junction (GEJ), which is defined as the imaginary line where the esophagus ends and the stomach begins. The Z-line has the appearance of a serrated line and is endoscopically recognized as the line defined by the junction of the pale pink epithelium that covers the esophagus and the red mucosa of the stomach. The GEJ is endoscopically recognized in the western world as the level of the most proximal extent of the gastric folds when the stomach is partially inflated with air (overinflating may obscure this landmark). For Japanese authors the distal limits of the palisade vessels are considered to be a precise marker of the GEJ. In a normal GEJ the two landmarks are coincident, which means that the Z-line coincides with the most proximal extent of the gastric folds (Fig. 1). When the Z-line is proximally located to the GEJ, there is a segment of the distal esophagus lined by a columnar

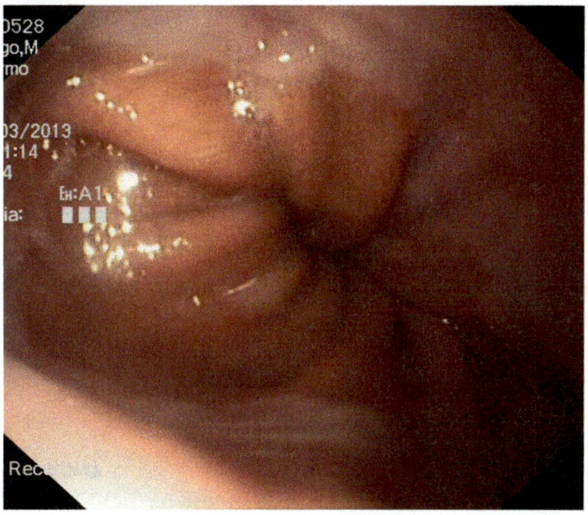

Esophageal Squamous Columnar Junction, Fig. 1 Normal Z-Line

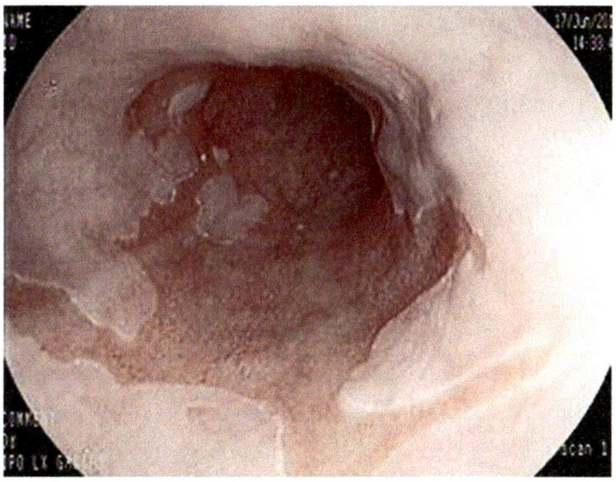

Esophageal Squamous Columnar Junction, Fig. 2 Proximally displaced Z-Line

epithelium or a columnar-lined esophageal segment (CLES) (Fig. 2). The endoscopic landmark to recognize the GEJ, the most proximal extent of the gastric folds, is a dynamic structure that varies with belching, respiratory movements, the degree of gastric distension, and the presence or absence of a hiatus hernia. Furthermore, since these endoscopic landmarks are mechanically manipulated, they cannot be used in surgical or autopsy specimens. Hence, the markers used macroscopically to distinguish a normal from an abnormal junction are complex and imprecise, being difficult to establish whether the Z-line normally is coincident or slightly proximal to the GEJ (Spechler

2004). A recent study showed that the endoscopically defined GEJ coincides with the anatomical GEJ. This is a particularly important issue in gastrointestinal (GI) pathology since the recognition of a normal vs. an abnormal Z-line is a key factor for the differential diagnosis in esophageal pathology. Regardless of the normal histology of the GEJ (see microscopy), intestinal metaplasia is undoubtedly a metaplastic epithelium in this location. The reported prevalence of intestinal metaplasia at a normal appearing GEJ is widely variable, ranging between 5% and 25%. Moreover, there is published evidence that the endoscopically Z-line appearance correlates to the prevalence of intestinal metaplasia (Wallner et al. 2000).

Microscopy

The microscopic picture of a normal Z-line is also an area under discussion. Today, it is consensual that the entire esophagus normally exhibits a stratified squamous lining whereas the gastric fundus is lined by oxyntic mucosa, which is characterized by a columnar lining with abundant mucous cells at the foveolar surface and numerous parietal and chief cells at the deep glands. It is also consensual that between these two epithelia there is a columnar-lined segment of mucosa known as *cardiac* epithelium, with a few millimeters to a few centimeters of extension that is characterized by tortuous tubular glands lined almost exclusively by mucus-secreting cells. The question is whether this is a congenital or an acquired epithelium. Traditionally, it was considered as congenital, mostly due to Hayward (Hayward 1961) who sustained that this structure is normally present at birth working as a buffer protector of the squamous esophageal lining against gastric acid digestion. However, the evidence on which this claim is supported is dubious. More recently, it was proposed that *cardiac* epithelium was an acquired structure (Chandrasoma et al. 2001) developed as a metaplastic response to long-standing gastroesophageal reflux (GER). In fact, Paull (Paull et al. 1976) had described the epithelia that integrated the spectrum of esophageal columnar metaplasia in patients with long-standing GER. He described three types of epithelia, *junctional*, *gastric atrophic fundic*, and *specialized columnar*, randomly distributed along the metaplastic segment. Paull further suggested that the *gastric atrophic fundic* epithelium was more frequent at the distal part of the metaplastic segment while the *specialized columnar* was more commonly observed at the proximal part. Nevertheless, he did not make any comment about the chronological relationship between the tree epithelia. Recently, Chandrasoma (Chandrasoma et al. 2001) sustained that *cardiac* epithelium, which was designated by Paull as *junctional*, is the initial step in the development of a columnar lining in response to GER. He also suggested that *cardiac* epithelium may progress to *oxyno-cardiac* or to *intestinal metaplasia*, the *gastric atrophic fundic* and *specialized columnar* epithelium, respectively, according to the nomenclature proposed by Paull.

Despite the controversy on the nature of *cardiac* epithelium, this is the columnar type of mucosa that meets the stratified squamous esophageal lining at the Z-line or squamous-columnar junction.

Immunophenotype

Not applicable.

Molecular Features

Not applicable.

Differential Diagnosis

Not applicable.

References and Further Reading

Chandrasoma, P. T., Deer, R., Dalton, P., et al. (2001). Distribution and significance of epithelial types in columnar-lined esophagus. *The American Journal of Surgical Pathology, 25*, 1188–1193.

Hayward, J. (1961). The lower end of the oesophagus. *Thorax, 16*, 36–41.
Paull, A., Trier, J. S., Dalson, M. D., et al. (1976). The histologic spectrum of Barrett's esophagus. *The New England Journal of Medicine, 295*, 476–480.
Spechler, J. S. (2004). Intestinal metaplasia at the gastroesophageal junction. *Gastroenterology, 126*, 567–575.
Wallner, B., Sylvan, A., Stenling, R., & Janunger, K. G. (2000). The esophageal Z-line appearance correlates to the prevalence of intestinal metaplasia. *Scandinavian Journal of Gastroenterology, 35*, 17–22.

Esophagitis, Chemotherapy Induced

Mário Ferraz de Oliveira[1] and Maria José Brito[2]
[1]Serviço Anatomia Patológica, Centro Hospitalar Lisboa Central EPE, Lisbon, Portugal
[2]Serviço Anatomia Patológica, Hospital Garcia de Orta, Almada, Portugal

Synonyms

Chemotherapy effect in esophagus

Definition

Esophagitis is a common side effect of chemotherapy and different degrees of mucosal toxicity depend on the number of drugs used, their dosage, and length of treatment and the presence of concomitant radiotherapy.

Many chemotherapeutic drugs damage directly the esophageal mucosa, in a similar way to other parts of gastrointestinal tract, acting primarily on mitotically active cells, leading to cell death, inflammation, and ulceration. The chemotherapeutic agents reported are dactinomycin, bleomycin, cytarabine, daunorubicin, 5-fluorouracil, methotrexate, and vincristine.

Clinical Features

Patients with chemotherapy esophagitis suffer from chest pain and discomfort. Symptoms are similar with different chemotherapeutic agents, and there is a synergistic effect with the frequent combination with radiation therapy, with more severe symptoms due to more severe damage.

Macroscopy

In acute phase, the macroscopic examination reveals friable mucosa with edema and coalescent ulcers (mucositis). Later, on an average 1 month after therapy, strictures may develop.

Microscopy

At first, less severe lesions are seen in a nonulcerated epithelium with alterations in the basal layer, namely, apoptotic bodies and enlarged atypical squamous cells with bizarre cytomegaly (Fig. 1) and atypical mitosis (Fig. 2). In the more severe cases, a nonspecific type of esophagitis develops with necrosis and formation of ulcers, associated with inflammation and granulation tissue. Stromal cells and submucosal glands also may appear atypical.

In more chronic cases, parakeratosis, acanthosis, and blood vessel hyalinization are seen.

Chemotherapy with cyclophosphamide, methotrexate, and 5-fluoroacil may cause associated Barrett esophagus.

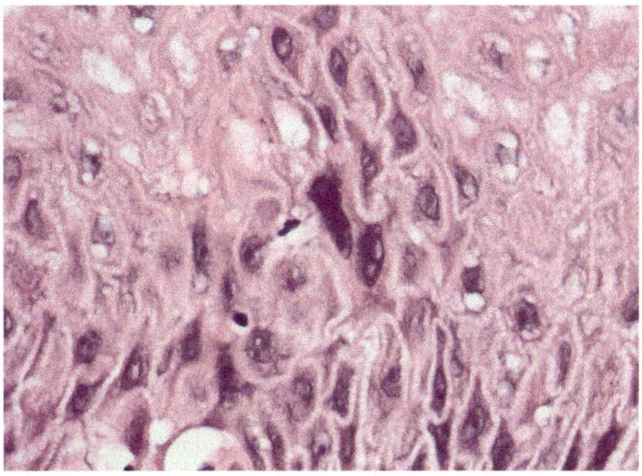

Esophagitis, Chemotherapy Induced, Fig. 1 Esophageal epithelium with atypical squamous cell (hematoxylin-eosin, X400)

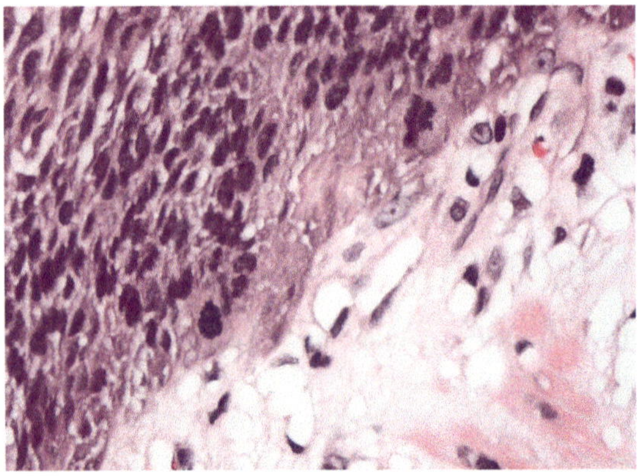

Esophagitis, Chemotherapy Induced, Fig. 2 Basal esophageal epithelium with atypical mitoses (hematoxylin-eosin, X400)

Long-term complications are mural scarring and strictures.

Differential Diagnosis

The main differential diagnoses are: infections (HSV and cytomegalovirus) and neoplasia.

High N/C ratio, mitosis, and hyperchromatism are seen in neoplasia, but bizarre cytomegaly and atypical mitosis are also seen in chemotherapy esophagitis.

Multinucleation seen in chemotherapy esophagitis should be distinguished from HSV infection.

If necessary, immunostains are recommended in the workflow of the differential diagnosis.

References and Further Reading

Montgomery, E., & Lacobuzio-Donahue, C. (2012). *Gastrointestinal and liver pathology* (2nd ed., pp. 29–31). Philadelphia: Elsevier.

Noffsinger, A. E. (2009). Update on esophagitis-controversial and underdiagnosed causes. *Archives of Pathology & Laboratory Medicine, 133*, 1087–1095.

Sonis, S. T., Elting, L. S., Keefe, D., et al. (2004 May 1). Perspectives on cancer therapy-induced mucosal injury: Pathogenesis, measurement, epidemiology, and consequences for patients. *Cancer, 100*(9 Suppl), 1995–2025.

Esophagitis, In Crohn's Disease

Paula Borralho Nunes
Hospital Cuf Descobertas and Escola Superior de Tecnologia da Saúde de Lisboa and Instituto de Anatomia Patológica, Faculdade de Medicina da, Universidade de Lisboa, Lisboa, Portugal

Synonyms

Esophageal Crohn's disease

Definition

Crohn's disease (CD) is a chronic, idiopathic, segmental transmural inflammatory disease arising from an interaction between genetic and environmental factors but observed predominantly in developed countries of the world. The precise etiology is unknown. The disease may involve one or more segments of the gastrointestinal (GI) tract from the mouth to the anus. The ileum, the colon, the rectum, and the perianal region are the most frequent locations of disease involvement. However, esophageal involvement can also be present in patients with Crohn's disease, even though CD involvement of the upper gastrointestinal tract is almost invariably accompanied by small or large bowel disease.

Histologic abnormalities found in the upper GI tract may be contributory in establishing a specific diagnosis of Crohn's disease. In the majority of cases, the proximal disease extends beyond the esophagus, involving the stomach and the duodenum too (Van Assche et al. 2010).

The complete anomalies observed in Crohn's disease are summarized elsewhere.

Clinical Features

The most common presenting symptom of esophageal Crohn's disease (CD) is dysphagia. The complaints of odynophagia, epigastric pain, chest pain, weight loss, and poor oral intake are frequently found in patients with esophageal involvement (Kaplan KM). Early lesions, however, can exist without any complaint. Sometimes the proximal involvement is silent, and the disease is diagnosed incidentally during endoscopy in an asymptomatic patient.

Coughing and aspiration pneumonia can be the result of a complicating esophagotracheal fistula. These symptoms can present before the usual intestinal manifestations have occurred. Usually the activity of CD in the esophagus parallels that of the disease of CD elsewhere in the GI tract.

- **Incidence**
  While involvement of the lower gastrointestinal (GI) tract has been studied in detail, CD of the upper GI tract has not been fully evaluated. The exact prevalence and incidence figures of CD of the upper GI tract are not known because large prospective studies, including both symptomatic and symptomatic patients, are lacking (Witte et al. 1998). Descriptions of the prevalence of CD in the esophagus, stomach, and duodenum vary significantly. Data concerning the prevalence of participation of the esophagus in CD are somewhat conflicting, not only as far as what concerns the different definitions of upper tract "involvement" used, but also concerning the different populations studied (adult or pediatric). Esophageal involvement in CD seemed to be much more frequent in children and adolescents, with some series reporting up to 30% of patients with esophageal lesions (Lenaerts et al. 1989). In adults, however, the incidence described was usually much lower (0.2% cases with esophageal involvement in one series of approximately 9,900 patients with CD). Most studies in the past, however, have been carried out retrospectively on symptomatic patients. Prospective radiological and endoscopic studies of the upper GI tract in both symptomatic and asymptomatic CD patients show a more frequent involvement (Annunziata et al. 2012).
- **Age**
  As mentioned, according to most series, children seem to have higher incidence of esophageal involvement in CD. However, data have to be interpreted with caution, as they may merely reflect differences in practice patterns: upper endoscopy and biopsy are more routinely performed in pediatric IBD centers, while in adults upper endoscopy is reserved for patients with symptoms suggestive of disease involvement. Recent publications suggest that upper GI involvement may occur with equal frequency in children and adults.
- **Sex**
  There is no gender predilection among patients with involvement of the esophagus in CD.
- **Site**
  The distal third of the esophagus alone is involved in majority of cases, with the middle and lower third in fewer patients. Rarely, the whole esophagus can be involved.

  The vast majority of patients with CD of the esophagus also have lesions in the stomach and duodenum and also in the intestine.
- **Treatment**
  The precise etiology is unknown and therefore a causal therapy is not yet available. In general, it appears that medical treatment for upper GI CD does not differ substantially from the classic distal CD. In fact, most patients are frequently on treatment for coexisting extra-esophageal disease.

  Current therapeutic strategies of upper GI CD are derived from extrapolation of efficacy data from clinical trials conducted predominantly in patients with more common phenotypes of CD. Treatment can also be specifically aimed at improving esophageal symptoms (namely, proton pump inhibitors and a few reports with "topical" treatment with ingestion of inhalable budesonide), if necessary together with systemic corticosteroids and azathioprine/mercaptopurine, or, if intolerant, with methotrexate. Infliximab is an alternative for refractory disease (Van Assche et al. 2010).

Dilatation or surgery is appropriate for obstructive symptoms, after failing medical and conservative therapy.

- **Outcome**
  Although old case reports suggest a poor outcome of esophageal CD with severe complications, often requiring esophagectomy, more recent publications describe a more benign prognosis (Decker et al. 2001). A clinical course seems to be variable, with some patients improving spontaneously or with first-line therapy and others being more difficult to manage, with a need of more aggressive immune modifier therapy or surgery.

Macroscopy

There are no pathognomonic features on endoscopy, but the most commonly described findings are aphthous ulcers, superficial erosions, and, at a later stage, stricturing and a more irregular cobblestone appearance to the mucosa. For the most part, the ulcers are the superficial, aphthous type. Because of the transmural nature of CD, spontaneous fistulae can be found. Pseudopolyps may be seen in the regenerative stage of severe inflammation (Witte et al. 1998). Huchzermeyer differentiated two stages in the esophageal inflammatory process: stage I, in which inflammatory changes predominate as a mild or more often erosive-ulcerative esophagitis, and stage II, in which a stenosing form is present (Huchzermeyer et al. 1976). These morphological changes are predominantly limited to the lower part of the esophagus.

Microscopy

There are no pathognomonic histologic features of esophageal CD. The transmural nature of the disease cannot be assessed accurately from the superficial mucosal biopsies obtained on endoscopy. Such specimens often show evidence of chronic inflammation without revealing its specific etiology. The most consistent finding is a lymphocytic infiltrate in the lamina propria (Fig. 1). Less commonly, however, a chronic inflammatory infiltrate and eventually noncaseating granulomas can be recognized. In fact, the histologic hallmark of Crohn's disease is the presence of a noncaseating granuloma. Although they are not routinely seen and are not considered essential (identified in about 20% of biopsy cases), their finding reinforces the diagnosis. The granuloma in CD is defined as a collection of epithelioid histiocytes (monocyte/macrophage cells), the outlines of which are often vaguely defined. Multinucleated giant cells are not characteristic but can be seen, and necrosis is usually not apparent (Figs. 2 and 3).

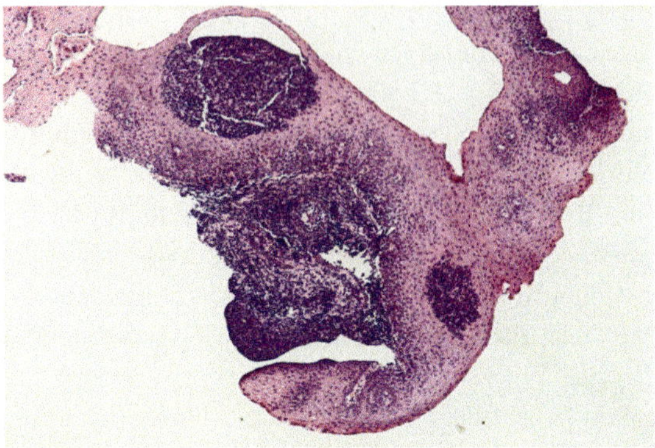

Esophagitis, In Crohn's Disease, Fig. 1 Low-power H&E stain demonstrates dense inflammatory infiltrate in the submucosa of an esophageal biopsy

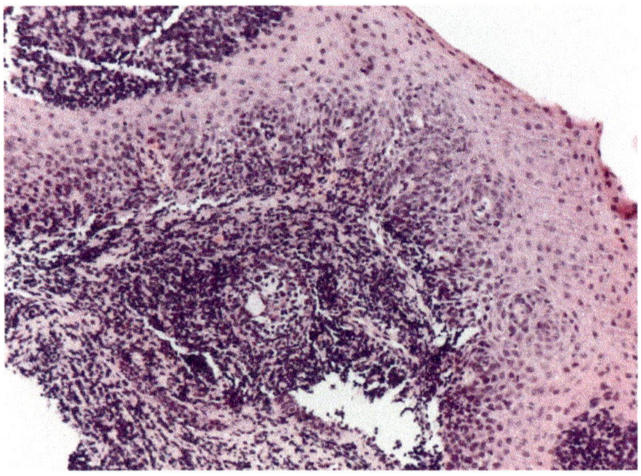

Esophagitis, In Crohn's Disease, Fig. 2 In a medium-power H&E stain, intense chronic inflammatory infiltrate with focal permeation of the epithelium and a granuloma in the lamina propria can be seen

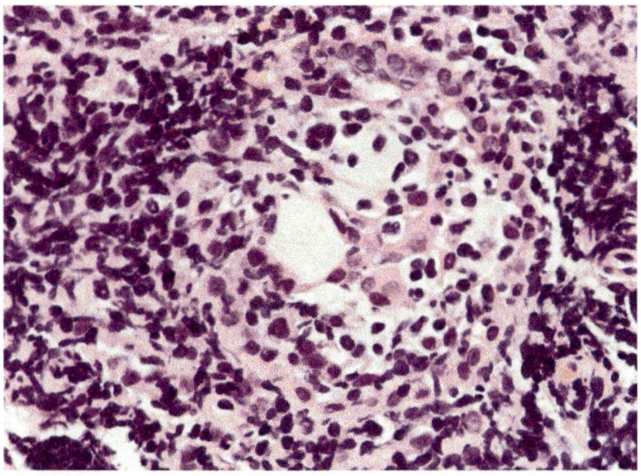

Esophagitis, In Crohn's Disease, Fig. 3 Higher power shows closer view of a noncaseating granuloma, with epithelioid histiocytes and multinucleated giant cells

Because granulomas are usually located in the deep submucosa and lamina muscularis, the low incidence of granulomas found in biopsy specimens probably is a function of the superficial nature of endoscopic biopsies and patchy distribution of lesions.

Immunophenotype

Immunohistochemistry is not very helpful in the diagnosis of esophageal involvement in Crohn's disease, except for the exclusion of conditions that may mimic or complicate it (e.g., bullous diseases, CMV infection).

Molecular Features

Some of the most recent developments in our understanding of the pathogenesis of IBD have been in the field of genetics. A decade ago, NOD2/CARD15 was identified as the first susceptibility gene for CD. NOD2 is a member of a family of intracellular proteins that respond to bacterial proteins and contribute to host defense. In one large study 50% of patients with CD were found to have at least one NOD2 gene mutation, with 17% having a double mutation. A number of other genes have been shown to be important for CD, namely, mutations in the interleukin (IL)-10 receptor and in genes encoding IL-27.

Differential Diagnosis

The differential diagnosis includes reflux esophagitis, involvement in gastrointestinal sarcoidosis (► Sarcoidosis, Gastro-Intestinal), Tuberculosis, Fungal Infections, chronic granulomatous disease, Behçet's syndrome, and bullous diseases (► Bullous Pemphigoid).

References and Further Reading

Annunziata, M. L., Caviglia, R., Papparella, L. G., et al. (2012). Upper gastrointestinal involvement of Crohn's disease: A prospective study on the role of upper endoscopy in the diagnostic work-up. *Digestive Diseases and Sciences, 57*(6), 1618–1623.

Decker, G. A., Loftus, E. V., Jr., Pasha, T. M., et al. (2001). Crohn's disease of the esophagus: Clinical features and outcomes. *Inflammatory Bowel Diseases, 7*(2), 113–119.

Huchzermeyer, H., Paul, F., Seifert, E., et al. (1976). Endoscopic results in five patients with Crohn's disease of the esophagus. *Endoscopy, 8*, 75–81.

Lenaerts, C., Roy, C. C., Vaillancourt, M., et al. (1989). High incidence of upper gastrointestinal tract in children with crohn's disease. *Pediatrics, 83*(5), 777–781.

Van Assche, G., Dignass, A., Panes, J., European Crohn's and Colitis Organisation (ECCO), et al. (2010). The second European evidence-based consensus on the diagnosis and management of Crohn's disease: Definitions and diagnosis. *Journal of Crohn's & Colitis, 4*(1), 7–27.

Witte, A. M. C., Veenendaal, R. A., & Van Hogezand, R. A. (1998). Crohn's disease of the upper gastrointestinal tract: The value of endoscopic examination. *Scandinavian Journal of Gastroenterology, 33*, 100–105.

F

Fundic Gland Polyp

Chella R. S. van der Post[1] and Fátima Carneiro[2]
[1]Department of Pathology, Radboud University Medical Center, Nijmegen, The Netherlands
[2]Faculty of Medicine of Porto University, Centro Hospitalar São João and Ipatimup/i3S, Porto, Portugal

Synonyms

Cystic hamartomatous epithelial (gastric) polyp; Elster's (gland) cyst; FGP; Fundic gland hyperplasia

Definition

Fundic gland polyps (FGPs) are small polyps typically located in the gastric corpus and fundus. Elster et al. first described them as a distinct pathological polyp in 1977. Their characteristic morphology shows cystically dilated glands lined by mucous neck cells, parietal cells, and/or chief cells. FGPs arise in two settings, namely, sporadic and familial adenomatous polyposis (FAP) syndrome-associated settings. FGPs are among the most common gastric polyps in both sporadic and FAP patients. In comparison to sporadic FGPs, FAP-associated FGPs are more likely to be multiple and to occur at younger age. Sporadic fundic gland polyposis ($\geq$10 FGPs) is occasionally observed in the non-FAP population.

The pathogenesis of FGPs is not well understood. FGPs have formerly been regarded as non-neoplastic lesions, either hamartomatous or hyperplastic/functional in nature. It has been suggested that they are retention cysts caused by corpus gland secretion impairment. However, the frequent finding of mutations in the *APC* and *β-catenin* genes indicates that FGPs are neoplastic growths.

Sporadic FGPs are presumably related to the use of proton pump inhibitors (PPI). Literature is not conclusive about the role of PPI use, but especially long-term PPI therapy seems to be associated with an increased risk of developing FGPs. The reason that acid suppression can lead to the development of FGPs may be a result of PPIs elevating serum gastrin, which is a growth factor for oxyntic mucosa and a downstream target of Wnt signaling. In gastric biopsies from patients on PPI therapy, there are often development of hyperplasia and protrusions of parietal cells, and this is thought to be an initial step. Protrusions are defined as hypertrophic parietal cells showing tonguelike protrusions of the apical membrane into the lumen of corpus glands. A second step in the development is the formation of fundic gland cysts. These intramucosal cysts are believed to form from glands that are dilated because of increased intraglandular pressure. This increase in pressure could be caused by increased resistance to outflow from the gland due to

F. Carneiro et al. (eds.), *Pathology of the Gastrointestinal Tract*, Encyclopedia of Pathology,
DOI 10.1007/978-3-319-40560-5

blockage of the isthmus by parietal cell protrusions. Interestingly, FGPs occur almost exclusively in patients without *Helicobacter pylori* infection. And, in addition, regression of sporadic polyps has been observed to coincide with the acquisition of *H. pylori*. It has been suggested that enzymatic degradation of gastric mucus by *H. pylori* protease may facilitate the glandular outflow and thus protect against retention and cystic dilation. This does not take place in *H. pylori*-negative patients, thus increasing the risk of fundic gland polyp development.

FGPs do not cause symptoms; sporadic FGPs are typically a coincidental finding detected during investigation for abdominal pain, dyspepsia, or chronic reflux. They are the most common gastric polyps in patients with familial adenomatous polyposis (FAP). FAP results from inherited germline mutations in the *adenomatous polyposis coli* (*APC*) gene, coupled with second somatic mutations. This leads to the inactivation of both copies of the *APC* tumor suppressor gene. In comparison to sporadic FGPs, FAP-associated FGPs are more likely to be multiple and occur at a younger age. Sporadic FGPs have very weak malignant potential, and the frequency of dysplasia is very low. This is in contrast with patients with FAP who often develop dysplasia (in 44–54% of cases) in FGPs; however, malignant transformation is extremely rare. The frequent finding of genetic alterations involving the *APC/β-catenin* pathway, either sporadic or arising in the setting of FAP, suggests that FGPs may be neoplastic.

Worthley et al. reported **three** families with an inherited syndrome which is associated with fundic gland polyposis, namely, gastric adenoma and proximal polyposis of the stomach (GAPPS). This unique gastric polyposis syndrome is characterized by the autosomal dominant transmission of fundic gland polyposis of especially fundic gland polyps. Occasional hyperplastic and adenomatous polyps can occur, and patients with this syndrome are at increased risk of developing dysplasia and intestinal-type gastric adenocarcinoma. The malignant potential of gastric polyps in GAPPS seems to be much higher than in FAP. Recently, it was discovered that these families have germline mutations in specifically the promoter 1B of the *APC* gene (Worthley et al. 2012; Li et al. 2016).

Clinical Features

- **Incidence**
  FGPs are currently the most common type of polyp identified in the stomach, accounting for approximately 50% of all endoscopically and histologically diagnosed benign gastric polyps. Most FGPs are non-syndromic and it has been estimated that sporadic FGPs occur in 0.8–5.9% of adults undergoing upper endoscopy. In FAP patients FGPs are thought to develop in 53–84% of mutation carriers. The incidence of FGPs seems to be increasing; reasons for this may be the expanded use of upper endoscopy, the increasing use of acid suppressive medications, and the decreasing prevalence of *H. pylori* infection.
- **Age**
  Most patients are of middle age; however, FGPs can be found during upper endoscopy at any age. FAP-associated FGPs are more commonly observed at a much younger age compared to sporadic polyps and may occur as early as 8 years of age in FAP.
- **Sex**
  FGPs are more commonly encountered in women.
- **Site**
  FGPs develop in the acid-secreting mucosa of the gastric corpus and fundus.
- **Treatment**
  Treatment consists of endoscopic removal of the polyp to confirm their identity and to exclude other lesions. FGPs have little malignant potential, but they serve as a marker for FAP, especially in patients with multiple lesions who are not taking proton pump inhibitors. The management of FGPs, therefore, centers more on the concern for FAP and exclusion of colorectal carcinoma than on concern for neoplastic progression in the gastric mucosa. Colonoscopy and subsequently genetic testing have to be considered in

patients with fundic gland polyposis or a relevant family history. Family history and patient age are not entirely reliable factors in excluding FAP since approximately 25% of patients with FAP have no relevant family history and are presumably caused by de novo mutations in the *APC* gene. There is no surveillance scheme defined, but usually in the setting of FAP, upper endoscopy is recommended every 1–3 years depending on polyp number and the presence of dysplasia or adenomas. It can be considered to discontinue PPI therapy; however, there is conflicting evidence regarding the role of acid suppression in the pathogenesis of FGPs, and the need for acid suppression may outweigh any concerns regarding these benign gastric polyps.

- **Outcome**
  Little is known about the natural behavior of FGPs. The number and size of FGPs have been shown both in the sporadic setting and in FAP to slowly increase, remain the same, or sometimes even decrease. Symptoms are rarely encountered. The incidence of gastric cancer is slightly increased in patients with FAP-associated FGPs. The lifetime risk of gastric cancer in FAP is estimated to be 0.6–4.2%. The exact risk of gastric cancer in GAPPS is unknown but appeared higher than in FAP. Sporadic FGPs have typically been regarded as benign lesions with no risk of malignant transformation. Low-grade dysplasia is diagnosed in approximately 1% of sporadic FGPs. There is a single case report of high-grade dysplasia, and there are no reports of gastric cancer arising from sporadic FGPs.

Macroscopy

FGPs may be single or multiple (fifty or more) but usually fewer than 10 polyps are observed in the sporadic setting; often they are solitary. In the setting of FAP and GAPPS, numerous FGPs are usually observed, and they may cover the entire surface of acid-secreting epithelium resulting in a carpet of several hundred polyps. The polyps are limited to the oxyntic mucosa (corpus and fundus) of the stomach. FGPs are usually glassy, transparent, small polyps, measuring 1–5 mm in diameter, although larger polyps are observed. They have a sessile base and a smooth dome-shaped surface. FGPs are the same pale pink color as the surrounding normal mucosa and often exhibit tiny surface blood vessels. These characteristic findings make FGPs endoscopically distinguishable from other types of gastric polyps.

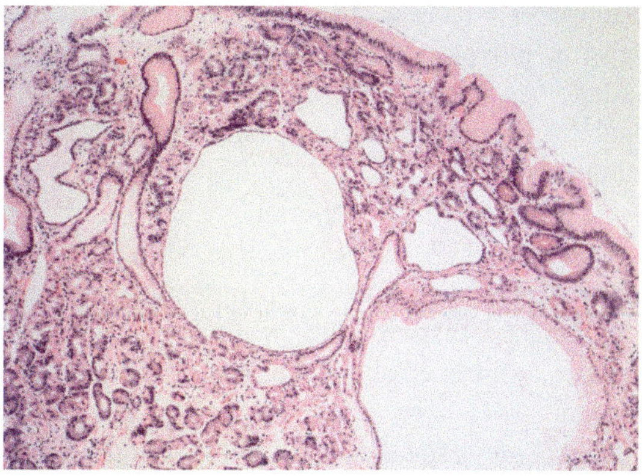

Fundic Gland Polyp, Fig. 1 Fundic gland polyp characterized by irregular dilated glands lined by mucous, parietal, and chief cells (H&E, original magnification 25×)

Microscopy

Histologically, FGPs are characterized by distorted glandular architecture with dilated and irregularly budded fundic glands. These microcystic oxyntic glands are lined by flattened parietal cells, chief cells, and variable numbers of mucous neck cells (Fig. 1). The overlying surface and foveolar gastric epithelium is normally without abnormalities and non-dysplastic. However, in some FGPs, dysplasia of the overlying foveolar epithelium is observed. Crowding of surface and neck mucin cells with enlarged hyperchromatic nuclei and loss of cytoplasmic mucin characterize dysplasia in FGPs. The underlying cystically dilated oxyntic glands in these polyps do not demonstrate epithelial dysplasia. The surrounding mucosa is uniformly normal, and concurrent glandular atrophy or intestinal metaplasia is seldom observed. Inflammatory infiltrate in these polyps is usually minimal or absent and there is no

H. pylori infection. This is in contrast to other gastric polyps, such as hyperplastic polyps or adenomas, that are often associated with a background of mucosal injury, atrophy, and intestinal metaplasia.

The morphology of sporadic FGPs is similar to syndromic FGPs in FAP patients. However, sporadic FGPs have little or no potential for (pre-) malignant transformation, while low- and high-grade dysplasias and even gastric adenocarcinoma have been associated with syndromic FGPs. Low-grade dysplasia involving the overlying foveolar epithelium is common and seen in up to approximately 50% of FAP-associated cases. Even in the pediatric population, low-grade dysplasia is often seen. High-grade dysplasia occasionally arises in FAP-associated FGPs. The risk of gastric adenocarcinoma in FAP patients is markedly elevated in Japanese and Korean patients. In Western countries there does not seem to be an increased risk of developing gastric carcinoma among FAP patients. Nevertheless, several well-documented cases of invasive adenocarcinoma arising from FAP-associated FGPs have been reported.

Immunophenotype

The diagnosis of FGPs is made on normal routine H&E staining. There are no typical immunohistochemical features of FGPs without dysplasia. Despite the frequent finding of *β-catenin* gene mutations in FGPs, studies showed normal expression and location of β-catenin in FGPs, with normal diffuse membranous positivity and without nuclear staining in any of the cases. In FGPs with dysplasia, studies showed abnormal nuclear β-catenin staining and higher rates of cell proliferation and apoptosis than non-dysplastic areas. Overexpression of p53 was not observed in FGPs with dysplasia.

Molecular Features

Most sporadic FGPs contain activating mutations on or near several phosphorylation sites in exon 3 of the *β-catenin* oncogene. In studies, activating *β-catenin* gene mutations were present in 64–91% of sporadic FGPs. In contrast, *β-catenin* gene mutations were not present in any of the (attenuated) FAP-associated FGPs. In sporadic FGPs with dysplasia, frequent *APC* alterations were identified.

FAP is caused by germline mutations in the *adenomatous polyposis coli (APC)* gene. FAP is estimated to occur in only 1 per 6,000–18,000 births. This syndrome is defined by the occurrence of hundreds to thousands of colonic adenomas. In the setting of FAP, FGPs, like colonic adenomas, arise through "second-hit" inactivating mutations in the *APC* gene or through chromosome 5q allelic loss. These second, somatic mutations lead to mutational inactivation of the *APC* gene.

The molecular basis of the different groups of FGPs involves the APC/β-catenin/Tcf signaling pathway, albeit being based on completely different molecular defects. The presence of clonal *APC* or *β-catenin* mutations in FGPs indicates that they are neoplastic growths, but they have limited potential for malignant transformation. Both genes are involved in the same cell growth-signaling pathway, which explains why mutations in either gene can give rise to FGPs that are histologically similar. Both types of mutations – inactivation of the *APC* tumor suppressor gene and activation of the *β-catenin* oncogene – result in stabilization of β-catenin protein and its abnormal accumulation in affected cells.

Differential Diagnosis

Endoscopically, FGPs may be difficult to differentiate from carcinoid tumors which, in a certain subgroup of patients, are also small, often multiple, and exclusively located in the corpus or fundic region. However, carcinoid tumors are usually yellowish and have a firm consistency.

Atrophic (autoimmune) gastritis with multiple persistent islands of oxyntic glands in the corpus mucosa may mimic FGPs. Histologically, FGPs are quite characteristic; however, focal foveolar hyperplasia may resemble FGPs.

References and Further Reading

Abraham, S. C. (2010). Fundic gland polyps: Common and occasionally problematic lesions. *Gastroenterol Hepatol (NY), 6*(1), 48–51.

Abraham, S. C., Nobukawa, B., Giardiello, F. M., Hamilton, S. R., & Wu, T. T. (2000). Fundic gland polyps in familial adenomatous polyposis: Neoplasms with frequent somatic adenomatous polyposis coli gene alterations. *American Journal of Pathology, 157*(3), 747–754.

Burt, R. W. (2003). Gastric fundic gland polyps. *Gastroenterology, 125*(5), 1462–1469.

Jalving, M., Koornstra, J. J., Boersma-van Ek, W., de Jong, S., Karrenbeld, A., Hollema, H., et al. (2003). Dysplasia in fundic gland polyps is associated with nuclear beta-catenin expression and relatively high cell turnover rates. *Scandinavian Journal of Gastroenterology, 38*(9), 916–922.

Lee, R. G., & Burt, R. W. (1986). The histopathology of fundic gland polyps of the stomach. *American Journal of Clinical Pathology, 86*(4), 498–503.

Li, J., Woods, S. L., Healey, S., et al. (2016). Point Mutations in Exon 1B of APC Reveal Gastric Adenocarcinoma and Proximal Polyposis of the Stomach as a Familial Adenomatous Polyposis Variant. *American Journal of Human Genetics, 98*(5), 830–842.

Torbenson, M., Lee, J. H., Cruz-Correa, M., Ravich, W., Rastgar, K., Abraham, S. C., et al. (2002). Sporadic fundic gland polyposis: A clinical, histological, and molecular analysis. *Modern Pathology, 15*(7), 718–723.

Worthley, D. L., Phillips, K. D., Wayte, N., et al. (2012). Gastric adenocarcinoma and proximal polyposis of the stomach (GAPPS): a new autosomal dominant syndrome. *Gut, 61*(5), 774–779.

F

G

Gangliocytic Paraganglioma, Duodenal

Saba Kiremitci
Department of Pathology, Ankara University Medical School, Sihhiye, Ankara, Turkey

Synonyms

Nonchromaffin paraganglioma of the duodenum

Definition

Gangliocytic paraganglioma is a rare and unique neuroendocrine neoplasm which is currently classified as an epithelial tumor according to the classification of tumors of the digestive tract by the World Health Organization (WHO). The tumor reveals histologic and immunohistochemical features of both neural and endocrine tissues, and histologic diagnosis requires the presence of three different cell lineages: epithelioid cells resembling paraganglioma or well-differentiated neuroendocrine tumor; spindle cells reminiscent of Schwann cells; and ganglion or ganglion-like cells.

Gangliocytic paraganglioma has been considered as a hyperplastic or hamartomatous counterpart to the neoplastic duodenal well-differentiated neuroendocrine tumor (carcinoid), both derived from the same embryonic anlage. Although it is regarded as a benign neoplasm, the benign nature of this tumor is controversial due to the several reports of lymph node and distant metastasis in the literature.

Major clinical symptoms of the tumor include abdominal pain, nausea, vomiting, and gastrointestinal bleeding.

Clinical Features

- **Incidence**
  It is considered as a rare tumor with an increased propensity in NF1 patients.
- **Age**
  Most patients are present in the fifth and sixth decades, with ages ranging from 17 to 80 years.
- **Sex**
  There is slight male predominance over females as 1.8:1.
- **Site**
  Most GPs arise in the medial aspect of the second part of the duodenum, especially at the ampulla of Vater. Jejunum, stomach, and appendix localizations may rarely be seen.
- **Treatment**
  Surgical treatment modalities vary from endoscopic excision to pylorus-preserving pancreaticoduodenectomy. The possibility of lymph node metastasis makes the optimal therapy controversial. Recent reports indicate that

F. Carneiro et al. (eds.), *Pathology of the Gastrointestinal Tract*, Encyclopedia of Pathology,
DOI 10.1007/978-3-319-40560-5

endoscopic polypectomy is the treatment of choice, except in cases where the tumor is >3 cm and/or there is active or recent bleeding. A follow-up endoscopy after 3–6 months is recommended to verify that the resection was complete. Surgical treatment is indicated for all GPs that are unresectable by upper gastrointestinal endoscopy and for all malignant forms.

- **Outcome**
  There is controversy over the nature of GPs because of their malignant potential. Though GPs usually follow a benign clinical course there are 23 reported cases with lymph node metastasis, one case of bone metastasis, and two cases of liver metastasis in the literature. Recurrences are possible in lesions that are incompletely excised. The 2010 WHO classification indicates tumor size (>2 cm) as the predictive factor for recurrences. There is, however, not sufficient data to label the tumor as malignant.

Macroscopy

Gangliocytic paraganglioma typically presents as a single pedunculated or sessile polypoid, submucosal lesion with a diameter varying from 5.5 to 100 mm (mean, 24.2 mm). The tumor is usually a well demarcated, un-encapsulated, solid mass with an infiltrative border, typically centered in the submucosal layer and frequently infiltrating the mucosal and/or muscularis layer. The overlying mucosa is typically ulcerated even when there is no mucosal invasion (Fig. 1).

Microscopy

Histopathologic diagnosis of GP requires the specification of three distinct cell lineages: (i) epithelioid cells arranged in an endocrine growth pattern, (ii) spindle cells with the appearance of nerve sheet cells, (iii) ganglion or ganglion-like cells. The proportion of the three characteristic cell types may vary widely. In many cases, epithelioid cells dominate the picture while ganglion cells and/or spindle areas may be scarce.

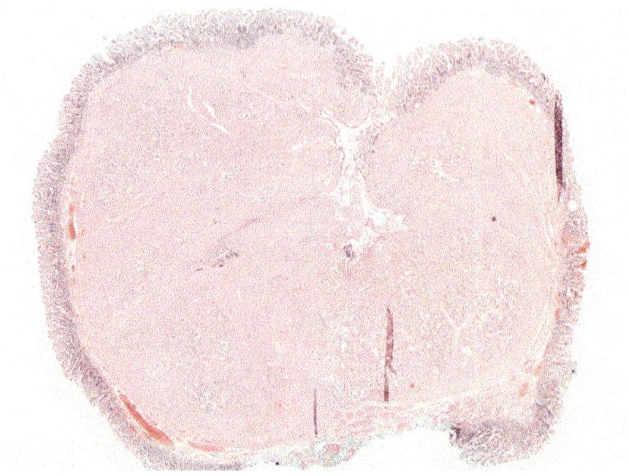

Gangliocytic Paraganglioma, Duodenal, Fig. 1 A polypoid tumor localized in the submucosal layer of the duodenum with well-demarcated borders (H&E; ×20)

The epithelioid cells may show varying growth patterns as nests, ribbons, trabeculae, pseudoglandular, and occasionally papillary structures in a vascular background, reminiscent of an endocrine tumor. These neuroendocrine cells have eosinophilic or amphophilic cytoplasm and ovoid nuclei with variations in size and nuclear shape, with low or no mitotic activity. Spindle cells show bland round to elongated nuclei and may form broad fascicles with proliferating nerve fibrils and Schwann cells typical of neurofibroma. The ganglion cells may be scattered singly or aggregated in clusters, intermixed with the epithelioid and spindle components. The ganglion-like cells may reveal a spectrum ranging from typical ganglion cells to larger cells with abundant often granular eosinophilic cytoplasm, small, inconspicuous, or even indiscernible nucleoli, in contrast to those in typical ganglion cells (Fig. 2).

Mitoses are rare (up to 3 per 10 high-power fields). Cytologic atypia is minimal and necrosis is absent. Rarely psammoma bodies are observed. Even in cases with lymph node metastasis, lymphatic invasions are rarely reported.

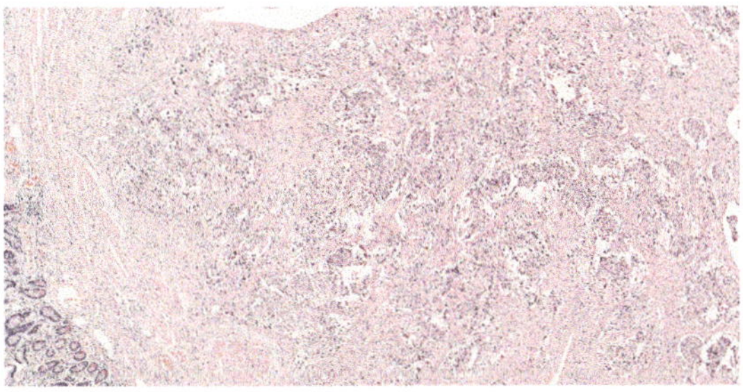

Gangliocytic Paraganglioma, Duodenal, Fig. 2 The epithelioid component arranged in nests and nodules resembling an endocrine tumor and the spindle cell component of the tumor with broad fascicles and palisading Schwann like cells is striking in low power examination (H&E; ×100)

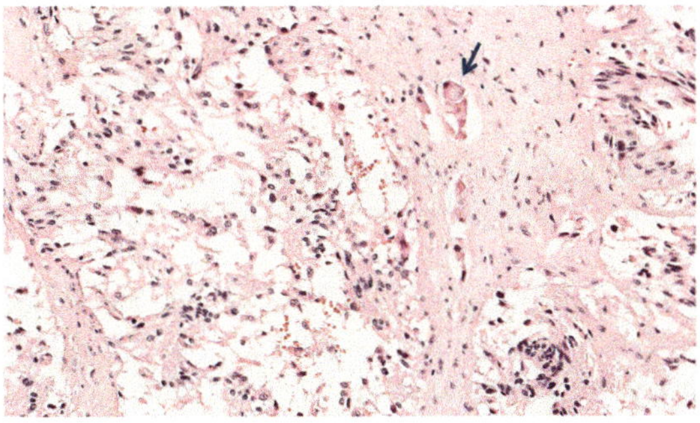

Gangliocytic Paraganglioma, Duodenal, Fig. 3 The ganglion-like cells scattered in the tumor begin to come apparent at high-power examination (H&E; ×200)

These tumors have the tendency to infiltrate the surrounding smooth muscle and mucosa of the duodenum, and those in the ampulla often show entrapment of pancreatic ducts.

Immunophenotype

Each of the three cellular components shows characteristic immunohistochemical staining. The epithelioid-neuroendocrine cells are immunoreactive for a variety of antibodies including principally cytokeratin, chromograninA, synaptophysin, neuron-specific enolase (NSE), and human pancreatic polypeptide (HPP) and followed in frequency by somatostatin and vasoactive intestinal peptide (VIP). The spindle cells are almost always immunoreactive for S100 protein and may also stain with NSE, neurofilament protein, and synaptophysin in varying degrees. The ganglion cells are frequently immunoreactive for synaptophysin, NSE, and neurofilament protein (Fig. 3).

There have been reports supporting the relation between bcl2 and/or p53 positivity with malignant behavior and Ki-67 (MIB-1) index as a prognostic indicator in neuroendocrine tumors. However, no sufficient data is present for GPs, and there is no reported immunohistochemical diversity between GPs with or without lymph node metastasis (Fig. 4).

Molecular Features

GPs have been associated with NF1. No specific immunophenotypic feature is reported for GPs.

Differential Diagnosis

The diagnosis of GP is achieved by routine H&E stained sections with its characteristic three cell lineages in typical cases. Immunohistochemical examination is also regarded as an important diagnostic tool to assist the definite diagnosis. The variation in the proportion of the cellular components and the infiltrative borders suggesting a malignant tumor may lead to misdiagnosis. The lesions that are most commonly mistaken for GPs are carcinoid tumors, paragangliomas, ganglioneuromas, nerve sheet tumors, smooth muscle tumors, gastrointestinal stromal tumors, and also adenocarcinomas, particularly in biopsy material.

A careful histologic examination uncovering the scarce ganglion-like cells and/or spindle component and the variation in size and nuclear shape in contrast to the uniform cells of duodenal carcinoids can help to differentiate the diagnosis towards GP (Fig. 5).

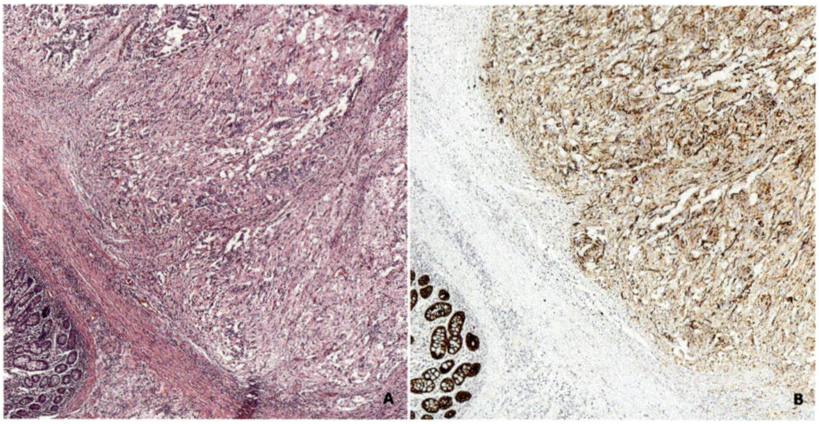

Gangliocytic Paraganglioma, Duodenal, Fig. 4 A gangliocytic paraganglioma with an epithelioid dominant cell lineage resembling a carcinoid or a paraganglioma (**a**) shows pancytokeratin (HMWCK + LMWCK) positivity (antiPANCK IHC; ×200)

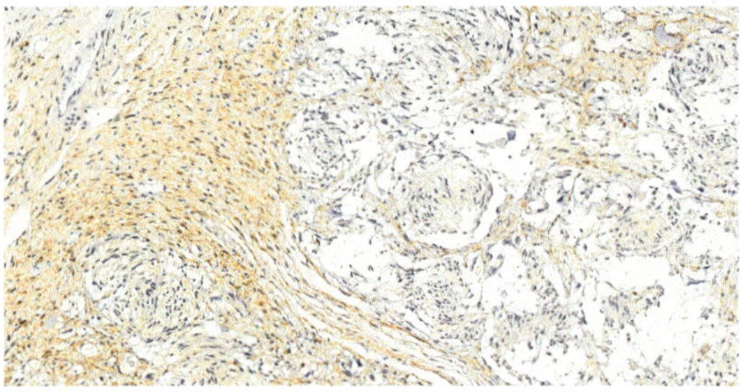

Gangliocytic Paraganglioma, Duodenal, Fig. 5 Spindle cell component of the tumor strongly immunoreactive with S100 antibody (antiS100 IHC; ×200)

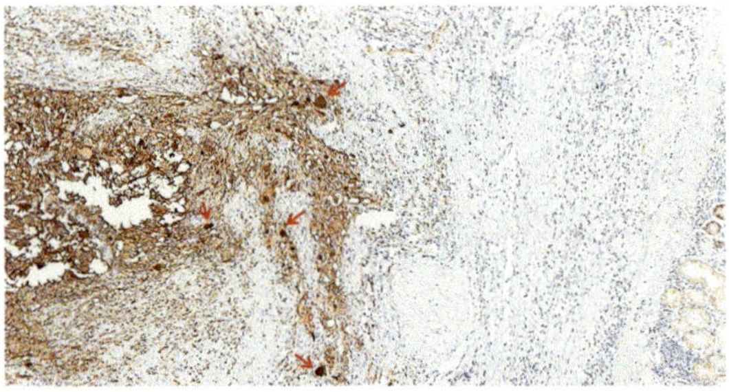

Gangliocytic Paraganglioma, Duodenal, Fig. 6 Diffuse Synaptophysin positivity both in the epithelioid component and the scattered ganglion-like cells (*arrows*) (antisynaptophysin IHC; ×200)

Extraadrenal paragangliomas which lack ganglion-like and spindle cells can occur in the mesentery of the bowel including that of the duodenum. Cytokeratin expression which is generally not found in paragangliomas can aid the differentiation of GP from that potentially malignant and extremely rare tumor (Fig. 6).

It is extremely rare for a GP to reveal an inconspicuous epithelioid component, even when the spindle cell component is predominant. Therefore, a careful search for epithelioid areas shall differentiate GPs from its mimickers like ganglioneuromas and the spindle cell tumors including nerve sheet tumors, smooth muscle tumors, and neurofibroma which consistently lack the epithelioid cells.

Misdiagnosis of carcinoma can be made because of the infiltrating borders of GP. GIST, smooth muscle tumors, and adenocarcinoma can easily be excluded by immunohistochemical positivity with NSE, S-100 protein, and synaptophysin.

References and Further Reading

Burke, A. P., & Helwig, E. B. (1989). Gangliocytic paraganglioma. *American journal of Clinical Pathology, 92*(1), 1–9.

Okubo, Y., Yokose, T., Tuchiya, M., et al. (2010). Duodenal gangliocytic **paraganglioma** showing lymph node metastasis: A rare case report. *Diagnostic Pathology, 5*, 27.

Okubo, Y., Nemoto, T., Wakayama, M., et al. (2015). Gangliocytic paraganglioma: A multi-institutional retrospective study in Japan. *BMC Cancer, 15*, 269.

Park, H. K., & Han, H. S. (2016). Duodenal gangliocytic paraganglioma with lymph node metastasis. *Archives of Pathology and Laboratory Medicine, 140*(1), 94–98.

Snover, D. C., Ahnen, D. J., Burt, R. W., & Odze, R. D. (2010). Serrated polyps of the colon and rectum and serrated polyposis. In F. T. Bosman, F. Carneiro, R. H. Hruban, & N. D. Theise (Eds.), *WHO classification of tumours of the digestive system* (4th ed.). Lyon: IARC.

Ganglioneuroma

Berna Savaş[1] and Arzu Ensari[2]
[1]Department of Pathology, Ankara University Medical School, Ankara, Turkey
[2]Department of Pathology, Ankara University Medical School, Sihhiye, Ankara, Turkey

Synonyms

Diffuse ganglioneuromatosis; Ganglioneuromatosis; Ganglioneuromatous polyposis; Isolated (solitary) polypoid ganglioneuroma; Mucosal ganglioneuroma

Definition

Ganglioneuroma (GN) of gastrointestinal tract is an extremely rare neuroectodermal tumor that is characterized by the presence of mucosal ganglion cells and spindled Schwann cells often with numerous eosinophils. Gastrointestinal GNs are divided into three groups defined as polypoid GN, ganglioneuromatous polyposis (GP), and diffuse ganglioneuromatosis (DG). The most common form is polypoid GNs form which show a mixture of ganglion cells and nerve fibrils within mucosa, extending to submucosa. In GP, most polyps resemble typical polypoid GN, whereas others show filiform mucosal projections containing groups of ganglion cells with little neural stroma. GP affects patients with familial adenomatous polyposis (FAP), Cowden's disease, tuberous sclerosis, multiple endocrine neoplasia type 2b (MEN type 2b) syndrome, colorectal carcinoma, and juvenile polyposis (JP). Patients with GP may develop multiple cutaneous lipomas and may have a family history of multiple intestinal polyps, adrenal myolipomas, and nodular goiter. DG is characterized by a poorly demarcated nodular or an exuberant proliferation of nerve fibers, ganglion cells, and supporting cells of the enteric nervous system. DG may be associated with MEN type 2b syndrome. In contrast to DG and GP, polypoid GNs do not usually have any evidence of multiple tumor syndromes or familial diseases (Fig. 1).

Clinical Features

- **Incidence**
  GNs of GI tract are extremely rare tumors. No figures for incidence available.
- **Age**
  Isolated polypoid GNs occur at any age, most patients are younger than 20 years. GP and DG have a higher mean age of over 30 years.
- **Sex**
  Isolated polypoid GNs develop equally in both sexes while GP and DG show a male predilection.
- **Site**
  In GI GNs mainly involve colon and rectum, unlike neurofibromas and neurofibromatosis, which occur more commonly in small intestine and stomach. Isolated polypoid GNs develop in the appendix, terminal ileum, duodenum, stomach, intestine, and anus. GPs are found in the colon ant terminal small bowel while DGs can be seen anywhere along the GI tract.
- **Treatment**
  Isolated GNs and GPs can be treated with polypectomy and/or mucosectomy. DGs, however, can be treated with total resection of the affected segment which is usually the entire colon.
- **Outcome**
  Isolated GN, GPs have favorable outcome after total excision, while DGs may cause severe morbidity.

Macroscopy

GNs and GPs typically develop in the mucosa or submucosa as a polypoid mass <1–2 cm or as multiple polyps. In DGs, the lesions vary in size from 1 to 17 cm with thickening of bowel wall with nodules leading to strictures (Fig. 2).

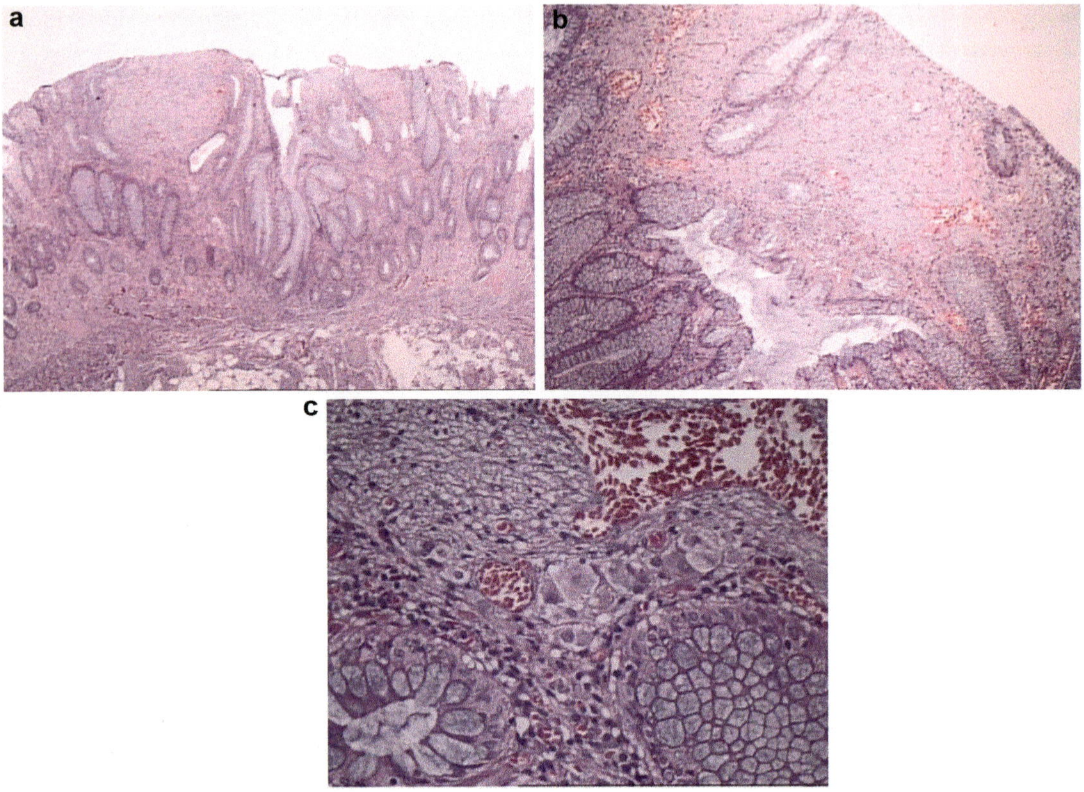

Ganglioneuroma, Fig. 1 (**a**, **b**) Mucosal polypoid ganglioneuroma with neurofibrillary matrix widening the lamina propria. (**c**) Clusters of ganglion cells within the neurofibrillary matrix (H&E; ×40, ×100, ×200, respectively)

Microscopy

GNs show a mixture of ganglion cells and nerve fibrils within mucosa, extending to submucosa. In GPs, many polyps are indistinguishable from the typical polypoid GN, while others show unusual filiform mucosal projections containing clusters of ganglion cells with little or no apparent neural component. Crypt architecture is disturbed with extension of the lamina propria by neural matrix and ganglion cells. In GPs, ganglion cell content shows grater variability in comparison to GPs. The surface of the lesions may be ulcerated. In DGs mucosa, submucosa, and submucosal plexuses may be involved. Unlike the polypoid GNs, these lesions are mostly ill-defined. DGs consist of transmural proliferation of nerve fibers, ganglion cells, and stromal cells.

Immunophenotype

The immunohistochemical stains used for confirming the diagnosis of GN also provide useful information about the mucosal and submucosal distribution of the lesion and highlight the presence of ganglion cells, nerve fibers, and supportive cells in all plexuses. All lesions suggestive of diagnosis of GN are stained for synaptophysin (SYN), chromogranin A (CHRA), S-100 protein, neuron specific enolase (NSE), and RET protein immunohistochemically. The ganglioneuromatous nature of proliferating spindle cells and supportive cells of the enteric system can be confirmed by strong immunoreactivity for S-100 protein, while ganglion cells stay nonreactive. SYN is present in ganglion cells and nerve fibers. CHRA shows only weak cytoplasmic staining in ganglion cells.

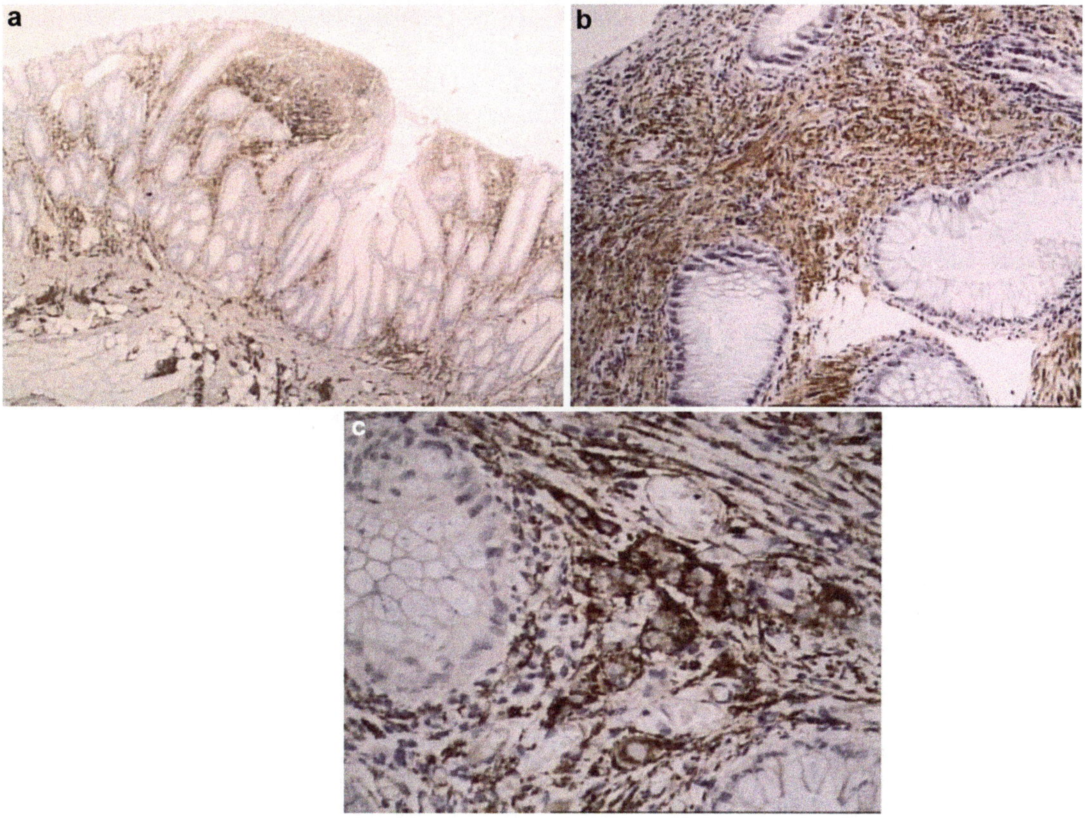

Ganglioneuroma, Fig. 2 (**a**, **b**) S100 protein positivity in neurofibrillary matrix. (**c**) Ganglion cells positively stained with SYNP (streptavidin-biotin peroxidase; ×40, ×100, ×200, respectively)

Molecular Features

In isolated GNs no specific molecular alteration has been described. GP and DP show mainly the molecular alterations with respect to the associated clinical syndrome such as Cowden's Syndrome, MEN2B, NF1 involving genes like PTEN, RET, NF1, etc.

Differential Diagnosis

Differential diagnosis varies for GNs, GPs, and DGs. GNs can resemble endoscopically and macroscopically any polypoid lesion of the GI tract. Microscopically these lesions should be differentiated from mucosal neuromas, schwannomas, perineuriomas, and GISTs, particularly when there is paucity of ganglion cells. GPs, on the other hand, should be distinguished from other GI polyposis syndromes. Hirschsprung's disease, intestinal neuronal dysplasia, and various other neuromuscular disorders of the GI tract should be considered in the differential diagnosis of DGs.

References and Further Reading

Al-Daraji, W. I., Abdellaoui, A., & Salman, W. D. (2005). Solitary polypoidal rectal ganglioneuroma: A rare presentation of a rare tumor. *Journal of Gastroenterology and Hepatology, 20*, 961–971.

Hechtman, J. F., & Harpaz, N. (2015). Neurogenic polyps of the gastrointestinal tract: A clinicopathologic review with emphasis on differential diagnosis and syndromic associations. *Archives of Pathology and Laboratory Medicine, 139*(1), 133–9.

Sayki Arslan, M., Ekız, F., Yilmaz, G., Çoban, Ş., Savaş, B., Ensarı, A., & Örmecı, N. (2012). Ganglioneuromatous polyposis of the colon in

a patient with multiple adenomatous polyps. *The Turkish Journal of Gastroenterology, 23*(6), 780–3.
Smith, V. V., Eng, C., & Milla, P. J. (1999). Intestinal ganglioneuromatosis and multiple endocrine neoplasia type 2B: Implications for treatment. *Gut, 45*, 143–146.
Vinitsky, A., Zaleski, C. A., Sajjad, S. M., & McPherson, E. W. (2013). Intestinal ganglioneuromatosis: Unusual presentation of Cowden syndrome resulting in delayed diagnosis. *American Journal of Medical Genetics Part A, 161A*(5), 1085–90.

Gastric Antral Vascular Ectasia (GAVE)

Francisco Ferro de Beça and
Elisabete Rios
Department of Pathology, Centro Hospitalar de São João, Porto, Portugal
Faculty of Medicine of the University of Porto, Porto, Portugal
IPATIMUP – Institute of Pathology and Molecular Immunology of the University of Porto, Porto, Portugal

Synonyms

Watermelon stomach

Definition

GAVE was firstly described in 1984, in a report of three cases, as referring to a condition with a characteristic endoscopic antral appearance in which the longitudinal antral folds had visible reddened vessels radiating from the pylorus and therefore resembling the stripes on a watermelon (Jabbari et al. 1984). Usual presentation ranges from occult bleeding (with possible transfusion-dependent anemia) to severe acute GI bleeding. Although etiology remains largely unknown, most patients with GAVE have chronic medical conditions with up to 30% of patients suffering from liver cirrhosis. In case of non-cirrhotic patients, autoimmune diseases have consistently been reported (Selinger and Ang 2008), being autoimmune connective tissue disorders, Raynaud's phenomenon, and sclerodactyly the most common.

Clinical Features

- **Incidence**
  GAVE is considered a rare medical condition that accounts up to 4% of all non-variceal upper GI bleedings.
- **Age**
  The mean age of presentation in non-cirrhotic is 73 years old. Cirrhotic patients are younger with a mean age of 65.
- **Sex**
  Classic non-cirrhotic GAVE is more common in women (71%) whereas cirrhotic GAVE patients are usually in men (1.5:2 ratio).
- **Site**
  The ectatic vessels are typically limited to the antrum of the stomach. There is a report of some patients with classical GAVE and similar lesions occurring also in the cardia.
- **Treatment**
  Several therapeutic modalities are used for GAVE. Symptomatic therapy for correction of chronic or acute blood loss includes fluids and blood transfusions as well as iron supplementation. Pharmacological therapy has been tried with corticosteroids and estrogen and progesterone with some successful reports. Tranexamic acid has also been tested in reducing bleeding episodes and transfusion requirements (Selinger and Ang 2008).

  Due to uncontrolled blood loss, treatment of GAVE often requires endoscopic therapy with thermal ablation. However, many patients will ultimately require a surgical resection (antrectomy or gastrectomy) to achieve cure and eliminate transfusion dependency (Selinger and Ang 2008).
- **Outcome**
  Although no exact proportions are reported, morbidity and mortality are high, particularly in patients with decompensated cirrhosis.

Macroscopy

The endoscopic appearance is usually characterized by visible columns of red tortuous ectatic vessels along the longitudinal folds of the antrum. When present, these macroscopic features are pathognomonic for GAVE (Montgomery and Voltagio 2012). In other cases, the endoscopic appearance only consists of a gastric diffuse erythema and may present a diagnostic challenge (see further discussion in Immunophenotype and Differential Diagnosis).

Microscopy

On microscopic examination, there are usually features of mucosal prolapse, with foveolar hyperplasia, fibromuscular hypertrophy, dilated mucosal capillaries, and focal fibrin thrombi. Interestingly this last feature allows the distinction from patients with portal hypertensive gastropathy (PHG), since these do not have fibrin thrombi in the dilated capillaries (Montgomery and Voltagio 2012). However, the described histological features for GAVE are not pathognomonic.

Immunophenotype

CD61 immunolabelling (platelet glycoprotein IIIa antigen) can be used to highlight the fibrin thrombi in the dilated capillaries. This marker has been reported as always positive in GAVE and therefore as a possible useful marker for differentiating GAVE from PHG (Westerhoff et al. 2010).

Differential Diagnosis

The main differential diagnosis to consider is portal hypertension gastropathy (PHG). However clinically, PHG occurs in a setting of portal hypertension, whereas GAVE does not, as previously referred, a significant proportion of patients with GAVE also have liver pathology (Burak et al. 2001). Furthermore, endoscopically, both conditions might have very similar presentations with considerable overlap in cases of GAVE with associated liver cirrhosis and severe PHG. Still, sometimes difficult, it is important to make the correct differential diagnosis between these two conditions due to critically different therapies.

Other causes of GI bleeding, specially upper GI bleeding, such as Dieulafoy's lesion, should also be considered as possible differential diagnosis of GAVE (Burak et al. 2001).

References and Further Reading

Burak, K. W., Lee, S. S., & Beck, P. L. (2001). Portal hypertensive gastropathy and gastric antral vascular ectasia (GAVE) syndrome. *Gut, 49*(6), 866–872.

Jabbari, M., Cherry, R., Lough, J. O., Daly, D. S., Kinnear, D. G., & Goresky, C. A. (1984). Gastric antral vascular ectasia: The watermelon stomach. *Gastroenterology, 87*(5), 1165–1170.

Montgomery, E. A., & Voltagio, L. (2012). Chapter 2, Stomach. In: *Biopsy interpretation of the gastrointestinal tract mucosa. Vol 1: Non-neoplastic.* 2nd ed. (pp. 88–89). Philadelphia: Lippincott Williams & Wilkins.

Selinger, C. P., & Ang, Y. S. (2008). Gastric antral vascular ectasia (GAVE): An update on clinical presentation, pathophysiology and treatments. *Digestion, 77*(2), 131–137.

Westerhoff, M., Tretiakova, M., Hovan, L., Miller, J., Noffsinger, A., & Hart, J. (2010). CD61, CD31, and CD34 improve diagnostic accuracy in gastric antral vascular ectasia and portal hypertensive gastropathy: An immunohistochemical and digital morphometric study. *The American Journal of Surgical Pathology, 34*(4), 494–501.

Gastric Antrum (Distal Stomach)

Chella R. S. van der Post and
J. Han van Krieken
Department of Pathology, Radboud University Medical Center, Nijmegen, The Netherlands

Synonyms

Antropyloric region; Distal stomach; Pyloric antrum

Anatomy

Anatomically, the stomach is divided from proximal to distal into the following regions: cardia, fundus, corpus or body and the antropyloric region; the latter is in this entry designated as antrum. The extent of the gastric regions varies between individuals, and in individuals, with age and with disease progress. The triangularly shaped antrum is demarcated from the corpus by a notch in the lesser curvature, the incisura angularis. A greatly thickened distal muscular wall forms the pyloric sphincter. A narrow lumen passes through the pyloric sphincter to the duodenum. Possibly due to chronic gastritis, many older adults have a reduction in the area of fundic mucosa, with expansion of the zone of pyloric mucosa. This results in proximal displacement of the pylorofundic junction, a change termed pyloric or pseudopyloric metaplasia.

Function

The stomach functions as reservoir, harbors a mucosal barrier function, hormonal functions, and initiates the digestive process by mixing and degradation of food and secretion of protein-digesting enzymes and acids to food. The antropyloric region is involved in hormonal regulation of gastric acid secretion and mechanical gastric emptying.

Neuroendocrine Functions

The stomach contains a wide variety of hormone-producing cells. In the antrum, the predominant endocrine cells, about 50% of the whole endocrine cell population are gastrin-producing (G) cells, 30% are enterochromaffin (EC) cells, and 15% are somatostatin-producing (D) cells. This is in contrast with the corpus where the majority of endocrine cells are enterochromaffin-like (ECL) cells, which secrete histamine. The hormone-producing cells in the antrum are mostly located in the neck region just below the foveolae. The hormones either enter the blood or modulate other locally situated cells (paracrine effect).

- The G cells secrete gastrin, which stimulates acid production and mucosal cell growth. There are two major forms of gastrin, G17 and G34, depending on the number of amino-acid residues. G17 is the major form found in the antrum. Its actions are mediated primarily through the CCK-2 receptor on ECL cells, a G protein-coupled receptor previously termed the CCKB or gastrin receptor. Gastrin release is stimulated either as a result of distention of the antrum (mechanical stimulus) or by direct stimulation from ingested food, due to increased pH and proteins (chemical stimulus). When the antrum becomes distended or alkalinized, G cells release gastrin that binds to gastrin receptors on ECL cells. This results in hyperplasia of ECL cells as well as histamine release, subsequently binding to histamine receptors on parietal cells, stimulating acid secretion. Gastrin also stimulates directly the acid secretion by binding to gastrin receptors on parietal cells. Acid secretion is further influenced by vagal stimuli. Consequently, the lower pH negatively regulates gastrin secretion through a feedback loop. The G cell population consists of approximately ten million but can increase and is influenced by disease. Hypergastrinemia, defined as a fasting serum gastrin concentration of >100 pg/mL, can be caused by gastrinoma, antral predominant *H. pylori* gastritis, gastric outlet obstruction, renal failure, atrophic gastritis, and antisecretory therapy. The highest amount of G cells is found in the antrum near the pylorus, the number gradually decreases proximally to the junctional zone between the antrum and corpus. G cells are normally not found in the corpus.
- The luminal pH-sensitive population of D cells secretes somatostatin. D cells inhibit acid secretion, gastrin and intrinsic factor secretion, and acetylcholine release by secretion of somatostatin. Somatostatin inhibits acid secretion in a paracrine fashion directly by inhibiting secretion from the parietal cell as well as indirectly by inhibiting histamine secretion from the ECL cell and gastrin secretion from the G cell.

- EC cells synthesize, store and secrete mainly serotonin; other products are tachykinins, enkephalins, and motilin. EC cells can be identified in all alimentary tract segments and are most numerous in the gut. They have regulatory functions including the initiation of peristalsis by stimulating gut motility and the regulation of gastrin release inhibition. Serotonin is released in response to an increase in intraluminal pressure or chemical stimuli, low pH, hypertonic glucose, amino acids, secretion, and peristalsis.

Gastric Mucin

The pH of gastric mucin is in the neutral or alkaline range, and therefore neutralizes the hydrochloric acid to some degree to prevent the gastric mucosa. The exact physiologic role of gastric mucin is not determined. Clearly, the soluble mucin plays a role in lubrication. The insoluble fraction acts as a surface laying, forming a barrier that, together with bicarbonate secreted by the superficial epithelial cells, prevents back-diffusion of acid and gastric autodigestion.

Pylorus

The pylorus is a muscular sphincter and regulates the movement of digested contents from the stomach into the duodenum. The muscle also functions as a sphincter by preventing backflow of duodenal contents into the stomach. When contracting, it narrows the diameter of the aperture, and when the cylinder is fully contracted, the aperture is closed.

Size, Weight

The entire stomach has a volume of 1,200–1,500 mL, but can extend to over 3,000 mL. The triangularly shaped antrum occupies the distal third of the stomach proximal to the pyloric sphincter. The antrum extends along the lesser curvature, around 5–8 cm and often almost reaches the cardia, while along the greater curvature, the extension is approximately 4–6 cm. The pyloric canal measures 2.5–5 cm in length.

Macroscopy

The antrum represents the distal third of the stomach proximal to the pyloric sphincter. The junction between the antrum and corpus is poorly demarcated. By external examination, the antrum comprises the portion of stomach distal to the incisura, a notch on the lesser curvature. The antrum is characterized grossly by mucosa that is flatter than the prominent gastric folds or rugae in the corpus. Furthermore, the antrum is more firmly anchored to the underlying submucosa. The muscular pyloric sphincteric cylinder is a tube of thickened muscularis externa, in adults approximately 2.5–5 cm in length when fully contracted. The pyloric ring (3–4 mm in width) is the aboral thickening of the cylinder.

Microscopy

Histologically the gastric mucosa is divided into three distinctive epithelial mucosa zones: cardiac, oxyntic (corpus and fundus), and antropyloric mucosa. The mucosa can be divided in three major epithelial compartments: the gastric pits and surface lining, the mucous neck region, and the glands. The nature and relative thickness of the glands and pits defines each gastric zone. The antropyloric mucosa constitutes the distal 20% of the stomach and consists of foveolae and antropyloric glands, both occupying about half of the mucosal thickness (Fig. 1).

Antropyloric glands are coiled tubular glands and resemble histologically cardiac glands and Brunner's glands of the duodenum (Fig. 2). However, they are more compact and there is less abundant lamina propria surrounding the glands compared to cardiac mucosa. Antropyloric glands are coiled and extensively branched, cystic dilation is usually absent. The glands are composed of two major cell types: tall columnar cells, which secrete neutral mucin, and scattered endocrine cells. The columnar cells of the antropyloric glands have ill-defined borders and a bubbly vesicular cytoplasm that is different from the foveolar and surface epithelium. Single or small groups of isolated parietal cells are frequently

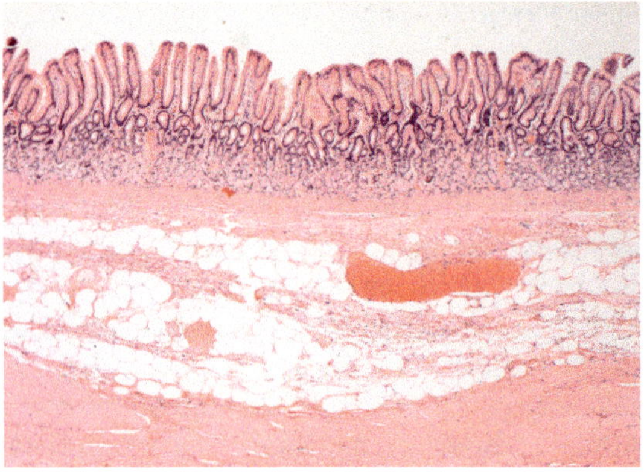

Gastric Antrum (Distal Stomach), Fig. 1 Gastric antropyloric mucosa, submucosa, and muscularis propria. The surface epithelium appears slightly villous. The antropyloric glands are loosely packed and occupy about half of the mucosa (H&E, original magnification 25×)

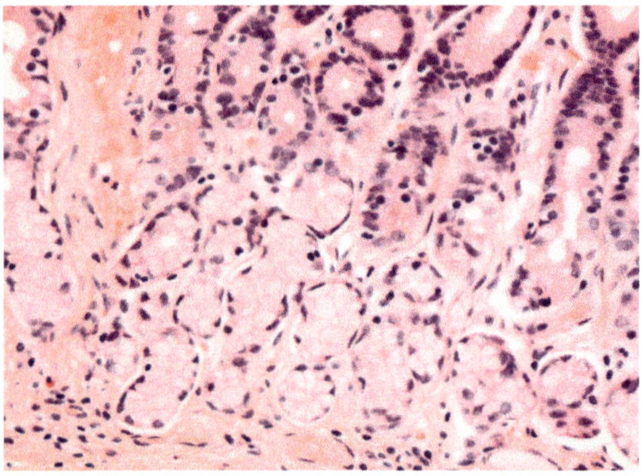

Gastric Antrum (Distal Stomach), Fig. 2 Antropyloric glands are coiled tubular glands and resemble cardiac glands and Brunner's glands of the duodenum. The cells have an eccentric nucleus and contain foamy cytoplasm (H&E, original magnification 200×)

found in the antrum, especially at the junctional zone next to the corpus. However, it is uncommon for chief or zymogenic cells to be present outside of the corpus and junctional area. The pyloric glands secrete neutral mucin only. Mucous neck cells reside in the neck and isthmic region of the gastric glands. They derive from mitotically active stem cells in the neck region. In the antropyloric region, the pits occupy approximately 40% of the mucosa. They branch and may not always lie perpendicular to the surface.

Neuroendocrine cells appear as cuboidal or short columnar cells scattered among the gastric epithelia, usually in the glands. In the antrum, approximately 50% of neuroendocrine cells are G cells, 30% are EC cells, and 15% are D cells. The remaining 5% consist of other endocrine cell types. G cells are large, round, or oval cells and lie predominantly in the neck region of the antral glands, trailing off toward the gland base. G cells normally have an irregular and random spatial distribution that ranges between one to four cells per gland. They contain variably dense cytoplasmic granules measuring 150–200 μm in diameter. EC cells are sparse in the mucous neck portion but are quite numerous in the lower half of the gland. Their overall distribution is patchy; areas with numerous EC cells alternate with areas containing few or none. They are especially numerous in areas of intestinal metaplasia. D cells are uniformly distributed throughout the antral and body mucosa. Most D cells are open cells that act as receptors, interacting with luminal contents. A feedback mechanism exists in which intraluminal acid stimulates somatostatin secretion. Antral D-cell hyperplasia can be observed in patients with duodenal ulcer disease. Antral G-cell hyperplasia is seen as a reaction in patients with autoimmune gastritis.

The lamina propria provides structural support, consisting of a fine meshwork of reticulin with occasional collagen and elastic fibers that are condensed underneath the basement membrane. The lamina propria is more abundant in the superficial portion of the mucosa between the pits, especially in the pyloric mucosa. It contains numerous cell types, including fibroblasts, histiocytes, plasma cells and lymphocytes, polymorphs, and mast cells. The lamina propria also contains capillaries, arterioles, and nonmyelinated nerve fibers. A few fibers of smooth muscle extend upward from the muscularis mucosa into the lamina propria, occasionally reaching the superficial portion of the mucosa, especially in the distal antrum. Small aggregates of lymphocytes can be found in the normal stomach.

At the junction of two different mucosal types, as in the junction of the antrum and corpus, there are transitional zones that share features of both

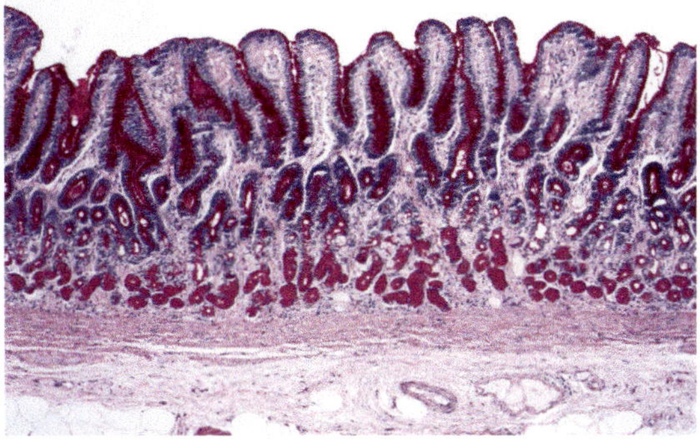

Gastric Antrum (Distal Stomach), Fig. 3 PAS staining highlights the mucin-containing cells (PAS, original magnification 50×)

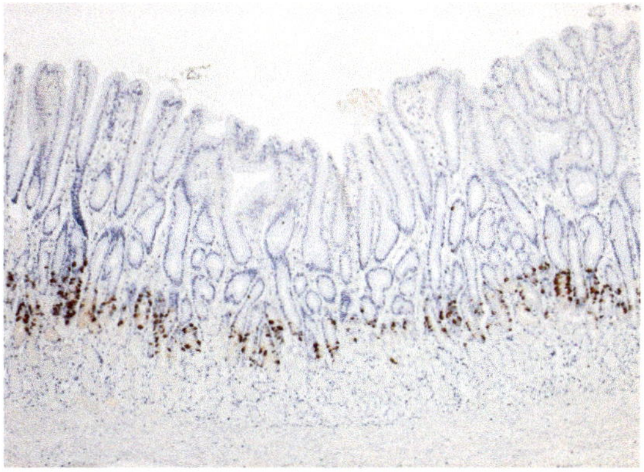

Gastric Antrum (Distal Stomach), Fig. 4 Immunohistochemical staining of gastrin shows the distribution of G cells in the neck region of the antral glands. G cells have an irregular and random spatial distribution that ranges between one to four cells per gland (Gastrin stain original magnification 50×)

mucosa types. This transitional mucosa usually has the structure of antral mucosa, with clustered glands and tall pits; the glands usually contain mucous cells and gastrin-producing cells of antral mucosa mixed with parietal and chief cells of oxyntic mucosa. As people age, transitional mucosa gradually creep proximally, especially along the lesser curvature. The border between the antrum and corpus may show a mixture of oxyntic and mucous glands for a variable length of mucosa. The most useful criteria to determine when one crosses from corpus into antrum are the absence of chief cells and the change from single tubular glands in the corpus to branched glands in the antrum. It may be difficult to determine the site of origin of the gastric mucosa, particularly when it is altered by inflammation, atrophy, and/or metaplasia. In particular, it may be difficult to differentiate between a nonatrophic antral gastritis and atrophic body gastritis with pseudopyloric metaplasia.

Immunophenotype/ Immunohistochemistry

Mucin stains such as (A)PAS, alcian blue, or combined PAS/alcian blue can be used to highlight the morphology (Fig. 3). Within the neuroendocrine cells, hormones are present as cytoplasmic granules located between the nucleus and basement membrane; but, because the granules are generally inconspicuous on H&E sections, special immunostains are required for their demonstration. The EC cells have argentaffin granules, which can be stained by Fontana, Masson, or the diazo technique. Individual hormones, for example, gastrin and somatostatin, may be demonstrated by immunohistochemistry with the use of specific antibodies (Fig. 4).

Table with Important Diseases (Links)

Gastric Adenoma
Gastric Stump
Gastritis Cystica Polyposa/Profunda
Goblet Cells
Hyperplastic Polyp
Neuroendocrine Tumors
Neuroendocrine Cell Hyperplasia

References and Further Reading

Fenoglio-Preiser, C. M., Noffsinger, A. E., Stemmerman, G. N., Lantz, P. E., & Isaacson, P. G. (2008). *Gastrointestinal pathology: An atlas and text* (3rd ed.). Philadelphia: Lippincott Williams & Wilkins.

Keet, A. D. (1982). The anatomical extent of the pyloric sphincteric cylinder, the pyloric mucosal zone and the

pyloric antrum. *South African Medical Journal, 62*(10), 329–333.
Owen, D. A. (1986). Normal histology of the stomach. *The American Journal of Surgical Pathology, 10*(1), 48–61.
Schubert, M. L. (2009). Gastric exocrine and endocrine secretion. *Current Opinion in Gastroenterology, 25*(6), 529–536.
Stave, R., Brandtzaeg, P., Nygaard, K., & Fausa, O. (1978). The transitional body-antrum zone in resected human stomachs. Anatomical outline and parietal-cell and gastrin-cell characteristics in peptic ulcer disease. *Scandinavian Journal of Gastroenterology, 13*(6), 685–691.

Gastric Cardia (Proximal Stomach)

Chella R. S. van der Post and
J. Han van Krieken
Department of Pathology, Radboud University Medical Center, Nijmegen, The Netherlands

Synonyms

Proximal stomach

Anatomy

The stomach is divided into four anatomic regions: cardia, fundus, corpus, and antropyloric. The gastric cardia is a narrow, ill-defined region and is not grossly distinctive or sharply demarcated. It represents the area of the mucosa located distal to the anatomic gastroesophageal junction and proximal to the body of the stomach (fundus/corpus) that is composed entirely of oxyntic glands. The cardia is a very short segment (<0.4 cm) of the mucosa that is typically composed of pure mucous glands or mixed mucous and oxyntic glands.

The extent of the cardiac mucosa and even its existence as a component of the normal stomach has been disputed. In many studies an attempt has been performed to delineate the normal histology of the true gastric cardia, using biopsies, resections, or autopsy specimens. Some studies, mainly in adults, reported the presence of gastric cardia in only 50% of the studied population. A significant proportion of patients with cardiac mucosa concomitantly had chronic active inflammation with variable amounts of intestinal metaplasia. Conclusions drawn were that the cardiac mucosa is an acquired, metaplastic lesion and probably results from gastroesophageal reflux disease (GERD). However, several histology studies in neonates, infants, and young pediatric patients have shown the existence of true gastric cardia as a normal component of the stomach. In these patient groups there is minimal or no confounding influences of diseases that increase in prevalence with age, such as gastric reflux or *Helicobacter pylori* infection. The presence of the cardiac mucosa in the proximal stomach, located between esophageal squamous and gastric fundic glands, has also been confirmed in the embryo-fetal stomach and at term delivery. This data establish the congenital nature of gastric cardia at this stage of human development. The discussion around the gastric cardia is ongoing and is related to the lack of precise, standardized, and reproducible definitions of the gastroesophageal junction. The exact location of retrieved biopsies in this area is often unclear due to a lack of clinical information and good endoscopic correlation.

Function

The mucinous columnar epithelium serves as a “buffer zone” between the squamous epithelium of the esophagus and the oxyntic glands of the stomach. Cardiac glands secrete mucus that forms a protective blanket on the gastric surface.

Size, Weight

The cardiac mucosa is concentrated in a narrow zone of the proximal stomach, and the length of the gastric cardia is generally considered to be smaller than 5 mm. There may be geographical or ethnic differences; ranges have been reported from 1 to 5 mm in Caucasian adults in Europe and North America, and ranges of 13–15 mm are reported in Japanese and Chinese studies. It is unclear whether this represents a true ethnic difference in the distribution of the amount of cardiac glands or that it results from the application of other definitions. However, the interesting difference of the amount of cardiac glands might be associated with different disease pathogenesis mechanisms among various ethnic patient groups.

Macroscopy

The transition point or Z-line separates the pearly white-gray esophageal squamous mucosa from the erythematous gastric columnar mucosa. The gastric cardia is defined as the proximal area of the stomach and is demarcated proximal by the squamocolumnar mucosal boundary (Z-line) and distal by the oxyntic mucosa from the fundus and corpus. Macroscopically, the cardiac mucosa has no distinctive features. For the evaluation of biopsies, it is important that the endoscopist describes the exact location where biopsies were acquired, especially with regard to the gastroesophageal transition.

Microscopy

The esophagus is lined by stratified squamous epithelium and contains scattered mucous glands within the lamina propria of the mucosa and salivary gland-like mixed mucous/serous glands in the submucosa (Fig. 1). Until recently, it was commonly believed that the distal 1–2 cm of esophagus is lined by mucinous columnar epithelium similar to the antropyloric region; however, it is now thought that this transition to columnar epithelium is in fact metaplastic in origin. The stomach is lined by mucinous columnar epithelium and contains either pure oxyntic glands in the fundus and corpus or pure mucous glands in the antropyloric region. The histology of the gastroesophageal junction is controversial and variable. In "normal" individuals, the anatomic gastroesophageal junction corresponds to the histologic transition point between the esophageal squamous epithelium and the gastric mucinous columnar epithelium.

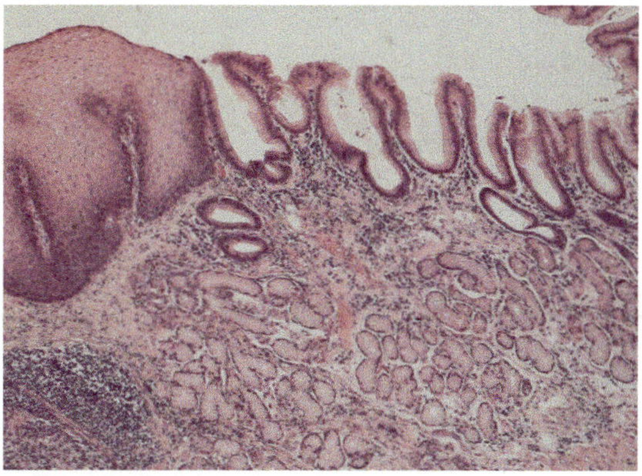

Gastric Cardia (Proximal Stomach), Fig. 1 Resection specimen demonstrates the gastroesophageal region with the transition of the squamous epithelium to the gastric glandular cardiac-type epithelium. Note the carditis with abundant inflammation marked by an increase in lymphocytes and plasma cells around the cardiac glands

The cardiac mucosa is composed of surface mucinous columnar epithelium and either pure mucous glands or a mixture of mucous and oxyntic glands in most individuals. The presence of mixed mucous and oxyntic glands in the gastric cardia is comparable to other regions of the tubal gut with histologic transitions from one functional gland type to another. For instance, the transition zone between the gastric corpus and the antrum is also a histologically variable area and often shows a mixture of antropyloric-type mucous glands and corpus-type oxyntic glands at this zone.

Cardiac glands are tubular, similar to antropyloric glands, or compound acinar or racemose, mimicking the duodenal Brunner glands. They consist predominantly of mucous cells with variable amounts of parietal cells, undifferentiated cells in the neck zone and endocrine cells in the base of the gland. Chief cells are generally not present in cardiac glands.

Carditis can be detected in 79–95% of patients undergoing upper endoscopy and seems to increase with age. Carditis is characterized by abundant inflammation with predominant neutrophil granulocytes and an increase in lymphocytes and plasma cells with or without formation of reactive lymphoid aggregates. Varying degrees of intestinal metaplasia, pancreatic metaplasia, and *Helicobacter pylori* organisms can be identified.

The length of cardia-type mucosa can increase and extend proximally above the level of the gastroesophageal junction into the distal esophagus. It is debatable whether these cardiac glands in the distal superficial esophagus underneath the squamous mucosa are metaplastic in nature or normal congenital tissue. Most commonly, this area is considered metaplastic and originates as a result of GERD; it is referred to as columnar metaplasia of the distal esophagus or Barrett's esophagus when goblet cells are identified.

Immunophenotype/ Immunohistochemistry

The cardiac glands secrete predominantly neutral mucin with small amounts of sialomucin. At the subcellular level, the mucus cells are equipped with short microvilli at the apical surface and possess secretory granules in the apical cytoplasm, which can be highlighted with periodic acid-Schiff (PAS) stain. The mucus cells are negative using Alcian blue stain at pH 2.5 or lower, which is similar to the staining pattern of mucus cells elsewhere in the stomach.

Table with Important Diseases (Links)

Carditis
Adenocarcinoma of the gastroesophageal junction
Intestinal metaplasia
Gastroesophageal reflux disease

References and Further Reading

Chandrasoma, P. (2005). Controversies of the cardiac mucosa and Barrett's oesophagus. *Histopathology, 46*(4), 361–373.

De Hertogh, G., Van Eyken, P., Ectors, N., & Geboes, K. (2005). On the origin of cardiac mucosa: A histological and immunohistochemical study of cytokeratin expression patterns in the developing esophagogastric junction region and stomach. *World Journal of Gastroenterology, 11*(29), 4490–4496.

Filipe, M. I. (1979). Mucins in the human gastrointestinal epithelium: A review. *Investigative & Cell Pathology, 2*(3), 195–216.

Huang, Q. (2011). Controversies of cardiac glands in the proximal stomach: A critical review. *Journal of Gastroenterology and hepatology, 26*(3), 450–455.

Odze, R. D. (2005). Unraveling the mystery of the gastroesophageal junction: A pathologist's perspective. *The American Journal of Gastroenterology, 100*(8), 1853–1867.

Gastric Epithelial Dysplasia

Xiaogang Wen
Centro hospitalar de Vila Nova de Gaia/Espinho, Institute of Molecular Pathology and Immunology of the University of Porto, Porto, Portugal

Synonyms

Gastric intraepithelial neoplasia, adenoma.

Definition

Gastric epithelial dysplasia represents unequivocal gastric epithelial neoplastic proliferation characterized by variable cytological and architectural atypia, without convincing evidence of invasive growth.

Clinical Features

- **Incidence**
  Incidence of gastric epithelial dysplasia shows considerable geographic differences and is usually associated with the regional prevalence of *Helicobacter pylori* infection. The incidence of dysplasia varies from 0.5% to 4% in western populations and from 9% to 20% in high-risk areas for gastric carcinomas.

- **Age**
  The incidence of gastric epithelial dysplasia increases with age. It is much more prevalent after sixth decade.
- **Sex**
  Gastric epithelial dysplasia is more frequent in males than in females, with a male to female ratio of 1.2–3:1.
- **Site**
  Gastric epithelial dysplasia occurs more frequently in the gastric antrum and incisura angularis, although it can involve the whole stomach.
- **Treatment**
  The low-grade dysplasia/adenoma can be treated by endoscopic resection or can just be kept under surveillance. High-grade dysplasia/adenoma should be resected endoscopically or surgically. The choice of the treatment should depend on the overall size of the lesion, the risk of invasion (as assessed endoscopically, radiologically, or ultrasonographically), and on general factors such as the patient's age and comorbidity conditions.
- **Outcome**
  In some studies, spontaneous regression of the low-grade dysplasia was observed in about 50% of the cases. However, without treatment, it was estimated that about 15% of the lesions would progress to high-grade dysplasia or invasive carcinoma. The risk of progression from high-grade dysplasia to invasive carcinoma was estimated up to 80~85%. The spontaneous regression was observed in less than 5% of the lesions.

Macroscopy

Gastric epithelial dysplasia can be polypoid (pedunculated or sessile), flat or slightly depressed. The flat and depressed lesions may display an irregular appearance on chromoendoscopy. In European countries and North America, the term "adenoma" has been applied when the neoplastic proliferation produces a discrete, protruding lesion. In Japan, however, "adenomas" include all gross types (i.e. flat, elevated, and depressed).

Microscopy

The gastric epithelial dysplasia lesions are characterized by cytological and architectural abnormalities, which include loss of surface maturation, glandular irregularity, nuclear pseudostratification, increased nuclear size and irregularity, heterogeneity of chromatin and mitotic activity. In the more acceptable two-tiered grading system, the dysplasia is divided into low-grade and high-grade.

The low-grade dysplasia lesions display minimal architectural disorganization and mild to moderate cytological atypia. The nuclei are elongated, polarized and basally located, with dense chromatin an mild to moderate nuclear pseudostratification. Figures of mitosis can be frequent, but they are usually confined to the basal half of the epithelium (Fig. 1).

The high-grade dysplasia lesions display severe glandular irregularity with intraluminal folding and, rarely, cribriform pattern. The nuclei are irregular and vesicular with clumping and heterogeneous chromatin, and prominent, sometimes, multiple nucleoli (Fig. 2). The nuclear pseudostratification and figures of mitosis frequently extend to the luminal aspect of the glands, although sometimes the large nuclear size and less crowded nuclear arrangement can give the lesion a "less pseudostratified appearance". Necrosis is

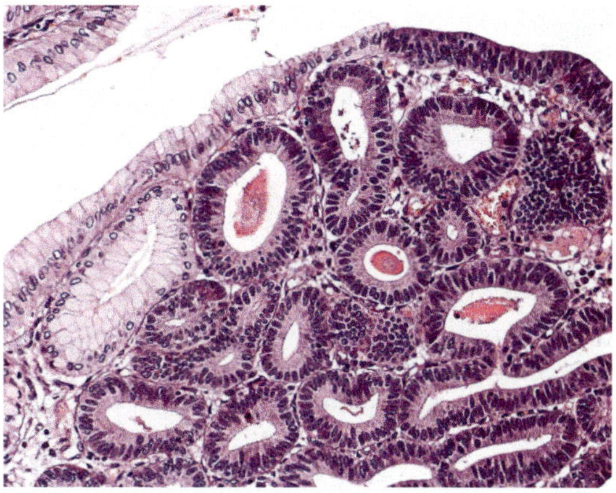

Gastric Epithelial Dysplasia, Fig. 1 Low grade dysplasia, intestinal type, the nuclei are hyperchromatic and elongated. The glands are relatively regular

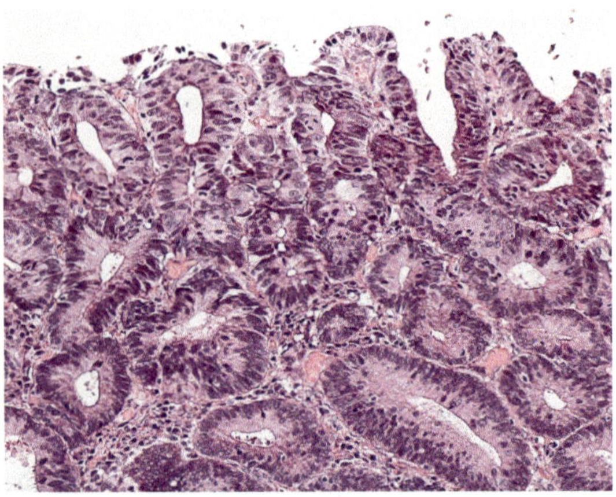

Gastric Epithelial Dysplasia, Fig. 2 High grade dysplasia, intestinal type, the loss of nuclear polarity and the glandular irregularity are evident

not infrequent. The nuclear basal orientation and polarity can be totally lost in the most severe lesions, which could be diagnosed as carcinoma *in situ* according to the criteria of the Japanese classification.

Gastric epithelial dysplasia can be morphologically and genetically categorized into intestinal phenotype (adenomatous type, type I) and gastric phenotype (foveolar type, type II). The former is more common and is constituted by cells with pencillated and pseudostratified nuclei, and expression of intestinal-type mucin, resembling colonic adenomas. The latter is less common and is frequently constituted of columnar cells with round to oval nuclei and eosinophilic or pale cytoplasm. The nuclear pseudostratification is not as prominent as in the former. The cells contain gastric-type mucin.

Immunohistochemistry

P53 protein, Bcl-2, Ki-67, CD44v6, and other markers were used in some studies and even in routine diagnostic work. Although these markers may be helpful in some circumstances, none of them can definitely distinguish gastric epithelial dysplasia from non-neoplastic proliferation. The adenomatous and gastric dysplasia can be distinguished by the expression of of mucin, CD10, and CDX2 (intestinal/adenomatous: MUC2, CD10, and CDX2; gastric/foveolar: MUC5AC, absence of CD10 and low expression of CDX2).

Molecular Features

Although many genetic and molecular events have been described in dysplasia, no specific alterations are helpful for routine diagnosis.

Differential Diagnosis

Gastric epithelial dysplasia should be distinguished from regenerative hyperplasia. The latter occurs frequently in the border of the benign ulcer with intense inflammatory reaction. The glands with regenerative hyperplasia usually have regular architecture and are composed of cuboidal or columnar cells, with basophilic cytoplasm. The nuclei are usually regular and round. The nuclear basal orientation and polarity are preserved, and the nuclear pseudostratification, if present, is less intense than in dysplasia. Cytological atypia is not uncommon, but should be confined in foveolae or lower part of the glands. The cells of the overlying surface epithelium should maintain the relatively normal morphology. In other words, there is a tendency of surface maturation in regenerative hyperplasia. This point is considered as one of the most important criteria to distinguish reactive hyperplasia from dysplasia.

For cases in which it is difficult or even impossible to evaluate the surface maturation and other criteria, for example, in small biopsies exhibiting inflammation, the term indefinite dysplasia can be used. In such cases, re-biopsy is encouraged, especially after treatment for the possible etiologies.

Gastric epithelial dysplasia should be differentiated also from invasive adenocarcinoma. The desmoplastic stromal reaction and existence of isolated or small solid group of atypical epithelial cells suggest invasion. Confluent growth pattern of the glands, such as aggregation of irregular glands without evident stroma, complex cribriform glands, and luminal necrosis are also indicators of invasion. It is not surprising that the invasion can't always be confirmed. In the *revised Vienna classification of gastrointestinal epithelial neoplasia* exist a subgroup within the group of high grade dysplasia, which is called "suspicious of invasive carcinoma."

References and Further Reading

de Vries, A. C., & Kuipers, E. J. (2007). Epidemiology of premalignant gastric lesions: Implications for the development of screening and surveillance strategies. *Helicobacter, 12*(Suppl 2), 22–31. Review. PubMed PMID: 17991173.

Dixon, M. F. (2002). Gastrointestinal epithelial neoplasia: Vienna revisited. *Gut, 51*(1), 130–131. PubMed PMID: 12077106; PubMed Central PMCID: PMC1773259.

Lauwers, G. Y., & Riddell, R. H. (1999). Gastric epithelial dysplasia. *Gut, 45*(5), 784–790. Review. PubMed PMID: 10517922; PubMed Central PMCID:PMC1727726.

Raftopoulos, S. C., Kumarasinghe, P., de Boer, B., Iacobelli, J., et al. (2012). Gastric intraepithelial neoplasia in a Western population. *European Journal of Gastroenterology and Hepatology, 24*(1), 48–54. PubMed PMID: 22081007.

You, W. C., Blot, W. J., Li, J. Y., Chang, Y. S., Jin, M. L., Kneller, R., Zhang, L., Han, Z. X., Zeng, X. R., & Liu, W. D. (1993). Precancerous gastric lesions in a population at high risk of stomach cancer. *Cancer Research, 53*(6), 1317–1321. PubMed Central PMCID: PMC1 8443811.

Gastric Graft-Versus-Host Disease

Wen-Yih Liang[1] and Gregory Y. Lauwers[2]
[1]Department of Pathology, Taipei Veterans General Hospital, Taipei, Taiwan
[2]Department of Pathology, Massachusetts General Hospital, Harvard Medical School, Boston, MA, USA

Synonyms

Graft-vs-host disease, GVHD

Definition

GVHD is the result of the activation of donor lymphocytes attacking and damaging the recipient tissues after allogeneic transplant.

Currently, acute and chronic GVHD are defined more along clinicopathologic features rather than time post transplant (previous classifications suggested a breakdown of <100 days for acute GVHD, 100 days for chronic GVHD). Some authors suggest that better terms would be *active* and *active/chronic* GVHD.

Clinical Features

- **Presentation**
  Gastrointestinal GVHD commonly presents 3 or more weeks after transplant. The classic triad of nausea, vomiting, and diarrhea detected in over 60% of patients represents the most common symptoms. Isolated diarrhea with or without abdominal pain is observed in 20% of patients, while nausea or vomiting without other symptoms is present in only 10% of the cases. Only 7% of GVHD patients experience abdominal pain alone.
- **Incidence**
  Autologous GVHD is described in up to 10% of patients receiving autologous hematopoietic stem cell transplantation. The incidence of gastrointestinal disease ranges from 4% to 16%. The higher incidences reported recently are likely due to increased awareness of the disease, which is typically classified as mild.
- **Site**
  The skin is the most common site, followed by the gastrointestinal tract and liver. In the gut, any site from oral mucosa to anus may be involved.

  It remains a matter of debate which gastrointestinal tract segment (e.g., duodenum, stomach, ileum, colon, sigmoid, rectum) offers the highest sensitivity for diagnosing gastrointestinal GVHD. Some series report that rectosigmoid biopsies have a higher sensitivity and negative predictive value, while other reports report similar accuracy in reviewing gastric biopsies.
- **Treatment**
  The mainstay of treatment is steroids, usually at a high dose, followed by a slow tapering of the dose. Other immunosuppression therapy

includes mycophenolate mofetil, tacrolimus, cyclosporine, infliximab, and daclizumab.

- **Outcome**
  A short course of steroids is effective in managing acute GVHD in the majority of patients (~80%), and many others respond to a second course of prednisone. However, up to 50% of patients develop chronic problems secondary to GVHD.

Macroscopy

The endoscopic appearance of the gastric mucosa affected by GVHD varies markedly. Surprisingly, in most cases, the mucosa is endoscopically normal. More severe alterations range from mucosal edema and erythema to nodularity, erosions/ulceration, and exudate. Overall, the correlation between the endoscopic appearance and a histological diagnosis of GVHD varies from moderate (40%) to excellent (80%).

Microscopy

- Universal gastrointestinal mucosal involvement has been reported, with similar diagnostic features recognizable throughout the length of the gastrointestinal tract.
- The same histological grading system is used for GVHD throughout the gastrointestinal tract (Table 1). An NIH Consensus report also has proposed recommendations for the reporting of biopsies performed to confirm GVHD (Table 2).
- The histological hallmark of acute GVHD in the entire gut is epithelial cell apoptosis (Figs. 1 and 2). However, some mitigating factors ought to be considered in making the diagnosis of GVHD when only a few apoptotic bodies are found. For example, conditioning chemotherapy may induce epithelial cell necrosis and apoptosis (Figs. 3 and 4). Therefore, a diagnosis of GVHD should not be based solely on the presence of apoptotic bodies

Gastric Graft-Versus-Host Disease, Table 1 Traditional grading of acute gastric GVHD

Grade 1	Isolated apoptotic epithelial cells, without gland loss
Grade 2	Loss of isolated glands, without loss of contiguous glands
Grade 3	Loss of two or more contiguous glands
Grade 4	Extensive glandular loss with mucosal denudation

Gastric Graft-Versus-Host Disease, Table 2 Reporting template of the National Institutes of Health

Not GVHD	No histologic evidence for GVHD
Possible GVHD	Evidence of GVHD but other possible etiologies for the findings, such as CMV infection, MMF-associated colitis, or other features suggesting a drug reaction
Consistent with GVHD	Histologic evidence of GVHD in association with mitigating factors, such as limited sampling; minimal findings (e.g., single/rare apoptotic epithelial cells); recent chemotherapy or radiotherapy; or a CMV-infected biopsy with abundant apoptosis not associated with the infection
GVHD	Unequivocal evidence of GVHD

MMF mycophenolate mofetil

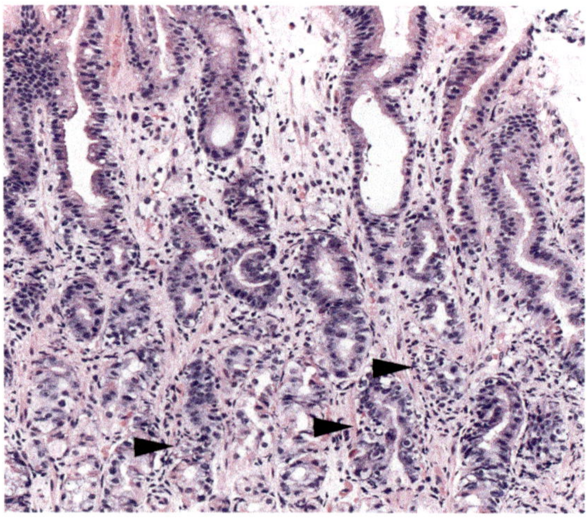

Gastric Graft-Versus-Host Disease, Fig. 1 This low power image illustrates preserved gastric mucosa with mild edema of the lamina propria and limited inflammation. However, multiple apoptotic bodies are identified predominantly in the neck region (*arrowhead*) (GVHD grade 1)

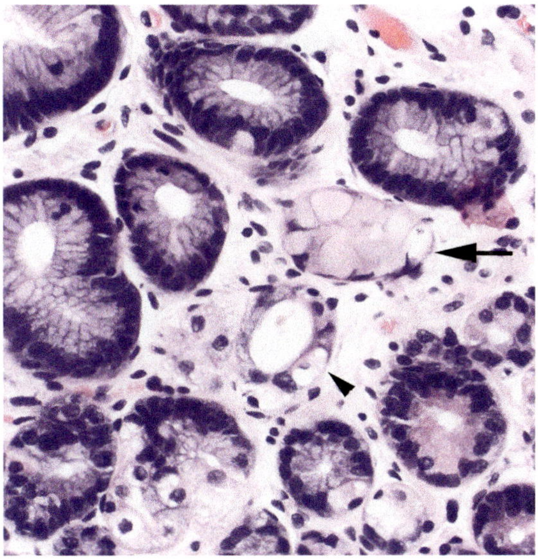

Gastric Graft-Versus-Host Disease, Fig. 2 While many of the gastric pits are preserved, subtle evidence consistent with GVHD grade 1 is noted. Please note in the center of the field the attenuated glandular structure, while in other pit regions, damage with ballooned epithelial cells can be noted

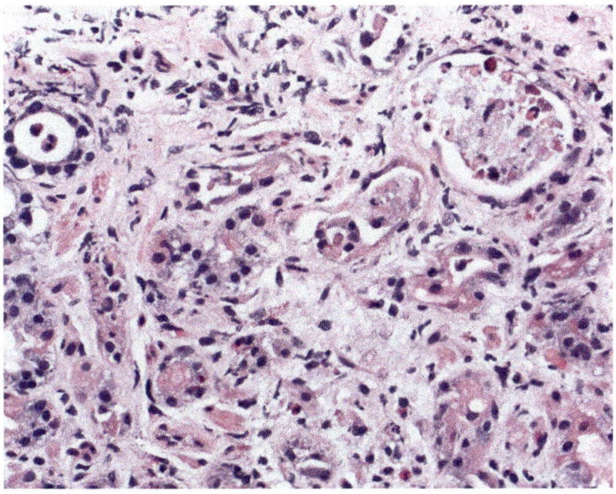

Gastric Graft-Versus-Host Disease, Fig. 3 Biopsy with unequivocal evidence of GVHD. Prominent apoptosis is readily identified, with several glands and pits variably involved with numerous apoptotic bodies. One gland is filled with necrotic debris and is identified only by a residual rim of attenuated epithelial cells (*right upper* quadrant) (GVHD grade 2)

within the first 3 weeks post transplantation. CMV infection, a common complication in immunosuppressed patients, also can induce apoptotic degeneration.

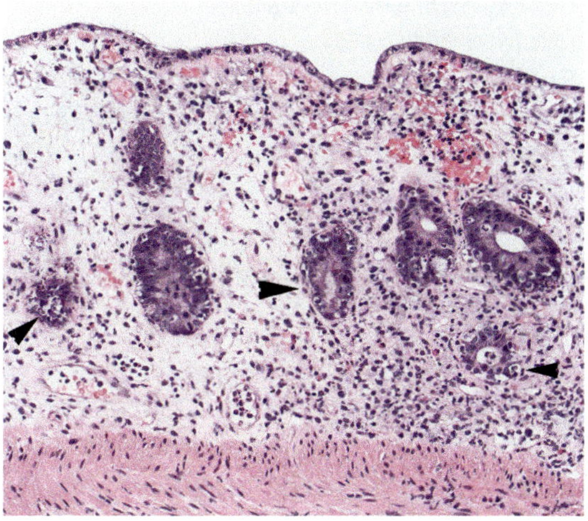

Gastric Graft-Versus-Host Disease, Fig. 4 Severe GVHD with markedly attenuated architecture. Only residual glands are identified. Numerous apoptotic bodies are identified (GVHD grade 3)

- The inflammatory infiltrate of the lamina propria is typically sparse and consists primarily of mononuclear cells; scattered eosinophils and neutrophils may be seen. A pattern of focally enhanced gastritis has been reported as well.
- Fibrosis of the lamina propria, marked architectural distortion, gland distortion and/or loss, and Paneth cell metaplasia develop with longstanding GVHD. Clusters of endocrine cell nests may be the only residual cells observed in advanced cases.
- Practically, it is worth underscoring that the microscopic features of GVHD can be patchy. Therefore, evaluation of multiple biopsy samples and evaluation of several levels are important before excluding such a diagnosis.

Immunophenotype

Immunohistochemical evaluation to exclude CMV infection is important to review in suspected cases. Caspase 3 immunohistochemistry has been used by some investigators for detecting apoptosis.

Differential Diagnosis

Several conditions ought to be ruled out when considering a diagnosis of gastric GVHD. These include

- Cytoreactive chemotherapy (conditioning)–induced gastritis and epithelial apoptosis. The damage is seen within the first 2–3 weeks after transplant.
- Mycophenolate mofetil effect. The histology can be identical to GVHD. Microscopically, the presence of dilated gastric glands with numerous eosinophils will favor this diagnosis.
- Infections. Cytomegalovirus, adenovirus, and cryptosporidiosis all can induce apoptosis. Proper use of special stains is helpful. The presence of neutrophils should alert to a possible bacterial infection

References and Further Reading

Cruz-Correa, M., et al. (2002). Endoscopic findings predict the histologic diagnosis in gastrointestinal graft-versus-host disease. *Endoscopy, 34*(10), 808–813.

Holmberg, L., Kikuchi, K., Gooley, T. A., et al. (2006). Gastrointestinal graft-versus-host disease in recipients of autologous hematopoietic stem cells: Incidence, risk factors, and outcome. *Biology of Blood and Marrow Transplantation, 12*, 226–234.

Ross, W. A., et al. (2008). Endoscopic biopsy diagnosis of acute gastrointestinal graft-versus-host disease: Rectosigmoid biopsies are more sensitive than upper gastrointestinal biopsies. *The American Journal of Gastroenterology, 103*(4), 982–989.

Shulman, H. M., et al. (2006). Histopathologic diagnosis of chronic graft-versus-host disease: National Institutes of Health Consensus Development Project on Criteria for Clinical Trials in Chronic Graft-versus-Host Disease: II. Pathology Working Group Report. *Biology of Blood and Marrow Transplantation, 12*(1), 31–47.

Thompson, B., et al. (2006). Prospective endoscopic evaluation for gastrointestinal graft-versus-host disease: Determination of the best diagnostic approach. *Bone Marrow Transplantation, 38*(5), 371–376.

Gastric Heterotopia

Helena Baldaia
Serviço de Anatomia Patológica, Centro Hospitalar de São João, Porto, Portugal

Synonyms

Inlet patch (upper esophagus)

Definition

Heterotopia is defined as the occurrence of normal tissue in an abnormal location. The presence of displaced gastric mucosa occurs throughout the gastrointestinal (GI) tract, from the tongue to the rectum (Hayama et al. 2010).

The precise pathogenic mechanism is yet unknown, although a congenital origin has often been advocated (Tang et al. 2004). Other authors defend, particularly in the upper esophagus, that the gastric mucosa originates as a metaplastic end-product in response to aggressive stimuli to the local mucosa (Fenoglio-Preiser et al. 2008a). In one study, esophageal gastric heterotopia was associated with Barrett's esophagus in 20% of the biopsies studied (Tang et al. 2004).

Gastric heterotopia can occur alone but is frequently associated with congenital anomalies. It occurs in association with duplications, diverticula (being commonly present in Meckel diverticulum), heterotopic pancreas, vertebral body defects, and megacolon (Fenoglio-Preiser et al. 2008b).

Gastric heterotopia is frequently asymptomatic. However, especially in the presence of parietal cells, symptoms such as dysphagia, intestinal obstruction, GI bleeding with ulceration, or stricture formation can occur (Fenoglio-Preiser et al. 2008c). When it occurs in the gallbladder, right upper quadrant abdominal pain, nausea, vomiting, or sometimes symptoms associated with biliary obstruction or jaundice can occur (Hayama et al. 2010).

Clinical Features

- **Incidence**
  The incidence of gastric heterotopia is variable. In the upper esophagus, it occurs in 1–21% of the population (Fenoglio-Preiser et al. 2008a), although meticulous autopsy studies have found an incidence in up to 70% of cases (Fu and Rueda-Pedraza 2012). In the colorectal area, it is very rare (Sousa et al. 2010), even if it is the most common heterotopia occuring in the large intestine (Fenoglio-Preiser et al. 2008b). In the gallbladder, it is extremely rare (Hayama et al. 2010).
- **Age**
  Gastric heterotopia is found in every age group, although, in the esophagus, it has been reported as being more common in the first year of life (Fu and Rueda-Pedraza 2012). One study found the median age of the patients with anorectal gastric heterotopia to be 21 years (Sousa et al. 2010).
- **Sex**
  There is no gender predilection in most of the reported cases (Fu and Rueda-Pedraza 2012), although in one study on anorectal gastric heterotopia, there was a slight male predominance (Sousa et al. 2010).
- **Site**
  As mentioned earlier, gastric heterotopia can occur throughout the GI tract (Hayama et al. 2010). In the esophagus, inlet patch refers to gastric heterotopic mucosa in the proximal portion of that organ (Fu and Rueda-Pedraza 2012). In the duodenum, the most common location is the bulb (Yantiss and Antonioli 2009).
- **Treatment**
  Treatment options depend on the localization of the lesion and the presence of symptoms or complications such as ulceration or strictures. In the esophagus, both medical therapies, such as proton pump inhibitors and histamine type 2 receptor antagonists (used in symptomatic patients), and endoscopic therapies, such as endoscopic mucosal resection (EMR), have been used with success (Basseri et al. 2009). In other locations, such as the gallbladder and the anorectum, surgical treatment is usually employed (Hayama et al. 2010; Sousa et al. 2010).
- **Outcome**
  Gastric heterotopia has a good outcome. Prognosis is dependent on the presence of complications, such as strictures or ulceration. The development of adenocarcinoma in heterotopic gastric mucosa has been reported, although very rarely (Fenoglio-Preiser et al. 2008a).

Macroscopy

The macroscopic appearance is variable. Inlet patch appears as a well-demarcated patch of salmon-colored mucosa (Fu and Rueda-Pedraza 2012). Small intestinal lesions are usually small (<1.5 cm) polypoid nodules (Yantiss and Antonioli 2009), and large intestinal lesions can also appear as polyps, masses, or hemorrhoids (Fenoglio-Preiser et al. 2008). In the gallbladder, gastric heterotopia appears as polypoid lesions measuring between 0.3 and 4 cm (Hayama et al. 2010).

Microscopy

Histologically gastric heterotopia (Fig. 1) appears as tightly packed antral and oxyntic glands, architecturally normal, covered by foveolar epithelium (Fenoglio-Preiser et al. 2008; Yantiss and Antonioli 2009). Chronic and acute inflammation and ulceration may occur (Fu and Rueda-Pedraza 2012). Sometimes, particularly in polypoid lesions, as a result of repeated trauma, reactive secondary changes such as submucosal fibrosis, prominence of the muscularis mucosae, and epithelial hyperplasia may occur (Yantiss and Antonioli 2009).

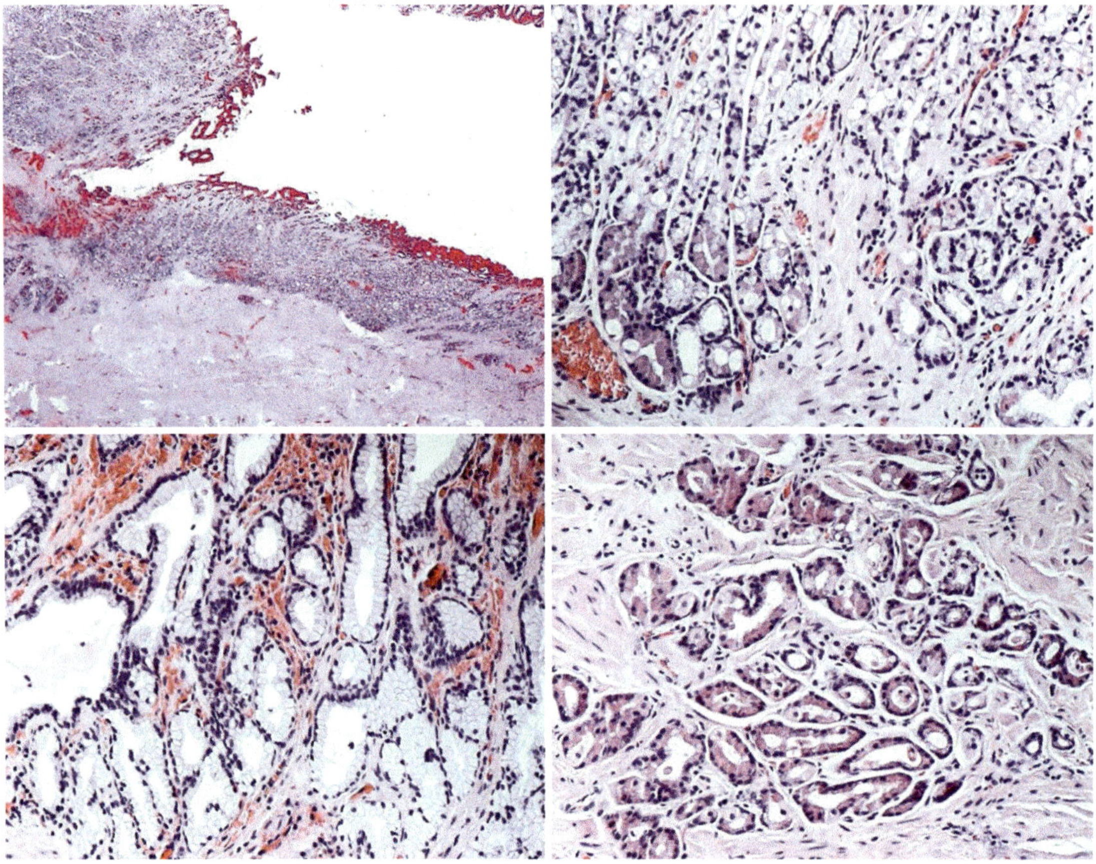

Gastric Heterotopia, Fig. 1 Gastric heterotopia in the tongue. Muscle layer of the tongue covered by tightly packed antral and oxyntic glands, architecturally normal

Molecular Features

Recent studies have suggested that the deregulation of selected homeobox genes in response to inflammatory stimuli can be involved in the pathogenesis of gastric heterotopia (Sousa et al. 2010).

Differential Diagnosis

In the esophagus, the main differential diagnosis is with Barrett's esophagus. In gastric heterotopia, however, goblet cells are not commonly present. Also, gastric heterotopia usually appears in the proximal esophagus (Fu and Rueda-Pedraza 2012).

In other locations, metaplasia is also the most important differential diagnosis. In small intestinal gastric heterotopia, the presence of oxyntic glands is a key feature to differentiate this entity from gastric metaplasia (Yantiss and Antonioli 2009). The same feature helps to distinguish metaplastic polyps from gastric heterotopia in the gallbladder (Hayama et al. 2010).

References and Further Reading

Basseri, B., Conklin, J., Mertens, R., et al. (2009). Heterotopic gastric mucosa (inlet patch) in a patient with laryngopharyngeal reflux (LPR) and laryngeal carcinoma: a case report and review of literature. *Diseases of the Esophagus, 22*, E1–E5.

Fenoglio-Preiser, C. M., Noffsinger, A. E., Stemmermann, G. N., Lantz, P. E., & Isaacson, P. G. (2008a). The nonneoplastic esophagus. In J. McGouh & J. Pine (Eds.), *Gastrointestinal pathology an atlas and text* (pp. 20–21). Philadelphia: Lippincott Williams & Wilkins.

Fenoglio-Preiser, C. M., Noffsinger, A. E., Stemmermann, G. N., Lantz, P. E., & Isaacson, P. G. (2008b). The nonneoplastic colon. In J. McGouh & J. Pine (Eds.), *Gastrointestinal pathology an atlas and text* (p. 747). Philadelphia: Lippincott Williams & Wilkins.

Fenoglio-Preiser, C. M., Noffsinger, A. E., Stemmermann, G. N., Lantz, P. E., & Isaacson, P. G. (2008c). The nonneoplastic small intestine. In J. McGouh & J. Pine (Eds.), *Gastrointestinal pathology an atlas and text* (pp. 312–313). Philadelphia: Lippincott Williams & Wilkins.

Fu, B., & Rueda-Pedraza, M. E. (2012). Non-neoplastic disorders of the esophagus. In C. A. Iacobuzio-Donahue, E. Montgomary, & J. R. Golblum (Eds.), *Gastrointestinal and liver pathology* (pp. 4–7). Philadelphia: Saunders.

Hayama, S., Suzuki, Y., Takahashi, M., et al. (2010). Heterotopic gastric mucosa in the gallbladder: Report of two cases. *Surgery Today, 40*, 783–787.

Sousa, J., Cabezuelo, L., Rodrigues, A., et al. (2010). Gastric heterotopia of rectum: A rare entity. *Acta Médica Portuguesa, 23*, 1151–1154.

Tang, P., McKinley, M. J., Sporrer, M., & Kahn, E. (2004). Inlet patch: Prevalence, histologic type, and association with esophagitis, Barrett esophagus, and antritis. *Archives of Pathology and Laboratory Medicine, 128*(4), 444–447.

Yantiss, R. K., & Antonioli, D. A. (2009). Polyps of the small intestine. In R. Odze & J. Goldblum (Eds.), *Surgical pathology of the GI tract, liver, biliary tract and pancreas*. Philadelphia: Saunders.

Gastric Stump

Chella R. S. van der Post[1] and Fátima Carneiro[2]
[1]Department of Pathology, Radboud University Medical Center, Nijmegen, The Netherlands
[2]Faculty of Medicine of Porto University, Centro Hospitalar São João and Ipatimup/i3S, Porto, Portugal

Synonyms

Gastric remnant; Gastroenterostoma

Definition

The gastric stump is defined as the part of the stomach that remains after partial resection. The gastroenterostomy area, either gastroduodenostomy (after Billroth-I) or gastrojejunostomy (after Billroth-II surgery), is important since there is an increased risk of developing (pre-)neoplastic conditions after remote partial gastrectomy. Gastric stump carcinoma or gastric remnant cancer is defined as a gastric carcinoma occurring in the gastric remnant at least 5 years after surgery for benign peptic ulcer disease. Many studies have confirmed the increased risk of developing gastric cancer in the gastric stump. Sometimes the term "gastric stump carcinoma" is used more broadly to refer to all cancers arising in the remnant stomach after partial gastrectomy, regardless of the initial disease or operation, and includes local recurrence in the gastric stump after prior partial gastrectomy for gastric cancer. In the latter, it seems better to refer to recurrence of cancer since malignant disease presumably originates from (pre-)cancerous conditions that already existed before the initial operation and these cancers are presumably metachronous lesions or recurrence of disease.

Peptic ulcer surgery has dramatically decreased because of the introduction of H2-receptor antagonists, proton pump inhibitors, and the discovery of *Helicobacter pylori* (*H. pylori*). Despite the fact that conservative medical therapy has long replaced partial gastrectomy for the treatment of ulcer, the incidence of gastric stump carcinoma is not yet declining, due to the long latency period. Since surgical therapy was still used frequently for the treatment of gastroduodenal ulcer disease until the 1970–1980s, and the fact that cancer develops with a time interval of 20–40 years, these cancers will be seen at least until 2015–2020 on a regular basis. Currently, there are still indications for distal gastric resection, such as distal carcinoma, perforation, refractory bleeding, or recurrent ulcer with outlet obstruction of the stomach. The risk of developing gastric stump cancer rapidly increases with time, leading to a 4–7 fold higher incidence than the general population. The time interval is one of the most important factors for the development of a gastric stump carcinoma, because the gastric remnant is constantly under carcinogenic influence.

Factors involved in the etiology of gastric stump carcinoma include:

- Chronic damage caused by duodenogastric reflux containing bile and pancreatic juice.
- Antrectomy, leading to decreased gastrin production and resulting in less acid production.
- Denervation by vagotomy, also leading to hypochlorhydria.
- Epstein-Barr virus positivity, which is more often seen in gastric stump carcinomas.
- Possible endogenous factors: The interleukin-1β 31T > C polymorphism is associated with an increased risk of developing gastric stump carcinoma.

Surgery performed for peptic ulcer disease include a two-third gastric resection with Billroth-II reconstruction with an antecolic short afferent jejunal loop without a Braun's anastomosis. The Billroth-I procedure was used less frequently. Changes to the anastomotic site are already apparent shortly after surgery, but less when a Roux-en-Y conversion has been carried out to avoid reflux.

The two main factors responsible for changes in the gastric remnant are chronic damage secondary to duodenogastric reflux of bile and pancreatic juice, and hypochlorhydria subsequent to denervation by vagotomy and antrectomy which lead to lower levels of gastrin important for the stimulation of acid production in the corpus. The chronic duodenogastric reflux initiates tumor progression with chronic atrophic gastritis and leads to intestinal metaplasia, dysplasia/adenoma, and eventually carcinoma. It is not yet known which specific components of the reflux are responsible for the damage in the remnant. Bile acids like deoxycholic bile acid show a co-carcinogenic effect and may contribute to the carcinogenesis in the gastric stump. The associated gastric atrophy causes hypochlorhydria and an increasing pH-value, resulting in growth of bacteria in the gastric stump. Especially anaerobic bacteria can reduce dietary nitrates to nitrites. Nitrites in the presence of substrates, such as proteins of food, can lead to the formation of potent carcinogens. This assumption of a circulating carcinogen is supported by the observation that there is an increased risk of developing cancer in locations other than the gastric stump, in particular the increased risk of developing colon and pancreas carcinoma after a time interval of 15–20 years.

The role of *H. pylori* in the development of gastric stump carcinoma seems to be minimal. The rate of infection ranges between 23% and 28% and is rather low compared to 54–71% in primary gastric carcinoma. The lower rate of infection is probably caused by the duodenal reflux that leads to a reduction of *H. pylori* in the gastric stump.

Clinical Features

- **Incidence**
  The proportion of gastric stump carcinoma ranges from 1% to 5% of all gastric carcinomas. In recent years, the incidence of gastric stump carcinoma has been increasing, because of the long latency period and the frequent performance of partial gastrectomy in the previous decades. When compared to a matched control population, the risk of developing gastric stump carcinoma is increased 4–7 fold after a time interval of at least 20 years.
- **Age**
  Most patients are above 60 years of age, and generally around 70–80 years, since the average latency time after surgery is around 20–40 years.
- **Sex**
  Men are four to nine times more frequently affected by gastric stump carcinoma than women. The reason for this could be the higher frequency of ulcer disease and resections in men, but until now, a definite explanation for this phenomenon could not be found.
- **Site**
  The gastric remnant and pouch are most at risk. Most carcinomas are diagnosed in the distal residual stomach and at the gastric stoma site. Accompanying dysplasia is often observed elsewhere in the residual pouch.

- **Treatment**
  Periodic screening by gastroscopy, initiating 15 years after partial gastrectomy, improves detection of tumors at a curable stage. The surgical treatment for gastric stump carcinoma should include complete resection of the carcinoma in the gastric remnant with an en-bloc resection of the prior gastroduodenal (Billroth-I) or gastrojejunal (Billroth-II) anastomosis. Another important factor for an adequate treatment is a radical lymph node dissection with regard to the altered lymph drainage of the gastric stump with particular attention to potential pathways along the left gastric, splenic arteries and jejunal mesentery. Roux and Y procedure is the recommended reconstruction method particularly for the patients with early gastric cancer and long life expectancy, since it best keeps duodenal contents away from the remnant stomach.
- **Outcome**
  Gastric stump carcinoma is often described as a tumor with a poor prognosis since most tumors are at presentation in advanced stage. This leads to a low resection rate (38–40%) because of extended lymph node metastases and infiltration of adjacent organs. The reported 5-year disease-specific overall survival ranges from 7% to 20% in literature.

Macroscopy

At endoscopy, various changes can be encountered in the gastric stump including redness, erosions, atrophy, and xanthelasmas that present as white-yellow nodules or plaques of a few millimeters. Gastric remnant cancer can present as an obstructive ulcerative or polypoid tumor, or as a diffuse carcinoma (Fig. 1).

Microscopy

Histological features that can be identified in the gastric stump preceding carcinoma include atrophy, foveolar hyperplasia, cystic dilation of glands, intestinal metaplasia, dysplasia, and adenoma (Figs. 2 and 3). The gastric stump is

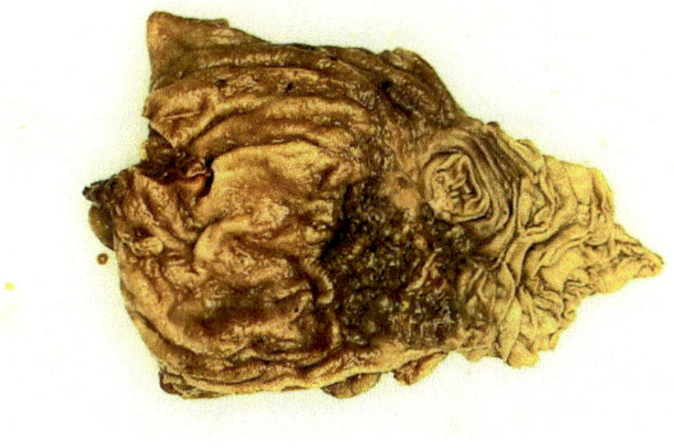

Gastric Stump, Fig. 1 Opened macroscopic resection of the anastomotic site, a brown, irregular tumor is present at the transition from stomach to jejunum

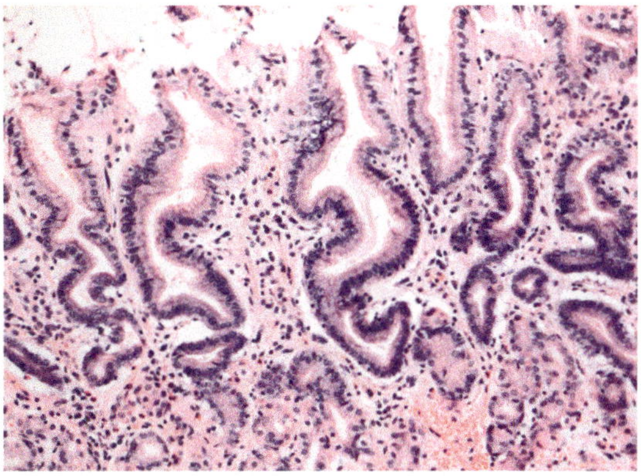

Gastric Stump, Fig. 2 Gastric stump with features of foveolar hyperplasia and mild chronic inflammation (H&E, original magnification 200×)

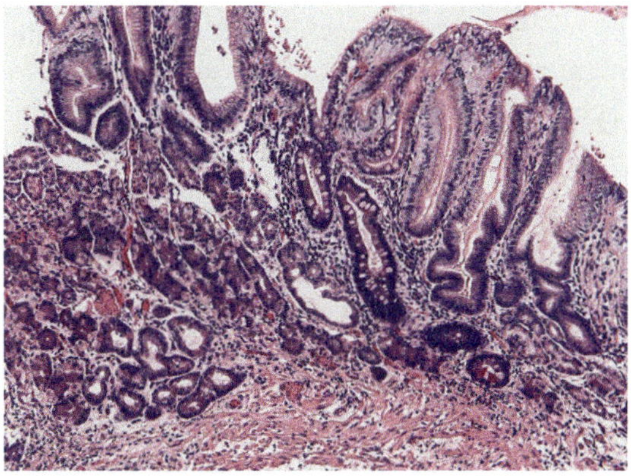

Gastric Stump, Fig. 3 Gastric stump with intestinal metaplasia, hyperchromasia of nuclei, and cystic dilation of glands (H&E, original magnification 100×)

most commonly associated with chronic gastritis and atrophy of the gastric mucosa, while the extent of intestinal metaplasia and the incidence of *H. Pylori* infections are less compared with usual gastric adenocarcinoma. It is thought that a microenvironment is created by bile reflux that is not suitable for *H. pylori* and this will eradicate the microorganisms from the anastomosis after surgery. The microscopy of the anastomosis will therefore change from the chronic active *H. pylori* gastritis picture into that of the typical reflux gastritis. The most important features of reflux gastritis are foveolar hyperplasia, congestion, paucity of inflammatory infiltrate, reactive epithelial change, and smooth muscle fiber proliferation. In the long run, other microscopic features are encountered in the operated stomach. Loss of parietal cells with subsequent disappearance of chief cells introduces an accelerated mucosal atrophy that is caused by vagotomy and the lack of the hormone gastrin. The specialized glandular mucosa is replaced by intestinal metaplasia and pseudopyloric metaplasia. Atrophy of the gastric mucosa may lead to vitamin B12 deficiency. At the anastomotic site, the glands often become cystically dilated, and sometimes these dilated glands herniate through the muscularis mucosae. This provides a nodular aspect to the anastomosis and gives rise to a microscopic picture known as gastritis cystica polyposa/profunda. Erosions may occur as a result of compromised vasculature due to the surgery, but in the case of persistent ulceration after surgery, Zollinger-Ellison-like syndrome or a retained antrum needs consideration; high gastrin levels accompany these conditions. The retained antrum is caused by resection that is too limited and G-cell hyperplasia in the stretch of antral mucosa left behind. Xanthelasmas, also known as gastric xanthomas or gastric lipid islands, are aggregates of foamy macrophages filled with lipids that can be seen more often after partial gastrectomy and need to be distinguished from signet ring cell carcinomas.

It has been hypothesized that depending on the localization of the tumor in the gastric stump, one of the following two pathogenetic mechanisms are more responsible for the outcome. In the region of the anastomosis, duodenogastric reflux is responsible for the development of premalignant lesions involving adenocystic proliferation. This lesion expresses the gastric phenotype and develops into diffuse type carcinoma. In the body of the gastric stump, dysplasia may develop, which progressively loses its gastric phenotype. As a result, intestinal type carcinoma develops. This process is especially promoted by the denervation of the gastric stump.

Differential Diagnosis

- In the differential diagnosis of gastric stump, carcinoma is a local recurrence or metastases in the gastric stump after prior partial gastrectomy for gastric cancer.
- Gastritis cystica polyposa is characterized by the presence of entrapped glands into the muscularis mucosa and submucosa, and can mimic carcinoma. Gastritis cystica polyposa generally will not penetrate into the deep muscularis propria or serosa. Other features to consider adenocarcinoma are presence of nearby dysplasia, marked pleomorphism in the glands, (intraluminal) necrosis, high proliferation, and stromal desmoplasia.

References and Further Reading

MacDonald, W. C., & Owen, D. A. (2001). Gastric carcinoma after surgical treatment of peptic ulcer: An analysis of morphologic features and a comparison with cancer in the nonoperated stomach. *Cancer, 91*(9), 1732–1738.

Offerhaus, G. J., van de Stadt, J., Huibregtse, K., Tersmette, A. C., & Tytgat, G. N. (1989). The mucosa of the gastric remnant harboring malignancy. Histologic findings in the biopsy specimens of 504 asymptomatic patients 15 to 46 years after partial gastrectomy with emphasis on nonmalignant lesions. *Cancer, 64*(3), 698–703.

Sinning, C., Schaefer, N., Standop, J., Hirner, A., & Wolff, M. (2007). Gastric stump carcinoma – epidemiology and current concepts in pathogenesis and treatment. *European Journal of Surgical Oncology, 33*(2), 133–139.

Sitarz, R., Maciejewski, R., Polkowski, W. P., & Offerhaus, G. J. (2012). Gastroenterostoma after Billroth antrectomy as a premalignant condition. *World Journal of Gastroenterology, 18*(25), 3201–3206.

Gastric Xanthelasma

Xiaogang Wen
Centro hospitalar de Vila Nova de Gaia/Espinho, Institute of Molecular Pathology and Immunology of the University of Porto, Porto, Portugal

Synonyms

Gastric xanthoma

Definition

Gastric xanthelasma is a sharply demarcated yellowish accumulation of lipid-containing macrophages (xanthomatous cells) within the gastric mucosa. They may develop in the setting of cholestasis and hypercholesterolemia.

Clinical Features

- **Prevalence**
  The reported prevalence of upper gastrointestinal xanthelasma is 0.23%. Approximately 76% of the lesions are located in the stomach, particularly in the antrum and the pyloric region (70%).
- **Age**
  The incidence increases with age, reaching the highest values between 40 and 60 years of age.
- **Sex**
  Xanthelasma seems to be more frequent in women, though there are some discrepancies in the literatures regarding gender predilection.
- **Site**
  Most lesions localize in the antrum and the pylorus.
- **Treatment**
  The lesion itself does not cause symptoms and does not need treatment. However, it is often associated with duodenal reflux, chronic gastritis, gastric surgery, or even cancer. The treatment of the primary gastrointestinal disorders may cure this disorder.

Macroscopy

The lesions have a circular-oval, yellowish-white appearance, are between 0.5 and 10 mm in size, and are multiple in 13–24% of the cases; 17% of the patients have more than five lesions.

Microscopy

The lesions consist of collections of lipid-containing macrophages (xanthomatous cells) arranged in pavement-like patterns in the upper lamina propria immediately beneath the surface epithelium (Fig. 1). The xanthomatous cells contain foamy, finely vacuolated cytoplasm and are PAS negative.

Immunohistochemistry

The lesion stains with the macrophage marker CD68 (KP1).

Differential Diagnosis

Signet ring cell carcinoma: signet ring cell carcinoma can mimic the xanthoma lesion especially in its early stage. However, signet ring cells

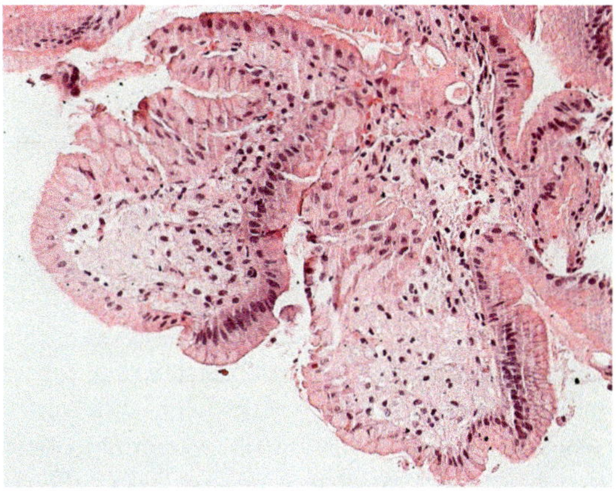

Gastric Xanthelasma, Fig. 1 The lesions consist of collections of xanthomatous cells, localized in the upper lamina propria immediately beneath the surface epithelium

contain more or less homogeneously stained mucin vacuoles and hyperchromatic (sometimes polymorphic) and eccentrically placed nuclei, which are different from the foamy cytoplasm and pyknotic, centrally placed nuclei of the xanthomatous cells. The cytokeratins and PAS staining are very useful in the differential diagnosis, which are positive in the carcinoma.

Granular cell tumor: the tumor cells contain eosinophilic granular cytoplasm and are positive for S100 protein staining and negative for CD68.

References and Further Reading

Gürsoy, S., Yurci, A., Torun, E., Soyuer, I., Güven, K., Ozbakir, O., & Yücesoy, M. (2005). An uncommon lesion: gastric xanthelasma. *The Turkish Journal of Gastroenterology, 16*(3), 167–170.

Gastritis Cystica Polyposa/Profunda

Chella R. S. van der Post[1] and Fátima Carneiro[2]
[1]Department of Pathology, Radboud University Medical Center, Nijmegen, The Netherlands
[2]Faculty of Medicine of Porto University, Centro Hospitalar São João and Ipatimup/i3S, Porto, Portugal

Synonyms

Gastritis cystica profunda; Gastritis cystica superficialis; Polypoid cystic gastritis; Stomal polypoid hypertrophic gastritis

Definition

Gastritis cystica polyposa is defined as a polypoid lesion or mass in the gastric wall, most often around a gastroenterostomy site, containing elongated gastric foveolae and cystically dilated glands extending into the muscularis mucosa and submucosa. In literature, similar findings are described under several synonymic terms. Gastritis cystica polyposa or profunda is the most commonly used name for this disorder. The lesion is better defined as "polyposa" when an intraluminal polyp is present and "profunda" when the bulk of the lesion is located in the wall of the stomach.

Gastritis cystica polyposa is considered to be a mucosal prolapsed condition caused by several factors, such as chronic inflammation, ischemia, presence of foreign material, and prior gastric surgery. Previous partial gastrectomy can lead to mucosal damage in the remnant stomach due to bile reflux, chronic inflammation, and ischemia. The lesion almost always occurs on the gastric side of the anastomosis. The chronic inflammation leads to a reactive proliferation with trauma-induced entrapment of epithelium in deep portions of the gastric wall. Direct surgical effects with an interruption of the muscularis mucosaes could also allow migration of epithelial elements into the submucosa. Gastritis cystica polyposa has been suggested to be a precancerous lesion, because dysplasia or carcinoma is frequently found in the superficial mucosa and the histological features of gastritis cystica polyposa resemble experimental stomal polyps preceding carcinoma after partial gastrectomy in rats.

The first report of gastritis cystica polyposa by Littler and Gleibermann in 1972 described a patient with clinical symptoms of obstruction caused by a cystic glandular mass at a gastroenteric anastomosis. Since then, numerous cases have been described of patients with gastritis cystic polyposa previously undergoing partial gastrectomy, especially for benign peptic ulcer disease. There are also case reports describing gastritis cystica polyposis in patients without previous gastric surgery. Some authors have suggested that this condition could be better termed "heterotopic submucosal cysts" or "mucosal prolapse." The mechanism of the development of gastritis cystica polyposa in the unoperated stomach is unclear; probably, it is also caused by chronic inflammation with weakening of the gastric wall that allows gastric gland migration into the submucosa. This lesion shares the same histological features of gastritis cystica polyposa and is also associated with development of gastric cancer probably due to chronic (*Helicobacter pylori*-associated) inflammation.

Clinical Features

- **Incidence**
  The exact incidence of gastritis cystica polyposa is unknown. It is considered to be a rare lesion and can develop 3–40 years after prior gastric surgery.
- **Age**
  Around or above 70 years of age.
- **Sex**
  There seems to be predominance in men.
- **Site**
  The lesions presents near gastroenterostomy stomal sites and can develop several years after gastroenterostomies (Billroth I and II surgeries) for benign peptic ulcer disease or adenocarcinoma.
- **Treatment**
  To exclude adenoma or adenocarcinoma, the lesion has to be removed. However, follow-up with endoscopy and biopsies for dysplasia and cancer surveillance is also a possible strategy.
- **Outcome**
  Gastritis cystica polyposa may result in substantial gastric bleeding, warranting acute surgical exploration. It has been associated with dysplasia and gastric stump carcinoma. However, it is still unclear whether gastritis cystica polyposa is a precancerous condition or just a combined phenomenon in the background of carcinogenic circumstances such as mucosal damage due to chronic atrophic gastritis.

Macroscopy

Gastritis cystica polyposa presents on CT scan as an exophytic or endophytic mass with cystic components around the stomal site. Grossly and endoscopically, single or multiple, soft, sessile 1–3-cm polypoid lesions are located around gastric anastomotic sites. These polyps can measure up to 10 cm in diameter and present as a confluent circumferential mass. The overlying mucosa is sometimes red, and often associated with enlarged rugal folds. A thickened gastric wall with numerous cystic glands is seen in cut sections.

Microscopy

Histologically, the most obvious feature is the presence of entrapped glands into disorganized strands of muscularis mucosa and submucosa (Figs. 1 and 2). The glands resemble pyloric glands and are lined by cuboidal to columnar, mucin-containing epithelium. Sometimes the glands contain parietal cells. They are often irregularly and cystically dilated and surrounded by lamina propria-like stroma. In the stroma, there is edema with chronic inflammation, fibrosis and scarring with thickened and splayed muscle bundles. The background gastric mucosa shows enlarged foveolae and an atrophic appearance with reactive changes, hyperplasia, and mucin depletion. There is often chronic active inflammatory infiltrate with

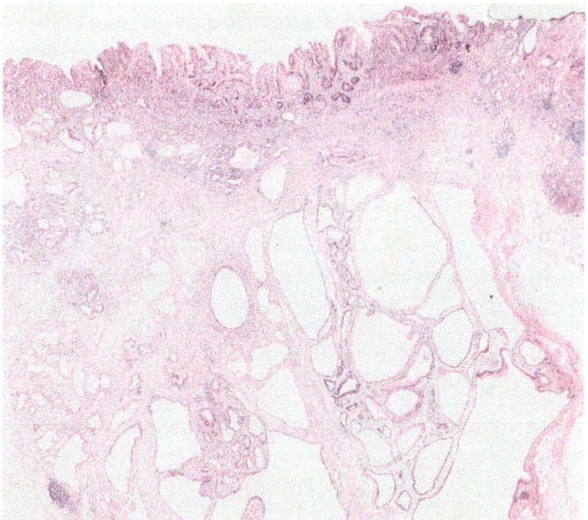

Gastritis Cystica Polyposa/Profunda, Fig. 1 Gastritis cystica profunda characterized by cystically dilated glands extending through the muscularis mucosa into the submucosa. The overlying mucosa shows features of gastric stump with enlarged foveolae, reactive changes, hyperplasia, and chronic active inflammatory infiltrate

G

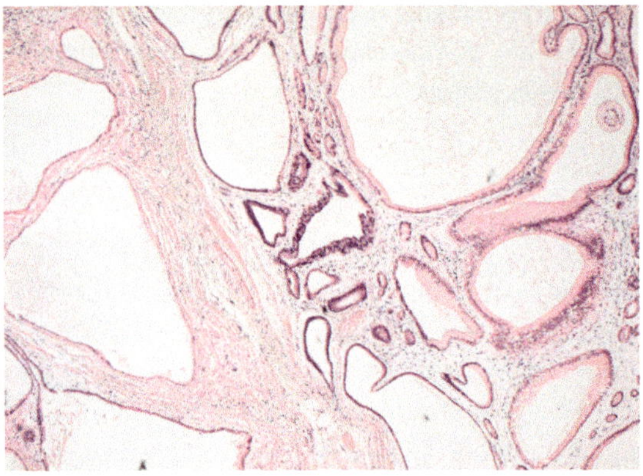

Gastritis Cystica Polyposa/Profunda, Fig. 2 High power shows dilated glands, between smooth muscle bundles, lined by cuboidal to columnar, mucin-containing epithelium without cytonuclear atypia, pleomorphism, or high mitotic activity

mononuclear cells and neutrophils and sometimes presence of *Helicobacter pylori*.

Dysplasia and carcinoma may develop in or near the herniated glands. But it is sometimes difficult to distinguish the cystically entrapped glands from invasive adenocarcinoma. Since patients with gastric stumps are at increased risk for developing both gastric carcinoma and gastritis cystica polyposa, this differentiation is important. Features to consider adenocarcinoma are presence of nearby dysplasia, marked pleomorphism in the glands, (intraluminal) necrosis, high proliferation, and stromal desmoplasia. Gastritis cystica polyposa generally will not penetrate into the deep muscularis propria or serosa. Gastric cancer in patients with gastritis cystica polyposa develops more often in older age and men. In these cancers, there is a possible association with Epstein Barr virus infection.

Differential Diagnosis

- Stump carcinoma: the presence of cystically dilated and irregular glands deep in the submucosa and muscularis propria can be mistaken for invasive adenocarcinoma. Histological features to differentiate are described above.
- Grossly, the polypoid lesion can resemble an adenoma or hyperplastic polyp.

References and Further Reading

Choi, M. G., Jeong, J. Y., Kim, K. M., Bae, J. M., Noh, J. H., Sohn, T. S., et al. (2012). Clinical significance of gastritis cystica profunda and its association with Epstein-Barr virus in gastric cancer. *Cancer, 118*(21), 5227–5233.

Kurland, J., DuBois, S., Behling, C., & Savides, T. (2006). Severe upper-GI bleed caused by gastritis cystica profunda. *Gastrointestinal Endoscopy, 63*(4), 716–717.

Littler, E. R., & Gleibermann, E. (1972). Gastritis cystica polyposa. (Gastric mucosal prolapse at gastroenterostomy site, with cystic and infiltrative epithelial hyperplasia). *Cancer, 29*(1), 205–209.

Park, C. H., Park, J. M., Jung, C. K., Kim, D. B., Kang, S. H., Lee, S. W., et al. (2009). Early gastric cancer associated with gastritis cystica polyposa in the unoperated stomach treated by endoscopic submucosal dissection. *Gastrointestinal Endoscopy, 69*(6), e47–e50.

Gastroesophageal Junction

Namrata Setia[1] and Gregory Y. Lauwers[2]
[1]Department of Pathology, Massachusetts General Hospital, Boston, MA, USA
[2]Department of Pathology, Massachusetts General Hospital, Harvard Medical School, Boston, MA, USA

Synonyms

EGJ; Esophagogastric junction; GEJ; Oesophagogastric junction; OGJ

Definition

The gastroesophageal junction (GEJ) is the point where the esophageal mucosa interfaces with the gastric mucosa. It has been defined anatomically, physiologically, radiologically, endoscopically, and histologically. Nevertheless, to date, there is no universally accepted definition of the GEJ, even though one is needed in order to diagnose Barrett esophagus appropriately. Physiologically, the GEJ corresponds to the lower esophageal sphincter (area of high pressure). In a healthy individual, it ideally will correspond to the endoscopic GEJ and the microscopic squamocolumnar junction (SCJ).

Macroscopy

Anatomically, in resection specimens and autopsy studies, the GEJ is defined as the line between the angles of the opened esophagus and the greater curvature of the stomach. Endoscopically, in most Western countries, the GEJ is defined as "the upper limit of the gastric longitudinal mucosal folds." In Japan, the GEJ is defined instead as "the lower limit of the palisade longitudinal vessels." Thus, following the Japanese approach, the detection of palisading vessels seen through salmon pink epithelium is diagnostic of Barrett esophagus.

However, both methods are fraught with limitations. The Japanese method is suboptimal in the setting of gastroesophageal reflux, which leads to mucosal cloudiness and redness limiting the detection of the palisading vessels. The use of the proximal end of the gastric folds as a defining criterion is also limited. The folds can be flattened artificially with overinflation of the stomach during endoscopy and changed during respiration, thus reducing their detection. This endoscopic landmark is also altered when a hiatal hernia has developed.

Microscopy

Histologically, the SCJ can be defined as the most distal end of the squamous epithelium and deep esophageal glands and ducts. Large veins exceeding 100 μm in diameter (corresponding to palisading vessels) are also observed in the lamina propria. In a healthy person, the histologic SCJ should correspond to the endoscopic GEJ. However, it has been seen that the endoscopic and histologic landmarks often do not correspond. This hiatus has been reported differently in Asian and Caucasian patients in two autopsy studies. In a series of 21 cases, Bombeck et al. reported a distance ranging from 5 to 21 mm (mean 11 mm) between the SCJ and the endoscopic GEJ, whereas in a Japanese series of 50 cases, this distance ranged from 0 to 10 mm. In pathologic states such as in patients with hiatal hernia or Barrett esophagus, the SCJ is displaced even further upwards from the GEJ.

The Z line, i.e., the line between the esophagus and stomach mucosa, is irregular. Three histologic junctional patterns have been reported: (1) an abrupt transition between the two mucosae; (2) a band of squamous epithelium overlapping the gastric cardiac glands that continuously extend into the distal esophagus, forming superficial esophageal cardiac glands (seen in most Japanese patients); and (3) an upward displacement of the SCJ proximally away from the GEJ, with the distance between the SCJ and the GEJ defining the length of the Barrett esophagus.

The histology of the most proximal segment of the stomach (the cardia) comprises either true gastric cardia (composed of compact mucin-secreting glands and short pit regions) or oxyntocardiac mucosa (composed of mixed mucous/oxyntic glands) (Fig. 1). In endoscopic

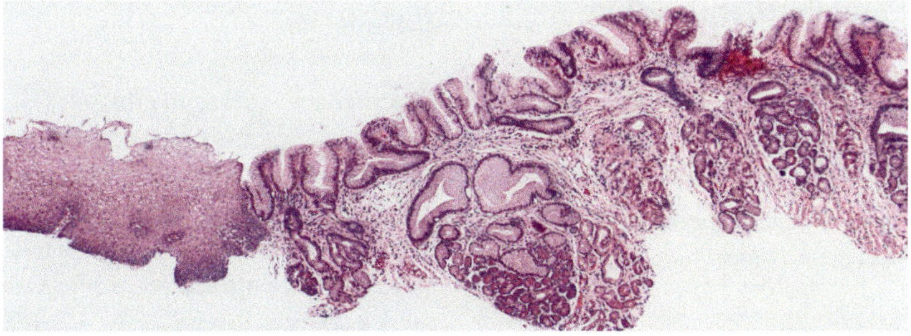

Gastroesophageal Junction, Fig. 1 Gastroesophageal junction (GE junction): an abrupt transition is seen at this GE junction, where the nonkeratinizing stratified squamous mucosa of the esophagus changes to gastric mucosa with foveolar epithelium on the surface and oxyntocardiac glands in the lamina propria

Gastroesophageal Junction, Table 1 Histologic characteristics of Barrett esophagus and gastric cardia with intestinal metaplasia

Histologic feature	BE	Carditis with IM
Squamous epithelium overlying crypts with IM	++	–
Crypt disarray	+++	++
Crypt atrophy	++	+
Incomplete IM	++++	++
Diffuse IM	++	+
Hybrid glands	+	–
Multilayered epithelium	++	+
Esophageal glands/ducts	+	–

biopsies taken from the SCJ of patients with suspected Barrett esophagus, the origin of a biopsy from the esophagus and not from the gastric cardia, with or without intestinal metaplasia, can be determined if the following histologic findings are detected: squamous islands, deep esophageal (cardial) glands and ducts, and multilayered epithelium (a stratified epithelium composed of basal squamoid cells and superficial mucin-secreting columnar cells). It usually develops at the ostium of the esophageal ducts and is considered to be a version of specialized columnar epithelium. Other histologic features more commonly associated with Barrett esophagus are architectural disarray, mucosal atrophy, and hybrid glands with intestinal metaplasia occurring only in the superficial portion of a mucous gland (Table 1).

References and Further Reading

Bombeck, C. T., Dillard, D. H., & Nyhus, L. M. (1966). Muscular anatomy of the gastroesophageal junction and role of phrenoesophageal ligament; autopsy study of sphincter mechanism. *Annals of Surgery, 164*(4), 643–654.

Odze, R. D. (2005). Pathology of the gastroesophageal junction. *Seminars in Diagnostic Pathology, 22*(4), 256–265.

Sharma, P., Dent, J., Armstrong, D., Bergman, J. J., Gossner, L., Hoshihara, Y., et al. (2006). The development and validation of an endoscopic grading system for barrett's esophagus: The prague C & M criteria. *Gastroenterology, 131*(5), 1392–1399.

Srivastava, A., Odze, R. D., Lauwers, G. Y., Redston, M., Antonioli, D. A., & Glickman, J. N. (2007). Morphologic features are useful in distinguishing barrett esophagus from carditis with intestinal metaplasia. *The American Journal of Surgical Pathology, 31*(11), 1733–1741.

Takubo, K., Arai, T., Sawabe, M., Miyashita, M., Sasajima, K., Iwakiri, K., et al. (2003). Structures of the normal esophagus and Barrett's esophagus. *Esophagus, 1*, 37–47.

Takubo, K., Aida, J., Sawabe, M., Arai, T., Kato, H., Pech, O., et al. (2008). The normal anatomy around the oesophagogastric junction: A histopathologic view and its correlation with endoscopy. *Best Practice & Research Clinical Gastroenterology, 22*(4), 569–583.

Gastroesophageal Reflux Disease (GERD)

Luis Novais[1] and Paula Chaves[2,3]
[1]Neurogastroenterology and Gastrointestinal Motility Laboratory, CEDE-Faculty of Medical Sciences, New University of Lisbon, Lisbon, Portugal
[2]Serviço de Anatomia Patológica, Instituto Português de Oncologia de Lisboa de Francisco Gentil, Lisbon, Portugal
[3]Faculdade de Ciências da Saúde, Universidade da Beira Interior, Covilhã, Portugal

Synonyms

GERD

Definition

Gastroesophageal reflux disease (GERD) includes chronic symptoms or mucosal damage caused by the abnormal reflux of gastric contents into the esophagus. Montreal consensus defined GERD as "a condition which develops when the reflux of stomach contents causes troublesome symptoms and/or complications."

Reflux esophagitis refers to a subset of GERD that has endoscopic or histological changes in the esophageal mucosa. Nonerosive reflux disease

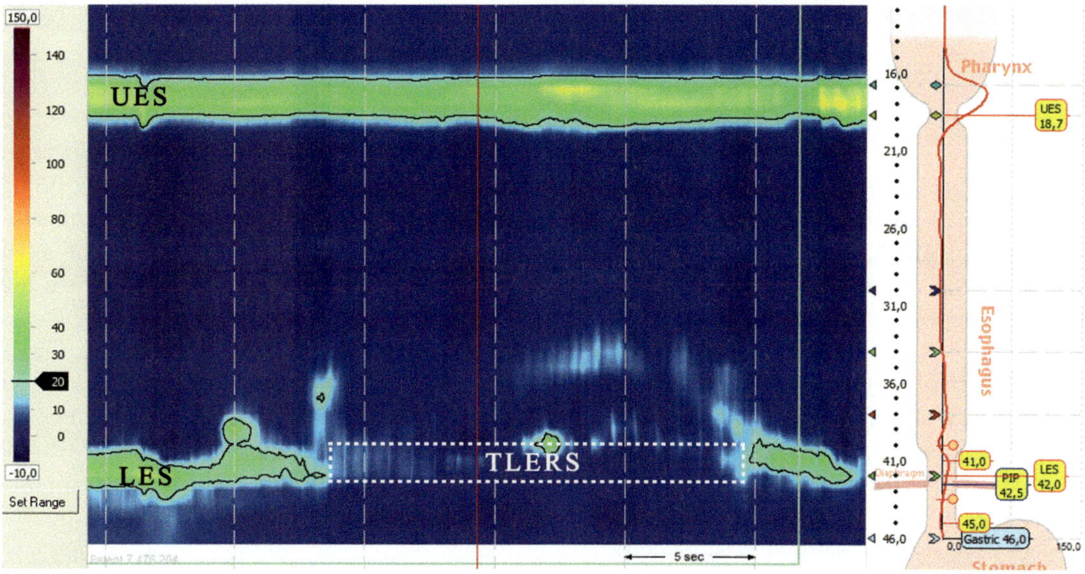

Gastroesophageal Reflux Disease (GERD), Fig. 1 Esophageal high-resolution manometry tracing. A spontaneous, transient lower esophageal sphincter relaxation (*TLERS*). The onset of TLERS is indicated by *vertical arrow*. Relaxation occurs in the absence of a swallow as manifested by the absence of pharyngeal pressure wave. The LES relaxation is complete to the level of intragastric pressure (Neurogastroenterology and Gastrointestinal Motility Laboratory, CEDE – Faculty of Medical Sciences, New University of Lisbon, Portugal). *UES* upper esophageal sphincter, *LES* lower esophageal sphincter, *TLERS* transient lower sphincter relaxation

(NERD) refers to a clinical condition that evolves with typical GERD symptoms but with normal upper endoscopic features. Barrett's esophagus (BE) is a complication of chronic GERD and is defined as an endoscopic alteration on the distal esophagus that shows intestinal metaplasia or columnar metaplasia at the biopsies, according to the American or British definition, respectively.

Clinical presentations of GERD vary considerably but can be logically grouped into three categories: typical symptoms, atypical symptoms, and complications that comprise the spectrum of GERD. Heartburn and regurgitation are typical symptoms, which are characteristically worsened after eating, by bending or stooping and by lying down in the bed at night. Atypical symptoms include angina-like chest pain, chronic hoarseness, nonallergic asthma, chronic cough, and protracted hiccups. A variety of other atypical symptoms have been suggested: globus sensation, erosion of dental enamel, and ear pain. GERD can also present with the complications of reflux, such as erosive or ulcerative esophagitis, peptic stricture, and BE.

The major mechanism of reflux in normal subjects and patients with GERD is spontaneous transient relaxation of lower esophageal sphincter (Fig. 1).

Clinical Features

- **Incidence**
  Population-based studies suggest that GERD is a common condition with a prevalence of 10–20% in Western Europe and South America, with a low prevalence in Asia and rare in Africa.
- **Age**
  Community-based studies suggest that the prevalence of reflux symptoms is much the same in adults of all ages, but the proportion of individuals who seek medical help for the symptoms increases with age.
- **Sex**
  GERD is equally prevalent in men and women; however, there is male predominance for

esophagitis (2–3:1) and BE (10:1). Pregnancy is associated with the highest incidence of GERD, with 48–79% of pregnant women complaining of heartburn.

- **Site**

  The effects of GERD are not limited to the esophagus, and esophagitis is the *sine qua non* of GERD. Erosions or ulcerations of the mucosa visualized through the endoscope are indications of reflux injury but may be subtle or absent, and it is clinically important, because many patients with GERD do not have esophagitis. The severity of reflux esophagitis is actually normally characterized by the Los Angeles classification: grade A, one or more mucosal breaks <5 mm and not contiguous with adjacent mucosal fold tops; grade B, one or more mucosal breaks >5 mm and not contiguous with adjacent mucosal fold tops; grade C, mucosal breaks contiguous between tops of two or more folds but involving <75% of esophageal circumference; and grade D, mucosal breaks contiguous between tops of two or more folds but involving >75% of esophageal circumference.

  Other sites could be affected by gastroesophageal reflux, such as the larynx, pharynx, lungs, teeth, and ears. The epithelium of the larynx is thin and is not adapted to accommodating injury from acid and pepsin. Potential laryngopharyngeal signs associated with gastroesophageal laryngitis include edema and hyperemia of larynx, hyperemia and lymphoid hyperplasia of posterior pharynx, contact ulcers, laryngeal polyps, granuloma, interarytenoid changes, subglottic stenosis, posterior glottic stenosis, Reinke's edema, and tumors. Pharyngitis, sinusitis, recurrent otitis media, and idiopathic pulmonary fibrosis were proposed as clinical conditions associated to GERD.

- **Treatment**

  The goals of any GERD therapy are to control symptoms, heal the esophageal mucosa, and prevent GERD-related complications. The management of GERD follows a hierarchy that advances through lifestyle modifications, the pharmacologic armamentarium (antacids, a mucosal protectant, a prokinetic agent, H2-receptor antagonist (H2RAs), and proton pump inhibitors (PPIs)), and surgery. Lifestyle modifications include head-of-bed elevation on 4–6" blocks, avoidance of tight-fitting garments, weight loss in obese subjects, cessation of cigarette smoking, reduction of size of meals, reduction of foods which are known to reduce basal LES tone (fatty foods, chocolate, alcohol, coffee), drinking fluids between meals rather than at meals, and avoiding eating within 2–3 h of reclining.

  For pharmacotherapy, the longer the control of intragastric acidity, the better the response. Antacids temporarily neutralize gastric contents and briefly improve reflux symptoms. Antacids should be used exclusively for symptom relief and rarely, if ever, are sufficient to adequately treat a patient with other than occasional heartburn. Sucralfate is a mucosal protective agent that bonds with inflamed tissue, perhaps protecting the esophageal mucosa by blocking diffusion of gastric acid and pepsin across the mucosal barrier. This compound has a minimal impact in actual medical therapy; there is value in special populations such as pregnant women. Prokinetic agents (metoclopramide, domperidone) should be used only in patients with gastroparesis and GERD symptoms refractory to antisecretory therapy, and stop if the patient has side effects. Antisecretory therapies in the form of H2-receptor antagonist (cimetidine, ranitidine, famotidine, nizatidine) or PPIs (omeprazole, lansoprazole, rabeprazole, pantoprazole, esomeprazole, OME-IR, dexlansoprazole) are the most commonly employed medications for GERD management. Treatment benefits for these agents are directly related to the duration of acid suppression over a 24-h period. Consequently a greater decrease in the degree of esophagitis healing is seen with PPIs that have more sustained periods of acid suppression than with most H2RAs regimens. Most patients responding to antisecretory therapy will require long-term management, as antisecretory medications do nothing to treat the underlying pathogenesis of GERD. The epithelium may heal, providing a delay before sufficient esophageal epithelial damage and symptoms recur.

Medical therapy of GERD is effective for symptom relief and mucosal healing, as well as long maintenance of remission. However, the need for continued daily administration, occasionally failure to provide complete symptom relief, and the possible side effects may limit its use in some patients who may be candidates for alternative treatment strategies. Antireflux surgery is an alternative to long-term medical therapy for GERD. The laparoscopy approach has been demonstrated to reduce perioperative and postoperative morbidity compared to the open surgical approach. The efficacy of surgery seems to decrease over time, with up to half of patients requiring medication to control recurrent reflux symptoms 10 years following surgery. Several endoscopic techniques for GERD are available, but endoscopic antireflux therapy is still in evolution.

- **Outcome**
  The currently available natural course studies suggest that lack of progression is more common than progression along the spectrum for GERD patients. GERD can present with the complications bleeding, peptic stricture, and BE. GERD is responsible for less than 10% of acute gastrointestinal bleeding. Strictures from GERD result from fibrosis in the area of chronic inflammatory change. The incidence of peptic strictures appears to be stable or even decreasing in recent years despite an increase in the prevalence of GERD, probably as result of the widespread use of PPIs which minimize esophageal injury. They occur more frequently in older, white males, who demonstrated GERD symptoms longer. The incidence of BE has increased in the last decades. It is estimated that it is observed in approximately 5–15% of patients undergoing endoscopy for symptoms of GERD. A variety of risk factors have been identified for the presence of BE, including frequent and long-standing reflux disease, smoking, male, age, and central obesity.

Macroscopy

Recurrent gastroesophageal reflux can damage the mucosa, resulting in inflammation, hence the term "reflux esophagitis." Findings of GERD include erosive esophagitis, strictures, and columnar lined esophagus. Upper endoscopy can grade the severity of esophagitis and also determine the presence or absence of Barrett's epithelium. The severity of reflux esophagitis is characterized by the grading systems Los Angeles classification and Savary–Miller classification.

Microscopy

In reaction to gastroesophageal reflux injury, the squamous esophageal lining develops basal cell hyperplasia and elongation of the papillae with concomitant epithelial permeation by inflammatory cells, namely, by eosinophils, and with or without erosive changes. These morphological alterations suggest the existence of a successive degenerative/regenerative process and are not restrict to peptic damage. Actually the esophageal mucosa has a limited range of morphological reaction to injury, and so the histological aspects of different etiologic entities are often overlapping. For the interpretation of the histological picture, the pathologist relies on the clinical information of GERD and on the endoscopic description of the macroscopic features which have to be correlated with the microscopic findings in order to achieve a correct diagnosis. As all along the gastrointestinal tract mucosa, the diagnosis on endoscopic biopsy samples is a clinicopathologic exercise in which the pathologist is responsible for the interpretation of the histological features on the setting of the macroscopic findings observed by the endoscopist.

Chronic GERD may lead to the development of BE, a complication of long-standing GERD which has characteristic endoscopic and morphological features (▶ Barrett's Esophagus).

Immunophenotype

Not applicable.

Molecular Features

Not applicable.

Differential Diagnosis

GERD must be distinguished from symptoms related to other disorders including infectious esophagitis, eosinophilic esophagitis, pill esophagitis, peptic ulcer disease, dyspepsia, biliary disease, esophageal motor disease, and coronary artery disease. The differential diagnosis of GERD in patients with atypical symptoms can be difficult and often will be performed in conjunction with the otolaryngologist, allergist, pulmonologist, or cardiologist. Patients whose gastrointestinal symptoms are accompanied by unexplained chest pain should have a cardiovascular evaluation, because it is important that coronary artery disease be given early consideration because of its potential lethal implications. The differential diagnosis can be addressed by PPI trial, upper endoscopy, laryngoscopy, abdominal ultrasonography, and ambulatory monitoring (ambulatory intraesophageal pH monitoring and impedance monitoring).

Ambulatory intraesophageal pH monitoring can detect and quantify gastroesophageal reflux and correlate symptoms temporally with reflux (Fig. 2). The two types of equipment are pH probe of monocrystal line catheters with antimony electrodes and Bravo wireless system.

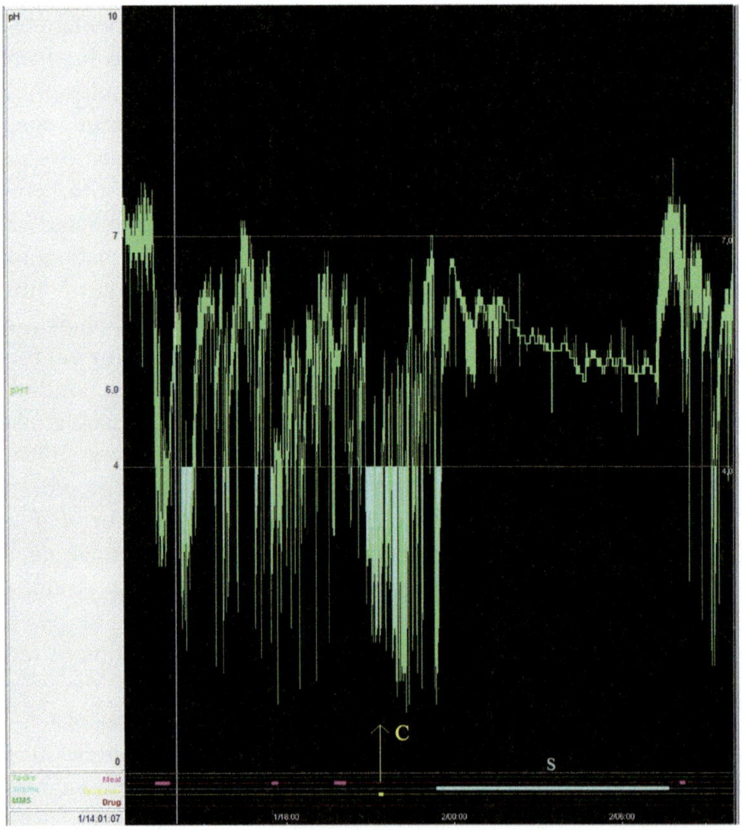

Gastroesophageal Reflux Disease (GERD), Fig. 2 pH monitoring can be used to evaluate the temporal sequence between acid reflux episode and symptoms. Example of 24-h ambulatory esophageal single probe pH tracing in a patient with an acid reflux period followed by chest pain (Neurogastroenterology and Gastrointestinal Motility Laboratory, CEDE – Faculty of Medical Sciences, New University of Lisbon, Portugal). *pH* ambulatory intraesophageal pH monitoring; *C* chest pain, *S* supine position

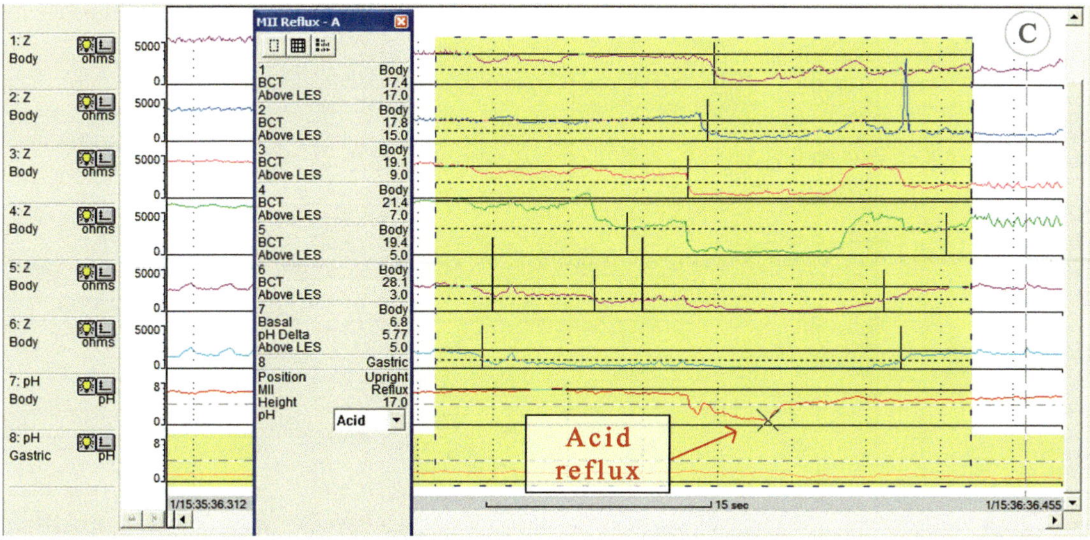

Gastroesophageal Reflux Disease (GERD), Fig. 3 Combined impedance-pH monitoring can be used to evaluate the temporal sequence between an acid reflux episode and symptoms. Example of reflux episode followed by cough (Neurogastroenterology and Gastrointestinal Motility Laboratory, CEDE – Faculty of Medical Sciences, New University of Lisbon, Portugal). Z 1–6 multichannel intraluminal impedance

The pH probe with one to two sensors is inserted into the esophagus via the nares, and a distal electrode is positioned 5 cm above the proximal border of the LES, normally using esophageal manometry, and 15 cm apart to detect pH at proximal esophagus. The pH electrodes are connected to a portable digital data recorder worn around the waist, which stores pH data samples every 4 s for up to 24 h. Patients are required to keep a diary of symptoms, mealtimes, time of lying down for sleep, and time of rising in the morning. They are instructed to perform normal daily activities and consume their usual diet without restrictions. Patients return on the following day to have the probes removed and diaries reviewed. Bravo pH is a wireless ambulatory pH monitoring system which employs a small pH capsule that transmits pH data to the receiver via radiotelemetry signals. The pH capsule is positioned 6 cm above the gastroesophageal junction (GEJ) with a special delivery system. The pH monitoring is performed over 24–48 h. The capsule is designed to drop off from the esophageal wall and pass through the GI tract.

Impedance monitoring (multichannel intraluminal impedance – MII) uses ring electrodes mounted along a catheter to detect the type (liquid, gas, or liquid–gas combination) and direction of bolus movement in the esophagus by measuring changes in intraluminal electric resistance. Combined MII and pH monitoring (MII-pH) can characterize reflux events such as liquid, gas, or mixed (liquid and gas), and acid, weak acid, acid re-reflux, or nonacid permits differentiation of the reflux as either acid or nonacid. MII-pH is useful for the evaluation of typical and atypical gastroesophageal reflux (Fig. 3), or symptoms refractory to aggressive acid-suppression therapy, and in elucidating the role of nonacid reflux in continued reflux symptoms (Fig. 4). Combined MII-pH catheter is a thin flexible 2.1 mm polyvinyl catheter similar to a standard pH catheter. On this catheter there are six impedance-measuring segments (four distal and two proximal) and one or two pH sensors. It is placed transnasally into the esophagus and positioned so that the distal esophageal pH sensor is 5 cm above LES. The impedance-measuring segments are located on the catheter so that when properly placed in the esophagus, impedance is measured at 3, 5, 7, 9, 15, and 17 cm above lower esophageal sphincter (LES). The MII-pH test is performed similar to 24-h ambulatory pH

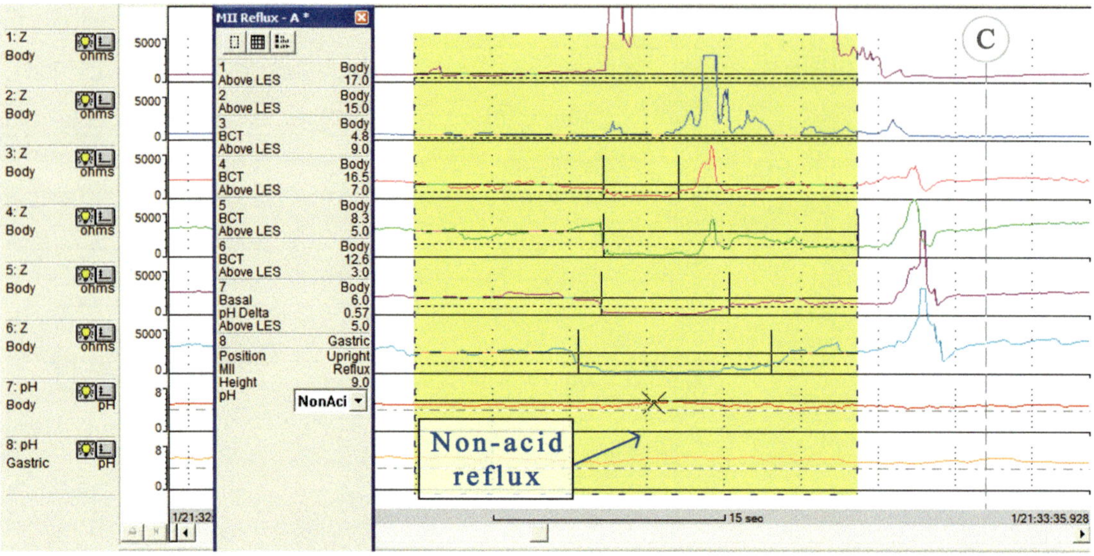

Gastroesophageal Reflux Disease (GERD), Fig. 4 Combined impedance-pH monitoring can be used to evaluate the temporal sequence between a nonacid reflux episode and symptoms. Example of impedance tracing showing a nonacid reflux episode followed by cough (Neurogastroenterology and Gastrointestinal Motility Laboratory, CEDE – Faculty of Medical Sciences, New University of Lisbon, Portugal). Z 1–6 multichannel intraluminal impedance

monitoring. During the monitoring period, the patients are instructed to perform normal daily activities, eat normally, and keep a diary of symptoms, mealtimes, time of lying down for sleep, time of rising in the morning, and time of acid-suppression medication. The patients return the following day to have their probe removed and diaries reviewed. The MII-pH data are downloaded, and the numbers, type, and distal and proximal reflux events are analyzed and attempt to correlate symptoms with reflux events, using a dedicated computer program.

References and Further Reading

Fass, R., Fennerty, M. B., & Vakil, N. (2001). Nonerosive reflux disease – Current concepts and dilemmas. *The American Journal of Gastroenterology, 96*, 303–314.

Lundell, L. R., Dent, J., Bennett, J. R., Blum, A. L., Armstrong, D., Galmiche, J. P., Johnson, F., Hongo, M., Richter, J. E., Spechler, S. J., et al. (1999). Endoscopic assessment of oesophagitis: Clinical and functional correlates and further validation of the Los Angeles classification. *Gut, 45*, 172–180.

Richter, J. E., & Castell, D. O. (2012). *The esophagus* (5th ed.). Chichester: Willey-Blackwell Publishing Ltd.

Vaezi, M. F. (2006). *An atlas of investigation and management: Esophageal diseases. Gastroesophageal reflux disease (GERD)* (pp. 69–85). Oxford: Clinical Publishing.

Vakil, N., van Zanten, S. V., Kahrilas, P., Dent, J., & Jones, R. (2006). The Montreal definition and classification of gastroesophageal reflux disease: A global evidence-based consensus. *The American Journal of Gastroenterology, 101*(8), 1900–1920.

Gastrointestinal Autonomic Nerve Tumor

José Manuel Lopes
Faculty of Medicine of the University of Porto and Institute of Molecular Pathology and Immunology of the University of Porto, Porto, Portugal

Synonyms

Gastrointestinal pacemaker cell tumor (GIPACT); Gastrointestinal stromal tumor (GIST); Plexosarcoma

Definition

Gastrointestinal autonomic nerve tumor (GANT) is considered a variant of the phenotypic spectrum of GISTs (Miettinen et al. 2010) displaying ultrastructural features of autonomic nervous system (enteric plexus) differentiation (Veloso et al. 2005) (e.g., neuritic processes, sparse synapses, and neurosecretory-type granules). Clinicopathological, histological, immunohistochemical, and molecular features of gastrointestinal autonomic nerve tumor indicate that they are similar to GIST (Lee et al. 2001). The small series of reported cases of this variant of GIST preclude validation of any specific implication regarding treatment, outcome, and management of patients with gastrointestinal autonomic nerve tumor diagnosis.

Clinical Features

- **Incidence**
  See ▶ C-Kit (CD117), Gastrointestinal Stromal Tumors (GISTs)
- **Age**
  See ▶ C-Kit (CD117), Gastrointestinal Stromal Tumors (GISTs)
- **Sex**
  See ▶ C-Kit (CD117), Gastrointestinal Stromal Tumors (GISTs)
- **Site**
  See ▶ C-Kit (CD117), Gastrointestinal Stromal Tumors (GISTs)
- **Treatment**
  See ▶ C-Kit (CD117), Gastrointestinal Stromal Tumors (GISTs)
- **Outcome**
  See ▶ C-Kit (CD117), Gastrointestinal Stromal Tumors (GISTs)

Macroscopy

See ▶ C-Kit (CD117), Gastrointestinal Stromal Tumors (GISTs)

Microscopy

See ▶ C-Kit (CD117), Gastrointestinal Stromal Tumors (GISTs)

Immunophenotype

See ▶ C-Kit (CD117), Gastrointestinal Stromal Tumors (GISTs)

Molecular Features

See ▶ C-Kit (CD117), Gastrointestinal Stromal Tumors (GISTs)

Differential Diagnosis

See ▶ C-Kit (CD117), Gastrointestinal Stromal Tumors (GISTs)

References and Further Reading

Lee, J. R., Joshi, V., Lasota, J., & Mittinen, M. (2001). Gastrointestinal autonomic nerve tumor: Immunohistochemical and molecular identity with gastrointestinal stromal tumor. *American Journal of Surgical Pathology, 25*, 979–987.

Miettinen, M., Fletcher, C. D. M., Kindblom, L.-G., & Tsui, W. M. S. (2010). Mesenchymal tumours of the oesophagus, stomach, small intestine, colon and rectum. In F. T. Bosman, F. Carneiro, R. H. Hruban, & N. E. Theise (Eds.), *WHO classification of tumours of the digestive system* (pp. 74–76). Lyon: International Agency for Research on Cancer (IARC).

Veloso, F. T., Pereira, P., Saraiva, A., Capelinha, A. F., & Lopes, J. M. (2005). Colonic gastrointestinal autonomic nervous tumor in a patient with Crohn's disease. *Digestive Diseases and Sciences, 50*, 1476–1480.

Gastrointestinal Stromal Tumor

José Manuel Lopes
Faculty of Medicine of the University of Porto and Institute of Molecular Pathology and Immunology of the University of Porto, Porto, Portugal

Synonyms

GIST is the English acronym for Gastro Intestinal Stromal Tumor

Definition

It is a mesenchymal tumor, generally with immunohistochemistry expression of CD117-cluster of differentiation molecule 117/KIT (kinase-tyrosine receptor of stem cell factor), driven frequently by *KIT* or *PDGFA* (platelet-derived growth factor alpha) activation mutations, that occurs along the gastrointestinal tract, rarely extra-gastrointestinal tract (E-GIST), and displays a spectrum of benign to malignant clinical behavior.

Clinical Features

- **Incidence**
  Annual incidence of GISTs is 11–19.6/million population (Corless et al. 2011).
- **Age**
  GISTs occur typically in middle age to old adults (median age: ~60–65 years), and rarely in childhood and young adults (Miettinnen et al. 2010).
- **Sex**
  No distinct differences in incidence by gender, probably slightly more common in males.
- **Site**
  GISTs occur most commonly in the stomach (60%), jejunum and ileum (30%), duodenum (5%), colon rectum (<5%), and rarely in other gastrointestinal tract or extra-gastrointestinal tract sites.
- **Treatment**
  Safe complete macroscopically surgical resection, including laparoscopic excision, aiming negative surgical margins (R0) (Gouveia et al. 2008), remains the treatment option with curative intent for primary localized GISTs. Tyrosine kinase inhibitor (TKI) imatinib mesylate [a small-molecule ATP – adenosine triphosphate analogue which inhibits both KIT and PDGFRA (platelet-derived growth factor receptor alpha)] is useful in the neoadjuvant setting to allow surgical resection of locally advanced GISTs. Adjuvant imatinib is useful in the control of tumor (free/overall) survival of higher risk tumors and ruptured tumors as well as in the (tumor progression/overall) survival of metastatic or unresectable GISTs. The tyrosine kinase inhibitor sunitinib malate [a small-molecule ATP analogue which inhibits KIT, PDGFRs, RET (glial cell-line derived neurotropic factor receptor rearranged during transfection), CSF-1R (colony-stimulating factor-1 receptor), and flt3 (fetal liver tyrosine kinase 3)] is useful in patients with intolerance to imatinib and GISTs with primary (10%) and secondary (up to 67% with primary *KIT* mutation, but none in wild-type tumors) resistance after initial response to imatinib. Considerable heterogeneity in secondary resistance to imatinib within an individual tumor and multiple metastatic tumors in the same patient affects efficacy of salvage tyrosine kinase inhibitor therapy and requires, namely, alternative targets of signaling cellular metabolic effectors and of tumor stem cells. New therapies, including tyrosine kinase inhibitors, HSP90 (heat shock protein 90) inhibitors, and monoclonal antibodies, are being tested for the treatment of GISTs (Corless et al. 2011).
- **Outcome**
  Five-year survival rates after resection of primary GISTs varies widely (32–76%) probably due to different clinicopathological features and management procedures (Gouveia et al. 2008). Recurrences (intra-abdominal: liver metastases, peritoneal sarcomatosis – splenic and hepatic capsules, or both; rarely to lymph nodes, lungs, bones of axial skeleton, and, preferentially to abdominal soft tissues) may occur during the first 2 years of follow-up. Location in gastrointestinal tract, tumor size, and mitotic rate (per 50 high power fields: 5 mm^2) are parameters included in the risk classification systems (National Health Institute, Armed Forces Institute, and Tumor Node Metastasis – TNM) that are useful to define (absent/very low, low, intermediate/moderate, and high) risk of (progression/metastatic) GIST behavior (Miettinnen et al. 2010). The mutational status [e.g., *KIT*/*PDGFRA*/*BRAF* (*v-raf murine sarcoma viral oncogene homolog B*)/*SDH* (*succinate dehydrogenase*)], and the genetic and immunohistochemical

features of GISTs may improve the accuracy of prognosis evaluation and therapy management of patients. Imatinib achieves control of disease in 70–85% of advanced KIT-positive GISTs with median progression-free survival of 20–24 months; median survival 5 years, 34% patients surviving >9 years (Corless et al. 2011). The probability of primary resistance (progression within 6 months) to imatinib treatment for *KIT* exon 11, *KIT* exon 9, and wild-type GISTs is 5%, 16%, and 23%, respectively (Heinrich et al. 2003). *PDGFRA* D842V (activation loop)-mutant GISTs are usually imatinib resistant. Gains on chromosomes 8q, 3q, and 17q associate to metastatic behavior. Malignant behavior of GISTs associates with loss of RKIP (raf kinase inhibitor protein) expression (Martinho et al. 2009), p27 (p27kip1) downregulation, overexpression of cyclins A and H, CDKN2A (cyclin-dependent kinase inhibitor 2 alpha) inactivation, *p53* (*tumor suppressor gene protein 53*) mutation, *MDM2* (*murine double minute 2*), and *CCND1* (*cyclin D1*) gene amplification. Tumors <1 cm (micro-GISTs) are usually benign incidental (up to 35% in gastrectomy for other reasons) tumors.

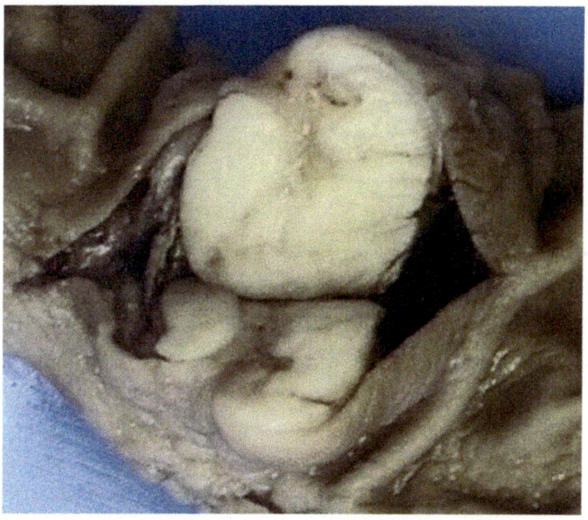

Gastrointestinal Stromal Tumor, Fig. 1 Macroscopy of submucosal gastric GIST

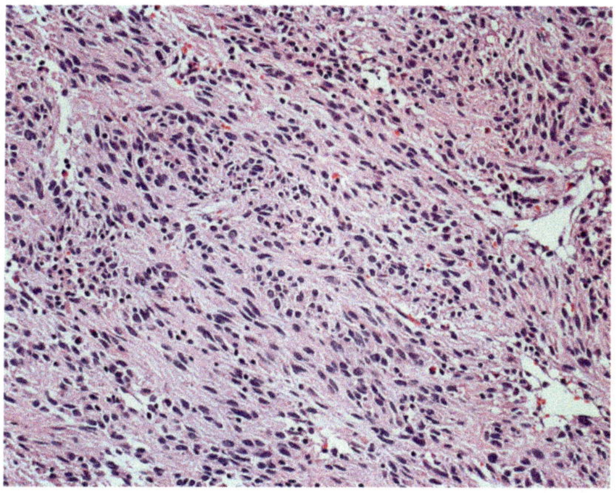

Gastrointestinal Stromal Tumor, Fig. 2 GIST with spindle tumor cells

Macroscopy

The tumors are usually well circumscribed uninodular (Fig. 1) or multinodular firm/fleshy, gray-white, and may disclose mural, polypoid intraluminal (occasionally ulcerated) or pedunculated serosal growth in the tubular gastrointestinal tract; cut surface may display cystic, myxoid, necrotic, and hemorrhage areas.

Microscopy

GISTs encompass a broad morphologic spectrum (Miettinnen et al. 2010) including spindle (~70%) (Fig. 2), epithelioid (Fig. 3) (~20–25%), and mixed (spindle and epithelioid) cell tumors. Tumor cell pleomorphism is rare. Histological patterns among spindle GISTs include several types: sclerosing, with collagenous matrix and dystrophic calcification; palisaded-vacuolated with nuclear palisading and perinuclear vacuolization, and extracellular skenoid fibers; hypercellular with high mitotic rate; and sarcomatous with high mitotic rate, nuclear atypia, and necrosis. Epithelioid types include: sclerosing; hypercellular; pseudopapillary; paraganglioma- or carcinoid-like; signet-ring change; microcystic (mucin pools) change; discohesive; pleomorphic; and sarcomatous. Myxoid and extensive hyaline change can occur in both spindle and epithelioid GISTs. Morphology after imatinib may disclose

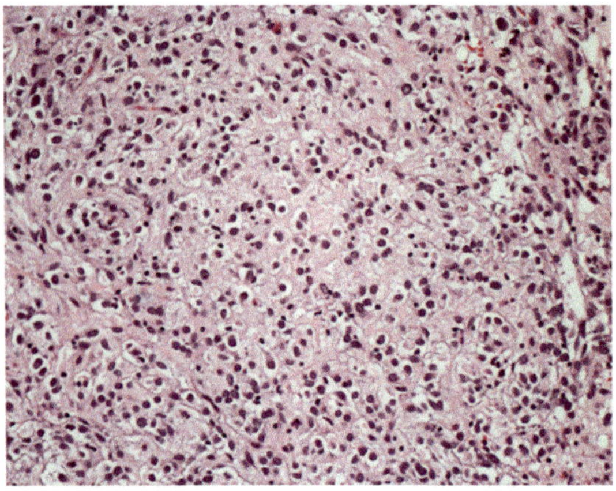

Gastrointestinal Stromal Tumor, Fig. 3 GIST with epithelioid tumor cells

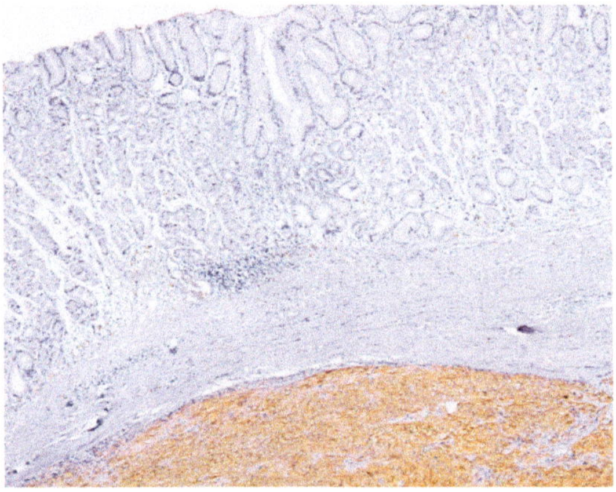

Gastrointestinal Stromal Tumor, Fig. 4 Low power features of diffuse expression of CD117 in gastric submucosa GIST

paucicellular hyaline or myxoid areas, with similar pretreatment tumor cell features, sometimes spindle to epithelioid change morphology, epithelioid pseudopapillary change, and rarely rhabdomyoblastic differentiation.

Immunophenotype

Immunohistochemical markers expressed in GISTs include (Miettinnen et al. 2010): CD117/KIT (95%) in the cytoplasm (Figs. 4 and 5a–c), sometimes with dot-like paranuclear pattern, being more focal and weaker in epithelioid cells which more frequently display membrane staining; CD34 – cluster of differentiation molecule 34 (70%) that may vary by tumor location and cell type; DOG1 -discovered on GIST-1 (90–95%) that may be useful in KIT-negative tumors; smooth muscle actin-SMA (40%) focal to diffuse; desmin rare and focal; h-caldesmon (50–60%); S100 protein (5%); cytokeratins (CK18 and CK 8) rarely. The diagnosis of KIT-negative GISTs should include a panel of biomarkers and molecular analyses, the microscopy, and clinical/imaging features of the tumors.

Molecular Features

Most GISTs harbor molecular alterations (Corless et al. 2011). The accuracy of diagnosis, prognosis, and the therapy management of patients can improve with the molecular analysis of tumors. *KIT* somatic mutations (75–80%) occur in exon 11 (67%) (deletions, insertions, substitutions, duplications) that affect the juxtamembrane domain, exon 9 (10%) extracellular domain, exon 17 (1%) activation loop, exon 13 (1%) ATP – adenosine triphosphate-binding region, and rarely exon 8; deletions of exon 11 associate with shorter progression-free and overall survival; mutations in exon 9 are more frequent in small and large intestine tumors. *PDGFRA* somatic mutations (5–8%) occur in exon 18 (6%) that affect the activation loop, exon 12 (1%) juxtamembrane domain, and exon 14 (<1%) ATP-binding domain; mutations in exon 18 and 14 are more common in gastric tumors; most common exon 18 D842V mutants are imatinib resistant. GISTs without somatic mutations of *KIT* and *PDGFRA* (12–15%) include cases with somatic *BRAF* (~7–13%) mutated tumors; most GISTs that occur in pediatric patients (~1%), tumors in the Carney triad (~1%) (GIST, paraganglioma-PGL, and pulmonary chondroma) are, so far, "wild-type" GISTs. Germline mutations were reported in GIST kindreds harboring mutations of *KIT* (exons 8, 11, 13 and 17), *PDFRA* (exon 12 and 18), and of *SDHA*/*SDHB*/*SDHC*/

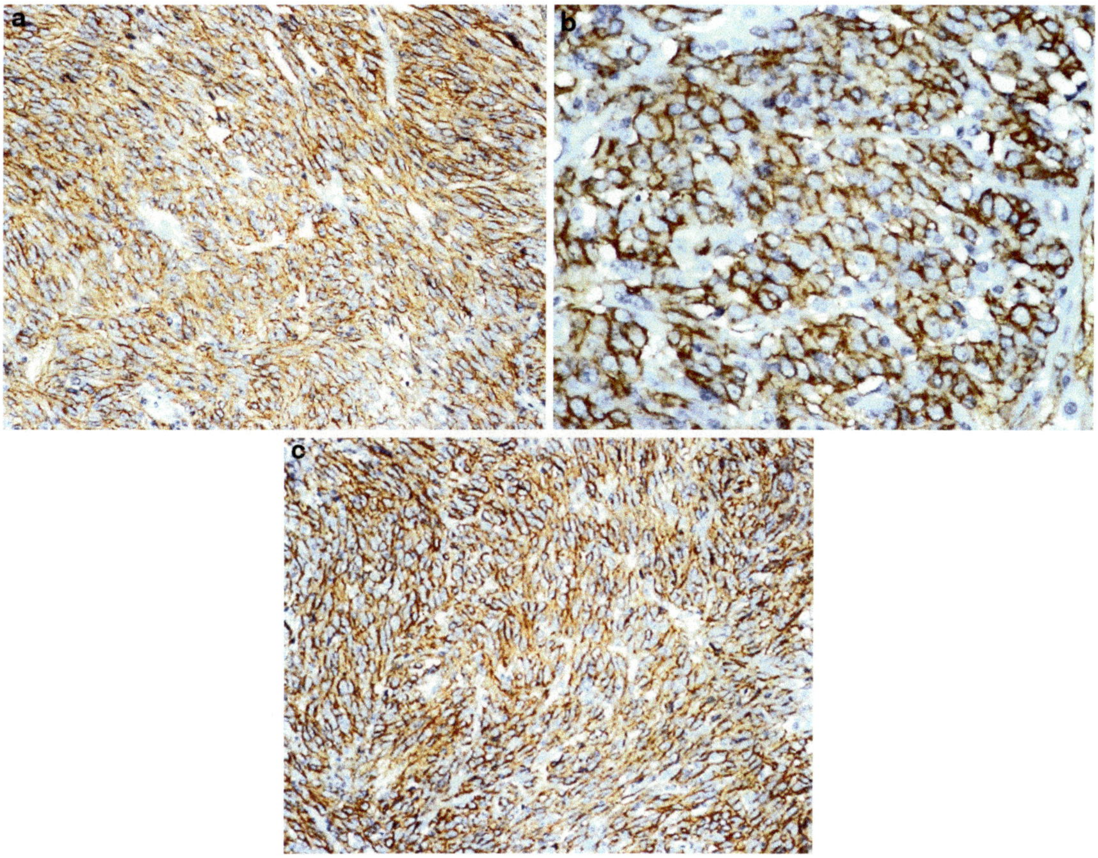

Gastrointestinal Stromal Tumor, Fig. 5 (**a**–**c**) Diffuse expression of CD117 in GIST tumor cells

SDHD (~2%) in Carney-Stratakis syndrome (GISTs and PGLs). GISTs occur in ~7% of neurofibromatosis 1 (NF1), are usually multiple, and located in the small intestine associated with hyperplasia of interstitial cells of Cajal; <10% GISTs in NF1 display *KIT* or *PDGFRA* mutations (Miettinnen et al. 2006). Most GISTs (none of pediatric-type) disclose either monosomy of chromosome 14 or partial loss of 14q. Genomic signatures may be useful for the risk evaluation/management decision of GISTs.

Differential Diagnosis

GISTs are the most common malignant mesenchymal tumors of the gastrointestinal tract that are considered to originate from interstitial cells of Cajal progenitor/stem cells. Interstitial cells of Cajal express KIT and DOG1. Several spindle and epithelioid neoplasms that occur in gastrointestinal tract should be considered in the differential diagnosis of GISTs. Leiomyoma (common in esophagus and colon/rectum) and leiomyosarcoma (rare, more common in colon/rectum) usually display diffuse expression of desmin and are KIT negative. Benign (rare schwannoma occur in gastrointestinal tract, more in stomach) and malignant nerve sheath tumors usually express S100 protein but are KIT negative. Intra-abdominal fibromatosis (rare, mostly extra gastrointestinal tract) and inflammatory myofibroblastic tumors (childhood, in stomach, intestines, and extra-gastrointestinal tract) express β-catenin and ALK (anaplastic lymphoma kinase), respectively, but are KIT negative. Inflammatory fibroid polyp (more common in stomach and small intestine) express CD34 but are KIT negative. Tumors expressing KIT [e.g., metastatic melanoma and small cell carcinoma, angiosarcoma, PNET (primitive neuroectodermal tumor)/Ewing sarcoma as well as other tumors (e.g., neuroendocrine neoplasms, glomus tumor, clear cell sarcoma)] that are KIT negative may simulate GISTs and should be ruled out with clinical, immunohistochemistry, and eventually molecular features.

References and Further Reading

Corless, C. L., Barnett, C. M., & Heinrich, M. C. (2011). Gastrointestinal stromal tumours: Origin and molecular oncology. *Nature Reviews Cancer, 11*(12), 865–878. doi:10.1038/nr3143.

Gouveia, A. M., Pimenta, A. P., Capelinha, A. F., de la Cruz, D., Silva, P., & Lopes, J. M. (2008). Surgical margin status and prognosis of gastrointestinal stromal tumor. *World Journal of Surgery, 32*, 2375–2382.

Heinrich, M., Corless, C. L., Demetri, G. D., von Mehren, M., Joensuu, H., McGreevey, L. S., Chen, C. J., Van den Abbeele, A. D., Druker, B. J., Roberts, P. J., Singer, S., Fletcher, C. D., Silberman, S., Dimitrijevic, S., & Fletcher, J. A. (2003). Kinase mutations and imatinib response in patients with metastatic gastrointestinal tumor. *Journal of Clinical Oncology, 21*, 4342–4349.

Martinho, O., Gouveia, A., Silva, P., Pimenta, A., Reis, R. M., & Lopes, J. M. (2009). Loss of RKIP expression is associated with poor survival in GISTs. *Virchows Archives, 455*, 277–284.

Miettinnen, M., Fetsch, J. F., Sobin, L. H., & Lasota, J. (2006). Gastrointestinal stromal tumors in patients with neurofibromatosis: a clinicopathologic and molecular genetic study of 45 cases. *American Journal of Surgical Pathology, 30*, 90–96.

Miettinnen, M., Fletcher, C. D. M., Kindblom, L.-G., & Tsui, W. M. S. (2010). Mesenchymal tumours of the oesophagus, stomach, small intestine, colon and rectum. In F. T. Bosman, F. Carneiro, R. H. Hruban, & N. E. Theise (Eds.), *WHO classification of tumours of the digestive system*. Lyon: International Agency for Research on Cancer (IARC) (pp. 35–36, 74–76,115–116, and 181–182, respectively).

Gastroparesis

Andreia Albuquerque
Serviço de Gastrenterologia, Centro Hospitalar de São João, Porto, Portugal

Synonyms

Delayed gastric emptying; Gastric stasis

Definition

Gastroparesis is a syndrome characterized by delayed gastric emptying in the absence of mechanical obstruction of the stomach. It is traditionally associated with nausea, vomiting, postprandial fullness, early satiety, bloating, and abdominal pain.

The etiology is multifactorial and the most common causes are diabetes, postsurgical status, and idiopathic. Other causes include medication, Parkinson's disease, collagen vascular disorders, thyroid dysfunction, liver disease, chronic renal insufficiency, intestinal pseudo-obstruction, and miscellaneous.

Gastroparesis may be due to abnormalities of the fundus (post-vagotomy state, diabetes mellitus, and functional dyspepsia), abnormalities in antroduodenal contraction (low amplitude, frequency, and decreased antral motor function or dysfunction), pyloric dysfunction (idiopathic hypertrophic stenosis and diabetes gastroparesis), or abnormalities in small bowel motility. Diabetic gastroparesis is believed to represent a form of neuropathy involving the vagus nerve. Hyperglycemia itself can also cause antral hypomotility, gastric dysrhythmias, and delayed gastric emptying in some patients. Idiopathic gastroparesis is present in many patients with functional dyspepsia and may in some cases occur after a viral infection.

Symptoms of gastroparesis are often persistent, but some patients experience episodic symptom flares that are separated by asymptomatic periods. There are several complications associated with gastroparesis, namely, deficiencies in vitamins A, B6, C, and K, as well as iron, potassium, and zinc; postprandial hypoglycemic reactions in diabetic patients, and bezoar formation.

The diagnosis is based on the presence of appropriate symptoms/signs, delayed gastric emptying, and the absence of an obstructing structural lesion in the stomach or small intestine. Routine laboratory is useful to identify diseases that are associated with gastroparesis, to rule out other disorders and to assess the nutritional sate of the patient. Patients should undergo an upper endoscopy or barium meal, mainly to exclude mechanical obstruction or mucosa disease as the cause. Gastric emptying scintigraphy of a radiolabeled solid meal is the best accepted method to test for diagnosis, the most useful parameters are gastric retention >10% at 4 h and >70% at 2 h. In patients who have evidence of gastric stasis by a scintigraphy study without an identifiable cause, gastroduodenal manometry can help differentiate myopathic from neuropathic process. Breath testing can also be performed and measure of gastric emptying using the nonradioactive isotope 13C to label octanoate, a medium-chain triglyceride, which can be bound into a solid meal and gastric emptying, can be indirectly determined. This test has been used primarily for clinical research and pharmaceutical studies.

Mild gastroparesis is thought to have a low mortality rate, but patients with decompensated gastroparesis are more likely to develop complications and have related mortality.

Clinical Features

- **Incidence**
  A study conducted to assess the incidence, prevalence, and outcomes of patients with gastroparesis in Olmsted County, Minnesota, from 1996 to 2006, revealed that gastroparesis is an uncommon condition in the community, but is associated with a poor outcome.

  The incidence of gastroparesis ranged from 6.3 to 17.2 cases per 100,000 person-years. The true prevalence is unknown, it is estimated to occur in 4% of the adult population, 20–40% of patients with diabetes mellitus, primarily those with long duration of type 1 diabetes mellitus with other complications, and may also be present in 25–40% of patients with functional dyspepsia.
- **Age**
  About 68% of patients are under 40 years of age at the time of initial presentation, with a mean age of 45 years.
- **Sex**
  There is a female predominance of gastroparesis, with a female: male ratio of 4:1.

  Several studies showed that female gender was associated with delayed gastric emptying in both functional dyspepsia and in patients with diabetes. There are several theories than can explain this, namely, a possible hormonal cause and female patients seem to seek health care more frequently than males.
- **Site**
  The stomach is the organ involved.
- **Treatment**
  Primary treatment of gastroparesis includes dietary manipulation and administration of antiemetic and prokinetic agents. Dietary recommendations include eating frequent smaller-size meals and replacing solid food with liquids, such as soups. Foods should be low in fat and fiber content. Antiemetic agents are administered for nausea and vomiting. The principal classes of antiemetic drugs are antidopaminergics, antihistamines, anticholinergics, and, more recently, serotonin receptor antagonists.

  Patients refractory to the initial treatment can be difficult to manage, treatment may involve switching prokinetic and antiemetic agents, combining prokinetic agents, injecting botulinum toxin into the pylorus, using gastrostomy/jejunostomy tubes, or implanting a gastric electric stimulator.

- **Outcome**

  The natural history of gastroparesis is largely unknown.

  The study performed by Soykan et al., including 146 patients with gastroparesis seen over 6 years, revealed that 74% required continuous prokinetic therapy, 22% were able to stop prokinetics, 5% had undergone gastrectomy, 6.2% went onto gastric electrical stimulation (pacing), and 7% died. At some point, 21% had required nutrition support with a feeding jejunostomy tube or periods of parenteral nutrition. A good response to pharmacological agents can be expected in the viral and dyspeptic subgroups, Parkinson's disease, and the majority of diabetics, whereas a poorer outcome to prokinetics can be expected in postgastrectomy patients, those with connective tissue disease, a subgroup of diabetics, and the subset of idiopathic gastroparesis dominated by abdominal pain and history of physical and sexual abuse. Appreciation of the different etiologies and psychological status of the patients may help predict response to prokinetic therapy.

  Community studies of the outcome of gastroparesis are lacking, and studies conducted in tertiary referral centers may not reflect findings encountered in the general population.

Macroscopy

Normally there are no macroscopic abnormalities described in association with gastroparesis.

Microscopy

Pathologic assessment of gastric tissue in patients with gastroparesis is limited.

Gastroparesis Clinical Research Consortium (GpCRC) recently described the cellular changes associated with diabetic (DG) and idiopathic (IG) gastroparesis. Full-thickness gastric body biopsies were obtained from 40 gastroparetics (20 diabetic) and matched controls. In this study, the majority of patients with gastroparesis (83%) had defined gastric wall cellular abnormalities. Hematoxylin and eosin staining was graded as normal in all 20 patients with diabetic gastroparesis and in 19 patients with idiopathic gastroparesis. Smoothelin immunolabeling was decreased in three patients with diabetic gastroparesis and in six with idiopathic gastroparesis. Presence of fibrosis as determined by trichrome staining was present in one patient with diabetic and two patients with idiopathic gastroparesis. All other patients had normal trichrome staining, including eight of the nine patients with abnormal smoothelin immunolabeling.

Histologic examination of gastric tissues from patients with severe gastroparesis reveals heterogeneous and inconsistent defects in the morphology of enteric neurons, smooth muscle and interstitial cells of Cajal, and increased levels of inflammatory cells.

Vagus nerves from patients with diabetes exhibit variable levels of myelin degeneration.

Immunophenotype

Gastroparesis Clinical Research Consortium (GpCRC) also showed that the most commonly observed findings were loss of interstitial cells of Cajal (ICC) and an immune infiltrate containing macrophages, characterized by an increase in CD45 and CD68 immunoreactivity in both DG and IG. A 14–17% decrease in the number of enteric nerve fibers as defined by Protein Gene Product 9.5 (PGP9.5) immunoreactivity was also seen. Less common were changes in nNOS, vasoactive intestinal peptide (VIP), substance P (SP), and tyrosine hydroxylase (TH).

Differential Diagnosis

1. Gastroparesis should be differentiated from delayed gastric emptying due to *mechanical obstruction* of the stomach. An upper endoscopy should be performed to exclude obstruction.

2. *Mucosal inflammation* due to infection or acid-peptic disease can exacerbate gastroparesis symptoms.
3. Idiopathic gastroparesis may be difficult to distinguish from *functional dyspepsia* in some cases. Presentation with predominant pain and less nausea is considered to be more typical of functional dyspepsia, whereas dominant nausea with minimal pain is more consistent with idiopathic gastroparesis.

So, other conditions potentially causative of symptoms, such as gastric outlet obstruction, peptic ulcer disease, neoplasm, small bowel obstruction, or IBD, should be excluded by endoscopy or contrast radiology prior to conferring a diagnosis of gastroparesis.

References and Further Reading

Parkman, H. P., Hasler, W. L., Fisher, R. S., et al. (2004). American Gastroenterological Association medical position statement: Diagnosis and treatment of gastroparesis. *Gastroenterology, 127*, 1589–1591.

Park, M. I., & Camilleri, M. (2006). Gastroparesis: Clinical update. *American Journal of Gastroenterology, 101*, 1129–1139.

Soykan, I., Sivri, B., Sarosiek, I., Kiernan, B., et al. (1998). Demography, clinical characteristics, psychological and abuse profiles, treatment, and long-term follow-up of patients with gastroparesis. *Digestive Diseases and Sciences, 43*, 2398–2404.

Jung, H. K., Choung, R. S., Locke, G. R., 3rd, et al. (2009). The incidence, prevalence and outcomes of patients with gastroparesis in Olmsted County, Minnesota from 1996 to 2006. *Gastroenterology, 136*, 1225–1233.

Grover, M., Farrugia, G., Lurken, M. S., et al. (2011). Cellular changes in diabetic and idiopathic gastroparesis. *Gastroenterology, 140*, 1575–1585.

Gastropathy, Portal Hypertension

Andreia Albuquerque
Serviço de Gastrenterologia, Centro Hospitalar de São João, Porto, Portugal

Synonyms

Congestive gastropathy; PHG; Portal hypertensive gastropathy

Definition

In 1985, MacCormack was the first to describe the condition “congestive gastropathy.” Actually, the term “portal hypertensive gastropathy” (PHG) is more frequently used and defines a wide spectrum of diffuse macroscopic lesions that appear in the gastric mucosa of patients with portal hypertension and therefore is commonly found in association to cirrhosis, but can also be found in non-cirrhotic causes of portal hypertension.

The pathogenesis is not well known but venous congestion and increased gastric blood flow in the upper stomach seems to be important factors for its development. It does not seem to be related with acid secretion or *Helicobacter pylori* presence in the gastric mucosa. Portal hypertension is a prerequisite for the development of PHG and it is defined by an increase in portal pressure gradient to a threshold above approximately 10 mmHg.

Typically, PHG displays a snake-skin mosaic pattern (mild PHG) that can be accompanied with flat or bulging red or brown spots (severe PHG).

Chronic anemia is the most common clinical manifestation, although acute gastrointestinal bleeding can occur. It is uncommon as an isolated cause of significant upper gastrointestinal bleeding in portal hypertension.

Clinical Features

- **Incidence**
  There are major controversies concerning the true incidence of PHG, ranging from 7% to 98% in the available studies. Primignani et al. showed that PHG is relatively low (56%) in patients with a new diagnosis of cirrhosis, higher (75%) in a previous diagnosis of cirrhosis and no prior bleeding, and even higher (91%) in patients with a previous variceal bleeding with current or prior sclerotherapy. The prevalence of PHG is correlated with the duration of disease, severity of portal hypertension, presence of esophagogastric varices, and a previous history of endoscopic variceal sclerotherapy. It has been suggested that

variceal obliteration results in hyperdynamic congestion, which gives rives to hypertensive gastropathy.

- **Age**
  PHG is common in middle-aged patients.
- **Sex**
  PHG occurs mainly associated with cirrhotic portal hypertension, so it is more common in males, over 60% of patients with chronic liver disease and cirrhosis are men.
- **Site**
  Diagnosis is endoscopic with mucosal abnormalities observed in the stomach; characteristically, PHG is located mainly in the fundus. Similar endoscopic lesions may be observed in other areas of the gastrointestinal tract, findings have been termed portal hypertensive duodenopathy, portal hypertensive enteropathy, or portal hypertensive colopathy, depending on the location of the characteristic lesions.
- **Treatment**
  The mainstay is based on portal-hypotensive pharmacological treatment, more invasive options should be reserved for refractory cases.

  The most frequent setting is finding PHG on a routine endoscopy performed to evaluate the presence of varices. Normally, the patient is asymptomatic with no evidence of chronic bleeding; prophylaxis of bleeding from PHG has not been evaluated in clinical studies and recommendations for therapy are not available yet.

  In some cases, when patients present with chronic anemia, treatment is based on portal pressure reduction. The use of non-selective beta-blockers, particularly propranolol, is recommended in the chronic setting. Most patients are started with propranolol at the initial dose of 20 mg twice a day (BID), although some cases require a lower dose. The dose is gradually escalated to a maximum of 160 mg BID or the maximum tolerated dose, provided heart rate is maintained around 50–55 bpm. Secondary effects associated to beta-blockers, such as light-headedness, fatigue, impotence, may limit further increases in dosage. In patients that requiring frequent transfusion, portosystemic shunt therapies should be considered, either surgical or through the placement of transjugular intrahepatic portosystemic shunt (TIPS).

  Rarely, PHG can lead to acute gastrointestinal hemorrhage, those patients should be adequately resuscitated with blood transfusions to maintain hemoglobin level between 7 and 8 g/dL, initiation of vasoconstrictor drug therapy (terlipressin or somatostatin or analogues), and prophylactic antibiotics. If refractory bleeding occurs, rescue therapies are the same as recommended in chronic bleeding.

  Liver transplantation is indicated if the patient has decompensated liver disease.

  Thermal coagulation, injection therapy, H2-blockers, sucralfate, and surgical resection are ineffective for controlling diffuse bleeding or for preventing rebleeding from extensive portal hypertensive gastropathy.
- **Outcome**
  Gastropathy can progress from mild to severe and vice versa or even disappear completely. Primignani et al. observed that during follow-up, PHG was stable in 29% of patients, deteriorated in 23%, improved in 23%, and fluctuated with time in 25%. Bleeding from PHG is uncommon and rarely severe. Acute bleeding occurred in 2.5% of patients, chronic bleeding in 10.8%, and bleeding-related mortality was 12.5%. There are few data concerning mortality rates of patients bleeding from PHG in comparison with those bleeding from esophageal or gastric varices.

Macroscopy

PHG includes several mucosal lesions which have been classified as mild or severe. The most accepted classification is from the New Italian Endoscopic Club for the study and treatment of esophageal varices (NIEC) and according to this classification, the elementary lesions of PHG are:

1. Mosaic-like pattern, defined by the presence of small polygonal areas surrounded by a whitish-yellow depressed border (Fig. 1). The mosaic is defined as mild when the areola is uniformly

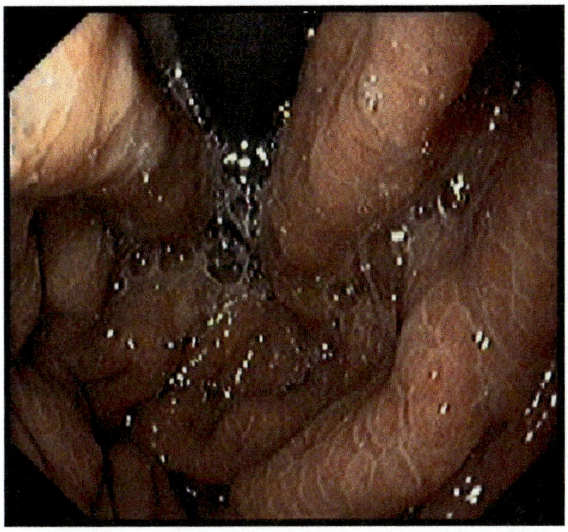

Gastropathy, Portal Hypertension, Fig. 1 Upper endoscopy revealing a mosaic-like pattern in the gastric fundus and proximal body suggesting mild portal hypertensive gastropathy

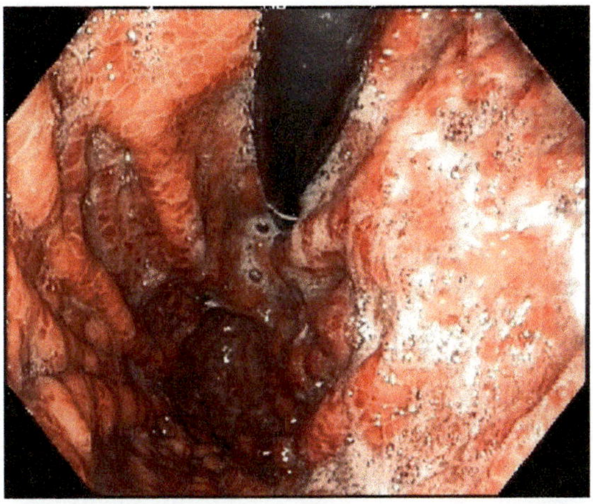

Gastropathy, Portal Hypertension, Fig. 2 Upper endoscopy revealing small, flat, red-point lesions in the gastric fundus and body suggesting severe portal hypertensive gastropathy

pink, moderate if the center is red, and severe if the areola is uniformly red.

2. Red-point lesions, that are small, flat, <1 mm in diameter (Fig. 2).
3. Cherry-red spots are red-colored, round lesions >2 mm in diameter, and slightly protrude into the lumen.
4. Black-brown spots are irregularly shaped flat spots, black or brown, persistently present after washing and cause intramucosal hemorrhage.

PHG is defined as mild when only mosaic-like pattern of any degree is present and severe when red-points, cherry-red, or black-brown spots are present.

Mild lesions are highly prevalent (65–90%), whereas severe lesions account for only 10–25% of the cases.

Microscopy

PHG is characterized by marked dilatation of the capillaries and collecting venules in the gastric mucosa. In addition, submucosal veins appear also with ectasia, irregular, and with areas of intimal thickening. These vascular alterations are present in the absence of any significant inflammatory cell infiltrate or erosion in the gastric mucosa, making incorrect the previous classification of these lesions as gastritis.

Routine endoscopic biopsies obtained by conventional forceps are often unhelpful because of the patchy nature of vessel dilatation. In contrast, large snare biopsies can easily ascertain the presence of dilatated vessels, but this procedure is not recommended for routine use. PHG seems not to be related to the presence of *Helicobacter pylori* in the gastric mucosa, the prevalence is similar in the cirrhotic patients than in the general population.

Differential Diagnosis

The most common differential diagnosis is with *gastric antral vascular ectasia* (*GAVE*). Both can cause acute or chronic bleeding in cirrhotic patients, but they have many distinctive features. GAVE is usually located in the antrum (Fig. 3) and although associated with liver disease (40% of the cases), it can also be observed in non-hepatic chronic diseases such as autoimmune diseases (autoimmune connective tissue disorders), bone

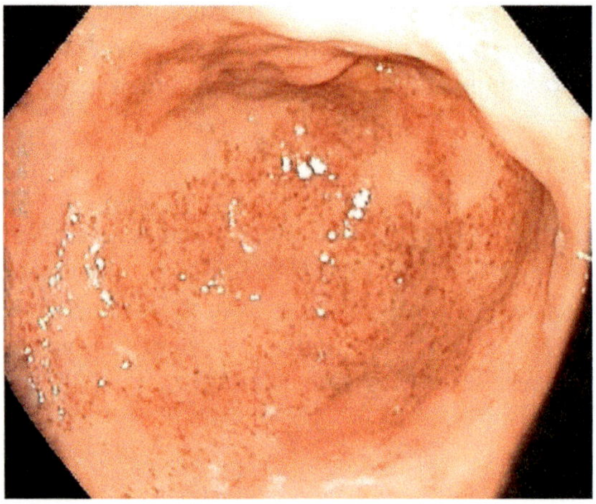

Gastropathy, Portal Hypertension, Fig. 3 Upper endoscopy revealing gastric antral vascular ectasia (GAVE), in the antrum

marrow transplantation, and chronic renal failure. GAVE is a less frequent condition, having been reported in only 2% of patients awaiting liver transplantation or 3% of patients with Hepatitis C virus and advanced fibrosis. It describes a vascular lesion of the gastric antrum that consists of tortuous, dilated vessels radiating outward from the pylorus-like spokes of a wheel and resembling the dark stripes on the surface of a watermelon. The typical histological appearance of GAVE includes marked dilatation of capillaries and collecting venules in the gastric mucosa and submucosa with areas of intimal thickening characterized by fibromuscular hyperplasia, fibrohyalinosis, and thrombi. Vasodilation mediators such as gastrin and prostaglandin E2 have been associated to the presence of GAVE. Mechanical stress and abnormal antral motility have also been associated to GAVE development. Similar to PHG, GAVE will most frequently present with chronic iron deficiency anemia due to chronic gastrointestinal bleeding. Acute gastrointestinal bleeding can also occur. Endoscopic treatment (argon-plasma coagulation) is the mainstay of treatment of symptomatic lesions. Although, PHG and GAVE have the same common clinical manifestations, they have distinct pathophysiology, endoscopic appearance, and therapeutic approach.

References and Further Reading

McCormack, T. T., Sims, J., Eyre-Brook, I., et al. (1985). Gastric lesions in portal hypertension: Inflammatory gastritis or congestive gastropathy? *Gut, 26*, 1226–1232.

Piqué, J. M. (1997). Portal hypertensive gastropathy. *Baillière's Clinical Gastroenterology, 11*, 257–270.

Primignani, M., Carpinelli, L., Preatoni, P., et al. (2000). Natural history of portal hypertensive gastropathy in patients with liver cirrhosis. The New Italian Endoscopic Club for the study and treatment of esophageal varices (NIEC). *Gastroenterology, 119*, 181–187.

Ripoll, C., & Garcia-Tsao, G. (2011). The management of portal hypertensive gastropathy and gastric antral vascular ectasia. *Digestive and Liver Disease, 43*, 345–351.

Thuluvath, P. J., & Yoo, H. Y. (2002). Portal hypertensive gastropathy. *American Journal of Gastroenterology, 97*, 2973–2978.

Giardiasis

Arzu Ensari
Department of Pathology, Ankara University Medical School, Sihhiye, Ankara, Turkey

Synonyms

Cercomonas intestinalis; *Giardia duodenalis*; *Giardia intestinalis*; *Giardia lamblia*; *Lamblia intestinalis*; *Megastoma enterica*

Definition

Giardiasis, caused by the intestinal parasite, *Giardia lamblia*, is the leading GI protozoan disease worldwide with an increase in summer and autumn. Many countries, especially developing countries show a high prevalence of giardiasis. Infection occurs by fecal-oral transmission, contaminated food and water, and person to person transmission, particularly in homosexuals. It is commonly observed in patients with selective IgA deficiency and in HIV-infected patients. Diarrhea, abdominal pain, bloating, nausea and vomiting, malabsorption, and weight loss are the main presenting symptoms. Giardia can be diagnosed by stool examination, examination of duodenal aspirates or duodenal biopsies. The taxonomy is giardiasis is complicated as there are seven known species including *G. duodenalis* which is divided into eight assemblages. They are based on phylogenetic analysis of nucleotide sequence of small-subunit rRNA and comprise of A, B, C, D, E, F, G, and H. Molecular testing using PCR can be used to accurately identify the subtypes of *Giardia*.

Clinical Features

- **Incidence**
  The exact incidence is unknown, but it is the leading GI protozoal disease with a prevalence of 2–7% worldwide, reaching up to 30% in developing countries.
- **Age**
  All age groups may be affected; in developed countries, the most common age groups affected are children aged 1–4 years and adults aged 20–40 years.
- **Sex**
  Infection occurs equally in both sexes.
- **Site**
  Although *G. lamblia* has a preference for the small intestines, colonization of the stomach and colon has also been reported.
- **Treatment**
  Anti-parasitic agents are used for the treatment. However, sanitation measures need to be taken to prevent outbreaks of giardiasis. Drugs such as Albendazole, Metronidazole, Nitazoxanide, Tand inidazole can be used for treatment.
- **Outcome**
  The infection may resolve spontaneously but often persists for weeks or months.

Macroscopy

Endoscopic appearance is generally normal.

Microscopy

Giardia exists in two forms: the motile trophozoite and the infective cyst. Following ingestion, the cyst forms two trophozoites in the duodenum. These are pear shaped with two nuclei, or sickle-shaped in sagittal plane appearing faintly basophilic on H&E sections. Trophozoites are typically found in the lumen near the surface or as attached to the surface of the enterocytes (Figs. 1 and 2). Giardiasis is a typical example of enteric infection which presents with normal or near-normal mucosa, although more severe change in the villous morphology resembling celiac disease may rarely be seen. In children, giardiasis can cause lymphoid hyperplasia in the small intestinal mucosa. Duodenal mucosa may either show no alterations despite the presence of the organism, or IELosis with normal villus morphology, or partial or complete villus atrophy

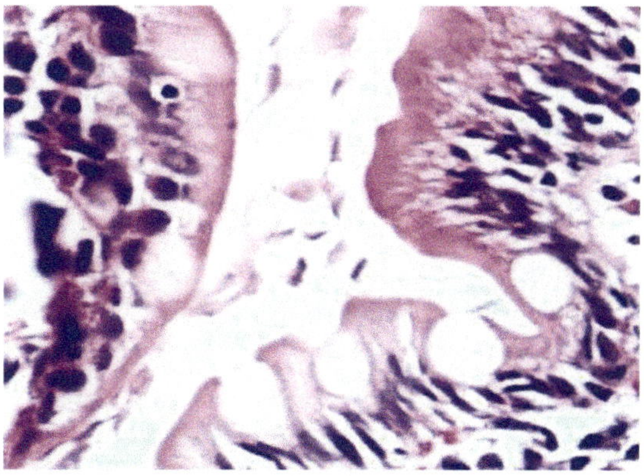

Giardiasis, Fig. 1 *G. lamblia* trophozoites in the lumen and attached to the surface (H&E; ×200)

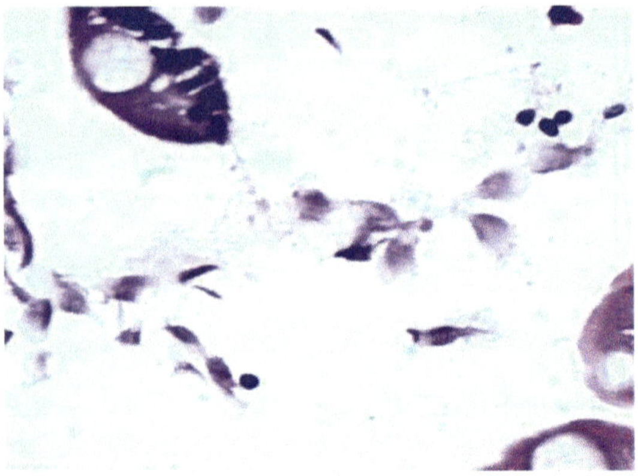

Giardiasis, Fig. 2 *G. lamblia* trophozoites with their pear-shape and two nuclei (H&E; ×400)

with increased IELs and lamina propria inflammatory cells.

Immunophenotype

No specific immunphenotypic feature is reported.

Molecular Features

No specific molecular feature is reported.

Differential Diagnosis

The differential diagnosis of giardiasis involves all other causes of malabsorption.

References and Further Reading

Barry, M. A., Weatherhead, J. E., Hotez, P. J., & Woc-Colburn, L. (2013). Childhood parasitic infections endemic to the United States. *Pediatric Clinics of North America, 60*(2), 471–485.

Muhsen, K., & Levine, M. M. (2012). A systematic review and meta-analysis of the association between *Giardia lamblia* and endemic pediatric diarrhea in developing countries. *Clinical Infectious Diseases, 55*(Suppl 4), S271–S293.

Nash, T. E. (2013). Unraveling how Giardia infections cause disease. *The Journal of Clinical Investigation, 123*(6), 2346–2347.

Oberhuber, G., Kastner, N., & Stolte, M. (1997). Giardiasis: A histologic analysis of 567 cases. *Scandinavian Journal of Gastroenterology, 32*, 48–51.

Ortega, Y. N., & Adam, R. D. (1997). Giardia: Overview and update. *Clinical Infectious Diseases, 25*, 545–550.

Glomus Tumor, Gastrointestinal

José Manuel Lopes
Faculty of Medicine of the University of Porto and Institute of Molecular Pathology and Immunology of the University of Porto, Porto, Portugal

Synonyms

Glomangioma; Glomangiomatosis; Glomangiomyoma; Glomangiopericytoma; Glomangiosarcoma; Malignant glomus tumor; Symplastic glomus tumor

Definition

Glomus tumors are mesenchymal neoplasm comprising cells that resemble the modified smooth muscle cells of the normal glomus body. The glomus body is a specialized form of arteriovenous anastomosis which is involved in temperature regulation. There is a central coiled canal known as Sucquet-Hoyer canal which is lined by plump endothelial cells. This is surrounded by longitudinal and circular muscle fibers containing epithelial appearing glomus cells.

Clinical Features

- **Incidence**
  Glomus tumors are rare in the gastrointestinal tract. The incidence of glomus tumor is estimated to be 1% of that of gastrointestinal tumors.

- **Age**
  The median age of gastrointestinal glomus tumors is 48–55 years (range 19–90 years) (Kang et al. 2012).
- **Sex**
  Gastrointestinal glomus tumors predominate in females (~ 3:1) (Miettinnen et al. 2010).
- **Site**
  Most gastrointestinal glomus tumors occur in the stomach (it is the second commonest site after the skin), occasionally in the esophagus, the small intestine, and the colon (Miettinen et al. 2002).
- **Treatment**
  Preoperative diagnosis of gastric glomus tumor is difficult. Safe treatment of gastrointestinal glomus tumors consists of adequate excision (e.g., wedge resection), depending on location, aiming R0 surgical margins status. Enucleation is not recommended for glomus tumors due to the potential of high recurrence rates. Traumatized or incompletely excised glomus tumor may lead to intra- and postoperative hemorrhage. Since the overall number of cases reported is small, there are not enough data to support an active follow-up.
- **Outcome**
  Most glomus tumors are benign; malignant behavior, namely, due to liver metastasis, lymph nodes and peritoneum, is rare and unpredictable (Miettinen et al. 2002, 2010). Features associated to malignant behavior of glomus tumors in deep soft tissues include size >2 cm, atypical mitotic figures, moderate to high nuclear atypia, and five mitoses per 50 high power fields (HPFs). However, there seems to be a marked difference in clinical behavior between glomus tumors in deep peripheral soft tissue and those in the stomach. The rate of malignant behavior of gastrointestinal glomus tumors is lower than for glomus tumors at deep soft tissues. Gastric glomus tumors are usually small, with median size ranging from 2 to 3 cm, but the tumors that metastasized were 6.5 and 8.5 cm. The evaluation of nuclear atypia may be subjective, and the described metastatic glomus tumors showed only mild nuclear atypia with a few mitoses (1–3/50 HPFs). Therefore, absence of nuclear atypia and paucity of mitotic activity do not rule out malignant potential, and the size greater than 5 cm might be a more appropriate indicator of risk for gastric glomus tumor (Kang et al. 2012).

Macroscopy

Most glomus stomach tumors locate in the antrum but may occur in other gastric sites. Rarely, they are multiple lesions located the lesser curve, anterior, and posterior wall of the gastric corpus. In some cases, the glomus tumors are incidental findings during clinical evaluation or abdominal operation. Glomus tumors are usually well circumscribed, round or oval, intramural, located in gastric submucosa or muscularis, endoluminal, sometimes ulcerated, or serosal. On sectioning, glomus tumors vary from soft to rubbery and are variably white, pink, red, or brown solid masses, with calcification and hemorrhagic foci. Pseudocapsule may form around the tumor. Median size of gastrointestinal glomus tumors is 2.0–3.0 cm (range, 0.8–22.0 cm) (Kang et al. 2012).

Microscopy

Glomus tumors comprise small uniform rounded or slightly polygonal epithelioid-like cells with sharp cellular borders and central small uniform round nucleus with fine chromatin and inconspicuous nucleoli and amphophilic to lightly eosinophilic cytoplasm, occasionally oncocytic or clear, and cells may be spindled (Figs. 1, 2–4). The tumor cells are outlined by PAS (periodic acid Schiff)-positive basement membranes. Mitotic index of gastrointestinal glomus tumors is low, usually <1/50 HPF and usually <5/50 high power fields in mitotically active tumors; nuclear atypia may be observed (symplastic glomus tumor); intramuscular tumors >2 cm in largest dimension with >5/50 HPF mitosis or atypical mitosis should be considered as having risk of malignant behavior (malignant glomus tumor, glomangiosarcoma) (Miettinnen 2010). Glomus

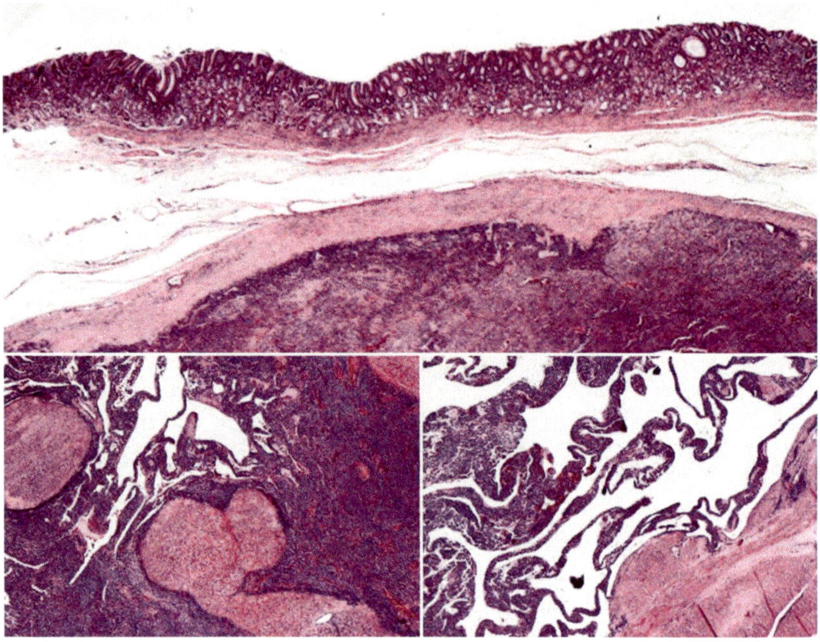

Glomus Tumor, Gastrointestinal, Fig. 1 Low power view and detailed features of gastric glomus tumor

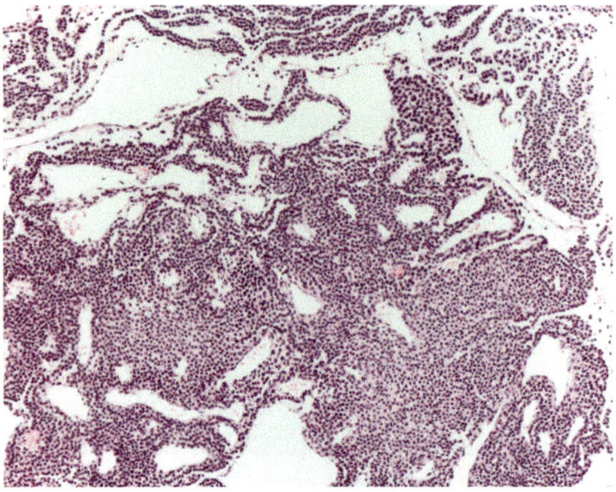

Glomus Tumor, Gastrointestinal, Fig. 2 Solid and angiomatous pattern

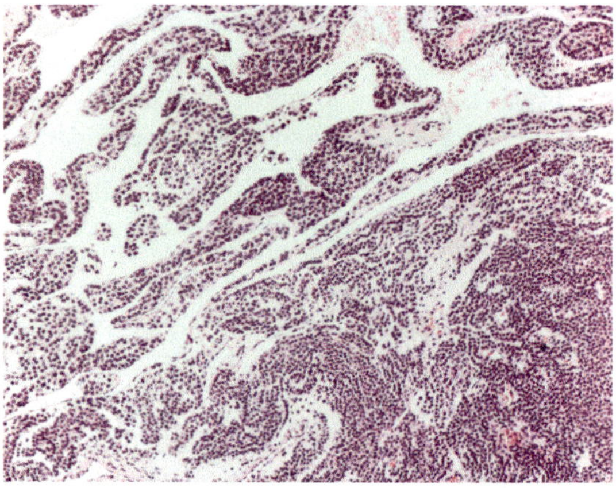

Glomus Tumor, Gastrointestinal, Fig. 3 Solid and angiomatous pattern (higher amplification)

tumor cells are surrounded by basal lamina and stroma may be myxoid or hyaline (Fig. 5) and contain sparse mast cells, small thin vessels, and sometimes hemangiopericytoma-like vessels (glomangiopericytoma). Glomus tumor cells may display solid patterns, that are separated by bands of gastric smooth muscle or surround dilated cavernous vessels (glomangiomas), and transition to elongated smooth muscle type cells (glomangiomyomas). The stroma may be hyalinized. Some tumors may have intravascular growth (glomangiomatosis type) without adverse prognostic significance (Miettinnen et al. 2010).

Immunophenotype

Glomus tumor cells display strong expression of vimentin, smooth muscle actin (Fig. 6), sometimes CD34, and variable h-caldesmon, calponin, and focal synaptophysin, in the absence of CD117-cluster of differentiation molecule

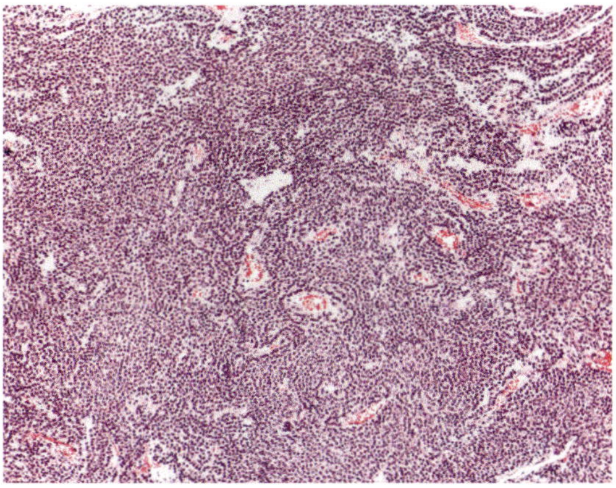

Glomus Tumor, Gastrointestinal, Fig. 4 Solid pattern

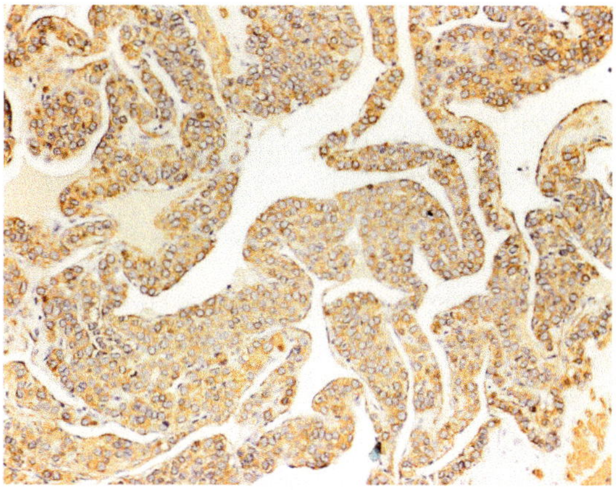

Glomus Tumor, Gastrointestinal, Fig. 6 Diffuse expression of smooth muscle actin in glomus gastric tumor cells

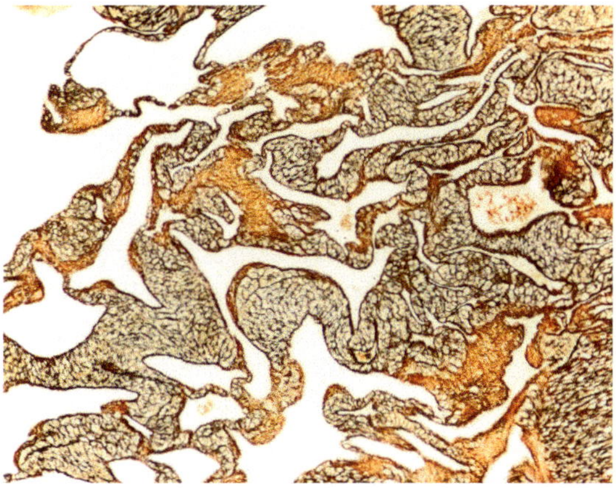

Glomus Tumor, Gastrointestinal, Fig. 5 Reticulin surrounding individual glomus gastric tumor cells

117/KIT (kinase-tyrosine receptor of stem cell factor), DOG1 (discovered on GIST-1), desmin, keratins, S100 protein, chromogranin, CD20 (cluster differentiation molecule 20), and CD 45 (cluster differentiation molecule 45). Laminin and collagen IV is expressed in the pericellular matrix (net-like pattern) of glomus tumors (Miettinnen et al. 2010; Miettinnen 2010).

Molecular Features

The current literature on sporadic glomus tumors records no molecular findings in gastrointestinal glomus tumors which lack *KIT (kinase-tyrosine receptor of stem cell factor)* and *PDGFRA (platelet-derived growth factor receptor alpha)* gene mutations that are characteristic of GISTs (gastrointestinal stromal tumors) (Miettinen et al. 2002).

Differential Diagnosis

Immunohistochemistry is essential in the differential diagnosis of glomus tumors. Glomangiopericytoma should be differentiated from other mesenchymal tissue tumors with hemangiopericytoma-like features, such as solitary fibrous tumor, and hemangiopericytoma which are usually negative for smooth muscle actin and from epithelioid GISTs that usually express CD117/KIT and DOG1. They should also be differentiated from NETs (neuroendocrine tumors) which display expression of keratins, synaptophysin, and chromogranin A in the absence of smooth muscle actin. Other differential diagnoses include tumors of smooth muscle, vascular, or nerve sheet origin, such as angioleiomyoma, hemangioma, or peripheral nerve sheet tumor. Occasionally, highly cellular glomus tumors may be mistaken for nevi or even malignant melanomas which express S100 protein and malignant lymphomas that express CD45.

References and Further Reading

Kang, G., Park, H. P., Kim, J. Y., Choi, D., Min, B. H., Lee, J. H., Kim, J. J., Kim, K.-M., Park, C. K., Sohn, T. S., & Kim, S. (2012). Glomus tumor of the stomach: A clinicopathologic analysis of 10 cases and review of the literature. *Gut and Liver, 6*, 52–57.

Miettinen, M., Paal, E., Lasota, J., & Sobin, L. H. (2002). Gastrointestinal glomus tumors: A clinicopathologic, immunohistochemical, and molecular genetic study of 32 cases. *American Journal of Surgical Pathology, 26*, 301–311.

Miettinnen, M. (2010). Glomus tumor, sinonasal haemangiopericytoma, and myopericytoma. In M. Miettinen (Ed.), *Modern soft tissue pathology: Tumors and non-neoplastic conditions* (pp. 648–656). Cambridge: Cambridge University Press.

Miettinnen, M., Fletcher, C. D. M., Kindblom, L.-G., & Tsui, W. M. S. (2010). Mesenchymal tumours of the oesophagus, stomach, small intestine, colon and rectum. In F. T. Bosman, F. Carneiro, R. H. Hruban, & N. E. Theise (Eds.), *WHO classification of tumours of the digestive system* (p. 76). Lyon: International Agency for Research on Cancer (IARC).

Glycogenic Acanthosis

Rita Canas Marques[1] and Ricardo Fonseca[2]
[1]Serviço de Anatomia Patológica, Instituto Português de Oncologia de Lisboa de Francisco Gentil and Faculdade de Ciências Médicas, Universidade Nova de Lisboa, Lisbon, Portugal
[2]Serviço de Anatomia Patológica, Instituto Português de Oncologia de Lisboa Francisco Gentil, Lisboa, Portugal

Synonyms

Hyperplasia; Leukoplakia

Definition

First named by Rywlin and Ortega (1970), glycogenic acanthosis is an esophageal disorder characterized by multifocal white plaques of hyperplastic squamous epithelium with abundant intracellular glycogen deposits (Lopes et al. 2010). Its pathogenesis remains unclear; no positive correlation has been made between glycogenic acanthosis and dietary habitus, the use of tobacco, or significant alcoholic intake (Glick et al. 1982). It has been suggested that this entity could be a nonspecific pattern of epithelial response to anatomical site-specific injury (Fyfe and Garcia 1998). However, an association between glycogenic acanthosis and gastroesophageal reflux disease has been reported (Berliner et al. 1981; Lopes et al. 2010), Cowden's syndrome (Coriat et al. 2011; Kay et al. 1997; Lashner et al. 1986; McGarrity et al. 2003), and Celiac disease (Suoglu et al. 2004). Unless there is a coexisting disease, patients with glycogenic acanthosis are asymptomatic (Glick et al. 1982).

Clinical Features

- **Incidence**
  Incidence: 5–15% in endoscopic series (Berliner et al. 1981; Glick et al. 1982; Lopes et al. 2010); 20–40% (Lee et al. 2007); 15–100% in autopsy series (Berliner et al. 1981; Glick et al. 1982).
- **Age**
  The incidence seems to increase with age. In the original study (Rywlin and Ortega 1970), patient's age ranged between 52 and 85 years old (Rywlin and Ortega 1970).
- **Sex**
  There is no gender predilection.
- **Site**
  May involve any segment of the esophagus but is more prominent in the distal third (Bender et al. 1973; Lee et al. 2007; Lopes et al. 2010; Stern et al. 1980). There is one case of glycogenic acanthosis reported in the larynx (Fyfe and Garcia 1998).
- **Treatment**
  No treatment is required.
- **Outcome**
  Glycogen acanthosis is a benign condition, clinically insignificant, that does not require surveillance (Belafsky 2004). An endoscopy should be used only when the appearance is atypical and/or the clinical suspicion of esophageal disease is high (Glick et al. 1982).

Macroscopy

At esophagoscopy, these lesions appear as slightly raised gray-white plaques, which are usually 2–10 mm in diameter ($<$50 mm), surrounded by normal mucosal. These whitish mucosal elevations may be discrete or extensive and confluent assuming a conglomerative pattern of growth giving a cobblestone-like appearance of the esophageal mucosa (Fig. 1) (Lopes et al. 2010). The larger lesions may appear to have a polypoid nature (Berliner et al. 1981).

Microscopy

Glycogenic acanthosis is characterized by a two- to three-fold increase of the epithelial layer due to epithelial hyperplasia and cellular hypertrophy through swelling of the more superficial cells due to increased intracellular glycogen (Fig. 2) (Berliner et al. 1981; Glick et al. 1982).

The esophagic mucosa is composed of squamous epithelium that is focally thickened by groups of enlarged and clear cells located in the upper layers of the epithelium which contain abundant cytoplasmatic glycogen and appear clear because of routine histological processing removal (Fig. 3) (Lopes et al. 2010).

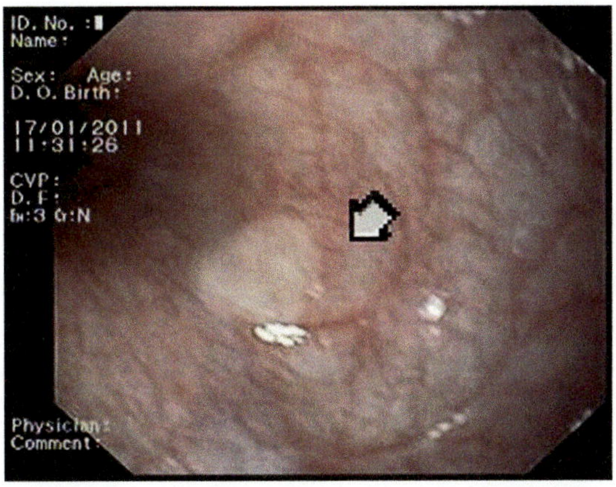

Glycogenic Acanthosis, Fig. 1 Endoscopic view of an esophagus with discrete raised whitish mucosal elevations that coalesce in a cobblestone-like appearance

Hyperkeratosis, cell atypia and, dysplasia are absent (Bender et al. 1973), and there is no malignant potential (Berliner et al. 1981).

Immunophenotype

There is no specific immunophenotype of this lesion. However, studies regarding its histochemical profile revealed that the epithelial esophageal cells in glycogenic acanthosis are positive with

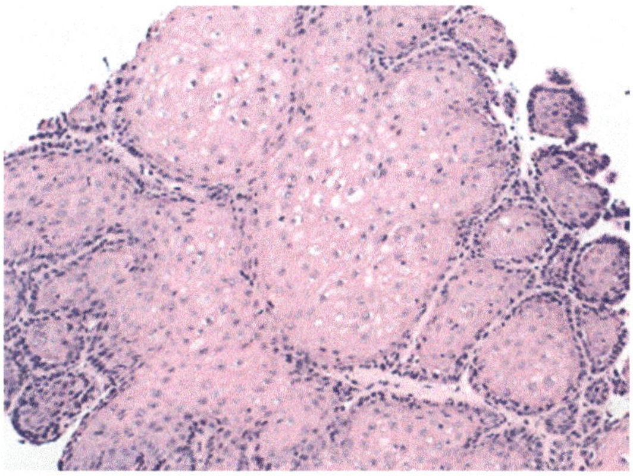

Glycogenic Acanthosis, Fig. 2 Low-power microscopic appearance (200×) of glycogenic acanthosis. Cellular hyperplasia and hypertrophy of the squamous epithelium due to swelling of cells mostly in the superficial cell layers

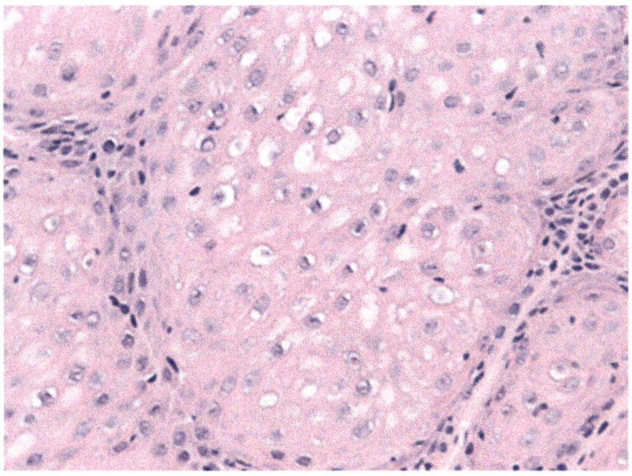

Glycogenic Acanthosis, Fig. 3 High-power microscopic appearance (400×) of glycogenic acanthosis. Groups of enlarged and clear cells are seen at the upper layers of the squamous epithelium which cells contain abundant cytoplasmatic glycogen that as a clear appearance with hematoxylin-eosin stain

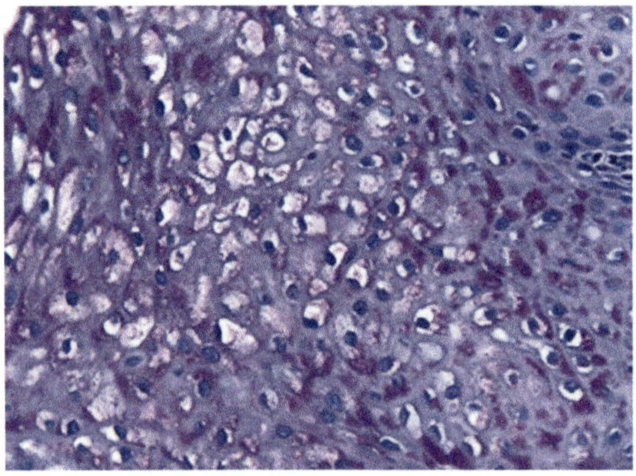

Glycogenic Acanthosis, Fig. 4 PAS stain at high-power view (400×). Positive PAS material is observed within the cytoplasm of the clear and enlarged epithelial squamous cells

Periodic Acid Schiff (PAS) (Fig. 4), and are diastase-sensitive, and are negative for Oil red O and Colloidal iron stainings.

Molecular Features

No molecular features have been studied in this condition.

Differential Diagnosis

This entity should be included in the differential diagnosis of superficial mucosal lesions of the esophagus (Berliner et al. 1981) such as esophageal leukoplakia, moniliasis, and bullous pemphigoid.

Leukoplakia, although rare in the esophagus, is characterized by inflamed edematous mucosa covered with a superficial white layer. Histologically, dyskeratosis, parakeratosis, and cellular atypia are typical features (Stern et al. 1980).

Moniliasis lesions are usually smaller and whiter lesions are surrounded by an edematous and hyperemic mucosa.

References and Further Reading

Belafsky, P. C. (2004). Glycogenic acanthosis. *Ear, Nose, & Throat Journal, 83*, 229.

Bender, M. D., et al. (1973). Glycogenic acanthosis of the esophagus: A form of benign epithelial hyperplasia. *Gastroenterology, 65*, 373–380.

Berliner, L., et al. (1981). Glycogen plaques (glycogenic acanthosis) of the esophagus. *Radiology, 141*, 607–610.

Coriat, R., et al. (2011). Endoscopic findings in Cowden syndrome. *Endoscopy, 43*, 723–726.

Fyfe, B. S., & Garcia, F. U. (1998). Laryngeal glycogenic acanthosis presenting as leukoplakia. *Archives of Otolaryngology – Head & Neck Surgery, 124*, 1029–1030.

Glick, S. N., et al. (1982). Glycogenic acanthosis of the esophagus. *AJR. American Journal of Roentgenology, 139*, 683–688.

Kay, P. S., et al. (1997). Diffuse esophageal glycogenic acanthosis: An endoscopic marker of Cowden's disease. *The American Journal of Gastroenterology, 92*, 1038–1040.

Lashner, B. A., et al. (1986). Ganglioneuromatosis of the colon and extensive glycogenic acanthosis in Cowden's disease. *Digestive Diseases and Sciences, 31*, 213–216.

Lee, J. K., et al. (2007). Education and imaging. Gastrointestinal: Glycogenic acanthosis. *Journal of Gastroenterology Hepatology, 22*, 1550.

Lopes, S., et al. (2010). Glycogenic acanthosis of the esophagus: An unusually endoscopic appearance. *Revista Espanola de Enfermedades Digestivas, 102*, 341–342.

McGarrity, T. J., et al. (2003). GI polyposis and glycogenic acanthosis of the esophagus associated with PTEN mutation positive Cowden syndrome in the absence of cutaneous manifestations. *American Journal of Gastroenterology, 98*, 1429–1434.

Rywlin, A. M., & Ortega, R. (1970). Glycogenic acanthosis of the esophagus. *Archives of Pathology, 90*, 439–443.

Stern, Z., et al. (1980). Glycogenic acanthosis of the esophagus. A benign but confusing endoscopic lesion. *American Journal of Gastroenterology, 74*, 261–263.

Suoglu, O. D., et al. (2004). Celiac disease and glycogenic acanthosis: A new association? *Acta Paediatrica, 93*, 568–570.

Goblet Cells

Chella R. S. van der Post[1] and Fátima Carneiro[2]
[1]Department of Pathology, Radboud University Medical Center, Nijmegen, The Netherlands
[2]Faculty of Medicine of Porto University, Centro Hospitalar São João and Ipatimup/i3S, Porto, Portugal

Synonyms

Mucus-producing cell

Anatomy

The number of goblet cells increases with distal progression along the bowel, from duodenum 4% to distal colon 16%, where they are most abundant in the sigmoid colon and rectum. Reflecting a dominant function in absorption and antigen processing, the right colon displays a higher colonocyte to goblet cell ratio (5:1) as compared to the left colon. Proceeding distally an increase in goblet cells are apparent, facilitating increased formation of gel-type mucin in the descending and sigmoid colon necessary for consolidation and transit of the increasingly formed fecal matter. Their broad shape creates the false impression that they constitute the majority of the cells; however, in the sigmoid colon and rectum, the ratio is approximately one goblet cell for every four columnar cells.

Goblet cells are also found in other epithelia and they are a normal component of the conjunctiva, respiratory epithelium of the nose and larynx, and in the bronchial epithelium. Goblet cells are sometimes encountered in the ductal epithelium of the pancreas, endocervix, and anal intramuscular glands. Goblet cell metaplasia can be seen in the gastroesophageal junction and stomach; however, goblet cells in the upper intestinal tract do not belong to the normal cell staff, and the presence of goblet cells is referred to intestinal metaplasia.

Function

Goblet cells in the gut play an important role in mucosal protection. They secrete mucus, ions, and water into the overlying mucous gel that protects the epithelial cell surfaces. Goblet cells also produce trefoil peptides, which are important in preventing intestinal injury and promoting wound healing. The mucus layer overlying the epithelium secreted by the goblet cells promotes the elimination of gut contents and provides the first line of defense against physical and chemical injury caused by ingested food, microbes, and the microbial products. The mucus layer coating the gastrointestinal tract is the front line of innate host defense, largely because of the secretory products of intestinal goblet cells. Goblet cells in the small intestine contain both neutral and acid mucin and function as secretory cells, sustaining a moist viscid environment within the lumen. The acid mucins of the small intestine are primarily sialomucins, in contrast to the colonic goblet cell, which contains predominantly acid sulfomucins. The number of goblet cells increases with distal progression along the bowel.

Goblet cells appear early in the development and are present at 9–10 weeks gestation in the human fetal small intestine. They synthesize and secrete bioactive molecules such as secretory and membrane-bound mucins, trefoil peptides, resistin-like molecule β, and Fc-γ binding protein that are components of mucus. Two pathways secrete these molecules, constitutive or basal secretion, which is low-level continuous secretion dependent on cytoskeletal movement of secretory granules, or stimulated or regulated secretion, which involves exocytosis of granules in response to external stimuli. Mucins are the main goblet cell product. Mucins are highly glycosylated large glycoproteins with protein backbone structures rich in serine and threonine, which are linked to a wide variety of O-linked oligosaccharide side chains.

Intestinal metaplasia in the stomach is defined as the replacement of gastric columnar epithelial cells by cells with intestinal morphology, which appears in the multistep progression of (especially intestinal type) gastric cancer. Next to, chronic atrophic gastritis and dysplasia, intestinal metaplasia is considered to be an important step in the progression of gastric cancer. Intestinal metaplasia is a common condition, the prevalence of which increases with age and is associated with chronic atrophic gastritis, peptic ulcer, and gastric cancer.

Intestinal metaplasia, characterized by the presence of goblet cells, is separated into two broad types termed "complete" and "incomplete." This classification system is based primarily on the histologic and biochemical resemblance of metaplastic epithelium to normal intestinal epithelium. Common to both groups are typical round or barrel-shaped goblet cells secreting acid mucins. Incomplete intestinal metaplasia is composed of mucinous columnar epithelium mixed with goblet cells. This type is further subdivided into two subgroups based on the presence or absence of colonic-type mucins (termed sulfomucins) in the cytoplasm of mucinous columnar cells. In contrast, complete (type I) intestinal metaplasia is composed entirely of surface absorptive enterocytes with a well-developed brush border admixed with goblet cells and sometimes Paneth cells resembling the normal gut, without mucinous columnar epithelium.

Barrett's epithelium is histologically and biochemically similar to the incomplete (type II or III) metaplasia in the stomach. Less commonly, Barrett's epithelium may show complete type I intestinal metaplasia. Subtyping of intestinal metaplasia has no practical clinical significance in diagnosing or treating patients with Barrett metaplasia. Gastroesophageal reflux disease and *Helicobacter pylori* infection are the major etiologic factors in the development of inflammation and intestinal metaplasia of the gastroesophageal junction.

Microscopy

True goblet cells have a rounded goblet shape, have clear or slightly blue-tingled cytoplasm, and contain an eccentrically located and sometimes compressed nucleus. Goblet cells contain acid mucin that stains intensely blue with Alcian blue at pH 2.5. The goblet cell secretes mucin derived from the carbohydrate protein complex synthesized in the rough endoplasmic reticulum, which is then glycosylated, sulfated, and packaged in the Golgi system. The cytoplasmic mucin contains a mixture of both sialomucins and sulfomucins, but sialomucins generally predominate. Goblet cells can be readily recognized in H&E-stained tissue sections.

Intestinal metaplasia/goblet cells in Barrett have to be distinguished from pseudogoblet cells that are distended mucinous cells. These are barrel shaped and contain distended cytoplasmic vacuoles that impart an appearance similar to goblet cells. Pseudogoblet cells usually stain less intensely than true goblet cells using Alcian blue at pH 2.5. However, morphology is used to make

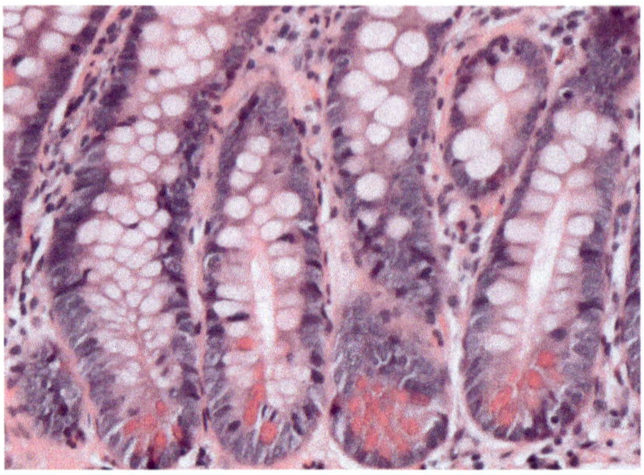

Goblet Cells, Fig. 1 Biopsy of the distal stomach shows glands with complete intestinal metaplasia with replacement of glands with goblet cells and Paneth cells

the distinction since the difference on Alcian blue is usually quite subtle. The acid mucins of the small intestine are primarily sialomucins, in contrast to the colonic goblet cell, which contains predominantly acid sulfomucins.

Intestinal metaplasia of the stomach or gastroesophageal junction can be easily recognized morphologically by the presence of goblet cells, absorptive cells, and cells resembling colonocytes by its enzyme or mucin content. Intestinal metaplasia has been categorized into complete and incomplete forms and using mucin histochemistry into three main types according to its morphology and glycoprotein content (Figs. 1 and 2). In type I complete intestinal metaplasia, goblet cells contain sialomucins and are interspersed between nonsecretory absorptive cells with well-delineated brush borders. In type II, sialomucin-containing goblet cells are scattered among gastric-type cells containing either neutral mucin or sialomucins. Type III is characterized by tortuous and branched crypts lined by tall columnar cells containing abundant sulfomucins with smaller numbers of goblet cells containing either sialomucins or sulfomucins.

Intestinal metaplasia is a condition predisposing to the development of carcinoma. Complete metaplasia is believed to carry the lowest risk of gastric cancer. However, there is not enough consensus or evidence; therefore, the performance of special stains to define the types of metaplasia and the assessment of gastric cancer risk is not regularly done.

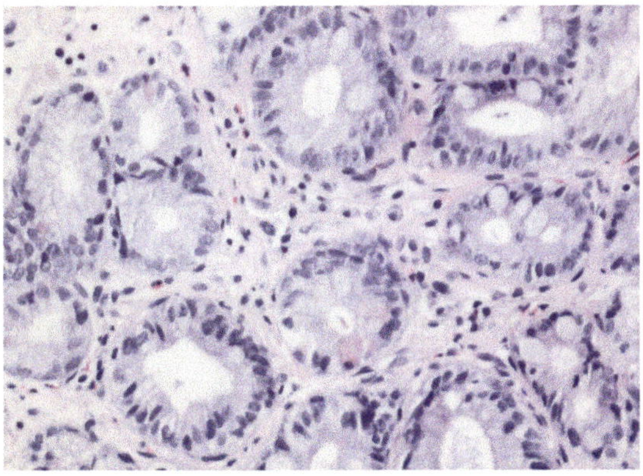

Goblet Cells, Fig. 2 Biopsy of the esophagus with Barrett's epithelium with irregular glands with scattered goblet cells and a few Paneth cells (incomplete metaplasia)

Immunophenotype and Immunohistochemistry

Goblet cells synthesize secretory mucin glycoproteins (MUC2) and bioactive molecules such as epithelial membrane-bound mucins (MUC1, MUC3, MUC17), trefoil factor peptides (TFF), resistin-like molecule β (RELMβ), and Fc-γ binding protein (Fcgbp).

Acidic glycoproteins are best demonstrated with the AB/PAS technique at pH 2.5 staining blue or purple, in contrast to the Schiff-positive neutral mucins present in the surface and foveolar epithelium and the mucous glands of the non-metaplastic gastric mucosa. In a combined Alcian blue/PAS stain, the droplets in goblet cells appear blue-purple.

Normal gastric mucosa produces mainly neutral mucins, except for the mucus-secreting cells of the neck glands that secrete acid mucins. Normal human stomach expresses MUC1, MUC5AC, and MUC6. MUC1 and MUC5AC are expressed in the superficial foveolar epithelium, whereas MUC6 is expressed in the mucous neck cells of the body and deeper glands of the antrum.

Complete intestinal metaplasia shows positive staining with MUC2 and CD10. Incomplete intestinal metaplasia is highlighted with MUC2, MUC1, MUC5AC, and MUC6.

Table with Important Diseases (Links)

Barrett's esophagus
Adenocarcinoma of the upper gastric tract
Goblet cell carcinoid

References and Further Reading

Filipe, M. I. (1979). Mucins in the human gastrointestinal epithelium: A review. *Investigative & Cell Pathology, 2*(3), 195–216.

Goldman, H., & Ming, S. C. (1968). Mucins in normal and neoplastic gastrointestinal epithelium. Histochemical distribution. *Archives of Pathology, 85*(6), 580–586.

Jass, J. R., & Filipe, M. I. (1981). The mucin profiles of normal gastric mucosa, intestinal metaplasia and its variants and gastric carcinoma. *The Histochemical Journal, 13*(6), 931–939.

Kim, Y. S., & Ho, S. B. (2010). Intestinal goblet cells and mucins in health and disease: Recent insights and progress. *Current Gastroenterology Reports, 12*(5), 319–330.

Odze, R. D. (2005). Unraveling the mystery of the gastroesophageal junction: A pathologist's perspective. *The American Journal of Gastroenterology, 100*(8), 1853–1867.

Silva, E., Teixeira, A., David, L., Carneiro, F., Reis, C. A., Sobrinho-Simoes, J., et al. (2002). Mucins as key molecules for the classification of intestinal metaplasia of the stomach. *Virchows Archiv, 440*(3), 311–317.

Granular Cell Tumor, Gastrointestinal

José Manuel Lopes
Faculty of Medicine of the University of Porto and Institute of Molecular Pathology and Immunology of the University of Porto, Porto, Portugal

Synonyms

Abrikossoff tumor; Granular cell myoblastoma; Granular cell nerve sheath tumor; Granular cell schwannoma

Definition

Granular cell tumors comprise a group of variable etiological and clinical tumors characterized by large cells with granular eosinophilic cytoplasm. Myoblasts, Schwann cells, histiocytes, perineural fibroblasts, and undifferentiated mesenchymal cells have been postulated as the origin of the tumor, while theories of the nonneoplastic nature of the lesion resulting from trauma, as a degenerative process or as a storage disorder involving histiocytes, have also been claimed. Recent reports support a peripheral nerve-related cell of origin for the majority of these tumors based on the findings of cytoplasmic granules with numerous membrane-bound vacuoles containing myelin-like tubules and “angulate bodies” that show close relation with preexistent axons at the ultrastructural level, found between granular cells. The expression of nestin in granular cell tumors suggests that these tumors may arise from a common multipotential stem cell in the gastrointestinal tract, which has the potential to differentiate along both interstitial cell of Cajal and peripheral nerve pathways. Despite remaining controversies about granular cell tumor histogenesis, Schwann cell derivation from multipotential stem cell is the most frequent and favored origin for this nonspecific cell lineage tumor type (Johnston and Helwig 1981; Parfitt et al. 2006; Radaeli and Minoli 2009).

Clinical Features

- **Incidence**
  Granular cell tumors are uncommon tumors and up to 8% occur in the gastrointestinal tract (Radaeli and Minoli 2009).
- **Age**
  The mean age of granular cell tumors is 41.8 years (range, 15–79 years) (Johnston and Helwig 1981). In the esophagus they occur in the fourth to sixth decades (range, 23–65), and colorectal granular cell tumors occur in the sixth decade (range, 22–79) (Parfitt et al. 2006; Johnston and Helwig 1981).
- **Sex**
  The male/female ratio of granular cell tumors is 1.4:1 (Johnston and Helwig 1981). In the esophagus, granular cell tumors are more common in women, whereas in the colorectal, they are more common in men (Parfitt et al. 2006).
- **Site**
  Most granular cell tumors occur in the submucosa of (distal) esophagus (some as multiple tumors), followed by colorectal (more in cecum and rectum, some as multiple tumors), stomach, appendix, and small bowel; duodenal granular cell tumors are extremely rare (Johnston and Helwig 1981; Parfitt et al. 2006).
- **Treatment**
  Surveillance endoscopy can be considered, after histological biopsy diagnosis, for asymptomatic small granular cell tumors whenever resection-related risks outweigh the potential benefits, thus avoiding the potential complications of surgical procedures. Otherwise, safe treatment is resection, by either endoscopy (polypectomy when <1 cm; mucosal resection or submucosal dissection for larger tumors) or surgery (Radaeli and Minoli 2009) aiming R0 margins, particularly in symptomatic patients with large tumors or those with tumors demonstrating rapid growth, having transmural infiltration, or suspected of malignancy. For larger tumors, the views concerning treatment have been changing over the years with the introduction of new therapeutic options including laser, diathermy loop, and endoscopic resection.
- **Outcome**
  Granular cell tumors usually follow a benign course, recurrence occurs in up to 10% (Parfitt et al. 2006) and malignancy in <2% of the cases (Parfitt et al. 2006). The features associated with the possibility of malignancy include local recurrence, fast growth to a size larger than 4 cm, tumor necrosis, increased cellularity, spindle tumor cells, cytologic atypia, high nuclear to cytoplasmic ratio, pleomorphism, vesicular nuclei with large nucleoli, mitotic index higher than two mitoses per high-power field, and infiltrative pattern of growth. Also a positivity rate of more than 50% for p53

(tumor suppressor protein 53) and a Ki-67 (proliferation-related antigen) labelling index higher than 10% indicates potential malignant behavior. There are reports of cases that have recurred or metastasized despite having a benign histological appearance. Regrowth may be common due to incomplete tumor resection.

Macroscopy

Granular cell tumors are nonencapsulated, usually submucosal, sometimes polypoid, yellow-white and solid nodules, rarely with transmural infiltration. Most are solitary, <2 cm in largest dimension, but synchronous presentations can occur in up to 20% of cases.

Microscopy

Granular cell tumors comprise plump, polygonal cells with abundant granular light eosinophilic cytoplasm, with round, small, and uniform hyperchromatic nuclei (Fig. 1). The most characteristic feature of these lesions is that the cytoplasm of the neoplastic cells demonstrates globular and diffuse periodic acid-Schiff positivity, which remains after diastase digestion. Nuclear pleomorphism, prominent nucleoli, and mitotic figures are uncommon. The tumors can display infiltrative (sometimes with remote satellite nodules) or expansive growth pattern, a lymphoid cuff, focal calcification, and reactive mucosal surface changes. The growth pattern varies with the age of the lesion; while the cells tend to form large nests surrounded by thin fibrous septa in younger lesions, the pattern of older lesions is characterized by marked desmoplasia with few scattered small nests of granular cells embedded in a dense collagenous stroma. While tumor cells are mainly polygonal or round, areas composed of spindle cells can be observed, especially in colonic granular cell tumors. In the esophagus, the overlying squamous epithelium may display pseudo-epitheliomatous hyperplasia. It is unclear whether the 3-tiered grading system used for soft tissue tumors – benign, atypical, and malignant – based on the presence of necrosis, nuclear atypia, and mitotic activity is useful in granular cell tumors of the gastrointestinal tract (Miettinen et al. 2010).

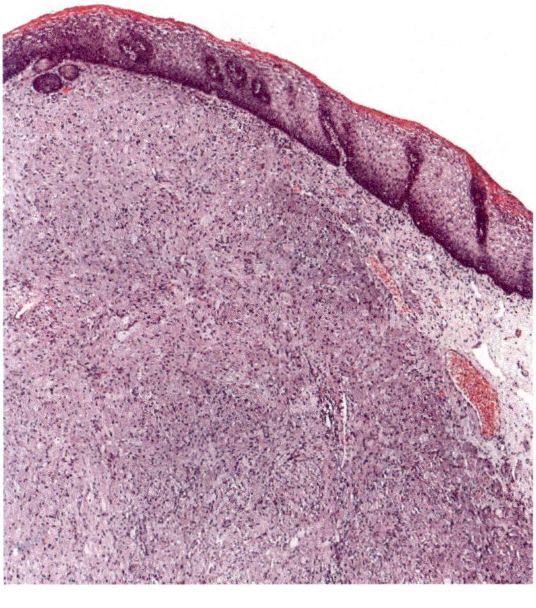

Granular Cell Tumor, Gastrointestinal, Fig. 1 Low power features of esophagus granular cell tumor

Immunophenotype

Granular cell tumor cells express S-100 protein (Fig. 2), vimentin, neuron-specific enolase, CD68 (cluster differentiation molecule 68), alpha1-antitrypsin, CD57 (cluster differentiation antigen 57) (Leu-7), myelin basic protein, PGP 9.5 (protein gene product 9.5), nestin (found normally in neuroectodermal stem cells and early skeletal muscle), inhibin-alpha, calretinin, laminin, NGFR (nerve growth factor receptor), and P2-P0 (peripheral nerve myelin proteins P2 and P0) in the absence of smooth muscle actin, desmin, neural filaments, CD117 (cluster differentiation molecule 117)/KIT (kinase-tyrosine receptor of stem cell factor), DOG1 (discovered on GIST-1), keratins, HMB45 (premelanosome glycoprotein present in melanomas and other tumors derived from

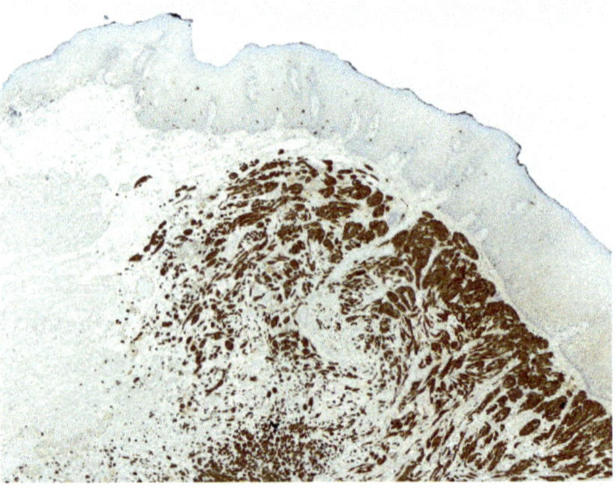

Granular Cell Tumor, Gastrointestinal, Fig. 2 Low power features of diffuse expression of S100 protein in esophagus granular cell tumor

melanocytes), Melan-A (protein antigen present in melanocytes), CD34 (cluster differentiation molecule 34), and GFAP (glial fibrillary acidic protein) (Parfitt et al. 2006).

Molecular Features

So far, there are no available data regarding molecular features of granular cell tumors.

Differential Diagnosis

The diagnosis of gastrointestinal granular cell tumors is usually straightforward based on adequate clinical/imaging evaluation, sampling, histology, and immunohistochemistry studies. Differential diagnoses may include gastrointestinal stromal tumor, leiomyoma, leiomyosarcoma, and carcinoma.

References and Further Reading

Johnston, J. M., & Helwig, E. B. (1981). Granular cell tumors of the gastrointestinal tract and perianal region. A study of 74 cases. *Digestive Diseases and Sciences, 26*, 807–816.

Miettinen, M., Fletcher, C. D. M., Kindblom, L.- G., & Tsui, W. M. S. (2010). Mesenchymal tumours of the oesophagus, and colon and rectum. In F. T. Bosman, F. Carneiro, R. H. Hruban, & N. E. Theise. (Eds.), *WHO classification of tumours of the digestive system* (pp. 35–36, and 182, respectively). Lyon: International Agency for Research on Cancer (IARC).

Parfitt, J. R., McLean, C. A., Joseph, M. G., Streutker, C. J., Al-Haddad, S., & Driman, D. K. (2006). Granular cell tumours of the gastrointestinal tract: Expression of nestin and clinicopathological evaluation of 11 patients. *Histopathology, 48*, 424–430.

Radaeli, F., & Minoli, G. (2009). Granular cell tumors of the gastrointestinal tract: Questions and answers. *Gastroenterology and Hepatology, 5*, 798–800.

Granulomatous Gastritis

Wen-Yih Liang[1] and Gregory Y. Lauwers[2]
[1]Department of Pathology, Taipei Veterans General Hospital, Taipei, Taiwan
[2]Department of Pathology, Massachusetts General Hospital, Harvard Medical School, Boston, MA, USA

Definition

Granulomatous gastritis is a descriptive diagnosis that encompasses a broad range of conditions characterized by the development of mucosal or submucosal granulomas.

Clinical Features

Etiology/Pathogenesis

The development of granulomatous gastritis can be associated with multiple etiologies, including infectious, immune-related, and foreign material, among others (Table 1).

- Crohn disease is the most common etiology in Western nations, representing 17–55% of cases. The patients tend to be of the pediatric age group and complain of nausea, vomiting, and upper abdominal pain. Endoscopic and microscopic involvement of the lower gastrointestinal tract is common but not obligatory.
- Gastric sarcoidosis may be detected in patients with an established diagnosis, or as a presenting manifestation of the disease. In

Granulomatous Gastritis, Table 1 Etiologies of granulomatous gastritis

Idiopathic	
Infectious agents	Tuberculosis (*Mycobacterium tuberculosis*)
	Histoplasma capsulatum
	Anisakis (*Anisakis simplex*)
	Taeniasis and *Strongyloides stercoralis*
	Syphilis (*Treponema pallidum*)
Systemic conditions	Sarcoidosis
	Crohn disease
	Langerhans cell histiocytosis
	Chronic granulomatous disease
	Common variable immunodeficiency
	Wegener granulomatosis
Foreign bodies	Impacted food, drug coatings
	Suture material, barium
	Drugs
Periphery of neoplastic process	Adenocarcinoma
	Lymphoma

North America, the disease is more common in African-Americans. The diagnosis remains a diagnosis of exclusion. Detection of hypercalcemia and granulomatous lesions of the lung, liver, and lymph nodes will be significant in confirming the diagnosis.

- It is now generally accepted, despite early publications, that *Helicobacter pylori* infection is not an etiology of gastric granuloma.
- Isolated granulomatous gastritis has been described as a distinct clinicopathologic entity. However, the diagnosis has been questioned due to lack of adequate clinical information and follow-up, which is especially important since some cases may in fact represent the first manifestation of sarcoidosis or Crohn disease. Thus, if no etiology is evoked, it is best to use a descriptive designation of "granulomatous gastritis of uncertain etiology" rather than idiopathic granulomatous gastritis.
- Other causes include foreign body granulomas (secondary to impacted food, suture material, or drugs) and rare causes of granulomatous inflammation, such as Langerhans cell histiocytosis, chronic granulomatous disease, common variable immunodeficiency, Whipple's disease, and systemic vasculitides. Gastric granulomas can also be diagnosed in association with neoplasia, i.e., adenocarcinomas and lymphomas likely representing an inflammatory response to the tumor proper or neoplastic antigens. Infectious etiologies, bacterial, fungal, and parasitic infections should always be considered.

Incidence

Granulomatous gastritis is uncommon. The incidence reported in various series ranges from 0.08% to 0.35%. The median age of the population studied, the geographic locale, and the socioeconomic factors play a role in the etiologies to be considered.

Presentation

Most cases are incidental with the discovery of a granuloma in a pinch biopsy evoking a series of various clinical conditions. However, in several conditions, inflammation of the gastric mucosa will be detected (see section "Macroscopy"). Abdominal pain, nausea, and vomiting with chronic diarrhea and weight loss can be observed in Crohn disease patients.

Treatment

In many instances, the detection of granulomatous gastritis is an accompanying feature that will not generate specific treatment. However, in systemic conditions, the treatment of the primary disease will be beneficial to the gastric manifestation. Antibiotic therapy is used for infectious etiologies and supportive care for noninfectious conditions.

Outcome

Except for infectious conditions, the diagnosis of granulomatous gastritis is frequently inconsequential, and the clinical course is related to the outcome and management of the underlying etiology.

Macroscopy

In many cases, the endoscopy is normal. However, various endoscopic features can be associated with a histologic diagnosis of granulomatous gastritis. These include erythema, mucosal nodularity, polyps, erosions, and ulcerations, as well as thickening of the gastric wall.

For example, changes associated with Crohn disease have been found predominantly in the antrum, including aphthoid-type erosions, cobblestone appearance, linear fissures, and thickened and nodular gastric folds (i.e., bamboo-like appearance) (Fig. 1). In tuberculosis, large nonhealing ulcers and stricturing fibrosis have been reported, while in syphilis, rugal hypertrophy, including linitis plastica, has been observed. In sarcoidosis, a similar pattern of mucosal nodularity, thickening, and linitis plastica-like (Fig. 2) involvement has been noted.

Microscopy

In general, the number, size, location, and composition of the granulomas are variable, and the morphology seldom points to a diagnosis. However, some specific features will be suggestive of certain etiologies. Large compact granulomas with Langerhans-type giant cells, a peripheral lymphocytic cuff, and mucosal scarring suggest sarcoidosis (Fig. 3). Necrotizing granulomas point toward infectious etiologies such as tuberculosis. Prominent eosinophilic infiltrate usually surrounds nematodes of *Anisakis*, other parasitic infections, and vasculitides. Crohn-associated granulomas are commonly antral

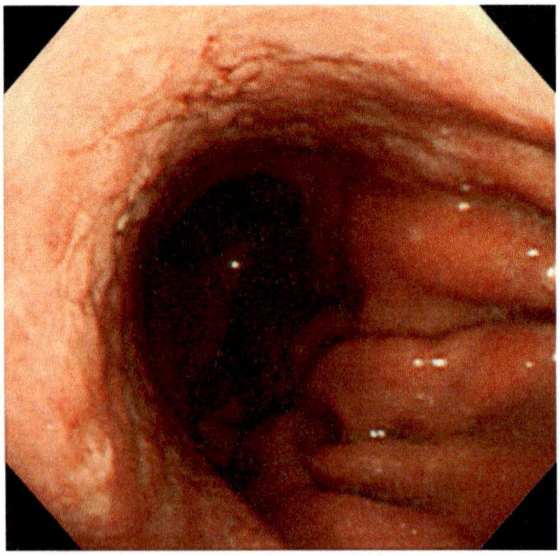

Granulomatous Gastritis, Fig. 1 Endoscopic picture of a patient with sarcoidosis. In this example, a diffuse mucosal infiltrate mimicking a neoplastic infiltrate was observed

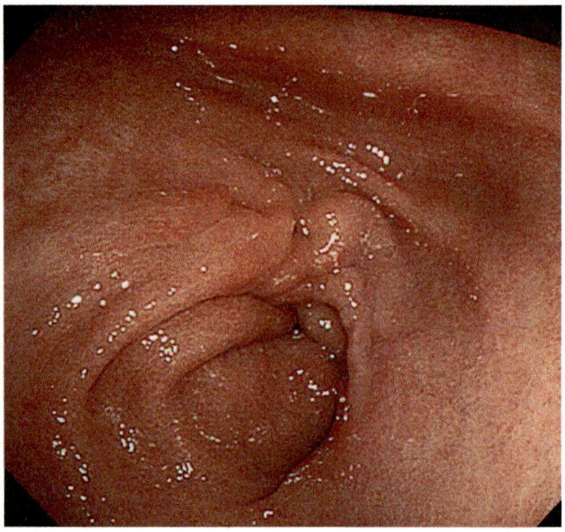

Granulomatous Gastritis, Fig. 2 Endoscopic picture of a case of involvement of the gastric mucosa with thickened and nodular gastric folds

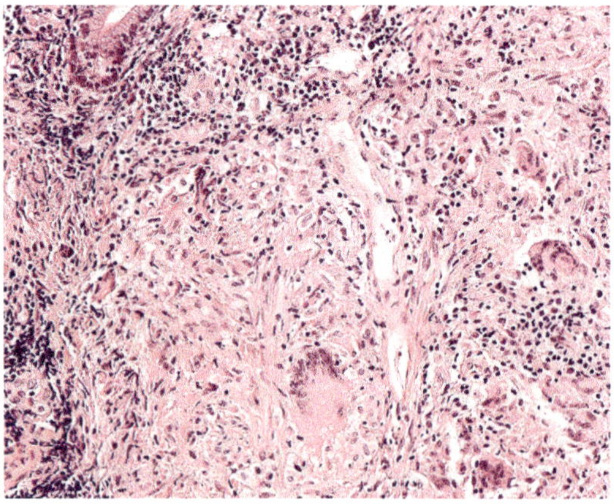

Granulomatous Gastritis, Fig. 3 Expansile and compact granuloma with distortion of the mucosal architecture in a patient with known sarcoidosis. Note the Langerhans-type giant cells and the (albeit minimal in this case) lymphocytic cuff

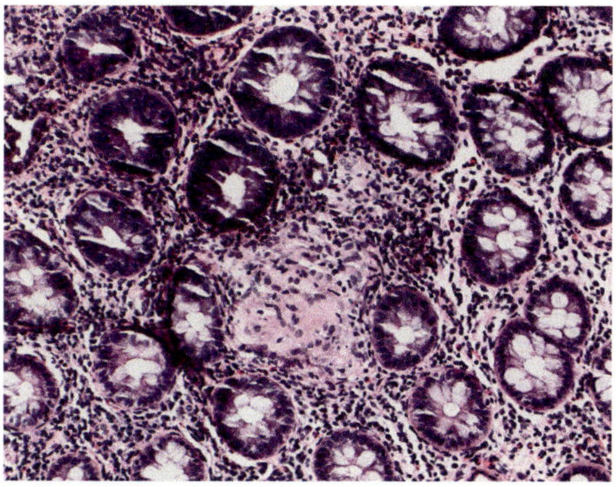

Granulomatous Gastritis, Fig. 4 Small non-necrotizing granuloma composed of clustered histiocytes in a patient with Crohn disease

and composed of small clusters of epithelioid histiocytes (Fig. 4). They are usually noted in the midzone close to the glandular isthmus and frequently are associated with focally enhanced gastritis.

Immunophenotype

No specific immunohistochemical stain is associated with a diagnosis of granulomatous gastritis.

Molecular Features

No single molecular feature is associated with a diagnosis of granulomatous gastritis. However, some PCR analysis, under certain conditions, will be helpful in ruling out or confirming some specific infectious diagnoses.

References and Further Reading

Daniels, J. A., et al. (2007). Gastrointestinal tract pathology in patients with common variable immunodeficiency (CVID): A clinicopathologic study and review. *The American Journal of Surgical Pathology, 31*(12), 1800–1812.

Ectors, N. L., et al. (1993). Granulomatous gastritis: A morphological and diagnostic approach. *Histopathology, 23*(1), 55–61.

Koyama, S., et al. (2003). Idiopathic granulomatous gastritis with multiple aphthoid ulcers. *Internal Medicine, 42*(8), 691–695.

Maeng, L., et al. (2004). Granulomatous gastritis: A clinicopathologic analysis of 18 biopsy cases. *The American Journal of Surgical Pathology, 28*(7), 941–945.

Sato, Y., et al. (2002). Gastric sarcoid without other sarcoid lesions. *Journal of Clinical Gastroenterology, 35*(4), 359.

Srivastava, A., et al. (2007). Pathology of non-infective gastritis. *Histopathology, 50*(1), 15–29.

H

Hamartomatous Polyps

Helena Baldaia
Serviço de Anatomia Patológica, Centro Hospitalar de São João, Porto, Portugal

Synonyms

Cowden syndrome; Hamartomatous polyposis; Juvenile polyposis; Juvenile polyps; Peutz-Jeghers polyps; Peutz-Jeghers syndrome

Definition

Hamartomatous polyps are malformations of tissue elements indigenous to the gastrointestinal (GI) tract that protrude into the visceral lumen (Fenoglio-Preiser et al. 2008). They are polypoid lesions characterized by a variable admixture of epithelial and mesenchymal elements that recapitulate the composition of normal gut.

Hamartomatous polyps can be found in almost any GI segment, either solitary sporadic lesions or part of hereditary polyposis syndromes. In the latter, in rare cases, their appearance is not specific, but in most, the histological features together with thorough clinical background will allow a proper diagnosis. This is of important prognostic importance since different polyposis syndromes have additional extra-GI manifestations and different association with the development of malignancy.

Peutz-Jeghers (PJ) polyps are part of the homonymous syndrome, an autosomal dominant disorder characterized by gastrointestinal hamartomatous polyps and pigmented mucosal and cutaneous macules, especially in orofacial location. These polyps can cause intussusception, bleeding, or pain. The occurrence of autoamputation is not rare. Patients with Peutz-Jeghers syndrome may present with hamartomas in the urogenital as well as the respiratory tract (Kopacova et al. 2009).

Juvenile polyps (JP) are the most frequent colorectal polyps in the pediatric population (Fenoglio-Preiser et al. 2008). They can occur as isolated lesions or in the context of Juvenile Polyposis syndrome which can be divided, clinically, into three subtypes (Hornick and Odze 2009). The rare juvenile polyposis of infancy is a fatal pediatric syndrome with polyps throughout the GI tract, diarrhoea, and protein-losing enteropathy. The juvenile polyposis coli and the generalized juvenile polyposis are autosomal dominant conditions presenting with juvenile polyps in the colon and rectum, in the former, and throughout the GI tract, in the latter. Extra-GI manifestations include a number of congenital birth defects, detectable in up to 15% of patients (Fenoglio-Preiser et al. 2008).

Juvenile polyps, associated with lipomas, ganglioneuromas, or lymphangiomas, can also

F. Carneiro et al. (eds.), *Pathology of the Gastrointestinal Tract*, Encyclopedia of Pathology,
DOI 10.1007/978-3-319-40560-5

occur in the setting of Cowden disease, part of the PTEN hamartomatous tumor syndrome. Cowden syndrome has numerous extra gastrointestinal features including mucocutaneous lesions, oesophageal glycogenosis, fibrocystic breast disease, and multinodular goiter (Calva and Howe 2008).

Cronkhite-Canada syndrome is a nonhereditary, adult onset, gastrointestinal polyposis syndrome (Fenoglio-Preiser et al. 2008). Hamartomatous polyps similar to juvenile polyps can occur in association with cutaneous hyperpigmentation, alopecia, and onychodystrophy. Clinical manifestations are similar to juvenile polyposis of infancy and include diarrhoea and an important protein-losing enteropathy (Fenoglio-Preiser et al. 2008).

Fundic gland polyps occur in the stomach and can be isolated, sporadic lesions, frequently associated with proton pump inhibitor therapy, or may occur in the setting of familial adenomatous polyposis (FAP). Although classically they have been categorized under hamartomatous polyps, the current WHO blue book considers them as neoplastic lesions (Lauwers et al. 2010) and they will be addressed in another chapter.

Clinical Features

- **Incidence**
  The incidence of hamartomatous polyps depends greatly on the context they appear in.
  Peutz-Jeghers sporadic polyps are very rare. PJ syndrome is estimated to occur in 1 in each 120,000 births (Fenoglio-Preiser et al. 2009).
  Isolated juvenile polyps occur in up to 2% of the pediatric population, constituting the most common hamartomatous GI polyps in infancy (Hornick and Odze 2009). Juvenile polyposis is rare, with an estimated incidence of 1 per 100,000 births (Fenoglio-Preiser et al. 2008).
- **Age**
  Sporadic Peutz-Jeghers polyps can occur at any age. The median time of appearance of polyps in PJ syndrome is 11–13 years (Kopacova et al. 2009).
  Juvenile polyps are most frequently diagnosed in the pediatric population, but they are also not rare in adults. One study reported a mean age of occurrence of 5.9 years (Hornick and Odze 2009).
- **Sex**
  There is no sex predilection for the occurrence of PJ polyps (Kopacova et al. 2009).
  In multiple juvenile polyps there is a male predilection. Isolated pediatric lesions occur with equal frequency in both genders (Fenoglio-Preiser et al. 2008).
- **Site**
  Peutz-Jeghers polyps can occur throughout the GI tract, affecting jejunum, ileum, colon, stomach (usually the antrum), duodenum, and appendix in decreasing order of frequency (Kopacova et al. 2009; Fenoglio-Preiser et al. 2008). Finding multiple polyps in the small bowel can be a diagnostic clue to PJ syndrome because other hamartomatous polyposis syndromes do not usually involve only this area (Hornick and Odze 2009).
  Sporadic juvenile polyps occur only in the colon or rectum, especially in the rectosigmoid colon (Hornick and Odze 2009). In juvenile polyposis coli besides appearing in the colorrectum, some polyps may arise in the small bowel. In generalized juvenile polyposis multiple polyps can occur in any segment of the GI tract (Hornick and Odze 2009).
- **Treatment**
  Treatment options depend mainly on the clinical context. Sporadic polyps can be excised with safety but lesions occurring in hereditary setting are not only much more numerous but associated with extra-gastrointestinal manifestations and an increased risk of malignancy such that management options should include symptomatic treatment and a surveillance protocol.
  In PJ syndrome screening protocols include colonoscopy since the beginning of symptoms or late teens, at least every 3 years, upper endoscopy biannually, and capsule or small bowel radiography annually. Also, screening for pancreatic neoplasia, breast cancer, and gynecological or testicular neoplasia should

be performed (Calva and Howe 2008; Fenoglio-Preiser et al. 2008).

In juvenile polyposis, all the polyps should be removed and analyzed. If the number is very high or if there is dysplasia or carcinoma, a colectomy or gastrectomy can be necessary. Colonoscopy and upper endoscopy screening for malignancy should start in the mid teens and continue annually if polyps are identified (Calva and Howe 2008).

Other hamartomatous polyposis syndromes, such as Cronkite-Canada syndrome that have associated anaemia and protein-losing enteropathy, may include the need for supportive therapy, such as transfusions and nutritional and electrolyte replacement therapy and/or removal of symptomatic segments of the GI tract (Calva and Howe 2008).

- **Outcome**
  The outcome of patients with hamartomatous lesions is variable.

  Solitary PJ polyps have no malignant potential (Hornick and Odze 2009). Peutz-Jeghers syndrome patients have an increased risk of developing a number of gastrointestinal and extragastrointestinal malignancies, particularly breast carcinoma (in both sexes) and ovarian, testicular, and biliary tumors. Ovarian sex cord tumor with annular tubules (SCAT) is particularly prevalent in this population. Also, mucinous ovarian tumors and adenoma malignum of the uterine cervix have been diagnosed in association with this syndrome (Fenoglio-Preiser et al. 2008). In the gastrointestinal tract, carcinoma occurs most commonly in the small intestine, particularly in the duodenum. 2–6% of PJ polyps can have foci of dysplasia or carcinoma (Yantiss and Antoniolli 2009). GI carcinomas in PJ syndrome patients develop in the second and third decade (Fenoglio-Preiser et al. 2008).

  Solitary juvenile polyps are not associated with malignancy or recurrence (Hornick and Odze 2009). In JP syndrome, however, the risk of upper or lower GI cancer has been estimated as 55%. In a study the mean age at diagnosis of carcinoma was 35.5 (range 4–60 years old), being the tumor stage advanced. Dysplasia and carcinoma occur both in juvenile polyps and in adenomatous lesions without evidence of juvenile polyp, mainly in larger lesions (>1 cm) and in villous polyps (Fenoglio-Preiser et al. 2008).

  JP syndrome patients also have an increased risk of developing gastric, duodenal, and pancreatic cancer (Calva and Howe 2008).

  Mortality in Cronkite-Canada syndrome can reach to as many as 60% of cases and derives mainly from hemorrhagic complications or malnutrition. Association with carcinoma, colonic or gastric, has been described in up to 20% of patients (Fenoglio-Preiser et al. 2008).

Macroscopy

Endoscopically, PJ polyps have a characteristic multinodular appearance and a thick stalk due to the abundance of smooth muscle fibers. They can be single or more than 100, carpeting the mucosa (Fenoglio-Preiser et al. 2008).

Juvenile polyps have a smooth surface and are usually small and pedunculated. Sometimes there is ulceration of the polyp surface. The cut surface frequently shows mucinous material filled cysts. In JP syndrome the number of polyps is usually between 50 and 200 and the mucosa between the polyps is usually spared. In Cronkite-Canada syndrome, lesions are usually indistinguishable from juvenile polyps but the intervening mucosa has edema and inflammatory features (Fenoglio-Preiser et al. 2008).

Microscopy

Peutz-Jeghers polyps have histological distinctive features (Fig. 1). They are lined by normal mucosa of the site of origin, such as villi with goblet and Paneth cells in the small bowel, colonic epithelium (sometime villous appearing) in the colon, or foveolar epithelium and endocrine cells in the stomach. In the duodenum, Brunner glands can be found. A feature distinctive to PJ polyps is the presence of dispersed arborizing thick smooth muscle bundles lined by indigenous epithelium

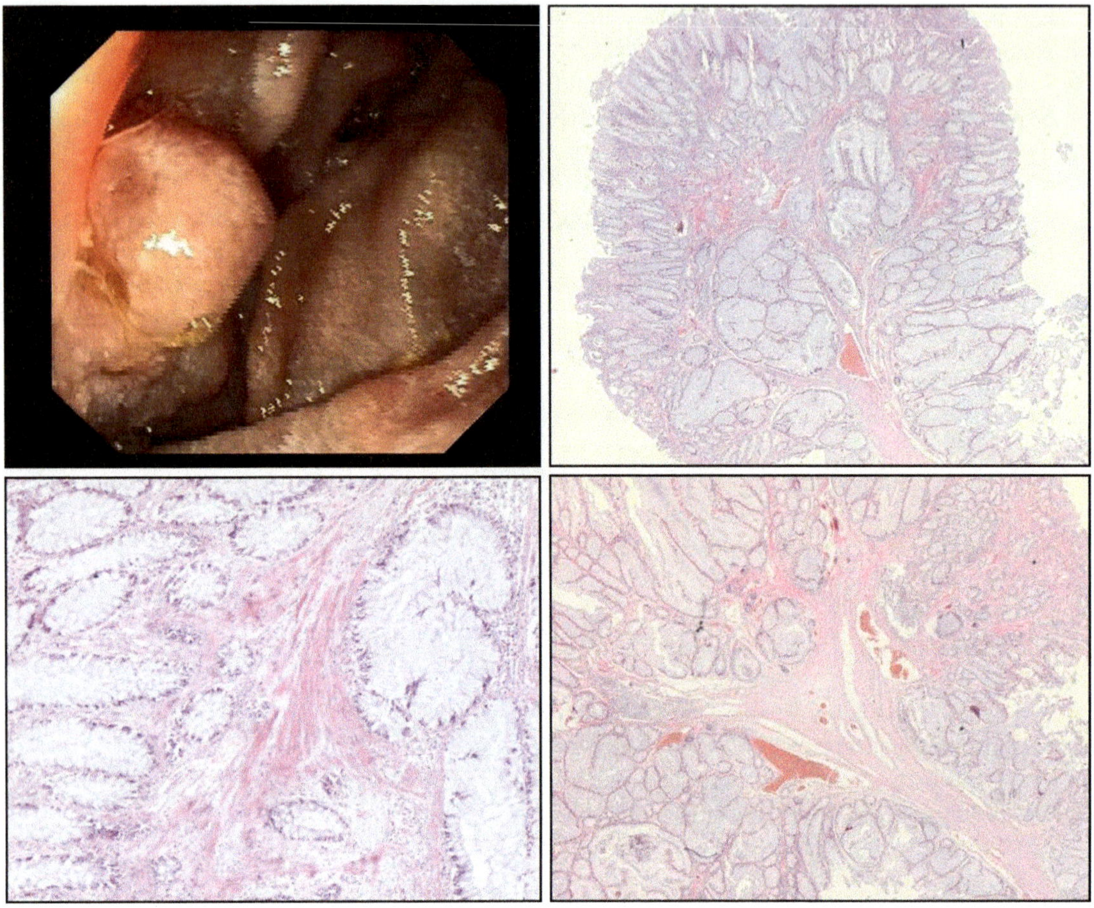

Hamartomatous Polyps, Fig. 1 Peutz-Jeghers polyp. Note the arborizing structure with prominent smooth muscle bundles in the lamina propria

(Kopacova et al. 2009). These bundles are usually inconspicuous in small bowel polyps but can be quite subtle in the colon or stomach. The lamina propria is usually uneventful but erosion and reactive aspects of the lining epithelium can occur. In larger polyps, the presence of displaced glands in the thickness of the polyp, a feature that can reflect the hamartomatous nature of the lesion or be secondary to trauma, can originate the problem of differential diagnosis with adenocarcinoma (Fenoglio-Preiser et al. 2008). As been stated previously, PJ polyps in the setting of PJ syndrome can harbor dysplasia and adenocarcinoma.

Juvenile polyps have mucus filled cystically dilated and tortuous glands (Fig. 2). The lamina propria is expanded by the presence of edema and inflammatory infiltrate with plasma cells, lymphocytes, neutrophils, and eosinophils (Hornick and Odze 2009). In JP syndrome polyps termed typical can be found intermingled with atypical polyps. The latter show a less stromal and more epithelial proliferation, frequently with a villiform appearance (Offerhaus and Howe 2010). Occasionally ganglioneuromatous proliferations and metaplastic alterations can be found (Fenoglio-Preiser et al. 2008). Ulceration of the surface epithelium is common. Gastric JP can sometimes be indistinguishable from hyperplastic polyps and clinical information is essential to the diagnosis. JP can also have associated dysplasia, usually low grade but also high grade, and adenocarcinoma (Hornick and Odze 2009).

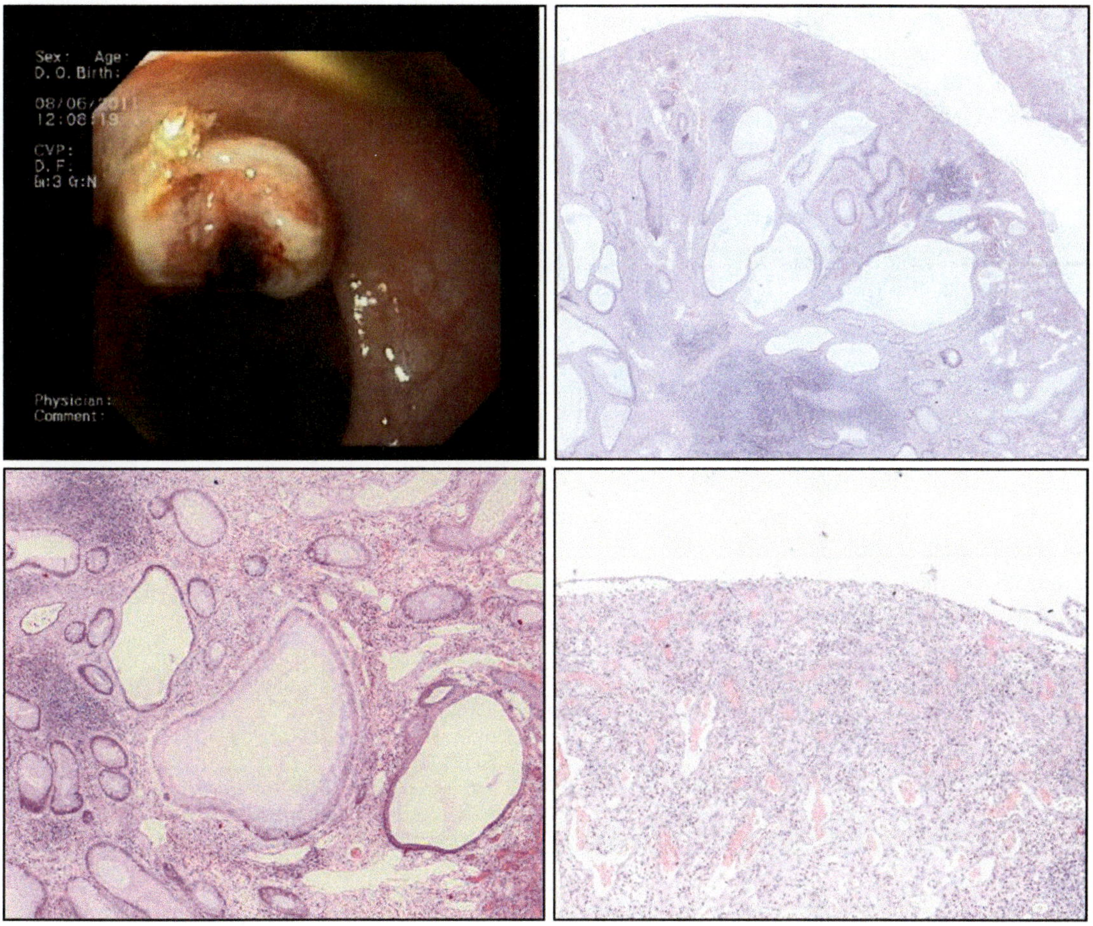

Hamartomatous Polyps, Fig. 2 Juvenile polyp. This sporadic juvenile polyp of a 2-year-old boy shows superficial ulceration, dilated glands, and prominent inflammation in the lamina propria

Cronkite-Canada polyps are very similar to hyperplastic polyps or juvenile polyps, but rather than being spared, the intervening mucosa has cystic glands. Once more, clinical information is of paramount importance. It is not clear whether dysplasia and carcinoma that have been reported in Cronkite-Canada syndrome arise from Cronkite-Canada polyps or from associated adenomatous polyps (Fenoglio-Preiser et al. 2008).

Molecular Features

More than half of the patients with Peutz-Jeghers syndrome harbor a mutation in a gene (*LKB1/STK11*) located on chromosome 19p13.3 that encodes a serine threonine kinase that normally inhibits cell growth by stimulating the promoter activity of *CDKNIB*. It has also been found to interact with p53 and some SMAD4 complexes and is involved in cell polarity, chromatin remodelling, and Wnt signalling (Calva and Howe 2008).

In juvenile polyposis syndrome the most common abnormality involves the TGF-β pathway. About 50% of patients inherit mutations in *SMAD4/DPC4* or *BMPR1A* in an autosomal dominant fashion, while in a percentage of cases, there is a de novo mutation. SMAD4 is a protein that functions as the common intercellular mediator of the TGF-β, bone morphogenic protein (BMP), and activin signalling pathways. BMPR1A is a transmembrane receptor involved in the same pathways that in the end regulate the transcription of various genes (Calva and Howe 2008; Fenoglio-Preiser et al. 2008).

Cowden disease results from mutations in the *PTEN* gene, which encodes a protein that affects apoptosis and inhibits cell spreading (Calva and Howe 2008).

Differential Diagnosis

The main differential diagnosis is between the different types of hamartomatous polyps and with hyperplastic polyps. In the stomach, for example, the distinction is frequently impossible. In other instances, location of the polyp (e.g., PJ polyps are more frequently located in the small bowel while JP only occur in the jejunum in rare occasions, in the context of a generalized syndrome) and some histological clues can help in the differential diagnosis. The presence of large branching smooth muscle fibers is distinctive of PJ polyps. However, in the stomach and colon, this feature can be very inconspicuous and JP can have sparse muscle bundles in the lamina propria. JP has an expanded lamina propria with inflammatory cells and edema, a feature that is not common in PJ polyps (Fenoglio-Preiser et al. 2008).

When PJ and JP have misplaced glands, sometimes a distinction from adenocarcinoma can be difficult. In the former however, even if the misplaced glands have dysplasia, there are usually some glands lacking atypia next to them, there is lack of stromal desmoplasia, and, frequently, lamina propria surrounding the displaced glands can be appreciated (Fenoglio-Preiser et al. 2008).

When hamartomatous polyps harbor dysplasia, they can be difficult to differentiate from adenomatous polyps. Usually dysplasia occurs in superficial areas of the polyp and other characteristics of the hamartomatous polyp can still be recognized. However in cases with diffuse dysplasia or adenocarcinoma, the distinction can be impossible.

A diagnosis of a polyposis syndrome is not advisable without proper clinical and endoscopical information that can fulfil the needed diagnostic criteria. For example, finding two JP cannot allow a diagnosis of juvenile polyposis. However if there is information about family history of juvenile polyposis, a diagnosis can be suggested. The finding of the same two juvenile polyps associated with the information that the patient has multiple colon polyps, facial tricholemmomas, and goiter can suggest the diagnosis of Cowden syndrome.

References and Further Reading

Calva, D., & Howe, J. (2008). Hamartomatous polyposis syndromes. *The Surgical clinics of North America, 88*(4), 779.

Fenoglio-Preiser, C. M., Noffsinger, A. E., Stemmermann, G. N., Lantz, P. E., & Isaacson, P. G. (2008). Polyposis and hereditary cancer syndromes. In J. McGouh & J. Pine (Eds.), *Gastrointestinal pathology an atlas and text* (pp. 704–724). Philadelphia: Lippincott Williams & Wilkins.

Hornick, J. L., & Odze, R. D. (2009). Polyps of the large intestine. In R. Odze & J. Goldblum (Eds.), *Surgical pathology of the GI tract, liver, biliary tract and pancreas*. Philadelphia: Saunders.

Kopacova, M., Tacheci, I., Rejchrt, S., & Bures, J. (2009). Peutz-jeghers syndrome: Diagnostic and therapeutic approach. *World Journal of Gastroenterology, 15*(43), 5397–5408.

Lauwers, G. Y., Carneiro, F., Graham, D. Y., Curado, M. P., Franceschi, S., Montgomery, E., Tatematsu, M., & Hattori, T. (2010). Gastric carcinoma. In F. T. Bosman, F. Carneiro, R. H. Hruban, & N. D. Theise (Eds.), *WHO classification of tumours of the digestive system* (pp. 48–58). Lyon: IARC.

Offerhaus, G. J. A., & Howe, J. R. (2010). Juvenile polyposis. In F. T. Bosman, F. Carneiro, R. H. Hruban, & N. D. Theise (Eds.), *WHO classification of tumours of the digestive system* (pp. 166–167). Lyon: IARC.

Yantiss, R. K., & Antoniolli, D. A. (2009). Polyps of the small intestine. In R. Odze & J. Goldblum (Eds.), *Surgical pathology of the GI tract, liver, biliary tract and pancreas*. Philadelphia: Saunders.

Helicobacter heilmannii Infection

Ceu Figueiredo
Department of Pathology, Faculty of Medicine of the University of Porto, Institute of Molecular Pathology and Immunology of the University of Porto (IPATIMUP), Porto, Portugal

Synonyms

Gastrospirillum hominis; Gastric non-*Helicobacter pylori Helicobacter* species; "*Helicobacter heilmannii*"-like organisms (HHLO)

Definition

The name "*Helicobacter heilmannii*" has been used for many years referring to uncultivable, long, spiral-shaped bacteria, morphologically distinct from *H. pylori*, observed in the stomach of humans and animals. These bacteria were initially designated as "*Gastrospirillum hominis*" and, based on sequence analysis of the 16S rRNA gene, were provisionally named "*Helicobacter heilmannii*," in honor of the German pathologist Konrad Heilmann who first studied the pathology associated with these microorganisms.

"*H. heilmannii*" was further subdivided into two taxa, as phylogenetic analysis of the 16S rRNA gene revealed two types that differed by more than 3% in their nucleotide sequence: "*H. heilmannii*" type 1, which are morphologically and genetically identical to *H. suis* (formerly designated "*Gastrospirillum suis*"), a species that colonizes the stomachs of pigs; and "*H. heilmannii*" type 2, which represents a group of species that have been isolated from the stomachs of cats and dogs, which include *H. felis*, *H. bizzozeronii*, *H. salomonis*, *H. cynogastricus*, *H. baculiformis*, and *H. heilmannii* sp. nov. The latter species was given in 2004 the provisional name "*Candidatus H. heilmannii*," based on taxonomic evaluation of the urease genes, and because it could not be cultured in vitro at that time. Only very recently was *H. heilmannii* formally recognized as a valid species name after successful in vitro isolation.

The nomenclature used to designate this expanding group of gastric non-*Helicobacter pylori Helicobacter* species is complex and confusing, but nevertheless essential as the pathogenicity to humans and susceptibility to antimicrobial agents is still largely unknown and may vary depending on the bacterial species.

To avoid further confusion in the nomenclature, the introduction of the terms *H. heilmannii* sensu lato (*H. heilmannii* s.l.) and *H. heilmannii* sensu stricto (*H. heilmannii* s.s.) has been recently proposed. The proposal is that *H. heilmannii* s.l. is used to refer to the whole group of non-*H. pylori Helicobacter* species detected in human or animal stomachs, and when only results of histopathology, electron microscopy, or crude taxonomic data are available, and that *H. heilmannii* s.s. or the other species names is used whenever bacteria are really identified to the species level. This nomenclature will be adopted in this entry.

In the great majority of "*H. heilmannii*"-related case reports, the species status is unknown and, as a consequence, it is not clear which species are associated with certain disease outcomes. The fastidious nature of these microorganisms has made their in vitro isolation difficult and hampered correct species identification for a long time. Although the only *H. heilmannii* s.l. species isolated from the human gastric mucosa so far is *H. bizzozeronii*, humans may also be colonized with *H. suis, H. felis*, *H. salomonis*, and *H. heilmannii* s.s. There are no reports on the presence of *H. cynogastricus* and *H. baculiformis* in the human gastric mucosa.

H. heilmannii s.l. infection in humans has been associated with chronic gastritis and occasionally with acute gastritis. Glandular atrophy or intestinal metaplasia may be present, but these lesions are less common in *H. heilmannii* s.l. infection than in *H. pylori* infection. Gastric erosions

H

mainly in the antrum, duodenal ulcers, gastric adenocarcinoma, and low-grade MALT lymphoma of the stomach have also been reported in association with *H. heilmannii* s.l. infections. The risk of developing MALT lymphoma is higher in infections with *H. heilmannii* s.l. than with *H. pylori.*

Data suggest that human infections with *H. heilmannii* s.l. likely originate from animal transmission. *H. heilmannii* s.l. are commonly found infecting dogs, cats, and pigs, and a higher incidence of *H. heilmannii* s.l. infection has been noted in humans that have had contact with these animals.

Clinical Features

- **Incidence**
  There are no data available regarding the incidence of *H. heilmannii* s.l. infection. The prevalence of *H. heilmannii* s.l. infection is low, ranging from <0.5% in developed countries to 1.2–6.2% in Eastern European and Asian countries.

  In gastric biopsy samples of humans with histological evidence of *H. heilmannii* s.l. infection, PCR-based techniques detect the following prevalences of the different species: *H. suis:* 14–37%; *H. felis*: 15–49%; *H. bizzozeronii*: 4–49%; *H. salomonis*: 21–49%; and *H. heilmannii* s.s.: 8–19%. Infection with multiple *H. heilmannii* s.l. species or with *H. heilmannii* s.l. and *H. pylori* has been reported.
- **Age**
  H. heilmannii s.l. has been reported infecting children and adults. Patients infected with *H. heilmannii* s.l. may not have clinical symptoms, or present acute or chronic epigastric pain and nausea. Other nonspecific symptoms include hematemesis, recurrent dyspepsia, vomiting, heartburn, and dysphagia, often accompanied by decreased appetite.
- **Sex**
  H. heilmannii s.l. infection occurs more frequently in males than in females (male to female ratio 2:1).
- **Site**
  H. heilmannii s.l. infects the stomach. In the human gastric mucosa, *H. heilmannii* s.l. colonization is mainly focal and is most frequently restricted to the antrum, with concurrent colonization of the corpus/fundus in only 20–30% of the cases.
- **Treatment**
  In patients that present severe pathology and clinical symptoms associated with *H. heilmannii* s.l. infection, treatment is indicated. Treatment regimens identical to those used to eradicate *H. pylori* infection, such as the triple therapy using combinations of a proton pump inhibitor and two antimicrobial agents selected from clarithomycin, metronidazole, amoxicillin, and tetracycline, have been used and were effective in most cases. However, the efficacy of such treatment is not easy to determine, as randomized trials are difficult to organize given the low prevalence of these infections in humans.

  Studies concerning antimicrobial susceptibility and acquired resistance of *H. heilmannii* s.l. have been hampered by the very low number of in vitro isolates available.
- **Outcome**
  H. heilmannii s.l. treatment results in resolution of the gastritis, healing of duodenal ulceration, and remission of primary gastric low-grade MALT lymphoma in the majority of patients.

Macroscopy

Macroscopic features observed during upper gastroscopy appear to correlate poorly with *H. heilmannii* s.l. status.

Microscopy

In gastric biopsy specimens, *H. heilmannii* s.l. appear as long (5–10 μm), spiral-shaped, sometimes tightly coiled, bacteria. Colonization is generally less dense than that observed for *H. pylori* infection. Microorganisms may occur isolated or in small groups, located within the mucus layer, above the surface cells, and in the gastric foveolar lumen. *H. heilmannii* s.l. do not show adherence to the surface cells nor colonize the intercellular spaces. Ultrastructurally, and in contrast to light microscopy, *H. heilmannii* s.l. microorganisms sometimes appear to be attached to the membranes of the surface cells.

Chronic gastritis in *H. heilmannii* s.l. infection presents less severe inflammatory scores than those observed in *H. pylori*-associated gastritis. *H. heilmannii* s.l.-associated gastritis generally features lymphocytic exudation into gastric foveolae. Lymphoid aggregates may be present in the mucosa. The presence of intracytoplasmic microorganisms in parietal cells has been reported.

Immunophenotype

No data is available.

Molecular Features

There is a big lack of knowledge regarding the main virulence characteristics and the bacterium-host interactions of *H. heilmannii* s.l. that colonize the human gastric mucosa, owing to the difficulties in obtaining in vitro cultures of this group of bacterial species.

The genomes of *H. felis, H, suis*, and *H. bizzozeronii* have recently been completed, all of them containing homologues of genes associated with colonization and virulence properties of *H. pylori* and other bacteria. In addition to complete urease gene clusters, homologues of genes encoding several outer membrane proteins, the neutrophil-activating protein NapA, the γ-glutamyl transpeptidase, as well as comB secretion systems required for DNA uptake by natural transformation, are present in the three genomes. All of the genomes lack homologues of the *H. pylori cag* pathogenicity island, including the gene encoding the cytotoxin-associated protein (CagA). The *H. suis* genome contains an homologue of the *H. pylori* vacuolating cytotoxin VacA, and both *H. felis* and *H. bizzozeronii* harbor homologues of the secreted serine protease HtrA that cleaves the extracellular domain of E-cadherin.

Further knowledge on other *H. heilmannii* s.l. genomes and the availability of pure isolates will expedite studies on the pathogenicity of the different species and facilitate the development of typing methods.

Differential Diagnosis

H. heilmannii s.l. are weakly stained by hematoxylin and eosin, and their structural characteristics are better observed using the Giemsa, and the Steiner and Whartin-Starry silver stains. *H. heilmannii* s.l. microorganisms may be two to three times longer and present higher number of spirals and tighter coils than *H. pylori*. However, morphology is not an accurate method for species identification, as different species may be morphologically very similar and also variation in morphology within a species may occur. There are no antibodies available for specific immunohistochemical detection of *H. heilmannii* s.l. Polyclonal anti-*H. pylori* antibodies show cross-reactivity with *H. heilmannii* s.l.

Rapid urease tests performed in the gastric biopsy specimen may not be sensitive due to the lower colonization density of *H. heilmannii* s.l. compared to that of *H. pylori* and also do not allow species identification.

In vitro culture cannot be used as a diagnostic tool. Only very few laboratories have succeeded in isolating *H. heilmannii* s.l. from the stomachs of cats, dogs, or pigs, and *H. bizzozeronii* has only been isolated two times from the human gastric mucosa.

For conclusive species identification, PCR with species-specific primers or followed by sequencing of the urease A and B genes are currently the most suitable methods, as sequences of these genes are available for all *H. heilmannii* s.l. species. Sequencing of the genes encoding heat shock protein 60 (*hsp60*) or gyrase subunit B (*gyrB*) may also be useful. Sequencing of the 16S or 23S rRNA-encoding genes is an

H

inappropriate tool for the discrimination of *H. heilmannii* s.l. species, although it allows differentiation of *H. suis* from the rest of the *H. heilmannii* s.l species.

Cross-References

▶ Chronic Gastritis
▶ *Helicobacter pylori* Infection

References and Further Reading

Haesebrouck, F., Pasmans, F., Flahou, B., Chiers, K., Baele, M., Meyns, T., Decostere, A., & Ducatelle, R. (2009). Gastric *Helicobacters* in domestic animals and nonhuman primates and their significance for human health. *Clinical Microbiology Reviews, 22*, 202–223.

Haesebrouck, F., Pasmans, F., Flahou, B., Smet, A., Vandamme, P., & Ducatelle, R. (2011). Non-*Helicobacter pylori Helicobacter* species in the human gastric mucosa: A proposal to introduce the terms *H. heilmannii* sensu lato and sensu stricto. *Helicobacter, 16*, 339–340.

Heilmann, K. L., & Borchard, F. (1991). Gastritis due to spiral shaped bacteria other than *Helicobacter pylori*: Clinical, histological, and ultrastructural findings. *Gut, 32*, 137–140.

O'Rourke, J. L., Grehan, M., & Lee, A. (2001). Non-pylori *Helicobacter* species in humans. *Gut, 49*, 601–606.

Stolte, M., Kroher, G., Meining, A., Morgner, A., Bayerdorffer, E., & Bethke, B. (1997). A comparison of *Helicobacter pylori* and *H. heilmannii* gastritis. A matched control study involving 404 patients. *Scandinavian Journal of Gastroenterology, 32*, 28–33.

Helicobacter pylori Infection

Ceu Figueiredo
Department of Pathology, Faculty of Medicine of the University of Porto, Institute of Molecular Pathology and Immunology of the University of Porto (IPATIMUP), Porto, Portugal

Synonyms

Campylobacter pylori; *Campylobacter pyloridis*

Definition

Helicobacter pylori are gram-negative, spiral-shaped, microaerophilic bacteria that colonize the human stomach. Although the presence of bacteria in the human stomach has been known for more than a century, only about 30 years ago, *H. pylori* was successfully isolated and cultured from a gastric biopsy specimen. This discovery, together with studies on the implication of *H. pylori* as an etiologic agent in gastritis and peptic ulcer disease, resulted in the awarding of the 2005 Nobel Prize in Physiology or Medicine to Barry Marshall and Robin Warren.

Before acquisition of its current name, the microorganisms were first named "*Campylobacter pyloridis*," then "*Campylobacter pylori*," and finally assigned to the genus *Helicobacter*. Since the discovery of *H. pylori*, many new species that infect human or animal hosts have been described, and the *Helicobacter* genus now includes at least 33 formally named species.

H. pylori is a very successful human pathogen and is considered as the most common chronic infection in man. *H. pylori* induces chronic gastritis in all individuals, a condition that lasts for life if the infection is not treated. A proportion of infected individuals may develop clinical disease, depending on *H. pylori* strain virulence, host susceptibility, and environmental factors.

H. pylori is the main etiologic factor of peptic ulcer disease. These microorganisms are found in approximately 95% of duodenal and 85% of gastric ulcers. It is estimated that the lifetime risk for peptic ulcer disease in *H. pylori*-positive subjects is three to ten times higher than in *H. pylori*-negative subjects, and that 10–15% of *H. pylori* infections result in peptic ulcer disease development.

H. pylori infection causes non-cardia gastric carcinoma. Data on the geographical associations between the prevalence of *H. pylori* and the incidence of gastric carcinoma, the development of gastric carcinoma in in vivo experimental animal models of infection, together with a considerable number of prospective observational studies, both nested case-control and cohort, provided results supportive of an association between *H. pylori* infection and non-cardia gastric carcinoma. The risk for non-cardia gastric carcinoma in the context of *H. pylori* infection was estimated to be threefold but more accurate methodologies now indicate the risk to be at least 20-fold. *H. pylori* infection is associated with the two main histological types of gastric carcinoma. The development of intestinal type gastric carcinoma follows a multistep cascade starting with *H. pylori*-induced chronic superficial gastritis through atrophic gastritis, intestinal metaplasia, and dysplasia. At variance, the pathway leading to the diffuse type gastric carcinoma is less clear, but nevertheless preceded by chronic *H. pylori*-associated gastritis.

H. pylori also plays an etiological role in gastric MALT lymphoma. The noninfected gastric mucosa has no MALT tissue and its acquisition depends upon infection with *Helicobacter* species, usually *H. pylori* (see also ► *Helicobacter heilmannii* Infection). Nearly all low-grade MALT lymphoma patients are infected with *H. pylori*.

H. pylori infection has now also been conclusively linked with the etiology of otherwise unexplained iron-deficiency anemia and idiopathic thrombocytopenic purpura (ITP).

Clinical Features

- **Incidence**
  H. pylori infects more than 50% of the population worldwide. The prevalence of *H. pylori* infection varies widely by geographic area, ranging from 20% to 50% in developed countries, to more than 80% in developing countries. In developed countries, and over recent decades, the prevalence of *H. pylori* has substantially decreased, probably as a result of improved hygiene and sanitation, and widespread use of antimicrobials for treatment of other common infections, especially during childhood. In developing countries, the prevalence of *H. pylori* infection has remained relatively stable.

  The exact mechanisms by which *H. pylori* is acquired are largely unknown, but direct person-to-person transmission is the most likely transmission route, via either oral-oral or fecal-oral routes or both.

  The best established risk factor for *H. pylori* infection is low socioeconomic status, and factors, such as education, income, hygienic conditions, household crowding, and the number of young children in the household, contribute to the inverse relation between *H. pylori* prevalence and socioeconomic status.
- **Age**
  H. pylori infection is mostly acquired during childhood. Prevalence rates differ by age, being highest in the older age groups. In developed countries, the prevalence of *H. pylori* is low early in childhood and slowly rises with increasing age. This increase does not result from *H. pylori* acquisition at later ages, but reflects a decrease in infection rates in childhood in successive birth cohorts over the past decades in these countries. In developing countries, *H. pylori* infection rates rise rapidly in the first years of life and persist constantly high throughout adulthood.
- **Sex**
  There are no significant gender differences in the prevalence of *H. pylori* infection in most studies. Some studies however point to a weak male predominance of the infection in adults.
- **Site**
  H. pylori infects the gastric mucosa. In the stomach, *H. pylori* colonizes both the antrum and the corpus. In conditions that decrease the number or inhibit the function of acid-secreting parietal cells, *H. pylori* may be observed predominantly colonizing the corpus.
- **Treatment**
  Guidelines published in Europe and North America recommend therapeutic regimens that achieve *H. pylori* cure rates >80% in an intention-to-treat basis. The triple therapy including a proton pump inhibitor (PPI) and two antibiotics (clarithromycin plus amoxicillin or metronidazole), and which had been recommended by all the consensus conferences worldwide, is now less efficacious and achieves cure rates of only about 70% of the patients. One of the most important reasons

underlying the decrease in efficacy of the standard triple therapy is the increase in *H. pylori* resistance to clarithromycin. The overall clarithromycin resistance rate increased in most parts of Europe in the last decade, and has reached a high prevalence (>20%) in the majority of Central, Western, and Southern European countries. In Northern European countries, clarithromycin resistance is <10%, which is considered a low resistance rate. Taking these findings into account, the Maastricht IV/Florence Consensus Report on the management of *H. pylori* infection recommends that the treatment regimen should be selected according to areas of low and high clarithromycin resistance.

In areas of low clarithromycin resistance, the standard PPI-clarithromycin-containing regimen is still recommended as the first-line treatment. Bismuth-containing quadruple treatment is also an alternative. However, in areas of high clarithromycin resistance, bismuth-containing quadruple therapies (containing bismuth salts, PPI, tetracycline, and metronidazole) are recommended for first-line treatment. If bismuth drugs are not available, a non-bismuth quadruple treatment (either sequential, using a PPI and amoxicillin for 5 days followed by a PPI with clarithromycin and metronidazole for the next 5 days, or "concomitant") is recommended.

To evaluate the success of eradication treatment, both the urea breath test (UBT) and laboratory-based validated monoclonal stool tests are recommended as noninvasive tests (see section "Differential Diagnosis").

- **Outcome**

  Eradication of *H. pylori* leads to peptic ulcer healing and reduces the risk of ulcer recurrence. It also reduces the recurrence of bleeding ulcers in those patients in whom the ulcer bleeding was due to *H. pylori* infection.

  H. pylori eradication may decrease the risk for development of non-cardia gastric carcinoma, especially in patients without precancerous conditions such as atrophic gastritis and intestinal metaplasia. While there is no evidence that *H. pylori* eradication can lead to regression of intestinal metaplasia, the same is not necessarily true for gastric atrophy.

  Complete remission of low-grade MALT lymphoma is achieved in 60–80% of patients following *H. pylori* eradication. Over 10% of those who initially reach complete remission show recurrent disease during further follow-up. In cases with the translocation t(11;18) leading to AP-12-MALT-1 fusion, *H. pylori* eradication is usually ineffective.

Macroscopy

Macroscopic features observed during endoscopy correlate poorly with *H. pylori* status.

Microscopy

In gastric biopsy specimens, *H. pylori* appear as curved or S-shaped bacilli (2.5–4 μm long and 0.5–1-μm wide). *H. pylori* can be observed free in the mucus layer, adhering to mucous cells, and in the intercellular spaces. The presence of intracellular microorganisms has been reported in a low number of cases. *H. pylori* may be present on gastric metaplastic cells outside the stomach, and although it does not colonize intestinal metaplasia, it can be seen adhering to areas of incomplete intestinal metaplasia. *H. pylori* may sometimes be observed assuming coccoid shapes.

The acute phase of *H. pylori* infection is rarely observed in gastric biopsy specimens. The chronic phase of the infection shows infiltration of the lamina propria with lymphocytes, plasma cells, and neutrophils. Neutrophils can also be seen permeating the foveolar epithelium, characterizing an active phase of the gastritis. In some cases of active *H. pylori* chronic gastritis, surface epithelial damage, mucous depletion, and erosions are observed. Lymphoid follicles are frequently present associated with *H. pylori* infection.

Immunophenotype

The systemic immune response to *H. pylori* shows an initial increase of the immunoglobulin M (IgM), followed by the rise of IgG and IgA specific antibody levels in serum. IgG is the predominant immunoglobulin class in *H. pylori* infection, being present in virtually all infected cases in the serum and at the mucosal level. IgM and IgA have little diagnostic utility in *H. pylori* infection. IgM is infrequently observed, as samples from the acute phase of *H. pylori* infection are rarely available. IgA is also elevated in the majority but not in all of the infected cases.

Antibodies anti-CagA, a highly immunogenic virulence-associated *H. pylori* protein, can be detected in the serum of patients infected with CagA-positive strains (please see section "Molecular Features").

After *H. pylori* eradication and in cases where *H. pylori* may no longer be present in the stomach, such as advanced gastric atrophy and gastric carcinoma, antibodies against *H. pylori*, especially against CagA, remain elevated and may take months or years before returning to baseline values.

Molecular Features

Differential pathogenic properties of *H. pylori* strains contribute to the discrepancy between the number of infected individuals and those that end up developing disease. *H. pylori* are genetically highly diverse bacteria. Among bacteria virulence factors that display genetic variation between strains and that are associated with the clinical outcomes of the infection, CagA and VacA are the most important.

CagA is present in about 60–70% of strains and is a marker for the presence of the *cag* pathogenicity island. This pathogenicity island encodes a type IV secretion system that allows the translocation of CagA into the host cells. CagA can activate multiple host signaling pathways leading to cell proliferation, cytoskeletal rearrangements, and disruption of cell-cell junctions. Transgenic expression of CagA was shown to lead to gastric carcinoma in mice.

CagA-positive strains increase the risk for peptic ulcer disease and for gastric carcinoma, and are more frequently found in patients with higher inflammatory scores, surface epithelial damage, gastric atrophy, and intestinal metaplasia, in comparison with CagA-negative strains. This holds true in Western populations but not in Asian populations, where almost all *H. pylori* strains are CagA-positive.

After translocation into the host cells, CagA can be phosphorylated at tyrosine residues in Glu-Pro-Ile-Tyr-Ala (EPIYA) amino acid motifs at the polymorphic carboxyl-terminus of the protein. Four different EPIYA motifs (A, B, C, and D) exist and can be present as repeats. *H. pylori* strains with high number of EPIYA-C motifs in the CagA protein are associated with increased risk for gastric atrophy, intestinal metaplasia, and gastric carcinoma, but not with duodenal ulcer.

VacA is a *H. pylori* toxin with multiple cellular activities. In mice, the administration of purified VacA induces gastric epithelial erosions, and in vitro the addition of VacA to epithelial cells results in cell vacuolation, membrane channel formation, disruption of endosomal/lysosomal function, and apoptosis.

The gene encoding VacA is present in all *H. pylori* strains, but is polymorphic and varies more significantly in the signal (s)-, the intermediate (i)-, and the mid (m)-regions, each with two major types. Infections with the more virulent *vacA* s1, i1, and m1 strains increase the risk for peptic ulcer disease and for gastric carcinoma, when compared with the less virulent *vacA* s2, i2, and m2 strains. The more virulent strains are frequently found associated with higher levels of inflammation, epithelial damage, gastric atrophy, and intestinal metaplasia. In East Asia, the great majority of *H. pylori* strains are *vacA* s1, i1, and m1, and are not associated with any particular clinical outcome.

When genotypes of CagA and VacA are combined with certain host genetic polymorphisms affecting the expression of pro-inflammatory cytokines important in the context of *H. pylori* infection, such as the interleukin-1β, the risk for gastric carcinoma may markedly increase.

Although the pathogenic properties of strains influence the outcome of *H. pylori* infection, no specific bacterial virulence markers are currently recommended for clinical practice.

Differential Diagnosis

Different invasive and noninvasive tests can be used for the diagnosis of *H. pylori*, each with specific advantages and disadvantages. Invasive methods require an endoscopy and the collection of gastric biopsy specimens for histology, culture, urease test, or molecular methods, whereas noninvasive tests are based on peripheral specimens, such as blood, breath, or stools for detection of antibodies, bacterial antigens, or urease activity. The choice of a specific test for an individual patient depends on the clinical setting. For routine diagnostic purposes, histology, urea breath test, and culture are currently most often used.

For histological detection of *H. pylori*, conventional hematoxylin and eosin stain is not well-suited because of the weak contrast between the bacteria and the mucus, and may be particularly difficult in cases with low colonization density. The modified Giemsa, as well as silver stains, such as the Warthin-Starry, facilitate the detection. Immunohistochemistry with specific anti-*H. pylori* antibodies increases sensitivity and specificity. Sensitivity also increases from the observation of multiple biopsy specimens in the antrum and corpus.

Culture of *H. pylori* from a gastric biopsy specimen is another method used to diagnose this infection. *H. pylori* is a fastidious microorganism and requires complex growth media, often supplemented with blood or serum, microaerobic conditions, and an optimum temperature of 37 °C. *H. pylori* can be identified as small (≈1 mm), round, and smooth colonies, that are oxidase, catalase, and urease positive, observed after 3–4 days after plating the biopsy specimen. In the case of negative culture, a 7–10 day incubation is recommended to ensure that the result is negative. Culture is time-consuming, requires expertise, and is not always successful, but has the advantage of allowing further antimicrobial susceptibility testing and bacteria typing.

The urease test allows the detection of *H. pylori* urease activity in gastric biopsy specimens. The introduction into a urea-rich medium of an infected biopsy results in the breakdown of urea into carbon dioxide and ammonia by the action of *H. pylori* urease. The increase in pH induced by the production of ammonia is reported by a pH indicator that changes the color of the medium, therefore indicating a positive infection.

Molecular approaches, such as polymerase chain reaction (PCR)-based methods, can be used directly in frozen or formalin-fixed paraffin-embedded gastric biopsy specimens, or in cultured bacteria isolates. For detection of *H. pylori*, and due to significant genetic diversity between strains, it is recommended that primers are directed to conserved areas of conserved bacterial genes. Sensitivity and specificity can be increased by probe hybridization methods after the PCR. PCR-based methods have the advantage of not only detecting, but also quantifying *H. pylori*, characterizing genes relevant to pathogenesis, as well as specific mutations associated with antimicrobial resistance.

Regarding noninvasive methods for *H. pylori* detection, the urea breath test (UBT) using ^{13}C urea is considered the best test due to its high accuracy and easiness to perform. It consists of the ingestion of ^{13}C labeled urea by the patient, which is hydrolyzed by *H. pylori* urease if the microorganism is present in the stomach. The labeled CO_2 is then absorbed by the blood and exhaled in expired air, which does not occur if the patient is not infected.

The stool antigen test (SAT) aims at the detection of *H. pylori* antigens in stool specimens. For using this test, the recommendation is to use an ELISA format with monoclonal antibodies, which provides a high accuracy both for initial and post-treatment diagnosis of *H. pylori*.

Serology can also be used to diagnose *H. pylori* infection and only validated commercial IgG ELISA tests should be used.

There are specific clinical settings in which awareness should be taken in the choice of the diagnostic tests. In patients treated with PPIs, the decrease in bacterial load, especially in the antrum, may cause false-negative results of histology, culture, urease test, UBT, or SAT, with the exception of serology. In these patients, if possible, PPI should be stopped for 2 weeks before testing.

Decisively, to determine the success of *H. pylori* eradication, both the UBT and validated monoclonal SATs are recommended as noninvasive tests. There is no role for serology in evaluating *H. pylori* eradication treatment.

Cross-References

- ► Adenocarcinoma, Upper Gastrointestinal Tract
- ► Chronic Gastritis
- ► Peptic Ulcer

References and Further Reading

Atherton, J. C. (2006). The pathogenesis of *Helicobacter pylori*-induced gastro-duodenal diseases. *Annual Review of Pathology, 1*, 63–96.

IARC Monographs on the Evaluation of Carcinogenic Risks to Humans. (2009). A review of human carcinogens: Biological agents (Vol. 100 – Part B). Lyon: International Agency for Research on Cancer.

Kusters, J. G., van Vliet, A. H., & Kuipers, E. J. (2006). Pathogenesis of *Helicobacter pylori* infection. *Clinical Microbiology Reviews, 19*, 449–490.

Malfertheiner, P., Megraud, F., O'Morain, C. A., Atherton, J., Axon, A. T., Bazzoli, F., Gensini, G. F., Gisbert, J. P., Graham, D. Y., Rokkas, T., El-Omar, E. M., Kuipers, E. J., & European Helicobacter Study Group. (2012). Management of *Helicobacter pylori* infection – The maastricht IV/ florence consensus report. *Gut, 61*, 646–664.

Mégraud, F., & Lehours, P. (2007). *Helicobacter pylori* detection and antimicrobial susceptibility testing. *Clinical Microbiology Reviews, 20*, 280–322.

Hemorrhoids

Gabriel Becheanu
Department of Pathology, Fundeni Clinical Institute, Carol Davila University of Medicine and Pharmacy, Bucharest, Romania

Synonyms

Anal cushions; Piles

Definition

Hemorrhoids or anal cushions are anatomical structures located in the distal portion of the rectum and the anus, composed of a network of vascular channels without muscular wall (sinusoids), elastic and connective tissue, and smooth muscle fibers (submucosal Trietz's muscle). The term "hemorrhoids" is currently not used for a pathological state and represents a normal feature of the anal region with a role in maintaining the anal canal closed and contributing to fecal continence.

Anal cushions become pathological when abnormal changes like swelling and inflammation (sometimes followed by hemorrhage and thrombosis) take place.

Internal hemorrhoids have their origins in the superior hemorrhoid plexus of the lower part of the rectum, while external hemorrhoids are located under the anorectal line or dentate line.

Symptomatic hemorrhoids are caused by increased intra-abdominal pressure such as that occurring in the straining of bowel movements, constipation or diarrhea, long-lasting sitting position, and different conditions such as pregnancy, chronic liver disease with ascites, or abdominal masses (Schubert et al. 2009). There is also evidence of a high resting sphincter pressure in patients with hemorrhoidal disease, which could affect the venous drainage of vascular structures. A host of other factors are believed to play an important role: low-fiber intake, lack of exercise, aging, obesity. There is no clear evidence of hereditary predisposition, but pathogenesis seems to be related to degenerative changes in the collagen structure of the vessels or supporting stroma, features which could have a genetic inheritance substrate.

Hemorrhoids are often presented as a type of varices or varicosities, but hemorrhoids and rectal varices are two separate conditions. Portal hypertension is not associated with hemorrhoidal presence, while rectal varices, which appear in these patients, are different entities defined as a collateral venous circulation.

Clinical Features

- **Incidence**
  Symptomatic hemorrhoids are common in adult persons, with an increased prevalence in the third decade of life. Epidemiological surveys indicate that hemorrhoidal disease affects between 5% and 36% of the general population, but the real incidence is thought to be hard to appreciate, because most people avoid medical examination.
- **Age**
  Hemorrhoids usually become abnormal in middle aged adults, with a peak between 45 and 65 years of age.
- **Sex**
  Both sexes are affected by this condition with a predilection for Caucasians and for people with high socioeconomic life conditions, the latter possibly related to their facile access to medical care.
- **Site**
  There are two types of hemorrhoids: internal – located above the dentate line, covered by rectal mucosa, and external – located under the dentate line and covered by anal skin. In the anal canal, they are typically situated in three regions: left lateral, right anterior, and right posterior position, but minor hemorrhoidal additional tissue can be found between these spaces. Anal cushions are important structures for continence and become pathological when they are exposed to high intra-abdominal pressure for long periods of time.

  The vascular structures grow to be engorged and prolapse together with the connective tissue. Some physicians suggest that rectal mucosal prolapse is a part of hemorrhoidal disease, while others consider this a distinct pathology.
- **Symptoms**
  Symptoms depend on the type and condition of the vascular structures involved. The most frequent symptom of internal hemorrhoids is painless rectal bleeding (due to their visceral innervation). The blood is of the "bright red" well-oxygenated type, comes at the end of bowel movements, and usually covers the fecal stool. External hemorrhoids, which are very well innervated with somatic nerves, usually become painful when exposed to high or low temperatures, thrombosed, strangulated, or when anal fissure is present. Bleeding from hemorrhoids is not so significant and rarely determines anemia, which, when present, should further be investigated. External hemorrhoids are sometimes associated with discomfort, irritation of the surrounding area (due to discharge of mucus), itchiness, and acute pain.
- **Treatment**
  Conservative treatment consists in: increased fiber intake, adequate hydration, and rest. Sitz bath and topical agents are considered to have a limited effect, and there is lack of evidence for their help. Oral drugs like flavonoid fraction are used for increasing the vascular tonus, lymphatic drainage, and capillary perfusion and resistance; nonsteroidal anti-inflammatory drugs help reduce inflammation and pain.

  Other useful simple procedures are rubber band ligation, sclerotherapy, infrared coagulation, diathermy, and laser therapy. Surgical hemorrhoidectomy is indicated only in cases where conservative management and simple techniques have failed, and is associated with some degree of complications like bleeding, anal strictures, infections, and urinary retention.
- **Outcome**
  The outcome in the long term is generally good with conservative treatment, but some persons

may have recurrence of symptoms. Surgical treatment is reserved only for cases where other procedures were unsuccessful, not tolerated, or in the final grades III–IV of mixed internal-external hemorrhoids.

Macroscopy

Internal pathologic hemorrhoids are swollen cushions located proximal to the dentate line (pectinate line) covered by rectal or transitional mucosa, while external anal cushions appear as blue or purple mucosal bulges or polyps lined by skin. On gross section, they present as vascular dilated spaces with thrombi, inside of a tissular area.

Internal hemorrhoids are graded using Goligher's classification according to their degree of prolapse and possibility of reduction:

Grade I – Protrusion inside of the anal canal but no prolapse
Grade II – Prolapse behind the external sphincter during defecation with spontaneous reduction
Grade III – Prolapse with manual reduction
Grade IV – Prolapsed and non-reducible

The grade of hemorrhoids is an important selection criterion for treatment choice, usually irreducibility being an indication for surgery; however, other symptoms like frequent bleeding, size, and discomfort should be taken into consideration when establishing the type of therapeutic procedure. Hemorrhoids in the acute thrombosis phase and incarcerated masses are also considered grade IV according to AGA (American Gastroenterological Association) criteria. Together with an increase in the availability of endoscopy, different endoscopical classification systems have been developed, which are correlated with the symptoms of hemorrhoidal disease.

Microscopy

Histologically, hemorrhoids are composed of connective tissue stroma which contains dilated vascular structures in the submucosa with different diameters (Fig. 1), frequently with inflammation of vascular wall, with ulceration and thrombosis, and often with hemorrhage extended in the surrounding tissue.

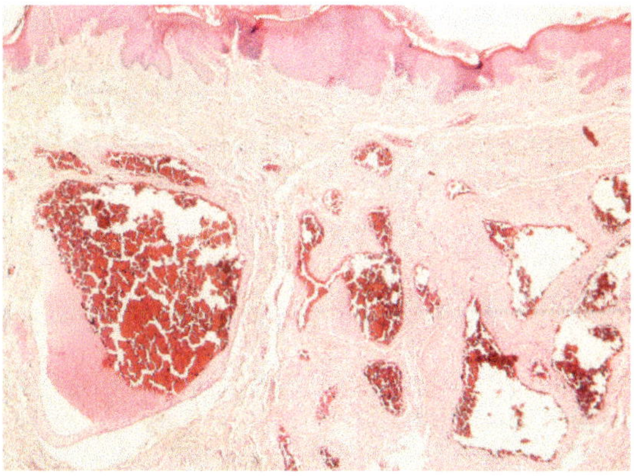

Hemorrhoids, Fig. 1 Hemorrhoids with dilated vascular structures, thrombosis, and chronic inflammation, H&E stain

Internal hemorrhoids are covered by columnar epithelium or a transitional epithelium (close to the dentate line), while external hemorrhoids are lined by squamous epithelium of anoderm and external anal skin.

The stroma may show fibromuscular hyperplasia, fragmentation of the anal subepithelial muscle fibers, or elastic fiber proliferation, with a chronic inflammatory background composed of mast cells, lymphocytes, and plasmocytes. Regenerative changes may be present such as metaplasia of the rectal mucosa or keratotic reactions. Dysplasia has occasionally been discovered in the rectal mucosa and anal area associated with hemorrhoidal tissue, without evidence for a direct correlation. Human papilloma virus (HPV) infection was confirmed in most of the cases with squamous changes.

Immunophenotype

In the mucosal and submucosal layers of pathological anal cushions, different immunohistochemistry studies revealed an increased expression of some markers responsible for differentiation and vascular development like: endoglin (CD105), EGFR, VEGF, COX-2, and notch-3.

Hemorrhoidal masses express some positive CD34 stroma cells, involved in repair and overgrowth, but their number is higher in anal fibroepithelial polyps, lesions which resemble hemorrhoids.

Molecular Features

Some mediators were studied as being involved in mechanisms as angiogenesis, inflammation, and tissue degeneration that determine hemorrhoidal disease. Researches revealed that matrix metalloproteinase-2 and -9 (MMP-2, MMP-9), enzymes with a role in degradation of extracellular proteins, were activated and overexpressed in hemorrhoidal tissue and could be responsible for elastin and collagen degeneration. Other studies have shown that endoglin (CD105), a cell membrane glycoprotein, VEGF (vascular endothelial growth factor), EGFR (epidermal growth factor receptor) and notch-3 (marker of vascular differentiation), involved in stromal blood vessel development, are highly expressed in symptomatic hemorrhoids and are possibly related to the increase in microvascular density, especially in areas of thrombosis. Also the high expression of NOS (nitric oxide synthase) and COX-2 present in hemorrhoidal pathologic tissue supports the implication of inflammatory mechanisms in the pathogenesis of this condition. Further studies are necessary to elucidate all of the processes involved in the development of piles.

Differential Diagnosis

Several different lesions with symptoms that mimic hemorrhoids can appear in the anal region: fistulas, fissures, abscesses, different masses (rectal or anal polyps, anal warts, carcinoma, melanoma, anal fibroepithelial polyps), inflammatory bowel diseases (perianal Crohn's disease), rectal prolapse.

Some authors consider fibrous anal polyps (fibroepithelial polyps) an end stage of thrombosed hemorrhoids despite the lack evidence for remnant vessels or signs of previous hemorrhages.

References and Further Reading

American Gastroenterological Association medical position statement. (2004). Diagnosis and treatment of hemorrhoids. *Gastroenterology, 126*, 1461–1462.

Kaidar-Person, O., Person, B., & Wexner, S. D. (2007). Hemorrhoidal disease: A comprehensive review. *Journal of the American College of Surgeons, 204*(1), 102–117.

Lohsiriwat, V. (2012). Hemorrhoids: From basic pathophysiology to clinical management. *World Journal of Gastroenterology, 18*(17), 2009–2017.

Schubert, M. C., Sridhar, S., Schade, R. R., & Wexner, S. D. (2009). What every gastroenterologist needs to know about common anorectal disorders. *World Journal of Gastroenterology, 15*(26), 3201–3209.

Hernias

Gabriel Becheanu
Department of Pathology, Fundeni Clinical Institute, Carola Davila University of Medicine and Pharmacy, Bucharest, Romania

Synonyms

Herniation; Rupture or break of the wall

Definition

Hernia represents a protrusion of an internal part of the body (organ or tissue) through a weakness in the muscular wall or in the surrounding tissue. The most common hernias are in the abdomen. Hernia could be congenital (as in umbilical hernia) or acquired when the pressure in the abdominal compartment is increased by different factors such as: heavy weight lifting, excessive coughing, chronic constipation, pregnancy, ascites, or obesity. Also the weakness of the membranes or muscular wall could be involved like in poor nutrition, losing weight, scars, or posttraumatic situations.

Study of thoraco-abdominal diaphragm reveals a volume reduction of the diaphragmatic muscle fibers with vasodilatation, perivascular inflammation, and an increase of interstitial space which appears edematous with hemorrhagias, especially in the crura muscular portion. Quantitative analysis suggests loss of elasticity and reduced functional capacity of diaphragm muscle.

Another research that focused on inguinal hernia observed that the mean diameter of the fascia lata fibers is decreased in the group of patients as compared with healthy controls, suggesting a multietiological connective tissue pathology involved in hernia pathogenesis. A chaotic arrangement of collagen fibers was discovered together with decreasing of elastic component in the tissue specimens from rectus muscle sheath in patients with inguinal hernia. Different researches confirm the fact that hernia formation and recurrence is associated with alteration of collagen metabolism. This change is manifested by a decreased type I: III collagen ratio with predominance of immature type III that contributes to a decrease of fiber strength.

Clinical Features

- **Incidence**
  The most common type encountered is inguinal hernia (up to 75% of all abdominal hernias).
  Congenital diaphragmatic hernia affects approximately 1:3,000 newborns and in almost 50% of cases is associated with other genetic anomalies.
- **Age**
  Hiatus hernia increases in incidence with age, more than 60% of patients being older than 50.
  Congenital umbilical hernia is a birth defect, usually in premature or low-weight birth newborn.
  Femoral hernias are more frequently encountered in adults than in children (usually before 1 year old).
- **Sex**
  Inguinal hernias are more common in men than in women, while femoral hernias are predominantly developed in women because of the larger bone structure of the pelvis. In children, almost 90% of inguinal hernias are encountered in boys.
  Femoral hernias usually appear in multiparous women because of the frequently high abdominal pressure which enlarges the femoral ring.
  Umbilical hernia is more often seen in African-American females and in premature babies.
- **Site**
  According to their site, hernias can be divided in different types.
  Hiatal hernia develops when the superior part of the stomach protrudes through a defect of the diaphragm in the mediastinum. It is part of diaphragmatic hernia which can involve also the intestine. Two types are described: *sliding* hiatus hernia (95%) when stomach and esophageal sphincter with few centimeters of the esophagus moves up through the hiatus and *para-esophageal or rolling* hiatus hernia when only the fundus of the stomach pushes up through the diaphragmatic hiatus while the esophago-gastric junction remains fixed.
  Epigastric hernia is a hernia above the umbilicus, through the linea alba.
  Congenital diaphragmatic hernia involves a failure in closure of the pleuroperitoneal canals between the eighth and tenth weeks of pregnancy.
  Umbilical hernia is a hernia presenting in the umbilical site. It can occur as a congenital malformation in the newborn but can also be acquired in adult life as a consequence of an increased abdominal pressure in obesity, chronic coughing, or multiple pregnancies.
  Paraumbilical hernia appears in adults and involves a defect in the midline, near the umbilicus.
  Spigelian hernia or latero-ventral hernia is a protrusion through an aponeurotic part of the transverse muscle of the abdomen (Spigelian fascia) usually on the right side. It may contain

an intestinal part or an empty sac and because it is interparietal, often it is hard to detect as swelling.

Inguinal hernia – abdominal content protrudes in the inguinal canal – direct or indirect – depends on its relationship with inferior epigastric vessels. Direct hernia protrudes through a weak point in the fascia of the abdominal wall and is located medial of the inferior epigastric vessels. Indirect inguinal hernia passes through the inguinal ring and is in a lateral relationship with vessels.

Femoral hernia – abdominal content enters the femoral canal below the inguinal ligament.

- **Treatment**

The clinical presentation of the hernia determines the intervention.

A reducible hernia can be pushed inside of the cavity, spontaneous or manual. Usually is painless and does not require surgery. An irreducible hernia is blocked and painful.

An obstructive hernia involves a part of the intestine which is incarcerated in the hole with obstruction of the lumen, with pain and vomiting.

A strangulated hernia blocks the blood of the organ which is protruded and when it is abdominal, it involves severe pain, nausea, and vomiting. This type of evolution is more common in femoral, spigelian, and inguinal hernia, because the hole could become small. It is considered an emergency, and surgery is an immediate option.

The umbilical hernias, even when they are large, usually are spontaneously resolved until 2–3 years age of life. For a small hernia (<2 cm), reducible and asymptomatic, usually no surgical intervention is necessary. Femoral hernia usually requires surgical intervention. Hiatus hernia can progress with severe complication (ischemia, necrosis, and breathing problems) if it is not surgically treated.

Treatment methods involve open surgery or laparoscopic techniques, muscle strengthening techniques like mesh prothesis placed over or under the defect.

- **Outcome**

The size of the hernia base is very important because of the risk of strangulation. An incarcerated hernia with gangrene has a great mortality rate, and evolution depends on how much the bowel is affected.

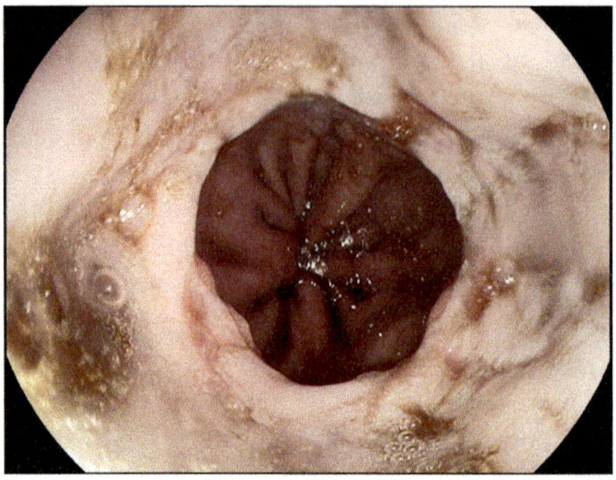

Hernias, Fig. 1 Hiatus hernia with reflux esophagitis – endoscopic view

The hiatus hernia could become complicated with gastroesophageal reflux disease, with esophagitis (Fig. 1) and rolling hernia can lead to obstruction of the gastrointestinal tract. A very large hernia in the mediastinum can push the pulmonary tissue and cause dysfunction of breathing.

Hernia recurrence represents the most frequent complication after repair and can appear in 2–3 years, usually following open surgery.

Macroscopy

In a strangulated abdominal hernia, necrosis and gangrene of the organ wall are the most important complications. Gangrenous segment present a dusty green to black color of the serosa. Sometimes only one side of the bowel wall can be trapped in the hernia, leading to ischemia and followed by perforation without obstruction – Richter's hernia – named after August Gottlieb Richter, a German surgeon.

Microscopy

Study of the herniated organ revealed an infarcted wall, with necrosis, hemorrhage and covered by fibrinous exudate. A diffuse fibrohyaline degeneration and fatty replacement of the muscular structures, inflammatory infiltrate, and hyperemia of the muscular frame with vascular congestion were described in the structures around the hernias. Edema, degenerative fibrosis, and atrophy of the nervous structures from the abdominal wall were also observed. Lesions graduate from partial mucosal necrosis of the intestinal wall with dilated vessels in first stages of reducible hernia, to transmural hemorrhagic infarction sometimes with intravascular thrombosis or vasculitis, in the strangulated hernia. In irreducible hernia the content of the sac become adherent to internal peritoneal wall due to a chronic inflammation.

Molecular Features

In abdominal hernias, an abnormal metalloproteinase (MMP) expression, especially MMP-1, MMP-2, MMP-9, and MMP-13, and an imbalance with their endogenous tissue inhibitors (TIMPs) has strongly correlated with direct abdominal hernia and recurrence. Some genetic alterations were discovered in children with congenital diaphragmatic hernia as haploinsufficiency of ZFPM2 with inherited deletions on some chromosomes. Other studies revealed the hypothesis that a disruption of the retinoid-signaling pathway may be involved in this hernia development.

Differential Diagnosis

Hernias must be differentiated from some abdominal wall diseases such as tumors (lipomas, hemangiomas, fibromas, metastases from lung and pancreatic tumors, desmoid tumors), hematomas, eventrations, enlarged abdominal vessels (in cirrhosis) and **lymph nodes**. Ingunial hernias should be clearly separated from undescended testicles, **abdominal aneurysm**, abscesses, hydrocele, lymphoma, while femoral hernia is different from large dilated varicose vein (saphena varix), cysts, abscess and lymph nodes, epididymitis, and testicular torsion. Hiatal hernia is important to be recognized and differentiated by similar symptoms related to angina pectoris, GERD (gastroesophageal reflux disease), pneumonia, gastric obstruction or atonia, esophageal motility disorders. Umbilical hernia should not be confused with omphalocele (exomphalos) that result from a defect of the umbilicus insertion and it is not covered by skin.

References and Further Reading

Aguirre, D. A., Santosa, A. C., Casola, G., & Sirlin, C. B. (2005). Abdominal wall hernias: Imaging features, complications, and diagnostic pitfalls at multi-detector row CT. *Radiographics, 25*(6), 1501–1520.

Antoniou, G. A., Tentes, I. K., Antoniou, S. A., Simopoulos, C., & Lazarides, M. K. (2011). Matrix metalloproteinase imbalance in inguinal hernia formation. *Journal of Investigative Surgery, 24*(4), 145–150.

Ardeleanu, V., Chebac, G. R., Georgescu, C., Vesa, D., Frâncu, L., Frîncu, L. D., & Păduraru, D. (2010). The modifications suffered by the peri-esophageal anatomical structures in the hiatal hernia disease: A qualitative and quantitative microanatomic study. *Romanian Journal of Morphology and Embryology, 51*(4), 765–770.

Szczesny, W., Glowacka, K., Marszalek, A., Gumanski, R., Szmytkowski, J., & Dabrowiecki, S. (2012). The ultrastructure of the fascia lata in hernia patients and healthy controls. *Journal of Surgical Research, 172*(1), e33–e37.

Hiatus Hernia, Acquired, Paraesophageal (Rolling)

Ana Lagos, Miguel Serrano and
Susana Mão de Ferro
Department of Gastroenterology, IPOLFG, E.P.E., Lisbon, Portugal

Synonyms

Hiatal hernia; Rolling hiatus hernia; Type II hiatus hernia

Definition

A hernia is a protrusion of the abdominal cavity beyond its fascial or muscular walls through fascial or muscular openings or defects.

The distal end of the esophagus, which is normally located in the abdominal cavity, is anchored to the diaphragm by the phrenoesophageal membrane, formed by the fused endothoracic and endoabdominal fascia. This elastic membrane inserts circumferentially into the esophageal musculature, very close to the squamocolumnar junction which resides within the diaphragmatic hiatus. However, these attachments are not firm and a limited longitudinal movement of the esophagus may still occur without alteration of the normal anatomy of the diaphragmatic hiatus.

In hiatal hernia, the upper portion of the stomach (rarely, the entire stomach, a segment of the colon, or the spleen) herniates through the esophageal hiatus of the diaphragm into the thorax.

Depending on the degree of failure of the anchoring mechanisms and the diameter of the hiatus, several type of herniation may occur. The most comprehensive classification scheme recognizes four types of hiatal hernia based on the location of the gastroesophageal junction (GEJ) and the hernia sac contents. Type I or sliding hiatus hernia (SHH) accounts for more than 95% of cases, while the remainder are paraesophageal (type II) or mixed (type III or IV).

Risk factors for the development of hiatus hernia include all the conditions that increase abdominal pressure, such as heavy lifting or bending over, frequent or hard coughing, hard sneezing, pregnancy and delivery, violent vomiting, straining with constipation, and obesity. Smoking, drug use (e.g., cocaine), and diaphragm weakness are also another risk factors.

SHH occurs when the GEJ and some portion of the stomach are displaced above the diaphragm. The orientation of the stomach axis is unchanged. The etiology of sliding hiatal hernias is not known, but there are instances in which trauma, congenital malformation, and iatrogenic factors can be clearly implicated. This type of hernia is characterized by widening of the muscular hiatal tunnel and circumferential laxity of the phrenoesophageal membrane, allowing a portion of the gastric cardia to herniate upward. The phrenoesophageal membrane remains intact and the hernia is contained within the posterior mediastinum. Most sliding hiatal hernias are small and of little clinical significance.

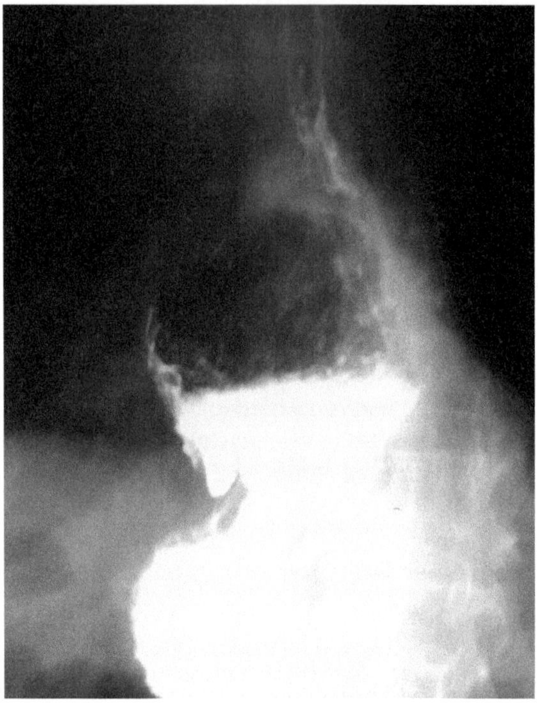

Hiatus Hernia, Acquired, Paraesophageal (Rolling), Fig. 1 Barium swallow radiography reveals a paraesophageal hernia

Hiatal hernias that are larger than 2 cm in axial span can be diagnosed easily by barium swallow radiography, endoscopy, or esophageal manometry (Figs. 1 and 2). By contrast, endoscopy and radiography are much less accurate for defining smaller hernias. Many patients with small simple sliding hiatal hernias are asymptomatic. The main clinical significance of the SHH is its contribution to gastroesophageal reflux disease. Type I hiatus hernia impacts on reflux both by affecting the competence of the GEJ in preventing reflux and in compromising the process of esophageal acid clearance once reflux has occurred. The likelihood of symptomatic gastroesophageal reflux increases with the size of the hiatal hernia. It is rare for complications other than reflux to occur as a result of a type I hiatal hernia. In addition to heartburn and regurgitation, patients with large sliding hiatal hernias may complain of dysphagia or discomfort in the chest or upper abdomen.

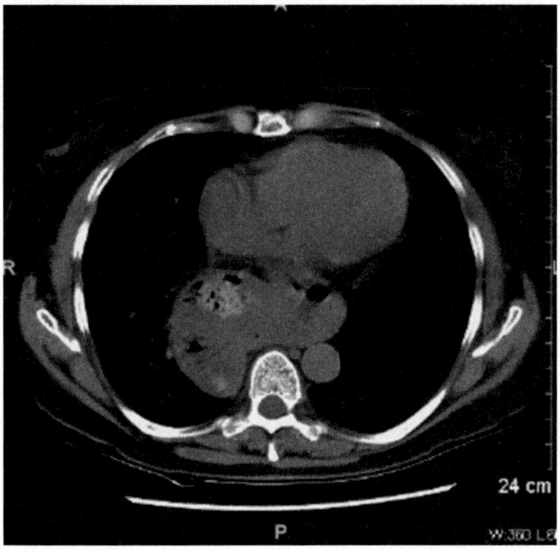

Hiatus Hernia, Acquired, Paraesophageal (Rolling), Fig. 2 CT reveals a large paraesophageal hernia

Ulcers or linear erosions (Cameron lesions) may develop in patients with sliding hiatal hernias, particularly large hernias. These mucosal lesions are usually found on the lesser curve of the stomach at the level of the diaphragmatic hiatus. Mechanical trauma, ischemia, and peptic injury have been proposed as the etiology of these lesions. The prevalence of Cameron ulcers among patients with hiatal hernias who undergo endoscopy has been reported to be about 5%, with the highest prevalence in the largest hernias. Cameron ulcers may cause acute or chronic upper gastrointestinal bleeding.

The paraesophageal hernia is defined by the protrusion of the stomach through the esophageal hiatus alongside the esophagus. The gastroesophageal junction typically remains in a normal position at the level of the diaphragm because there is preservation of the posterior phrenoesophageal ligament with normal anchoring of the gastroesophageal junction. Type II hernia results from a localized defect in the phrenoesophageal membrane, while the GEJ remains fixed to the preaortic fascia and the median arcuate ligament. Thus, the gastric fundus serves as the leading point of herniation. Either as cause or effect, paraesophageal hernias are associated with abnormal laxity of structures normally preventing displacement of the stomach – the gastrosplenic and gastrocolic ligaments. Frequently, the herniation is progressive with migration of increasing amounts of the stomach into the chest. Since the greater curvature always protrude first, large herniations result in an inversion of the stomach with its greater curvature lying uppermost. In extreme cases, the entire stomach may enter the thorax and present as an "upside down stomach." This unusual condition is identical to an organoaxial volvulus in which the stomach has twisted along its longitudinal axis.

Although their etiology is usually unclear, paraesophageal hernias are a recognized complication of surgical dissection of the hiatus as occurs during antireflux procedures, esophagomyotomy, or partial gastrectomy.

Types III and IV hiatal hernias are variants of the type II (purely paraesophageal) hernia. Type III hernias have elements of both types I and II. With progressive enlargement of the hernia through the hiatus, the phrenoesophageal membrane stretches, displacing the GEJ above the diaphragm, thereby adding a sliding element to the type II hernia. Type IV hiatus hernia is associated with a large defect in the phrenoesophageal membrane, allowing other organs, such as the colon, spleen, pancreas, and small intestine, to enter the hernia sac.

Patients with paraesophageal or mixed hiatal hernias are rarely completely asymptomatic but can be diagnosed incidentally when the chest X-ray reveals an air-fluid level in the mediastinum or the left chest. Almost half of the patients with this type of hernia have symptoms related to gastroesophageal reflux. Esophageal complication are rare; however, a hiatal hernia may be responsible for intermittent bleeding from associated esophagitis, Cameron ulcers, or a discrete esophageal ulcer, leading to iron deficiency. The prevalence of large hiatal hernias in patients with iron deficiency is 6–7%. Nonesophageal complications are also rare; incarceration of a hiatal hernia is observed only with paraesophageal hernia. When this occurs, it can present abruptly, with a sudden onset of vomiting and pain, sometimes requiring immediate surgery.

Paraesophageal hiatus hernia can be diagnosed on a chest radiograph as an abnormal soft tissue density (often with a gas bubble) in the mediastinum or left chest. The best diagnostic study is an upper gastrointestinal radiography; the typically findings are that the mucosal folds are seen going up into the chest, next to the esophagus, and gastroesophageal junction remains below the diaphragm. Paraesophageal hernias can also be detected on upper gastrointestinal endoscopy. Computed tomography scanning can also demonstrate that part of the stomach is in the chest.

Clinical Features

- **Incidence**
  Estimates of the incidence of hiatal hernia vary widely due to inconsistencies in definition, widespread confusion regarding the clinical implications of a hiatal hernia, and the normal function of the GEJ. True incidence is difficult to determine because a large number of patients are asymptomatic. Hiatal hernias are more common in Western countries, probably secondary to a state of chronic constipation and straining during bowel movement due to a fiber-depleted diet. The frequency of SHH increases with age, from 10% in patients younger than 40 years to 70% in patients older than 70 years.

  Of these, 9% are symptomatic, depending on the competence of the LES. 95% of these are sliding hiatus hernias and only 5% are the paraesophageal type.
- **Age**
  The majority of SHH occur beyond the fifth decade of life and the frequency then increases with advancing age.

  People of all ages can have paraesophageal hiatus hernia, but this condition also increases with age. Patients with symptomatic paraesophageal hernia are most often middle-aged to older adults.
- **Sex**
  Hiatal hernias are twice as likely to occur in women, and the incidence in women increases with advancing age.

  Paraesophageal hernia affects both sexes equally.
- **Site**
  Paraesophageal hernias generally tend to enlarge with time, and sometimes the entire stomach is found within the chest.
- **Treatment**
  Simple and asymptomatic SHH does not require treatment. When symptoms are due to gastroesophageal reflux, the goals of treatment include modifying lifestyle factors, neutralizing or inhibiting acid production, and enhancing esophageal and gastric motility. Surgery is necessary only in the minority of patients with complications of gastroesophageal reflux despite aggressive treatment with proton pump inhibitors.

  Regarding paraesophageal hernias, many experts suggest that surgery should be offered to all patients with because some complications will develop in about 30% of patients left untreated. In general, a select approach to patients with large paraesophageal is warranted.

  The principles of surgery for SHH and paraesophageal hernia includes three main elements: reduction of the hernia from the mediastinum or chest with excision of the hernia sac, reconstruction of the diaphragmatic hiatus with simple closure or use of prosthetic mesh, and fixation of the stomach in the abdomen with a wrap, gastropexy, or gastrostomy tube. These elements can be accomplished laparoscopically or via open surgery and may be approached through the abdomen and/or chest. Opinion varies as to whether or not an antireflux procedure (Nissen fundoplication) is necessary if concomitant pathologic reflux has not been demonstrated.
- **Outcome**
  The prognosis is excellent following surgical repair of a type I hiatal hernia. The recurrence after paraesophageal hernia repair is 25–30%; however, the clinic impact of a recurrence may be minimal, as most of these patients remain symptom free.

Macroscopy

A paraesophageal hernia, a true hernia with a hernia sac, is characterized by an upward dislocation of the gastric fundus alongside a normally positioned gastroesophageal junction. The gastric fundus and abdominal viscera protrude into the mediastinum through the defect in the diaphragm.

Microscopy

Biopsies from hiatus hernia include the presence of variably inflamed cardiac or oxyntic mucosa with edema, lymphatic dilation, and pronounced muscle hyperplasia, splaying, or stranding. Squamous metaplasia may be present.

Differential Diagnosis

Paraesophageal hernias commonly mimic ischemic heart disease or respiratory ailments such as pneumonia and asthma due to compression of the lung.

References and Further Reading

Jeyarajah, D. R., & Harford, W. V. (2010). Abdominal hernias and gastric volvulus. In *Sleisenger and Fortrans's gastrointestinal and liver disease* (pp. 379–395). Philadelphia: Saunders/Elsevier.

Mori, T., Nagao, G., Sugiyama, M. (2012). Paraesophageal hernia repair. Annals of Thoracic and Cardiovascular Surgery. http://www.ncbi.nlm.nih.gov/pubmed/22850094.

Preiser, C. M. F, Noffsinger, A., Stemmermann, G. et al. The nonneoplastic stomach. In *Gastrointestinal pathology an atlas and text* (pp. 135–231). Lippincott.

Schieman, C., & Grondin, S. C. (2009). Paraesophageal hernia: clinical presentation, evaluation, and management controversies. *Thoracic Surgery Clinics, 19*, 473–484.

Hirschsprung's Disease

Erdener Özer
Department of Pathology, Dokuz Eylül University School of Medicine, Izmir, Turkey

Synonyms

Aganglionic megacolon; Congenital megacolon

Definition

Hirschsprung's disease is a common cause of neonatal intestinal obstruction due to improper muscle movement in the bowel. Patients are unable to defecate because of the lack of ganglion cells. It is a congenital condition; therefore, it is present from birth. Newborns will often have abdominal distension, while older children may suffer from chronic constipation. Hirschsprung's disease results from the absence of ganglion cells within the myenteric and submucosal plexus of the rectum and/or colon. Colonic ganglion cells are derived from the neural crest and migrate caudally with the vagal nerve fibers along the intestine. These ganglion cells arrive in the proximal colon by 8 weeks of gestation and in the rectum by 12 weeks of gestation. The arrest in ganglionic migration leads to an aganglionic segment. This results in clinical Hirschsprung's disease.

Clinical Features

- **Incidence**
  Its incidence is estimated to be 1 in 5,000 births, ranging from 1 in 2,000 to 1 in 12,000 live births.
- **Age**
  Nearly all children with Hirschsprung's disease are diagnosed during the first 2 years of life. Approximately one half of children affected with this disease are diagnosed before the age of 1 year. A small number of children with Hirschsprung's disease are not recognized until much later in childhood or adulthood.
- **Sex**
  Hirschsprung's disease is four times more common in males than in females.
- **Site**
  The aganglionic segment in Hirschsprung's disease begins at the anal sphincter and extends proximally. In 80% of cases, aganglionosis is limited to the rectum and distal sigmoid colon; this situation is sometimes referred to as short-segment Hirschsprung's disease. In the remaining patients, the aganglionic segment is longer (long-segment Hirschsprung's disease) and extends as far proximally as the splenic

H

flexure or transverse colon in 10% and the cecum in 5% (total colonic aganglionosis). In rare cases, aganglionosis extends into the small intestine and may reach as far as the proximal duodenum. A small percentage of patients have ultrashort-segment Hirschsprung's disease, a controversial entity in which the aganglionic segment is confined to the anal sphincter. Some authors suggest this condition to be an abnormality of the anal sphincter that should not be diagnosed as true Hirschsprung's disease, but others accept it as one end of the spectrum of Hirschsprung's disease. Ultrashort-segment Hirschsprung's disease is a manometric diagnosis; therefore, microscopic examination cannot demonstrate any abnormality.

- **Treatment**
  Before surgery, a procedure called serial rectal irrigation helps to relieve the pressure in the bowel. The abnormal section of colon must be removed with surgery. The healthy part of the colon is then pulled down and attached to the anus. The surgery is often done in two sessions. A colostomy is performed first, and another procedure is performed later in the child's first year of life.
- **Outcome**
  The symptoms improve in most children after surgery. A small number of children may have constipation or problems controlling defecation. Children who get treated early or who have a shorter segment of bowel involved have a better outcome. Possible complications are enterocolitis occurring before surgery, and sometimes during the first 1–2 years afterward, perforation or rupture of the intestine and short bowel syndrome, a condition that can lead to malnourishment and dehydration. The overall mortality of Hirschsprung enterocolitis is 25–30%, which accounts for almost all of the mortality from Hirschsprung's disease.

Macroscopy

Although macroscopically is normal, the affected gut is unable to relax, causing a functional bowel obstruction with dilation of the proximal segment.

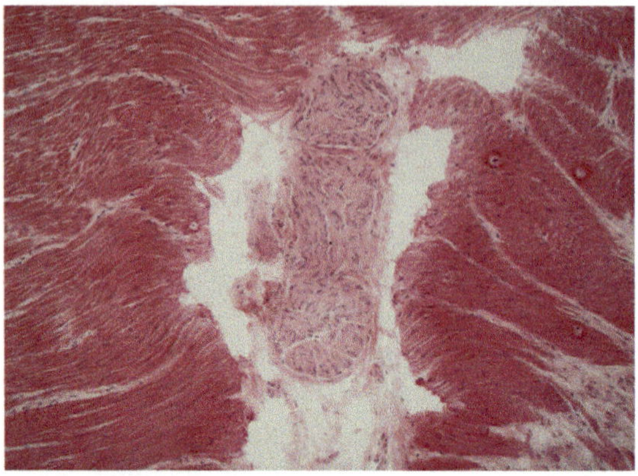

Hirschsprung's Disease, Fig. 1 In this medium power H&E stained section of muscular wall from the aganglionic portion of the colon, the myenteric plexus in the middle displays hypertrophic nerve fibers but no ganglion cells (i.e., aganglionosis)

Microscopy

Hirschsprung's disease is characterized by the following easily identifiable features: absence of ganglion cells in the submucosal (Meissner) and myenteric (Auerbach) plexus (Fig. 1), and typical increase in acetylcholinesterase (AChE) activity in the parasympathetic nerve fibers of the lamina propria mucosa and muscularis mucosa of the aganglionic segment (Fig. 2). AChE staining is an effective screening method for Hirschsprung's disease, but false-negative results have been encountered. This problem is more likely when the biopsy does not include muscularis mucosa or is taken too high in very-short-segment disease. In addition, acetylcholinesterase-positive fibers may be absent in the early neonatal period.

Immunophenotype

Although no immunohistochemical staining is considered currently equal to the diagnostic value of enzyme histochemistry (AChE staining), the absence of calretinin immunostaining in the nerve fibers may serve as a diagnostic tool in the diagnosis of aganglionic segments.

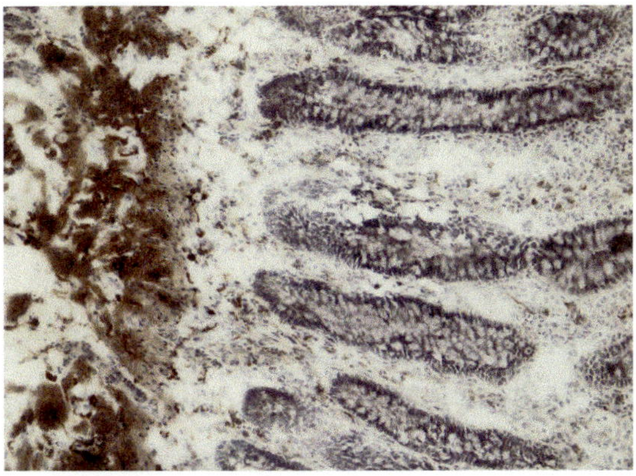

Hirschsprung's Disease, Fig. 2 An enzyme histochemical stain for acetylcholinesterase (*AchE*) may be helpful in establishing the diagnosis by demonstrating numerous dark staining AChE-positive nerve fibers in the lamina propria

Molecular Features

The disease is generally sporadic, although incidence of familial disease has been increasing. Multiple loci appear to be involved, including chromosomes 13q22, 21q22, and 10q. Mutations in the Ret proto-oncogene have been associated with multiple endocrine neoplasia and familial Hirschsprung's disease. Other genes associated with Hirschsprung disease include the glial cell-derived neurotrophic factor gene, the endothelin-B receptor gene, and the endothelin-3 gene. About 15% of patients with Hirschsprung's disease have Trisomy 21 (Down syndrome). Other associations include Waardenburg syndrome, congenital deafness, malrotation, gastric diverticulum, and intestinal atresia.

Differential Diagnosis

Normally there is a 2–3-cm-long aganglionic zone immediately above the mucocutaneous junction of the anus. Biopsies taken from this physiological aganglionic zone may be wrongly diagnosed as Hirschsprung's disease. In addition, it should be noted that the transitional zone of variable length, comprising hypoganglionosis and thickened nerve fascicles, often intervenes between distal aganglionic segment and normally innervated bowel. Another differential diagnostic challenge is the presence of immature ganglion cells. These cells have sparse cytoplasm, lack prominent nucleoli, form rosette-like structures, and may be overlooked. These appearances may persist until the end of the first year of life. Intestinal neuronal dysplasia is a poorly defined condition that clinically may simulate Hirschsprung's disease. Its status as a distinct clinicopathological entity is under discussion as the histological features originally described such as hyperplasia of the intramural plexuses and giant ganglia have been found to be nonspecific.

References and Further Reading

Gershon, M. D., & Ratcliffe, E. M. (2004). Developmental biology of the enteric nervous system: Pathogenesis of Hirschsprung's disease and other congenital dysmotilities. *Seminars in Pediatric Surgery, 13*, 224–235.
Kapur, R. P. (2009). Practical pathology and genetics of Hirschsprung's disease. *Seminars in Pediatric Surgery, 18*, 212–223.
Kenny, S. E., Tam, P. K., & Garcia-Barcelo, M. (2010). Hirschsprung's disease. *Seminars in Pediatric Surgery, 19*, 194–200.
Moore, S. W., & Johnson, G. (2005). Acetylcholinesterase in Hirschsprung's disease. *Pediatric Surgery International, 21*, 255–263.
Swenson, O. (2002). Hirschsprung's disease: A review. *Pediatrics, 109*, 914–918.

Hyperplastic Polyps (Stomach)

Chella R. S. van der Post[1] and
Fátima Carneiro[2]
[1]Department of Pathology, Radboud University Medical Center, Nijmegen, The Netherlands
[2]Faculty of Medicine of Porto University, Centro Hospitalar São João and Ipatimup/i3S, Porto, Portugal

Synonyms

Gastritis polyposa; Hyperplasiogenic polyp; Inflammatory polyp; Regenerative polyp

Definition

Hyperplastic polyps are localized, non-neoplastic mucosal expansions consisting of elongated, tortuous, and cystically dilated foveolae supported by an edematous lamina propria and distended vessels. Hyperplastic polyps arise probably as a result of reparative and regenerative responses to mucosal injury. First there is ongoing healing and a reparative response in the form of foveolar hyperplasia after mucosal injury and erosion. This hyperplastic reaction can end or persist and progress with the formation of a hyperplastic polyp. The common causative agents of mucosal injury are *Helicobacter pylori* and autoimmune gastritis leading to chronic gastritis, although any agent causing chronic gastritis may be a predisposing condition. *H. pylori* has been shown to increase the expression of cyclooxygenase-2 (COX-2), interleukin 1-beta, and hepatocyte growth factor in stromal cells, which are increased in number at sites of inflammation. This increased expression and inflammation has been suggested to play a role in the development of hyperplastic polyps by increasing epithelial cell turnover. *H. pylori* eradication has been shown to cause complete regression or significant decrease in size of these polyps. Likewise, the polyps can recur with recurrence of *H. pylori* infection. It remains to be shown whether other putative agents also cause hyperplastic polyps by the same mechanism. Hypergastrinemia has also been implicated in the causation of hyperplastic polyps as it has a trophic effect on the gastrointestinal mucosa. Interestingly, gastric hyperplastic polyps have been shown to develop in up to 15% of post-transplant patients, both solid organ and bone marrow transplant. All these patients had no evidence of chronic gastritis. The pathogenesis of these polyps appears to be different, whether and through which mechanism the immune suppressed state of these patients is related to the development of hyperplastic polyps has to be clarified.

Gastric hyperplastic polyps were, like colorectal hyperplastic polyps, considered initially to be completely banal and inconsequential. However, it has been shown that dysplasia and carcinoma develop within hyperplastic polyps with rates of occurrence varying from 1.5% to 4.5%. There should be a thorough search and sampling for dysplasia in large polyps, since especially in polyps with a diameter of >2 cm, the risk of developing carcinoma increases. Carcinomas arising in relation to hyperplastic polyps are well differentiated, although some cases of poorly differentiated and signet-ring cell carcinomas have been reported. The overall risk of developing carcinoma in hyperplastic polyps is very low, and most often, these polyps are not considered premalignant; however, it is important to examine the surrounding background mucosa for abnormalities. Patients with hyperplastic polyps are at increased risk of developing gastric cancer. It seems that not the hyperplastic polyps themselves but rather the associated conditions, the chronic atrophic gastritis, is responsible for this risk.

Most hyperplastic polyps occur as a single lesion, but multiple polyps are discovered in approximately 20% of patients. Gastric hyperplastic polyposis has been defined as a syndrome comprising equal to or more than 50 hyperplastic polyps. There have only been a few reports of this condition, with also familial risk. No particular germline mutations have been identified. Gastric hyperplastic polyposis has been associated with gastric carcinomas and colorectal adenomas and carcinomas. Hypergastrinemia as a result of *H. pylori* infection and subsequent atrophy has been suggested to be the possible link between gastric hyperplastic polyposis and colorectal neoplasia.

Clinical Features

Patients may be asymptomatic and the polyps may be an incidental finding at upper GI endoscopy done for some other reason. If symptomatic, patients usually complain of dyspepsia, heartburn, abdominal pain, or upper gastrointestinal bleeding, leading to anemia; sometimes hyperplastic polyps have been the cause of gastric outlet obstruction.

- **Incidence**
  Hyperplastic polyps are among the most frequently observed gastric epithelial polyps and comprise 28–75% of all gastric polyps. Due to the increased use of proton pump

inhibitors, the incidence of fundic gland polyps is nowadays likely to be higher than the incidence of hyperplastic polyps.

- **Age**
  Hyperplastic polyps are mostly detected in older patients with peak incidence in the sixth and seventh decades of life. They can develop at any age and are also observed in children.
- **Sex**
  There is no definite gender predilection. There is a slight predominance in women noted in most studies; however, there are also studies showing a higher incidence among men.
- **Site**
  Hyperplastic polyps develop throughout the stomach, slightly preferentially located in the gastric antrum.
- **Treatment**
  Preferably hyperplastic polyps are endoscopically removed in order to determine their nature and to prove that the lesions are benign. If there are a large number or big polyps, there is controversy whether gastric hyperplastic polyps should be entirely removed due to the risk of gastric polypectomy. In hyperplastic polyps, there can be development of intestinal metaplasia, dysplasia, and even carcinoma. Biopsy sampling may miss dysplastic foci within a hyperplastic polyp; therefore, some authors recommend polypectomy of all polyps. Others recommend that only large hyperplastic polyps should be removed since neoplastic transformation usually occurs in bigger polyps. Surveillance of hyperplastic polyps that are not removed because of number or size is probably safer than multiple polypectomies. A single repeat endoscopy at 1 year is reasonable, but there is no evidence for repeated surveillance. There is often a background of atrophic autoimmune gastritis or inflammatory gastritis. It is important to test for *H. pylori* and eradicate when present. In view of associated background pathology, the endoscopist should always examine and sample the surrounding nonpolyp gastric mucosa.
- **Outcome**
  Hyperplastic polyps are mostly regarded as benign lesions. The risk of developing adenocarcinoma within a hyperplastic polyp is approximately 2% and depends on size; especially, polyps larger than 1 cm are at risk of malignant transformation.

Macroscopy

Hyperplastic polyps are generally less than 2 cm in diameter. They can range from a few millimeters up to many centimeters in diameter; sizes of up to 12 cm may be reached. The polyps are usually solitary, small, smooth, lobulated, sessile, or pedunculated lesions. Multiple polyps that may appear confluent occur in approximately 20% of patients. They tend to be softer and shinier than other polyps, and their surface is almost always eroded or may show central umbilication. Hyperplastic polyps cannot be separated reliably from small adenomas endoscopically.

Microscopy

Histologically, hyperplastic polyps are characterized by an elongation, branching, and cystic dilatation of the foveolae. There is crowding of cells and infolding of the epithelium which gives a tortuous or corkscrew appearance (Figs. 1–4).

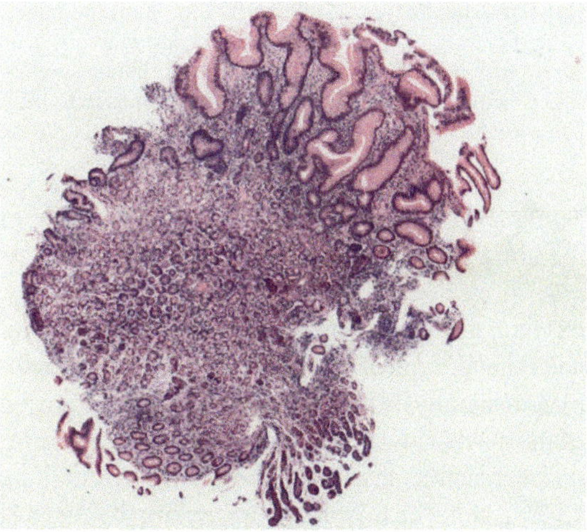

Hyperplastic Polyps (Stomach), Fig. 1 Gastric biopsy with a hyperplastic polyp with elongated pits with mucinous cytoplasm and stromal inflammation (H&E, original magnification 25×)

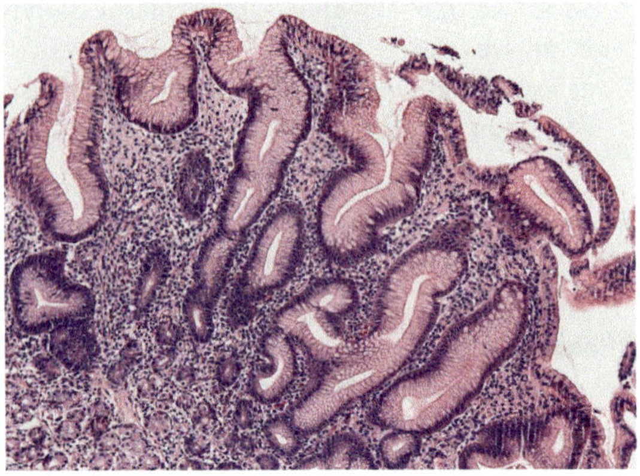

Hyperplastic Polyps (Stomach), Fig. 2 More detailed image of Fig. 1 (H&E, original magnification 100×)

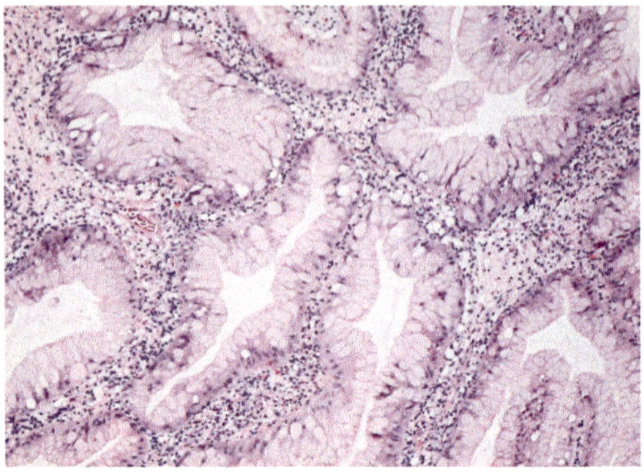

Hyperplastic Polyps (Stomach), Fig. 4 Detail of glands showing foveolar epithelium with prominent globoid cells and chronic inflammation (H&E, original magnification 200×)

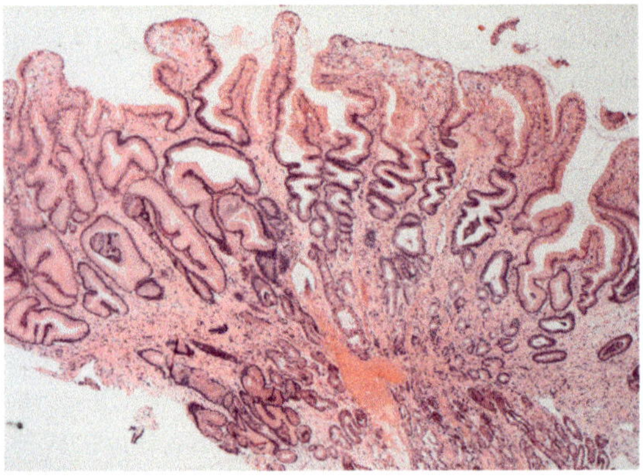

Hyperplastic Polyps (Stomach), Fig. 3 Hyperplastic polyp showing elongated, dilated, and tortuous pits with focal erosion on the surface. The fibrotic lamina propria shows hemorrhage and chronic inflammation (H&E, original magnification 25×)

The glands in hyperplastic polyps are usually of the antral or pyloric type, even when the polyps arise in the body or fundus, although occasionally, oxyntic glandular mucosa is seen. The foveolar cells have typically abundant mucinous cytoplasm but may be mucin-depleted focally. Erosion of the surface, with subsequent regeneration, produces reactive atypia in the lining epithelium. Cytoplasmic eosinophilia, an enlarged nucleus, prominent nucleoli, and a cuboidal cell shape characterize this. The prominent edematous stroma separating the glands in hyperplastic polyps sometimes mimics sarcoma or spindle cell carcinoma. The stroma often becomes fibrotic and shows reactive mesenchymal cells and a mixed inflammatory infiltrate of plasma cells, lymphocytes, histiocytes, neutrophils, and eosinophils. Smooth muscle fibers may also be apparent in the lamina propria and extend upward from the splayed muscularis mucosae. Most hyperplastic polyps arise on a background of mucosal abnormality. The surrounding gastric mucosa often shows signs of chronic atrophic gastritis.

In some cases, it may be difficult to distinguish the regenerating foveolar epithelium from adenomatous epithelium. Small foci of intestinal metaplasia are seen in around 15% of hyperplastic polyps, and infrequently dysplasia or carcinoma is encountered. The microscopic appearance of dysplasia in hyperplastic polyps is similar to that in other areas of the GI tract and is categorized as either low- or high-grade dysplasia. In low-grade dysplasia, the epithelium is composed of cells with hyperchromatic elongated nuclei, clumped chromatin, and pseudostratification (Fig. 5). These changes always involve the surface epithelium but may also occur in the deep glands. Mitotic activity is brisk. The architecture is more complex in high-grade dysplasia, with the formation of cribriform profiles and tubular budding. Moreover, features of cellular differentiation such as cytoplasmic mucin are progressively lost in high-grade dysplasia.

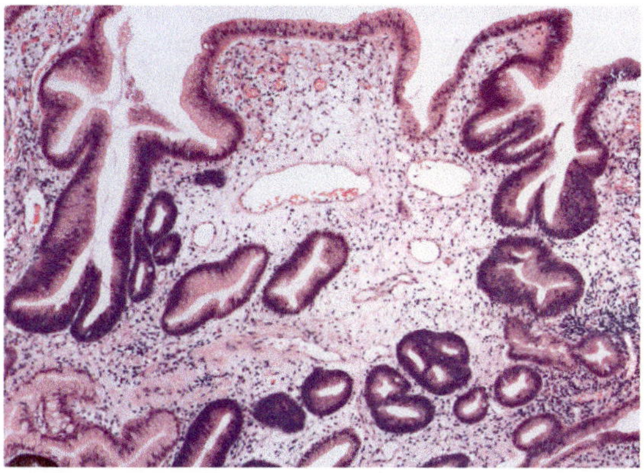

Hyperplastic Polyps (Stomach), Fig. 5 Hyperplastic epithelium with low-grade dysplasia showing enlarged, hyperchromatic, stratified nuclei (H&E, original magnification 50×)

Immunophenotype

Immunohistochemistry for p53 and Ki-67 can be performed to confirm increased staining in hyperplastic polyps with dysplastic or carcinomatous foci.

Molecular Features

Some data suggest that *TP53* mutations, *KRAS* mutations, microsatellite instability, chromosomal loss, and chromosomal gain may all be important in the development of dysplasia and carcinoma in gastric hyperplastic polyps, but further research is needed to better define the molecular biology of neoplastic transformation in these lesions. Although there have been several studies trying to implicate markers for malignant transformation in gastric hyperplastic polyps, a marker identifying which hyperplastic polyp will undergo malignant transformation has not yet been found.

Differential Diagnosis

- Fundic gland polyps are also among the most common gastric polyps. These have a different histology with cystically dilated glands lined by chief, parietal, or mucous cells with a normal mucosal background without inflammation.
- Ménétrier's disease involves the gastric body and fundic mucosa diffusely with oxyntic glandular atrophy. In Ménétrier's disease, there is prominent foveolar hyperplasia associated with protein-losing gastropathy and lacking significant inflammation.
- Gastritis cystica polyposa/profunda arise in the gastric anastomotic site after partial gastrectomy. These lesions contain prominent features of mucosal prolapse with irregular dilated glands in the submucosa.
- Juvenile polyps are more commonly found in children. They contain a smooth rounded surface with erosion and granulation tissue. Cystically dilated glands are often with neutrophilic granulocytes.
- Polyps arising in patients with Peutz-Jeghers, Cowden, or Cronkhite-Canada syndrome are associated with a typical clinical history. Correct diagnosis requires clinical, endoscopic, and histological correlation. Peutz-Jeghers polyps most often arise in the small bowel. Gastric Peutz-Jeghers polyps may resemble hyperplastic polyps and frequently lack the characteristic arborizing bundles of smooth muscle in the stroma. Clinical signs typical for Peutz-Jeghers include pigmented macules involving the mucous membranes (lips) and skin. In Cowden's syndrome, multiple hamartomatous polyps arise from the esophagus to colon. Typical clinical features of Cowden's disease include facial trichilemmomas, acral keratosis, papillomatous papules, and mucosal lesions. Cronkhite-Canada syndrome is associated with diffuse GI polyposis, abnormal skin pigmentation, and nail dystrophy. In the stomach, Cronkhite-Canada syndrome polyps are histologically similar to hyperplastic polyps.

References and Further Reading

Abraham, S. C., Singh, V. K., Yardley, J. H., & Wu, T. T. (2001). Hyperplastic polyps of the stomach: Associations with histologic patterns of gastritis and gastric atrophy. *American Journal of Surgical Pathology, 25*(4), 500–507.

Carneiro, F., David, L., Seruca, R., Castedo, S., Nesland, J. M., & Sobrinho-Simões, M. (1993). Hyperplastic polyposis and diffuse carcinoma of the stomach. A study of a family. *Cancer, 72*, 323–329.

Carneiro, F., Santos, L., & Sobrinho-Simões, M. (1995). Carcinoma arising in gastric hyperplastic polyps. *Gastrointestinal Endoscopy, 41*, 178–179.

Goddard, A. F., Badreldin, R., Pritchard, D. M., Walker, M. M., Warren, B., & British Society of Gastroenterology. (2010). The management of gastric polyps. *Gut, 59*(9), 1270–1276.

Hattori, T. (1985). Morphological range of hyperplastic polyps and carcinomas arising in hyperplastic polyps of the stomach. *Journal of Clinical Pathology, 38*(6), 622–630.

Jain, R., & Chetty, R. (2009). Gastric hyperplastic polyps: A review. *Digestive Diseases and Sciences, 54*(9), 1839–1846.

Yao, T., Kajiwara, M., Kuroiwa, S., Iwashita, A., Oya, M., Kabashima, A., et al. (2002). Malignant transformation of gastric hyperplastic polyps: Alteration of phenotypes, proliferative activity, and p53 expression. *Human Pathology, 33*(10), 1016–1022.

I

Imperforate Anus

Andrzej Mróz
Department of Gastroenterology and Hepatology, Histopathology Unit, Medical Center for Postgraduate Education, Warsaw, Poland

Synonyms

Anorectal malformation

Definition

Imperforate anus can be defined as the defect of the development of the lowest portion of intestinal and urogenital tracts. Imperforate anus is a result of cloacal membrane imperforation. Anus and rectum develop from dorsal portion of the hindgut by forming urorectal septum which separates rectum and anal canal from bladder and urethra. It is believed to complete by the 7th week of gestation. The anus develops from anal tubercles and proctodeum, the external invagination which communicates with proximal parts after disintegration of anal membrane at 8th weeks' gestation. The cause and genetic background for abnormal development is not fully elucidated, and no definite risk factors are known. As a result, rectum opens in abnormal locations in the perineum or female genitals. Stenosis, occlusive membranes, or agenesis of rectum and anal canal ensue with or without fistulas in perineal skin, urethra, prostate, bladder, vulva, or vagina.

Historically, imperforate anus is divided into four groups (Fig. 1): stenosis alone (11%); imperforate anus with the thin membrane separating the anus and rectum (4%); imperforate anus with a widely separated anus and rectum (76%); and normal anus with rectum ending at some level above it (9%). Fistulas occur most often in groups 3 and 4. In males, the fistulas are most often urinary (urethra 25%, bladder 33%, perineum 42%) and in females, urinary and genital (vaginal 84%, perineum 14.5%, bladder 1.5%). This scheme refers also to Wingspread classification which divides anorectal malformations to high (anorectal agenesis, rectovaginal fistulas, retroprostatic urethral fistulas, rectal atresia), intermediate (rectobulbar and rectovaginal fistulas, anal agenesis without fistulas) and low (anocutaneous and anovestibular fistulas, anal stenosis) malformations. This division was related to the muscle levator ani position.

The newer staging is the anatomic classification which connects malformation with its anatomical site and reflects the severity of symptoms:

- Perineal fistula: good prognosis, in either sex, closed anus with the small connection opening on the perineal body, sometimes with small loop of skin at the anal opening (so-called bucket-handle pathognomonic for perineal fistula)

F. Carneiro et al. (eds.), *Pathology of the Gastrointestinal Tract*, Encyclopedia of Pathology,
DOI 10.1007/978-3-319-40560-5

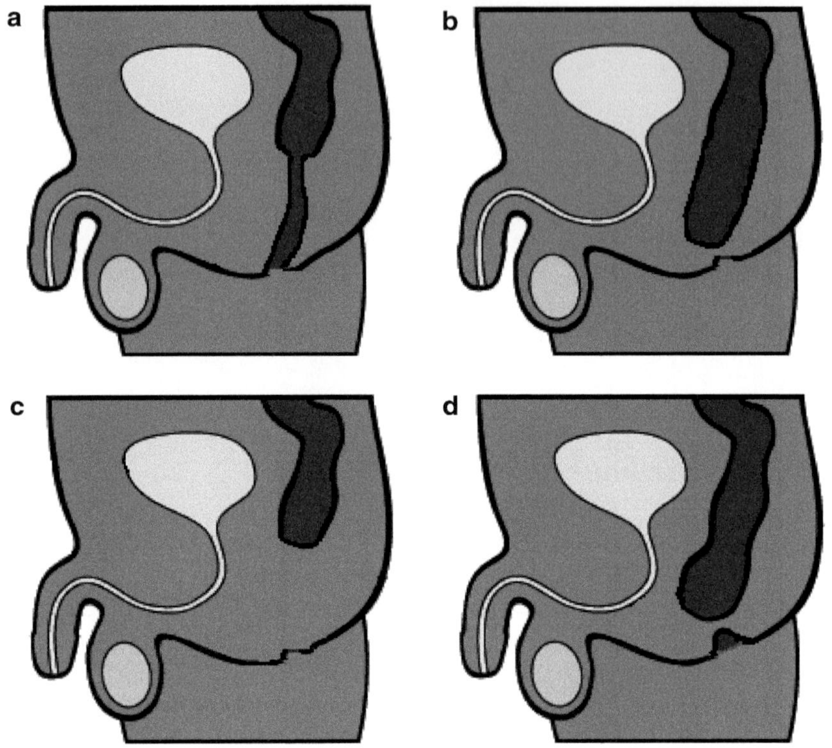

Imperforate Anus, Fig. 1 OEIS syndrome (Omphalocele-Exstrophy-Imperforate Anus-Spinal Defects) – It affects 1 in 200,000–400,000 pregnancies, its cause is unknown, sometimes in trisomy 18, male: female ratio is 3:1. Cloacal exstrophy is a result of breakdown and mesodermal invasion of cloacal membrane. The exstrophy of the urinary bladder and small intestines, anal atresia, hypoplasia of the colon, omphalocele, and anomalies of external genitals are seen. It can be accompanied by meningocele, spina bifida, unilateral hypoplasia of the kidney, single umbilical artery, Meckel's diverticulum, and colonic duplication

- Vestibular fistula: good prognosis, small opening at the posterior aspect of the vestibule externally to hymen
- Cloaca: common channel incorporating urethra, vagina, and rectum, prognosis is connected with the length of the channel (the shorter the channel, the better prognosis)
- Bulbar urethral fistula: relatively common malformation in boys, visualization of the fistula requires additional radiographic methods
- Prostatic fistula: rare type with poorer prognosis
- Bladder-neck fistula: 10% of boys, very poor prognosis
- Absent fistula: best prognosis, rare, common in children with trisomy 21, determined on exclusion of fistulas, amenable to primary correction
- Cloacal exstrophy: extremely rare, extremely poor prognosis, part of *OEIS syndrome*

Imperforate anus and anorectal abnormalities can be associated with other malformations:

- Cardiovascular malformations in 12–22% of patients including Fallot's tetralogy, ventricular septal defects, transposition of the great arteries, and hypoplastic left heart syndrome
- Gastrointestinal abnormalities: annular pancreas, duodenal atresia or/and obstruction, midgut malrotation, esophageal atresia, intestinal atresia, Townes-Brocks syndrome, VATER and VATERL syndromes, CHARGE syndrome, and others
- Vertebral anomalies: lumbosacral defects in patients with high lesions
- Spinal abnormalities: dysraphism (tethered spinal cord), cord lipomas, and syringohydromyelia
- Gynecological anomalies: bicornate uterus, and uterus didelphus may be present in up to 35% females with imperforate anus, vaginal septum (most common malformation in females with anorectal abnormalities), vaginal duplication and agenesis sometimes associated with ipsilateral absent ovary and kidney

Clinical Features

- **Incidence**
  Imperforate anus (anorectal malformations) affects 1 in 5,000 live-born infants.
- **Age**
  Most of the cases are identified at the time of birth upon routine physical examination. Delayed diagnosis may result from incomplete initial examination or from the subtle nature of the malformation like perineal fistula not visible at the first glance. These patients may present months or years after birth.
- **Sex**
  No sex predilection is reported (previous studies pointed to male sex predilection).
- **Site**
  Anorectum is the primary site.
- **Treatment**
  Newborns with imperforate anus should not be fed. Intravenous broad-spectrum antibiotics should be administered in order to avoid infection and sepsis. Cardiac defects must be ruled out prior further diagnostic and surgical interventions are performed.

  Thorough diagnostic process should be undertaken in order to select patients for surgical care. This includes sacral radiography, abdominal ultrasonography, spinal ultrasonography or MRI, lateral pelvic radiography, augmented-pressure distal colostography CT scanning, and others.

  Some patients may undergo primary repair in the neonatal period (pull-through methods), but most of them may reach definite repair in staged fashion including colostomy usually in the left lower quadrant, followed by reconstructive surgery varying upon the type of malformation, the general concept is to separate rectum from other structures, divide and ligate fistulas, fully reconstruct pelvic anatomy within adequate muscle complex, and colostomy closure.
- **Outcome (Prognosis)**
  Children with no life-threatening comorbidity should survive. Prognosis depends on severity of malformation and its amenability to surgical correction. Children with imperforate anus and anorectal anomalies are endangered with injury to surrounding organs (mainly during operative procedures) as well as are at greater risk of infection.

  Main complication of anorectal abnormalities which influence prognosis in these patients is fecal and urinary incontinence. The more severe form of anomaly (e.g., common channel cloaca, bladder-neck, and prostatic fistulas) the poorer nerve and muscle formation which may result in fecal and urinary incontinence. Children with imperforate anus and no fistulas should have voluntary bowel movements in at least ¾ cases, whereas boys with bladder-neck fistulas achieve voluntary bowel movements in 15%. Medical and psychological care for these patients is mandatory.

Macroscopy

Anal region may be flat or has only small excavation with no obvious orifice. Perineal fistulas may be visible as small openings, for vestibule fistulas separation of labia may be needed. Gentle pressure on suprapubic region may result in evacuation of meconium from urethra in boys or from vagina in girls. Fourchette type of fistula combines the features of vestibule and perineal fistula, giving the velvety mucosal appearance from vestibule side and dry anoderm from posterior perineal side.

In girls with cloaca only, one opening between the shortened labia is visible usually with no fistulas.

The abdomen may be distended due to palpated masses such as dilated kidney or bladder, hydrocolpos, ectopic kidney, duplication, or other cystic structures.

Microscopy

Microscopy can be sometimes utilized in searching for meconium elements in urine or vaginal discharge.

Differential Diagnosis

Other reasons of delayed meconium evacuation must be ruled out. Intestinal atresia with Hirschsprung disease may come in differential diagnosis, although in these cases, perineal region is not changed.

References and Further Reading

Fenoglio-Preiser, C., et al. (1999). *Gastrointestinal pathology plus: An atlas and text*. Philadelphia: Lippincott Williams & Wilkins.

Mirza, B., Ijaz, L., Sharif, M., & Sheikh, A. (2011). Anorectal malformations in neonates. *African Journal of Paediatric Surgery, 8*, 151–154.

Pena, A. (1995). Anorectal malformations. *Seminars in Pediatric Surgery, 4*, 35–47.

Rosen, N. G., & Cuffari, C. (2012). Pediatric imperforate anus. In *Medscape reference drugs, diseases & procedures*. www.emedicine.medscape.com/article/929904-clinical.

Infarction, Intestinal

Maria Sotiropoulou
Department of Pathology, Alexandra Hospital, Athens, Attica, Greece

Synonyms

Dead bowel; Dead gut; Intestinal necrosis; Ischemic bowel

Definition

Intestinal infarction is damage or death of a part of the intestine due to reduction in the blood flow or decreased blood flow. There are several causes of infarction involving either arterial or venous impairment. Possible causes include hernia and adhesions from a previous surgery when the intestine becomes trapped in scar tissue. Arterial insufficiency is the most common cause of intestinal infarction and is divided in nonocclusive (central) and occlusive (peripheral) ischemia.

Nonocclusive ischemia represents up to 25% of acute mesenteric infarction and is characterized by low blood flow and insufficient oxygen supply to the tissue without arterial obstruction. Hypotension, cardiac failure, and shock of any etiology are the main causes. Hypotension in elderly patients who have atherosclerotic disease often causes nonocclusive stenosis of the major arteries.

In occlusive arterial insufficiency, there is obstruction of the blood flow, which may be due to extramural causes like volvulus, torsion, intussusception, or compression by a tumor. Of the luminal causes, vascular emboli or thrombi are the most common. Emboli may travel from the heart in a patient with atrial fibrillation, whereas thrombi can block arteries with arteriosclerotic disease. Mural causes include dissecting aneurysms, radiation injury, tumors, and amyloidosis. Drugs and toxins like potassium salts, cocaine, and venoms from snakes and scorpions can cause arterial occlusions. Vasculitis and arteriopathies can also cause ischemia.

Venous insufficiency accounts for 5.15% of causes of intestinal ischemia and is related to external venous compression, thrombosis or pathologic intramural processes, hypercoagulative states, and less commonly inflammation, portal hypertension, or trauma.

Small intestinal blood supply must be reduced in more than 25–50% for the intestinal viability to be lost. The resulting ischemic injury is dependent not only on the degree of vascular obstruction but also on the collateral circulation and the presence of contributing diseases.

Acute mesenteric ischemia is a syndrome in which inadequate blood flow causes ischemia or gangrene of bowel. The superior mesenteric artery supplies small intestine, and proximal mid-colon and inferior mesenteric artery supplies distal colon and rectum. Superior mesenteric vein is responsible for venous drainage. Embolic phenomena account for 5% of all clinical cases and arterial thrombosis for about 25%. Nonocclusive mesenteric ischemia is the cause of 20% and mesenteric venous thrombosis of less than 10%. The superior mesenteric vessels are more frequently involved than inferior mesenteric vessels. Damage ranges from reversible ischemia to transmural infarction with necrosis and perforation. Bowel necrosis leads to peritonitis and can occur in 8–12 h after the onset of the symptoms. The vascular occlusion from emboli is sudden, and patients do not have time to develop collateral flow. Mesenteric venous thrombosis in more than 80% of cases develops secondary to a clot in the mesenteric circulation. It may affect a younger population, and patients may have prolonged symptoms, sometimes exceeding 30 days.

Only angiography or exploratory surgery makes early diagnosis possible, which is the best way to improve patient survival.

Clinical Features

- **Incidence**
  The overall prevalence of acute mesenteric infarction is 0.1% of all hospital admissions and is more common in countries where individuals have higher life expectancy.
- **Age**
  This is a disease of people older than 50 years old. In younger people, there are risk factors like atrial fibrillation, oral contraceptive use, or hypercoagulative states.
- **Sex**
  Overall, no sex preference exists in the different causes of mesenteric venous thrombosis, except for a predilection for women that take oral contraceptives or are pregnant.
- **Site**
  The location and extent of ischemic lesions depend on the anatomy and physiology of the blood supply which is relatively poor in the colon and particularly on the left side. Moreover, colon has poorer collateral vascular network than the small bowel. In a review of 1,000 cases, the distribution of lesions was 8% in the right colon and 73% in the splenic flexure, descending colon and sigmoid in total. The superior mesenteric artery is affected more commonly than the inferior mesenteric artery. The most severe atherosclerotic lesions affect the proximal 2 cm of the superior and inferior mesenteric arteries. Approximately 95% of all mesenteric thromboses involve the superior mesenteric vein leading to infarction of the small intestine or proximal colon. The combined involvement of small and large bowel is not infrequent.
- **Treatment**
  The initial treatment includes resuscitation and infusion of papaverine and thrombolytics. After thrombolysis, in a small proportion of patients who have atherosclerotic plaques in the superior mesenteric artery, angioplasty can be performed, but with a high rate of restenosis (20–50%). On the other hand, in mesenteric venous thrombosis, the main treatment is heparin.

  If signs of peritonitis develop, the resection of the necrotic bowel is the treatment of choice in all types of acute mesenteric infarction. Intraoperative fluorescein administration can differentiate the viable from the nonviable bowel. For embolic acute mesenteric infarction, a transverse arteriotomy may be performed or a bypass, if thrombectomy is unsuccessful. For thrombotic acute mesenteric ischemia and if the gut is not gangrenous, revascularization with arteriomesenteric bypass is the appropriate management.
- **Outcome (Prognosis)**
  Approximately 15–20% of patients develop gangrene or perforation. The prognosis is poor when bowel wall infarction has occurred and the mortality rate is 90% and falls slightly even with proper treatment. In a long-term follow up of patients who had surgery, the 2 and 5 year survival were 70% and 50%, respectively. Colonic ischemia is transient in half of the patients, with the rest 20–25% having chronic colitis or deep colonic infarction and between 10% and 15% developing ischemic strictures.

Macroscopy (Gross)

Resection specimens for ischemia may be evaluated for ischemic damage extension, estimation of the viability of the margins, and, if possible, revealing the etiology. The length of time before the examination of the surgical specimen or autopsy is responsible for differences in appearance. Acute ischemic injury may be patchy or diffuse. At first the bowel is dilated and dark with red edematous mucosa which may have ulcerations superficial or, sometimes, deep. The serosa has lost its shiny smooth appearance and appears rough and cyanotic. The bowel wall is friable and thinner than normal, and sometimes, there is perforation. The lumen is filled with blood, and in some cases, there is complete necrosis with the appearance of gangrene. The mesentery appears thick, hemorrhagic with thrombosed veins, while arteries usually appear normal. Moreover, organizing recanalized thrombi will be observed in mesenteric venous vasculature. If there is recovery, the bowel reestablishes normal thickness, induration, and contraction. Sometimes the formation of an ischemic stricture is a complication.

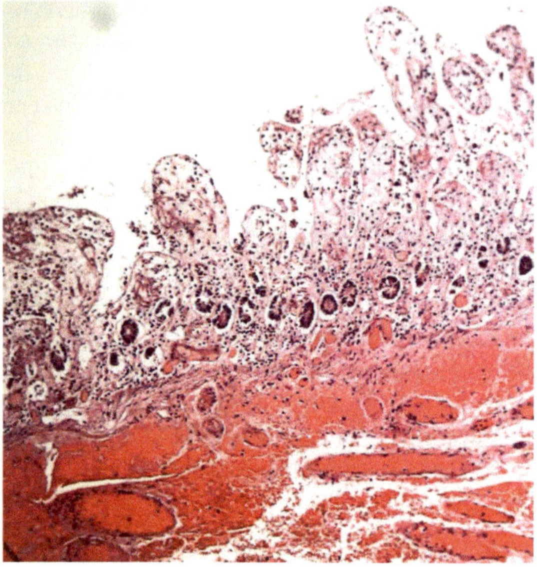

Infarction, Intestinal, Fig. 1 Acute ischemia of the small bowel with hemorrhage in mucosa with proteinaceous material, dilated and congested vessels in the submucosa, and glandular dropout loss of epithelium

Microscopy

In acute ischemia, there is hemorrhage in the mucosa and later in submucosa. The upper mucosa is relatively hypoxic and consequently particularly vulnerable and becomes necrotic, while the lower mucosa remains intact. The crypts in the upper parts often appear necrotic and the remaining in the lower mucosa are more preserved (Fig. 1). In severe cases, the whole mucosa remains as a shadow of the normal histology. In milder cases, the upper halves of the crypts show varying degree of degeneration and sloughing. The remaining epithelium is attenuated with goblet cell loss and regenerative hyperchromatism. Moderate inflammatory cell infiltration is usually present, and fibrin plugs may be noted in mucosal capillaries. Necroinflammatory exudate mimicking pseudomembranes may be seen in some cases (Fig. 2).

The lamina propria has various degrees of edema and congestion with coexistence of pink proteinaceous material and contains a moderate acute inflammatory exudate at an early stage,

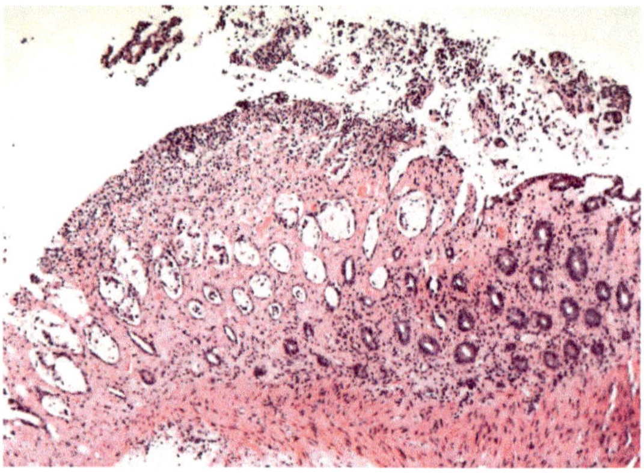

Infarction, Intestinal, Fig. 2 Large bowel biopsy with pseudomembranes covers the surface

which increases later. Submucosa is edematous with vessel dilatation. If a recovery phase follows, subacute and chronic inflammation with the formation of granulation tissue and fibrosis alternate with islands of hyperplastic mucosal folds and mimic Crohn's disease or fulminant ulcerative colitis (Fig. 3). The presence of

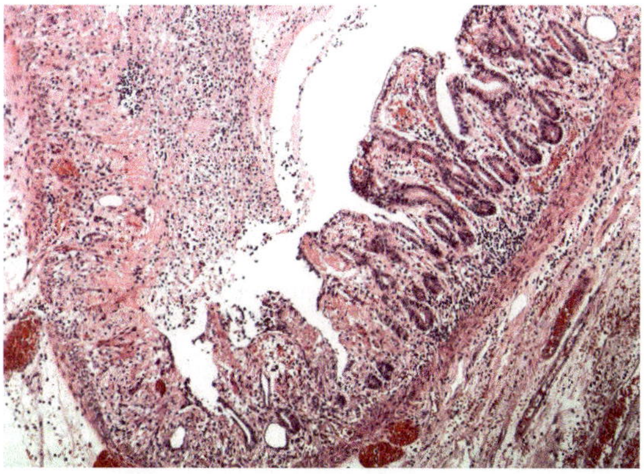

Infarction, Intestinal, Fig. 3 Regenerative changes following ischemic damage with architectural distortion and hyperchromatic nuclei with intense nucleoli

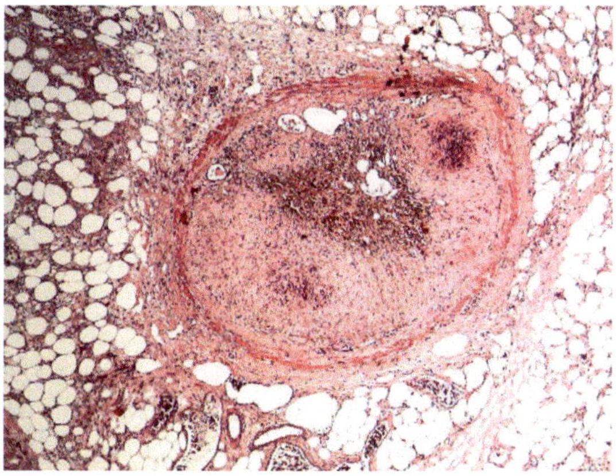

Infarction, Intestinal, Fig. 4 Submucosa showing congestive and thrombosed vein with organization and revascularization

iron-laden macrophages in the mucosa and submucosa is important in differential diagnosis from inflammatory bowel disease. If the degree and extension of injury are not severe, mucosa may reverse to normal. The presence of thrombi in mesenteric vessels must be estimated with caution, because thrombi may develop as a response to stasis and congestion. The organization of thrombi is the evidence of true thrombosis and is clinically significant (Fig. 4).

Strictures are rare because severe infarction of the colon is accompanied by small bowel involvement and the patient usually dies. Strictures are relatively frequent in the left colon and are tubular or fusiform with fibrosis, which extends through the entire thickness of the wall till the pericolic tissue. Ulcers may develop, which affect only the mucosa or extent to all parts of the bowel wall with perforation.

Immunophenotype

There is not any specific marker in intestinal infarction.

Molecular Features

There are not molecular features that contribute to the diagnosis of intestinal infarction.

Differential Diagnosis

The differential diagnosis includes pseudomembranous colitis, acute ulcerative colitis, toxic megacolon, and Crohn's disease.

References and Further Reading

Fenoglio-Preiser, C., Noffsinger, A., Stemmermann, G., et al. (2008). *Gastrointestinal pathology. An atlas and text* (3rd ed., pp. 327–340). Philadelphia: Lippincott, Williams and Wilkins.

Herbert, G. S., & Steele, S. R. (2007). Acute and chronic mesenteric ischemia. *The Surgical Clinics of North America, 87*(5), 1115–1134.

Rosenblum, G. D., et al. (1997). The mesenteric circulation. Anatomy and physiology. *The Surgical Clinics of North America, 77*(2), 289–306.

Tendler, D. A. (2003). Acute intestinal ischemia and infarction. *Seminars in Gastrointestinal Disease, 14*(2), 66–76.

West, B., & Mitchell, K. (2009). In R. Odze & J. Goldblum (Eds.), Vascular disorders of the GI tract. *Surgical pathology of the GI tract, liver, biliary tract and pancreas* (2nd ed., pp. 207–211). Philadelphia: Saunders/Elsevier.

Infectious Colitis

Anne Jouret-Mourin
Department of Pathology, Cliniques Universitaires St. Luc, UCL, Brussels, Belgium

Synonyms

Acute infectious colitis (AIC); Acute infectious-type colitis (AITC); Acute self-limited colitis (ASLC); Dysentery

Definition

Infectious colitis corresponds to the inflammation of the colon caused by an infectious agent including bacteria, viruses, protozoa, fungus, or parasites.

Epidemiology

In western countries, infectious colitis is most commonly due to bacterial and viral pathogens but it may also be caused by protozoa, fungus, and parasites. The last three pathogens are mostly observed in immune-compromised patients or travellers coming from developing countries. Infection caused by bacteria or viruses usually resolves within a few weeks without residual histologic findings.

Many enteric infections are transmitted to humans through contaminated food and water. Populations in less developed countries often live in ramshackle housing without sanitary environment, which facilitates greatly the occurrence of colonic infections. In industrialized countries, other and different practices facilitate germ transmission. These include large-scale food production, fast-food chains, traveling, etc. Furthermore, the populations of patients with immune-compromising conditions such AIDS or transplantation increase in number and these are more susceptible to develop infectious colitis. The most frequently identified bacterial pathogens are *Salmonella*, *Campylobacter*, *Shigella*, *Clostridium difficile*, *Yersinia*, *Escherichia coli*, and *Klebsiella oxytoca*. The latter three were most significant during the last decade. Noroviruses are major viral pathogens and an important cause of diarrhea in both children and adults, as well in immune-competent patients as in immune-compromised individuals.

Infection by adenovirus is another common cause of childhood diarrhea and also an important cause of diarrhea in immune-compromised patients (AIDS, transplant patients. . .). Other possible causative agents are protozoa (Giardia) and parasites.

Pathogeny

Watery diarrhea is the result of a disturbed balance between intestinal secretion and absorption. Viruses can infect and kill villous tip enterocytes, thereby disturbing absorption. Bloody diarrhea is most often of bacterial origin. Production of bloody stools means a mucosal breakdown caused by entero-invasive bacteria such as *Shigella*, *Campylobacter coli* or *jejuni, Salmonella*, *Yersinia*, or by cytotoxin-producing pathogens such as *C. difficile* and protozoa such as Amoebae. *E. coli*, *Vibrio cholerae*, *Salmonella*, *C. perfringens* type A, and *Klebsiella* can also cause acute bloody diarrhea, Cytomegalovirus and Herpes virus as well as protozoa can also provoke bloody diarrhea. Acute bloody diarrhea, however, usually begins with watery diarrhea. The most common causes for acute infectious watery diarrhea are viral, and most frequently involve the small intestine. Rotavirus represents the most common cause of childhood diarrhea, in addition to adenovirus. Noroviruses are recognized as playing a major role in enterocolitis. It is the second most common cause of watery diarrhea in children and an important cause in adults (see ► Viral Gastroenteritis).

Clinical Features

- **Incidence**
  The risk for developing infectious colitis varies considerably throughout the world and

depends on local conditions. The incidence steadily increases, and infectious colitis is responsible for significant morbidity and mortality worldwide. In industrialized countries, most incidents of infectious colitis are acute self-limited colitis and mostly due to bacterial colitis.

- **Site**
  Any level of the colon may be involved but the site of the lesion can be helpful for diagnosis. Several bacteria such as *Yersinia pseudotuberculosis*, *Campylobacter jejuni*, and *Salmonella* species can induce infections of the small and large intestine. Other bacteria such as *Shigella* species and enterohemorrhagic *E. coli* induce infections of the large intestine alone. Some pathogens are located preferentially at the appendix, caecum, and right colon such as *Salmonella* sp. Viral infections like rotavirus and noroviruses are most often localized in the small bowel.
- **Age**
  Infectious colitis affects persons of all ages with no gender differences. Children, elderly patients, and immune-compromised patients are more susceptible to contract infectious colitis as well as travelers in undeveloped countries.
- **Clinical Symptoms**
  Most enteric infections are self-limited. The most common symptom is a history of less than 1 week watery diarrhea with blood or mucus (dysentery), usually with acute onset. Watery diarrhea is more often of viral etiology and at routine bacteriological investigation cultures will be negative. Sometimes abdominal cramps, bloating, and tenesmus may also be observed. The frequency of the diarrhea can lead to dehydration.

  Chronic diarrhea with three or more loose stools for more than 30 days can also be seen in infectious colitis of viral (rotavirus, cytomegalovirus, adenovirus), bacterial (*Campylobacter*, *Clostridium difficile*, *Aeromonas*, *E. coli*, *Salmonella*, *Yersinia*), or protozoal (*Entamoeba histolotyca*, *Isospora*) origin.
- **Treatment**
  The treatment is determined by the specific agent. Supportive care is important. Antibiotics may help treat bacterial infectious colitis if needed while specific drugs are available for parasitic infections.

Macroscopic Features

Endoscopic features are nonspecific with erythema, friability, variable hemorrhage, and sometimes erosions of the mucosa being present. The specific findings of bacterial infections are described in the chapter of bacterial colitis. Viral infections may be macroscopically normal. Sometimes, specific features are seen. These are described with each virus.

Microscopic Findings

The microscopic features of infectious colitis are highly variable. They depend upon the responsible agent, the immune status of the patient, and the duration of the disease. In the majority of the cases, there is no specific pattern. The spectrum of microscopic features includes a normal biopsy, samples showing only edema, samples showing active inflammation with neutrophils which can be mild or severe, fulminant disease with bowel wall necrosis, and samples showing residual lesions.

Three microscopic features can be observed most frequently:

The majority of infections cause minimal or no inflammatory change. This is seen in infections induced by agents such as toxigenic *Vibrio cholerae*, *Nesseiria gonorrhea*, Enteroadherent *E. coli*, and many viruses. In adenovirus infection, some smudgy inclusions within surface epithelial cells, mostly in goblets cells, may be observed together with apoptosis of crypt epithelial cells and surface damage.

Acute self-limited colitis (ASLC) is the most common pattern in enteric infections. The term of "ASLC" refers to such histologic presentation, which is associated with a rapid spontaneous positive evolution. However, in some cases, the infection may not be self-limited and even can be fatal. For this reason, the synonymous term "acute infectious-type colitis" is also proposed.

Infectious Colitis, Fig. 1 ASLC/AITC: Presence of inflammatory infiltrate in the middle and upper levels of the crypts and, more frequently in the lamina propria with cryptitis, in a background of preserved crypt architecture

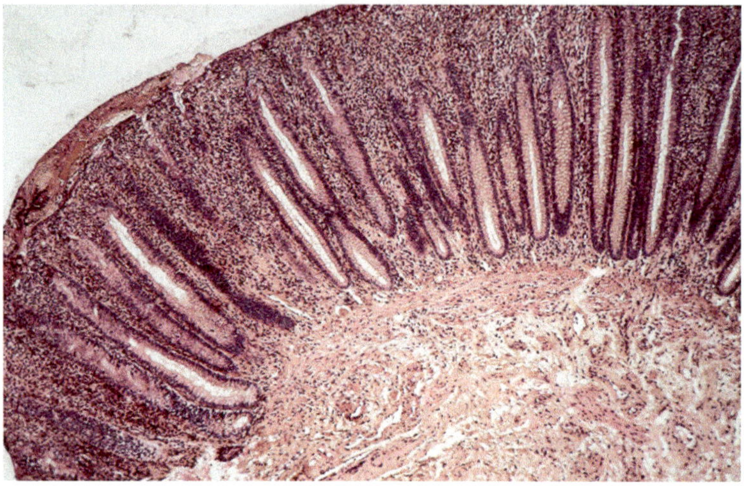

ASLC corresponds to the presence of an increased inflammatory infiltrate in the middle and upper levels of the crypts, more frequently in the lamina propria with cryptitis in a background of preserved crypt architecture. Neutrophils are more common in the early phase of the disease, and they can be either numerous or very few. They can invade the surface and crypt epithelium, inducing cryptitis and sometimes crypt abscesses. The crypts remain parallel, but they are often smaller at the upper part. The surface and crypt epithelial cells may show mucin depletion and can appear flattened or cuboidal due to epithelial damage by cytotoxins. The lamina propria may contain mononuclear cells including lymphocytes, histiocytes, and plasma cells, but basal plasmocytosis should not be present (Figs. 1 and 2). Morphologic changes show a focal or patchy but rarely diffuse distribution. Erosions can be observed. The diagnosis of acute self-limited colitis relies mainly on the presence of active superficial inflammation and the absence of features suggestive for IBD.

The term "focal active colitis (FAC)" is used to describe the isolated finding of focal crypt injury, varying from a single crypt abscess to rare foci of cryptitis or crypt abscesses. These features may correspond to resolving infectious colitis, but recent studies have shown that it may also correspond to other causes such as Crohn's disease particularly in children, and adverse drug

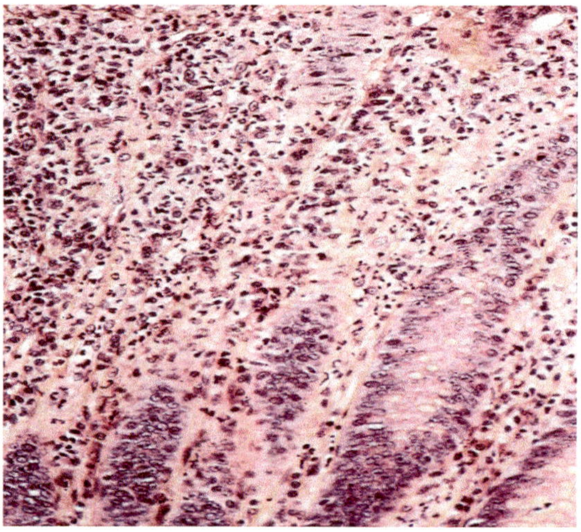

Infectious Colitis, Fig. 2 Neutrophils invade crypt epithelium causing cryptitis. The crypts remain parallel but there are often smaller at the upper part

reactions or that it can be observed incidentally (bowel preparation artifact).

Nonspecific mucosal injury as well as ASLC or AITC or FAC may be seen with many bacterial infections including *Campylobacter*, *Aeromonas*, non-typhoid *Salmonella*, *Shigella*, etc. Various bacteria induce slightly different localizations of the lesions which can be recognized and can be used for diagnostic purposes.

Some pathogens can be specifically identified in tissue sections or produce specific features allowing a microscopic diagnosis such as a pseudomembranous pattern (*Clostridium difficile*, enterohemorrhagic *E. coli*), granulomatous pattern (Mycobacterium tuberculosis or avium in immune-competent patients, *Yersinia*), a diffuse histiocytic pattern (*Rhodococcus equi*, *Mycobacterium avium* in immune-compromised patients, histoplasmosis, Whipple disease), a predominantly lymphohistiocytic pattern (lymphogranuloma venerum, *Salmonella typhimurium*) or viral inclusions such as Cytomegalovirus infection.

Differential Diagnosis

The differential diagnosis between infectious colitis and other types of colitis is sometimes difficult. Most often, the diagnosis of infectious colitis does not require intestinal biopsies, since the evolution is usually rapidly favorable. Clinical findings may help the diagnosis. Travelers coming from tropical or subtropical countries or whenever more than one person is acutely ill at the same moment are situations that favor an infectious colitis.

When sampling is performed, the histological aspect of infectious colitis can mimic other intestinal diseases.

Acute self-limited infectious colitis should especially be distinguished from chronic idiopathic inflammatory bowel disease (IBD) including ulcerative colitis and Crohn's disease, ischaemic colitis, or other types of colitis such as lymphocytic colitis or adverse drug reaction, because the treatment is different.

Patients with acute infectious-type colitis may present with the same symptoms as those with acute onset IBD.

Numerous authors have tried to establish criteria to distinguish an infectious colitis from an IBD at the time of the first biopsies. One of the most important studies was performed by Surawicz who showed that features with a high predictive value (87–100%) of diagnosing IBD were distorted crypt architecture, a villous surface, epithelioid granuloma, crypt atrophy, and basal lymphoid aggregates. Pointers to an infective cause were the presence of edema and a neutrophil polymorph infiltrates. The neutrophil aggregates were usually conspicuous in the lamina propria and surrounded or infiltrated the upper crypt epithelium. Diffuse, regional, or focal active colitis without crypt architectural distortion and prominent cryptitis favor the diagnosis of infectious colitis. But this is less useful and not that specific. So, biopsy diagnosis of acute infectious disease is based on the absence of histological criteria, favoring IBD and the lack of features of chronicity.

Schumacher in 1994 carried out a prospective study and confirmed the significant features of IBD. In this study, the strongest predictor of IBD was the basal plasmocytosis followed by crypt branching, crypt distortion, and the presence of a villous surface. In the same paper, the authors showed that structural changes were dependent on the duration of symptoms: Basal plasmocytosis seems to be the earliest sign of IBD which appears in the first week, while crypt distortion is found only after two or more weeks.

Giant cells are also observed in infectious-type colitis but are more present in the upper part of the lamina propria.

The difficulty of the differential diagnosis is even greater if one realizes that many enteric pathogens can reveal the first attack of IBD or may cause exacerbations or relapses of IBD.

The resolving phase of infectious colitis which shows an increase of lymphocytes and plasmocytes in the lamina propria with focal cryptitis or an increase of intraepithelial lymphocytosis may also be more difficult to diagnose and to differentiate from Crohn's disease or lymphocytic colitis. Stool culture may help.

Ischaemic patterns can be observed following an infection with some bacteria such as *Escherichia coli* or *Clostridium difficile* in the later phase. Both may present as pseudomembranous colitis. The presence of a hyalinized lamina propria and small or atrophic crypts are more specific features of ischemia. Pseudomembranes are more diffuse in *clostridium difficile* colitis but they are patchy in ischemic colitis. An ischaemic pattern with pseudomembranes and fibrin thrombi may also be observed in enterohemorrhagic *E. coli* infection.

Drug abuses are also a common cause of acute diarrhea and they can mimic either infectious colitis or IBD.

Useful Tests

Stool culture may be essential to diagnosis.

Some complementary special histological stainings can be used for diagnostic purposes such as the Warthin starry stain or periodic Acid-Schiff for spirochetosis and microsporidium.

Immune histochemistry (specific antibodies against CMV, adenovirus, *E. coli, Campylobacter, Samonella*, etc.) can also help confirm the diagnosis.

Molecular biology tests are also available for some infectious lesions such as for *Campylobacter, Yersinia*, Adenovirus, and Norovirus.

Bacterial Infections

See entry "▶ Bacterial Enterocolitis"

Viral Infections

Many viruses may affect the colon and the small bowel. Their clinical features vary according to the type of virus and the immune status of the patient. Cytomegalovirus (CMV), Herpes, Adenovirus, and Norovirus are the most frequent viral colonic infections.

CMV

- **Incidence**
  CMV occurs in both immune-compromised and immune-competent patients, but it affects most commonly immune-compromised patients (AIDS, transplant patients). It can also occur in the context of patients with IBD.
- **Site**
  CMV may be found anywhere in the colon.
- **Clinical Symptoms**
  The most common symptom is bloody or watery diarrhea with abdominal pain and fever.
- **Prognosis**
  In healthy patients, primary infections are often self-limited. Sometimes, CMV can cause a surinfection in cases of chronic intestinal disease such as ulcerative colitis, Crohn's disease or can also cause an exacerbation of the IBD. CMV infection can also lead to toxic megacolon in IBD, which is a dangerous complication.
- **Macroscopic Features**
  CMV causes a wide variety of lesions in the colon. Ulcers are the most common lesion, either superficial or deep, linear, single or multiple. Hemorrhagic colitis, erosions, or pseudomembranes may also be seen.

  The lesion may be segmental.
- **Microscopic Findings**
  The histologic features are very variable. Edema, mucosal erosions, diffuse inflammatory changes, vasculitis, and deep and large ulcers as well as ischaemic changes can be observed. The characteristic feature is the owl's eye eosinophilic intranuclear inclusion preferentially found in endothelial cells; sometimes in stromal cells, macrophages of the lamina propria, or rarely in glandular epithelial crypt (Fig. 3). These inclusions are preferentially localized in the ulcer base. They may be present in intact mucosa as well as in granulation tissue.
- **Differential Diagnosis**
  The differential diagnosis of CMV predominantly includes other viral infections.

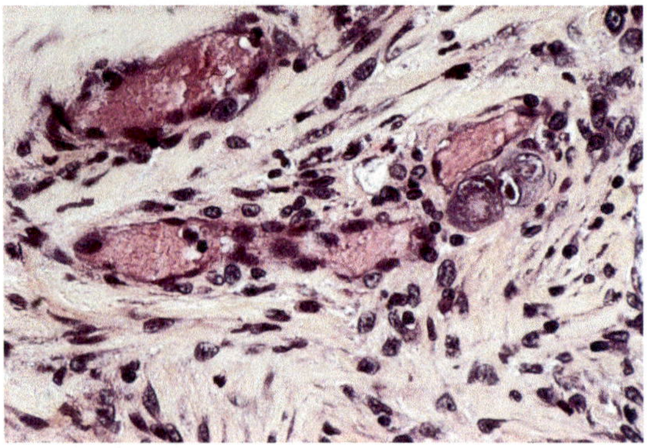

Infectious Colitis, Fig. 3 Characteristic owl's eye" CMV inclusions within endothelial cells

Adenovirus inclusions are more frequently located within surface epithelium and the inclusion is usually round to crescent-shaped and exclusively nuclear. Histologic features of CMV infections can mimic IBD, ischaemic colitis, or sur-infected IBD.

- **Useful Test**
  Immune histochemical staining and the use of probes against early specific antigens may increase the sensitivity of the diagnosis.

Herpes Virus

Herpes virus infections are most commonly seen in the anorectum, rarely in the colon and in this case, it is more frequently seen in immune-compromised patients. Herpes proctitis is the most common cause of nongonoccal proctitis in homosexual patients.

- **Clinical Symptoms**
  Severe anorectal pain, tenesmus, and discharge are the common symptoms.
- **Macroscopic Features**
  A typical finding is an anorectal ulceration. Ulcers are often multiple and confluent. Perianal vesicles may be seen as well as anorectal erosions and friable mucosa. In herpetic colitis, the most common lesion is an ulceration with a generally hemorrhagic and friable surrounding mucosa.
- **Microscopic Findings**
  Characteristic viral inclusions consisting of a "ground glass" nucleus with peripheral marginated chromatin are seen at the edges of ulcers and in sloughed cells.
- **Prognosis**
  In immune-competent patients, it is a self-limited disease. Immune-compromised patients may be at risk for complications.
- **Useful Test**
  Viral culture is the most helpful test to diagnose the virus, but immune histochemistry may also be useful.
- **Differential Diagnosis**
  The differential diagnosis predominantly includes other viral infection such as CMV and varicella. Morphology and localization of the inclusions may help for the diagnosis. Similarly to CMV, Herpes may superinfect and complicate preexisting IBD.

Adenovirus

Adenovirus infection is the second most frequent cause of self-limited childhood diarrhea.

It may be also seen in immune-compromised patients or transplant patients.

- **Site**
  Anywhere in the colon.
- **Clinical Symptoms**
  Diarrhea, fever, and abdominal pain associated sometimes with ileal or ileocolic intussusception, particularly in children.
- **Macroscopic Features**
  The colonic mucosa is often normal or erythematous and friable.
- **Microscopic Findings**
  The surface epithelial cells show degenerative changes with focal acute inflammation and characteristic smudgy crescent-shaped inclusion or apoptotic crypt epithelial cells.
- **Useful Tests**
  Immunohistochemistry and in situ hybridization can be helpful for diagnosis.

Norovirus

- **Incidence**
  Noroviruses are nowadays the most common cause of acute gastroenteritis in adults and represent the second major cause of severe diarrhea in infants and young children. Norovirus are estimated to become the predominant cause of diarrhea in all age groups worldwide, especially in infants younger than 5 years of age.
- **Epidemiology**
  Feco-oral spread is the primary mode of transmission. The infectious dose (18–1,000) viral particles is low. It can be detected in water or foods (fruit, vegetable, etc.).
- **Age**
  Norovirus disease involves patients of all ages and targets high-risk groups such as young children, elderly travelers, and immune-compromised patients.
- **Site**
  The small intestine is usually involved.

I

- **Clinical Symptoms**
  Vomiting and watery diarrhea are the most common symptoms with an acute onset with fever. The duration of the illness is short (only 2–3 days) but can last longer (particularly in children or immune-compromised persons). Association of norovirus with necrotizing enterocolitis in newborns, as well as exacerbations of IBD has been described.
- **Microscopic Findings**
  Pathologic studies are limited. The colonic mucosa shows most often no histological changes.
- **Differential Diagnosis**
  The differential diagnosis includes other viral infections. Sometimes, it may be difficult to distinguish norovirus infection from graft-versus-host disease (GVHD) since the pathological characteristics of norovirus infections may be similar. Computed tomography may be of help since in norovirus-infected patients, a bowel wall edema is observed, restricted to small intestine which is infrequently seen in patients with GVHD.
- **Prognosis**
  The illness is self-limited and less severe than many other infections but is more severe in children <5 year of age and adults >65 years of age.
- **Useful Tests**
  PCR can help in the diagnosis.

See also ► Viral Gastroenteritis.

Fungal, Protozoal, and Helminthic Infections

Fungal, protozoal, and helminthic infections can more easily be diagnosed especially when the pathogenic agents are seen on histological slides.

The percentage of fungal infections increase in parallel with the number of transplant patient or immune-compromised (AIDS) patients. Clinical symptoms include usually diarrhea, melena, abdominal pain, and fever. Fungal infections, such as histoplasmosis, aspergillosis, cryptococcosis, candidiasis, and mucormycosis, can be diagnosed morphologically. The PAS, Gomori methenamine silver stain, or Warthin starry special stain can help to discover the pathogen. The differential diagnosis includes other types of infectious colitis as well as Crohn's disease, ulcerative colitis, and ischaemic colitis. Culture and immunohistochemistry can be of help for the diagnosis.

The most common protozoal infection in the large bowel in developed countries is amoebiasis. The trophozoites are most numerous at the ulcer edges or in the overlying fibrinous exudates (Fig. 4). They are large, round to ovoid, varying in diameter from 6 to 40 μm, and contain ingested red blood cells (Fig. 5). The nucleus is rounded with a dense nuclear membrane and a clear nucleoplasm. The adjacent mucosa shows a chronic inflammatory infiltrate containing lymphocytes, histiocytes, plasma

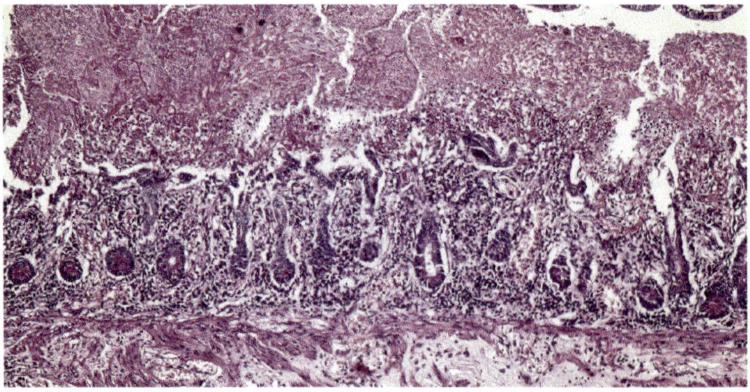

Infectious Colitis, Fig. 4 *Entamoeba histolytica* colitis. The trophozoite are present in the overlying fibrinous exudate of the mucosa

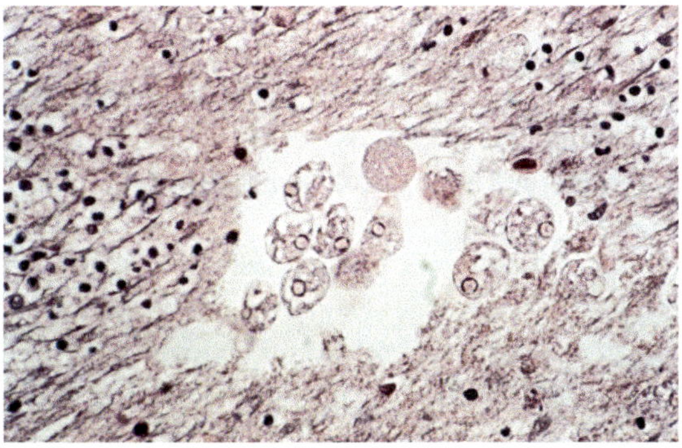

Infectious Colitis, Fig. 5 *Entamoeba histolytica* trophozoites with foamy cytoplasm, round eccentric nucleus and ingested red blood cells

cells, lymphoid follicles, pronounced edema, congestion, few crypt abscesses as well as minimal inflammation and necrosis. Amoebic ulcers usually develop slowly allowing cellular proliferation and fibrosis, thereby, preventing perforation.

References and Further Reading

Bok, K., et al. (2012). Norovirus gastroenteritis in immunocompromised patients. *The New England Journal of Medicine, 367*, 2126–2132.

Jouret-Mourin, A., & Geboes, K. (2002). Infectious colitis. *Acta Endoscopica, 32*, 167–184.

Kumar, N. B., et al. (1982). The histopathologic spectrum of acute self-limited colitis (acute infectious-type colitis). *The American Journal of Surgical Pathology, 6*, 523–529.

Lamps L. W. (2009). In LW Lamps (Ed.), *Surgical pathology of the gastrointestinal system: Bacterial, fungal, viral and parasitic infections*. New York: Springer.

Schumacher, G., et al. (1994). A prospective study of first attacks of IBD and infectious colitis. *Scandinavian Journal of Gastroenterology, 29*, 318–332.

Surawicz, C. M., et al. (1984). Mucosal biopsy diagnosis of colitis; acute self-limited colitis and idiopathic inflammatory bowel disease. *Gastroenterology, 107*, 755–763.

Udayakumar, N., et al. (2011). Infectious colitis. *Current Opinion in Gastroenterology, 27*, 66–71.

Infectious Esophagitis

Paula Borralho Nunes
Hospital Cuf Descobertas and Escola Superior de Tecnologia da Saúde de Lisboa and Instituto de Anatomia Patológica, Faculdade de Medicina da, Universidade de Lisboa, Lisboa, Portugal

Synonyms

Infective esophagitis

Definition

Infectious esophagitis is a relatively uncommon condition as normal esophageal mucosa is remarkably resistant to infection. Invasive esophageal infections can present in association with distinct clinical conditions but occur with few exceptions in immunocompromised patients, specifically those with AIDS, leukemia, lymphoma, and other cancers. Although immunosuppression from any condition or therapy can potentially lead to esophageal infections, the individuals at highest risk for infectious esophagitis are those with HIV infection and low CD4 counts and leukemia or lymphoma (especially during chemotherapy) (Mulhall and Wong 2003).

Some significant risk factors are iatrogenic, with some cases presenting in the context of chemotherapy, broad-spectrum antibiotics, immunomodulators, and high-dose corticosteroid administration. There are though important risk factors other than immunosuppression. The prevention of esophageal pathogen adherence is also an important aspect of host defense, and conditions in which the clearance of organisms is impaired can result in esophageal infection. Impairment in salivation, reduction in physiologic reflux or gastric acid production, injury to esophageal mucosa, alterations of esophageal motility, or defects in esophageal clearance can thus result in infection or colonization of the human esophagus. Patients with hypochlorhydria, progressive systemic sclerosis, or achalasia are consequently at risk. Moreover, when equilibrium amongst commensal organisms is disrupted (as with antibiotic therapy), organisms with pathogenic potential can also result in opportunistic infections. Individuals with conditions like diabetes mellitus, alcoholism, and adrenal insufficiency may also have alterations in their immune system that can increase the risk for infectious esophagitis. Finally, as the population ages, host defense mechanisms weaken, predisposing the elderly patients to infectious esophagitis.

Infectious agents involved depend considerably on the background conditions and exposure and include fungi (primarily *Candida species, Aspergillus, Blastomyces, Cryptococcus, Histoplasma, Coccidioides*), viruses (*herpes simplex* [HSV], *cytomegalovirus* [CMV], *varicella zoster virus* [VZV], *Epstein-Barr virus* [EBV], *human papillomavirus* [HPV], or human immunodeficiency virus [HIV]), bacteria (e.g., *Staphylococcus aureus, Streptococcus epidermidis*, *Bacillus species*, and *Mycobacterium species*), and parasites (*Trypanosoma cruzi, Leishmania species*). The likelihood of a specific infectious agent varies with the clinical situation, but Candida is generally the most common, especially in the modestly immunocompromised individual (Mulhall and Wong 2003). A decreased T-cell helper or suppressor ratio due to an increase in the number of suppressor cells in solid transplant recipients is often associated with CMV esophagitis. In those individuals who are profoundly immunocompromised, the full spectrum of listed agents (and sometimes more than one agent) can be the offending pathogens.

Candida is a commensal organism that is present as flora in the mouth, gastrointestinal tract, and vagina in normal individuals and is easily found in the environment. There are numerous fungal species that are less common inhabitants of the oropharynx and gastrointestinal tract (e.g., *Candida glabrata, Candida krusei, Candida parapsilosis*, and *Candida tropicalis*), but they can be significant pathogens in the right clinical setting. For a fungal infection to take place, host defenses must be overcome, including impairment of the host's ability to clear the pathogenic organism and problems with cellular immunity, which allows fungal invasion. Fungal infections may be (and often are) superimposed to other types of infections.

Viral pathogens can occur as a primary infection or as reactivation of previously latent infection especially in the immunocompromised patient, particularly in the cases of EBV, CMV, and HSV.

Human immunodeficiency virus, though a risk factor for many of the other infections noted earlier, is believed to be a direct pathogen, with HIV itself leading to esophageal ulcerations. Symptoms can be variable but often appear during the viral prodrome of early HIV infection and include severe dysphagia and odynophagia, as well as general symptoms (fever, malaise, weight loss).

Infectious CMV esophagitis can result from either new exposures or reactivation of latent virus. Patients with CMV infection have esophageal symptoms (dysphagia or odynophagia) and usually nonspecific symptoms (nausea and vomiting, abdominal pain, anorexia, and fevers), perhaps owing to frequent systemic or multiorgan involvement.

Esophageal herpes simplexes (human herpesviruses 1 and 2) are early and recurrent causes of morbidity in immunocompromised patients but can also be found in patients with diminished mucosa defenses by other pathologic conditions (i.e., eosinophilic esophagitis). Presumptive diagnosis can be made from cytologic scraping of the lesion or biopsies of the active border.

Bacterial infections of the esophagus can have significant clinical impact. The pathogenesis of bacterial esophagitis often involves previous injury that damaged the integrity of the mucosal barrier. They are more commonly seen in patients undergoing chemotherapy, because granulocytopenia (especially in combination with hypochlorhydria or acid suppression) is the greatest risk factor. Infection is generally polymicrobial, consisting predominately of oral and upper respiratory flora (e.g., *Staphylococcus aureus, Staphylococcus epidermidis,*

Streptococcus viridans, and *Bacillus*). Patients can present with dysphagia, odynophagia, nausea, and chest pain. The clinical course can be progressive and catastrophic, but more often, it is mild and asymptomatic.

Infrequently, esophagus can be involved in systemic infections, with symptomatic esophagitis and the initial diagnosis made on esophageal biopsies. Esophageal tuberculosis usually represents a secondary manifestation of a disseminated disease. Patients present frequently with dysphagia, resulting from compression of enlarged mediastinal lymph nodes. Individuals at risk for developing esophageal tuberculosis include immunocompromised patients as well as people from countries were tuberculosis is still endemic.

Protozoal infection of the esophagus is very rare but has been described. Visceral *leishmaniasis* may rarely involve the *esophagus*. The reported cases have been described in HIV-infected patients.

In a few cases, infectious esophagitis can result in "black esophagus" or acute necrotizing esophagitis (Trappe et al. 2007), a rare entity most often reported in debilitated patients, particularly in postoperative cancer patients, or during severe infections, with ischemia and exposure of the esophageal mucosa to acid playing probably an important role. Several pathogens have been implicated in this condition.

Clinical Features

- **Incidence**
  Infectious esophagitis is clearly uncommon in normal esophageal mucosa. However, because of the increased use of steroids and cytotoxic agents as well as the increase in acquired immunodeficiency syndrome, the incidence of opportunistic infections in the esophagus has increased.

  The prevalence of esophageal infections varies according to the agents involved and to the underlying condition of the patient (i.e., immune status and other pathologic disorders present). For instance, infectious esophagitis has been reported to occur in 46% of patients undergoing upper endoscopy following bone marrow transplantation and in 24% of the patients following orthotopic liver transplantation (Alexander et al. 1988). The individuals at highest risk for infectious esophagitis are those with HIV infection with low CD4 counts. For instance, CMV affects 40% or more of HIV-infected patients with CD4+ T-cell lymphocyte counts less than 100 cells//xL. *Candida albicans* is one of the most frequent causes of infectious esophagitis, especially in patients with AIDS, and is found in approximately 50% of symptomatic individuals (Lewin-Smith et al. 1998).
- **Age**
  The age distribution of infectious esophagitis depends of the underlying predisposing condition.
- **Sex**
  Infectious esophagitis is a very heterogeneous condition with no predilection for gender in general.
- **Site**
  The affected segment of the esophagus will depend mainly of the pathogen and the underlying condition. For instances, with herpetic esophagitis the lesions develop in the middle and distal thirds of the esophagus in about 90% of the cases.
- **Treatment**
  The treatment will vary according to the pathogen involved. General measures include limit use of antibiotics, corticosteroids, and other immunosuppressant as much as possible as well as strive to reduce exposure to pathogens, particularly in immunocompromised patients.

  For patients at risk for fungal esophagitis (especially patients with AIDS) presenting with dysphagia or odynophagia, oral systemic therapy is most appropriate. Initiation of fluconazole is the accepted standard in the United States and Europe; itraconazole is a reasonable alternative, especially in cases that demonstrate fluconazole resistance. For patients with more significant systemic symptoms, granulocytopenia, or an inability to tolerate oral medications, parenteral therapy may be required.

When infection with other pathogens has been excluded and esophageal lesions are consistent with HIV alone, therapy with oral corticosteroids may be warranted. If this therapy fails or other comorbidities dictate, oral dexamethasone, sucralfate, or thalidomide can be tried.

Patients with herpetic esophagitis should be considered for treatment with acyclovir, although results comparable to its use in the treatment of labial HSV have not been documented. However, the use of acyclovir, with its limited side effect profile, appears acceptable in symptomatic individuals. Parenteral acyclovir should be initiated until the patient can be converted to oral therapy (when dysphagia or odynophagia is resolved).

In CMV infection of the esophagus, parenteral therapy with ganciclovir or foscarnet is warranted. Both regimens may require maintenance therapy until immunosuppression resolves or indefinitely. Prophylaxis against CMV infection is accepted practice for those patients undergoing immunosuppression for organ transplantation. It should be considered in the appropriate setting for all individuals who are immunosuppressed and at risk for CMV infection.

For patients with bacterial esophagitis, usually with polymicrobial infections, appropriate therapy must be broad spectrum. If resistant organisms are discovered, these findings should help refine therapy. Otherwise, broad-spectrum monotherapy or combination therapy should be initiated.

- **Outcome**
  Depending on the pathogen involved and the immune status of the patient, this condition can have significant morbidity and mortality, if unrecognized. In severe cases esophagitis can become invasive with necrosis and esophageal perforation, leading to life-threatening sepsis due to mediastinitis, aspiration pneumonia, or pleural contamination. In some cases (i.e., HSV esophagitis), submucosal fibrosis can lead to subsequent esophageal stricture formation.

Macroscopy

The macroscopic aspects of esophageal infection are usually assessed by endoscopy and depend mainly on the pathogen implicated, although in some cases the lesions are nonspecific. In rare circumstances the macroscopic lesions have been described as acute esophageal necrosis or "black esophagus," an uncommon entity defined as a dark pigmentation of the esophagus associated with histologic mucosal necrosis.

Endoscopy favors the diagnosis of candida infection when whitish mucosal plaques are found, especially with underlying esophagitis and mucosal erythema, hyperemia, and friability (generally without ulcerations). In advanced cases the esophagus becomes narrowed, with a cobblestoned appearance. Rarely, fungal esophagitis assumes a polypoid or multinodular shape.

In HIV esophagitis discrete mucosal aphthoid lesions are usually found, but can coalesce and deepen, leaving large areas of ulceration ("giant esophageal ulcers") and predisposing the patient to secondary infection, esophageal bleeding, fistulae, or mucosal perforation.

In esophageal herpes simplex, "punched-out" ulcers are typical, often large and multiple, and frequently recur and persist, particularly in severely immunocompromised patients. Early in the course of herpetic infection, vesicular lesions develop, but vesicles do not last long, and the more common findings are the typical discrete ulcers with white exudates in their bases and erythematous or yellow raised margins. Large areas of denuded mucosa develop in severe disease.

In CMV esophagitis endoscopic lesions are often described as superficial and longitudinal or serpiginous in the mid- to distal esophagus, but they can vary greatly in their appearance. Ulcers can coalesce and diffuse ulceration has been described.

Patients with bacterial esophagitis usually present with ulcerations, discrete plaques, or pseudomembranes in the esophageal mucosa; diffuse mucosal friability is common.

In rare cases of *Leishmania* esophagitis, diffuse erythematous mucosa with extensive shallow and deep linear ulceration and sometimes Candida-like plaques can be seen on endoscopy.

Microscopy

The histologic diagnosis of infectious esophagitis relies mainly on the identification of an agent or of characteristic aspects (particularly with viral esophagitis). The microscopic features depend of the implicated pathogen, although in some cases findings can be nonspecific, mainly when biopsies are superficial or involve only the base of ulcers. The immune status of the patient also influences histologic findings, as in general in immunocompetent patients only a small number of typical lesions are present (e.g., viral inclusions), whereas in immunosuppressed patients these are usually numerous cells presenting diagnostic features. Another characteristic of infectious esophagitis in immunosuppressed individuals is the presence of multiple agents. Fungi and bacteria can coexist with HSV esophagitis, as well as CMV.

Diagnosis of infectious esophagitis related to *Candida* requires that biopsies demonstrate sloughing of epithelial cells with fungal invasion into the epithelium. Mycelia (hyphae), pseudomycelia, and budding yeasts are more characteristic of infection than colonization, and they should be demonstrated histologically to make the diagnosis of candidal infectious esophagitis. The mucosa and lamina propria appears acutely and chronically inflamed with areas of ulceration and granulation tissue in severe cases. When candida becomes pathogenic, it invades the underlying tissues. The yeasts and pseudohyphae (with no true branching) have poor staining with H&E but a strong magenta stain with PAS, sometimes useful, especially in cases with lots of debris and inflammation. Other special stains such as Grocott or silver methenamine (Fig. 1) also highlight the fungal presence.

In HIV esophagitis the esophagus exhibits variable inflammatory infiltrates, erosions, and ulcerations, although in some cases there are only focal edema and rare apoptotic cells. The submucosa usually becomes densely infiltrated with neutrophils, and a few mononuclear cells may extend into the muscularis propria. The ulcers can become quite large.

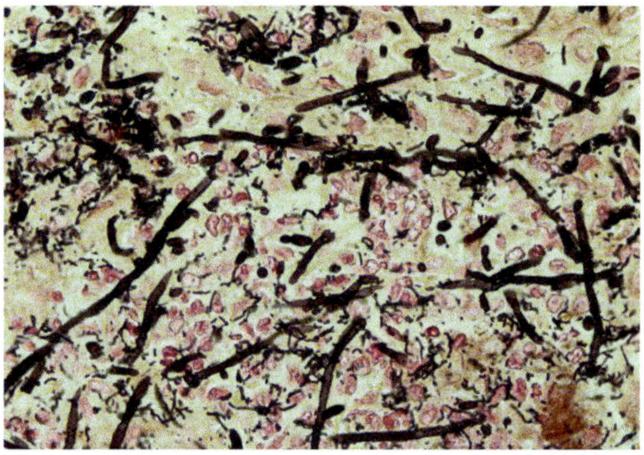

Infectious Esophagitis, Fig. 1 In this high-power Grocott stain, mycelia, pseudomycelia, and budding yeasts can be seen admixed with debris and inflammatory cells

Cytomegalovirus induces cytomegaly, forms inclusions, and exhibits a predilection for growth in endothelial and mesenchymal cells. CMV induces cytopathic effect in glandular cells, fibroblasts, and endothelial cells making particularly important to take biopsies from the base of ulcers to evaluate for this pathogen. Vasculitis with subsequent thrombosis and ischemia accounts for much of the significant pathology. Rarely, CMV may induce pseudotumors composed of granulation tissue and fibrosis with areas of acute and chronic inflammation. The enlarged nucleus of an infected cell possesses an oval ground-glass inclusion with a peripheral halo, the so-called "owl-eye" intranuclear inclusion (Fig. 2). Cytoplasmic inclusions are coarse and granular. Atypical ground-glass inclusions may be present, and the diagnosis can then be confirmed by immunohistochemistry or in situ hybridization. However, macrophage aggregates may be the only clue, and the diagnosis should be confirmed with immunohistochemical stains for antigens at the various stages of infection or viral culture.

On biopsy specimens from patients with herpes simplex esophagitis, there is acantholysis, erosions, vesicles and/or ulcers, as well as a variable degree of acute and chronic inflammation. Herpes simplex virus infects the squamous epithelium and infected cells are often multinucleated with ground-glass or eosinophilic (Cowdry type A)

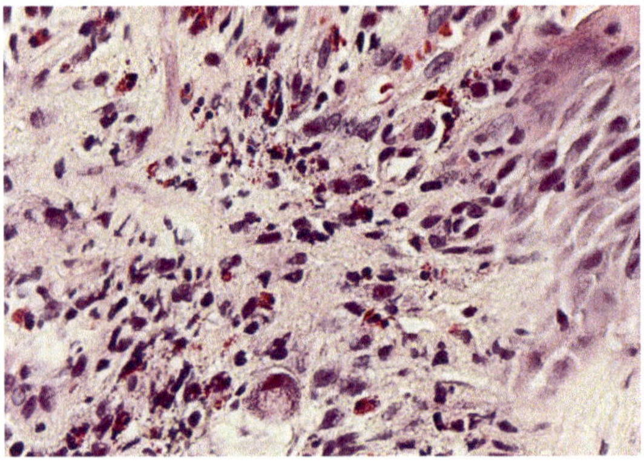

Infectious Esophagitis, Fig. 2 High-power H&E stain of CMV esophagitis. Characteristic cytopathic effect on an infected mesenchymal cell, with enlarged nucleus and oval eosinophilic inclusion

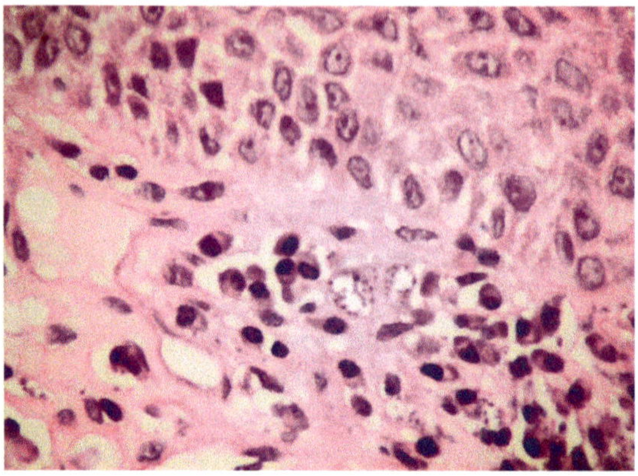

Infectious Esophagitis, Fig. 4 High-power H&E stain. Amastigotes on a biopsy of *Leishmania* esophagitis

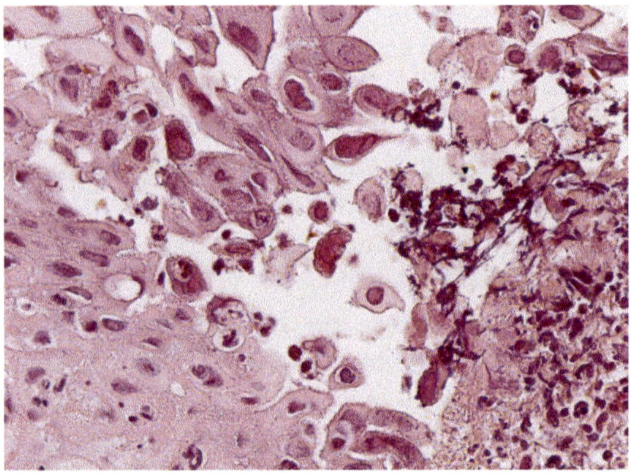

Infectious Esophagitis, Fig. 3 High-power H&E stain of herpes simplex esophagitis. Biopsies taken from herpetic ulcers reveal presence of squamous infected cells, often multinucleated with ground-glass (Cowdry type A) intranuclear inclusions as well as inflammatory infiltrates, necrosis, and granulation tissue

intranuclear inclusions (Fig. 3). Biopsies taken from the base of herpetic ulcers only reveal presence of nonspecific inflammatory infiltrates, necrosis, and granulation tissue. The histologic features are not specific for herpes simplex virus but also develop in patients with herpes zoster infection. If necessary, viral culture, in situ hybridization, or immunohistochemistry can be used to differentiate herpes simplex from zoster.

Diagnosis of bacterial esophagitis requires biopsies that show numerous bacteria on Gram's stain, with histologic evidence of bacterial invasion into the subepithelium without concomitant fungal or viral disease. Bacterial infections can produce a diffuse necrotizing process characterized by the presence of a dense neutrophilic exudate, necrosis, and cellular degeneration. Cultures of biopsies may not be informative given the high likelihood of growing non-pathologic bacteria as well, but they may help detect patterns of antibiotic resistance.

The histologic features of tuberculosis resemble those seen elsewhere in the gastrointestinal tract, with the presence of caseating granulomas containing epithelioid histiocytes, giant cells, and acid-fast bacilli.

Diagnosis of *Leishmania* depends on the identification of amastigotes on the biopsy of the esophageal ulcers, usually in macrophages in the submucosa (Fig. 4).

Immunophenotype

Ancillary techniques, such as immunohistochemistry or in situ hybridization, can be particularly valuable to confirm suspected viral esophagitis. Especially when CMV inclusions (Fig. 5) or HSV are atypical, immunohistochemistry is useful and usually reveals the presence of many positive cells that would not have been predicted by the examination of H&E stained slides only.

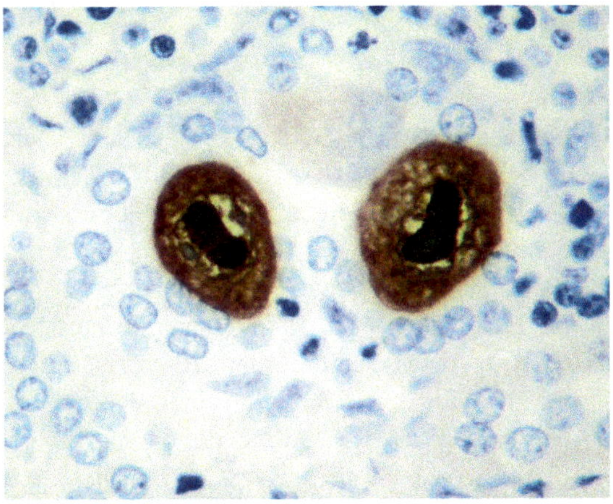

Infectious Esophagitis, Fig. 5 Immunohistochemistry can be useful in some cases of viral esophagitis, as shown in this high-power picture of an esophageal biopsy stained with CMV antibody

In HIV esophagitis, biopsies may demonstrate HIV viral particles and genomic sequences (Lewin-Smith et al. 1998).

Molecular Features

There are no significant molecular aspects concerning infectious esophagitis.

Differential Diagnosis

The differential diagnosis of infectious esophagitis includes reflux esophagitis, inflammation caused by lodging of medicinal agents ("pill" esophagitis), and esophagitis after the ingestion of corrosive agents. The correct diagnosis relies on correct clinical information, on endoscopic data, and on the identification of a causative agent.

References and Further Reading

Alexander, J. A., Brouillette, D. E., & Chien, M. C. (1988). Infectious esophagitis following liver and renal transplantation. *Digestive Diseases and Sciences, 33*(9), 1121–1126.

Fenoglio-Preiser, C. M., Noffsinger, A. E., Stemmermann, G. N., & Lantz, P. E. (1999). The Nonneoplastic esophagus. In *Gastrointestinal pathology: An atlas and text* (2nd ed., pp. 31–91). Philadelphia: Lippincott-Raven.

Lewin-Smith, M. R., Klassen, M. K., Frankel, S. S., et al. (1998). Pathology of human immunodeficiency virus infection: Infectious conditions. *Annals of Diagnostic Pathology, 2*(3), 181–194.

Mulhall, B. P., & Wong, R. K. H. (2003). Infectious esophagitis. *Current Treatment Options in Gastroenterology, 6*(1), 55–70.

Trappe, R., Pohl, H., Forberger, A., et al. (2007). Transpl Acute esophageal necrosis (black esophagus) in the renal transplant recipient: Manifestation of primary cytomegalovirus infection. *Infectious Diseases, 9*(1), 42–45.

Inflammatory Bowel Disease

Karel Geboes
Department of Pathology, N. Goormaghtig Institute, University Gent, Gent, Belgium
Department of Pathology, KU Leuven, Leuven, Belgium

Synonyms

Chronic idiopathic inflammatory bowel diseases; IBD

Definition

Inflammatory bowel diseases (IBD) is a group of chronic idiopathic inflammatory conditions that affect mainly the small intestine and the colon. The two major types are ulcerative colitis (UC) and Crohn's disease (CD). There is a genetic predisposition for IBD, and patients with this condition are more prone to the development of malignancy. Further types to be considered are indeterminate colitis (IC) and inflammatory bowel disease unclassified (IBDU). These are essentially "temporary diagnoses" when the difference between UC and CD cannot be established definitely at the time of presentation. IC should be used when examination of surgical samples is available together with clinical, serological, and imaging data, while IBDU is used for patients from whom only endoscopic biopsy samples are available. Many of the patients classified as "Indeterminate Colitis" present clinically with severe disease. Other chronic inflammatory conditions that are however not always classified as IBD are collagenous colitis, lymphocytic colitis, and variants together often called "microscopic colitis" and diversion colitis.

CD and UC must be considered in the differential diagnosis of clinically acute colitis because of differences in treatment strategies between infections and IBD. The differential diagnosis is particularly important when the complaints are persisting, when the diarrhea is excessive, when the patient is severely ill and in patients presenting with chronic bloody diarrhea with three or more loose stools for more than 30 days (persistent diarrhea; children more than 14 days). Disease severity at its onset, disease extent, and patient age at the time of diagnosis, along with other patient variables, determine overall disease severity and the likelihood of subsequent morbidity and mortality. Once established, IBD patients suffer episodic acute attacks that become superimposed on chronic disease. As a result, the patient is likely to suffer from potentially disabling disease for decades.

Since the large intestine is frequently involved and since it is accessible for biopsy, the colon is a major source of tissue for diagnosis of IBD and other forms of colitis. The differential diagnosis between IBD and infectious colitis and other types of colitis may be difficult: in patients coming from tropical or subtropical countries where infections are more likely. A diagnosis of IBD must be made cautiously, whenever more than one person has been acutely ill at the same moment. In such a situation, food poisoning has to be considered.

Despite years of intensive research, the etiologies of CD and UC are unknown. The current understanding of the pathogenesis of IBD implies a dysfunction of the interplay between genetic factors, environmental factors (the inciting agent may be environmental such as a bacterial infection), and the immune system.

Clinical Features

- **Incidence**

  Neither UC nor CD is a new disease. There were case series of patients with ulcerative colitis published already during the nineteenth century and a patient presented by Lesniowski in Poland (1904) and a series published by Kenneth Dalziel in 1913 constitute cases of Crohn's disease more than 20 years before Dr. Burrill B. Crohn's original description. UC and CD afflict individuals in many parts of the world. Studies assessing the incidence show an increase in both diseases after the Second World War, especially in the United States, Great Britain, and Scandinavia. They also show a strong correlation in the occurrence of UC and CD. Areas or populations with a high incidence attributable to UC also have a high incidence due to CD and vice versa. There is also a strikingly consistent pattern with regard to temporal trends for both diseases. An increasing incidence of UC generally precedes an increase in CD with a time lag of approximately 15–20 years. In most instances, the incidence figures of UC are higher than for CD. In the case of CD, the incidence seems to level off around 6.0 per 100,000. For UC, the incidence is approximately 15–20 per 100,000 although higher figures have been reported. The increase has involved all age groups except early childhood (<11 years) and old age (>80 years). A global north–south variation in the incidence of IBD has also been documented. Standardized incidence rates of 10.9–12.8 for ulcerative colitis and 6.0–7.0 for Crohn's disease have been reported from northern California and Scandinavia. Rates of 2.0–6.3 for ulcerative colitis and 0.9–3.1 for Crohn's disease have been observed in the southern hemisphere. The results from a major study in Europe, including 20 different centers in the early 1990s to test this hypothesis, suggest however, that the north–south gradient could be more a historic phenomenon.

  In surgical series, the percentage of cases difficult to classify ranges between 10%

and 16%. Accordingly, these patients are classified as IC. In newly diagnosed patients, analysis of multiple endoscopic biopsies of colon and ileum allows a correct diagnosis and classification in 66–75%. The addition of endoscopic and clinical data allows a final diagnosis in approximately 90% of the cases. In children, 4–23% of new-onset cases present with an equivocal diagnosis. Patients with uncertain diagnosis are classified as IBDU.

Epidemiologic studies show that "microscopic colitis" is almost as common as classic IBD. It may be diagnosed in 10% of patients investigated for chronic non-bloody diarrhea. Incidence rates of 2.6/100,000–10.8/100,000 inhabitants have been reported for collagenous colitis and 2.2 –14 per 100,000 inhabitants for lymphocytic colitis.

- **Age**
  From a population-based cohort from Copenhagen county, it appears that approximately 7% of the patients diagnosed with ulcerative colitis and 6% of the patients with Crohn's disease had an onset before 15 years of age. The median age at diagnosis was 12 years, indicating a steep increase in incidence around puberty. During the 26 years of the study, the mean incidence of IBD in children remained low at 2.2 per 10^5. Ulcerative colitis occurs in all ages, but the major peak is in the 15–25 age range, but some suggest a second smaller peak in the 1960s. It is extremely uncommon above age 75. IBDU is more prevalent in younger age (<12 years).

  Microscopic colitis is mainly observed at older age, being diagnosed in approximately 20% of patients older than 70 years presenting with non-bloody diarrhea. It is a rare phenomenon in childhood.
- **Sex**
  The sexes are affected approximately evenly, although there may be a female predominance for Crohn's disease with female-to male ratios being 1.3–1.89 to 1.0. In Japan, however, the male predominance for Crohn's disease is generally accepted. The incidence is 0.51 per 100,000 (male : 0.71; female : 0.32). The situation is reversed for ulcerative colitis (Binder 2004).

  Microscopic colitis typically affects elderly woman. The female predominance is less pronounced for lymphocytic colitis.
- **Site**
  Crohn's disease can affect the whole gastrointestinal tract although the terminal ileum and right colon are the sites most frequently involved. The stomach and esophagus can also show typical features. Ulcerative colitis is limited to the colon. In patients with pancolitis, the terminal ileum may be affected in continuity. Indeterminate colitis and IBDU are equally limited to the colon, because involvement of the colon would orient toward CD. In patients with IC or IBDU, involvement of the stomach can also be an argument for a definite diagnosis of CD, although even in UC, gastric inflammation can be present, especially in young children. Collagenous colitis and lymphocytic colitis primarily involve the colon, although in a minority of patients, the terminal ileum may be involved too.

  A large percentage of IBD patients suffer from one or more extraintestinal complications such as musculoskeletal complications and hepatobiliary disorders at some time during the course of their disease. In CD, up to 30% of patients are affected. These complications affect many organ systems and may be of little clinical consequence, or they may be severe and be critical determinants in directing therapy.
- **Treatment**
  The goal of medical treatment in IBD is to reduce the inflammation and by doing so induce symptom relief and eventually long-term remission. Anti-inflammatory treatment consists of aminosalicylates, topical or systemic corticosteroids, and immune system suppressors, including biologicals. Antibiotics can be used for complications. Other medications such as antidiarrheals and pain relievers can help for symptoms. If medical treatment, diet, and life style changes are insufficient, surgery may be indicated. Microscopic colitis can by treated with topical steroids.

- **Outcome**
  The typical course of IBD includes periods of remission interspersed with flare-ups. The course of CD is more variable The annual colectomy rate after the first year is 1% for all persons with UC. Surgery for UC generally is performed for the complications such as strictures and fistulas. Microscopic colitis is usually a more benign disease although surgery was needed in occasional cases.

Macroscopy

UC is a colonic disease. It starts from the rectum, spreading proximally and in continuity and involving a variable length of the colon (Fig. 1). It is characteristically a left-sided disease. CD is more frequently a right-sided disease. The terminal ileum and proximal colon are the commonest sites involved, followed by the anorectum and colon. Perianal disease is common. In IC, one finds extensive ulcerations, involvement of transverse and right colon, with usually diffuse disease (less severe in the distal colon). In microscopic colitis, classically, the endoscopic pattern is normal.

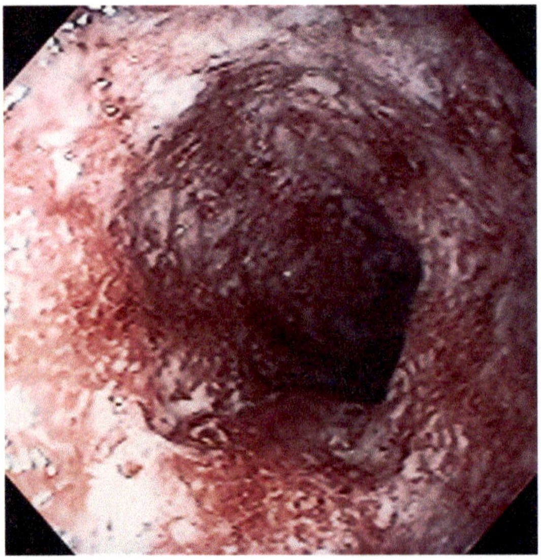

Inflammatory Bowel Disease, Fig. 1 Endoscopic picture of ulcerative colitis showing diffuse mucosal disease

Microscopy

The mucosal lesions of IBD consist of epithelial alterations and a cellular inflammatory response. The former includes cytological and architectural changes, indicative of damage and repair. Structural changes in the colon include the presence of an irregular surface, sometimes called pseudovillous or villiform surface and a disturbed crypt architecture. Crypt distortion (abnormalities in shape) includes shortened crypts that become widely separated from the underlying muscularis mucosae, crypt drop-out, and especially prominent crypt budding (branching crypts, bifid crypts) (Fig. 2). Mucosal atrophy (synonym: crypt atrophy) is a combination of crypt drop-out and shortening of crypts. Several other features may help to establish a diagnosis of IBD. These include mucosal ulcerations and erosions, mucin depletion, Paneth cell metaplasia, and alterations of the muscularis mucosae. The cellular inflammatory response consists of changes in density of the infiltrate, alterations in composition, and changes in the distribution pattern. Accumulation of plasma cells near the mucosal base or in between the crypt base and the muscularis mucosae (basal plasmacytosis) is a common and early feature.

The pathological diagnosis of IC on resected specimens relies on the presence of "overlapping features" or the absence of a "clear diagnostic

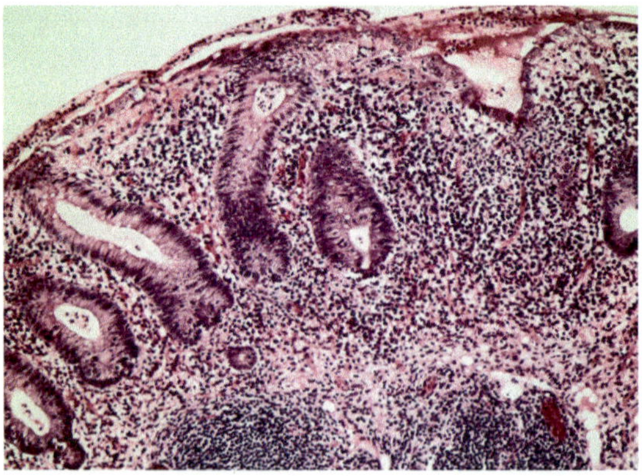

Inflammatory Bowel Disease, Fig. 2 Microphotograph of mildly active ulcerative colitis showing disturbed crypt architecture (shortened crypts) and basal location of cellular infiltrate

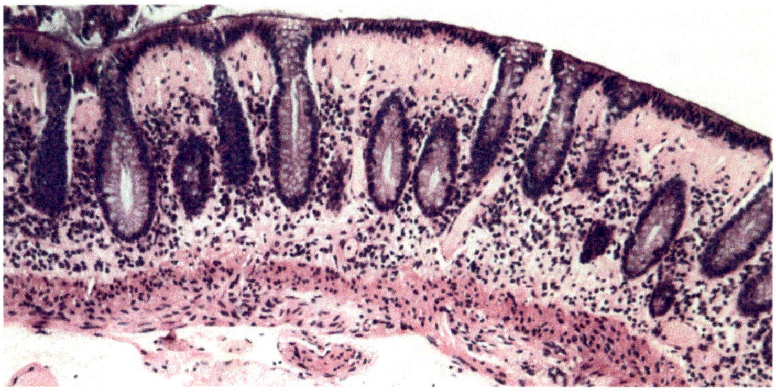

Inflammatory Bowel Disease, Fig. 3 Microphotograph of a biopsy from a patient with collagenous colitis showing the irregular thickening of the subepithelial collagen band

pattern." It is not a real "positive" diagnosis. IC usually is characterized by extensive ulceration with a sharp transition to normal adjacent mucosa and multiple V-shaped ulcers lacking surrounding inflammation. Overlapping features between UC and CD are "severe mucosal and wall involvement," including none aggregated transmural inflammation, fissures reaching the muscularis propria, and a discontinuous pattern. No clear histological features have been reported for a positive diagnosis of IBDU on endoscopic biopsies.

The diagnosis of collagenous colitis on routinely hematoxylin and eosin stained sections is based on the presence of a thick amorphous hyaline eosinophilic band immediately beneath the superficial epithelium of the mucosa (Fig. 3). This layer has an irregular, jagged aspect of the lower edge. The thickness is >10 μm. Its presence is associated with inflammation. The diagnosis of lymphocytic colitis is based upon a diffuse increase of intraepithelial lymphocytes (IELs) (>20 IELs per 100 epithelial cells) in the superficial epithelium without associated thickening of the subepithelial collagen accompanied by an increase of lamina propria inflammatory cells.

Immunophenotype

In animal models, inflammation generally occurs as a result of T lymphocytes. $CD4^{+}$ T helper (H) cells regulate critical aspects of the acquired immune response. They have been classified as either TH1 or TH2 on the basis of function and according to their ability to elaborate specific cytokines. TH1 cells orchestrate cell-mediated immune responses and are characterized by the ability to secrete interleukin (IL)-2, IL-12, and interferon-γ (IFN-γ). TH2 cells, in contrast, mediate humoral responses and secrete IL-4, IL-5, IL-6, IL-10, and IL-13. This dichotomy between TH-1 and TH-2-like mucosal inflammation is partly seen in human IBD in that the histopathological features of UC resemble those of experimental TH-2 cell-mediated colitis while CD would be more a TH-1 response. Cytokine patterns in these diseases are in accordance with these distinct mechanisms although the cytokine pattern in UC is less clear. It does not fit entirely into the TH1/TH2 dichotomy but more closely resembles, at least in established disease, a modified TH2 response. The immune response may also change during the course of the disease.

Molecular Features

Classifying IBD patients is important for decisions on the intensity of follow-up and therapy. The most recent classification Montreal classification is based on clinical grounds: for CD, the age at diagnosis and disease location and behavior and for UC, the age at diagnosis and the extent of disease. A molecular reclassification using serology and/or genetic markers is still premature, but might in the future become important for disease stratification, the

I

prediction of prognosis at the time of diagnosis, and the prediction of therapy outcome.

Differential Diagnosis

IBD must be differentiated from acute usually infectious colitis. In addition, there are several chronic conditions which can mimic IBD. These include chronic infections such as intestinal tuberculosis due to Mycobacterium tuberculosis or unusual types of mycobacteria and amoebic colitis which can mimic both UC and CD, some drug-related types of colitis such as NSAIDs induced colitis, diverticular-disease associated colitis, intestinal endometriosis which can mimic CD or be associated with CD, the solitary rectal ulcer syndrome.

References and Further Reading

Binder, V. (2004). Epidemiology of IBD during the twentieth century: An integrated view. *Best Practice & Research Clinical Gastroenterology, 18*, 463–479.
Geboes, K., Colombel, J. F., Greenstein, A., Jewell, D., Sandborn, W., Vatn, M., Warren, B., & Riddell, R. H. (2008). Indeterminate colitis: A review of the concept – What's in a name? *Inflammatory Bowel Diseases, 14*, 860–867.
Jenkins, D., Balsitis, M., Gallivan, S., Dixon, M. F., Gilmour, H. M., Shepherd, N. A., Theodossi, A., & Williams, G. T. (1997). Guidelines for the initial biopsy diagnosis of suspected chronic idiopathic inflammatory bowel disease. The British Society of Gastroenterology Initiative. *Journal of Clinical Pathology, 50*, 93–105.
Münch, A., Aust, D., Bohr, J., Bonderup, O., Fernandez Banares, F., Hjortswang, H., Madisch, A., Munck, L. K., Ström, M., Tysk, C., & Miehlke, S. (2012). Microscopic colitis: Current status, present and futures challenges. *Journal of Crohn's and Colitis, 8*, 932–945.
Silverberg, M., Satsangi, J., Ahmad, T., Arnott, I. D. R., Bernstein, C. N., Brant, S. R., Caprilli, R., Colombel, J. F., Gasche, C., Geboes, K., Jewell, D., Karban, A., Loftus, E. V., Pena, A. S., Riddell, R. H., Sachar, D. B., Schreiber, S., Steinhart, A. H., Targan, S. R., Vermeire, S., & Warren, B. F. (2005). Toward an integrated clinical, molecular and serological classification of inflammatory bowel disease: Report of a working party of the 2005 Montreal World congress of Gastroenterology. *Canadian Journal of Gastroenterology, 19*(Suppl A), 5–36.
Vermeire, S. (2012). Towards a novel molecular classification of IBD. *Digestive Diseases, 30*, 425–427.

Inflammatory Cloacogenic Polyp

Chatelain Denis[1] and Jean-François Fléjou[2]
[1]Service d'Anatomie Pathologique, Centre Hospitalier et Universitaire du Nord, Amiens, France
[2]Faculté de Médecine Pierre et Marie Curie, Service d'Anatomie et Cytologie Pathologiques, Hôpital Saint-Antoine, Paris, France

Synonyms

Polypoid variant of solitary rectal ulcer

Definition

The inflammatory cloacogenic polyp is a benign polypoid lesion of the anal transitional zone (ATZ). It is included into the mucosal prolapse syndrome with other conditions, with which it shares some histological and pathogenic features, such as the solitary rectal ulcer, the colitis cystic profunda, the inflammatory myoglandular polyp, and the cap polyp and polyposis.

Cloacogenic polyp is considered as a result of nonspecific regenerative changes of the anorectal mucosa caused by recurrent prolapse, or mucosal injury. It could result from mucosal ischemia and regenerative changes secondary to anal mucosal prolapse, caused by constipation, chronic disorders of defecation, and inappropriate puborectalis muscle contractions. The same type of changes can also be seen in other situations with mucosal prolapse, such as colonic intussusceptions, prolapsed colostomies, prolapsed hemorrhoids, prolapsing polyps in association with diverticular disease, and altered colonic mucosa adjacent to tumors.

Inflammatory cloacogenic polyp is discovered in patients presenting with various clinical symptoms. Rectal bleeding is the most common symptom, but patients can complain of tenesmus, mucoid stools, sensation of incomplete evacuation, and mucosal prolapse during defecation and constipation. It can be fortuitously discovered during rectoscopy performed for other conditions. Digital rectal examination can show a palpable polyp at the level of the dentate line.

Clinical Features

- **Incidence**
  The frequency of this rare entity is difficult to assess, but its prevalence could be similar to that of solitary rectal ulcer, 1 in 10,000 persons per year.
- **Age**
  Inflammatory cloacogenic polyp is reported in children and in elderly patients, but it predominantly affects adults aged between 30 and 50 years.
- **Sex**
  Inflammatory cloacogenic polyp is diagnosed equally in males and females.
- **Site**
  Inflammatory cloacogenic polyp is typically located in the transitional mucosal zone of the anal canal, the so-called ATZ for anal transitional zone.
- **Treatment**
  Treatment of inflammatory cloacogenic polyp consists of excision of the polyp by mucosectomy or endoscopic polypectomy.

  If present, constipation and anorectal mucosal prolapse can be treated by conservative therapy, with high-fiber diet and laxative medication. Surgical treatment is reserved for recurrent prolapse that does not respond to medical treatment, and includes submucosal injection of sclerosing agents, Thiersch cerclage, transanal excision of prolapsing anterior rectal mucosa, perineal rectopexy with or without sigmoid resection. Patients with inappropriate contraction of the puborectalis muscle can be offered biofeedback.
- **Outcome**
  The natural history of inflammatory cloacogenic polyp is uncertain, but it does not seem to recur after polypectomy. Inflammatory cloacogenic polyp is a non-neoplastic condition, but anal intraepithelial neoplasia and in situ squamous cell carcinoma have been described, fortuitously discovered in an inflammatory cloacogenic polyp. There are very rare cases of rectal adenocarcinoma occurring in prolapsed anorectal mucosa and fortuitously associated with an inflammatory cloacogenic polyp.

Macroscopy

Inflammatory cloacogenic polyp usually consists of a pale, friable, sometimes villiform polyp at the anal transitional zone. It has a smooth surface devoid of coarse lobulation and irregular nodularity, which are common features in dysplastic rectal adenomas. It can have a red color due to hyperemia or congestion and can be ulcerated.

I

Microscopy

Inflammatory cloacogenic polyp has a tubulovillous pattern of growth (Fig. 1). The surface epithelium consists of squamous, columnar (lined with enterocytes and goblet cells), or transitional epithelium, and may be ulcerated. Cytologically, the epithelium is usually normal but can show regenerative atypia with increased mitoses, nuclear pseudostratification, and a varying amount of goblet cell depletion. The crypts are elongated and hyperplastic and can show serrated

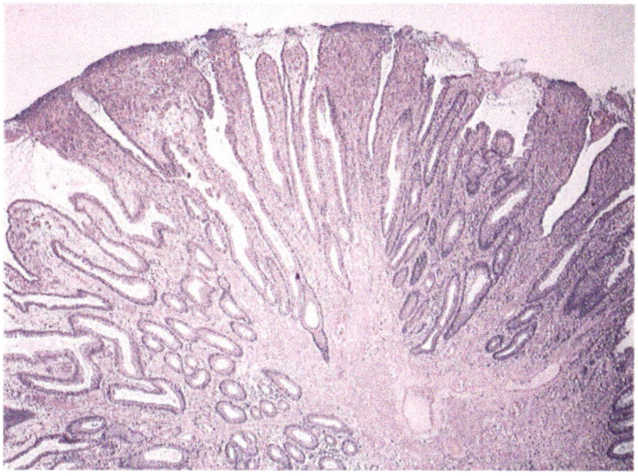

Inflammatory Cloacogenic Polyp, Fig. 1 Villous pattern of cloacogenic polyp with inflammation and regeneration

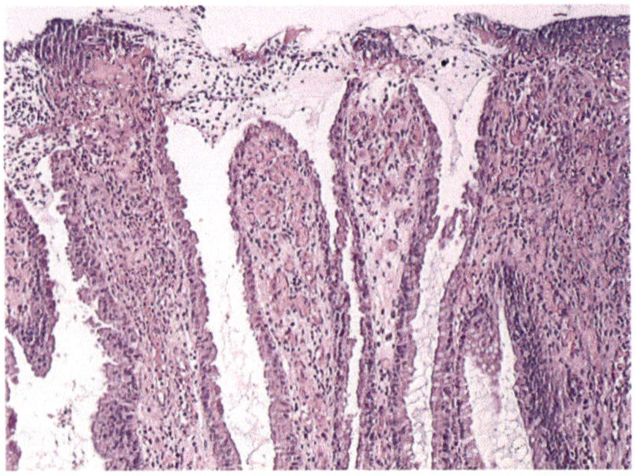

Inflammatory Cloacogenic Polyp, Fig. 2 Surface erosion in the upper part of cloacogenic polyp, with dilated capillaries in the lamina propria

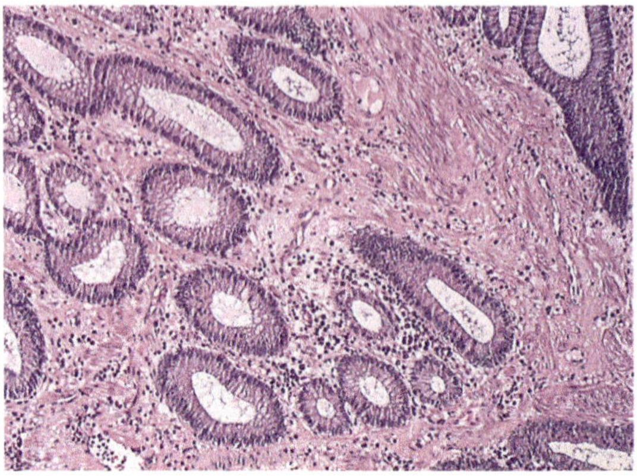

Inflammatory Cloacogenic Polyp, Fig. 3 Distorted groups of glands, some of which are diamond-shaped, and fibromuscular obliteration of the lamina propria

changes, and distortion with branching and shortening. There may be displaced groups of crypts into the submucosa, with dilated angular "diamond-shaped" crypts.

The lamina propria is edematous and shows an increased number of fibroblasts and chronic inflammatory infiltrate, with sometimes deposition of excess collagen and elastin. There is often an increase of dilated capillaries beneath the surface epithelium, with hemorrhage and hemosiderin deposition (Fig. 2). The muscularis mucosa is disorganized, thickened, and hyperplastic with upward extension of smooth muscle fibers into the lamina propria, between the crypts, resulting in characteristic fibromuscular obliteration of the lamina propria with disorientation of muscle fibers (Fig. 3).

Immunophenotype

The diagnosis of inflammatory cloacogenic polyp is performed on microscopic examination of H&E stains, and there is no need of immunohistochemical stains for the diagnosis or to exclude differential diagnoses.

Molecular Features

No specific genetic abnormalities have been described in inflammatory cloacogenic polyps.

Differential Diagnosis

Macroscopically, inflammatory cloacogenic polyp may mimic anorectal carcinoma or adenoma.

On microscopic examination, the tubulovillous architecture of the inflammatory cloacogenic polyp, with regenerative epithelial atypia, may sometimes cause diagnostic difficulties. It may mimic a villous adenoma, but dysplasia with crowded glands, lined by cylindrical basophilic cells with pseudostratified nuclei and increased mitotic activity, is absent in inflammatory cloacogenic polyp. Serrated architectural changes of crypts may mimic a sessile serrated adenoma or traditional serrated adenoma, but in inflammatory cloacogenic polyp, the glands are not typically dilated at the base with an L or T appearance, and there are numerous muscle fibers elongating from the muscularis mucosae between the crypts. The presence of misplaced glands with or without mucus lakes, within the submucosa (proctitis cystic profunda), may simulate mucinous adenocarcinoma, but the absence of carcinomatous cells in the mucus lakes, often surrounded by fibro-inflammatory changes, and the typical appearance on the surface of the lesion are key features for the differential diagnosis.

References and Further Reading

Du Boulay, C. E., Fairbrother, J., & Isaacson, P. G. (1983). Mucosal prolapse syndrome – A unifying concept for solitary ulcer syndrome and related disorders. *Journal of Clinical Pathology, 36*, 1264–1268.

Hanson, I. M., & Armstrong, G. R. (1999). Anal intraepithelial neoplasia in an inflammatory cloacogenic polyp. *Journal of Clinical Pathology, 52*, 393–594.

Lobert, P. F., & Appelman, H. D. (1981). Inflammatory cloacogenic polyp. A unique inflammatory lesion of the anal transitional zone. *The American Journal of Surgical Pathology, 5*, 761–766.

Saul, S. H. (1987). Inflammatory cloacogenic polyp: Relationship to solitary rectal ulcer syndrome/mucosal prolapse and other bowel disorders. *Human Pathology, 18*, 1120–1125.

Singh, B., Mortensen, N. J., & Warren, B. F. (2007). Histopathological mimicry in mucosal prolapse. *Histopathology, 50*, 97–102.

Inflammatory Fibroid Polyp, Lower Gastrointestinal Tract

Berna Savaş
Department of Pathology, Ankara University Medical School, Ankara, Turkey

Synonyms

Eosinophilic submucosal granuloma; Vanek's tumor

Definition

Inflammatory fibroid polyp (IFP) is a rare mesenchymal lesion of the gastrointestinal tract first described by Vanek in 1949. In 1953, Helwig and Ranier proposed the term "inflammatory fibroid polyp," which is generally accepted at present. IFPs are most commonly found in the stomach but can occur throughout the GI tract and in one series were more prevalent in the small bowel. IFPs have been reported in different sites, such as the esophagus, duodenum, and ileoanal pouch, but they occur relatively rare in colorectum.

Presenting symptoms can vary and may include abdominal pain, weight loss, and symptoms of GI obstruction or intussusception. IFP may also present as an incidental finding on routine endoscopic examination. IFPs may be associated with concurrent neoplastic (carcinoma, adenomatous polyps) and non-neoplastic (usually inflammatory) lesions of the GI tract.

Clinical Features

- **Incidence**
  IFPs are very rare tumors. The exact incidence of lower GI tract IFPs is not known. In a review of 76 cases, Johnstone and Morson found a relative incidence of 75% gastric, 18% small intestinal, 7% colonic, and 1% esophageal.
- **Age**
  IFPs occur mostly in adults but can occur in the pediatric cases, with a wide age range (2–90 years). The peak incidence is between fifth and sixth decades.
- **Sex**
  Though there is no significant sex predilection, in two reviews, a slight male predominance has been noted.
- **Site**
  In the lower GI tract, the most common reported site is the small intestine (10.5%), while 0.5% of the cases were in the colon. In the colon, most of the lesions tend to be found in the right colon.
- **Treatment**
  Local excision is usually curative. For larger lesions or in case of GI obstruction and intussusception, surgical excision can be applied.
- **Outcome**
  IFP is a benign lesion that does not metastasize and rarely recurs.

Macroscopy

IFPs represent as sessile or polypoid, solitary or multiple masses ranging in size from <1 to

7.5 cm. IFPs originate from submucosa where they appear as circumscribed oval-to round nodules of firm, gray-tan connective tissue that protrude into the intestinal lumen. In the majority of cases, the overlying mucosa is either eroded or ulcerated.

Microscopy

Colonic and small intestinal IFPs have similar appearance. IFPs are submucosal tumors, but they can infiltrate into the overlying mucosa and the muscularis propria or serosa. Histologically, it is distinguished as a localized proliferation of spindle, stellate, and cytologicaly bland cells centered in the submucosa accompanied by an inflammatory reaction predominantly composed of eosinophils and lymphocytes, with lymphatic vessels, capillaries, and vascular channels in an edematous or myxoid stroma (Figs. 1–3). The vascular network ranges from capillaries to larger vessels, which may be occluded. Stromal cells tend to be arranged in an onion skin pattern around the vessels and crypts. Mitotic figures are rare but may occasionally be found in the deeper parts of the lesion. Atypical mitoses are never found. Larger lesions may have collagen deposition and smooth muscle proliferation in the mucosa.

Immunophenotype

Stromal cells of IFP positively stained with vimetin, CD34, fascin, CD35, cyclin D1, and calponin. Smooth muscle actin positivity can be found in a small portion of polyps. IFP is negative for CD117 (ckit) and DOG1.

Molecular Features

Most investigators considered this lesion to be of non-neoplastic, benign, and reactive origin. However, recently, mutations in platelet-derived

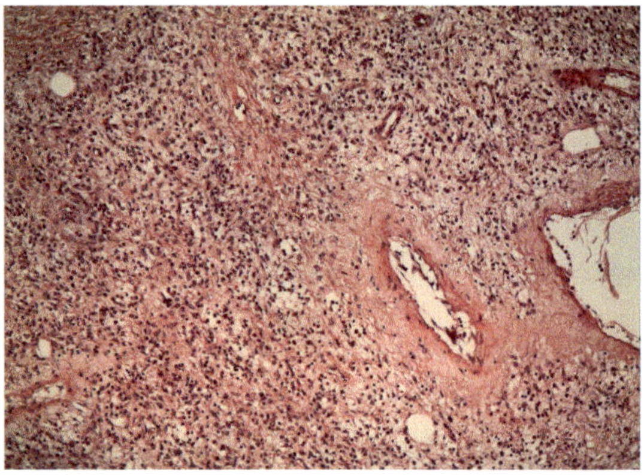

Inflammatory Fibroid Polyp, Lower Gastrointestinal Tract, Fig. 2 Tumor is composed of bland mesenchymal cells with prominent inflammatory cells and blood vessels (H&E, ×100)

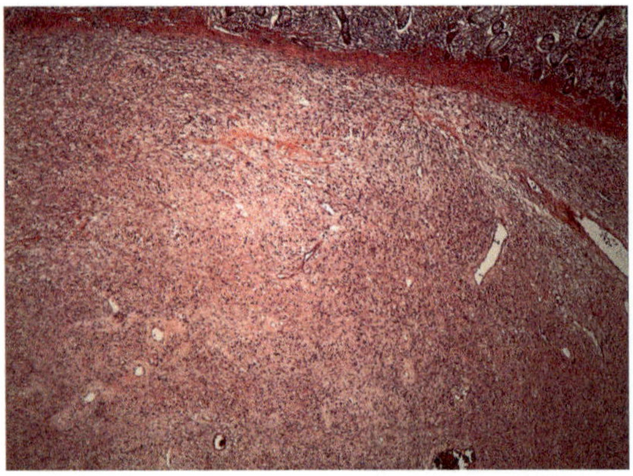

Inflammatory Fibroid Polyp, Lower Gastrointestinal Tract, Fig. 1 Submucosal polypoid tumor in ileum (H&E, ×40)

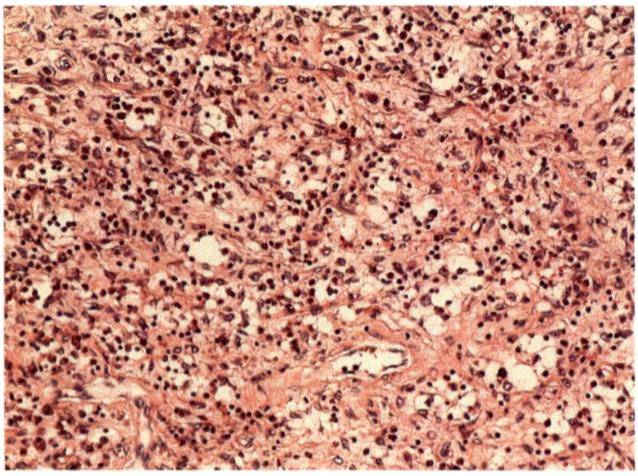

Inflammatory Fibroid Polyp, Lower Gastrointestinal Tract, Fig. 3 Prominent eosinophil and lymphocyte infiltration (H&E, ×400)

growth factor receptor alpha (PDGFRA) were reported in IFPs of the stomach and small intestine, raising suspicion of a possible neoplastic origin and relationship between PDGFRA-mutated gastrointestinal stromal tumors (GISTs) and IFPs.

Differential Diagnosis

It is important to distinguish eosinophilic gastroenteritis, especially its localized forms. Eosinophilic gastroenteritis affects mostly younger people with a personal and family history of allergic disorders, peripheral blood eosinophilia, and tends to be multifocal. Primary and metastatic polypoid mesenychmal lesions of lower GI tract should be considered in the differential diagnosis of IFPs. Accordingly, an important differential diagnostic consideration may represent ▶ gastrointestinal stromal tumor (GIST). GIST tends to be more cellular, composed of spindle and/or epithelioid cells showing positivity with the antibody against KIT protein. Hemangioendothelioma and hemangiopericytoma are rare tumors should be considered in the differential diagnosis of IFP. Both of the tumors consist of oval-to-spindle cells showing factor VIII-related antigen and factor XIIIa positivity, respectively, as well as lack of stoma with prominent inflammatory cells. Inflammatory myofibroblastic tumor which generally affects younger patients, and lacks prominent infiltration of eosinophils, is an another differential diagnostic consideration. Immunohistochemically, inflammatory myofibroblastic tumor cells are often positive for anaplastic lymphoma kinase (ALK), and variably for SMA.

References and Further Reading

Daum, O., Hes, O., Vanecek, T., et al. (2003). Vanek's tumor (inflammatory fibroid polyp). Report of 18 cases and comparison with three cases of original Vanek's series. *Annals of Diagnostic Pathology, 7*, 337–347.

Daum, O., Hatlova, J., Mandys, V., et al. (2010). Comparison of morphological, immunohistochemical, and molecular genetic features features of inflammatory fibroid polyp (Vanek's polyp). *Virchows Archiv, 426*, 491–496.

Miettinen, M., Fletcher, C. D. M., Kindblom, L. -G., & Tsui, W. M. S. (2010). World Health Organization classification of tumours. Pathology & genetics. Tumours of the digestive system. In F. T. Bosman, F. Carnerio, R. H. Hruban, & N. D. Theise (Eds.), *Mesencymal tumours of the small intestine* (pp. 115–118). Lyon: International Agency for research on cancer (IARC).

Ozolek, J. A., Sasatomi, E., Swalsky, P. A., et al. (2004). Inflammatory fibroid polyps of the gastrointestinal tract clinical, pathologic, and molecular characteristics. *Applied Immunohistochemistry & Molecular Morphology, 12*, 59–66.

Inflammatory Fibroid Polyp, Upper Gastrointestinal Tract

José Manuel Lopes
Faculty of Medicine of the University of Porto and Institute of Molecular Pathology and Immunology of the University of Porto, Porto, Portugal

Synonyms

Eosinophilic granuloma; Eosinophilic pseudotumor; Granuloblastoma; Submucosal granuloma with eosinophilic infiltration; Vanek's polyp/tumor

Definition

Inflammatory fibroid polyp is a benign submucosal tumor composed of bland spindle and/or stellate mesenchymal cells and edematous/myxoid stroma with prominent vasculature and inflammatory cells comprising eosinophils, lymphocytes, plasma cells, and mast cells (Bhattacharya 2012; Turner and Odze 2009). Despite many ultrastructural and immunohistochemical studies suggesting dendritic, fibroblastic, fibrohistiocytic, histiocytic, myofibroblastic, neural, and vascular differentiation, an origin of spindle cells comprising these polyps remains controversial. The consistent PDGFRA (platelet-derived growth factor receptor alpha) expression seen in gastric and small intestinal inflammatory fibroid polyps points to the fact that these tumors might develop from a subset of PDGFRA-positive mesenchymal cells (Lasota et al. 2009).

Clinical Features

- **Incidence**
  Inflammatory fibroid polyps are uncommon. In the stomach, they comprise ~3–4% of all gastric polyps (Bhattacharya 2012).
- **Age**
  Most of inflammatory fibroid polyps occur in adults; the mean age is 64 years (range, 7–92 years) (Bhattacharya 2012).
- **Sex**
  Male-to-female ratio of inflammatory fibroid polyps is 1:1.2 (Bhattacharya 2012); apparently, they occur more commonly in females (Turner and Odze 2009).
- **Site**
  Inflammatory fibroid polyps occur anywhere in the gastrointestinal tract. The stomach is the most frequent (70%) site (antrum, 67.3%; body, 8.2%; pylorus, 2.4%; incisura, 1.7%; and cardia and fundus, 1%) (Bhattacharya 2012; Solte and Finkenzeller 1990). Other sites in decreasing order of frequency: ileum, colon, jejunum, duodenum, and esophagus (Bhattacharya 2012).
- **Treatment**
  Safe treatment of inflammatory fibroid polyps includes endoscopic or surgical complete excision (Turner and Odze 2009), depending on size and site, and treatment of associated conditions is standard of care for inflammatory fibroid polyps.
- **Outcome**
  Inflammatory fibroid polyps are benign tumors; persistence/regrowth after incomplete resection may occur, particularly in large inflammatory fibroid polyps, but they do not metastasize.

Macroscopy

Inflammatory fibroid polyps make up solitary sessile or polypoid submucosal well-circumscribed non-capsulated (single, rarely multiple) tumors (Fig. 1), with gray-tan firm surface, most <3 cm (median size: 1.5 cm), some >5 cm (Bhattacharya 2012; Turner and Odze 2009), that may ulcerate the overlying mucosa or obliterate the gastrointestinal lumen.

Microscopy

See Definition. Inflammatory fibroid polyps (Figs. 2 and 3) display perivascular or

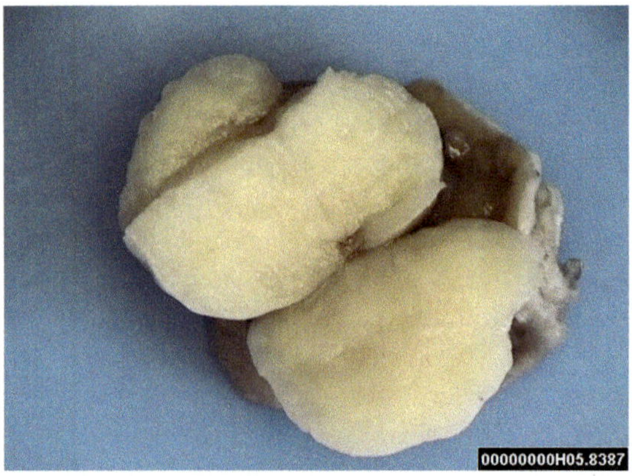

Inflammatory Fibroid Polyp, Upper Gastrointestinal Tract, Fig. 1 Macroscopy of gastric inflammatory fibroid polyp

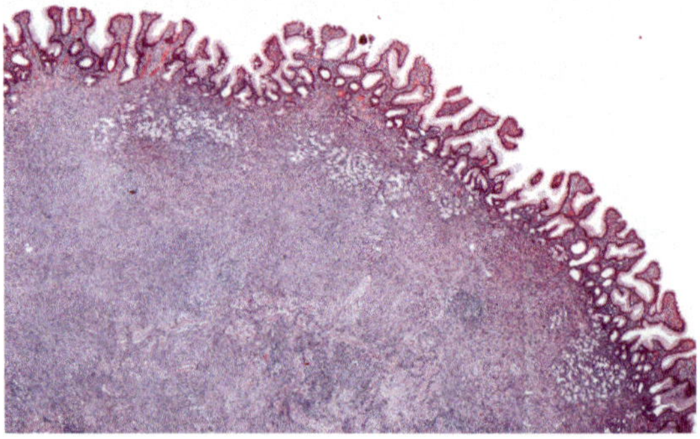

Inflammatory Fibroid Polyp, Upper Gastrointestinal Tract, Fig. 2 Low power features of gastric inflammatory fibroid polyp

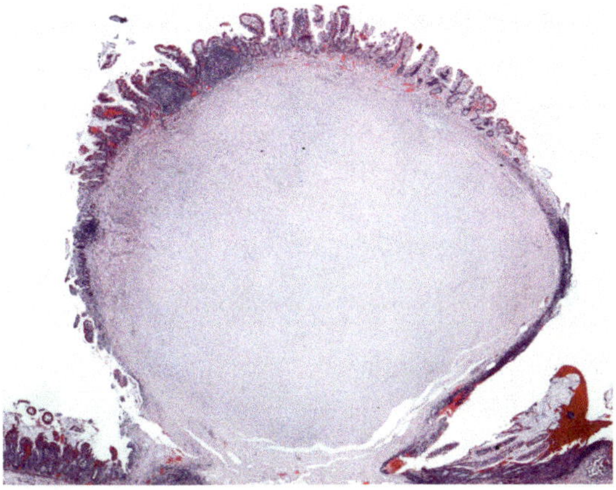

Inflammatory Fibroid Polyp, Upper Gastrointestinal Tract, Fig. 3 Low power view of ileal inflammatory fibroid polyp

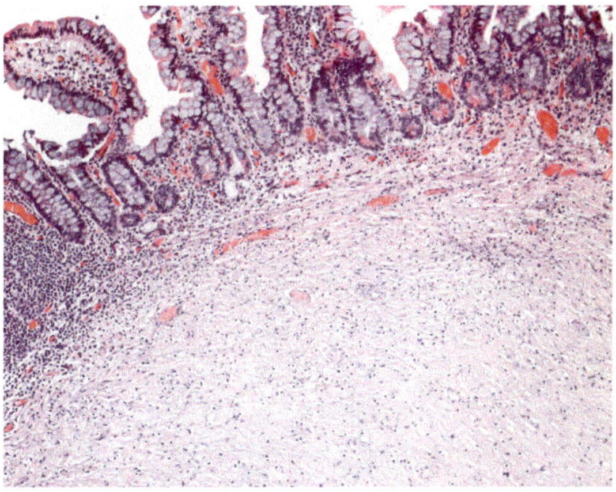

Inflammatory Fibroid Polyp, Upper Gastrointestinal Tract, Fig. 4 Ileal inflammatory fibroid polyp displaying collagenous stroma

periglandular spindle cells with onion-skin pattern around blood vessels and mucosal glands, and may have collagenous stroma, more frequent in ileal tumors (Fig. 4). The tumor cells have oval, stellate, or spindle nuclei with finely granular chromatin, small nucleoli, and eosinophilic cytoplasm (Fig. 5). Multinucleated giant cells, with floret-like arrangement, are frequent. Mitotic index is low with no atypical mitotic figures. Gastric inflammatory fibroid polyps tend to be smaller, seem to originate at the base of the lamina propria, extending through and disrupting the muscularis mucosa. They have a sharp, well-

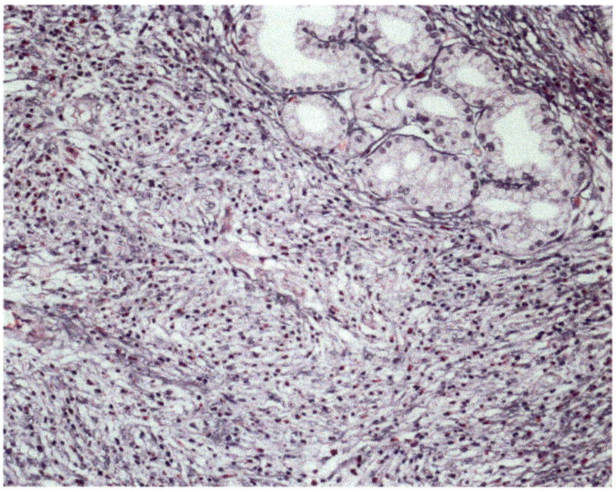

Inflammatory Fibroid Polyp, Upper Gastrointestinal Tract, Fig. 5 Gastric inflammatory fibroid polyp displaying bland spindle cells and inflammatory cells including eosinophils and lymphocytes

circumscribed, lower border in the submucosa. The ileal inflammatory fibroid polyps tend to be larger and are intramural proliferations that push against the muscularis mucosae, eventually disrupting it and extending into the mucosa, often ulcerating. They obliterate the submucosa and muscularis propria and often invade the mesentery (Bhattacharya 2012).

Immunophenotype

The spindle cells of inflammatory fibroid polyps express vimentin, CD34 (cluster differentiation molecule 34) (Figs. 6 and 7), PDGFRA, fascin, SMA (smooth muscle actin), calponin, CD 68 (cluster differentiation molecule 68), CD35 (cluster differentiation molecule 35) (focal), in the absence of CD117-cluster of differentiation molecule 117/KIT (kinase-tyrosine receptor of stem cell factor), DOG1 (discovered on GIST-1), keratins, EMA (epithelial membrane antigen), desmin, S-100, bcl-2 (B-cell chronic lymphocytic leukemia/lymphoma 2), HMB-45 (premelanosome glycoprotein present in melanomas and other tumors derived from melanocytes), GLUT-1 (glucose transporter 1), claudin-1, ALK (anaplastic lymphoma kinase), and collagen IV (Bhattacharya 2012; Daum et al. 2010; Lasota et al. 2009; Schildhaus et al. 2008; Turner and Odze 2009).

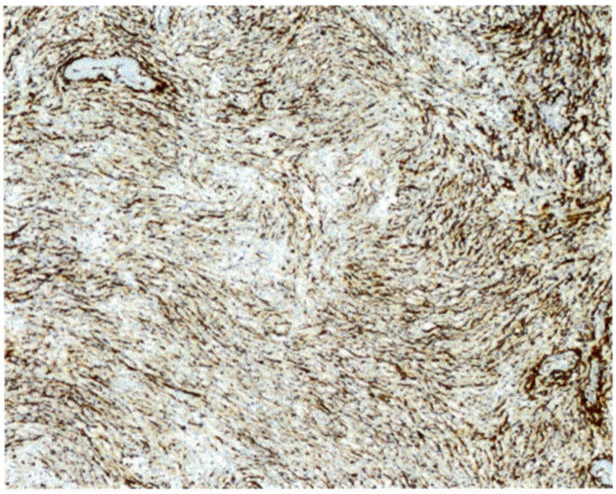

Inflammatory Fibroid Polyp, Upper Gastrointestinal Tract, Fig. 6 Expression of CD34 in spindle cells of inflammatory fibroid polyp

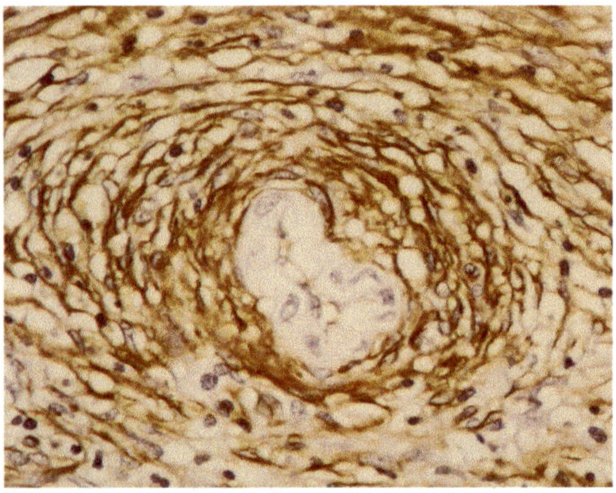

Inflammatory Fibroid Polyp, Upper Gastrointestinal Tract, Fig. 7 Onion-skin pattern of inflammatory fibroid polyp spindle cells expressing CD34

Molecular Features

Inflammatory fibroid polyps harbor activating mutations (up to 70% of cases) in the platelet-derived growth factor receptor alpha (*PDGRFA*, chromosome 4q12) gene (Daum et al. 2010; Lasota et al. 2009; Schildhaus et al. 2008) with a localization-specific pattern: Exon 12 mutations predominate in the small intestine, while exon 18 mutations occur frequently in the stomach (Huss et al. 2012).

Differential Diagnosis

Differential diagnosis of inflammatory fibroid polyps may include non-neoplastic lesions (eosinophilic gastroenteritis and parasitic infections that should be ruled out by clinical and laboratorial features) and other tumors based on clinical, histopathological, immunohistochemical (see Immunophenotype; e.g., schwannoma: S100+; leiomyoma: desmin+; solitary fibrous tumor: bcl-2+; perineurioma: EMA+, GLUT-1+, and claudi-1+; inflammatory myofibroblastic tumor-IMT: ALK+ and gastrointestinal stromal tumors-GISTs: CD117+ and DOG1+), and molecular (see "Molecular Features"; e.g., IMT: gene fusions involving ALK gene) features.

References and Further Reading

Bhattacharya, B. (2012). Non-neoplastic disorders of the stomach. In C. A. Iacobuzio-Doahue & E. Montgomery (Eds.), *Gastrointestinal and liver pathology* (pp. 130–133). Philadelphia: Saunders Elsevier.

Daum, O., Hatlova, J., Mandys, V., Grossmann, P., Mukensnabl, P., Benes, Z., & Michal, M. (2010). Comparison of morphological, immunohistochemical, and molecular genetic features of inflammatory fibroid polyps (Vanek's tumors). *Virchows Archiv, 456*, 491–497.

Huss, S., Wardelmann, E., Goltz, D., Binot, E., Wolfgang Hartmann, W., Merkelbach-Bruse, S., Buttner, R., & Schildhaus, H.-U. (2012). Activating PDGFRA mutations in inflammatory fibroid polypsoccur in exons 12, 14 and 18 and are associated with tumour localization. *Histopathology, 61*, 59–68.

Lasota, J., Wang, Z.-F., Sobin, L. H., & Miettinen, M. (2009). Gain-of-function PDGFRA mutations, earlier reported in gastrointestinal stromal tumors, are common in small intestinal inflammatory fibroid polyps. A study of 60 cases. *Modern Pathology, 22*, 1049–1056.

Schildhaus, H.-U., Cavlar, T., Binot, E., Buttner, R., Wardelmann, E., & Merkelbach-Bruse, S. (2008). Inflammatory fibroid polyps harbour mutations in the platelet-derived growth factor receptor alpha (*PDGFRA*) gene. *Journal of Pathology, 216*, 176–182.

Solte, M., & Finkenzeller, G. (1990). Inflammatory fibroid polyp of the stomach. *Endoscopy, 22*, 203–207.

Turner, J. R., & Odze, R. D. (2009). Polyps of stomach. In R. D. Odze & J. R. Goldblum (Eds.), *Surgical pathology of the GI tract, liver, biliary tract, and pancreas* (pp. 439–441). Philadelphia: Saunders Elsevier.

Inflammatory Myofibroblastic Tumor, Upper Gastrointestinal Tract

José Manuel Lopes
Faculty of Medicine of the University of Porto and Institute of Molecular Pathology and Immunology of the University of Porto, Porto, Portugal

Synonyms

Inflammatory myofibroblastoma; Inflammatory myofibrohistiocytic proliferation; Inflammatory pseudotumor; Plasma cell granuloma; Plasma cell pseudotumor

Definition

The inflammatory myofibroblastic tumor comprises spindle or polygonal fibroblast-/myofibroblast-type cells, which often express anaplastic lymphoma kinase (ALK), and stromal lymphoplasmacytic inflammatory cells. Some authors have differentiated inflammatory myofibroblastic tumors from reactive pseudosarcomatous processes and other neoplasms based on ALK immunoreactivity or evidence of the ALK translocation, but many consider ALK-negative inflammatory myofibroblastic tumors a valid diagnostic category.

Clinical Features

- **Incidence**
  Inflammatory myofibroblastic tumors (IMTs) are rare in the upper gastrointestinal (GI) tract.
- **Age**
  Inflammatory myofibroblastic tumors mean age (range) is 41 years (0.75–84) (Makhlouf and Sobin 2002).
- **Sex**
  The male to female ratio of inflammatory myofibroblastic tumors is 1.1:1 (Makhlouf and Sobin 2002).
- **Site**
  Inflammatory myofibroblastic tumors occur in the stomach (up to 25% of GI IMTs) and rarely in the esophagus (Makhlouf and Sobin 2002).
- **Treatment**
  Safe treatment requires complete excision in most inflammatory myofibroblastic tumors. Anti-inflammatory drugs, chemotherapy, anti-tumor necrosis factor antibody, and ALK inhibitor crizotinib (Kelleher and McDermott 2010) may be considered for unresectable/malignant cases.
- **Outcome**
  Most inflammatory myofibroblastic tumors pursue a benign clinical behavior, spontaneous resolution after incomplete resection may occur, and up to 25% may recur and rarely may develop metastases. Only about half of inflammatory myofibroblastic tumors harbor an ALK translocation, and these may behave more indolently than their ALK-negative counterparts, although this may not be the case for all ALK-rearranged tumors. There are no definitive prognostic clinical and pathological parameters.

Macroscopy

Inflammatory myofibroblastic tumors form white, tan, or yellow to white fleshy solid circumscribed (solitary, sometimes multiple) lesions with infiltrative borders (Fig. 1) and foci of myxoid change, mean size (range): 8 cm ± 5.2 (0.3–20) (Makhlouf and Sobin 2002).

Microscopy

See definition. Inflammatory myofibroblastic tumors can display several patterns: fasciitis-like, with vascular, myxoid, and inflammatory stroma with plasma cells; fascicular malignant fibrous histiocytoma or leiomyosarcoma-like spindle cell areas with inflammatory cells; and scar or sclerotic desmoid-like areas with calcification; these patterns may be found within the same tumor; eosinophils can be prominent in

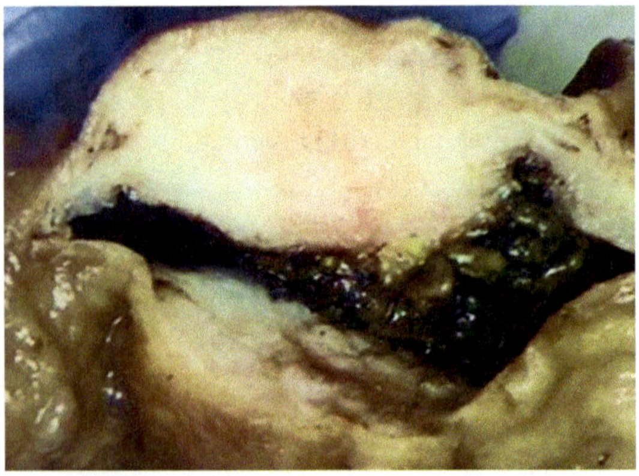

Inflammatory Myofibroblastic Tumor, Upper Gastrointestinal Tract, Fig. 1 Macroscopic features of gastric myofibroblastic tumor

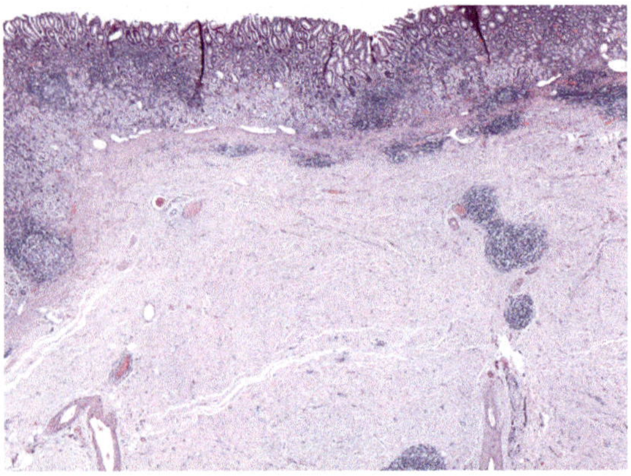

Inflammatory Myofibroblastic Tumor, Upper Gastrointestinal Tract, Fig. 2 Low power features of inflammatory myofibroblastic tumor below gastric mucosa

inflammatory myofibroblastic tumors, especially in fasciitis-like subtype, but plasma cells are the most common inflammatory cells overall (Coffin et al. 1995) (Figs. 2–4). The spindle cells have usually oval to elongated nuclei, variable prominent eosinophilic nucleoli, and amphophilic abundant cytoplasm reminding skeletal muscle cells or ganglion cells. Mitotic activity varies but is usually low (atypical mitosis are rare). Focal necrosis is rarely seen. Vascular invasion can be found but without adverse prognostic significance.

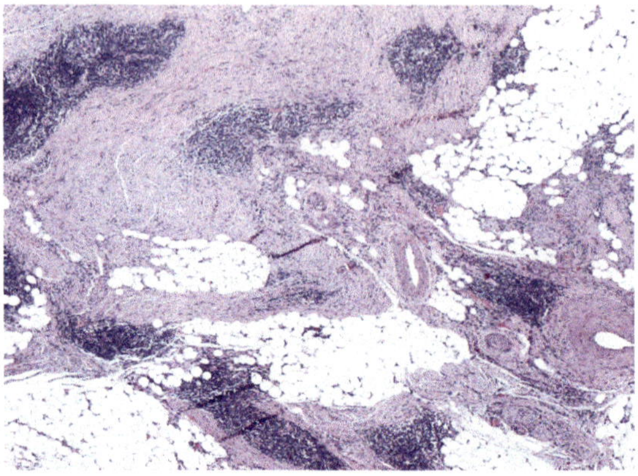

Inflammatory Myofibroblastic Tumor, Upper Gastrointestinal Tract, Fig. 3 Low power features of infiltrative growth pattern of inflammatory myofibroblastic tumor

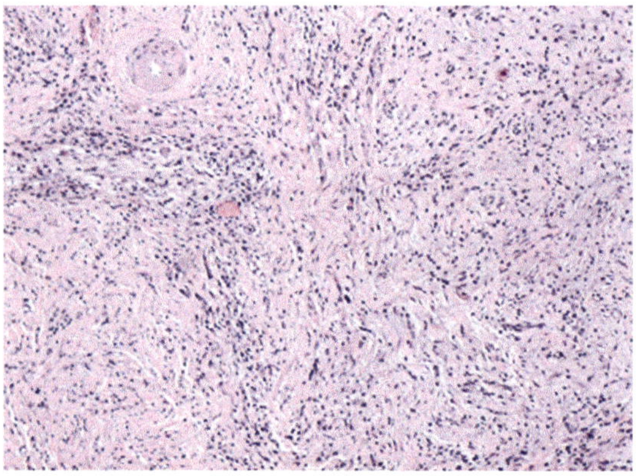

Inflammatory Myofibroblastic Tumor, Upper Gastrointestinal Tract, Fig. 4 High power features of inflammatory myofibroblastic tumor

Immunophenotype

Inflammatory myofibroblastic tumors express vimentin, ALK (cytoplasmic, 35–60% of cases), focal SMA (smooth muscle actin), CD34 (cluster differentiation molecule 34), cytokeratin, desmin (Fisher 2011), CD68 (cluster differentiation molecule 68), calponin, AE1/AE3 (keratins 1–8, 10, 14–16, and 19), and CAM 5.2 (keratins 7 and 8) in the absence of expression of S100 protein, CD117 (cluster of differentiation molecule 117)/ KIT (kinase-tyrosine receptor of stem cell factor), beta-catenin, myoglobin, myogenin, MyoD1 (myogenic basic muscle-specific protein), caldesmon, MDM2 (murine double minute 2), CDK4 (cyclin-dependent kinase 4), and calretinin.

Molecular Features

Cytogenesis banding studies have shown that approximately 50% of inflammatory myofibroblastic tumors have clonal rearrangements of chromosome 2, and recurrent involvement of 2p23, the locus for ALK, occurs in inflammatory myofibroblastic tumors. Inflammatory myofibroblastic tumors may harbor gene fusions involving the *ALK* (chromosome 2p23) and other genes (e.g., *ATIC, inosine monophosphate synthase; CARS, cysteinyl-tRNA synthetase; TPM3, tropomyosin 3; TPM4, tropomyosin 4; CLTC, clathrin, heavy chain; RANB2, ran-binding protein 2;* and *SEC31L, SEC31-like 1, Saccharomyces cerevisiae*) (Patel et al. 2007). Tropomyosin TMP3 and TMP4 fusion oncoproteins have been recognized as the most frequent gene rearrangement partners with the anaplastic lymphoma kinase gene (ALK) leading to constitutive activation: TMP3–ALK or TMP4–ALK t (1; 2), CLTC–ALK t (2; 17), and CARS–ALK t (2; 11), i.e., cysteinyl-tRNA synthetase (CARS) gene in inflammatory myofibroblastic tumors (Kelleher and McDermott 2010). ALK along with its fusion partner tends to localize to the cytoplasm, but ALK/RANBP2 localizes to the nuclear membrane.

Differential Diagnosis

Inflammatory myofibroblastic tumors encompass a spectrum of inflammatory pseudotumor to inflammatory fibrosarcoma type lesions (see outcome). Differential diagnosis of inflammatory myofibroblastic tumors may include fibroinflammatory proliferations and spindle cell tumors that contain inflammation (e.g., granulation tissue, IG4-related sclerosing disease, inflammatory fibroid polyp, fibromatosis, solitary fibrous tumor, embryonal rhabdomyosarcoma, GIST (gastrointestinal stromal tumor), dedifferentiated liposarcoma, leiomyosarcoma, sarcomatoid carcinoma, or sarcomatoid mesothelioma) and should be based on clinical, histological, immunohistochemical, and molecular features. Leiomyosarcomas are most often morphologically distinctive, with their non-tapered cells with eosinophilic cytoplasm and squared-off nuclei, arranged in cellular fascicles in a distinctive rectilinear pattern. Immunohistochemically, desmin, SMA (smooth muscle actin), muscle-specific actin, h-caldesmon, calponin, and smooth muscle myosin are expressed in the majority of leiomyosarcomas. Some examples coexpress cytokeratins (CKs) (frequently with a dot pattern), EMA (epithelial membrane antigen), and S100 protein, but usually only when the muscle-specific antigens are present. CD99 (cluster differentiation molecule 99) can also be seen in a paranuclear dot pattern. CD34 expression is variable but generally negative in leiomyosarcomas, and CD117 is absent from smooth muscle tumors. Dedifferentiated liposarcoma express CDK4 and MDM2. Fibromatosis are focally positive for smooth muscle actin (SMA) and occasionally for desmin in scattered cells. S100 protein can be focally positive, but CD34 is negative. Nuclear immunoreactivity for beta-catenin is found in variable numbers of nuclei. Nuclear beta-catenin positivity can also be found in solitary fibrous tumors. It is absent from GISTs, leiomyosarcomas, and inflammatory myofibroblastic tumors, and this is of use in the differential diagnosis of intra-abdominal spindle cell neoplasms. Fibromatosis is negative for h-caldesmon, anaplastic lymphoma kinase (ALK), CD34, CD117, and DOG1. Sarcomatoid carcinomas can express CKs focally, especially those of high molecular mass, but can also be negative for CKs. The diagnosis can be facilitated by finding areas of epithelial differentiation or surface dysplasia, or a nested reticulin pattern. Spindle cell carcinomas can also express SMA, but desmin, h-caldesmon, CD34, and S100 protein are absent. Spindle cell rhabdomyosarcomas are diffusely positive for desmin, and at least focally in nuclei for myogenin and MyoD1. Immunophenotypically, inflammatory myofibroblastic tumors react more commonly than inflammatory fibroid polyp for smooth muscle markers but fail to express CD34. GIST typically does not have the inflammatory background seen in inflammatory myofibroblastic tumors. In addition, some GIST cells have cytoplasmic vacuoles, a feature not seen in the inflammatory myofibroblastic tumors. Immunohistochemically, GIST is typically positive for CD117 but negative for ALK, whereas inflammatory myofibroblastic tumor shows an opposite profile.

References and Further Reading

Coffin, C. M., Watterson, J., Priest, J. P., & Dehner, L.-P. (1995). Extrapulmonary inflammatory myofibroblastic tumor (inflammatory pseudotumor). A clinicopathologic and immunohistochemical study of 84 cases. *The American Journal of Surgical Pathology, 19*, 859–872.

Fisher, C. (2011). Immunohistochemistry in diagnosis of soft tissue tumours. *Histopathology, 58*, 1001–1012.

Kelleher, F. C., & McDermott, R. (2010). The emerging pathogenic and therapeutic importance of the anaplastic lymphoma kinase gene. *European Journal of Cancer, 46*(13), 2357–2368.

Makhlouf, H. R., & Sobin, L. H. (2002). Inflammatory myofibroblastic tumors (inflammatory pseudotumors) of the gastrointestinal tract: How closely are they related to inflammatory fibroid polyps? *Human Pathology, 33*, 307–315.

Patel, A. S., Murphy, K. M., Hawkins, A. L., Cohen, J. S., Long, P. P., Perlman, E. J., & Griffin, C. A. (2007). RANBP2 and CLTC are involved in ALK rearrangements in inflammatory myofibroblastic tumors. *Cancer Genetics and Cytogenetics, 176*, 107–114.

Intestinal Atresia

Andrzej Mróz
Department of Gastroenterology and Hepatology, Histopathology Unit, Medical Center for Postgraduate Education, Warsaw, Poland

Synonyms

Intestinal atresia and stenosis

Definition

Intestinal atresia is a complete blockage of intestinal passage caused by mucosal diaphragm which totally occludes the lumen. Stenosis is formed by narrowed segment of the intestine or the mucosal diaphragm with small opening. Intestinal atresia and stenosis are responsible for most cases of bowel obstruction in newborns.

There are three major theories explaining development of intestinal atresia:

(i) Failed recanalization of the intestine during 12-th fetal week
(ii) Retarded epithelial growth during intestinal elongation which is slower than mesenchymal growth
(iii) Vascular abnormalities in utero leading to ischemia and segmental necrosis with subsequent scaring and development of atresia

Intestinal atresia differs in its clinical picture, diagnosis, and treatment methods, depending on the site of the involvement, which can be divided in duodenal, ileojejunal, and colon atresia. This condition is connected with prematurity in half of the cases, two-thirds of babies have abnormalities of the heart, and genitourinary or intestinal tract. Nearly 40% of patients have Down syndrome. Ileojejunal atresia includes obstruction of jejunum or ileum. The proximal part of the intestine distends to sometimes severe degree. In 10–15% of infants with ileojejunal atresia, part of the intestine dies during fetal development. Accompanying congenital abnormalities affect about 10% of patients and include mainly intestinal malrotation and malfixation and cystic fibrosis. Ileojejunal atresia may be sporadic or familial as monozygotic twins have higher risk due to possibly in utero vascular disruption. Colonic atresia is the rarest form of intestinal atresia (15%). It may be connected with small bowel atresia, Hirschsprung disease, and gastroschisis. Table 1 summarizes the abnormalities associated with intestinal atresia.

Intestinal Atresia, Table 1 Abnormalities associated with intestinal atresia

Malrotation of the gut
Meckel's diverticulum
Volvulus
Esophageal atresia
VACTERL syndrome
Other intestinal atresias including biliary atresia, annular pancreas, and imperforate anus
Pancreatic lipomatosis
Ocular anomalies
Microcephaly
Spina bifida
Immunodeficiency states
Hirschsprung's disease
Congenital heart failure
Cytogenetic changes: deletion of chromosome 13, ring chromosome 4, trisomy 21
Maternal lesions: polyhydramnios, intrapartum hemorrhage

Clinical Features

- **Incidence**
  Intestinal atresia affects 1:2,500–1:6,000 live births with duodenal atresia being the most common.
- **Age**
  Most cases are diagnosed in neonatal period. In distal atresias (particularly colonic), it may take few days for symptoms to develop.
- **Sex**
  No sex predilection has been reported.
- **Site**
  Duodenum, jejunum, ileum, and colon depending on the type of intestinal atresia. Most of the cases locate in postampullary region or at ampulla of Vater.
- **Treatment**
  All types of intestinal atresias require surgical treatment. Depending on length and level of intestinal involvement, proximal distention of the bowel, and general length of the intestine different types of operation are performed. Additional pre- and postoperative management must be instituted with evacuation of excess intestinal contents and gas, fluid, and electrolytes supplementation. Sometimes temporary gastrostomy must be created in case of duodenal atresia and colostomy in case of colonic atresia. In most cases of ileojejunal atresia, excision of affected segment may be performed instantly (jejunoplasty or excision of bowel segment with cut ends being sutured together).
- **Outcome (Prognosis)**
  Overall survival rate is about 90%, with operative mortality less than 1%. The survival rate improves with distal lesions reaching 100% in colonic atresia and decreases in multiple atresias (57%), apple peel atresia (71%) and if the atresia coexists with meconium ileus (65%), meconium peritonitis (50%) and gastroschisis (66%). Short-term complications are rare and include postoperative leakage of intestinal contents and subsequent infection and peritonitis.

  Long-term complications include malabsorption syndromes with short bowel syndrome, functional obstruction, and biliary hepatic cirrhosis in patients with total parenteral nutrition (TPN).

Macroscopy

Types of jejunoileal atresia:

- Atresia type I – there is a membrane (web) of mucosa at the internal aspect of the intestine. The intestine preserves normal length.
- Atresia type II – the segment of the intestine ends blindly and is connected with distal part (usually narrower) by a fibrous scar. The intestine also preserves normal length.
- Atresia type III – the blind ends are separated and the defect of vascular supply to intestinal wall occurs. Type IIIa has distended proximal and narrower distal parts of the intestine. In type IIIb, multiple stenoses with abnormal mesenteric formation take places (so called apple peel atresia). In type III, the length of the intestine is significantly shortened.

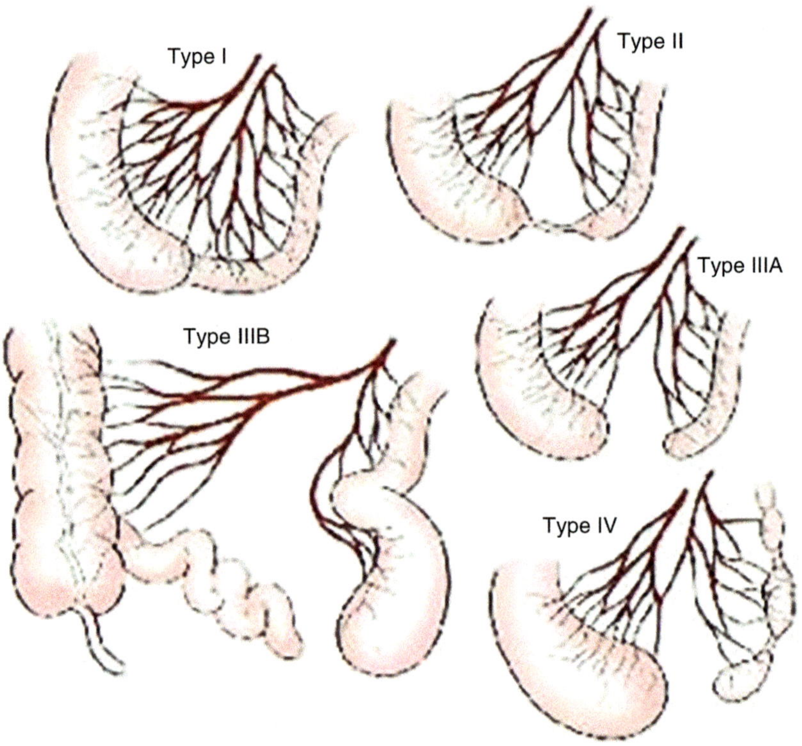

Intestinal Atresia, Fig. 1 Types of intestinal atresia (Source: www.cincinnatichildrens.org)

– Atresia type IV – there are multiple obstructed segments, resulting in severe shortening of bowel length.

The types of intestinal atresia are presented in Fig. 1.

Microscopy

In blind proximal segment, circular folds are widened. The villi may be shorter. Villi and crypts are sometimes necrotic and granulation, and ulceration may be the case. In the mucosa, one may find granulation tissue, granulomas, foreign body giant cells, fibroblasts, and resorptive macrophages. Muscularis mucosae may partially disappear, and prominent fibrosis of the submucosal layer is visible. Muscularis propria may be thickened and hypertrophic with inflammatory changes within myenteric plexus. The mucosa between atretic areas seems histologically normal.

Immunophenotype

There is no specific immunophenotypic feature.

Molecular Features

There is no specific molecular feature.

Differential Diagnosis

In multiple distal colonic atresias, Hirschsprung's disease comes into differential diagnosis.

References and Further Reading

Dalla Vecchia, L. K., Grosfeld, J. L., et al. (1998). Intestinal atresia and stenosis: 25-year experience with 277 cases. *Archives of Surgery, 133*, 490.

Fenoglio-Preiser, C., et al. (1999). *Gastrointestinal pathology plus: An atlas and text.* Philadelphia: Lippincott Williams & Wilkins.

Intestinal atresia and stenosis. www.cincinnatichildrens.org/health/i/obstructions/
Prasad, T. R., & Bajpai, M. (2000). Intestinal atresia. *Indian Journal of Pediatrics, 67*, 671–678.

Intestinal Lymphangiectasia

Arzu Ensari
Department of Pathology, Ankara University Medical School, Sihhiye, Ankara, Turkey

Synonyms

Primary intestinal lymphangiectasia (PIL); Waldmann's disease

Definition

Intestinal lymphangiectasia is defined as the presence of dilated lymphatics within the intestinal mucosa. The form, known as secondary intestinal lymphangiectasia, is associated with a local neoplastic or inflammatory condition causing lymphatic obstruction. Conditions associated with secondary intestinal lymphangiectasia include lymphoma, carcinoma, Crohn's disease, systemic lupus erythematosus, Behçet's disease, radiation therapy, trauma, heart disease, and liver transplantation. Primary intestinal lymphangiectasia, on the other hand, is a rare congenital disorder characterized by severe protein-losing enteropathy, peripheral edema, steatorrhea, and lymphocytopenia. Effusions may develop in pleural, pericardial, and peritoneal cavities with gross chylous ascites. There is a major structural abnormality of the lymphatic system consisting of dilatation and tortuosity of lymphatic vessels resulting in lymphatic stasis in the intestinal wall. The patients present with growth retardation, malabsorption, and severe hypoalbuminemia, while secondary form affects one side of the body resulting in unilateral edema but not protein-losing enteropathy. In the primary form, when large segments of the bowel are affected, secondary edema may occur as a result of protein-losing enteropathy and malabsorption. The edema is usually generalized in the primary form. Protein loss also causes immunoglobulin deficiency resulting in an immunodeficient state. In most histologically confirmed intestinal lymphangiectasia cases, however, clinical features may be very limited, and the classical "textbook" recorded changes may be more reflective of the most severe end of the clinicopathological spectrum in adults. Very rare familial forms of Waldmann's disease have also been reported.

Clinical Features

- **Incidence**
  The prevalence of clinically overt PIL is unknown.
- **Age**
  Primary intestinal lymphangiectasia is a disease of the newborn, whereas secondary form can occur in any age group. PIL primarily affects children (generally diagnosed before 3 years of age) and young adults but may be diagnosed later in adults.
- **Sex**
  The male-to-female ratio of PIL is 3:2.
- **Site**
  Though the entire small intestine can be involved, duodenum is the most commonly affected part of small intestine.
- **Treatment**
  Medical treatment comprises of a high-protein, low-fat diet with added medium-chain triglycerides (MCT). Octreotides have been reported to decrease intestinal protein loss. It is likely that the absence of fat in the diet prevents engorgement of the intestinal lymphatics with chyle, thereby preventing their rupture with its ensuing protein and T-cell loss. MCT are directly absorbed into the portal venous circulation and thus provide nutrient fat but avoid lacteal engorgement. In patients not responding to a low-fat diet, enteral nutritional therapy may be required.
- **Outcome**
  The long-term course is variable but progresses slowly with intermittent remissions. Lower

limb lymphedema requires specific long-term management (low-stretch bandage, manual lymph drainage, skin care, elastic hosiery). PIL outcome may be severe and even life-threatening when malignant complications (lymphoma) or serous effusion(s) (pleural, pericardial) occurs.

Macroscopy

Radiologically there is diffuse nodular thickening of the bowel wall with ascites. The mucosa shows features of lymphangiectasia on endoscopy as numerous white spots or nodules. The density of lymphangiectasia varies and their size ranges from mm to cm. Endoscopy may be negative when intestinal lesions are segmental or localized.

Microscopy

The white spots on endoscopy correspond to the dilated lymphatics in superficial mucosa involving the villus tips with formation of "lacteals." These are dilated lymphatic vessels with endothelial lining and pale basophilic material of lymph fluid in their lumen (Figs. 1 and 2). Foamy macrophages are also frequently present in the lamina propria together with amorphous deposits which are PAS positive. There is no associated inflammation in the surrounding mucosae. Histological examination of duodenum, jejunum, or ileum biopsies confirms the presence of lacteal juice, dilated mucosal (from moderate to severe), and submucosal lymphatic vessels (and also in the serosa) with polyclonal normal plasma cells. Intestinal lymphatics may be dilated in many villi or only a few.

Immunophenotype

There is no specific immunophenotypic feature of PIL.

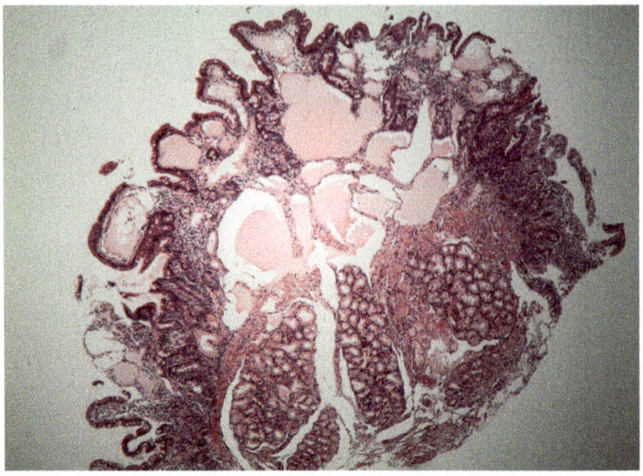

Intestinal Lymphangiectasia, Fig. 1 Small intestinal wall showing dilated lymphatics with proteinous material in their lumina (H&E; ×100)

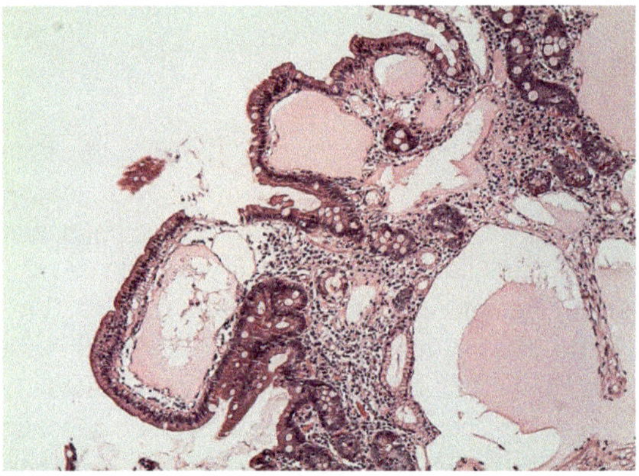

Intestinal Lymphangiectasia, Fig. 2 Lacteals within the tips of the villi (H&E; ×200)

Molecular Features

Several genes, such as *VEGFR3* (vascular endothelial growth factor receptor 3), prospero-related homeobox-transcriptional factor *PROX1*, and forkhead transcriptional factor *FOXC2* and *SOX18*, are implicated in the development of the lymphatic system. Recently, inconsistently changed expressions of regulatory molecules for lymphangiogenesis in the duodenal mucosa of PIL patients have been reported.

Differential Diagnosis

The differential diagnosis of primary intestinal lymphangiectasia is the secondary form caused by extramural obstruction or infections like Whipple's disease, mycobacterial enteritis, Crohn's disease, sarcoidosis, systemic sclerosis, radiation, and/or chemotherapy with retroperitoneal fibrosis, an isolated lymphangioma, and pneumatosis intestinalis. The changes in PIL may be patchy, thereby making multiple biopsies necessary for diagnosis. The diagnosis is thus a clinicopathologic one. However, it should also be born in mind that focally dilated lymphatics may also be present in normal mucosal biopsies. In addition, tissue artifacts may lead to detachment of the surface epithelium from the underlying basement membrane which can be mistaken for a dilated lymphatic vessel.

References and Further Reading

Braamskamp, M. J., Dolman, K. M., & Tabbers, M. M. (2010). Clinical practice. Protein-losing enteropathy in children. *European Journal of Pediatrics, 169*(10), 1179–1185.

Vignes, S., & Bellanger, J. (2008). Primary intestinal lymphangiectasia (Waldmann's disease). *Orphanet Journal of Rare Diseases, 3*, 5.

Wen, J., Tang, Q., Wu, J., Wang, Y., & Cai, W. (2010). Primary intestinal lymphangiectasia: Four case reports and a review of the literature. *Digestive Diseases and Sciences, 55*(12), 3466–3472.

Xinias, I., Mavroudi, A., Sapountzi, E., Thomaidou, A., Fotoulaki, M., Kalambakas, A., Karypidou, E., Kollios, K., Pardalos, G., & Imvrios, G. (2013). Primary intestinal lymphangiectasia: Is it always bad? Two cases with different outcome. *Case Reports in Gastroenterology, 20*, 153–163.

Intestinal Malrotation

Maria Sotiropoulou
Department of Pathology, Alexandra Hospital, Athens, Attica, Greece

Synonyms

Bowel malrotation; Malrotation of the gut

Definition

Intestinal malrotation (IM) is a congenital anomaly characterized by a disturbed topography within the abdominal cavity, involving primarily the duodenojejunal and ileocolic loops. It includes abnormalities of both rotation and fixation of the intestinal tube and, generally, results from the disordered embryonic counterclockwise rotation of the gut around the superior mesenteric artery (SMA) leading to a more or less unanchored bowel, a narrow base mesentery, and various acute and chronic presentations of disease.

The basic intestinal movement inside the abdomen of the developing embryo consists of a two- to three-stage anticlockwise rotation of the two segments of the initially symmetrically suspended midgut, meaning the more rapidly elongating cranial (prearterial) limb and the more slowly elongating caudal limb (postarterial) around the axis of the SMA. The first stage, beginning at the 5–6 weeks, consists of a 90° twist of the U-shaped midgut around the SMA, so that the duodenojejunal loop moves to the right and the ileocolic segment to the embryo's left. After the temporary herniation of the intestinal loops into the stalk of the yolk sac, the rotation continues at about 10–12 weeks when the sliding of the intestine back into the abdomen allows a further 180° counterclockwise rotation to be added to the previous one making a total of 270°. As a result, the third portion of the duodenum is placed horizontally, caudal and dorsal to the SMA and the ileocolic segment ventral and cranial to the proximal loop, with the cecum lying to the right abdomen near the liver. The final stage includes the descent of the cecum to the right lower quadrant and fixation of the mesenteries to the parietal peritoneum which last through fetal life.

According to the position of the third portion of the duodenum relative to the SMA and the misplacement of the intestine within the abdominal cavity, a simplified classification of IM is the following:

Non-rotation or complete failure of rotation, considered an arrest at an early stage, which

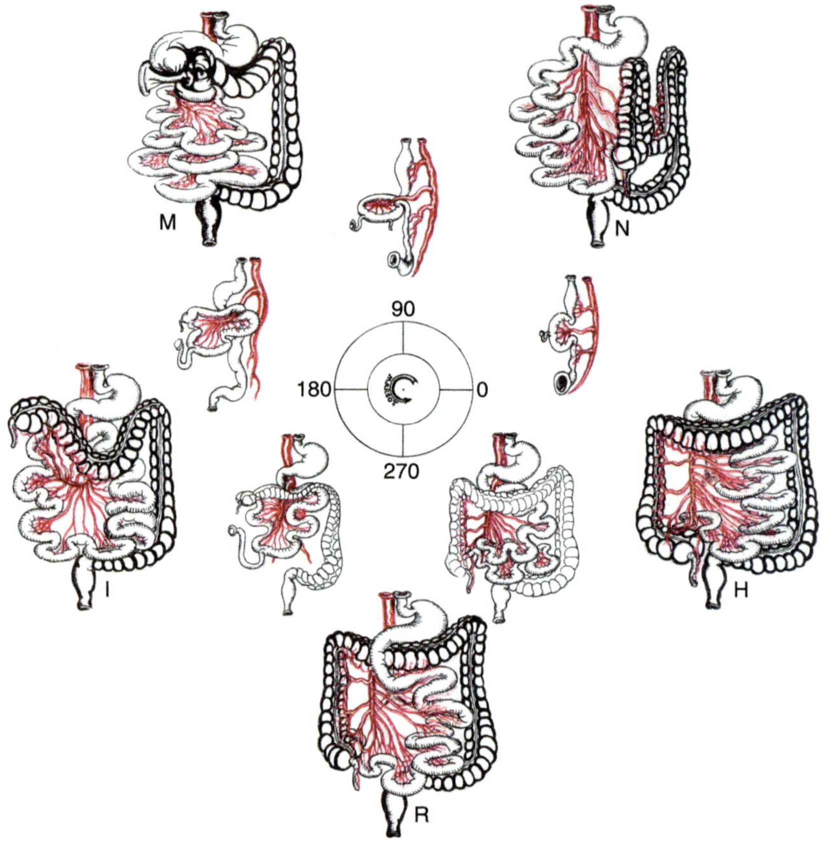

Intestinal Malrotation, Fig. 1 *N*, non-rotation; *M*, mixed rotation; and volvulus (fibrous adhesions of the cecum compress the third portion of the duodenum; *I*, incomplete rotation; *R*, reverse rotation; *H*, hyperotation

results in a right-sided jejunum and ileum and a left-sided colon

Incomplete, mixed, or partial rotation, which is the most common and results from the disrupted at stage II rotation having the small bowel mainly on the right side of the abdomen and the cecum in the right upper quadrant

Reverse rotation which is the rarest type and its occurrence follows two errors of reentry of the bowel loops after the combined 270° counterclockwise rotation outside the abdominal cavity

Abnormal fixation and abnormal mesenteries result in unfixed segments and form internal pouches such as right and left mesocolic hernias with possible entrapment of the neighboring small bowel (see section "Macroscopy" for more details) (Fig. 1)

Infants nearly always present with emesis, whereas in adults abdominal pain is the most common symptom, followed by emesis or nausea. Misplacement of the cecum and appendix may lead to delayed diagnosis of acute appendicitis. Intestinal malrotation may also present with volvulus, the incidence of which declines with age, abdominal distension, intraluminal bleeding due to persistent vascular compromise, acute or chronic duodenal obstruction due to Ladd bands, and forceful vomiting, bile stained or not, depending on location of obstruction. Additionally, in infants, malabsorption with steatorrhea and protein-losing enteropathy due to mesenteric lymphatic obstruction is a possible complication.

Upper GI series is the most common imaging study performed in infants and children and the study of choice (with barium as contrast) in stable patients or those that have chronic symptoms. Lower GI series is useful in indentifying the location of cecum and in cases where upper series is indeterminate for the location of the duodenal junction and in excluding the presence of colonic obstruction and ileal atresia. Ultrasonography is almost 100% sensitive in detecting neonatal malrotation and demonstrating a possible coiling of the superior mesenteric venous around the homonymous artery, a characteristic sign of possible volvulus. CT is the most common imaging study in adults, probably due to nonspecific clinical presentation.

- **Incidence**
  IM affects approximately 1/6,000 live births with the asymptomatic cases 12–30 times more prevalent (≈1/500).
- **Age**
  Seventy-five percent of patients with malrotation are diagnosed by the age of 1 year and 40% of them present within the first week of life. The remaining 25% of patients present after 1 year and into the late adulthood although there is at least one study that claims that nearly half of the patients present during adulthood in contrast to traditional teaching.
- **Sex**
  Intestinal malrotation is found primarily in males during the neonatal period with a male–female ratio of 2:1, though the age range extends through adulthood, but with no sexual predilection in patients older than 1 year.
- **Treatment**
  Medical management is directed toward stabilizing the patient and immediate surgical intervention whenever volvulus or obstruction is suspected. The Ladd procedure remains the basic surgical procedure for treatment of IM and includes:
  Reduction of volvulus and mobilization of the bowel
  Division of mesenteric bands
  Widening of the mesenteric base Appendectomy
- **Outcome**
  In general, older children are reported to have a better outcome than infants, for which the mortality rate ranges from 2% to 24% largely depending on the presence of necrotic bowel at surgery and association with other congenital anomalies (over 20 times higher risk). The most common complication of midgut volvulus is short bowel syndrome with patients having longer delays to recovery of bowel motility and function and higher risk for malabsorption and long-term parenteral nutrition. Other complications include wound infection, sepsis, and postsurgical ones such as adhesive small bowel obstruction, recurrent volvulus, and persistent gastrointestinal symptoms including constipation, intractable diarrhea, abdominal pain, vomiting, and feeding difficulties.

Macroscopy (Gross)

Macroscopy is the reflection of failure in any stage of intestinal rotation in combination with any superimposed complication, meaning obstruction, ischemia, necrosis, or peritonitis. Non-rotation results in a right-sided jejunum and ileum and a colon residing in the left abdomen, but may rarely affect only the duodenum with the small intestine, cecum, and colon assuming a normal anatomic location. Incomplete or mixed rotation which is more common results in the small bowel occupying mainly the right side of the abdomen with the cecum generally residing in the right upper quadrant. Typically, peritoneal fibrous bands running from the mispositioned cecum to the mesentery compress the third portion of the duodenum, most likely resulting in duodenal obstruction and midgut volvulus. In reversed rotation, which is the rarest type, depending on which segment, the postarterial or the prearterial, returns first to the abdomen and the rather clockwise than anticlockwise rotation of the duodenum, the small bowel respectively lies ventral to the colon and SMA, or in the left side with the colon occupying the right abdomen. These cases can be associated with situs anomalies of other organs and internal hernias, of which the left paraduodenal are the most common. Internal hernias are also a complication of abnormal fixation and unusually long mesenteries of various segments with the right and left mesocolic hernias being two common forms, where entrapment and strangulation of the small bowel may occur.

Microscopy

Normal histology is the rule, unless altered by vascular compromise and ischemia, necrosis, or peritonitis.

Immunophenotype

There is not any specific immunohistochemical stain concerning malrotation.

Molecular Features

The majority of children do not have any predisposing syndrome or genetic susceptibility, and little is known of the cause in the non-syndromic cases. Certain chromosomal abnormalities seem to be involved in the etiology of malrotation. Among them the most notable are trisomy 16 (FoxF1 at 16q24), ring chromosome 4 in midgut volvulus, and deletions of the long arm of 13, in the rare association of malrotation with Hirschsprung disease.

Differential Diagnosis

Malrotation should be differentiated from other causes of bowel obstruction in the newborn (atresia, diverticulum, intussusception and volvulus) and conditions such as gastroesophageal reflux, necrotizing enterocolitis, and sepsis, and the distinction is based on clinical features and imaging studies, although many patients are recognized intraoperatively during other procedures or at autopsy.

References and Further Reading

Bass, K. D., Rothenberg, S. S., & Chang, J. H. (1998). Laparoscopic Ladd's procedure in infants with malrotation. *Journal of Pediatric Surgery, 33*(2), 279–281.
Dietz, D. W., Wals, R. M., Grundfest-Broniatowski, S., et al. (2002). Intestinal malrotations: A rare but important cause of bowel obstruction in adults. *Diseases of the Colon and Rectum, 45*(10), 1381–1386.
Martin, V., & Shaw-Smith, C. H. (2010). Review of genetic factors in intestinal malrotation. *Pediatric Surgery International, 26*(8), 769–781.
Pickhardt, P., & Bhalla, S. (2002). Intestinal malrotation in adolescents and adults. Spectrum of clinical and imaging features. *American Journal of Roentgenology, 179*, 1429–1435.
Russo, P., & Huff, D. (2009). In R. Odze & J. Goldblum (Eds.), Congenital and development Disorders of the GI tract. *Surgical pathology of the GI tract, liver, biliary tract and pancreas* (2nd ed., pp. 162–163). Philadelphia: Saunders/Elsevier.

Intestinal Metaplasia

Rita Barros[1] and Raquel Almeida[1,2]
[1]Institute of Molecular Pathology and Immunology of the University of Porto (IPATIMUP), Porto, Portugal
[2]Faculty of Medicine, University of Porto, Porto, Portugal

Synonyms

IM

Definition

Metaplasia is a reversible change in which one adult cell type (epithelial or mesenchymal) is replaced by another adult cell type. Intestinal metaplasia (IM) of the stomach is a relatively frequent preneoplastic lesion resulting from the replacement of the gastric epithelium by an intestinal-like epithelium as a result of chronic injury. Colonization of the gastric mucosa with ► *Helicobacter pylori* is the main risk factor for IM and gastric cancer development, and it has been categorized by the International Agency for Research on Cancer as a type I carcinogen. This is one of the most common bacterial infections in humans with a prevalence that reaches 90% in many developing countries and a lower prevalence in developed ones that, nevertheless, varies between 30% and 50%.

IM appears following *H. pylori* infection and chronic inflammation, as part of a multistep precancerous process that was first described in 1975, by Pelayo Correa, based on observations in Colombian populations with high risk of gastric cancer development (Correa et al. 2010). This cascade of progressively more severe lesions usually starts with a non-atrophic chronic gastritis that may last for decades, unless the bacterium is eradicated. In a subset of individuals, multifocal atrophic gastritis will occur followed by the development of intestinal metaplasia, and a small proportion of these individuals will eventually develop dysplasia and gastric adenocarcinoma. Thus, IM is a step in a prolonged process, whose characterization may contribute to patient stratification and earlier diagnosis of gastric cancer and consequently better prognosis of this disease.

Histopathology

IM is a morphologically well-defined lesion, easily recognized in histologic sections with hematoxylin and eosin (HE) staining. IM displays alone or in combination the main intestinal cell types: enterocytes, goblet and Paneth cells (Fig. 1). In addition, ectopic intestinal glands show a complete reorganization, with displacement of the proliferative zone from the neck region down to the base of the crypt, resembling the normal intestinal architecture, concomitant with alterations in the extracellular matrix surrounding the metaplastic glands. The classification of IM, most widely used by pathologists, discriminates between complete and incomplete IM based on morphologic characteristics. Thus, IM is classified into complete type when the epithelium resembles the small intestine, displaying absorptive enterocytes with brush border, well-developed goblet cells and Paneth cells. On the other hand, the incomplete type resembles a colonic epithelium phenotype displaying goblet cells of variable size, absence of brush border, and absence of Paneth cells (Correa et al. 2010). Other classifications, used in research but not in the clinical practice, combine the previously described morphologic features with analysis of ▶ mucins. One of these classifications is based on histochemical methods that allow the discrimination between the neutral gastric mucins, that stain magenta with periodic acid-Schiff (PAS), and the acidic mucins present in IM which stain blue with Alcian blue at pH 2.5. Furthermore, high-iron diamine stains only acidic mucins that are sulfated as opposed to those that are sialylated. With this classification, IM is divided into three distinct types: Type I (complete) when only sialomucins are expressed; Type II (incomplete) when gastric and intestinal mucins (sialylated) are present, and Type III (incomplete) when sulfomucins are present (Correa et al. 2010). IM may also be classified into complete intestinal type or incomplete/mixed gastric-intestinal type based on mucin characterization using antibodies. In this case, the complete type is characterized by absence of gastric mucins and de novo expression of the intestinal mucin MUC2 in goblet cells (Fig. 2), whereas the incomplete IM expresses gastric mucins (MUC1, MUC5AC, and MUC6) in addition to MUC2 (Fig. 2). Multiple evidences support that incomplete IM (or Type III) is more associated with increased risk of gastric cancer, particularly of the intestinal type (Reis et al. 1999).

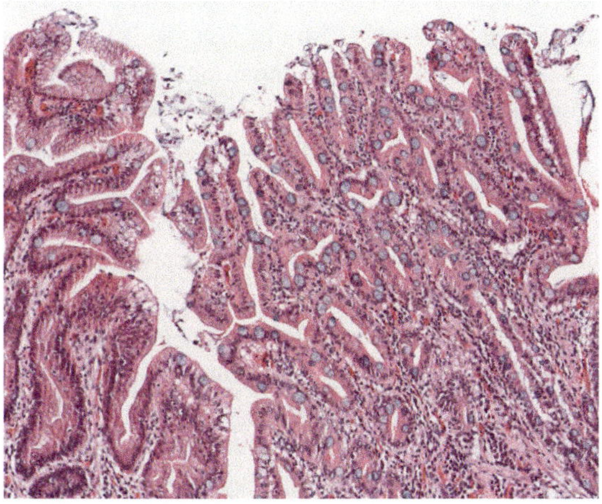

Intestinal Metaplasia, Fig. 1 H&E staining of a gastric mucosa, depicting intestinal metaplasia glands. Goblet cells are readily identifiable by the presence of blue vacuoles

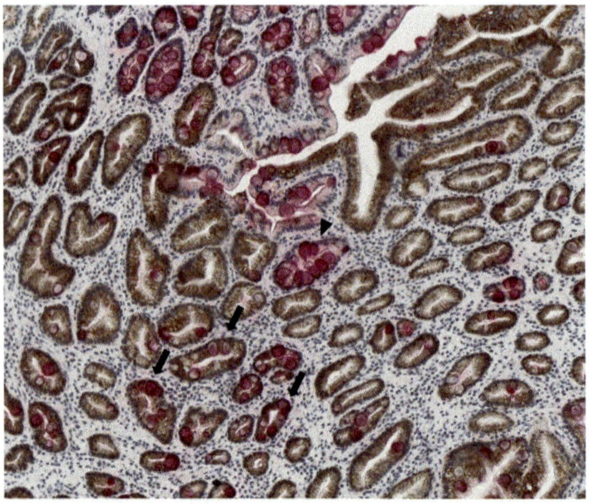

Intestinal Metaplasia, Fig. 2 Intestinal metaplasia stained for MUC2 (*red*) and MUC5AC (*brown*). Intestinal metaplasia of the complete type (*arrowhead*) expresses only the intestinal mucin MUC2, whereas intestinal metaplasia of the incomplete type expresses both MUC2 and the gastric mucin MUC5AC (*arrows*)

Risk Factors

The main risk factor for IM development is *H. pylori* infection but high salt intake, smoking, alcohol consumption, and chronic bile reflux might also play a role, although current evidences of their involvement are not as conclusive as for *H. pylori*. However, it is likely that the diversity of clinicopathological presentations of *H. pylori*–associated conditions/lesions might be related to the interaction of these environmental factors with bacterial virulence characteristics and the host genetic susceptibility since it is well known, from epidemiological studies, that only a fraction of individuals infected with this bacterium will develop IM. Furthermore, it is also well established that, in some countries particularly in Africa, gastric premalignant conditions/lesions, especially IM, and also gastric cancer are less frequent than expected considering the high prevalence of infection, which is known as the African enigma. This favors the hypothesis that other factors may be involved in the gastric carcinogenic cascade, in addition to *H. pylori* infection (Mesquita et al. 2006).

Different *H. pylori* strains vary in their association to gastric preneoplastic conditions, including IM, with those containing the virulence factor CagA inducing higher degree of inflammation and more severe lesions. It has also been demonstrated that, in individuals infected with CagA + strains, IM tends to be more difficult to revert. In addition, strains carrying babA2 and the vacA s1m1 genotypes are associated to increased risk of IM development. In contrast, IM was rarely associated with strains with a cagA–, babA2–, vacA s2m2 genotypes. More recently, it has been shown that strains carrying the CagA forms encoding multiple EPIYA-C type segments are also associated with a poorer outcome.

A vast number of studies have addressed the issue of the host susceptibility, particularly genetic variations, in the development of gastric premalignant conditions and cancer. In favor of the relevance of the host genetic makeup in gastric carcinogenesis is the finding that first-degree relatives of patients with gastric cancer have an increased prevalence of premalignant conditions/lesions including IM, as well as an increased risk for gastric cancer. One of the best studied addresses the role of interleukin polymorphisms particularly those that are involved in the inflammatory response to *H. pylori* infection leading to gastric atrophy. These include IL-1β pro-inflammatory polymorphisms as well as polymorphisms in the IL1-receptor antagonist, IL-8, IL-10 and in TNF-α. Polymorphisms of MUC1 mucin gene, namely, "small" VNTRs, predispose to the development of incomplete type IM in Portuguese and Colombian populations, and polymorphisms of the insulin-like growth factor binding protein-3 (IGFBP-3), leading to lower serum levels of IGFBP-3, have been associated with increased risk for the development of antral IM (Mesquita et al. 2006).

Conversely, a protective effect of some environmental exposures, particularly the relevance of antioxidants, has also been addressed but the results obtained are heterogeneous. A protective effect for fruits or vegetables consumption was identified in a few studies but not in others, thus remaining controversial, but overall suggestions are that antioxidants have a small or a null effect.

Spasmolytic Polypeptide–Expressing Metaplasia

Recently, another pattern of metaplasia, termed spasmolytic polypeptide–expressing metaplasia (SPEM), has been described. This is characterized by the expression of the TFF2 spasmolytic polypeptide that is associated with oxyntic atrophy. SPEM, which characteristically develops in the gastric body and fundus, appears to share some characteristics with pseudopyloric metaplasia, has a strong association with chronic infection with *H. pylori* and with gastric adenocarcinoma, and may represent another pathway to gastric neoplasia. However, at present, identification of SPEM is considered only an investigational parameter.

Clinical Features

- **Incidence**
  The incidence of gastric IM in the general population is a parameter impossible to assess since this condition remains asymptomatic and therefore undetected in the majority of the individuals. IM is thus only studied in terms of prevalence, which varies widely with the geographical location, displaying a trend analogous to the gastric cancer rates and defining low-risk areas such as North-American and most European countries, and high-risk areas such as Asian and South-American countries. Even prevalence data in the general population is scarce, since IM can only be diagnosed with endoscopic evaluation and histologic analysis; therefore, data on asymptomatic individuals is rare. A Japanese study showed that the prevalence of IM in individuals infected with *H. pylori* was about 37% as opposed to 0% in noninfected individuals (Uemura et al. 2001). Two recent studies performed in The Netherlands showed that the prevalence of IM is higher in symptomatic individuals referred for upper gastrointestinal endoscopy, in this case being around 30% than in asymptomatic individuals, where the prevalence is around 7% (de Vries et al. 2008).
- **Age**
  Most epidemiological studies are concordant in showing that IM prevalence increases with age. The same study performed in The Netherlands found that IM prevalence was significantly higher in patients aged more than 50 years old (31.9%) compared to those younger than 50 years old (10.4%). In addition, it was detected in 46.6% of the individuals older than 80 years and in only 5.2% of those less than 40 years old (de Vries et al. 2008).
- **Sex**
  In the same study, the distribution of IM was found to be similar in males and females; however, it was shown that the age at the initial diagnosis was significantly higher in women (68.7 vs 64.6). Furthermore, men with IM showed faster progression to gastric cancer. These findings suggest that male patients with IM have a higher risk of gastric cancer development than female patients (de Vries et al. 2008).
- **Site**
  In the distal stomach, IM tends to appear first at the ► antrum–corpus junction, especially at the incisura angularis and as the process advances, the foci extend to the neighboring mucosa in both the antrum and the corpus. IM might also develop in gastric ► cardia although this process is less well understood and is not only associated to *H. pylori* infection but also to gastroesophageal reflux.
- **Treatment**
  No specific treatment for gastric IM, other than eradication of *H. pylori* infection, is currently in use. However, in contrast to gastritis and atrophy, the effect of *H. pylori* eradication on gastric IM is controversial, with many studies showing that IM does not reverse but showing, nevertheless, that *H. pylori* eradication may slow the progression to gastric cancer; therefore, this treatment is recommended. In some cases, when the extension of IM is high, in young patients or in countries with a high prevalence of gastric preneoplastic and neoplastic diseases, endoscopic surveillance might be recommended.

- **Outcome**
  IM confers increased risk for dysplasia and gastric cancer development since it is one of the main precancerous conditions of the stomach, constituting the background in which these lesions develop. It remains an open discussion whether IM foci are the ones that progress to the more severe lesions. However, IM is a stable condition in most individuals. As a consequence, gastric cancer risk in patients with IM is too low to recommend surveillance of all patients. The types of metaplasia as well as the extension of metaplastic changes are determinants of the gastric cancer risk. These parameters have recently been incorporated in a staging system, the operative link for gastritis assessment (OLGA) now known as OLGIM, that instead of staging atrophy uses the histological assessment of IM which is easier and confers better interobserver agreement (Capelle et al. 2010).

  Data on the actual cancer risk in the presence of IM is very heterogeneous mostly due to the different types of studies that are employed, different sample selection and number of individuals enrolled in the studies, and also due to heterogeneous populations. In a large study performed in Japan in 2001, it was observed that 6.5% of the individuals harboring IM lesions developed gastric cancer as opposed to only 0.8% of those without IM (Uemura et al. 2001). This also shows that about 80% of the individuals that develop gastric cancer have previously developed IM. More recently, in the study performed in The Netherlands with a cohort of 92.250 patients, it was observed that 0.3%, 0.7%, 2.1%, and 24.9% of patients with atrophic gastritis, IM, low-grade dysplasia, and high-grade dysplasia, respectively, were diagnosed with gastric cancer within 1 year, and an additional 0.5%, 1.1%, 1.8%, and 7.8% of patients within 10 years of follow-up (de Vries et al. 2008).

Macroscopy

It is presently accepted that gastric IM does not produce significant macroscopic alterations. IM may appear as thin, white mucosal deposits on an endoscopic observation; however, the value of these or other endoscopic signs for the diagnosis of IM remains inconclusive due to poor interobserver agreement and low sensitivity and specificity. For this reason, the diagnosis of IM requires biopsy specimens which are collected randomly or in predefined locations. Nevertheless, efforts have been put on trying to improve the endoscopic diagnosis of IM, using magnification chromoendoscopy or narrow-band imaging, since it would increase the capacity of early detection of this lesion.

Microscopy

Gastric IM is easily recognized in histologic sections stained with hematoxylin and eosin. It appears as multiple microscopic foci of glands that resemble, morphologically, the intestine displaying, alone or in combination, the three main intestinal cell types, goblet, Paneth, and absorptive cells. Due to its multifocal nature, at least four non-targeted biopsies of two topographic sites, at the lesser and greater curvatures of both the antrum and corpus, are recommended in order to avoid misdiagnosis due to sampling errors.

Immunophenotype

The main characteristic of IM is obviously its intestinal differentiation, appearing de novo in the stomach. Due to this differentiation switch, IM foci express a high number of molecules that are very specific and completely absent from the gastric mucosa. These include intestinal proteins such as sucrase-isomaltase, carbonic anhydrase, lactase, alkaline phosphatase and villin, as well as the intestinal mucin MUC2, which is expressed in goblet cells, and the transcription factor CDX2 (Fig. 3) which is normally only present in intestine but appears aberrantly expressed in IM (Mesquita et al. 2006). The ones that are more frequently used to characterize IM foci, particularly for research purposes, are antibodies against MUC2 and the homeoprotein CDX2. Both

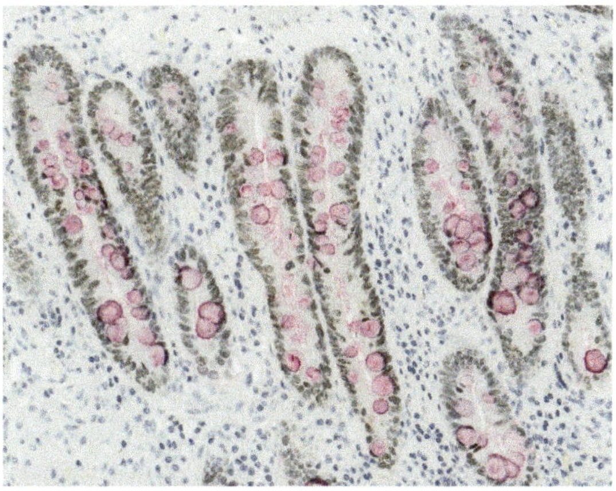

Intestinal Metaplasia, Fig. 3 Intestinal metaplasia glands with MUC2 mucin expression in the goblet cells (*red*) and CDX2 expression in the nuclei of all cells (*brown*)

antibodies stain all types of IM and do not stain the normal gastric mucosa (Fig. 2). In addition, double staining for MUC2 and for the gastric mucin MUC5AC allows the subtyping of IM into incomplete, whenever both mucins are present, or complete when only MUC2 is expressed.

Molecular Features

The most prominent molecular feature of gastric IM is the expression of intestinal proteins, which, in many cases, can be detected using antibodies. CDX2 is an early marker of this intestinal transdifferentiation, as well as many of its targets, particularly MUC2, LI-cadherin, sucrase-isomaltase, carbonic anhydrase, lactase, alkaline phosphatase, and villin. Mucin glycans are also modified in gastric IM. The Sialyl-Tn antigen, a carbohydrate structure normally expressed in intestinal mucosa, is aberrantly expressed in goblet cells of IM. In addition, IM also shows abnormal expression of Lewis antigens, namely, increased expression of Le^a and de novo expression of Sialyl-Le^a. Trefoil peptides are other tissue differentiation markers often modified in IM. Decreased expression of the trefoil peptide pS2 (TFF1) and increased expression of the intestinal trefoil factor (TFF3) have been consistently described in these lesions (Mesquita et al. 2006).

Differential Diagnosis

Gastric IM is a lesion very well defined morphologically. Differential diagnosis of IM is applied to distinguish between IM, particularly when it is hyperproliferative, from low-grade dysplasia.

References and Further Reading

Capelle, L. G., de Vries, A. C., Haringsma, J., Ter Borg, F., de Vries, R. A., Bruno, M. J., van Dekken, H., Meijer, J., van Grieken, N. C., & Kuipers, E. J. (2010). The staging of gastritis with the OLGA system by using intestinal metaplasia as an accurate alternative for atrophic gastritis. *Gastrointestinal Endoscopy, 71*, 1150–1158.

Correa, P., Piazuelo, M. B., & Wilson, K. T. (2010). Pathology of gastric intestinal metaplasia: Clinical implications. *American Journal of Gastroenterology, 105*, 493–498.

de Vries, A. C., van Grieken, N. C., Looman, C. W., Casparie, M. K., de Vries, E., Meijer, G. A., & Kuipers, E. J. (2008). Gastric cancer risk in patients with premalignant gastric lesions: A nationwide cohort study in the Netherlands. *Gastroenterology, 134*, 945–952.

Mesquita, P., Almeida, R., Lunet, N., Reis, C. A., Silva, L. F., Serpa, J., Van Seuningen, I., Barros, H., & David, L. (2006). Metaplasia–a transdifferentiation process that facilitates cancer development: The model of gastric intestinal metaplasia. *Critical Reviews in Oncogenesis, 12*, 3–26.

Reis, C. A., David, L., Correa, P., Carneiro, F., de Bolós, C., Garcia, E., Mandel, U., Clausen, H., & Sobrinho-Simões, M. (1999). Intestinal metaplasia of human stomach displays distinct patterns of mucin (MUC1, MUC2, MUC5AC, and MUC6) expression. *Cancer Research, 59*, 1003–1007.

Uemura, N., Okamoto, S., Yamamoto, S., Matsumura, N., Yamaguchi, S., Yamakido, M., Taniyama, K., Sasaki, N., & Schlemper, R. J. (2001). *Helicobacter pylori* infection and the development of gastric cancer. *The New England Journal of Medicine, 345*, 784–789.

Intestinal Obstruction

Maria Sotiropoulou
Department of Pathology, Alexandra Hospital, Athens, Attica, Greece

Synonyms

Bowel obstruction; Ileus

Definition

Intestinal obstruction is a partial or complete mechanical blockage of the bowel that prevents the contents, food, and fluid from passing through the intestinal lumen. The most common cause of mechanical intestinal obstruction in industrialized countries is scar tissue – intra-abdominal adhesions – from previous operations and accounts for approximately 65–75% of cases. Other causes include foreign bodies (items that were eaten), rarely gallstones, hernias (portion of intestine protruding into a structure or muscle), intussusception where a part of bowel telescopes and is trapped by an adjacent portion of the intestine. Other causes are bowel tumors or external tumors, inflammatory bowel disease such as Crohn's disease and twisted intestine called volvulus. Impairs of venous drainage or arterial flow caused by colon twist on its mesentery is the mechanism of obstruction in volvulus.

The leading cause of small bowel obstruction is the postoperative adhesions (60%), followed by malignancies, Crohn's disease, and hernias. Lower abdominal and pelvic surgery such as colorectal surgery, gynecologic surgery, hernia repair, and appendectomy lead to obstruction, more often than upper gastrointestinal surgeries. The risk of obstruction ranges from 1–10% after appendicectomy to 17–25% after restorative proctocolectomy. In large bowel, repetitive episodes of diverticulitis cause muscular hypertrophy and subsequent fibrosis and thickening of the colonic wall, leading to narrowing. The most common causes in pediatric cases are congenital atresia (imperforate anus) and intussusceptions. Of the latter, which mainly occurs in pediatric patients, 5–16% in the western world (2/3 are caused by tumors) occurs in adults as well Luminal obstructions may be endogenous in origin such as meconium in infants and rare in older children or even adults with cystic fibrosis. Meconium is tenacious and liable from abnormally viscid mucus due to decreased fluid and increased chloride iron secretion. The obstruction in these cases is in mid or terminal ileum. Gallstone ileus is a disease of adults and often elderly women. 1–2% of small intestine obstructions occur due to gallstones that enter the small intestine lumen through a cholecystoduodenal fistula or in rare cases due to a small stone that passes the biliary tree and may grow within intestinal lumen (enterolith) until it reaches the size that can cause obstruction.

The complete obstruction or a strangulated a surgical emergency. Small bowel obstruction leads to proximal dilatation with subsequent more than usual fluid accumulation by stimulation of cell secretory activity. The pathogenesis of obstructive ileitis additionally to a mechanism similar to that of obstructive colitis includes also a functional disorder of the ileocecal valve, due to tumor. Failure of the valve's functionality leads to ischemia, bacterial overgrowth, and deep ulceration by regurgitation of the contents and dilatation of the lumen. The bowel distention leads to increased intraluminal pressure and lymphedema by compression of mucosal lymphatics. Increased hydrostatic pressure in the capillary network is caused by higher intraluminal hydrostatic pressure. The concurrent distension (by adhesions) and twisting of the bowel on its mesenteric pedicle leads to strangulation with arterial occlusions and subsequent bowel ischemia and necrosis. In addition, the dilated intestinal lumen may cause vasospasm causing nonocclusive mesenteric ischemia. The possible reason for the higher incidence of obstruction on the left side, than on the right, is the relatively smaller caliber of the left segment.

Clinical Features

- **Incidence**
  Malignancies are the most common cause of colonic obstruction (about 60%) followed by diverticular disease (20%) and volvulus (5%). Colorectal cancer causes intestinal obstruction in 7–29% of patients.
- **Age**
  Bowel obstruction can affect individuals of any age, and different conditions occur with higher percentages in certain age groups.
- **Sex**
  The proportion of male and female is close to each other, and is 1.2:1.

- **Site**
  Small bowel is more commonly affected than large bowel (75% vs. 25%, respectively). If the reason of the obstruction is a malignant tumor, the incidence is 61% in the small bowel and 33% in large bowel. Left colon is affected more commonly than the right.
- **Treatment**
  Surgical intervention is the treatment of choice in acute intestinal obstruction because of the mechanical nature of the disease. In selected patients, conservative therapy is still considered in cases of incomplete adhesive obstruction, because some adhesions loosen up and the bowel lumen will open. Radiologic imaging of small bowel allows to discriminate between cases that can be treated conservatively and obstructions that are surgical emergencies. However, conservative therapy may increase the rate of strangulation, the risk of intestinal necrosis, and perforation. When surgery is performed, the cause of obstruction is removed with lysis of adhesions or excision of the damaged bowel. Small bowel obstruction cases due to peritoneal carcinogenesis, Crohn's disease, or sclerosing peritonitis are typically treated conservatively. In fetal and neonatal bowel obstruction, where the cause is intestinal atresia, the treatment is laparotomy and removing the damaged portion.
- **Outcome**
  Incomplete obstruction with early diagnosis and treatment has good prognosis, whereas complete obstruction, if treated conservatively, has a higher incidence of recurrence than if treated with an operation. If surgery is performed within 36 hours, the mortality is low (8%), while untreated strangulated obstruction is fatal in 100% of patients.

Macroscopy

Obstructive ileocolitis is an ulcerative and inflammatory lesion that occurs proximal to the obstruction from which it is separated by a variable length of normal mucosa. The lesion measures 0.5–2.5 cm. in length and is separated from the obstructed area by 2.5–35 cm. The changes vary and depend on the duration of obstruction. The lesions in obstructive colitis are erosions, shallow ulcers, and pseudopolyps, that may have a patchy distribution and must be distinguished from inflammatory bowel disease in cases of slowly developing lesions that are confined to the mucosa or submucosa. Rapidly developing lesions develop in the right colon and range from ulcers to fulminant colitis and necrosis. On the contrary, obstructive ileitis's ulcer may be deeply penetrating into the subserosal layer and occasionally perforating.

I

Microscopy

Obstructive colitis or ileitis refers to ischemic or gangrenous colitis or ileitis proximal to an obstructive colorectal lesion. Biopsy of obstructive colitis is not specific and has similar features with other disorders, particularly ischemia. The histologic changes are those of ischemic colitis with most common microscopic findings the necrosis of the mucosa with denudation of epithelial cells, hemorrhage, congestion, and prominent neutrophilic infiltration (Fig. 1).

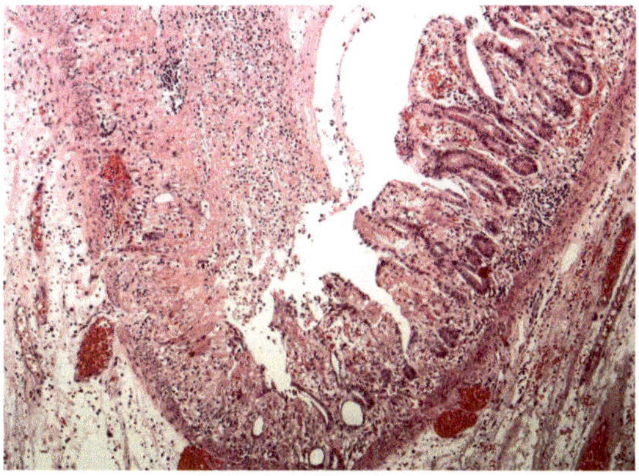

Intestinal Obstruction, Fig. 1 Gangrenous ileitis due to obstruction by hernia: part of the small bowel is completly necrotic with coagulative necrosis

Immunophenotype

There are not any specific immunohistochemical stains in intestinal obstruction.

Molecular Features

There are not any specific molecular features.

Differential Diagnosis

Intestinal pseudo-obstruction due to neuromuscular abnormalities is the main differential diagnosis. Among the latter, Hirschsprung disease can resemble colonic obstruction.

References and Further Reading

Cappell, M. S., & Bakke, M. (2008). Mechanical obstruction of the small bowel and colon. *The Medical Clinics of North America, 92*(3), 575–597.

Kahi, C. J., & Rex, D. K. (2003). Bowel obstruction and pseudo-obstruction. *Gastroenterology Clinics of North America, 32*(4), 1229–1247.

Khaikin, M., Schneidereit, N., Cera, S., et al. (2007). Laparoscopic vs open surgery for acute adhesive small bowel obstruction: Patients outcome and cost effectiveness. *Surgical Endoscopy, 21*(5), 742–746.

Morson, B. C., & Shepherd, N. A. (2003). *Morson and Dawson's gastrointestinal pathology* (4th ed., pp. 544–545). Hoboken: Blackwell.

Turnage, R. H., & Heldmann, M. (2010). Intestinal obstruction. In *Sleisenger and Fordtran's gastrointestinal and liver disease* (9th ed.). Philadelphia: Saunders Elsevier. Chap 119.

Intestinal Pseudo-Obstruction

Maria Sotiropoulou
Department of Pathology, Alexandra Hospital, Athens, Attica, Greece

Synonyms

Paralytic ileus

Definition

Intestinal pseudo-obstruction describes a syndrome in which the clinical presentation of mechanical obstruction occurs in the absence of any obvious reason. This can affect the colon or small bowel and based on clinical presentation is divided into acute and chronic. Acute colonic pseudo-obstruction appears with symptoms, signs, and radiologic findings similar to those of mechanical intestinal obstruction. Ogilvie, who described in 1948 two cases of massive colonic dilatation without mechanical obstacle and with malignant infiltration of the celiac axis and semilunar ganglion, concluded that the condition is an imbalance in the autonomic nerve supply. The clinical picture of the patients with pseudo-obstruction, despite etiology, is the same with that observed in intestinal obstruction.

Acute colonic pseudo-obstruction usually develops in elderly, hospitalized patients with a variety of problems such as neurological diseases, cardiac failure, chronic alcoholism, and malignancy. In general, the most common conditions in patients with pseudo-obstruction include trauma, burns, pregnancy, or cesarean delivery and severe conditions. The cardiothoracic, orthopedic, or pelvic surgery are common causes.

The pathophysiology of intestinal pseudo-obstruction remains unknown. The theory of an imbalance in the autonomic nervous system is in power, but new theories focus on the increased sympathetic and decreased parasympathetic tone or a combination. The increase of sympathetic tone leads to inhibition of colonic motility. This theory is supported by the successful treatment of patients by using epidural anesthesia to block the splanchnic sympathetic. Distally to the splenic flexure, the parasympathetic innervation is via the lumbar nerves, so if the sacral innervations become disrupted, the colon may be atonic and this can result in colonic pseudo-obstruction. Pathophysiology of Ogilvie syndrome has been studied in rats. Mechanical stretch induces the expression of COX-2 which plays an important role in suppression muscle contractility. Changes in the autonomic nervous function are produced by arrest of stimulation of the splanchnic sympathetic system or from damage to cholinergic fibers, due to surgical manipulation of the mesentery. Cofactors are electrolytic imbalance and anesthetic agents. In acute peritonitis, toxins absorbed through the peritoneal surface and anoxia due to vascular stasis lead to muscle disfunction.

Symptoms in acute colonic pseudo-obstruction are similar to acute mechanical obstruction and perforation, usually of the cecum.

Chronic colonic pseudo-obstruction occurs secondary to underlying systemic disease and rarely is a primary disorder (Tables 1 and 2). Chronic constipation that leads to megacolon is its usual presentation, while perforation is rare.

Intestinal Pseudo-Obstruction, Table 1 Idiopathic chronic intestinal pseudo-obstruction

Myopathic forms	Familiar visceral myopathy, sporadic visceral myopathy
Neuropathic forms	Familiar visceral neuropathies, sporadic visceral neuropathies, developmental abnormalities (Hirschsprung's disease, etc.)
Disorders of interstitial cells of Cajal	With visceral myopathy-type changes or without
Disorders of neurohormonal peptides	

Intestinal Pseudo-Obstruction, Table 2 Secondary chronic intestinal pseudo-obstruction

Systemic disorders	Progressive systemic sclerosis, SLE, etc.
Endocrine and metabolic disorders	Diabetes mellitus, hypothyroidism, etc.
Infiltrative disorders	Amyloidosis, diffuse lymphoid infiltrate, etc.
Paraneoplastic	Small cell carcinoma, etc.
Infections	Chagas disease, herpes virus, etc.
Miscellaneous	Ceroidosis, small intestine diverticulosis, etc.
Toxins and pharmacologic agents	Antidepressants, opiates, etc.

Clinical Features

- **Incidence**
  Acute colonic pseudo-obstruction occurs in 0.65–1.3% of patients undergoing orthopedic surgery, but the true incidence remains unknown, because of possibility of spontaneous resolution. 95% of the cases of acute colonic pseudo-obstruction occur due to medical or surgical conditions and only 5% are idiopathic.
- **Age**
  Most recent reports indicate that the intestinal pseudo-obstruction occurs in the seventh or eighth decade of life in contrast to the late 1980s, in which the mean age was the sixth decade.
- **Sex**
  The male to female ratio is 1.5/4.1.
- **Treatment**
  Conservative management may be attempted, if there are no signs of peritonitis or abdominal distention. Sometimes, repeated colonoscopic decompression is effective in 85% of the patients. If an operation is performed, the tube cecostomy is the procedure of choice with right colectomy as the alternative treatment in case of perforation or ischemia. An urgent laparotomy is indicated, if signs and symptoms of colonic ischemia or perforation are present, or if colonoscopy confirms ischemia. Secondary chronic intestinal pseudo-obstruction is managed by treating the underlying condition.
- **Outcome**
  Acute colonic pseudo-obstruction can recur. Recurrent or persistent colonic distension may cause ischemia or perforation. The mortality rate is 14% with conservative management and 30% with the surgical one. Evidence of poor prognosis-perforation is a distended cecum with a diameter more than 14 cm, delay in colonic decompression, and advanced age.

Macroscopy (Gross)

In familiar disorders, where there is atrophy of the colonic muscle, the intestine is dilated with a thin wall. In acquired muscle disorders, as scleroderma, there are large multiple sacculations in the antimesenteric border due to patchy fibrosis. The colonic innervation leads (not always) to hypertrophy of the colonic smooth muscle in a dilated megacolon, and on the other hand, drugs and toxins cause neurologic lesions which are accompanied by atrophy of the smooth muscle (megacolon with thin wall). Secondary due to stasis and extensive dilatation, the colon may have inflammation, ulceration, and ischemia.

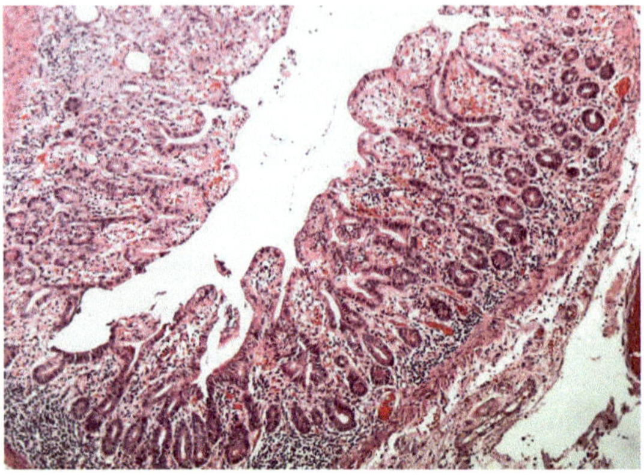

Intestinal Pseudo-Obstruction, Fig. 1 Intestinal pseudo-obstruction with features similar to ischemia due to intramural pressure: capillary congestion, loss of epithelium of the villi focally, and regenerative lesions

Microscopy

When the cause of intestinal pseudo-obstruction is a smooth muscle disorder, such as familiar visceral myopathy, the muscularis mucosa or muscularis propria are degenerated with nuclear enlargement, pleomorphism, increased mitotic figures, and a characteristic cytoplasmic vacuolation which is periodic acid stain (PAS) positive. At an early stage, fibrosis is not easily recognizable, so a trichrome stain can be helpful. Ultrastructurally, intracytoplasmic inclusions represent aggregates of degenerated myofibrils. In electron microscopy, mitochondrial vacuolation may be the only diagnostic feature. In final stage, there is progression to fibrosis and complete fibrous replacement of both muscular coats. The longitudinal layer tends to be more severely involved. In acquired damage of smooth muscle, as in dermatomyositis or scleroderma, the muscle coats are replaced patchily by collagen and elastic fibers. In advanced stage, fibrosis is diffuse with results in obliteration of the bowel. The difference from familiar conditions is the cytoplasmic vacuolation of the muscle fibers. Sometimes, arteries show lesions as such intimal proliferation, elastosis, and narrow lumen.

The surprising feature in myotonic dystrophy and progressive muscular dystrophy is the lymphocytic infiltration of the muscularis mucosa. When the cause is an infective agent as in Chagas disease, there is inflammatory reaction consisting of lymphocytes and plasma cells with destruction of the myenteric plexus, neuronal loss, and often Schwann cell hyperplasia with consequent smooth muscle hypertrophy. In paraneoplastic syndromes, the key finding in the diagnosis is the presence of numerous lymphoid cells and plasma cells within the myenteric plexus.

In acute intestinal pseudo-obstruction (paralytic ileus), no specific histopathologic changes are recognized and the picture mimics ischemia secondary to increased intramural pressure (Fig. 1).

Immunophenotype

Immunohistochemical markers which may be helpful in neuropathic forms of chronic intestinal pseudo-obstruction are VIP, substance P-related tachykinins, nitric oxide synthase, neuropeptide Y, calcitonin gene-related peptide, and Bcl-2. These markers cannot differentiate primary from secondary changes. Increased neural apoptosis revealed by Bcl-2 supports the idea of neuropathic changes. In cases of interstitial cells of Cajal abnormalities, loss of normally C-kit-positive cells or abnormal network is diagnostic, although difficult to estimate on formalin-fixed tissue.

Molecular Studies

Many genes have been indentified in syndromic forms of intestinal pseudo-obstruction including thymidine phosphorylase (endothelial cell growth factor-1), DNA polymerase gamma gene, and SOX10 (transcription factor). Decreased Bcl-2 gene product in some cases provokes decreased ganglion cell survival.

Differential Diagnosis

Intestinal obstruction acute or chronic due to mechanical reason is the main differential diagnosis. Ischemia from intestinal infarction can have some similar features.

References and Further Reading

Amiot, A., Cazals-Hatem, D., Joly, F., et al. (2009). The role of immunohistochemistry in idiopathic Chronic Intestinal Pseudo-Obstruction (CIPO): A case-control study. *The American Journal of Surgical Pathology, 33*(5), 749–758.

Antonucci, A., Fronzoni, L., Cogliadro, L., et al. (2008). Chronic intestinal pseudo-obstruction. *World Journal of Gastroenterology, 14*(19), 2953–2961.

Day, D. W., & Morson, B. C. (2003). *Morson and Dawson's gastrointestinal pathology* (4th ed., pp. 451–464). Malden: Blackwell.

Saunders, M. D., & Kimmey, M. B. (2005). Systemic review: Acute colonic pseudo-obstruction. *Alimentary Pharmacology & Therapeutics, 22*, 917–925.

Stranghellini, V., Cogliandro, R. F., De Giorgio, R., et al. (2005). Natural history of chronic idiopathic intestinal pseudo-obstruction in adults. A single centre study. *Clinical Gastroenterology and Hepatology, 3*, 449–458.

Intestinal Tuberculosis

Andrzej Mróz
Department of Gastroenterology and Hepatology, Histopathology Unit, Medical Center for Postgraduate Education, Warsaw, Poland

Synonyms

Intestinal caseating granulomas disease

Definition

Intestinal manifestation of tuberculosis, infectious disease caused by *Mycobacterium* species mainly *Mycobacterium tuberculosis*. Most of the cases represents secondary spread of pulmonary tuberculosis via swallowing of infected sputum, hematogenous, spread or direct extension from adjacent structures. Ileocaecal and jejunoileal segments are most commonly involved sites followed by duodenal, appendiceal, and anal/perianal sites. Peritoneal tuberculosis may be the case in substantial number of patients with ascites and clinically relevant adhesions. In rare cases, intestinal tuberculosis may be primary due to ingestion of infected milk from contaminated cows. This situation may take place in countries where milk pasteurization is not performed. Apart from intestines, primary tuberculosis may also localize in oral mucosa and tonsils. In these cases, *Mycobacterium bovis* species must be taken into account. Extrapulmonary localization is also more prevalent in immunocompromised AIDS patients. These patients present with *Mycobacterium avium-intracellulare* species infection.

Intestinal tuberculosis involves intestinal wall and regional lymph nodes. Lymph nodes may undergo caseous necrosis and be fixed in groups (tabes mesarrhaica). Clinical features of intestinal tuberculosis include: weight loss, fever, abdominal pain, diarrhea, and palpable abdominal mass. It is commonly accompanied by night sweats, malaise, anorexia, GI bleeding, and malabsorption.

Clinical Features

- **Incidence**
  Incidence of intestinal tuberculosis in developed countries is on the rise due to AIDS epidemic and increasing number of immunocompromised persons. Tuberculosis occurs also endemically in Asia and Africa regions. In addition to HIV-positive patients, homeless, incarcerated, alcoholics, people of poor socioeconomic standard also have the increased rate of infection. The incidence rate of intestinal

tuberculosis varies between 1.6% and 5% of pulmonary tuberculosis cases (up to 24% in advanced generalized tuberculosis). The risk of developing tuberculosis in HIV-positive patients is 5–10% per year. (Specific data for intestinal tuberculosis in these patients are not given.)

- **Age**
  In some series, peak incidence of intestinal tuberculosis occurs between 20 and 40 years of age. In general, morbidity is rather connected with living conditions and immune competency.
- **Sex**
  No evident sex predilection is reported. Blacks and Asians are more prone to develop tuberculosis.
- **Site**
  Ileocecal region in 90% of cases followed by ascending colon, appendix, jejunum, duodenum, sigmoid, and rectum. Peritoneal secondary tuberculosis is more common than intestinal tuberculosis.
- **Treatment**
  Long-lasting antimicrobial therapy is the treatment of choice in patients with intestinal tuberculosis. Surgical treatment is needed in case of complications – mainly obstruction, perforation, or fistula formation.
- **Outcome**
  Complications: severe enterocolitis, hemorrhage, perforation, obstruction, fistula formation, strictures, malabsorption, and severe secretory diarrhea due to bacterial overgrowth.

Macroscopy

Strictures and ulcers (or combination of both) are the most common findings. Ulcers are usually circumferential and located perpendicularly to intestinal axis. Mucosal folds may be thickened. Ileocaecal valve is often deformed and gaping. The wall is thickened, fibrotic, and strictured. The lesions may be segmental with skip areas mimicking Crohn's disease. The inflammatory lesions may form masses called "tuberculomas."

Macroscopically three forms of intestinal tuberculosis occur:

- Ulcerative form (60% of cases): multiple superficial ulcers
- Hypertrophic form (10%): mimics Crohn' disease and includes scarring, fibrosis, and mass lesion formation
- Ulcero-hypertrophic form (30%): intestinal wall is thickened and ulcerated, inflammatory mass is concentrated around ileocecal valve mimicking malignancy.

Endoscopic and gross view of ileocecal tuberculosis is presented in Figs. 1 and 2.

Mycobacterium avium-intracellulare (MAI) infections: endoscopy may be normal, 2–4 mm raised granular white mucosal nodules with reddish rim, ulcers and hemorrhages may also be present, mesenteric lymph nodes are enlarged, firm, solid, with foci of necrosis.

Microscopy

The wall of the bowel is thickened and edematous. Chronic inflammation may be present in all layers of intestines, typically lymphoid hyperplasia develops in later stages of the disease as also the wall fibrosis does.

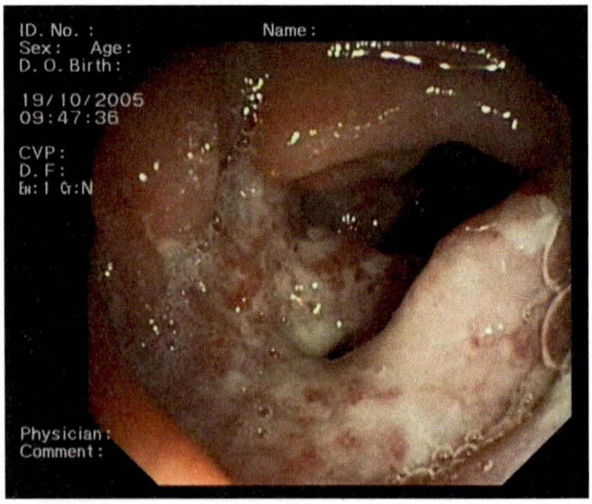

Intestinal Tuberculosis, Fig. 1 Ileocaecal tuberculosis – endoscopic view (Courtesy of dr Pachlewski from my department)

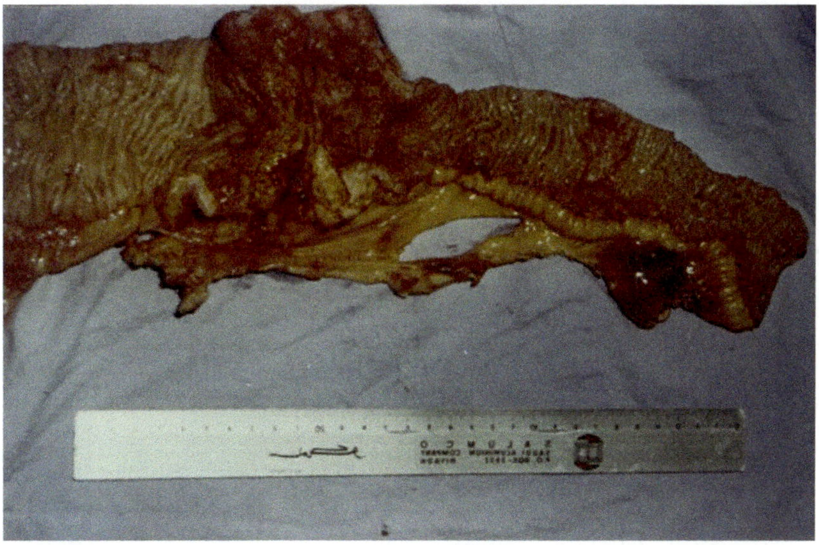

Intestinal Tuberculosis, Fig. 2 Ileocaecal tuberculosis causing ulcero-vegetant mass (Courtesy of prof. Ensari form Department of Pathology, Univeristy of Ankara)

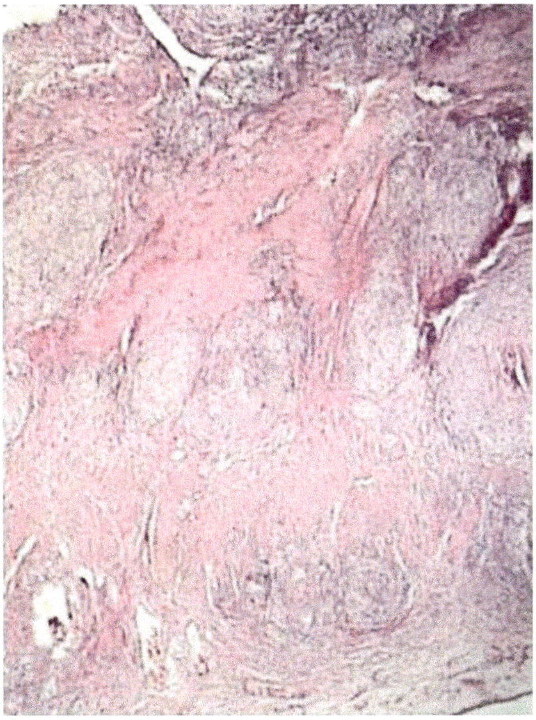

Intestinal Tuberculosis, Fig. 3 Multiple granulomas throughout the bowel wall (H&E; ×100) (Courtesy of prof. Ensari form Department of Pathology, Univeristy of Ankara)

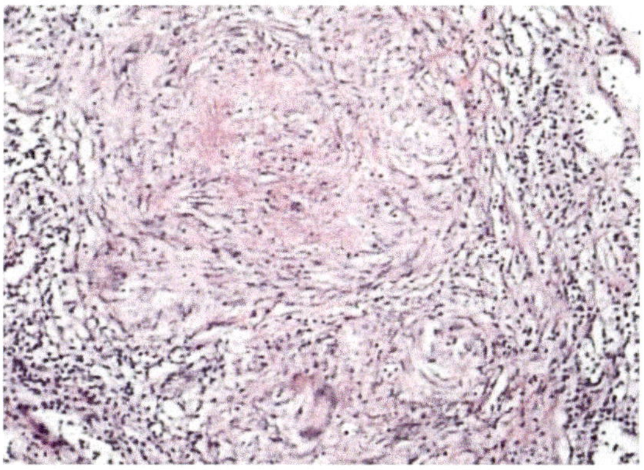

Intestinal Tuberculosis, Fig. 4 A caseating granuloma with Langhans type giant cell (H&E; ×200) (Courtesy of prof. Ensari form Department of Pathology, Univeristy of Ankara)

Ulcers are situated perpendicularly to long axis of the intestine, they may be superficial or deep. The necrotic area may overlie the Peyer's patches giving pattern of aphthoid ulcers.

The most characteristic feature of intestinal tuberculosis is the caseating granuloma. Granulomas may be isolated or confluent and are found in all layers of the wall, with submucosa being the most common location (Figs. 3 and 4). The lymphocytic rim at the periphery of the granuloma is sometimes present, giant cells may occur. As granuloma gets older it hyalinizes and calcifies to the extent it can be hardly spotted. Even though tuberculosis connects with granulomas, they may be also present in other intestinal conditions like

Intestinal Tuberculosis, Table 1 Comparison of histological features in differentiation of *M. tuberculosis*, *Yersinia*, and Crohn's disease (Taken from reference 2 with changes)

	M. tuberculosis	Yersinia	Crohn's disease
Caseating granulomas	Frequent	Rare	Absent
Confluent granulomas	Frequent	Frequent	Absent
Numerous granulomas	Common	Common	Rare
Lymphoid rim	Frequent	Frequent	Uncommon
Lymphoid hyperplasia	Common	Very common	Uncommon
Ulcers (deep and aphthous)	Common	Common	Common
Architectural distortion	May be present	May be present	Common
Chronic mucosal changes away from granulomas	Absent	Absent	Common
Multiple sites of involvement	Common	Rare	Common
Mucosal cobblestoning	Uncommon	Uncommon	Common
Fistulas	Uncommon	Rare	Common
Anal/perianal disease	Rare	Absent	Common

sarcoidosis, Crohn's disease, tularemia, yersiniosis, schistosomiasis, foreign bodies, malakoplakia, and others. Classical granulomas are also present in lymph nodes.

The mucosa between the ulcers is somewhat edematous and hemorrhagic, but in contrast to inflammatory bowel disease, the architecture of the crypts is usually well preserved. The slight architectural distortion may be however present in areas above caseating granulomas.

Acid-fast stains (mainly Ziehl-Neelsen stain) are used to show bacilli of *M. tuberculosis* mainly within necrotic areas or macrophages. These organisms are rod-shaped and have beaded morphology. They are usually numerous in immunocompromised patients, while in immunocompetent individuals, they may be very few and hardly detectable. Anti-tubercular therapy decreases the number of bacilli. PCR methods may be helpful but are also dependent on number of organisms. Microorganisms culturing remains the gold standard in diagnosis but is both time consuming and expensive.

MAI infection: in immunocompetent patients, typical granulomas are formed.

In immunocompromised patients, villi are distended and the diffuse infiltration of macrophages containing bacilli occurs. Such collections cause just sparse reactive inflammation. Bacilli stain with acid-fast stains and with PAS and GMS stains.

Differential Diagnosis

All entities with granuloma formation may enter the differential diagnosis, but in real clinical setting, yersiniosis and Crohn's disease are sometimes very difficult to differentiate from tuberculosis. Ulcers in Crohn's disease are linear not circumferential, deep fissures and fistulas may be present, and mucosal changes of chronic type away from ulcers and granulomas are also present. Yersinia granulomas are not usually caseating, and lymph aggregates may have collections of neutrophils in their centers. The following table summarizes histological features which may be of help in differentiating intestinal tuberculosis from yersiniosis and Crohn's disease (Table 1).

MAI infections require differentiation from Whipple's disease. Acid-fast stains and PCR assays may add in distinguishing mycobacterial infections from *T. whippeli*.

References and Further Reading

Fenoglio-Preiser, C., et al. (1999). *Gastrointestinal pathology plus: An atlas and text.* Philadelphia: Lippincott Willialms & Wilkins.

Lamps L. (2009). *Surgical pathology of the gastrointestinal system: bacterial, fungal, viral, and parasitic infections*. Springer Science+Business Media.

Rolo, R., Campainha, S., & Duarte, R. (2012). Crohn's disease and intestinal tuberculosis: A clinical challenge. *Revista Portuguesa de Pneumologia, 18*(04), 205–206.

Intussusception

Gabriel Becheanu
Department of Pathology, Fundeni Clinical Institute, Carol Davila University of Medicine and Pharmacy, Bucharest, Romania

Synonyms

Infolding; Introversion; Invagination

Definition

Intussusception occurs when a part of the intestine (*intussusceptum*) telescopes or is invaginated into the distal segment (*intussuscipiens*) and drags the mesentery with it. It was first described in 1674 by Barbette and was first treated successfully by surgery in 1831. This condition represents one of the four major causes of obstruction: herniation, adhesion, volvulus, and intussusception. Usually, in children, invagination is idiopathic, but there are a lot of points of traction that can determine invagination of the bowel segments like tumors or different intraluminal masses. In adults, intussusception in the small bowel generally has as a lead point a benign or inflammatory lesion, while that occurring in the large bowel is more likely of malignant etiology.

Alteration of intestinal motility (hyperperistalsis; irregular, retrograde, or reduced peristalsis) is considered to be responsible for intussusception in some cases. The primary symptoms include abdominal pain and vomiting.

Clinical Features

- **Incidence**
  Intussusception represents one of the most common causes of obstruction in children and toddlers, with an incidence of 2,000 infants in the first year of life, in the United States, that peaks between 4 and 9 months of age. Some authors suggest that seasonal gastroenteritis appears to have important roles in a seasonal incidence with a peak in spring, summer, and middle of the winter, but ecological studies indicate no correlation in the Unites States. In West Africa, cecocolic intussusception appears to be the most common form of invagination.
- **Age**
  Intussusception is usually present in infants and little children (2/3 younger than 1 year), while in adults, it represents only approximately 1% of the cases of intestinal obstruction; in the latter age group, a tumoral mass is the most common lead point.
- **Sex**
  It is more frequent in male than in female infants with a score of 3:1, and in older children (over 4 years old), the incidence is even higher for males, with a ratio of 8:1. In adults, a male preponderance has also been usually observed.
- **Site**
  Most of the cases (80–90%) are ileo-colic intussusception, usually in children, followed by ileo-ileal, colo-colic, ileo-ileo-colic, and sigmoido-rectal sites. Jejunal intussusceptions are rare, described in children, and commonly related to an anatomical malformation. Appendiceal intussusception occurs mostly in childhood, and different predisposing factors and lesions have been described. According to the segments of invagination, a few related types of appendiceal intussusception have been described: distal apex invagination, proximal apex invagination, base in cecum, or entire appendix.

  Rectal prolapse through the anal sphincter, considered an antegrade intussusception of the rectal wall, mainly presents in 1–3 year old children and elderly nulliparous women.

  Gastroduodenal intussusception is by far very rare, usually related to a tumoral mass.

  Typically intussusception is the distal propulsion of the invaginated segment, but retrograde intussusception has also been described.
- **Treatment**
  Barium intake may reduce intussusception in infants and young children, while older

patients usually require surgical treatment. Evidence of intestinal perforation represents a contraindication of bowel enema. The intussusception can spontaneously resolve in children.

- **Outcome**
  Untreated, the intussusception may progress to vascular obstruction, ischemia, and subsequent bowel infarction with necrosis of the bowel wall, 10% of surgery-treated patients requiring intestinal resection because of irreversible damage to these structures. The final stage is perforation of the bowel and sepsis, followed by death in 2–5 days. For these reasons, intussusception should be considered an emergency and treated as rapidly as possible in order to avoid ischemia of the intestinal mucosa and progression to perforation.

Macroscopy

Approximately 10% of intussusceptions have an anatomic lead point – a piece of bowel tissue that draws the proximal part inward, to be further propelled by peristalsis into the immediately distal part of the intestine. In older children and adults, the presence of an intraluminal mass or tumor is responsible as background for intussusception. Sometimes hypertrophied Peyer's patches, a consequence of viral infections (adenovirus or rotavirus), are considered to be involved in this condition. The key points (lead points) where the intussusception process starts could be represented by: Meckel's diverticulum, Peutz-Jeghers polyps or other intestinal polyps, intestinal duplication, adhesions, surgical scars, meconium, tumor masses (lymphomas, hemangioma, sarcoma), tuberculosis, endometriosis, heterotopic pancreas. Invagination could also appear associated with pain and melena in Henoch-Schönlein purpura due to the development of submucosal hematoma usually in the small bowel. In cystic fibrosis, an adherent, inspissated bowel content was described to be responsible for an increased incidence of intussusceptions. In children, the invagination could also be determined by an adherent bolus of ingested material (bezoars).

On macroscopy, the longitudinal section through the specimen reveals three layers: *intussuscipiens* wall, and entering and returning layers of the *intussusceptum* part which appears edematous and enlarged; congestion of the blood vessels on the serosal surface and black areas of infarction may be present. Cut sections may show pus or fecal material (sometimes calcified) in the lumen and a polypoid or tumoral mass, when present.

Microscopy

In the incipient stage of intussusception, the intestinal mucosa shows edema secondary to vascular obstruction, but continuous obstruction of arterial flow leads to ischemia with acute inflammatory changes and hemorrhagic necrosis. Histological features of intestinal prolapse can also be present with smooth muscle proliferation, fibrosis, and chronic inflammatory infiltrate. The position of the mucosal layers is changed with the mucosa in the external layer and muscularis in the internal part. The lamina propria in appendiceal intussusception can be obliterated by follicular hyperplasia with reactive germinative centers.

The apex of the *intussusceptum* should be carefully examined in order to find the lead point and to exclude a tumoral mass.

Molecular Features

A genetic predisposition with a familial anatomical tendency has been described by a study conducted in Japan. Other studies discovered an infiltration with CD3 positive lymphocytes in the nervous plexus of children with adenovirus infection as a possible mechanism involved in the pathophysiology of ileo-cecal intussusception associated with this disease. A research by Cserni and colleagues revealed that the inflammatory reactions that precede intussusception may lead to an increased production of nitric oxide (NO) and nitrergic neurons which may be followed by relaxation of the ileo-cecal valve, thus favoring invagination.

Differential Diagnosis

Different entities should be considered for a differential diagnosis of intussusception, most of them being causes of intestinal obstruction: hernia, volvulus, intestinal duplication, inflammatory diseases, appendicitis, polypoid lesions, and rectal prolapse.

References and Further Reading

Cserni, T., Paran, S., & Puri, P. (2007). New hypothesis on the pathogenesis of ileocecal intussusception. *Journal of Pediatric Surgery, 42*(9), 1515–1519.

Gayer, G., Zissin, R., Apter, S., Papa, M., & Hertz, M. (2002). Pictorial review: Adult intussusception–a CT diagnosis. *British Journal of Radiology, 75*(890), 185–190.

Kaemmerer, E., Tischendorf, J. J., Steinau, G., Wagner, N., & Gassler, N. (2010). Ileocecal intussusception with histomorphological features of inflammatory neuropathy in adenovirus infection. *Gastroenterology Research and Practice, 2009*, 579501. doi:10.1155/2009/579501. Epub 2010 Feb 11.

Oshio, T., Ogata, H., Takano, S., & Ishibashi, H. (2007). Familial intussusception. *Journal of Pediatric Surgery, 42*(9), 1509–1514.

Ischemic Bowel Disease

Ann Driessen
Department of Pathology, University Hospital Antwerp, Edegem, Belgium
Maastricht University Medical Centre, Maastricht, The Netherlands

Synonyms

Intestinal ischemia

Definition

Ischemic bowel disease, which may affect whole or parts of the gastrointestinal tract, is due to an imbalance between the blood supply, which is decreased, and the metabolic demands of the gastrointestinal tract. Ischemic bowel disease rarely involves the esophagus or the stomach, but mainly affects the small intestine and the colon.

The gastrointestinal tract is nearly completely supplied by three arteries, namely the coeliac axis, the superior mesenteric artery, and the inferior mesenteric artery. The coeliac axis, originating from the anterior aortae, gives rise to three blood vessels: the left gastric artery, the splenic artery, and the common hepatic artery. The coeliac axis and its branches supply the distal part of the esophagus, the stomach, the liver, the proximal duodenum, and the pancreas.

The superior mesenteric artery nourishes the small intestine beginning from the distal duodenum, the head of the pancreas, and the ascending and the proximal two third of the transverse colon. The inferior mesenteric artery supplies the distal part of the transverse colon with the splenic flexure, descending colon, and sigmoid, and the superior rectal (hemorrhoidal) artery, branching from the inferior mesenteric artery, provides the rectum.

Due to the well-developed collateral blood circulation, ischemia is rare in the esophagus, the stomach, or duodenum. In contrast, ischemic events are more commonly situated distally, especially at the splenic flexure and sigmoid.

In quiescent phase, the gut receives 20–25% of the cardiac output, but postprandial, it may increase up to 35% of the cardiac output.

According to the American Association of Gastroenterology, intestinal ischemia can be classified into acute mesenteric ischemia, chronic mesenteric ischemia or intestinal angina, and ischemic colitis or colon ischemia. Ischemic colitis will be discussed separately.

Acute mesenteric ischemia (95% of cases) is mainly due to mesenteric arterial embolism (50%), but may also occur in order conditions namely non-occlusive mesenteric ischemia

(20–25%), mesenteric arterial thrombosis (10–25%), mesenteric venous thrombosis (5–10%), and focal segmental ischemia (5%). Emboli may have a cardiac origin, such as atrial fibrillation, a recent myocardial infarct with mural thrombus formation, valvular vegetations secondary to a bacterial endocarditis. Mesenteric arterial thrombosis is due to atherosclerosis, hypercoagulability, hypovolemia, shock, or vasculitis. Mesenteric arterial emboli and thrombi are frequently situated in the superior mesenteric artery.

Different conditions, namely, hematological conditions, hypercoagulable states, diseases associated with intra-abdominal inflammation and sepsis, a parasitic infection, or blunt abdominal trauma, are associated with mesenteric venous thrombosis.

In non-occlusive mesenteric ischemia, the intestinal infarction is not the result of an occlusion, but involves a low cardiac output, leading to a decreased perfusion with vasoconstriction of the splanchnic bed, due to cardiac disorders such as congestive heart failure, myocardial infarction, aorta insufficiency, or increased blood viscosity from dehydration or hematological disorders.

Acute mesenteric ischemia is associated with severe tissue damage and necrosis, which is not only related to the reduced blood supply, but also due to the reperfusion, inducing a decreased tissue oxygenation with increased microvascular permeability. Prolonged ischemia will cause a breakdown of the mucosal barrier with intestinal necrosis, ileus, sepsis, and multiorgan failure, possibly resulting in death of the patient.

Chronic mesenteric ischemia (5% of the cases) is caused by an occlusion of the mesenteric vessels, commonly due to arteriosclerosis (35–70%). Occlusion of a single vessel rarely causes symptoms, except in case the mesenteric arterial interconnections between the superior and inferior mesenteric artery are less well developed. Chronic mesenteric ischemia will become symptomatic in patients with multivessel involvement. Uncommon causes of chronic mesenteric ischemia are fibromuscular dysplasia, Buerger disease, and aortic dissection.

Acute or chronic intestinal ischemia may also be the result of a vascular injury of small blood vessels, namely, venules, arterioles, or capillaries, in the mucosa. This microvascular insufficiency is caused by different, uncommon diseases, such as amyloidosis, vasculitis, thrombotic thrombocytopenic purpura, and diabetes mellitus.

Independent of etiology, the damage in the bowel is due to a dysfunction of the microcirculation, causing a failure in supply of nutrients such as oxygen, with secondary a local inflammatory cell response with release of mediators. Loss of the epithelial integrity results in a bacterial translocation, causing a systemic inflammatory response with eventually organ failure at a distance. In order to restrict the extent of bowel infarction and hence to improve the prognosis of the patient, early diagnosis is necessary.

The diagnosis of acute mesenteric ischemia is difficult and requires a high index of suspicion of the clinician for early diagnosis. Due to the acute ischemia, patients will present with nonspecific symptoms, such as nausea, vomiting, diarrhea, vague central abdominal pain, and rectal blood loss. The symptoms differ in function of the cause of the ischemia. Patients with mesenteric ischemia due to emboli present with an abrupt onset of severe abdominal pain. In case of chronic atherosclerotic lesions, the patients will have symptoms, such as postprandial pain, food fear, and weight loss pointing toward intestinal angina. The disproportion between the severity of the abdominal pain and the physical findings must make the clinician aware of the possibility of mesenteric ischemia. No definitive diagnostic test is available. Laboratory tests are applied to evaluate the condition of the patient. Plain abdominal X-rays reveal nonspecific findings. Moreover, in approximately 25% of the patients, normal findings are found on plain abdominal X-rays. Doppler ultrasonography is a highly specific technique for detection of occlusions or severe stenosis of the splanchnic bed, but this method has no value in the detection of emboli or in diagnosing non-occlusive ischemic mesenteric ischemia. CT scan, which has a significant high sensitivity (96%) and specificity (94%), is the golden standard for diagnosing of mesenteric ischemia. This method is more adequate in the assessment of venous thrombi.

Mesenteric angiography is used to differentiate embolic from thrombotic arterial occlusions and to assess the narrowed and irregular major branches of the superior mesenteric arteries, characteristic for non-occlusive mesenteric ischemia.

Chronic mesenteric ischemia is a clinical diagnosis based on symptoms. If there is clinically a high suspicion for chronic mesenteric ischemia, patients should undergo a screening with duplex ultrasonography, CT, or MRA to visualize the mesenteric vessels and to identify significant stenoses.

Clinical Features

- **Incidence**
  Acute mesenteric ischemia is significantly more common than chronic mesenteric ischemia, with 1 in 1,000 hospital admissions. A Swedish study has shown that there is a significant difference in incidence of acute mesenteric ischemia (12.9/100,000 persons-years) compared to mesenteric venous thrombosis (2.7/100,000 persons-years). The etiology is mainly due to an acute occlusion of the superior mesenteric artery (67.2%), whereas a mesenteric venous thrombosis (15.7%) and non-occlusive mesenteric ischemia (15.4%) are significantly less common.

  In contrast to acute mesenteric ischemia, the incidence and prevalence of chronic mesenteric ischemia is difficult to determine. Although population-based studies have shown that the prevalence of chronic mesenteric occlusive disease varies between 1% and 8%, in which approximately 2% of the patients show arteriosclerotic lesions in more than one vessel, the majority of these patients are asymptomatic. Therefore, it is estimated that chronic mesenteric ischemia accounts for less than 1 per 100,000 hospital admissions, which is likely an underestimation.
- **Age**
  Acute mesenteric ischemia occurs in elderly with slight variation in age distribution according to the cause: arterial embolism median age 74 year (range 61–96), arterial thrombosis 74 year (range 45–91 year); venous thrombosis 65 year (43–85 year). Non-occlusive ischemia happens in young people and is mostly associated to drug-intake (e.g., cocaine) or related to an inherited disorder of lipid metabolism. Similar to acute mesenteric ischemia, chronic mesenteric ischemia is a disease of the elderly, occurring in patients over 60 years of age.
- **Sex**
  Acute mesenteric ischemia is characterized by a gender predominance, in which women are affected, with three times the frequency of males.

  Similar to acute mesenteric ischemia, the classic presentation of chronic mesenteric ischemia is a female with postprandial abdominal pain, that results in significant weight loss. This disease is more common in women (70%) than in man.
- **Site**
  In acute as well as chronic mesenteric ischemia, the most common involved artery is the superior mesenteric artery. This artery is more prone to receive emboli because of its oblique origin from the visceral aortic segment. The majority of thromboemboli tend to stick in to the middle colic artery, a branch of the superior mesenteric artery, causing an ischemic infarction of the distal part of the colon with sparing of the first part of the small intestine and the ascending colon. Because of their small size, atheroemboli occlude distally the tiny branches of the artery, resulting in more localized areas of ischemia.
- **Treatment**
  Because of its poor outcome, acute mesenteric ischemia is an emergency in diagnosis and treatment. Patients have a better outcome if the time between symptoms and treatment is limited. Treatment consists of supportive therapy to stabilize the hemodynamic status and anticoagulation, eventually followed by surgery. Surgery, corresponding to an emergency laporatomy, is indicated as the patient present with signs of peritonitis, signifying bowel

infarction. Surgical treatment consists of a visceral revascularization (embolectomy, thrombectomy, endarterectomy, or bypass) and resection of the necrotic bowel segment, with achievement of vital section margins. If the condition of the patient does not improve, a second-look laporatomy should be performed.

In case of chronic mesenteric ischemia, revascularization, consisting of endovascular therapy with stenting, is performed. Patients with atherosclerosis should alter their life style by smoking cessation, aggressive lipid-lowering therapy, optimization of blood pressure, diabetes control, and antiplatelet therapy with aspirin.

- **Outcome**

  The prognosis varies in function of the etiology of acute mesenteric ischemia: Mortality in venous thrombosis 50–70%, arterial thrombosis 70–80%, and even higher in non-occlusive mesenteric ischemia, more than 80%. The surgical approach also influences the prognosis: patients have a better prognosis after surgical resection of the necrotic bowel segment, with revascularization than surgical resection or revascularization alone. In elderly, the prognosis is not dependent of their age, but is determined by the delay between the first presentation of their symptoms and surgery. If the time delay is more than 12 h, prognosis becomes worse due to complications such as peritonitis and sepsis.

  In contrast to acute mesenteric ischemia, patients with chronic mesenteric ischemia have a significant better prognosis with a low mortality (3.56–7.23%). However, chronic mesenteric ischemia is a progressive disease with finally failure of the collateral circulation and the development of a fatal mesenteric infarction with high mortality rates.

Macroscopy

Due to the delay in diagnosis because of the nonspecific symptoms, suggestive for more common diseases such as diverticulitis, appendicitis, pancreatitis, ileus, the diagnosis of acute mesenteric ischemia is frequently delayed. Diagnosis is not made on biopsies, but on a resection specimen or during autopsy. The diagnosis requires a systematic examination of the resection specimen with adequate sampling of the section margins in order to determine their viability. In the serosal and mesenterial fat, several blood vessels are sampled to determine the cause of ischemia, e.g., atherosclerotic changes, the presence of thrombi, or vasculitis. Biopsies of the most affected area are taken to determine the severity of the ischemia.

In contrast to venous embolism, the transition from normal to ischemic intestine is more sharp, with arterial embolism or thrombosis. Whereas in mesenteric occlusive ischemia, the distribution of the ischemia will be segmental, uniform in severity, involvement of the bowel due to non-occlusive mesenteric ischemia will be patchy, variable in severity, and frequently widespread. In early stage ischemia, an affected bowel shows an edematous and pale mucosa, with mucosal sloughing and a congestive submucosa. If the ischemia progresses, the bowel wall becomes dark purple and dusky (Fig. 1). At the level of the mucosa, erosions and ulcers are seen due to the necrosis. Ulcers may become deeply infiltrating, resulting in a perforation of the bowel wall. Patients with chronic mesenteric ischemia present with mural fibrosis and strictures.

Autopsy will show ischemia or an infarction of the small intestine without signs of a mechanical

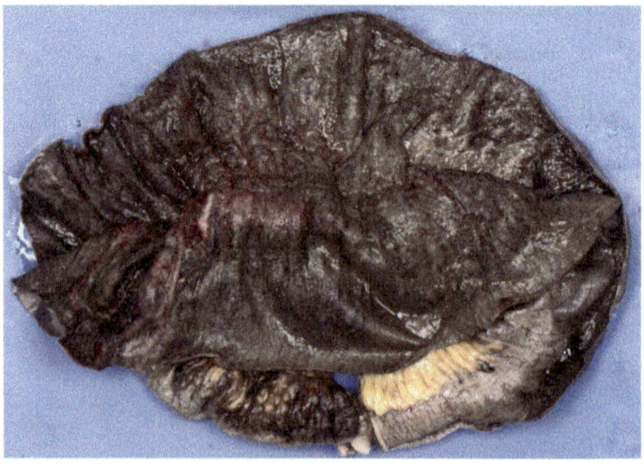

Ischemic Bowel Disease, Fig. 1 Necrotic small intestine with disappearance of the normal folding pattern and a dusky black mucosa

reason of obstruction such as a herniation. Mesenteric emboli and thrombi are usually found within the superior mesenteric artery, eventually with significant atherosclerotic lesions in case of arterial thrombosis. The latter however is not uncommon as approximately 10% of the population will have 50% stenosis in the mesenteric artery at autopsy. Venous thrombosis involves more commonly the superior mesenteric veins than the inferior mesenteric veins, resulting in a hemorrhagic infarction of the bowel.

Microscopy

The histologic features of ischemia will depend on the time period and the extent of the ischemic injury, on the degree of reperfusion of the affected area, on the delay between occurrence of the ischemic insult and surgical intervention. Intestinal ischemia is more commonly diagnosed on a resection specimen, than on biopsies. Biopsies are available for the pathologist if the clinical presentation is not clear and other diseases should be excluded.

Morphological changes, due to ischemia, occur initially at the level of the mucosa with detachment of the epithelium, first at the top of villi and later on extending to the base of the crypts (Fig. 2). Degenerated surface epithelium will show mucus depletion and reactive changes.

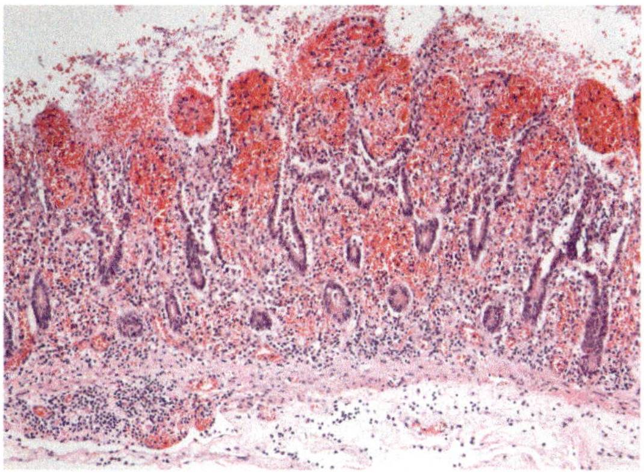

Ischemic Bowel Disease, Fig. 2 The villi of the small intestine are necrotic with sloughing and loss of the epithelium. The lamina propria has a hemorrhagic appearance (H/E, 200×)

At first instance, epithelial loss is not complete at the level of the crypts, which remain delineated by attenuated epithelium, but if the ischemia progresses, remnants of crypts, so-called crypt ghosts, are seen. Other morphologic features are congestive blood vessels eventually containing fibrin thrombi, hemorrhages, hyalinization, and a scarce inflammatory infiltrate in the lamina propria. The submucosa shows edema and congestion of the blood vessels, eventually with hemorrhages. In time, the reperfusion of the damage tissue causes an infiltration of the mucosa by neutrophils, with formation of pseudomembranes, composed of fibrinopurulent material with necrotic epithelium. If the ischemia perseveres or begins suddenly due to an acute occlusion of an artery, the damage will extend in depth inducing a transmural necrosis, eventually with a perforation. Occasionally pneumatosis intestinalis is observed in the necrotic wall as a result of the invasion of bacteria, producing gas.

Depending on the degree of recovery of the blood supply of the ischemic bowel, restoration occurs either up to a normal villous architecture, to a small intestinal mucosa resembling the colon, or to a flat mucosa without villi or crypts. In time however, the intestine will show a nearly normal morphology. The reparative phase of ischemia is characterized by a chronic inflammation, in which the lamina propria is infiltrated by lymphocytes and plasma cells. Proliferation of fibroblasts will result in a hyalinization of the stroma. The surface epithelium may show features of reepithelialization.

Differential Diagnosis

Based on the clinical and radiological presentation, several diseases may mimic intestinal ischemia such as infectious diseases like cytomegalovirus, Mycobacterium avium, Whipple disease, inflammatory bowel disease, especially Crohn's disease, coeliac disease, graft versus host disease, radiation enteritis, rare intestinal tumors, e.g., an adenocarcinoma or lymphoma of the small intestine, and amyloidosis. The clinical information and eventually pathological examination may solve this differential diagnostic problem.

Cytomegalovirus may affect the endothelial cells of the blood vessels, causing damage to the mucosa resembling ischemia. The virus causes typical viral inclusions, which can be highlighted by performing an immunohistochemical staining or molecular analysis. Mycobacterium avium infection and Whipple disease are both characterized by the presence of foamy macrophages, in which micro-organisms can be detected by applying either a Ziehl-Nielsen or PAS stain.

The disturbed villous architecture with presence of inflammation may give rise to a differential diagnostic problem between intestinal ischemia and Crohn's disease. However, in contrast to Crohn's disease, the inflammation is less pronounced with a limited number of neutrophils in early stage. Beside the different clinical presentation, intestinal ischemia may involve the deeper layers of the bowel wall with a scarce inflammatory infiltrate with a limited number of neutrophils, which differ from ulcerative colitis.

Radiation enteritis shows some microscopic features similar to intestinal ischemia, such as loss of surface and gland epithelium with an increased cellularity in the edematous and hyalinized stroma. However, the presence of telangiectatic vessels, atypical endothelial cells, and atypical fibroblasts are diagnostic for radiation enteritis.

References and Further Reading

Brandt, L. J., & Boley, S. J. (2000). AGA technical review on intestinal ischemia. American Gastrointestinal Association. *Gastroenterology, 118*, 954–968.

Fenoglio-Preiser, C. M., Noffsinger, A. E., Stemmermann, G. N., Lantz, P. E., & Isaacson, P. G. (2008). *Gastrointestinal pathology. An atlas and text* (3rd ed.). Philadelphia: Lippincott, Williams & Wilkins.

Odze, R. D., & Goldblum, J. R. (2009). *Surgical pathology of the GI tract, liver, biliary tract, and pancreas* (2nd ed.). Philadelphia: Saunders/Elsevier.

Umphrey, H., Canon, C. L., & Lockhart, M. E. (2008). Differential diagnosis of small bowel ischemia. *Radiologic Clinics of North America, 46*, 943–952, vi–vii.

Vollmar, B., & Menger, M. D. (2011). Intestinal ischemia/reperfusion: Microcirculatory pathology and functional consequences. *Langenbeck's Archives of Surgery/Deutsche Gesellschaft fur Chirurgie, 396*, 13–29.

Ischemic Colitis

Ann Driessen
Department of Pathology, University Hospital Antwerp, Edegem, Belgium
Maastricht University Medical Centre, Maastricht, The Netherlands

Synonyms

Acute large bowel ischemia; Colon ischemia; Lower gastrointestinal ischemia

Definition

Ischemic colitis or lower gastrointestinal ischemia, for the first time described by Boley et al. in 1963, is a vascular condition of the lower gastrointestinal tract, in which the colon is injured due to an inadequate blood supply. The extent of damage of the colon will depend on the duration and cause of the ischemic injury, the involved blood vessel type and its localization as well as the degree of collateral blood supply. The insufficient blood supply induces an inflammation of the colon, evolving from mucosal damage to full-thickness or transmural necrosis.

The vascular supply of the colon consists of three arteries, namely, the superior mesenteric artery, distributing the ascending and the proximal two thirds of the transverse colon, the inferior mesenteric artery, nourishing the distal part of the transverse colon with the splenic flexure, descending colon and sigmoid, and the superior rectal (hemorrhoidal) artery, branching from the inferior mesenteric artery, supplying the rectum. The latter part of the colon is also supplied by the internal iliac arteries. In contrast to the small intestine, the colon is more prone to ischemia due to the low blood flow and the less well-developed microvasculature. Areas at risk for ischemia are the so-called watershed zones, in which two circulations meet each other with limited collateral networks. These watershed areas are the splenic flexure (Griffith's point), an area situated between the superior and inferior mesenteric artery, the distal sigmoid (Sudeck's point), in between the inferior mesenteric artery and the superior rectal artery, and the right colon, where the marginal vessel is poorly developed in nearly half of the population.

According to the technical review on intestinal ischemia, published by the American Association of Gastroenterology, intestinal ischemia can be classified into acute mesenteric ischemia, chronic mesenteric ischemia or intestinal angina, and ischemic colitis or colon ischemia. The pathogenesis of ischemic colitis is very heterogeneous, but is based on two different mechanisms. The most common mechanism is a reduced blood supply, causing an imbalance between the blood supply and the required metabolic needs of the bowel. This non-occlusive form of mechanism is due to a low cardiac output in patients with cardiac failure or shock, either hypovolemic, hemorrhagic, or septic of origin. Other causes of non-occlusive ischemia are a colonic obstruction, caused by volvulus, colon cancer, fecal impaction, strangulated hernia, or pseudo-obstruction. In these conditions, the blood supply may be diminished as a result of the distension of the gut with increase of the intraluminal pressure. Drugs, such as NSAIDs, diuretics, or cocaine, may also be responsible for non-occlusive ischemic changes due to their vasoconstrictive effects. Ischemic colitis is also observed in patients, having major vascular surgery, such aorto-iliac reconstructive surgery (7%) or open aortic aneurysm repair (1–7%). The prevalence of ischemic colitis is significantly higher in patients having a ruptured aneurysm (24–44%). The occlusive form is mostly arterial of origin, of which an embolus (50%) is the most common cause. Other causes of vascular occlusion are small vessel occlusion (20%), a mesenteric arterial (10%), or venous thrombosis (10%). Patients with a hypercoagulable state, either congenital, e.g., factor V Leiden mutation of protein C or S deficiency, or acquired, e.g., antiphospholipid syndrome, are at risk of developing thrombotic occlusion of small vessels, causing colonic ischemia, in 28–74% of patients. A hypercoagulable state is more likely the cause in young patients with recurrent or chronic ischemia.

Clinical Features

- **Incidence**
  Ischemic colitis is the most common cause of ischemic disease of the gastrointestinal tract, affecting more than half of the cases (50–60%). In the general population worldwide, the incidence of this disease is difficult to determine and most likely underestimated because of the mild and transient nature of the disease, which is not uncommonly misdiagnosed as an acute self-limiting colitis or inflammatory bowel disease. According to literature, the incidence of ischemic colitis varies between 4.5 and 9.9 per 100,000 person years, with the highest published incidence of 44 cases per 100,000 person years. The disorder is responsible for 1–3 per 1,000 acute hospital admissions.
- **Age**
  The incidence of ischemic colitis is related to age with a significantly higher incidence in the elderly, aged over 65 years (119 per 100,000 person years) compared to individuals in their fourth decade of life (0 per 100,000 person years). The higher incidence in elderly is related to the high comorbidity rate such as coronary artery disease, hypertension, diabetes, chronic obstructive disease (COPD), and renal insufficiency. Chronic obstructive lung disease is associated with a higher incidence of ischemic colitis (9.2 per 100,000 person years) compared to the non-COPD control population (4.5 per 100,000 person years). Although ischemic colitis is more common in the elderly, a young age is not an exclusion criterion for the diagnosis of this disorder. In contrast to elderly in which ischemic colitis occurs in association with congestive heart

failure, coronary artery disease, or atherosclerosis, in young age patients, ischemia is mostly related to medications or extreme efforts such as marathon running, in which the extreme effort causes shunting of the blood away from the splanchnic circulation.

The clinical presentation is very heterogeneous and will depend on the etiology, the degree of blood flow reduction, the speed of the ischemic insult, the extent of collateral vascularization. In the non-gangrenous form (80–85%), which is more frequent than the gangrenous form (15–20%), the lesions are more transient and reversible, resolving within 1–3 months. If the ischemic injury is more pronounced, progression to chronic and irreversible strictures (10–15%), causing obstruction, or chronic segmental ischemic colitis (20–25%) occurs. An acute ischemic insult may cause either gangrene or a fulminant universal colitis. Important is the awareness of the clinician for this disorder, as the gangrenous stage has a high mortality rate of more than 60%.

Ischemic colitis is the second most common cause of a low gastrointestinal bleeding in patients presenting with a sudden onset of abdominal pain, usually in the lower left quadrant, and bloody diarrhea. Hematochezia occurs most commonly within one day after the onset of the abdominal pain. Other clinical symptoms are fever, urge for defecation, abdominal tenderness, situated at the level of the affected bowel segment. In case of full-thickness necrosis of the bowel wall, patients will have symptoms of peritonitis and eventually septic shock.

The diagnosis of ischemic colitis however remains a challenge as the symptoms are often nonspecific. Work-up starts with an anamnesis and physical examination. Laboratory values, such as leukocytes, lactate dehydrogenase (LDH), alkaline phosphatase, creatinine phosphokinase, may be abnormal but are nonspecific markers for identification of this disorder. Findings with radiological examination such as plain radiographs, computed tomography, on air contrast or barium/air contrast may suggest an ischemic colitis, but are not conclusive. Ultrasonography can be useful in the distinction between inflammation and ischemia, but its low sensitivity restricts its use as primary diagnostic tool. Colonoscopy is the golden standard for the diagnosis of ischemic colitis as this method has the highest sensitivity and specificity to detect mucosal alterations with as additional advantage tissue sampling. This routinely used technique however visualizes only the mucosal ischemia without assessment of the full-thickness ischemia of the bowel wall. Endoscopy is contraindicated in case of full-thickness necrosis because of the increased risk of perforation.

- **Sex**
  The risk of ischemic colitis is also gender determined with a higher incidence rate in women (58 per 100,000 person years) than in males (32 per 10,000 person years).
- **Site**
  Ischemic colitis is a segmental disease, which may affect any part the colon. However, watershed areas are more prone to ischemic injury than other parts of the colon. Studies have shown that the risk of ischemia is variable in these watershed areas, namely, in the right colon (33.3–46%), the rectosigmoid (25.6–40%), and the splenic flexure (15.4%). The distal part of the colon, consisting of the descending colon, sigmoid, and rectosigmoid, is more frequent involved that the proximal part, in which the right colon is more commonly affected. The rectum is more resistant to ischemia due to the dual blood supply by the superior rectal artery, branching from the inferior mesenteric artery and the internal iliac arteries.
- **Treatment**
  Because of its favorable prognosis with spontaneous resolution of the ischemic lesions, the treatment is mostly supportive in early stage disease. This therapy consists of intravenous fluid, broad-spectrum antibiotics, decompression of the distended bowel, bowel rest. Surgery is only acutely indicated in case of peritoneal signs, massive bleeding, or universal fulminant colitis, eventually associated

with a toxic megacolon. Subacute indications for surgery are persistence of the symptoms for more than 2–3 weeks, suggesting unresponsiveness to the supportive therapy, protein-losing colopathy, or patients with recurrent attacks of sepsis. Elective surgery is only indicated in patients with a symptomatic colon stricture or symptomatic segmental ischemic colitis. During laparotomy, the surgeon resects the gut involved, with achievement of vital section margins.

- **Outcome**

  The prognosis of ischemic colitis will depend on the etiology, the localization and extent of the involved gut segment, and the comorbidities. Patients with a transient ischemic colitis, treated with supportive therapy, have a significant lower risk of mortality (9%), than those, presenting with an acute abdomen, requiring immediate surgery (48%). Right-sided colitis has a less favorable prognosis because of its distinct severity, requiring surgery in approximately 60% of the patients with a mortality of around 25%.

Macroscopy

The appearance of the ischemic mucosa varies in function of the severity of the ischemic insult and the delay between this insult and the endoscopical examination (Fig. 1). In transient ischemic colitis, endoscopic examination reveals a pale and edematous mucosa with segmental erythema, petechial hemorrhages, superficial erosions, and linear ulcerations. Characteristically, there is sharp demarcation between the involved segment of the gut and the normally vascularized bowel segment. Progression of the disease is associated with hemorrhages and submucosal edema, presenting as luminal protruded bluish-black blebs or nodules. These lesions are responsible for the characteristic thumbprinting sign on radiologic investigations. Due to delay in the performance of this technical examination, this thumbprinting sign will fade away as a result of resorption of the submucosal hemorrhages or disappearance of these lesions when the mucosa ulcerates and sloughs. The chronic stage of the disease is characterized by strictures, disappearance of the haustrations and mucosal granularity. With increase in severity, the mucosa becomes dark or cyanotic with presence of pseudomembranes and pseudopolyps.

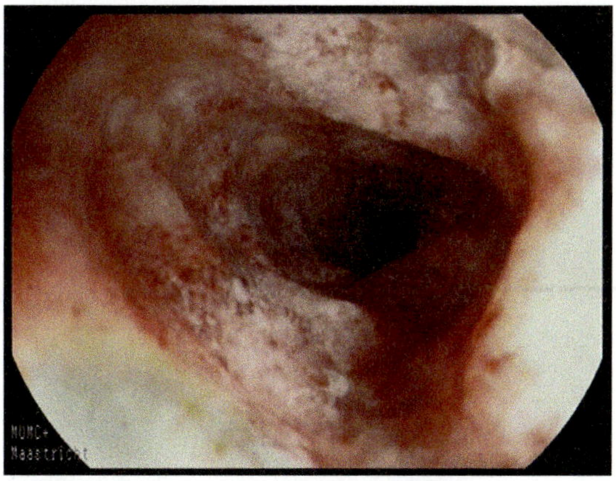

Ischemic Colitis, Fig. 1 Endoscopic view of a colon with an ischemic colitis, characterized by a loss of the normal folding pattern due to necrosis and ulcerations of the surface mucosa

Thorough examination of a resection specimen for ischemia is necessary in order to determine the extent of the ischemic injury, the viability of section margins, and the etiology of the injury by investigating the blood vessels to detect a vascular occlusion due to a thrombosis or arteriosclerotic changes.

Microscopy

Microscopical examination is rarely performed in transient ischemic colitis, because time will heal the ischemic lesions if the ischemic injury is mild. Moreover, the diagnosis is a clinical one. In case biopsies are performed, the morphological alterations will point either to an acute ischemia or a reparative phase. Acute ischemia has a patchy distribution with involved areas separated by a normal mucosa. It is characterized by necrosis of the superficial part of the crypts, whereas the remnants of the crypts have an atrophic appearance with a dilated lumen, lined by an attenuated epithelium (Fig. 2). The lamina propria is

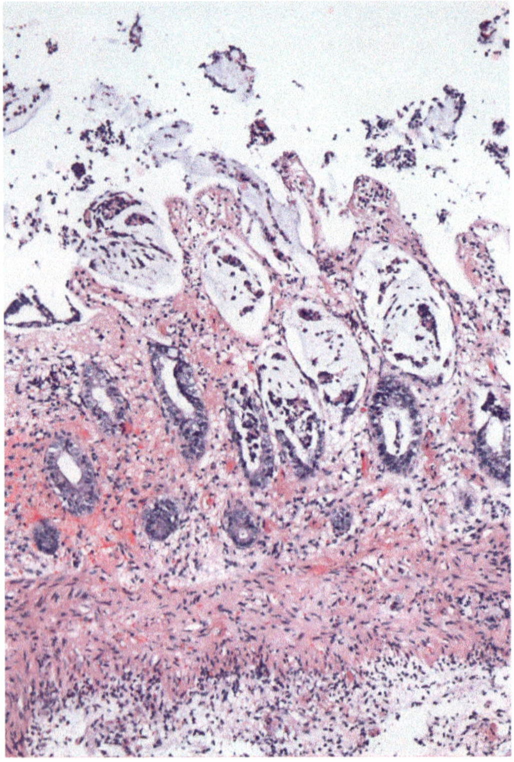

Ischemic Colitis, Fig. 2 Dilated crypts with necrotic and sloughed crypt epithelium at the surface of the mucosa, in a paucicellular stroma with microthrombi (H/E, ×150)

edematous with presence of congested blood vessels and lymphatic vessels. In the early phase of ischemia, the inflammation is restricted with a sparse number of neutrophils. These inflammatory cells may eventually infiltrate the atrophic crypts, causing cryptitis and crypt abscesses. At the surface pseudomembranes, consisting of fibrinopurulent material and necrotic epithelium, are seen. Breakdown of the surface epithelium will increase the permeability with an invasion of bacteria, inducing a neutrophilic infiltration. In more severe ischemia, the submucosa shows pronounced edema with capillary and lymphatic congestion, hemorrhages, and inflammation. If thrombi are present in blood vessels, necrosis of the mucosa occurs with development of superficial or linear ulcers. Deeply infiltrating ulcers, extending in to the serosa, may cause a perforation. The damage is not only the result of ischemia but is also induced by the reperfusion of the bowel wall. Although reperfusion may cause a reoxygenation of tissue, the increase in oxygen supply is associated with a release of cytotoxic oxidants. These oxidants are responsible for an inflammatory response, in which neutrophils are activated. Adhesion of neutrophils to endothelial cells may cause the formation of fibrin thrombi. Due to the occlusion of the blood vessels, necrosis may extend throughout all the layers of the wall, finally resulting in a transmural necrosis.

In the reparative phase, the ulcer base will be replaced by granulation tissue and fibrosis. The acute inflammation with neutrophils will change into a chronic inflammation with presence of lymphocytes and plasma cells. Due to the proliferation of fibroblasts, the mucosa becomes fibrotic with hyalinization of the lamina propria. This hyalinized stroma contains hemosiderin-containing macrophages. Regeneration of the epithelium will result in a reepithelialization and restoration of the crypts, be it that the crypt architecture will not completely normalize. Chronic inflammation with pronounced fibrosis in the submucosa may initiate stricture formation.

Molecular Features

Molecular data on the topic ischemic colitis are limited. According to the study of Theodoropoulou and Koutroubakis (2008), genetic predisposition may play an important role in the pathogenesis of ischemic colitis in young patients. They have shown that some polymorphisms of the genes FV R506Q en PAI-1 are associated with the development of ischemic colitis in young patients without serious illness. FVL is a thrombophilic factor, whereas the PAI-1 is an important inhibitor of the fibrinolytic system. The detection of FV 506Q and PAI-1 polymorphisms in young patients with ischemic colitis suggests that coagulation disorders play a role in the pathogenesis of this disease.

Differential Diagnosis

The differential diagnosis of ischemic colitis, based on its clinical presentation, is unlimited and includes vascular disorders, such as mesenteric artery insufficiency, mesenteric venous thrombosis, inflammatory disorders such as inflammatory bowel disease, infectious colitis, diverticulitis, pseudomembranous colitis, peptic ulcer disease, pancreatitis, or different causes of bowel obstruction.

Based on the morphological features, several diseases belong to the differential diagnosis such as pseudomembranous colitis, inflammatory bowel disease, collagenous colitis, radiation colitis.

Pseudomembranous colitis, caused by *Clostridium difficile*, and ischemic colitis are both characterized by the presence of pseudomembranes. Pseudomembranes are however patchy in ischemic colitis, whereas in pseudomembranous colitis, these pseudomembranes are diffusely distributed. Microscopic features diagnostic for ischemic colitis is the presence of a hyalinized mucosa and cryptatrophy. Other features are less specific, but are more pronounced in ischemic colitis, such as hemorrhages in the lamina propria and full-thickness mucosal necrosis. As a result of the severe submucosal edema, ischemic colitis may present endoscopically as a polyp or mass.

In hemorrhagic enterocolitis, the endothelium of the capillaries is injured due to bacterial toxins, produced by enterohemorrhagic *Escherichia coli* or *Klebsiella oxytoca*. This causes hemorrhages of the lamina propria with loss of the epithelium at the surface and the crypts. In contrast to ischemic colitis, the inflammation is more pronounced with numerous neutrophils at first instance and later on an infiltrate consisting of lymphocytes and plasma cells.

The chronic inflammation in the submucosa in a later stage of ischemic colitis with involvement of the left colon may give rise to a differential diagnostic problem with inflammatory bowel disease. In ischemic colitis however, infiltration of the crypts with cryptitis and crypt abscesses is less prominent than in inflammatory bowel disease. Granulomas, present in Crohn's disease, are not found. Hemosiderin-containing macrophages in the hyalinized stroma are diagnostic for ischemia, which in contrast to ulcerative colitis are also characterized by involvement of the deeper layers of the bowel wall.

The hyalinized stroma in collagenous colitis and radiation colitis may mimic ischemic colitis but with a different clinical presentation. Radiation colitis shows some microscopic features similar to ischemic colitis, such as loss of surface and gland epithelium with an increased cellularity in the edematous and hyalinized stroma. However, the presence of telangiectatic vessels, atypical endothelial cells, and atypical fibroblasts are diagnostic for radiation colitis. In collagenous colitis, the inflammation is more pronounced with presence of a mixed infiltrate of neutrophils, lymphocytes, and plasma cells.

References and Further Reading

Brandt, L. J., & Boley, S. J. (2000). AGA technical review on intestinal ischemia. American Gastrointestinal Association. *Gastroenterology, 118*, 954–968.

Fenoglio-Preiser, C. M., Noffsinger, A. E., Stemmermann, G. N., Lantz, P. E., & Isaacson, P. G. (2008). *Gastrointestinal pathology. An atlas and text* (3rd ed.). Philadelphia: Lippincott, Williams & Wilkins.

Georgescu, E. F., Carstea, D., Dumitrescu, D., Teodorescu, R., & Carstea, A. (2012). Ischemic colitis and large bowel infarction: A case report. *World Journal of Gastroenterology: WJG, 18*, 5640–5644.

Odze, R. D., & Goldblum, J. R. (2009). *Surgical pathology of the GI tract, liver, biliary tract, and pancreas* (2nd ed.). Philadelphia: Saunders/Elsevier.

Theodoropoulou, A., & Koutroubakis, I. E. (2008). Ischemic colitis: clinical practice in diagnosis and treatment. *World Journal of Gastroenterology, 14*(48), 7302–8.

Vollmar, B., & Menger, M. D. (2011). Intestinal ischemia/reperfusion: Microcirculatory pathology and functional consequences. *Langenbeck's Archives of Surgery/Deutsche Gesellschaft Fur Chirurgie, 396*, 13–29.

I

Ischemic Gastritis

Helena Baldaia
Serviço de Anatomia Patológica, Centro Hospitalar de São João, Porto, Portugal

Synonyms

Gastric ischemia

Definitions

When blood flow in the rich gastric vasculature is disrupted, ischemic damage to the stomach occurs. There is a wide array of causes associated with this disruption, and the severity of the effects is related to the underlying cause. The most commonly present risk factors are the association of diffuse and severe atherosclerosis, hypertension, and smoking (Fenoglio-Preiser et al. 2008). The mechanic impairment of blood flow by the presence of a volvulus or previous surgery is also listed as a cause of gastric ischemia. Furthermore, systemic alterations in circulation (such as shock or trauma induced hypotension or hypoxemia) eventually affect mesenteric blood flow. Thrombus or even emboli from the aorta may lodge in the arteries supplying the gastric wall and cause ischemic damage. A recently recognized cause of ischemic gastritis is the embolization, to the vasculature of the stomach, of radiologically placed beads used to perform embolization of hepatic metastases. This mandates the realization of an arteriography prior to the procedure (Mitchell 2009).

The symptoms associated with gastric ischemia are nonspecific. Nausea, vomiting, weight loss, and upper gastrointestinal bleeding are the most commonly reported clinical manifestations (Haberer et al. 2003).

Clinical Features

- **Incidence**
  Ischemic gastritis is very rare, accounting to the rich gastric blood supply provided by multiple anastomoses (Mitchell 2009). The variability of incidence reflects the multiplicity of causes and their own incidence.
- **Age and Sex**
  Adults are the mainly affected age group. In one study of 41 patients with upper gastrointestinal ischemia, the mean age was 60 (17–86) years, with a slight male predominance (Van Noord et al. 2010).
- **Treatment**
  The treatment options differ with the severity of the lesions and the underlying cause. Medical conservative treatment with proton pump inhibitors and electrolyte therapy can be used as first-line treatment (Haberer et al. 2003). Chronic vascular insufficiency can lead to gastroparesis that is typically reversible if the blood flow is re-established (Mitchell 2009). In large acute necrotizing lesions with perforation or sepsis, gastrectomy is warranted (Force et al. 1980).
- **Outcome**
  The extent of the lesions and the reversibility of the ischemia are the main factors that affect prognosis. In transmural necrotizing lesions, the mortality is very high (Mitchell 2009).

Macroscopy

Macroscopic findings (Fig. 1) vary, reflecting the severity and duration of the ischemia. Initial lesions demonstrate superficial erosions or ulcers. In some cases, the stomach can be entirely necrotic and exhibit perforation (Mitchell 2009).

Microscopy

The basic histological lesion is coagulative necrosis. In early lesions, however, the findings can be

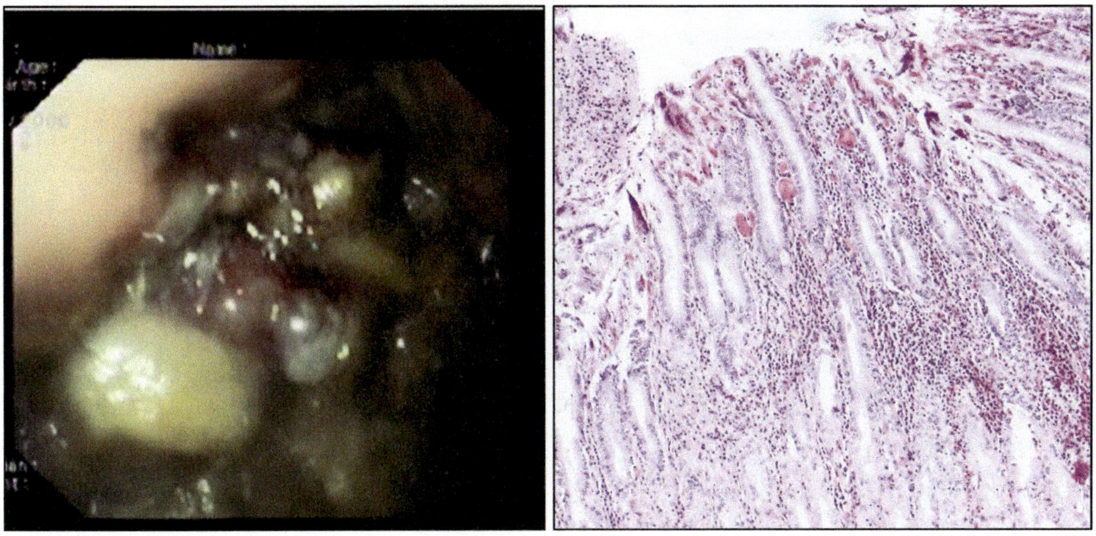

Ischemic Gastritis, Fig. 1 Ischemic gastritis. Endoscopic view of ischemic gastritis (*left photo*) and microscopic aspects (*right photo*), showing erosion/ulceration of the epithelial lining and reactive aspects of the epithelium. Lamina propria with prominent inflammatory infiltrates and vascular congestion

very scarce and nonspecific, with only superficial epithelial necrosis and congestion of the mucosa (Fig. 1). In more advanced lesions, there can be mucosal necrosis with hemorrhage, erosions, ulceration, and reactive changes of the remaining superficial epithelium. Sometimes microthrombi can be identified in the mucosal capillaries. In chronic vascular insufficiency, there can be a variable lamina propria fibrosis. In most truly severe cases, there is transmural coagulative necrosis. This finding is associated with a grim prognosis (Fenoglio-Preiser et al. 2008).

Differential Diagnosis

In superficial, early lesions, the histological findings in ischemic gastritis are nonspecific. In these cases, a degree of clinical suspicion and information can be very important to achieve a diagnosis. Peptic ulcer disease can be very difficult to distinguish from ischemic gastritis, especially in small biopsy material. Sometimes the presence of necrobiotic "withering" glands and vessel microthrombi, associated, once more to clinical and endoscopic correlation, can be important in the differential diagnosis (Van Noord et al. 2010).

References and Further Reading

Fenoglio-Preiser, C. M., Noffsinger, A. E., Stemmermann, G. N., Lantz, P. E., & Isaacson, P. G. (2008). The nonneoplastic stomach. In J. McGouh & J. Pine (Eds.), *Gastrointestinal pathology an atlas and text* (pp. 167–168). Philadelphia: Lippincott Williams & Wilkins.

Force, T., MacDonald, D., Eade, O., et al. (1980). Ischemic gastritis and duodenitis. *Digestive Diseases and Sciences, 25*(4), 307–310.

Haberer, J., Trivedi, N., Kohlwes, J., & Tierney, L. (2003). Clinical problem-solving. A gut feeling. *The New England Journal of Medicine, 349*(1), 73–78.

Mitchell, K. A. (2009). Vascular disorders of the GI tract. In R. Odze & J. Goldblum (Eds.), *Surgical pathology of the GI tract, liver, biliary tract and pancreas*. Philadelphia: Saunders.

Van Noord, D., Biermann, K., Moons, L., et al. (2010). Histological changes in patients with chronic upper gastrointestinal ischaemia. *Histopathology, 57*(4), 615–621.

J

Juvenile Polyp, Upper Gastrointestinal Tract

Helena Baldaia
Serviço de Anatomia Patológica, Centro Hospitalar de São João, Porto, Portugal

Definition

Juvenile polyps are hamartomatous polyps of the gastrointestinal (GI) tract. As such, they are composed of indigenous elements to the site of origin, although arranged in a malformed manner.

Juvenile polyps can appear as solitary sporadic polyps of the colon or, less frequently, in the context of a generalized polyposis syndrome, juvenile polyposis (JP). The diagnostic criteria established for juvenile polyposis are:

1. More than three to five juvenile polyps of the colorectum
2. Juvenile polyps throughout the gastrointestinal tract
3. Any number of juvenile polyps with a family history of juvenile polyposis (Offerhaus and Howe 2010)

JP can be clinically divided into three subtypes. The rare *juvenile polyposis of infancy* is a generalized polyposis syndrome usually diagnosed before the age of 2. These infants suffer from diarrhea, hemorrhage, malnutrition, and intussusception. Death occurs at an early age, and many of these patients have associated congenital anomalies (Brosens et al. 2011).

The *generalized juvenile polyposis* and *juvenile polyposis coli* seem to be a continuum of the same disease. In the latter, as the name implies, the polyps are confined to the colorectum. These forms may be inherited in an autosomal dominant manner or may be sporadic and are characterized by the presence of juvenile polyps and an increased risk of gastrointestinal cancer (Brosens et al. 2011). The most frequent clinical presentation is painless rectal bleeding (Iacobuzio-Donahue 2012). Congenital birth defects such as malrotation of the gut and cardiac and genitourinary defects are reported in 15% of JP patients (Hornick and Odze 2009), particularly in the nonfamilial cases (Fenoglio-Preiser et al. 2008).

Symptoms such as telangiectasia, epistaxis, and arteriovenous malformations, consistent with Osler-Rendu-Weber syndrome have been reported in individuals with JP syndrome, leading to the hypothesis that some cases can be a part of a combined syndrome of JPs – Osler-Rendu-Weber (Fenoglio-Preiser et al. 2008; Gammon et al. 2009).

Polyps similar to juvenile polyps can also be part of the phosphatase and tensin homolog [PTEN] hamartomatous tumor syndrome, although associated with other manifestations (Fenoglio-Preiser et al. 2008).

F. Carneiro et al. (eds.), *Pathology of the Gastrointestinal Tract*, Encyclopedia of Pathology,
DOI 10.1007/978-3-319-40560-5

Clinical Features

- **Incidence**
  Juvenile polyps are the most common pediatric GI polyps, accounting for 2% of the polyps in this population. JP syndrome, however, is rare (ten times less common than familial adenomatous polyposis) and the estimated incidence is 1 per 100,000 births (Fenoglio-Preiser et al. 2008).
- **Age**
  Patients with sporadic juvenile polyps usually range from 1 to 10 years of age. Juvenile polyposis syndrome patients are usually older, with a mean age at diagnosis of 9.5 years (Iacobuzio-Donahue 2012) and clinical presentation in the first and second decades (Fenoglio-Preiser et al. 2008).
- **Sex**
  Solitary juvenile polyps occur with no sex predilection. In the JP syndrome, there is a slight male predominance (Iacobuzio-Donahue 2012).
- **Site**
  Solitary juvenile polyps occur exclusively in the colorectum and predominantly (54%) in the rectosigmoid colon (Hornick and Odze 2009). In polyposis coli, the rectosigmoid area is also the most affected, with as few as five to as much as hundreds of polyps. In the context of generalized polyposis, polyps can also occur in the stomach (83%, particularly in the antrum but also throughout the gastric mucosa in one study), duodenum (33% in one study), jejunum, and ileum (Brosens et al. 2011). Rarely, polyps are confined to a diffuse carpeting of the gastric mucosa without colic involvement (Brosens et al. 2011).
- **Treatment**
  Solitary juvenile polyps can be resected without further complications.

  In the setting of juvenile polyposis, therapy is dependent on the severity of the clinical manifestations and pattern of polyp distribution, and management of these patients must always include an appropriate surveillance protocol in view of the increased risk of gastrointestinal malignancy.

  Patients at risk or high suspicion of JP syndrome should have endoscopic surveillance, initiating at 15 years of age or since the beginning of symptoms. This screening should be repeated annually (if any polyps are found) or every 2–3 years (if no polyps are identified) (Gammond et al. 2010). Every polyp should be sent for pathologic examination to exclude dysplasia or malignancy (Hornick and Odze 2009). If the polyp burden in the colon or stomach cannot be managed with endoscopic removal (usually >50–100 polyps) or in those patients with severe gastrointestinal bleeding or diarrhea, polyps with dysplasia or in patients with a strong family history of colorectal cancer, surgery is indicated (colectomy, gastrectomy, or small intestinal resection) (Brosens et al. 2011; Gammond et al. 2010). Recurrence of rectal polyps in patients with subtotal colectomy is frequent (Brosens et al. 2011).

  Given the rarity of JP of infancy, there are no approved guidelines of management, being supportive (transfusional, nutritional) measures the mainstay of therapy (Fenoglio-Preiser et al. 2008; Gammond et al. 2010).
- **Outcome**
  Sporadic solitary juvenile polyps have no increased risk of malignancy (Hornick and Odze 2009). In generalized juvenile polyposis or juvenile polyposis coli, the primary outcome is affected by the presence of malignancy. A cancer risk analysis calculated a cumulative life-time risk for colorectal cancer in JP syndrome of 39% and a relative risk of colorectal cancer of 34 (Offerhaus and Howe 2010). In one study, the mean age at cancer diagnosis was 35.5 years, with a range of 4–60 years (Fenoglio-Preiser et al. 2008). The majority of carcinomas are diagnosed in the colon and rectum, but cases in the stomach, duodenum, and pancreas have been reported (Brosens et al. 2011). It is believed that carcinoma can arise both from juvenile polyps with dysplasia and from adenomatous polyps that can also be encountered in juvenile polyposis (Fenoglio-Preiser et al. 2008).

  Cases of juvenile polyposis of infancy are usually accompanied by very severe anemia and protein-losing enteropathy, and children usually die before the age of 2 (Offerhaus and Howe 2010).

Macroscopy

Juvenile polyps are usually small pedunculated lesions with a smooth rounded shape and superficial ulceration. In juvenile polyposis, there are frequently hundreds of polyps, but the mucosa between them is usually spared (Fenoglio-Preiser et al. 2008). In the stomach, polyps are less often pedunculated and more commonly diffuse (Offerhaus and Howe 2010) (Fig. 1). Larger lesions are somewhat more lobulated due to repeated ulceration. Cut surface frequently exhibits variably sized mucin-filled cysts (Fenoglio-Preiser et al. 2008).

Microscopy

Typical juvenile polyps consist of gastrointestinal glands indigenous to the site of origin surrounded by a prominent stroma (Fig. 1). The glandular component is frequently branched, irregular, or dilated, originating cysts containing mucus or inflammatory cells. The stroma is edematous and

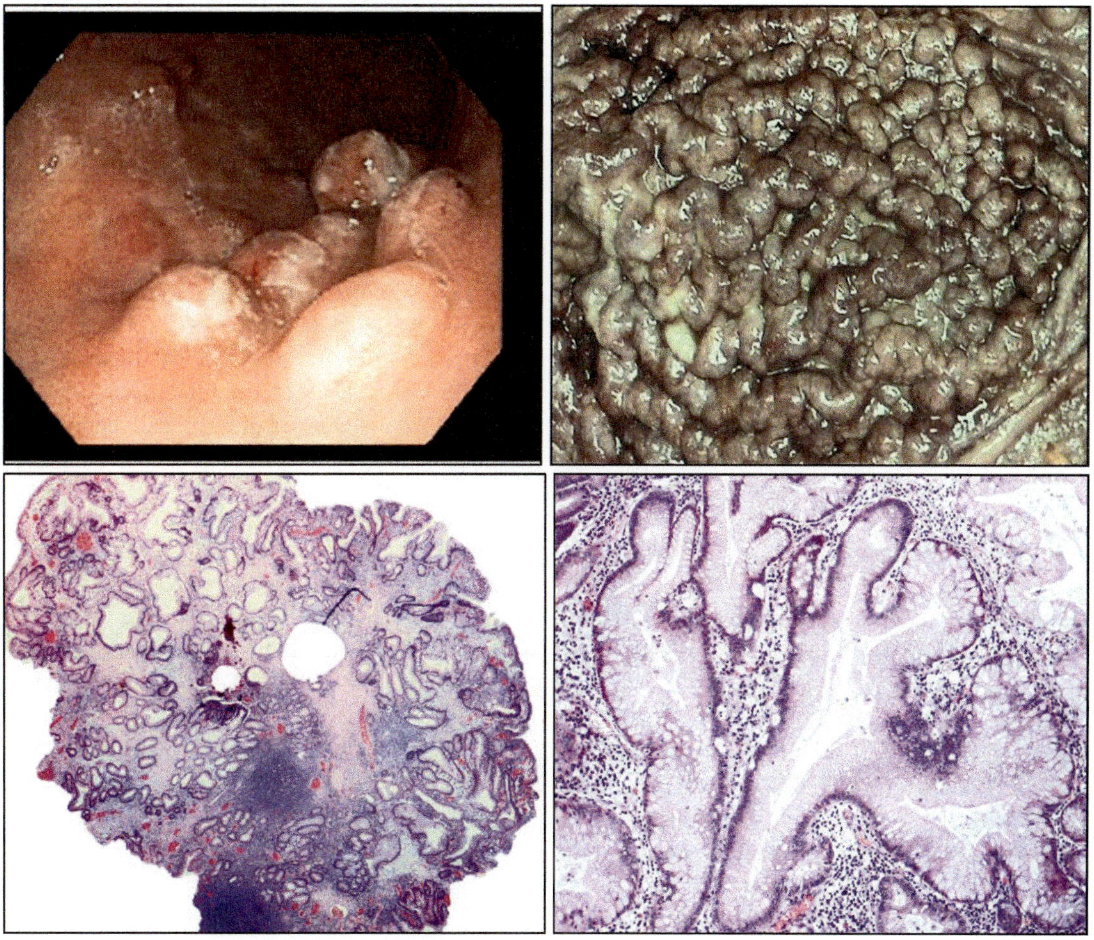

Juvenile Polyp, Upper Gastrointestinal Tract, Fig. 1 Juvenile polyposis with prominent gastric involvement. The gastric mucosa is carpeted with polypoid lesions. Histologically, these polyps show branching and dilation of the glandular component and prominent stromal inflammation. This patient had similar findings in the colon and a proven *SMAD4* mutation very rich in inflammatory cells including plasma cells, lymphocytes, and neutrophils. Smooth muscle bundles are usually inconspicuous. The smooth contour perceived macroscopically is due to ulceration of the surface epithelium which is usually prominent, forming a granulation tissue cap (Fenoglio-Preiser et al. 2008). Atypical juvenile polyps, more commonly encountered in a syndromic context, appear to have a more lobulated, finger-like surface with prominent glandular serration and irregularity and less cystic dilation (Offerhaus and Howe 2010). Gastric juvenile polyps are very similar to hyperplastic polyps with prominent foveolar hyperplasia and an inflammatory stroma (Fenoglio-Preiser et al. 2008). The important inflammatory background of juvenile polyps confers, very commonly, reactive changes to the epithelium. Dysplasia however is found in approximately 46.7% of atypical juvenile polyps and 9% of typical polyps (Fenoglio-Preiser et al. 2008). This diagnosis implies the presence of the established criteria for dysplasia such as nuclear enlargement, hyperchromasia, pseudostratification, and mitosis. Dysplasia is found more frequently in juvenile polyps exceeding 1 cm in diameter (Iacobuzio-Donahue 2012).

Juvenile polyps containing metaplastic and ganglioneuromatous components have been described (Fenoglio-Preiser et al. 2008).

Molecular Features

A germ-line mutation in the *SMAD4* or *BMPRA1* gene is found in about 50–60% of juvenile polyposis syndrome (Brosens et al. 2011). Both of these genes are involved in the TGF-β pathway. SMAD4 is a protein that functions as the common intercellular mediator of the TGF-β, bone morphogenic protein (BMP), and activin signaling pathways. BMPR1A is a transmembrane receptor involved in the same pathways that in the end regulates the transcription of various genes (Fenoglio-Preiser et al. 2008). The absence of known mutations in a large percentage of cases has led to an investigation of other potentially important genes, particularly those involved in the TGF-β pathway, such as the TGF-β coreceptor endoglin, which was reported to be mutated in two cases (Offerhaus and Howe 2010). Patients with *SMAD4* mutations are more likely to have upper gastrointestinal polyps and a family history of juvenile polyps than those with *BMPR1* mutations (Fenoglio-Preiser et al. 2008).

Differential Diagnosis

The main differential diagnosis of juvenile polyps is with other hamartomatous polyps, namely, Peutz-Jeghers (PJ) polyps and with inflammatory pseudopolyps and hyperplastic polyps.

The presence of a prominent inflammatory stroma and absence of smooth muscle bundles may allow a differential diagnosis of juvenile polyp with PJ polyps.

Although the differential diagnosis in a biopsy specimen can be difficult, inflammatory pseudopolyps arise in an inflamed mucosa and usually, in juvenile polyposis, the adjacent mucosa is spared (Iacobuzio-Donahue 2012).

The distinction, in gastric lesions, between hyperplastic and juvenile polyps is very difficult and frequently not possible. A diagnosis of juvenile polyposis can only be made with an in-depth knowledge of clinical and endoscopic findings (Fenoglio-Preiser et al. 2008).

References and Further Reading

Brosens, L. A., Langeveld, D., van Hattem, W., et al. (2011). Juvenile polyposis syndrome. *World Journal of Gastroenterology, 28*(17), 4839–4844.

Calva, D., & Howe, J. (2008). Hamartomatous polyposis syndromes. *The Surgical Clinics of North America, 88*(4), 779.

Fenoglio-Preiser, C. M., Noffsinger, A. E., Stemmermann, G. N., Lantz, P. E., & Isaacson, P. G. (2008). Polyposis and hereditary cancer syndromes. In J. McGouh & J. Pine (Eds.), *Gastrointestinal pathology an atlas and text* (pp. 704–724). Philadelphia: Lippincott Williams & Wilkins.

Gammon, A., Jasperson, K., Kohlmann, W., & Burt, R. W. (2009). Hamartomatous polyposis syndromes. *Best Practice & Research Clinical Gastroenterology, 23*(2), 219–231.

Hornick, J. L., & Odze, R. D. (2009). Polyps of the large intestine. In R. Odze & J. Goldblum (Eds.), *Surgical pathology of the GI tract, liver, biliary tract and pancreas*. Philadelphia: Saunders.
Iacobuzio-Donahue, C. A. (2012). Gastrointestinal polyposis syndromes. In C. A. Iacobuzio-Donahue, E. Montgomary, & J. R. Golblum (Eds.), *Gastrointestinal and liver pathology* (pp. 399–402). Philadelphia: Saunders.
Offerhaus, G. J. A., & Howe, J. R. (2010). Juvenile polyposis. In F. T. Bosman, F. Carneiro, R. H. Hruban, & N. D. Theise (Eds.), *WHO classification of tumours of the digestive system* (pp. 166–167). Lyon: IARC.

Juvenile Polyposis Syndrome, Lower Gastrointestinal Tract

Özgür Ekinci
Department of Pathology, Gazi University, Ankara, Turkey

Synonyms

Combined JP/hereditary hemorrhagic telengiectasia (Osler-Weber-Rendu) syndrome; Gastric JP; Generalized juvenile polyposis (JP); JP coli

Definition

JP is an autosomal dominant hereditary syndrome in which the affected individuals characteristically have multiple juvenile polyps in one or more parts of the GI tract: stomach, small bowel, or colorectum. The patients have increased risk of carcinomas of the stomach and small and large bowel. The juvenile polyps in these patients have the potential to transform to carcinoma.

The syndrome occurs in patients with no family history in roughly half of the cases.

It has been proposed that an individual has JP if at least one of the following criteria is met:

1. >3 or 5 juvenile polyps in the colorectum
2. Juvenile polyps present in throughout the GI tract
3. Any number of juvenile polyps in an individual with positive family history

Clinical Features

- **Incidence**
  The incidence is about 0.6–1/100,000 in western countries.
- **Age**
  While the syndrome presents most commonly in the first two decades, the outset can be at infancy to geriatric ages.
- **Sex**
  JP is considered not to show a sex predilection.
- **Site**
  The most common and the classical case has juvenile polyps in the colorectum. There are fewer patients that bear polyps of the stomach and less frequently the small bowel.
- **Treatment**
  The mainstay of the management is prevention and/or early diagnosis of dysplasia or carcinoma. Options include endoscopic surveillance or prophylactic surgery. Surgery is performed if dysplasia is discovered in a juvenile polyp or there are multiple individuals with JP-related carcinomas in the pedigree.
- **Outcome**
  The prognosis is solidly related to the early diagnosis of the syndrome and developing dysplasia, frequent follow-up endoscopy, and prophylactic surgery. Once a malignant tumor is developed, the prognosis will be that of the similar malignancy in a sporadic case.

  Patients that have extraintestinal conditions (congenital anomalies of the heart, nervous system, etc.) or hereditary hemorrhagic telangiectasia (Osler-Weber-Rendu syndrome) will suffer from these in addition to the GI neoplasia.

Macroscopy

By endoscopy or in a resection specimen, there can be one to hundreds of juvenile polyps. Polyps can be sessile or pedunculated, with a size of several centimeters. A classical juvenile polyp has a sphere-like, roundish luminal aspect. The so-called atypical juvenile polyps have more than one lobe, i.e., they are multilobated. These polyps are considered to be unique to the syndromic cases.

Microscopy

A juvenile polyp is generally an ulcerated polyp with overlying active inflammation with budding and cystically dilated glandular structures of varying size and shape. The lamina propria of the lesion is edematous and heavily populated by a mixture of inflammatory cells, mainly neutrophil leukocytes, especially at the top of the polyp (Fig. 1).

In most cases, there are signs of regenerative activity (especially at the bottom of the glands) in the epithelial cells which should not be confused with dysplasia. It is not unusual to observe few, cystic glandular elements that are mostly located more deeply, close to the base of the polyp, due to the overlying erosion and ulceration.

Sporadic juvenile polyps are commonly encountered in the daily pathology practice. In syndromic samples, around 20% of the polyps tend to be larger and multilobated with more crowded epithelial elements; these are termed atypical juvenile polyps.

Dysplasia, when detected in a syndromic juvenile polyp, has features of well-known intestinal adenomatous epithelium. The diagnosis should rely on the abrupt appearance of the pseudostratified pencil-like hyperchromatic cells, lack of maturation (i.e., in contrast to the proliferative regeneration at the basal aspect of the epithelial lining, the presence and persistence of dysplastic cells in the upper parts of the lesion), and possible structural alterations such as cribriform, labyrinthine, anastomosing, or solid patterns of dysplastic cells – high-grade dysplasia. It is imperative to seek for and report these findings in the pathology report as they would indicate a surgical resection.

Carcinoma can be seen as an ordinary adenocarcinoma with no evidence of a residual juvenile polyp; still, in many patients the malignant tumor can be observed to be originating from a juvenile polyp. There does not seem to be a differing phenotype of a JP-related carcinoma than its sporadic counterparts.

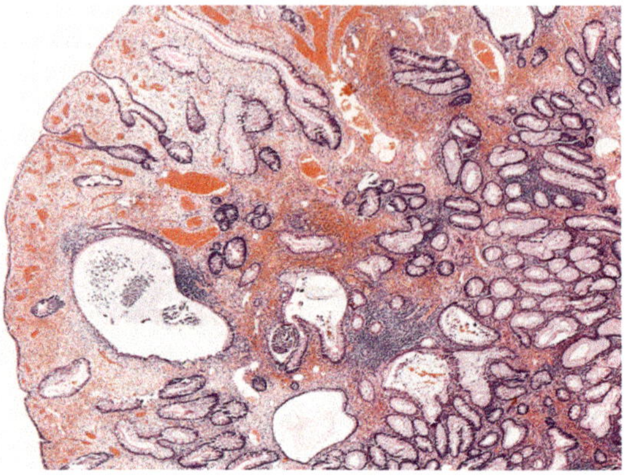

Juvenile Polyposis Syndrome, Lower Gastrointestinal Tract, Fig. 1 An ulcerated juvenile polyp with budding and cystically dilated glandular structures of varying size and shape and an edematous land inflamed lamina propria (H&E; ×200)

Immunophenotype

The juvenile polyps in syndromic patients do not exhibit a specifying immunohistochemical profile. Be that as is, it may be of interest to expect distinct immunophenotypes by antibodies being generated in the future, relying on the following molecular features.

Molecular Features

The present data indicates that the molecular defect lies in the TGFβ/BMP pathway. Loss-of-function germline mutations in SMAD4 or BMPR1A (components of the TGFβ/BMP pathway) are present in about half of the patients. The defects are because of point mutations or deletions. In the rest of the cases, the molecular basis is elusive.

As there is a conjunction with hereditary hemorrhagic telangiectasia (Osler-Weber-Rendu syndrome) in some cases, it is not surprising the latter syndrome is believed to be related to defects in the TGFβ/BMP pathway and SMAD genes.

It has been proposed that disruption of BMP signaling leads to a landscaper defect and crypts start to bud off or they grow perpendicular to the crypt-villus axis.

Differential Diagnosis

The distinction of a juvenile polyp from an inflammatory polyp or an inflamed hyperplastic polyp may be problematic. When in a patient with multiple GI polyps the pathologist is left with just one excised polyp, he/she should consider the clinical, endoscopic, and, if present, molecular findings. If these are not provided, for a hamartomatous-looking polyp, the pathologist may not safely give a diagnosis of a juvenile polyp. Still, there are ancillary considerations as follows.

A hyperplastic polyp virtually always – even irritated and/or ulcerated – bears a resemblance to the basic colorectal organization of the cryptic and stromal elements. That is, in a hyperplastic polyp, there is an expansion of the already-present epithelial and stromal components, a proliferation of the crypts: their "hyperplasia." The most expectable confusion would be between an inflamed goblet cell or microvesicular-type hyperplastic polyp and a juvenile polyp. The only clue to make a distinction between these two might be in that juvenile polyps do not show any organized dispersion of glandular structures. Juvenile polyps oftentimes contain a very exaggerated amount of inflammation and few residual glandular structures leading the microscopist to the contemplation that the active inflammation and surface ulceration had been causing a loss of the epithelial elements and their subsequent attempt at renewal. In addition, juvenile polyps have a greater inclination to have stalks, which is generally not valid for hyperplastic polyps, in that they are mostly sessile.

Inflammatory polyps are lesions deriving from the excessive regenerative activity of the GI mucosa. While they can be sporadic, they are most frequently associated with a chronic injurious condition of the GI wall, such as inflammatory bowel disease, ischemic states, persistent enteroinvasive infections, etc. The main response of the GI tract to injury is regeneration, not scarring or fibrosis. These taken into account, any etiology can cause an inflammatory polyp. These lesions can be very large so as to be called "giant" inflammatory polyps. Their microscopic features include an inflamed and edematous stroma, proliferating cryptic elements with distorted shapes, and frequently ulcerated luminal sides. These are the reasons why they are the number one lesion to be confused with juvenile polyps. The pathologist should question the presence of inflammatory bowel disease, chronic ischemic enterocolitis, drug use – especially NSAIDs – and any other known insult to the GI tract.

Juvenile polyps, by their morphology, generally are not prone to be confused with Peutz-Jeghers polyps, which have much more crowded glandular elements and a classically described tree-like smooth muscle proliferation in between the glands. Peutz-Jeghers polyps also may be sporadic, but in the syndromic samples, the polyps – especially in the stomach – can look much like a nonspecific hamartomatous polyp and, not unexpectedly, a juvenile polyp. The same is also true with Cowden's, Bannayan-Riley-Ruvalcaba, and Cronkhite-Canada syndromes, in which a given polyp may be indistinguishable from a juvenile polyp. As a rule of the thumb, in a patient with a proven hamartomatous polyposis syndrome, any hamartomatous polyp is to be diagnosed as a manifestation belonging to the relevant syndrome. In cases with no proven syndromes, the pathological diagnosis should convey to the clinicians that the present polyp is a hamartomatous polyp which can be present in many hamartomatous polyposis syndromes, and, if required, necessary investigations be pursued. With these in mind, the pathologist should be aware that a hamartomatous polyp cannot, sometimes, precisely be categorized or grouped to a specific syndromic entity.

As there can be a combination of JP and hereditary hemorrhagic telangiectasia (Osler-Weber-Rendu syndrome), in a given patient with ectatic, abnormally located vascular structures in GI resection specimen, the pathologist must keep in mind that the patient might also have JP or vice versa.

References and Further Reading

Coburn, M. C., Pricolo, V. E., DeLuca, F. G., & Bland, K. I. (1995). Malignant potential in intestinal juvenile polyposis syndromes. *Annals of Surgical Oncology, 2*, 386–391.

Howe, J. R., Roth, S., Ringold, J. C., Summers, R. W., Järvinen, H. J., Sistonen, P., Tomlinson, I. P., Houlston, R. S., Bevan, S., Mitros, F. A., Stone, E. M., & Aaltonen, L. A. (1998). Mutations in the SMAD4/DPC4 gene in juvenile polyposis. *Science, 280*, 1086–1088.

Howe, J. R., Bair, J. L., Sayed, M. G., Anderson, M. E., Mitros, F. A., Petersen, G. M., Velculescu, V. E., Traverso, G., & Vogelstein, B. (2001). Germline mutations of the gene encoding bone morphogenetic protein receptor 1A in juvenile polyposis. *Nature Genetics, 28*, 184–187.

Jansen, M., de Leng, W. W. J., Baas, A. F., Myoshi, H., Mathus-Vliegen, L., Taketo, M. M., Clevers, H., Giardiello, F. M., & Offerhaus, G. J. A. (2006). Mucosal prolapse in the pathogenesis of Peutz-Jeghers polyposis. *Gut, 55*, 1–5.

Jass, J. R., Williams, C. B., Bussey, H. J., & Morson, B. C. (1988). Juvenile polyposis – A precancerous condition. *Histopathology, 13*, 619–630.

L

Lewy Bodies, Achalasia

Manuela Mafra
Centro Hospitalar Lisboa Central-H.S.J,
Lisbon, Portugal

Synonyms

Achalasia cardiae; Cardiospasm; Esophageal achalasia; Esophageal aperistalsis; Megaesophagus

Definition

Achalasia is an esophageal motility disorder involving the smooth muscle layer of the esophagus and the lower esophageal sphincter (LES).

Though the disease was first described more than 300 years ago (Willis 1674), its exact pathogenesis still remains poorly understood. Pathophysiologically, achalasia is caused by loss of inhibitory ganglion in the myenteric plexus of the esophagus. In the initial stage, degeneration of inhibitory nerves in the esophagus results in unopposed action of excitatory neurotransmitters, such as acetylcholine, resulting in high amplitude non-peristaltic contractions (vigorous achalasia). Progressive loss of cholinergic neurons over the time results in dilation and low-amplitude simultaneous contractions in the esophageal body (classical achalasia).

The most common form of achalasia is primary, which has no underlying cause. Since the initial description, several studies have attempted to explore initialing agents that may cause the disease, such as viral infection (measles virus, herpes zoster virus, herpes virus), other environmental factors, autoimmunity, and genetic factors. A small proportion of cases occur secondarily to other conditions, such as Chagas disease and esophageal cancer. Both lead to destruction of myenteric plexus, but available evidence suggests that infection may not be an independent cause of primary achalasia. A genetic basis for achalasia is supported by reports showing occurrence of the disease in monozygotic siblings and other first-degree relatives and occurrence in association with other genetic diseases such as Down's syndrome and Parkinson's disease.

As a fact, one of the primary pathological observations in achalasia was simply loss of ganglion cells. New insights into the mechanism (s) underlying the disorder were given by Qualman et al. (1984) who reported the presence of Lewy bodies in degenerating ganglion cells.

Lewy bodies were first described by Frederic Lewy, in 1912, in the brains of patients with "paralysis agitans," commonly known as Parkinson's disease.

Nowadays, Lewy bodies are abnormal aggregates of protein that develop inside nerve cells, not only in Parkinson's disease but also in Lewy body dementia and some other disorders

F. Carneiro et al. (eds.), *Pathology of the Gastrointestinal Tract*, Encyclopedia of Pathology,
DOI 10.1007/978-3-319-40560-5

(aging brain, senile dementia, Parkinsonism-dementia complex, Alzheimer's disease, Hallervorden-Spatz syndrome, striatonigral degeneration supranuclear palsy).

They consist of a heterogeneous mixture of more than 90 molecules, including Parkinson's disease-linked gene products (alpha-synuclein, DJ-1, LRRK2, parkin, and PINK-1), mitochondria-related proteins, and molecules implicated in the ubiquitin-proteasome system, autophagy, and aggresome formation.

They represent an alteration in neuronal cytoskeleton structure and are identified under the microscope as spherical eosinophilic cytoplasmic inclusion that displaces other cell components. They are found on the brain and may also be seen in the peripheral nervous system myenteric plexus of the upper and lower intestinal tract in achalasia and Parkinson's disease.

Parkinson's disease and achalasia share many common features neurologically. Both have Lewy bodies in the esophageal myenteric plexuses and the substantia nigra, in addition to evidence of degeneration of the dorsal motor nucleus of the vagus. The esophageal features radiologically and manometrically are also similar.

Because its major component is alpha-synuclein, Lewy bodies can be detected by immunocytochemistry. The presence of this protein is the hallmark of neurodegenerative diseases, now known as synucleinopathies.

For a practical point of view, at the present moment, the identification of Lewy bodies on a biopsy during myotomy for megaesophagus may identicate a relative early degenerative phase of achalasia, prior to massive ganglion loss, or coincidental (or presymptomatic) Parkinson's disease (or other age-related neurofibrillary degenerations).

Lewy bodies formation has been considered to be a marker of neuronal degeneration because neuronal loss is found in the predilection sites for Lewy bodies. However, recent studies (Wakabayashi et al. 2013) have indicated that non-fibrillar alpha-synuclein is cytotoxic and that fibrillar aggregates of alpha-synuclein may represent a cytoprotective mechanism in Parkinson's disease.

Considerable work is being developed, in the last few years, to understand alpha-synuclein secretion, its function, and its correlation to cell dysfunction and death, which may open new therapeutic strategies.

Clinical Features

Achalasia is characterized by progressive dysphagia and regurgitation. Diagnosis is reached with esophageal manometry and barium swallow radiographic studies. Manometry shows aperistalsis, partial or incomplete relaxation of LES, and increased basal tone of LES. Barium swallow radiography reveals dilation of esophagus with a narrowed segment at the end of the esophagus.

- **Incidence**
  Achalasia affects about one person in 100,000 per year.
- **Age**
  Achalasia affects mainly adults, between 20s and 60s, but may appear in infancy and childhood (fewer than 5% of cases).
- **Sex**
  No sex predilection (male-to-female ratio: 1/1).
- **Site**
  Esophagus.
- **Treatment**
  There is no cure for this condition. Symptoms can usually be controlled with treatment. Drugs such as calcium channel blockers and nitrates may be useful for some time. Botulinum toxin (Botox) injections in LES have temporary effect. More permanent relief can be achieved by esophageal dilatation and surgical cleaving of the muscle (Heller myotomy).
- **Outcome**
  Even with successful treatment, dysphagia my still deteriorate over the time. Annual checkup and repeating treatments may be needed. Gastroesophageal reflux, peptic ulceration, fibrous stricture, and Barrett's esophagus may associate. The most serious complications of achalasia are the hazard of development of aspiration pneumonia of undigested food and

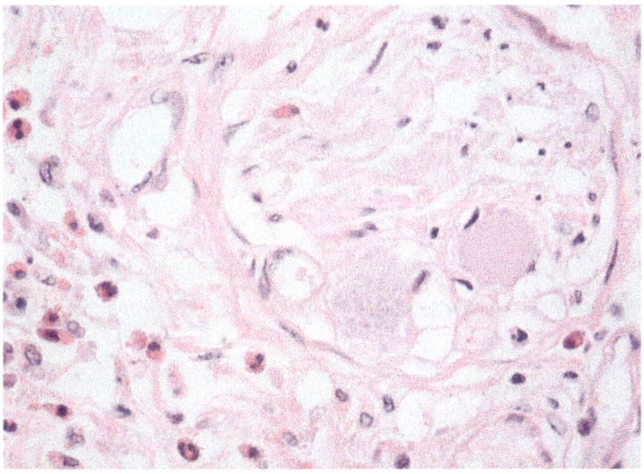

Lewy Bodies, Achalasia, Fig. 1 Eosinophilic infiltrate around and in a myenteric plexus with ganglion cells. (megaesophagus accidentally found in a forensic autopsy case (personal case)) (H&E 400×)

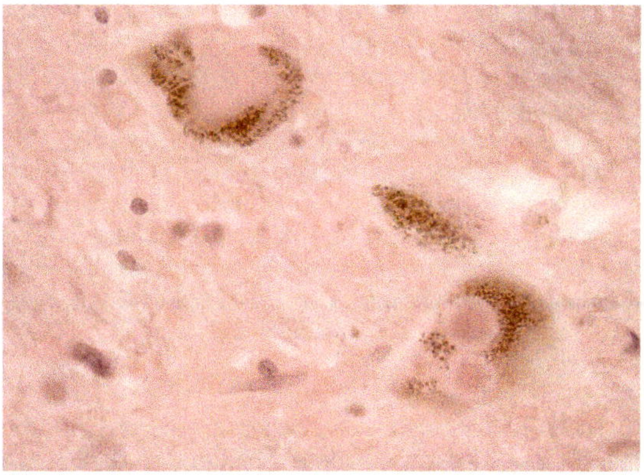

Lewy Bodies, Achalasia, Fig. 2 Three Lewy bodies in a pigmented neuron from substantia nigra. (necropsy case study from a patient with Parkinson's disease) (Courtesy of Dr. Olinda Rebelo, Coimbra; H&E 1,000×)

esophageal carcinoma (2–7% of cases), usually at a younger age than individuals without the disease, and of squamous cell type.

Macroscopy

Esophagus is dilated above the level of lower sphincter. Its wall may be of normal thickness, thicker than normal owing to hypertrophy of muscularis, or thinned out by dilation.

Microscopy

Histological examinations of the esophageal wall in achalasia reveal decreased numbers of neurons in the myenteric plexuses. The ganglion cells that remain often are surrounded by lymphocytes and eosinophils. T-cell inflammatory infiltrate of myenteric plexus with fibrosis is inversely correlated with the number of preserved ganglia. Eosinophils are found in the muscularis propria (not in the epithelium, as in eosinophilic esophagitis) (Fig. 1).

Lewy bodies can be seen in neurons of the myenteric plexus, in some achalasia patients at an early degenerative phase of the disease. They are identified as spherical eosinophilic cytoplasmic inclusion that displaces other cell components. They can be single or multiple, within a neuron, and their size may vary (Fig. 2).

Immunophenotype

Lewy bodies are identified by alpha-synuclein immunocytochemistry (its major component). Due to their heterogeneity, other proteins studied by immunocytochemistry (like ubiquitin, tyrosine hydroxylase, neurofilaments, tau) can reveal them.

Molecular Features

A mutation in the alpha-synuclein gene on chromosome 4 can be found in a few families with an autosomal dominant form of Parkinson's disease. Polymorphisms in genes encoding for nitric oxide synthase, receptors for vasoactive intestinal peptide, interleukin 23, and the ALADIN gene have been reported.

Differential Diagnosis

It does not apply.

References and Further Reading

Dichson, D., Fujishiro, H., DelleDonne, A., Menke, J., Ahmed, Z., Klos, K., Josephs, K., Frigerio, R., Burnett, M., Parisi, J., & Ahlskog, J. (2008). Evidence that incidental Lewy body disease is pre-symptomatic

Parkinson's disease. *Acta Neuropathologica, 115*, 437–444.
Ghosthal, U., Daschakraborty, S., & Singh, R. (2012). Pathogenesis of achalasia cardia. *World Journal of Gastroenterology, 18*(24), 3050–3057.
Giuli R, McCallum R. W., & Skinner, D. B. (1991). *Primary motility disorders of the esophagus*. Achalasia (hypomotility) is the best known entity.http://www.hon.ch/OESO/vol_4_Prim_Motility/400_chapters.html
Marques, O., & Outeiro, T. F. (2012). Alpha-synuclein: From secretion to dysfunction and death. *Cell Death and Disease, 3*(7), e350.
Qualman, S. J., Haupt, H. M., Yang, P., & Hamilton, S. R. (1984). Esophageal Lewy bodies associated with ganglion cell loss in achalasia. Similarity to Parkinson's disease. *Gastroenterology, 87*(4), 848–856.
Wakabayashi, K., Tanji, K., Odagiri, S., Miki, Y., & Takahashi, H. (2013). The Lewy body in Parkinson's disease and related neurodegenerative disorders. *Molecular Neurobiology, 47*(2), 495–508. (Epub ahead of print in 2012).
Wakabayashi, K., Mori, F., Tanji, K., Orimo, S., & Takahashi, H. (2010). Involvement of the peripheral nervous system in synucleinopathies, tauopathies and other neurodegenerative proteinopathies of the brain. *Acta Neuropathologica, 120*(1), 1–12.
Willis, T. (1674). *Pharmaceutice Rationalis Sive Diatribe de Medicamentorum Operationibus in Human Corpore*. London, England: Hagae Comitis.

Lymphocytic Colitis

Arzu Ensari
Department of Pathology, Ankara University Medical School, Sihhiye, Ankara, Turkey

Synonyms

Microscopic colitis; Microscopic colitis with intraepithelial lymphocytosis

Definition

Lymphocytic colitis (LC) is characterized by a diffuse increase of intraepithelial lymphocytes (IELs) (>20 IELs per 100 epithelial cells) in the surface epithelium accompanied by an increase of lamina propria inflammatory cells. By definition, no subepithelial collagen deposition should be present. The diagnosis of LC should be made in conjunction with clinical, endoscopic, and histological findings. Patients typically present with chronic watery diarrhea with normal or near-normal endoscopy.

Clinical Features

- **Incidence**
  The incidence of LC is approximately 3.1 in 100,000.
- **Age**
  It is common in middle-aged to older adults with a mean age of 51 years.
- **Sex**
  Female predominance is less in LC with nearly equal sex distribution.
- **Site**
  There are reports that suggest nonuniform colonic involvement, with less inflammation in the left colon compared with the right colon.
- **Treatment**
  Most patients respond to symptomatic or anti-inflammatory therapy.
- **Outcome**
  In some patients spontaneous recovery can be seen, while others may require 5-ASA compounds or immunosuppressants. The overall prognosis is good.

Macroscopy

The endoscopy is normal in the majority of patients. A few may show erosions or superficial ulcers.

Microscopy

The histological triad of increased IELs, surface epithelial injury, and increased lamina propria cellularity is characteristic of lymphocytic colitis (Figs. 1 and 2). The required number of intraepithelial lymphocytes varies between 10 and 20 per 100 surface epithelial cells (normal number = 4–10). The number can vary among

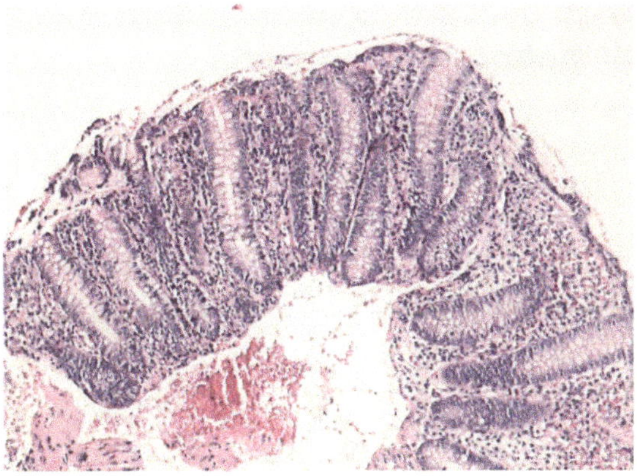

Lymphocytic Colitis, Fig. 1 Colonic mucosa with increased IELs and lamina propria inflammatory cells (H&E; ×100)

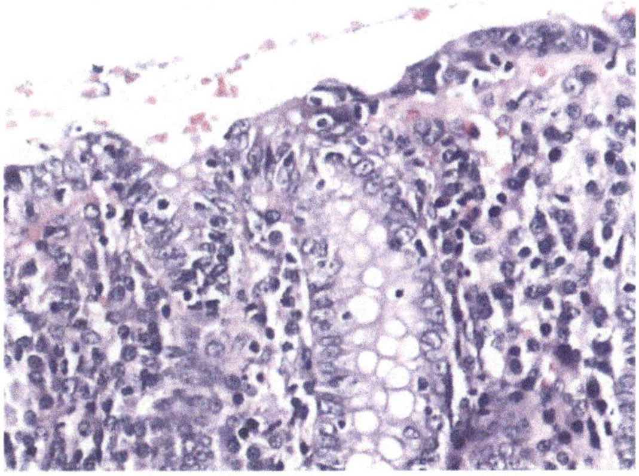

Lymphocytic Colitis, Fig. 2 Surface epithelial flattening and increased IELs (H&E; ×200)

biopsy samples between 10 and 65 (median 30). A second component is surface epithelial injury, which consists of a loss of the normal columnar shape, mucin depletion, and a flat or syncytial appearance of the surface epithelium. The crypt epithelium shows nuclear enlargement and a slight increase in mitotic activity. The lamina propria shows increased cellularity, due primarily to increased plasma cells with a fewer number of lymphocytes, eosinophils, and rarely neutrophils. Several variants or atypical forms of LC have been described. The clinical presentation is usually similar to the classic form of LC but the histology is different.

Cryptal Lymphocytic Colitis

Rubio and Lindholm (**49**) recently reported a series of patients with symptoms similar to those of LC and increased IEL count, not in the surface epithelium, but within the cryptal epithelium. Therefore, the authors proposed the name "cryptal lymphocytic colitis," in distinction to classic "surface" lymphocytic colitis. The mean number of IELs was 46/100 cryptal epithelial cells. In contrast, the mean number recorded in the surface columnar cells was 7 IELs/100 surface epithelial cells. Immunohistochemistry revealed a similar (CD3+ CD8+) phenotype as seen in classic LC. Special stains revealed a normal basement membrane underneath the surface epithelium. Similar to the classic form, all patients with cryptal lymphocytic colitis had long periods of watery diarrhea of unknown etiology. At endoscopy the colon showed either normal or mild patchy changes such as erythema. There was no indication that these patients suffered from celiac disease or from chronic inflammatory bowel disease, infectious colitis, or parasitic colitis.

Paucicellular Lymphocytic Colitis

The distinctive histologic features that separate paucicellular LC from classic LC are its patchiness and a lower density of surface IELs such that the morphologic criteria of classic LC are not fulfilled. Goldstein and Bhanot (**51**) recently reported 19 such cases. Colonic biopsies showed foci of mildly increased lamina propria lymphoplasmacytic inflammation and increased surface intraepithelial lymphocytes separated by foci or tissue fragments of normal mucosa. The mean surface IEL counts were 11.1 per 100 epithelial cells for paucicellular lymphocytic colitis and 29.3 IELs per 100 enterocytes for classic lymphocytic colitis. Clinical features of the paucicellular lymphocytic colitis, including endoscopy, are similar to those seen in classic LC. Therefore the authors suggested that paucicellular lymphocytic colitis should be considered as part of the morphologic spectrum of lymphocytic colitis. Some authors regard this condition as "colonic epithelial lymphocytosis" or "microscopic colitis, not otherwise specified (NOS)."

Immunophenotype

Immunohistochemical analysis shows that the increased IELs retain the normal CD3/CD8-positive T cell phenotype. The predominant cell type in the lamina propria is the CD4-positive T helper cell.

Molecular Features

There is no known molecular feature attributed to LC.

Differential Diagnosis

The differential diagnosis of LC includes fewer entities compared to CC. Among these, infectious colitis, the resolving phase in particular, chronic constipation, Crohn's colitis, drugs such as omeprazole, normal mucosa overlying a lymphoid follicle, and celiac disease may all cause histopathologic features resembling LC.

References and Further Reading

Beaugerie, L., Luboinski, J., Brousse, N., et al. (1994). Drug induced lymphocytic colitis. *Gut, 35*, 426–428.

Fernández-Bañares, F., Salas, A., Esteve, M., et al. (2003). Collagenous and lympho-cytic colitis: Evaluation of clinical and histological features, response to treatment, and long-term follow-up. *The American Journal of Gastroenterology, 98*, 340–347.

Langner C, Aust D, Ensari A, Villanacci V, Becheanu G, Miehlke S, Geboes K, Münch A; Working Group of Digestive Diseases of the European Society of Pathology (ESP) and the European Microscopic Colitis Group (EMCG) (2015) Histology of microscopic colitis-review with a practical approach for pathologists. *Histopathology, 66*(5), 613–626.

Lazenby, A. J., Yardley, J. H., Giardiello, F. M., et al. (1989). Lymphocytic ('microscopic') colitis: A comparative histopathologic study with particular reference to collagenous colitis. *Human Pathology, 20*, 18–28.

Wang, N., Dumot, J. A., Achkar, E., et al. (1999). Colonic epithelial lymphocytosis without a thickened subepithelial collagen table: A clinicopathologic study of 40 cases supporting a heterogeneous entity. *The American Journal of Surgical Pathology, 23*, 1068–1074.

Lymphocytic Esophagitis

Paula Borralho Nunes
Hospital Cuf Descobertas and Escola Superior de Tecnologia da Saúde de Lisboa and Instituto de Anatomia Patológica, Faculdade de Medicina da, Universidade de Lisboa, Lisboa, Portugal

Definition

Lymphocytic esophagitis (LE) is defined as a histologic phenotype of esophagitis, which is characterized by an excess of intraepithelial lymphocytes (IELs) in the peripapillary fields, with spongiosis and no or only rare intraepithelial granulocytes. The patients present with chronic dysphagia, odynophagia, and motility disorders.

There have been conflicting studies on the true existence of lymphocytic esophagitis, a condition first described by Rubio et al. in 2006. Controversy still exists over whether LE is a true pathologic entity with a corresponding specific clinical correlate or whether LE is merely a nonspecific histologic finding, eventually representing an extreme in the spectrum of gastroesophageal reflux disease or an involvement in other inflammatory conditions (e.g., Crohn's disease, celiac disease). In fact, in some cases of histologic diagnosis of LE, there is an associated Crohn's disease, and this seems to be is a relatively common finding particularly in the pediatric patients with CD. However, only one-fifth of these patients present with gastroesophageal reflux disease, as opposed to almost half of those with normal esophagus or other types of esophagitis. The prevalence of other possibly relevant concurrent pathological changes in other parts of the gastrointestinal tract was also studied. Helicobacter pylori infection has similar prevalence in patients with lymphocytic esophagitis who have simultaneous gastric biopsies and in patients with a normal esophageal mucosa. In contrast, the prevalence of Helicobacter pylori is significantly lower in patients with esophageal eosinophilia. There is no association with lymphocytic gastritis, but celiac sprue was diagnosed in 2 of 39 patients with lymphocytic esophagitis who also had duodenal biopsies (7.7%), in contrast to 1.1% in patients with normal esophagus and 1%.

The true causes for this apparently site-related chronic mucosal inflammation remain elusive. Some authors suggest this is because there are multiple etiologies, with IELs and spongiosis in the squamous epithelium of the esophagus representing nonspecific findings and a response to a variety of pathogenic stimuli, similar to the intraepidermal lymphocytes and spongiosis seen in spongiotic dermatitis of the skin. Although many patients described with LE had some type of allergy, no association was found in the literature between LE, seasonal allergies, asthma, or celiac disease. The possibility exists that some patients have unrecognized food allergies. LE could also be due to a nonallergic reaction to an ingested substance, such as a drug, causing topical injury to the esophageal mucosa.

In conclusion, no definite clinical associations have been detected in adults. As most published results are based on retrospective chart review, there may be important clinical information omitted that would only be apprehended with prospective and larger studies.

Clinical Features

- **Incidence**
  There is scant demographic data and the worldwide exact incidence of lymphocytic esophagitis is not known. Lymphocytic esophagitis is nevertheless a rare condition, reported with an incidence of 0.1%, in a large series of esophageal biopsies from a large gastrointestinal pathology practice covering 43 states in the USA (Haque and Genta 2012). However, LE seems to increase in its incidence (Cohen et al. 2012).
- **Age**
  There is wide age distribution in the published cases of LE and control cases (2–81 years in one series, with mean ages of 44 years (Purdy et al. 2008)).
- **Sex**
  Lymphocytic esophagitis seems to have a slight predilection for the female gender in the adult population.
- **Site**
  In the majority of published series, there is no reference to the exact location of the affected segment of the esophagus. In one series, biopsy specimens from LE cases were from the proximal (3/22 [14%]), mid (6/22 [27%]), and distal (16/22 [73%]) esophagus (Purdy et al. 2008).
- **Treatment**
  Being a condition where the true causes for this lymphocytic mucosal inflammation remains obscure, there is no specific strategy for treatment of LE. Corticosteroids have been noted to be beneficial in other gastrointestinal lymphocytic or autoimmune phenomenon, rendering a course of a topical corticosteroid agent (e.g., fluticasone) probably appropriate. Swallowed fluticasone in particular has been found to induce histological remission in closely related esophageal autoimmune conditions like eosinophilic esophagitis.
- **Outcome**
  LE seems to have a benign natural history, with most patients reporting an improvement in symptoms and satisfaction with their health-related quality of life (Cohen et al. 2012). Prospective studies are needed to better characterize the natural history and potential treatments for this clinical entity.

Macroscopy

Endoscopic examination of the esophagus reveals signs of esophagitis in about half the cases. Some reports describe endoscopic features similar to those seen in eosinophilic esophagitis, i.e., rings (Fig. 1), mucosal fragility, mucosal splitting, and even perforation. In fact, an endoscopic impression of eosinophilic esophagitis is reported in one-third of the patients. An impression of esophageal motility disorder was noted in some patients.

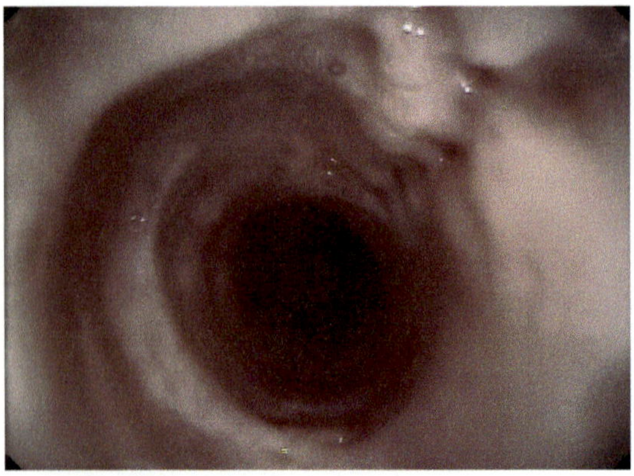

Lymphocytic Esophagitis, Fig. 1 Endoscopy showing rings throughout the length of the esophagus; these are common in lymphocytic esophagitis (Courtesy of Dr. Pedro Pinto Marques)

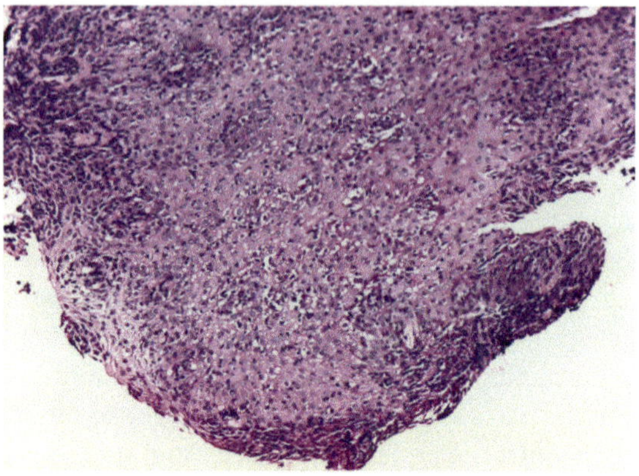

Lymphocytic Esophagitis, Fig. 2 Low power H&E stain demonstrates esophageal mucosa showing peripapillary intraepithelial lymphocytosis with basal zone hyperplasia and intercellular edema. No significant population of eosinophils or neutrophils is identified

Microscopy

Lymphocytic esophagitis is a histologic phenotype of esophagitis defined histopathologically as the presence of a dense lymphocytic infiltrates in the peripapillary esophageal squamous mucosa and marked spongiosis, in the absence of significant numbers of neutrophils or eosinophils. Lymphocytic infiltrates seem to be patchy: while in nonaffected areas often only scattered lymphocytes can be found, the counts can easily exceed 50 and even 100 in the affected peripapillary zones. There is a significant difference between the number of IELs in peripapillary and interpapillary fields.

Biopsies also show usually marked edema of the intercellular spaces of the squamous epithelium in the esophageal squamous mucosa ("spongiosis"). In fact, the peripapillary location of lymphocytes and association with spongiosis are more important and reliable criteria than the exact number. Spongiosis is a nonspecific inflammatory response that may also occur in patients with gastroesophageal reflux and eosinophilic esophagitis; however, in neither of these two conditions does the intensity of the inflammatory response approach that found in association with peripapillary lymphocytic infiltrate (Fig. 2).

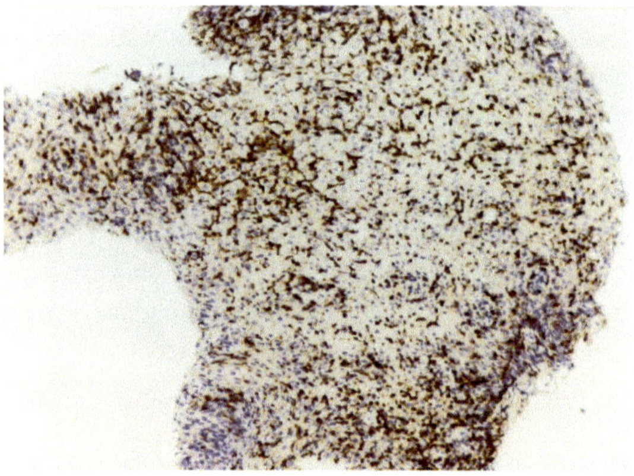

Lymphocytic Esophagitis, Fig. 3 Low power CD3 immunostain showing squamous epithelium of the esophagus infiltrated by high numbers of CD3+ intraepithelial lymphocytes

Immunophenotype

The immunostains show presence of CD3 and CD8 lymphocytes (T cell markers) in the epithelium, without significant amounts of lymphocytes expressing B cell markers (i.e., CD 20, CD79) (Figs. 3–5).

Molecular Features

There are no molecular anomalies associated with lymphocytic esophagitis.

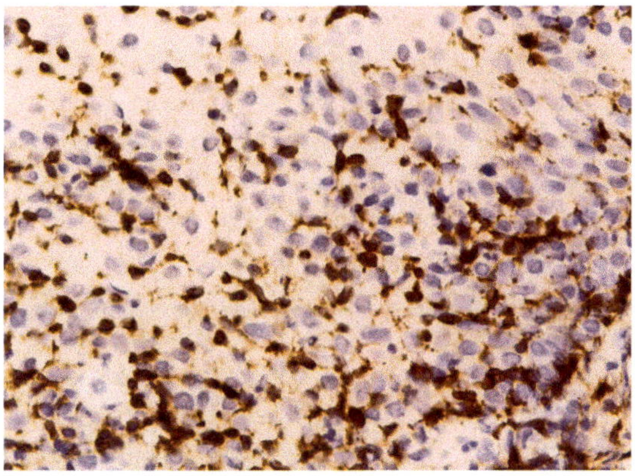

Lymphocytic Esophagitis, Fig. 4 Medium power CD8 immunostain. Numerous intraepithelial CD8+ lymphocytes can be identified

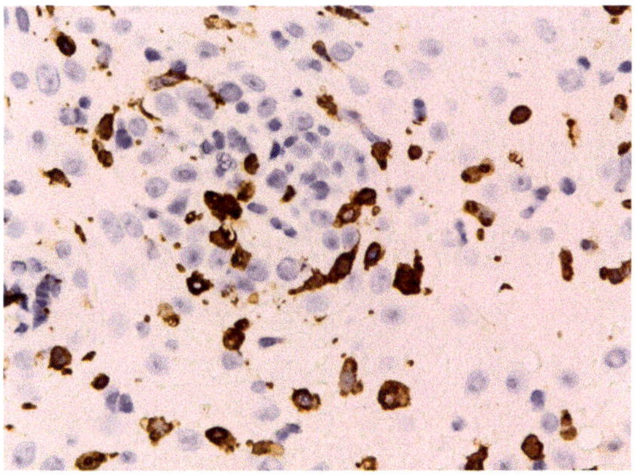

Lymphocytic Esophagitis, Fig. 5 High power CD8 immunostain showing intraepithelial lymphocytes around peripapillary fields

Differential Diagnosis

Endoscopically, lymphocytic esophagitis can be mimicked by reflux esophagitis or eosinophilic esophagitis.

On histology, drug-induced esophagitis has to be ruled out, as well as involvement of the esophagus with lichen planus and other dermatologic conditions, Crohn's disease, and lymphoma. In order to exclude the possibility of other underlying gastrointestinal disorder, esophageal, gastric, and duodenal biopsies as well as scrutiny of the past medical history are recommended, as lymphocytic esophagitis is a diagnosis of exclusion.

References and Further Reading

Cohen, S., Saxena, A., & Waljee, A. K. (2012). Lymphocytic esophagitis: A diagnosis of increasing frequency. *Journal of Clinical Gastroenterology, 46*(10), 828–832.

Ebach, D. R., Vanderheyden, A. D., Ellison, J. M., et al. (2011). Lymphocytic esophagitis: A possible manifestation of pediatric upper gastrointestinal Crohn's disease. *Inflammatory Bowel Diseases, 17*(1), 45–49.

Haque, S., & Genta, R. M. (2012). Lymphocytic oesophagitis: Clinicopathological aspects of an emerging condition. *Gut, 61*(8), 1108–1114.

Purdy, J. K., Appelman, H. D., Golembeski, C. P., et al. (2008). Lymp hocytic esophagitis: A chronic or recurring pattern of esophagitis resembling allergic contact dermatitis. *American Journal of Clinical Pathology, 130*(4), 508–513.

Rubio, C. A., Sjödahl, K., & Lagergren, J. (2006). Lymphocytic esophagitis. A histologic subset of chronic esophagitis. *American Journal of Clinical Pathology, 125*(3), 432–437.

Lymphocytic Gastritis

Helena Baldaia
Serviço de Anatomia Patológica, Centro Hospitalar de São João, Porto, Portugal

Synonyms

Varioliform gastritis

Definition

Lymphocytic gastritis is a pathological reaction pattern common to a variety of entities (Lash et al. 2009). It is characterized by an intense lymphocytic infiltrate in the gastric mucosa with permeation of the foveolar epithelium. It is mainly associated with celiac disease and *H. pylori* infection but it also complicates Crohn's disease, HIV infection, Menétrier disease, hypersensitivity reactions, autologous hematopoietic cell transplantation, lymphoma, and esophageal carcinoma (Fenoglio-Preiser et al. 2008).

The etiology is still unknown. The strong association with celiac disease and the fact that the intraepithelial lymphocytes are CD8+ T cells have raised the hypothesis of an allergic or autoimmune pathogenesis (Lash et al. 2009).

The most common symptoms are weight loss and anorexia (Lash et al. 2009).

Clinical Features

- **Incidence**
  It is seen in 1–4% of patients who undergo upper endoscopy (Lash et al. 2009).
- **Age**
  The most frequently affected individuals are middle-aged and elderly (Fenoglio-Preiser et al. 2008).
- **Sex**
  There is a male predominance (Lash et al. 2009).
- **Site**
  The site of involvement depends mainly on the disease association. In *H. pylori* infection, the infiltrate is more prominent in the corpus; in celiac disease, the lesions are more striking in the antrum (Fenoglio-Preiser et al. 2008).
- **Treatment**
  Currently, there is not a specific therapy available. Proton pump inhibitors are sometimes used and *H. pylori* eradication is indicated when the infection is encountered (Lash et al. 2009).
- **Outcome**
  Although very few cases of spontaneous regression have been reported, the course of the disease is usually chronic (Lash et al. 2009).

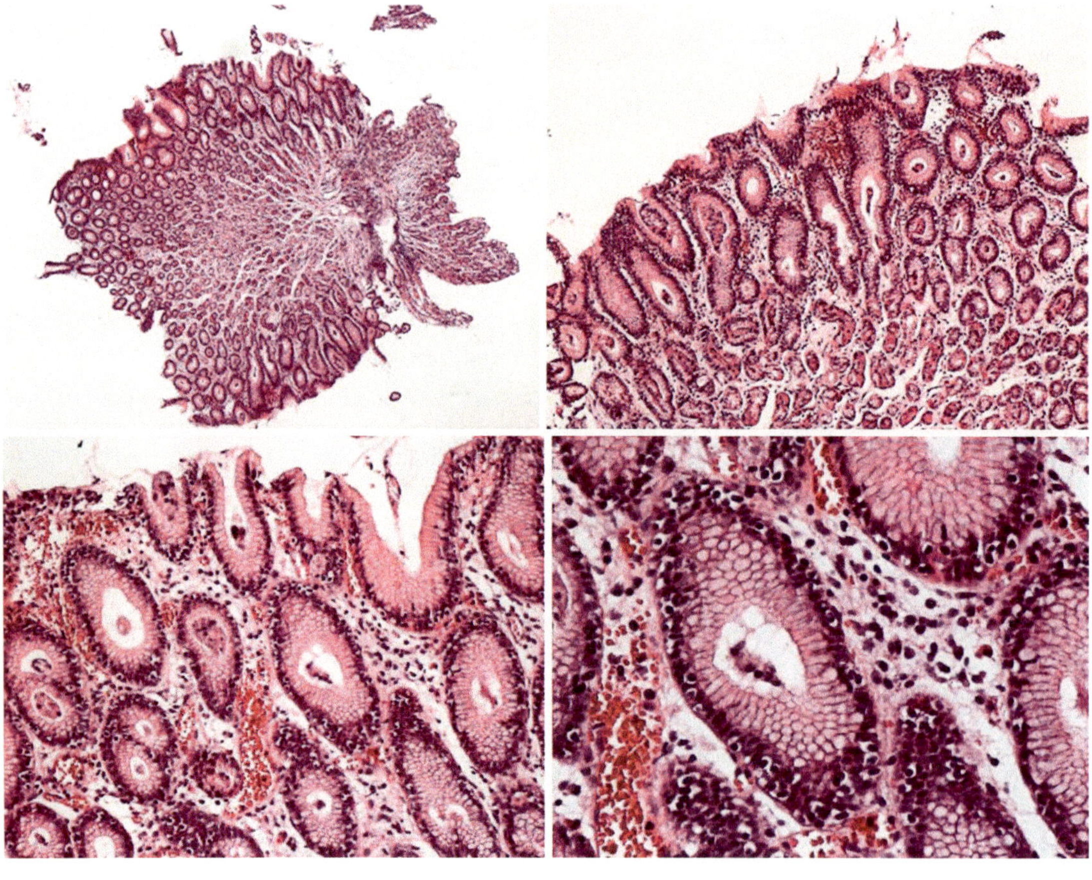

Lymphocytic Gastritis, Fig. 1 Lymphocytic gastritis. Prominent intraepithelial lymphocytosis

Macroscopy

Endoscopically, the gastric mucosa frequently presents with nodular elevations with central umbilications covered with mucus which are responsible for the name varioliform gastritis first attributed to this condition (Lash et al. 2009). Also, there can be thickening of the gastric folds, multiple erosions, or ulcers. The mucosa can appear endoscopically normal (Fenoglio-Preiser et al. 2008).

Microscopy

In lymphocytic gastritis (Fig. 1), there is epithelial lymphocytosis with at least 25 lymphocytes per 100 epithelial cells. The mucosal changes vary greatly in severity and are frequently patchy. There can be an inflammatory infiltrate in the lamina propria composed of lymphocytes, plasma cells, eosinophils, and mast cells. Neutrophilic infiltrate is usually scarce but can be moderate with erosions or ulcers (Fenoglio-Preiser et al. 2008).

Other histological findings are foveolar hyperplasia, degenerative changes of the epithelium, and increased mitoses. The degree of these associated changes depends on the underlying cause of lymphocytic gastritis. In celiac disease, the degree of gastric intraepithelial lymphocytosis correlates with the histological severity of the intestinal disease (Fenoglio-Preiser et al. 2008).

Immunophenotype

Intraepithelial lymphocytes in lymphocytic gastritis are CD8+ T cells (Lash et al. 2009).

Differential Diagnosis

The differential diagnosis with MALT (mucosa-associated lymphoid tissue) lymphoma is based on the morphology of the lymphocytes (in lymphocytic gastritis, there is no cytologic atypia), on the immunophenotype of the cells (B cells versus T cells), and on the degree of infiltration of the lamina propria which is more diffuse in lymphoma (Fenoglio-Preiser et al. 2008).

In typical *H. pylori* gastritis, the intraepithelial lymphocytosis is much less pronounced (Carmack et al. 2009).

References and Further Reading

Carmack, S. W., Lash, R. H., Gulizia, J. M., & Genta, R. M. (2009). Lymphocytic disorders of the gastrointestinal tract: A review for the practicing pathologist. *Advances in Anatomic Pathology, 16*(5), 290–306.

Fenoglio-Preiser, C. M., Noffsinger, A. E., Stemmermann, G. N., Lantz, P. E., & Isaacson, P. G. (2008). The nonneoplastic stomach. In J. McGouh & J. Pine (Eds.), *Gastrointestinal pathology an atlas and text* (pp. 197–199). Philadelphia: Lippincott Williams & Wilkins.

Lash, R. H., Lauwers, G. Y., Odze, R. D., & Genta, R. M. (2009). Inflammatory disorders of the stomach. In R. Odze & J. R. Goldblum (Eds.), *Surgical pathology of the GI tract, liver, biliary tract, and pancreas.* Philadelphia: Saunders.

L

Lymphoepithelioma-Like Carcinoma

Helena Baldaia
Serviço de Anatomia Patológica, Centro Hospitalar de São João, Porto, Portugal

Synonyms

Gastric carcinoma with a lymphoid stroma; Lymphoepithelial-like carcinomas; Medullary carcinoma with lymphocytic infiltration; Undifferentiated carcinoma with lymphoid stroma

Definition

Lymphoepithelioma-like carcinoma (LELC) is an undifferentiated carcinoma with prominent lymphoid stroma (Glickman and Odze 2009), which is similar to nasopharyngeal carcinomas. This type of tumor has been described in a number of extragastrointestinal sites, such as thyroid or breast, and also along the gastrointestinal tract (Delaney and Chetty 2012). In the latter, the most commonly reported site is the stomach, but cases arising in the esophagus and colon have been described (Delaney and Chetty 2012). Rarely, this type of tumor has been reported in the liver and biliary tree (Ishida et al. 2011).

LELC has been classically associated with Epstein-Barr virus (EBV) infection. In the stomach, more than 80% of cases have evidence of EBV infection, while in esophageal LELC, in one study, only 3% were positive for EBV by in situ hybridization or immunohistochemistry (Glickman and Odze 2009). In the biliary tree, evidence of EBV infection has been reported in some studies but not in others. EBV is a gamma-herpes virus with known oncogenic properties. The carcinogenic mechanism in LELC is unknown, but one study focusing in gastric LELC suggests that global CpG island methylation of promoter region of many associated cancer genes and abnormalities in signal transduction mediated by LMP2A as putative oncogenic EBV associated mechanisms in these tumors (Fukayama and Ushiku 2011).

In colorectal LELC, EBV association is obscure, with positivity frequently reported in stromal lymphocytes but weak or absent in epithelial cells. In one case of LELC of the colon, the patient had ulcerative colitis (Kojima et al. 2007). In one study, the tumor cells showed loss of expression of MLH-1 and PMS-2, thereby making it an MSI (microsatellite instability)-high LELC (Delaney and Chetty 2012). The authors suggest that LELC in the GI tract outside of the stomach is different in that it does not have the strong association with EBV like gastric cases, and may in fact be more strongly associated with MSI (Delaney and Chetty 2012).

The mechanism for the abundant lymphocytic infiltrate in LELC remains unclear. The lymphoid reaction could be a direct response either to the virus or virally induced antigens expressed by the neoplastic cells. In cases associated with a MSI-high profile, some have proposed that the inflammatory infiltrate represents an effective host response against the tumor cells (Delaney and Chetty 2012).

Clinical Features

- **Incidence**
  Lymphoepithelioma-like carcinoma of the GI tract is rare. In the stomach, it represents approximately 8% of all gastric carcinomas (Lauwers 2009). In the esophagus, less than 20 cases have been reported (Nakasono et al. 2007). In the colorectum, six cases have been reported so far (Delaney and Chetty 2012). In the liver and biliary tree, less than 20 cases have been described (Ishida et al. 2011). The majority of cases have been reported in Oriental countries, which are known endemic areas of EBV infection (Lee 2011).
- **Age**
  These tumors occur more commonly in the sixth decade. The mean age at diagnosis of gastric LELC was, in one study, 61.5 years (range 51–75) (Wang et al. 1999). In the esophagus, in the reported cases, age ranged from 54 to 79 years (mean 63.1) (Nakasono et al. 2007). One study reported LELC of the colon in a 25-year-old patient with ulcerative colitis (Kojima et al. 2007). The remaining colorectal LELCs were diagnosed in an age range 44–85 years. The age range of the reported cases of LELC of the biliary tract was 19–79 years.
- **Sex**
  There seems to be a male predominance, particularly in gastric and esophageal lymphoepithelioma-like carcinomas (Lauwers 2009; Nakasono et al. 2007).
- **Site**
  As already mentioned, GI lymphoepithelioma-like carcinomas have been described with variable incidences in the stomach, esophagus, and colon. Liver and biliary tract carcinomas have also been reported. In the stomach, LELC more commonly involves the proximal segments (gastric cardia/body) and is also frequently diagnosed in post-gastrectomy

remnants (Lauwers 2009; Fukayama and Ushiku 2011).

In the biliary tree, LELC is more commonly diagnosed in intrahepatic location (Ishida et al. 2011).

- **Treatment**
  Most of the cases described in the literature were surgically removed with variable adjuvant therapy. In the stomach, LELCs associated with EBV infection frequently display PD-L1 overexpression and are putative candidates for targeted therapy directed to the immune checkpoint (PD1/PD-L1).
- **Outcome**
  Although this is controversial, the prognosis of LELC is considered somewhat favorable. Survival rates close to 77% after 5 years have been reported in gastric LELC (Lauwers 2009). Esophageal LELC also seems to represent a relatively good prognosis (Nakasono et al. 2007). Local immune reaction may play an important role in suppression of tumor growth (Nakasono et al. 2007). The presence or absence of EBV has no prognostic significance in LELC of various organs (Ishida et al. 2011). The reduced number of cases of colorectal and hepatobiliary LELC carcinomas reported makes a prognosis assessment difficult.

Macroscopy

Lymphoepithelioma-like carcinomas usually appear as submucosal tumors, covered with normal appearing mucosa, frequently with central erosions or ulceration (Nakasono et al. 2007). In gastric LELC, there is also a degree of gastric wall thickening (Fukayama and Ushiku 2011). In colic LELC, polypoid tumors have been described (Kojima et al. 2007). Biliary tumors can appear as intrahepatic non-encapsulated well-circumscribed nodules with pushing borders (Lee 2011).

Microscopy

The characteristic histological appearance of lymphoepithelioma-like carcinoma is of irregular sheets, or syncytia, of polygon-shaped cells embedded within a prominent lymphocytic infiltrate, with occasional lymphoid follicles (Fig. 1). Plasma cells and even giant cells can be part of the infiltrate (Lauwers 2009). Granulomas have been occasionally reported (Tamura et al. 2010). Epithelial cells have eosinophilic cytoplasm, large vesicular nuclei, irregular nuclear profiles, and prominent nucleoli (Delaney and Chetty 2012). Unlike carcinomas of other organ sites, the majority of lymphoepithelioma-like cholangiocarcinomas are composed of two different components – an adenocarcinoma and a lymphoepithelioma-like carcinoma (Lee 2011).

Immunophenotype

Tumor cells stain with cytokeratin cocktails such as CAM5.2 and AE1/AE3. EMA staining has also been reported (Tamura et al. 2010; Nakasono et al. 2007). One colic tumor stained with cytokeratin and EMA, but the tumor cells were negative for CK7, CK20 and CDX-2 (Delaney and Chetty 2012).

Biliary neoplastic cells stain focally with CK7and CK19, and the rare hepatocellular tumors stain at least focally with HepPar-1 (Ishida et al. 2011).

The lymphocytic stroma is mainly composed of T lymphocytes (CD3 positive), usually CD8-positive. Also some CD4-positive T-cells and CD20-positive B lymphocytes are present and, sometimes, CD138-positive plasma cells can also be encountered (Lauwers 2009).

Immunohistochemical staining of tumor cells for EBV can also be performed, and intranuclear expression of EBV-encoded non-polyadenylated RNA-1 can be demonstrated by in situ hybridization (Lauwers 2009).

Molecular Features

There have been reports of losses of chromosomes 4p, 11p, and 18q, which seem to indicate a pathogenetic pathway different from other usual types of gastric carcinoma (Lauwers 2009). Also, CpG island methylation of the promoter region of

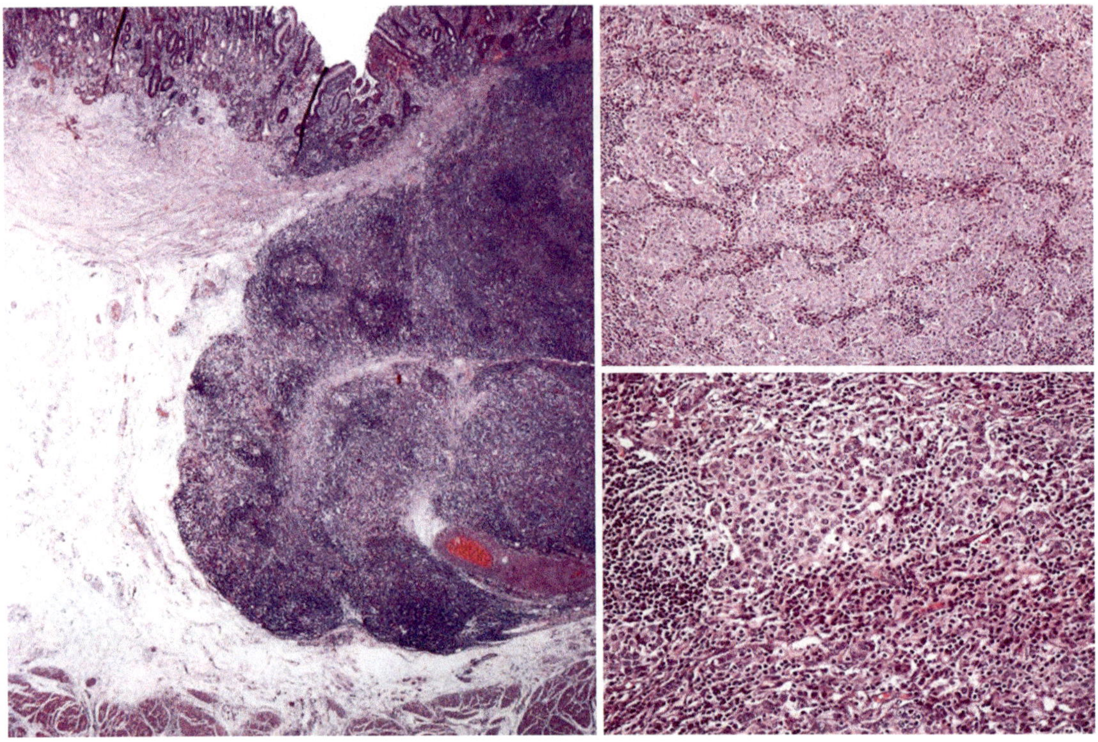

Lymphoepithelioma-Like Carcinoma, Fig. 1 Lymphoepithelioma-like carcinoma of the stomach. Syncytial aspect with nests of epithelial cells with abundant eosinophilic cytoplasm embedded in a lymphocytic stroma

many cancer-related genes with repression of tumor suppressor genes such as PTEN has been demonstrated in gastric LELC cells (Fukayama and Ushiku 2011). One colic tumor has shown a MSI-high phenotype with loss of expression of MLH-1 and PMS-2. The authors hypothesize there was a sporadic epigenetic hypermethylation of MLH-1 and its partner dimmer PMS-2, leading to a MSI-high colon cancer which attracted the dense lymphocytic population and the LELC phenotype (Delaney and Chetty 2012).

Differential Diagnosis

Gastrointestinal lymphoepithelioma-like carcinoma must be distinguished from *lymphoma*. Neoplastic atypical epithelial cells can usually be easily encountered, but immunostaining with cytokeratin can be of help in highlighting these cells. Also, the lymphocytes in LELC are usually small T lymphocytes.

Colic LELC can be difficult to distinguish from *medullary carcinoma* (which can be encountered in Lynch syndrome). In medullary carcinoma, there are more peritumoral than intratumoral lymphocytes; it has a pushing rather than infiltrative margin, and the tumor cells are uniform rather than pleomorphic, as seen in LELC (Delaney and Chetty 2012).

Biliary intrahepatic LELC may be morphologically indistinguishable from hepatocellular LELC. The latter, however shows at least focal HepPar1 positivity in the tumor cells.

When approaching lymphoepithelioma-like carcinoma, particularly in the liver, differential diagnosis of *metastatic* LELC from other organs must be considered (Ishida et al. 2011).

References and Further Reading

Delaney, D., & Chetty, R. (2012). Lymphoepithelioma-like carcinoma of the colon. *International Journal of Clinical and Experimental Pathology, 5*(1), 105–110.

Fukayama, M., & Ushiku, T. (2011). Epstein-Barr virus-associated gastric carcinoma. *Pathology, Research and Practice, 207*(9), 529–537.
Glickman, J., & Odze, R. D. (2009). Epithelial neoplasms of the esophagus. In R. Odze & J. Goldblum (Eds.), *Surgical pathology of the GI tract, liver, biliary tract and pancreas*. Philadelphia: Saunders.
Ishida, M., Mori, T., Shiomi, H., et al. (2011). Non-Epstein-Barr virus associated lymphoepithelioma-like carcinoma of the inferior common bile duct. *World Journal of Gastrointestinal Oncology, 3*(7), 111–115.
Kojima, Y., Mogaki, M., Takagawa, R., et al. (2007). A case of lymphoepithelioma-like carcinoma of the colon with ulcerative colitis. *Journal of Gastroenterology, 42*(2), 181–185.
Lauwers, G. Y. (2009). Epithelial neoplasms of the stomach. In R. Odze & J. Goldblum (Eds.), *Surgical pathology of the GI tract, liver, biliary tract and pancreas*. Philadelphia: Saunders.
Lee, W. (2011). Intrahepatic lymphoepithelioma-like cholangiocarcinoma not associated with Epstein-Barr virus: A case report. *Case Reports in Oncology, 4*(1), 68–73.
Nakasono, M., Hirokawa, M., Suzuki, M., et al. (2007). Lymphoepithelioma-like carcinoma of the esophagus: Report of a case with non-progressive behavior. *Journal of Gastroenterology and Hepatology, 22*(12), 2344–2347.
Tamura, T., Hamada, T., Sako, T., et al. (2010). Lymphoepithelioma-like carcinoma of the stomach with epithelioid granulomas. *Case Reports in Gastroenterology, 4*(3), 361–368.
Wang, H., Wu, M., Shun, C., et al. (1999). Lymphoepithelioma-like carcinoma of the stomach: A subset of gastric carcinoma with distinct clinicopathological features and high prevalence of Epstein-Barr virus infection. *Hepato-Gastroenterology, 46*(26), 1214–1219.

Lymphoma and Immunoproliferative Small Intestinal Disease (IPSID)

Başak Doğanavşargil
Department of Pathology, Ege University Medical School, Bornova, Izmir, Turkey

Abbreviations

BL	Burkitt lymphoma
DLBCL	Diffuse large B-cell lymphoma
DLBCL/BL, unclassifiable	Lymphoma, unclassifiable, with features intermediate between DLBCL and BL
EATL/EATL-I	Enteropathy-associated T-cell lymphoma-type-I
EATL-II	Enteropathy-associated T-cell lymphoma, type II (synonym with “Monomorphic epitheliotropic intestinal T-cell lymphoma”)
EBV+ DLBCL of elderly	EBV-positive diffuse large B-cell lymphoma of elderly
ENKTL	Extranodal NK/T-cell lymphoma
FL	Follicular lymphoma
IPSID	Immunoproliferative small intestinal disease
MALT lymphoma	Mucosa-associated lymphoid tissue lymphoma
MCL	Mantle cell lymphoma
MEITL	Monomorphic epitheliotropic intestinal T-cell lymphoma
NHL	Non-Hodgkin lymphoma
PBL	Plasmablastic lymphoma

Synonyms

Intestinal lymphoma: “Western-type” intestinal lymphoma

Immunoproliferative small intestinal disease (IPSID): Alpha chain disease; Mediterranean lymphoma; Seligmann disease

Monomorphic epitheliotropic intestinal T-cell lymphoma: Defined as “Enteropathy-associated T-cell lymphoma type” in World Health Organization (WHO) classification of tumors of haematopoietic and lymphoid tissues in 2008 and as “Monomorphic CD56 (+) intestinal T-cell lymphoma” in WHO Classification of Tumours of the Digestive System in 2010. The 2016 revision of the classification of lymphoid neoplasms defines the entity as “Monomorphic epitheliotropic intestinal T-cell lymphoma.”

Definition

Intestinal Lymphoma (IL)

The definition of “intestinal lymphoma (IL)” varies among the authors as it can occur as a primary lesion or in a secondary fashion in a substantial portion of the cases. Usually a "primary" gastrointestinal (GI) lymphoma is considered when the main bulk of disease is located in GI tract with involvement of only contiguous lymph nodes in the immediate vicinity of the primary mass but without involvement of liver or spleen. Additional criteria are normal levels of total and differential white blood cell count and absence of peripheral or mediastinal lymph node involvement at the time of presentation. In this context, "secondary" IL refers to lymphomas where the GI tract is additionally involved in a disseminated disease. However, some of the lymphomas concurrently occur in nodal and extranodal sites or show bone marrow infiltration simultaneously. Therefore, some series on ILs in the literature keep a unifying approach to all lymphomas arising in GI tract unless its primary gastrointestinal system origin is confirmed clinically or unless it is a type of lymphoma that exceptionally arise in GI tract as EATL or IPSID.

ILs are mature B, T, or NK/T-cell derived neoplasms; the clinical features, involvement patterns, treatment, and outcome of which differ from their nodal counterparts.

They usually present with abdominal pain, mass, lower GI bleeding, hematochezia, obstruction, perforation, or intussusceptions. Nausea, vomiting, weight loss, diarrhea, and clubbing are more common in small ILs. Malabsorption and malnutrition related symptoms usually accompany IPSID and EATL. Asymptomatic patients also exist or the lymphomatous infiltration can be clinically occult although rare.

Detailed information on lymphoma types can be found in related entries of this volume and World Health Organization monograph on tumors of the hematopoietic and lymphoid tissues.

Most commonly encountered intestinal B-cell lymphomas as DLBCL, MALT L, IPSID, BL, FL, MCL and less common but lower GI tract involving lymphomas *as* EBV+ DLBCL of elderly, PBL, DLBCL/BL, unclassifiable, and T or NK/T cell lymphomas as EATL, MEITL, or ENKTL, nasal type will be covered in this entry while the ones which rarely encountered in lower GI tract or only occur as a dissemination of a systemic disease will not be discussed in detail (Fig. 1).

IPSID is a variant of low grade extranodal marginal zone B-cell lymphoma of MALT type which typically presents as a malabsorption syndrome in young adults. It is characterized by marked plasma cell differentiation and dense lymphoplasmacytic infiltration and also called as "alpha chain disease" as it secretes defective alpha heavy chains unable to bind light chain (Fig. 2).

Clinical Features

Clinical features of ILs are given in Table 1.

- **Incidence**

  GI lymphomas are very rare and account for less than 4% of all gastrointestinal malignancies. On the other hand, GI tract is the commonest extranodal site, accounting for about 4–18% of all NHL's.

  The incidence of small intestinal lymphoma (23–30%) and colorectal lymphoma (6–23%) among GI lymphomas is less than stomach (60–75%) but much higher than in esophagus (1%) throughout the GI tract.

  The incidence of ILs and proportion of small intestinal ones among them show geographic variations due to increased frequency of IPSID in Mediterranean basin and the Far East or increased prevalence of EATL in Northern Europe due to coeliac disease. Colorectal lymphomas show almost equal prevalence around the world, but their incidence is increasing in relation with increasing prevalence of acquired or iatrogenic immunodeficiency conditions.

  Most of the ILs are NHL's and most of them are B-cell lymphomas; DLBCL (or regionally IPSID) is the most common form of lymphoma followed by BL or FL or MALT lymphoma in different series reported from different parts of the world. Recent reports also show increasing detection of small diminutive intestinal FLs due to enhancement in endoscopic techniques as double-balloon enteroscopy and capsule endoscopy. T-cell lymphomas are less common

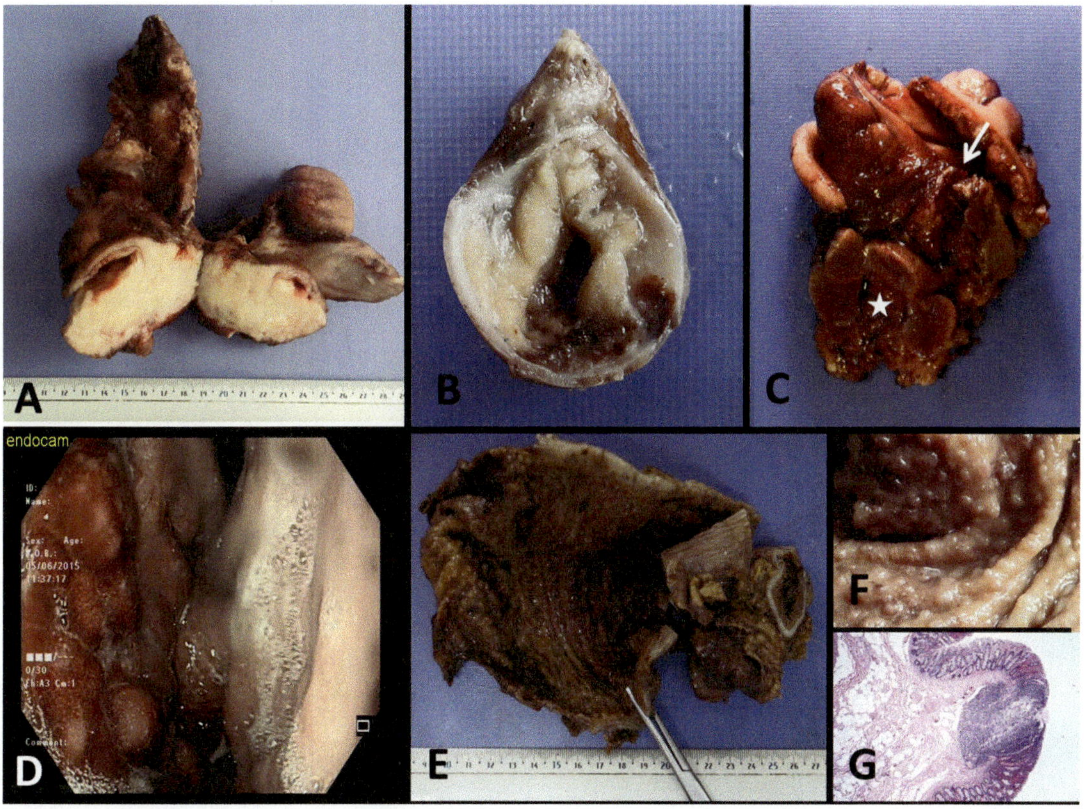

Lymphoma and Immunoproliferative Small Intestinal Disease (IPSID), Fig. 1 **Macroscopic appearance** (**a**) Large ileocecal mass (Burkitt Lymphoma). The cut-surface has a gray-white, soft, fish-flesh appearance. (**b**) Smaller Burkitt lymphoma located in cecum-appendix orifice, showing mucosal thickening, ulceration, hemorrhage, and submucosal invasion. (**c**) Diffuse large B-cell lymphoma presented with intussusception, early perforation (*arrow*), and lymph node involvement (*star*). (**d**) Endoscopic view of Mantle cell lymphoma with "multiple lymphomatoid polyposis" (also seen in MALT lymphoma and follicular lymphoma) (Courtesy of Prof. Dr. O. Ozutemiz from Ege University School of Medicine Department of Gastroenterology). (**e–f**) Multiple small nodulary/polypoid lesions incidentally found in a case with Hirschsprung's disease. (**g**) The histological view is consisted with nodular lymphoid hyperplasia (Haematoxylin-Eosin, ×4)

and accounts for approximately 10–25% of primary ILs (Fig. 3).

Incidence of IPSID: In 1980s, IPSID constituted up to 78% of all small intestinal malignancies and most common lymphoma in young adults in the Middle East, North and South Africa, and the Far East; however, recent reports show a decline in its prevalence, probably due to improvement in sanitary conditions, eventually reducing repeated infections leading to lymphoma-inducing chronic antigenic stimulations.

- **Risk factors**

  Some of the ILs occurs in the setting of chronic GI disease, bacterial or viral infections, and immunodeficiency conditions. The physiopathological mechanisms leading to this predisposition have not been well established for all types of lymphomas. However, chronic inflammation induced ongoing antigenic stimulation has a role in clonal expansion of lymphoid cells and eventually lymphoma development especially in MALT lymphoma and IPSID or in lymphomas related with viral

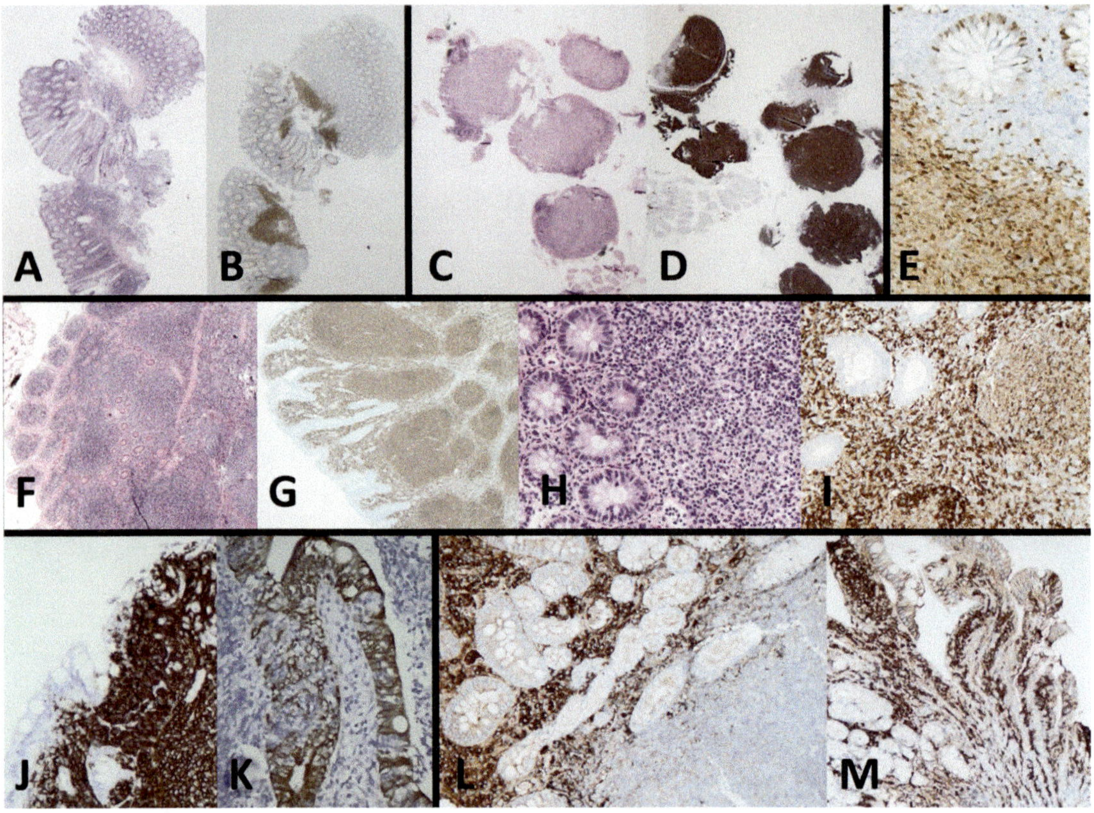

Lymphoma and Immunoproliferative Small Intestinal Disease (IPSID), Fig. 2 Small B-cell lymphomas. **(a–e) Mantle cell lymphoma (a)** Mantle cell lymphoma in an endoscopically normal mucosa (colon) (H&E, ×2). **(b)** Note the cyclin-D1 expression in deeper parts of mucosa highlighting the lymphoma infiltration (Cyclin-D1, ×2). **(c)** Mantle cell lymphoma in an endoscopically suspected case showing "nodular lymphomatoid polyposis" (colon) (H&E, ×2). **(d)** CD 20 positivity (CD20, ×2). **(e)** Nuclear cyclin-D1 expression (Cyclin-D1, ×20). **(f–i) Follicular lymphoma (f)** Mucosal involvement by follicular lymphoma. Note the broadened finger-like villi (H&E, ×4). **(g)** Follicular growth pattern which is more common than diffuse involvement in GI tract (CD 20, ×4). **(h)** Admixture of centrocytic and centroblastic cells (H&E, ×20). **(i)** BCL-2 expression (BCL-2, ×20). **(j–k) MALT lymphoma (j)** Small, CD 20 positive lymphocytes invading the epithelium of cecum (anti CD 20, ×10). **(k)** Lymphoepithelial lesion which is less frequent than gastric MALT lymphomas (Cytokeratin, ×10). **(l–m) IPSID: (l)** IgA positive cells in lamina propria (IgA, ×20). **(m)** Duodenal villi showing epithelial invasion with plasma cells (CD138, ×10)

infections. The following list summarizes the most common associations.

GI diseases

The relative risk of EATL(EATL-I) is approximately 1000-fold increased in ► Coeliac disease especially in refractory coeliac disease type II. The role of ► inflammatory bowel disease (IBD) is controversial; whether the disease itself or the immunosuppressive treatment alters this propensity remains unelucidated. Large, population-based cohort studies do not favor an evidence-based association for ulcerative colitis. However, the observations on Crohn's disease are more contradictory and suggest a possible relationship with EATL, EBV-positive Hodgkin lymphoma, or some B-cell NHLs (Fig. 4).

Infectious agents

► *Helicobacter pylori* (*H. pylori*) infection has an approved role in development of gastric MALT lymphoma; however, its contribution in extragastric locations where it does not normally colonize is questionable. Its role in immunodeficiency associated BL is also

Lymphoma and Immunoproliferative Small Intestinal Disease (IPSID), Table 1 Intestinal lymphomas at a glance: clinical features

	Incidence	Risk factors	Age	Sex	Site	Clinical behavior	Outcome
DLBCL	Most common IL in most series	Transformation from MALT L, FL	Broad range (8–88 years) (peak in 6th decade)	M	Ileocecal region	Aggressive	Potentially curable. (GCB-subtype more favorable than ABC-subtype)
MALT L	Frequent (its rank varies in different series)	Role of *H. pylori* in ILs is controversial	Middle-aged to older adults (peak in 7th decade)	M	Ileocecal region-rectum (Colon > small intestine)	Indolent (may transform into DLBCL)	Complete regression in early stage, may transform into DLBCL
IPSID	Most common IL in Mediterranean basin and the Far East.	*C. jejuni*/repeated polymicrobial infections	Older children and younger adults	M	Proximal small intestine (rarely reported in colon)	Indolent (may transform into DLBCL in stage C)	Potentially curable in Stage A. Risk of life-threatening malabsorption, In Stage C, needs long-term treatment, frequent follow-ups
MCL	Rare (<10% of IL). But most MCL show microscopic (88%) to overt (20%) GI involvement.	Solvents, GI infections	Older adults (>50 years)	M	Terminal ileum, jejunum, colon (more severe)	Aggressive	High recurrence rate despite treatment in most cases
FL	Less than 5% of GI lymphomas (common in North America, the UK, South Africa)	Western-type diet, sedentary life, immunosuppression	Middle-aged adults	F	Second part of duodenum (especially for duodenal-type FL), ileum, colon	Indolent (may transform into DLBCL, BL)	Localized polypoid forms and "duodenal type-FL" have excellent survival even without treatment
Burkitt L	Frequent (its rank varies in different series)	Endemic BL (EBV, malaria); Sporadic BL (30% EBV), Immunodeficiency-associated BL (Polymicrobial?)	Children and young adults	M	Ileocecal region	Aggressive and rapidly fatal if untreated	High remission rates with chemotherapy

(*continued*)

Lymphoma and Immunoproliferative Small Intestinal Disease (IPSID), Table 1 (continued)

	Incidence	Risk factors	Age	Sex	Site	Clinical behavior	Outcome
DLBCL/BL, unclassifiable	Very rare	HIV (in rectum)	Adults (rarely in children)	M	Ileocecal region	Aggressive	Depends on response to chemotherapy
EBV + DLBCL, elderly	Very rare. Common in East Asia, South America	EBV, Immunosenescence (Any known immunodeficiency/ lymphoma)	Classically older adults (>50 years), may also occur in younger patients	M[a]	Ileocecal region	Aggressive	Poorer than EBV (−) tumors
PBL	Very rare	Immunodeficiency (IBD?, HIV,EBV, HHV8)	Broad range (immuno-deficiency related in children) (peak in 6th decade)	M	Small intestine-anal region-cecum	Aggressive	Poor prognosis despite anti-HIV treatment
EATL (EATL-I)	Most common T-cell IL. Common in Northern Europe.	Coeliac disease (Refracter coeliac disease Type II)	Older adults (>50 years)	M[a]	Jejunum-proximal ileum (rarely duodenum-colon)	Aggressive	Poor prognosis, death from uncontrolled malabsorption, abdominal complications.
MEITL (EATL-II)	Less frequent. Common in Asians and Hispanic populations.	Unknown	Older adults (>50 years)	M	Ileocecal region, colon	Aggressive	Similar to EATL. Early lung spread
ENKTL, nasal type	Rare. More frequent in Asia and South America (Peru).	EBV infection	Middle-aged to older adults	M	Small intestine, ascending colon	Aggressive	Poor response (multidrug resistance)

Abbreviations: *IBD* inflammatory bowel disease, *HIV* human immunodeficiency virus, *EBV* Epstein-Barr virus, *HHV8* human herpesvirus-8, *GCB-subtype* germinal center like subtype, *ABC-subtype* activated B-cell like subtype

[a]Almost equal in some series

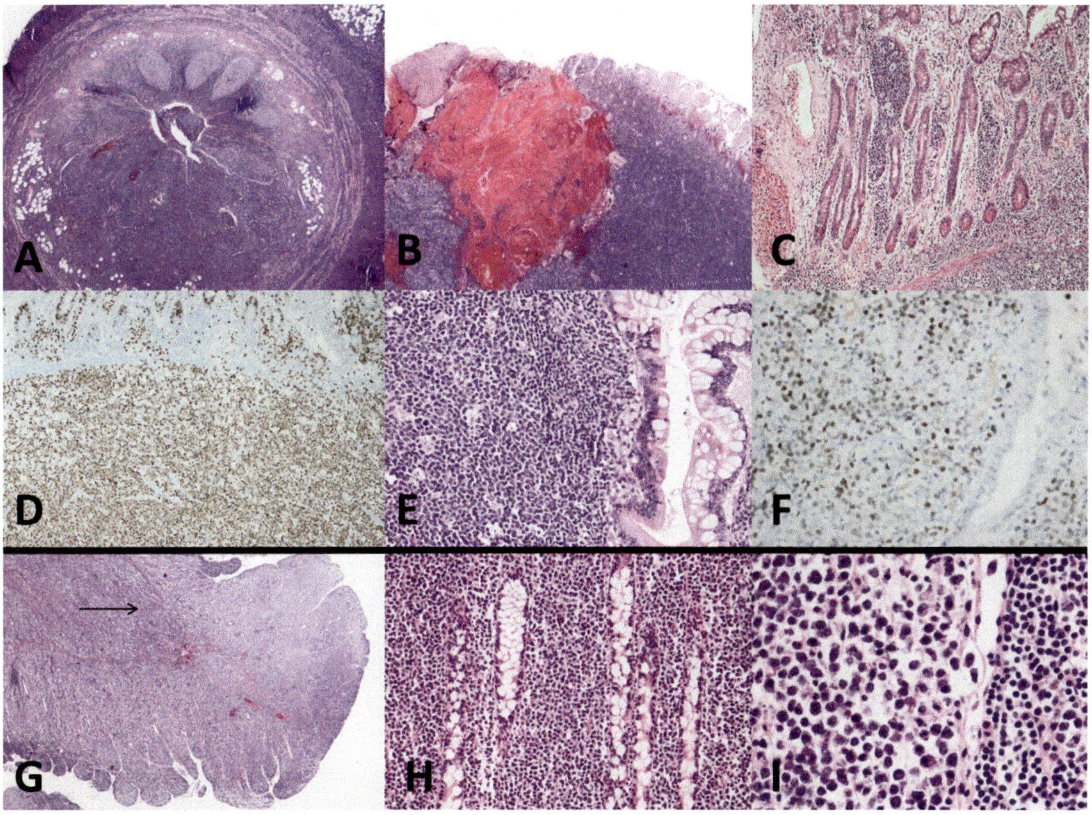

Lymphoma and Immunoproliferative Small Intestinal Disease (IPSID), Fig. 3 (**a–f**) **Burkitt lymphoma** (**a**) Appendiceal Burkitt lymphoma (H&E, ×2). (**b**) Terminal ileum involvement presented with penetrating ulceration and massive bleeding (H&E, ×4). (**c**) Mucosal involvement in case presented with large submucosal mass (H&E, ×10). (**d**) Ki-67 positivity (100%) (Ki-67, ×10). (**e**) Starry sky appearance (H&E, ×20). (**e**) c-Myc immunoexpression in lymphoma cells (c-MYC, ×20). (**g–i**) **Diffuse large B-cell lymphoma** (**g**) Full thickness bowel wall invasion totally effacing the mucosal architecture. Note the barely visible muscularis mucosa infiltrated by (**h**) Mucosal infiltration (**i**) Large cells with centroblastic and immunoblastic morphology. Note the adjacent smaller reactive lymphocytes

controversial. *Campylobacter jejuni* (*C. jejuni*) is the potential etiological factor for development of IPSID. A polymicrobial interference due to repeated intestinal infections (i.e., *Escherichia coli*, *Giardia lamblia*, *Ascaris lumbricoides*, *Vibrio cholera*, *Strongyloides stercoralis*) were also suspected for IPSID. ▸ Epstein-Barr virus (EBV) is the most common virus shown in different types of lymphomas, listed as the major etiological agent for development of BL (mostly the endemic form), EBV-positive DLBCL, MCL, ENKTL-nasal type, AIDS-associated immunoblastic lymphoma, anorectal DLBCL, and lymphomatoid granulomatosis. Although EBV-related lymphomas are heterogeneous group diseases, they all harbor *latent* EBV within tumor cells. Human immunodeficiency virus (HIV) has a role in development of PBL but of DLBCL and BL as well. Role of Hepatitis viruses (particularly HCV) is controversial, but there are reports pointing to regression of lymphomas (particularly lymphoplasmacytic lymphoma/ Waldenstrom macroglobulinemia) following antiviral treatment. *Plasmodium falciparum* malaria is potentially related with endemic BL (Fig. 5).

Immunodeficiency

Acquired immunodeficiency disease (AIDS): One third of AIDS-related NHLs involve the

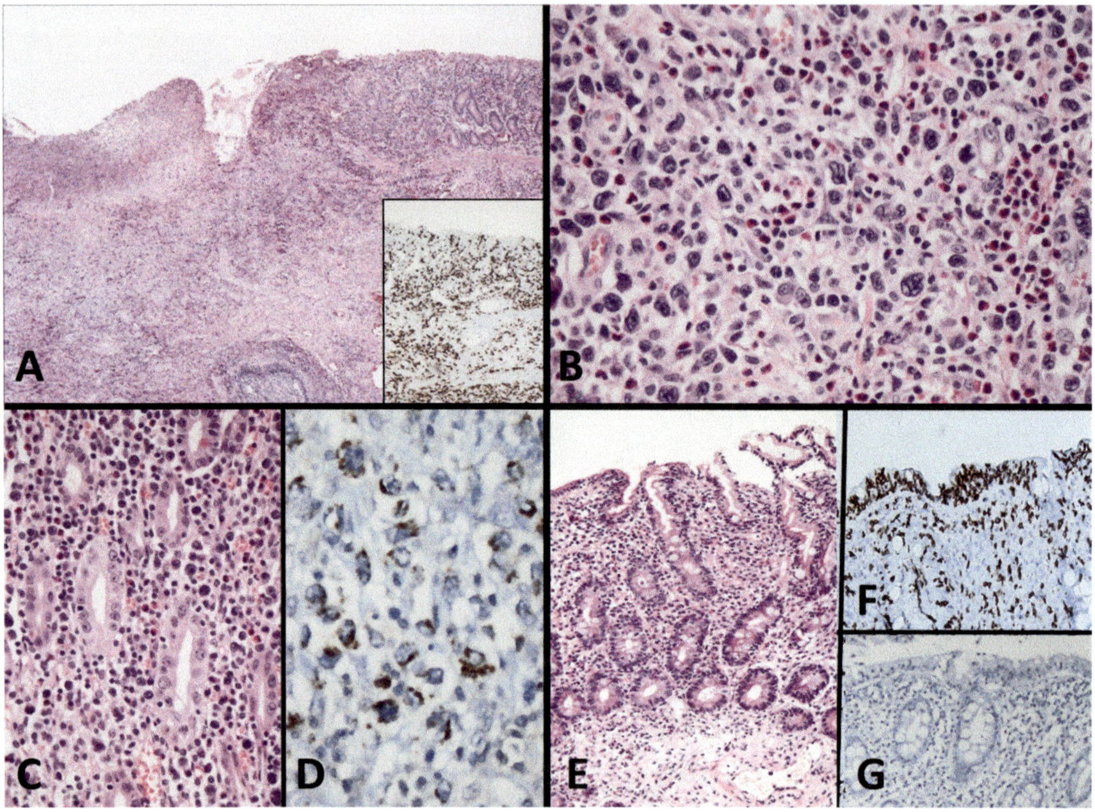

Lymphoma and Immunoproliferative Small Intestinal Disease (IPSID), Fig. 4 **T-cell lymphoma.** EATL (**a**) Mucosal ulceration and transmural neoplastic infiltration (H&E, ×4) (*inset*: CD7 immunoexpression in neoplastic cells, ×4). (**b**) Medium to large sized neoplastic cells, with irregular, pleomorphic vesicular nuclei, distinct nucleoli, pale cytoplasm. Background is rich in eosinophils (H&E, ×20). (**c**) Infiltration of mucosa, note the scattered cells with more irregular nuclei (H&E, ×20). (**d**) Granzyme-B staining cytotoxic granules in the cytoplasm of neoplastic cells (Granzyme-B, ×40). (**e**) Adjacent mucosa with enteropathic changes. Note architectural irregularity, villous shortening, and flattening (H&E, ×10). (**f**) Intraepithelial lymphocytosis (CD3, ×10). (**h**) Loss of CD8 staining in intraepithelial lymphocytes (CD8, ×10)

GI tract (especially colon and anorectal region) at presentation. Most of them are B-cell lymphomas, mostly occur in later stages of HIV infection, frequently show EBV association, present with multifocal involvement, and follow an aggressive course with increased frequency of complications as perforation and massive bleeding. On the other hand, the reported frequency of lymphoma is declining due to wide usage of antiretroviral treatments, in recent years.

Declined immune defense due to senescence: stands as the major etiopathogenetic mechanism in development of EBV+ DLBCL of elderly.

Immunosuppressive drugs: are responsible for most of IBD associated lymphomas. Corticosteroids and TNF-α inhibitors are the potential agents. Immunodeficiency is a risk factor particularly for development of BL.

- **Age**

  Age distribution varies between types of lymphomas. DLBCL has the broadest spectrum of age among all NHL's. Colorectal lymphomas are seen one or two decade earlier than small intestinal lymphomas. NHL's seen in immunocompromised or EBV-positive patients also occur earlier than expected in immunocompetent and EBV-negative

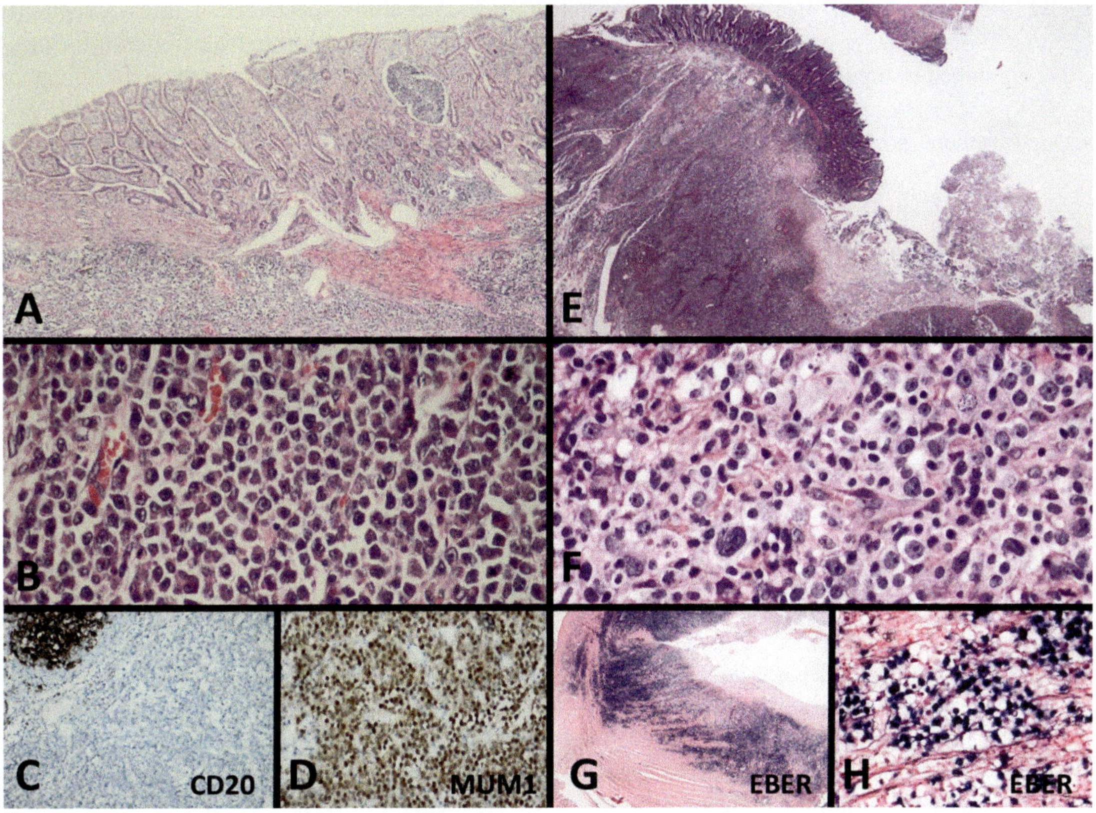

Lymphoma and Immunoproliferative Small Intestinal Disease (IPSID), Fig. 5 Rare entities. (**a–d**) **Plasmablastic lymphoma** (**a**) Mucosal and submucosal invasion in terminal ileum. Note the eroded surface (H&E, ×4). (**b**) Cell aggregates of plasmablastic cells and cells with immunoblastic features (H&E, ×40). (**c**) CD20 negativity (CD20, ×20). (**d**) Plasmablastic cells with MUM1 positivity (MUM1, ×20). (**e–h**) **EBV+ DLBCL of elderly** (**e**) Ileocecal tumor with penetrating mucosal ulceration (H&E, ×2). (**f**) Admixture of small and large cells, immunoblast-like cells, Hodgkin Reed-Sternberg like cells (H&E, ×40). (**g–h**) Extensive EBER positivity throughout the tumor by chromogenic in situ hybridization. (EBER CISH probe, ×2). (**h**) EBER positivity in neoplastic lymphocytes (EBER CISH probe, ×40)

population. Most frequently encountered age groups for most common lymphomas are given below.

First two decades: BL, IPSID, rarely FL, DLBCL, PBL

3rd–5th decades: MCL, FL, PBL, IPSID, DLBCL

5th–7th decades: EBV+ DLBCL of elderly (over 50 years old), MCL, FL, PBL, DLBCL

>7th decade: DLBCL, MALT lymphoma, MCL

- **Sex**

  Males predominate (two- to fourfold) in almost all subtypes of ILs. FL and MALT lymphoma (in some series) are slightly more frequent in females while EBV + DLBCL of elderly, and EATL are almost equally reported in both sexes in some series.
- **Site**

  Small intestinal lymphomas are more frequently reported than colorectal lymphomas probably due to regional high frequency of IPSID. In small intestine, ileum is the most commonly involved site (60–65%) followed by jejunum (20–25%) and duodenum (6–8%) involvement of other sites is less than 10%. For colonic lymphomas, ileocecal region, which harbors greater amount of lymphoid tissues, is the most frequently involved area followed by ascending colon and rectum. Anorectal lymphomas are rare (3%) and commonly encountered in immunocompromised patients, HIV, or EBV infected cases. Multifocal involvement is more common in MALT lymphoma and MCL.

Predilection site for special types of lymphomas are given below.

Duodenum: FL

Jejunum: IPSID (proximal jejunum), EATL, T-cell lymphomas, MCL

Ileum: IPSID, DLBCL, EATL-I (proximal ileum)

Ileocecal region: Most of ILs (BL, DLBCL, PBL, MEITL, MCL, EBV+ DLBCL of elderly, MALT lymphoma)

Appendix: BL (and less frequently DLBCL, MALT lymphoma)

Colon and rectum: DLBCL, MALT lymphoma, MCL, PBL, FL

Anorectal region: DLBCL, PBL

- **Treatment**

The treatment strategies are controversial and mostly but not only dependent on the histological type of the lymphoma. Different modalities can be applied alone or in combination according to the localization, stage or extent of the disease, age of patient, and accompanying disorders or complications..

"Wait and watch" approach can be chosen for early stage indolent lymphomas as FL (especially in duodenal-type FL). *Antibiotherapy* is a treatment option for early stage IPSID and duodenal/rectal MALT lymphoma, although the role of *H. pylori* in ILs is debated. Nevertheless, there are occasional reports of DLBCL transformed from MALT lymphomas, IPSID, and even BL regressed after eradication therapy for *H. pylori*, probably due to elimination of other bacterias contributing in disease progression. *Antiretroviral drugs* reduce the risk of lymphoma development in HIV-infected patients. *Radiotherapy* is beneficial for solitary tumors or for debulking large masses and is most effective when done prior to the chemotherapy. Surgery is preferred for mass forming or localized disease. Surgical intervention is also indicated for complications as obstruction, perforation, intussusceptions, stricture formation, and ulceration with massive bleeding. Chemotherapy with single or multiagent modalities or combined with surgery, radiotherapy, or immunotherapy is one of the main options especially for aggressive cases or for advanced disease. The "CHOP" regimen (cyclophosphamide, hydroxydaunorubicin, vincristine (Oncovin), and prednisone) or other anthracycline-based agents are the most commonly used combinations/agents. Rituximab (anti CD20 antibody) is either added to chemotherapy (R-CHOP) or used as a stand-alone effective targeted therapeutic agent. Notably, PBL, which typical lacks CD20, does not benefit from rituximab. Different protocols are used for more aggressive lymphomas as BL. Stem cell transplantation with high-dose chemotherapy can also be considered for aggressive lymphomas as EATL, BL, or MCL. Supplementary treatment is indicated for malabsorption due to IPSID or enteropathy-associated lymphomas although their effect to overall survival is controversial.

Treatment of IPSID: Antibiotherapy for early stage (Stage A) disease. Surgery and chemotherapy for advanced stages with addition of supplementary treatment.

- **Outcome**

The outcome of lymphomas is mainly dependent to histological subtype, the site, stage, grade, extent of disease, and certain molecular alterations. Case-dependent factors as declined immunity, presence of accompanying EBV or HIV infection, higher International prognostic index (IPI), and complications as initial presentation with bowel perforation, intractable massive bleeding, malnutrition are also significant adverse factors independently interfering with prognosis.

Staging of ILs is debated because of various staging systems. "Paris staging system" is also relevant for prognosis as the "modified Ann Arbor classification" and feasible for GI tract for minding the level of bowel wall invasion and presence of lymph node involvement similar to TNM system. Intestinal lymphomas have usually poorer outcome than their counterparts in stomach partly due to higher frequency of complications.

Most of the B-cell lymphomas even the more aggressive ones are potentially curable with different treatment modalities, while most T-cell lymphomas confer a poor prognosis with aggressive clinical behavior with frequent recurrences despite intense treatment.

- Lymphomas showing indolent course are Low grade B-cell lymphomas as FL (especially the "duodenal-type FLs"), IPSID, or MALT lymphoma.
- Aggressive lymphomas with poor prognosis are T-cell lymphomas, PBL, EBV+ DLBCL of elderly, MCL.
- Aggressive lymphomas with variable outcome (or potentially curable) are BL and DLBCL

Outcome of IPSID: The disease course in stage A is indolent and can last for years with vague symptoms and may respond to antibiotherapy and show remission if discovered in this stage. Stage B lesions do not respond to antibiotics and represent a transition to advanced disease. Stage C follows an aggressive clinical course similar to DLBCL requiring a systemic therapy and correction of malnutrition related symptoms.

Macroscopy

Macroscopic appearances of ILs are diverse and despite attempts for endoscopic or macroscopic classification of them, there is neither a standard classification nor a specific feature that can distinguish them from other benign or malignant GI lesions. Invasive forms may show early mesenteric invasion with extraluminal masses. But ILs do not necessarily present with intraluminal masses. Short or long segment involvement and multifocality can be seen. Although macroscopic presentation may change depending on the stage at the time of diagnosis and mixed forms can occur in an index case, there is some correlation between histological types of ILs and most common macroscopic appearances as follows:

- Endoscopically normal mucosa/overlooked lesions: MCL (Microscopic evidence can be found in up to 85% endoscopically normal cases)
- Diffuse infiltration: MCL, T-cell lymphomas, IPSID, MALT Lymphoma, PBL
- Multiple lymphomatous polyposis (multiple polyps/small nodules throughout GI tract, measuring 0.2–2 cm): Classically defined in MCL but also encountered in FL and MALT Lymphoma
- Large bulky masses: BL, DLBCL (rapidly growing)
- Obstruction and intussusception: DLBCL, BL, FL (less common)
- Ulceroinfiltrative lesions: DLBCL, EATL, T-cell lymphomas
- Transmural infiltration MALT lymphoma, EATL, DLBCL
- Ulcers-Strictures: More common in EATL, DLBCL, BL. T-cell lymphomas may mimic Crohn's disease with fistulization.
- Perforation: EATL, ENKTL, nasal type, EBV+ DLBCL of elderly, DLBCL (rarely forming aneurysms)

Macroscopy of IPSID: Stage A: Diffuse mucosal fold thickening with or without mesenteric lymph node involvement. Stage B: Slightly irregular, nodular mucosa, multiple lymphomatous polyposis, circumscribed small masses, submucosal invasion. Stage C: Large masses with overt mesenteric lymph node involvement.

Microscopy

Histological features of ILs are similar to their nodal counterparts with minor changes and can be found in related entries in more detail. Brief histopathological features of common ILs are summarized in Table 2.

EATL and IPSID are two exclusive types of lymphomas arising in GI tract solely. Therefore, they will be discussed in more detail herein as well as "duodenal-type FL" which is separately emphasized as a distinctive variant of FL in 2016 revision of the WHO classification of

Lymphoma and Immunoproliferative Small Intestinal Disease (IPSID), Table 2 Intestinal lymphomas at a glance: macroscopic and microscopic features

	Macroscopy	Microscopy
DLBCL	Large masses, ulceration, transmural infiltration, obstruction and intussusception, stricture, ulcer formation	Diffuse infiltration of large cells with basophilic cytoplasm. *Centroblastic* variant with round to oval vesicular nuclei (mostly in colon), *immunoblastic* with prominent central nuclei, or *anaplastic* with pleomorphic nuclei (mostly in immunosuppressive conditions) or *mixture* of all
MALT L	Solitary mass/nodule (more common in ileocecal region to rectum). Diffuse infiltration. May also present as multiple lymphomatous polyposis. Multicentricity is reported	Heterogenous population with predominantly centrocyte-like marginal zone cells or monocytoid cells with pale cytoplasm and small lymphocytes, scattered immunoblasts, centroblast-like cells, plasmacytic differentiation. LEL's are less prominent than in stomach. "Naked-follicle" appearance with obliteration of mantle zone and colonization of germinal centers by lymphoma cells. Muscularis mucosa disruption and submucosal invasion is apparent
IPSID	Stage A: Normal mucosa; Stage B: Thickened mucosal folds; Stage C: Mass forming lesions, lymph node involvement	*Stage A:* Blunt, broadened, and shortened villi. Plasma cell dominant lymphoplasmacytic infiltration confined to the mucosa and mesenteric lymph nodes. No cytological atypia. The overlying epithelium is usually intact, the crypts are sparse. *Stage B:* Nodular mucosal infiltrates similar to MALT lymphoma with follicular colonization, LELs and extension to the submucosa. *Stage C:* Immunoblastic and plasmablastic cells dominate, cytological atypia is frequent, mitoses are brisk. Risk of transformation to DLBCL
MCL	Multiple lymphomatous polyposis (classical presentation) (polyps are larger in ileocecal region). May also present as solitary mass or endoscopically normal mucosa with or without diminutive tumoral infiltrates	Diffuse involvement is more common than nodular or true mantle zone pattern. Monotonous centrocyte-like small to medium sized cells with angular/slightly to markedly irregular nuclei and scant cytoplasm. Mitotic figures, epitheloid histiocytes, finely hyalinized vessels are apparent. Glands/crypts are destroyed but no LELs. *Variants:* Blastoid (aggressive), pleomorphic (aggressive), rare small cell, marginal zone like types
FL	Multiple small polyps/nodules (multiple lymphomatous polyposis). Mucosal nodularity (more frequent in jejunum and ileum). Ulceroinfiltrative masses. Colonic FLs invade submucosal to subserosal areas	Mucosal involvement with follicular growth pattern (more common than diffuse infiltration in GI tract). Glove balloon-like villous hypertrophy. Monomorphic infiltration of small- to medium-sized centrocytes admixed with centroblasts. Lack of reactive germinal center tingible body macrophages
	Duodenal-type FL: multiple small submucosal polypoid lesions (1–5 mm) some clustering around the papilla Vateri	**Duodenal-type FL**: Centrocytes and few centroblasts packed together in usually well-circumscribed neoplastic follicles without starry sky appearance
Burkitt L	Bulky right lower quadrant mass. Intussusception, Stricture, ulcer formation	Diffuse monotonous infiltration. Medium-sized round to oval cells showing "squared-off" borders. Finely clumped chromatinized nuclei with multiple basophilic nucleoli. Deeply basophilic cytoplasm bearing multiple lipid vacuoles. Frequent mitosis, "starry sky" appearance with tingible body macrophages
DLBCL/BL, unclassifiable	Submucosal/mucosal nodule/mass. Rare lymphomatous polyposis	Morphological features intermediate between BL and DLBCL. The infiltration is composed of medium- to large-sized cells. More like BL with frequent mitosis, apoptosis, and starry sky appearance
EBV+ DLBCL of the elderly	Diffuse infiltration or mass forming. Perforation and multifocality reported	"Large cell" variant with monotonous immunoblast or HRS-like cells and "polymorphic" variant with scattered large cells

(*continued*)

Lymphoma and Immunoproliferative Small Intestinal Disease (IPSID), Table 2 (continued)

	Macroscopy	Microscopy
		in a mixed cellular small lymphocytic, plasmacytic, and histiocytic background, with geographic necrosis in both forms
PBL	Diffuse bowel thickening, exophytic mass, deep bowel wall invasion with serosal infiltration and perforation	Nodular and diffuse infiltration of cohesive cell aggregates of plasmablastic cells or cells with immunoblastic to more mature plasmacytic features. Mitotic activity and apoptotic bodies are frequent
EATL (EATL-I)	Thickened folds, multiple raised, ulcerated nodules/exophytic mass. Strictures. Stenosis, perforation, and multifocality reported. Ulcerative jejunitis in the prodromal period	Polymorphous infiltration of predominantly medium to large cells with irregular, angular, vesicular nuclei, distinct nucleoli, faint cytoplasm. Background rich in histiocytes, plasma cells, and numerous eosinophils, which may obscure neoplastic cells. Necrosis is common. Adjacent mucosa show enteropathic changes with villous atrophy, crypt hyperplasia, and intraepithelial lymphocytes
MEITL (EATL-II)	Similar to EATL-I	Monomorphic infiltration of small, round cells with dark nuclei and scant cytoplasm. Villi in the near vicinity of neoplastic infiltration show villous shortening and atypical intraepithelial lymphocytes while the distant zones preserve normal villous architecture without intraepithelial lymphocytes
ENKTL, nasal type	Multifocal or diffuse pleomorphic ulcers. Perforation	Diffuse polymorphous infiltration effacing the mucosal architecture. Variety of cells: small, medium, large sized, or anaplastic cells. Pleomorphic neoplastic cells with irregular, convoluted vesicular nuclei, indistinct nucleoli, pale moderate to abundant cytoplasm admixed with inflammatory cells. Angiocentric and angiodestructive growth pattern with necrosis and mucosal ulceration

GI gastrointestinal, *LEL* lymphoepithelial lesion, *MLP* multiple lymphomatoid polyposis, *HRS-like* Hodgkin Reed-Sternberg like cells

lymphoid neoplasms, which appears to have an indolent nature and an excellent outcome. Recent monograph recognizes "GI tract FL" as a variant.

Microscopic findings of duodenal-type FL: It is a low grade (grade 1–2) FL composed of centrocytes and fewer centroblasts that were packed together usually in well-circumscribed neoplastic follicles without tingible body macrophages (starry sky appearance) and mantle zones. Sheets of small lymphoid cells with round, dark nuclei are seen outside the follicles and the follicular structures occupy at least some duodenal villi. The neoplastic infiltration has overlapping features with "in situ follicular neoplasia" and MALT lymphoma.

Microscopic findings of EATL (EATL-I): The neoplastic lymphoid population is polymorphous, most commonly composed of medium to large sized cells with irregular, angulated, vesicular nuclei, prominent nucleoli, and moderate to ample pale staining cytoplasm. The predominant cell population can have an "immunoblastic," "pleomorphic," or "anaplastic" morphology. Anaplastic lymphoma-like appearance with multinucleated cells is also encountered in rare cases. Usually, there is an inflammatory background typically rich in eosinophils or histiocytes and plasma cells and may even obscure neoplastic cells. *Adjacent mucosa* characteristically shows varying degree of enteropathic changes reminiscent of coeliac disease with total or partial villous atrophy, intraepithelial lymphocytosis, and crypt hyperplasia or display normal architecture with only intraepithelial lymphocytosis showing the same abnormal immunophenotype with lymphoma.

Microscopic findings of MEITL (EATL-II) (CD 56+ Intestinal T-cell lymphoma): It is characterized by monotonous infiltration of small to medium sized cells with scant cytoplasm and hyperchromatic nuclei typically invading the crypt and surface epithelium. Villi in the close peripheral zone of neoplastic infiltration show villous shortening and infiltration of atypical intraepithelial lymphocytes while the distant zones are characterized with normal villous architecture and normal counts of intraepithelial lymphocytes.

This entity, which formerly regarded as EATL-type II, was renamed as "monomorphic epitheliotropic intestinal T-cell lymphoma" in the 2016 revision of WHO classification of lymphoid neoplasms (in press) and segregated from type I EATL (EATL) due to its distinctive nature and lack of association with coeliac disease.

Microscopic findings of IPSID: Resembles a MALT lymphoma with marked plasma cell differentiation and show variations in different stages of the disease.

Stage A: Lamina propria shows overwhelming infiltration of plasma cells with few monocytoid marginal zone B-cells. Cytological atypia is not observed. The lymphoplasmacytic infiltration is confined to mucosa; the overlying epithelium is usually intact but the infiltration may obliterate villous architecture and may cause mucosal flattening with blunting, broadening and shortening of villi, and crypt hyperplasia. Mesenteric lymph nodes can be involved even in Stage A.

Stage B: Mucosal infiltration is usually nodular. Classical MALT lymphoma histology with follicular colonization is observed. Minimal cytological atypia is usually present. Mucosal folds are thickened macroscopically and the infiltration extends beyond muscularis mucosa. This stage is a transformational stage where most of the cases are diagnosed.

Stage C: is characterized by marked cytological atypia, increased mitosis, immunoblastic and plasmablastic cells, Reed Sternberg-like cells and conversion to DLBCL. Large masses and extensive mesenteric lymph node involvement is evident. The rate of evolution from Stage A, B to stage C is not known.

Immunophenotype

Immunphenotypic features are detected either by immunohistochemistry (IHC) or by flow cytometry, and its determination is crucial for subtyping and differential diagnosis of lymphomas, prediction of disease outcome, and selection of cases for targeted therapy (i.e., anti CD20 immunotherapy). Table 3 summarizes the most frequently observed/expected immunophenotypic features of common ILs although variations may occur in an index case.

The best immunohistochemical diagnostic workup may vary depending on the suspected lymphoma subtype. A panel consisting of CD3 (for T-cell lineage and NK cells), CD20 (for B-cell lineage), CD5 (T cells and aberrant expression in small B-cells), CD23 (for dendritic cells), CD43 (T cells, aberrant expression in some small B-cells, plasma cells, and myeloid cells), CD10 (for follicular/Germinal Center–GC B-cell origin), BCL6 (for GC B-cells), BCL2 (for identifying neoplastic GC cells), and Cyclin D1 (for identifying MCL) will be of help in distinguishing many cases of B-cell lymphomas and provide clues to the diagnosis of T-cell or NK/T-cell lymphomas to some extent.

Other Pan B-cell markers (CD19, CD22, CD79A, PAX5/BSAP), Plasma cell markers (CD138, CD38, VS38c, kappa, lambda, IgG, IgM, IgA, IgD), or markers for plasmablastic differentiation (i.e., IRF4/MUM-1), Cytotoxic markers (Granzyme B, perforin, TIA1), NK/T-cell markers (CD4, CD7, CD8, TCRδ, CD16, CD103 and NK-cell associated markers as CD56 and CD57) can be added to the panel when needed. Assessment of Ki-67 proliferation index (i.e., virtually 100% positive in BL). EBV-related markers as latent membrane protein-1 (LMP1) and/or EBV nuclear antigen-2 (EBNA2) are also crucial in diagnosis of some ILs. Notably EBV-related EBV encoded RNA (EBER) gene product is not translated into proteins detectable by IHC, therefore evaluated only by in situ hybridization methods.

The distribution of positively stained cells whether they represent the true neoplastic compartment or the reactive background should be carefully evaluated and interpreted, as well as the host "gut-associated lymphoid tissue" (i.e., Peyer's patches or rectal tonsils) to avoid misdiagnosis.

IHC can also be used to reveal some clinically important subgroups in different types of

Lymphoma and Immunoproliferative Small Intestinal Disease (IPSID), Table 3 Intestinal lymphomas at a glance: immunphenotypic and molecular features

	Immunphenotypic features	Molecular features	Variants and pitfalls in differential diagnosis
	Positive: Pan-B (CD19, CD20, CD22, CD79a, PAX5/BSAP). High Ki-67	BCL6, BCL2, c-MYC rearrangements (non-Ig gene partner arrangements are more common in GI tract)	*Hans classification (immunohistochemical):* "GCB" subgroup (more favorable) (CD10+ or CD10-, BCL6+,IRF4/MUM1-) and "Non-GCB" subgroup (IRF4/MUM1+)
DLBCL	*Variably positive*: CD30 (anaplastic variant), CD5 (10%, especially in de novo cases), CD10, BCL2, BCL6, IRF4/MUM1, FOXP1	Gene expression profiling identifies two subgroups "GCB-like" and "ABC-like"	de novo GCB-like DLBCLs are (BCL6 +, CD10 +, BCL2 +) versus transformed MALT lymphomas (BCL6 +, CD10 -, BCL2 -)
	"Double-expressor lymphoma": DLBCL with concomitant MYC and BCL2 protein expression. (worse than the others but less aggressive than high grade double hit/triple hit lymphomas)	Both have common or distinctive alterations or mutations, clinical implications of which are not fully understood	Intestinal lymphomas are more likely to have GCB-like immunophenotype than gastric DLBCLs
MALT L	*Positive:* CD20, CD79a, IgM (rarely > IgA, >IgG). CD21, CD23, and CD35 staining FDC meshworks	*t (11;18)*(q21;q21): Most common, not related with *H. pylori* (Trisomy 18q21 associates with shorter survival time in t (11;18) negative ILs)	Variants: CD5 positive MALT lymphomas, MALT lymphoma with plasmacytic differentiation
	Variably positive: CD43 , BCL2. *Negative:* CD5, CD10, CD23, cyclin D1, BCL6, IgD (very occasionally +)	t (14;18)(q32;q21): rare	t (11;18) and t (1;14) are related with antibiotic resistance in gastric MALT lymphoma, but their impact is not well established in ILs
	Negative: CD5, CD10, CD23, cyclin D1, BCL6, IgD (very occasionally +)	t (1;14)(p22;q32): rare	Cyclin D1 and CD 10 negativity is valuable in differentiating from MCL and FL, respectively
	Low Ki-67	t (3;14)(q27;q32): Less frequent but reported in MALT Lymphoma transformed to DLBCL	
IPSID	*Positive*: CD19, CD20 (in small lymphoid cells), CD79a, CD138 (in CD20 negative plasmacytic cell component). Cytoplasmic Immunoglobulin (IgA) alpha heavy chain (both in atypical lymphocytic and plasmacytic components) with absence of light chain staining	Deletions of alpha heavy chain gene	Differential diagnosis: Chronic inflammatory process, coeliac disease, parasitic infestations, sprue, and lymphomas other than IPSID
	Negative: CD5, CD10, CD23		
MCL	*Positive:* CD19, CD20, CD 5 (weak), CD 43 (weak), sIgM, sIgD (mostly lambda light chain restricted), SOX11, Cyclin-D1	Cyclin D1 over expression, t(11;14) (q13;q32), leading to CCND1 gene up-regulation is characteristic	CD5 (−) phenotype. Cyclin-D1 (−) variant (SOX11 positivity valuable for diagnosis)
	Negative: CD10, BCL6, CD23, CD15, CD30.	Also have CCND2 translocations and ATM, NOTCH1 and NOTCH2 gene mutations	Cyclin D1 positivity is utmost important in differentiating from other small cell B-cell lymphomas. Higher Ki-67 index (>30%) is an important adverse predictive marker

(*continued*)

Lymphoma and Immunoproliferative Small Intestinal Disease (IPSID), Table 3 (continued)

	Immunphenotypic features	Molecular features	Variants and pitfalls in differential diagnosis
FL	*Positive*: Pan-B (CD19, CD20, CD22, CD79a, PAX5/BSAP), CD10, BCL2, BCL6, sIgM (IgD, IgG, IgA). CD21, CD23, and CD35 (staining FDC meshworks)	t (14;18) and BCL2 gene rearrangement is the hallmark of FL (may show geographic variation)	bcl-2 positivity distinguishes from reactive follicles
	Negative: CD3, CD5, CD23, CD43, IRF4/MUM1	CREBBP, MLL2, and EZH2 mutations (potential therapeutic targets)	
	Duodenal-type FL: CD20+, strong CD10+, BCL-6+, BCL-2+, Ki-67 (low). In contrast to nodal counterparts, FDC meshwork may be redistributed (i.e., compact networks or condensed at the periphery of the neoplastic follicles) or unusually diminished	Intestinal FLs more frequently express the mucosa homing receptors a4b7 integrin and chemokine receptor-9 (related with lymphocyte trafficking to the small intestinal mucosa)	
Burkitt L	*Positive:* Pan-B (CD19, CD20, CD22, CD79a) CD10, BCL6, CD38, CD43, c-myc, sIgM+, show light chain restriction. Ki-67 (100%)	c-MYC rearrangement t (8;14) (q24;q32) is typical	Pitfalls in differential diagnosis: c-MYC expression, Ki-67:100%
	Negative: CD5, CD23, CD15, CD30, CD45RO, BCL2, and TdT	t(2;8)(p11;q24) involving IGK and t(8;22)(q24; q11) IGL are variably encountered among endemic and sporadic cases. TCF3 or ID3 mutations are found in up to approximately 70% of cases	EBER+ (90% of endemic, 20–30% of sporadic cases)
DLBCL/ BL	Mixed morphology with BL-like immunophenotype: Pan B +, CD10+, BCL6+, BCL2-IRF/MUM1 – (or weak+). Or BCL2 positivity but BL-like morphology. Ki-67 > 90%	**DLBCL/BL**: BCL2-positive, Ki-67 < 95%, IG-MYC rearrangement, non-IG-MYC rearrangement, MYC, BCL2-, and/or BCL6 rearrangements (double-hit/triple-hits, complex karyotype)	Features favoring *diagnosis of **BL***: BCL2-negativity, Ki-67 > 95%, IG-MYC rearrangement (simple karyotype) **DLBCL/BL**: BCL2-positivity, Ki-67 < 95%, IG-MYC rearrangement, non-IG-MYC rearrangement, MYC and BCL2-rearrangements (double-hit, complex karyotype) **DLBCL**: BCL2-positivity, Ki-67 < 90%, MYC-negative rearrangement, BCL6-rearrangement, BCL2-rearrangement
EBV+ DLBCL-e	Similar to DLBCL except for EBV positivity; often CD10 and BCL6 negativity; variable expression of IRF4/MUM1 and CD30	Clonality of Ig genes and EBV	

PBL	*Positive:* CD138, CD38, Vs38c, MUM1, cIgG, EMA, CD30, EBER, high Ki-67	Clonality of IgH genes	CD20 is negative (does not respond to rituximab)
	Negative: CD20, PAX5, CD79a (may be positive in half of the cases), BCL6, EBNA-2, and LMP1	Characteristically EBER (+), but EBNA-2 or LMP1 (−)	
EATL-I (EATL)	*Positive*: CD3, CD7, CD103 and granzyme B, perforin, and/or TIA	Clonal rearrangements of TCRB and TCRG. Complex chromosomal aberrations; Gains at 5q or gains or partial trisomy of 1q (in EATL-I) gains at 9q or deletions in 16q (common in EATL-I and EATL-II)	IELs in the adjacent enteropathic mucosa: CD3+, CD5-, CD8-, CD4-
	Variably positive: CD8, CD30 and TCRB	The HLA-DQ8 and HLA-DQ2 or HLA-DQB1 genotype (common in coeliac disease and EATL-I)	IELs in Refractary coeliac disease type II: Similar immunophenotype with monoclonal TCR gene rearrangements and gains in 1q and 5 q (suggesting their perception as EATL in situ)
	Negative: CD4, CD5, CD56		Cases with anaplastic morphology (Anaplastic variant): CD30 +, CD3-, CD4- and CD8-
EATL-II (MEITL)	Similar to EATL, except for CD56/NCAM1 and MAPK positivity. CD8 positivity and TCR$\alpha\beta$ expression is also more frequent	Similar to EATL with rearrangements of TCRB and TCRG. Amplification of MYC (8q24) is more common in EATL-II. STAT5B were only associated with $\gamma\delta$ MEITL	EBER (−)
ENKTL, nasal type	*Positive*: CD2, CD56, cCD3 and granzyme B, perforin, and/or TIA, EBER. *Variably positive*: CD7 and CD30 (in anaplastic variant)	Clonal TCR rearrangement (in minority of cases). Deletions and inversions in Chr 6. Abnormal methylation of promoter CpG domains of the p73 gene, mutation of TP53, KRAS, KIT or β-catenin, and partial deletion of FAS gene	EBER negativity should raise suspicion for diagnosis
	Negative: surface CD3, CD4, CD5, CD8, TCRδ, CD16 and CD57		

Abbreviations: *GCB-subtype* Germinal center like subtype, *ABC-subtype* Activated B-cell like subtype, *FDC* Follicular dendritic cell, *IEL* Intraepithelial lymphocytes lymphomas as in DLBCL (i.e., distinction of GCB and Non-GCB subgroups by Hans's algorithm which uses CD10, BCL6, and IRF4/MUM1 antibodies) (See Table 3).

Immunophenotypic features of common ILs is summarized in Table 3 with emphasis on minor variations from their nodal counterparts.

Immunophenotypic features of duodenal-type FL: CD20+, strong CD10+, BCL-6+, BCL-2+, Ki-67 (low). FDC meshwork (revealed by CD21, CD23, CD35 expression) may be unusually diminished in contrast to nodal counterparts or redistributed, with compact networks or a condensed rim of enhanced staining at the periphery of the neoplastic follicles.

Immunophenotypic features of EATL (EATL Type I): The neoplastic T cells are positive for: CD3, CD7, CD103, and cytotoxic markers such as granzyme B, perforin, and/or TIA.

Variably positive for: CD8, CD30, and TCRβ. Typically *negative for:* CD4, CD5, and CD56

Variants: *Anaplastic variant* (CD30 +, CD3-, CD4-, and CD8-).

Pitfalls in differential diagnosis The adjacent mucosa with or without enteropathic changes also show CD3 positivity but loss of CD4, CD5, and CD8 expression in intraepithelial lymphocytes. The intraepithelial lymphocytes in cases with Refractary ► Coeliac disease type II (RCD-II), especially the ones subsequently develop into EATL, also show similar immunophenotypic features with monoclonal TCR gen rearrangements suggesting their perception as EATL *in situ.*

Immunophenotypic features of MEITL (EATL-II, Monomorphic CD56 (+) Intestinal T-cell lymphoma): Similar immunophenotypic features with EATL in respect to neoplastic infiltration except for presence of CD56/NCAM1 and MAPK expression and more frequent TCRαβ expression than EATL (EATL-I). TCRα and TCRγ expressions are similar.

Immunophenotypic Features of IPSID

Positive for: CD19, CD20 (in atypical monocytoid-small lymphoid cells), CD79a, CD138 (in plasmacytic cell component which is CD20 negative), IgA will stain strongly with heavy chain (both in atypical lymphocytic and plasmacytic components) with absence of light chain staining.

Negative for: CD5, CD10, and CD23.

Molecular Features

Molecular diagnostic tests are primarily used either to demonstrate monoclonality of the lesion (neoplastic rather than reactive nature) or to reveal a specific chromosomal translocation or to elaborate a viral association.

Karyotypic changes are less frequently evaluated in routine practice. Flow cytometry can be used as an adjunct to IHC in detection of immunophenotypic features or may even give better results than IHC, i.e., by enabling simultaneous evaluation of several surface antigens or by detecting clonality especially in B-cell lymphomas. PCR-based clonality analyses, for B-cell clonality; targets immunoglobulin (Ig) gene rearrangements on certain localizations as Ig heavy chain (IGH) on 14q32, Ig kappa light chain (IGK) on 2p11, and Ig lambda light chain (IGL) on 22q11, while T-cell clonality analysis targets T-cell receptor (TCR) genes rearrangements as TCR beta (TCRβ) on 7q32–35; TCR gamma (TCRγ) on 7p15; or TCR delta (TCRδ) within the TCR alpha (TCRα) loci in chr 14. Fluorescence in situ hybridization (FISH) analysis is valuable in detecting typical chromosomal aberrations as translocations, rearrangements, and less frequently amplifications or deletions for certain subtypes of lymphomas. Some of these alterations are also detectable in formalin fixed paraffin embedded tissues by IHC. EBER *in situ* hybridization (ISH) is preferred over IHC as EBER gene (which is not translated into IHC detectable-protein) is expressed in all latency programs of latent EBV infection, hence regarded more sensitive than LMP1/EBNA-2 detected by IHC. Moreover, EBV-positive intestinal NK/T cell lymphomas and BLs may be negative by IHC (i.e., LMP). On the other hand, EBER must be carefully interpreted, as higher frequency of latent EBV infection in adults may cause positivity in non-neoplastic lymphoid compartment.

Common molecular features encountered in common ILs are overviewed below and summarized in Table 3 in respect to different types of lymphomas.

Gene rearrangements: IGH and IGK rearrangements virtually occur in all mature B-cell lymphomas. TCRβ and TCRγ rearrangements are present in both EATL and MEITL but detected only in minority of cases of ENKTL nasal type.

Translocations: Translocations are usually observed in B-cell ILs. The t(2;5)(p23;q35) is the only recurring translocation routinely evaluated in T-cell lymphomas, but it is particularly observed in anaplastic large cell lymphoma which is uncommon in GI tract. Most frequent translocations, involved genes, and associated B-cell lymphomas are as follows:

Cyclin-D1(CCND1, IGH): t(11;14)(q13;q32) → MCL (60–95%)
BCL2, IGH: t(14;18)(q21;q32) → FL (>90%), DLBCL, DLBCL/BL, unclassifiable
API2/MLT: t(11;18)(q21;q21) → MALT lymphoma
BCL-6: t(3;n)(q27;n) → DLBCL, MZL
MYC: →BL (80–90%), DLBCL (0–20%), DLBCL/BL, unclassifiable (25–50%, with a non-Ig gene partner)
Translocations MYC- IGH t(8;14)(q24;q32); MYC-IGK t(2;8)(p11;q24) MYC-IGL t(8;22) (q24;q11) differ among sporadic and endemic cases of BL

Lymphomas with concurrent MYC and BCL2 translocations and MYC, BCL2, and BCL6 translocations are called "Double-hit lymphomas" and "Triple-hit lymphomas," respectively. In the 2016 revision of WHO classification of lymphoid neoplasms, all "double/triple hit" lymphomas other than FL or lymphoblastic lymphomas are categorized under "High grade B-cell lymphoma, with MYC and BCL2 and/or BCL6 translocations."

Virus Associated Changes

EBER positivity is observed in BL (90% of endemic, 20–30% of sporadic cases), ENKTL, nasal type, EBV+ DLBCL, PBL, and lymphomatoid granulomatosis. Note that EBER (+) PBL is characteristically negative with EBNA-2 or LMP1, especially in colorectal HIV-associated cases. For T-cell lymphomas, EBER positivity is associated with poor prognosis.

DLBCL is molecularly subclassified as "germinal center B-cell-like (GCB)" and "activated B-cell-like (ABC)" subgroups based on gene expression profiling (GEP). Both have common or distinctive alterations or mutations; clinical implications of which are not fully understood. As GEP is not a routine clinical test, IHC algorithms to differentiate the cases as GCB and non-GCB subgroups (i.e., Hans algorithms) can be used for stratification although it does not show "exact correlation" with the molecular categories.

EATL: Rearrangements of TCRβ and TCRγ are present in both EATL (EATL-I) and MEITL (EATL-II).

Cases with EATL are characterized with HLA-DQ8, HLA-DQ2, and HLA-DQB1 genotype which is shared with coeliac disease.

EATL and MEITL also harbor 9q31.3-qter gains and 16q12.1 deletions. EATL additionally displays gains at 5q or gains or partial trisomy of 1q, while MEITL more commonly express MYC gains at 8q24 locus instead. Cases with refractory coeliac disease also show 1q and 5q gains in intraepithelial lymphocytes indicating a genetic link with EATL.

Molecular features of IPSID: Deletions in the variable (VH) and the first constant domain (CH1) of the alpha heavy chain gene are typical. This faulty heavy chain detains binding of light chain so the plasma cells bear abnormal (truncated) alpha heavy chains. This anomalous alpha heavy chain protein can also be detected in the serum. Translocations with breakpoints involving the IGH or IGL loci were also described. Although considered a subtype of MALT lymphoma IPSID lacks t(11;18) frequently present in other MALT lymphomas.

Differential Diagnosis

The major concerns in differential diagnosis of ILs are:

1. **Differentiating small cell lymphoma types** (see Table 2).

Before further evaluation, the cell size should be compared with macrophage nuclei to avoid mistaking large/intermediate lymphoid cells for small cell infiltration, especially in suboptimal fixed tissues.

2. **Distinguishing a small cell lymphoma from host lymphoid tissue or/reactive lymphoid hyperplasia which may extensively be present throughout the lower GI tract.**

Peyer patches are ring-forming organized lymphoid tissues located in lamina propria and submucosa of ileum. Their size and distribution show great individual variations. They can endoscopically form tan-white nodular mucosal tumefactions measuring 0.1–0.5 cm and mimic early stage lymphoma. The presence or "spilling over" of marginal zone B-lymphocytes in the surface epithelium, at the broader luminal aspect of marginal zone, or "Lymphoepithelium" formation which are also seen in crypt epithelium adjacent to lymphoid follicles should not be misinterpreted as lymphoepithelial lesions observed in MALT lymphoma.

Rectal tonsil (Lymphoid follicular hyperplasia of rectum) is a localized rectal mucosal or submucosal lymphoid proliferation which may present as slightly raised, endoscopically delineated/polypoid lesions. It may cause rectal bleeding and can mimic a lymphomatous proliferation with mild architectural distortion and overlying cryptitis.

Nodular lymphoid hyperplasia (NLH) (Reactive follicular hyperplasia) is characterized with variably sized follicles with well-defined mantle zones, brisk mitosis, and tingible body macrophages; architecture is preserved in contrast to mucosal effacement or obliteration observed in FLs. Reactive changes can be florid in ileocecal region and appendix especially in children and can be related with viral infection, food allergies, or chronic constipation or accompany AIDS, common variable immunodeficiency (CVID), selective IgA deficiency, and *Giardia lamblia* infestation especially in duodenum. BCL2 is negative in follicles of NLH, and therefore presence of BCL2 expression can be a valuable aid in diagnosis of a lymphoma. However, BCL2 expression is not restricted to FL and must be carefully evaluated as reactive T-cells may also show positivity. Similarly, CD43 should also be cautiously interpreted in GI tract as normal B-cells in Peyer's patches may also be positive. *Reactive lymphoid proliferations* (i.e., accompanying appendicitis) typically present with mixed inflammatory background.

3. **Distinguishing a large cell lymphoma from other malignancies:**

Malignant melanoma, poorly differentiated adenocarcinoma, or myeloid sarcoma are the major concerns, but the distinction is less troublesome by the aid of IHC once the possibility of a nonlymphoid malignancy is considered.

4. **Differentiating a lymphoma from benign diseases:**

NK-cell enteropathy: A recently described, rare entity of unknown etiology, characterized with atypical proliferation of NK-cells limited to the GI tract (duodenum, colon, and stomach). Cellular infiltration causes glandular architectural distortion (in early stages) or destruction (in advanced disease). The disease course is indolent and differentiated from aggressive ENKTLs by absence of epitheliotropism, angiocentric angiodestructive growth pattern, and EBV positivity.

Lymphoid follicular proctitis: Characterized with rectal bleeding and endoscopically nodular mucosa. Atypical lymphoid cells can be observed and should not be confused with lymphoma.

CVID: Presence of NLH in duodenum especially in children should raise suspicion for CVID, which shows paucity or absence of plasma cells. The endoscopic appearance NLH is quite typical with small mucosal nodular protrusions, prominent especially in duodenum.

Morphology based immunphenotypical or molecular differential diagnosis of different types of lymphomas are given in Table 2 and elsewhere in different entries of this volume. Only distinct lymphoma types exclusively encountered in lower GI tract will be discussed herein.

Differential diagnosis of EATL and MEITL: mainly rely on clinical background and cellular morphology. Both are associated with enteropathic changes and show similar ulceroinfiltrative pattern with strictures and intestinal perforation. Clinical course is poor in both disease with frequent recurrences and resistance to chemotherapy.

EATL: Common in Northern Europe, associated with coeliac/refractory coeliac disease, and share similar HLA-DQ8, HLA-DQ2 genotype; it is characterized by medium to large sized cells, with irregular nuclei and prominent nuclei, necrosis is frequent with background inflammatory reaction. Neoplastic cells are CD3 +, CD7 +, TCRβ ±, CD8-, and CD 56 – and frequently displays chromosomal 1q and 5q gains.

MEITL: Common in Asia, occurs sporadically, not necessarily associated with coeliac disease, characterized by monomorphic small, round cells. Necrosis is rare, inflammatory reaction is minimal. CD56 is typically positive hence formerly also called as "monomorphic CD56+ intestinal T-cell lymphoma," CD 8 positivity is more common, segmental chromosomal 1q and 5q gains are usually lacking.

ENKTL, nasal type, may show necrosis as EATL and CD56 positivity as MEITL. But ENKTL typically exhibit EBER positivity and angiocentric and angiodestructive growth pattern lacking in both types of EATLs.

Lymphomatoid granulomatosis, which primarily involves pulmonary system, is also reported in small intestine and colon. It should be differentiated from ENKTL, nasal type as it is also an angiocentric and angiodestructive lymphoproliferative disorder characterized with polymorphous lymphoid infiltrate, necrosis, granulomatous features, and EBV positivity. The distinction is made by immunohistochemical demonstration of mature CD20+ B cell population, in a background of reactive T cells.

Differential diagnosis of IPSID includes chronic inflammatory processes in early stages of the disease though the distinction may even not be possible without clonal studies for IGH chain gene rearrangement. Coeliac disease is also listed in differential diagnosis as both are characterized by villous atrophy and lymphoplasmacytic infiltrate. Immunophenotypic features, clinical, and serological findings with response to gluten free diet favor coeliac disease. The distinction of IPSID from other small B-cell lymphomas is given in Tables 2 and 3.

References and Further Reading

Al-Saleem, T., & Al-Mondhiry, H. (2005). Immunoproliferative small intestinal disease (IPSID): A model for mature B-cell neoplasms. *Blood, 105*, 2274–2280.

Arora, N., Manipadam, M. T., Pulimood, A., Ramakrishna, B. S., Chacko, A., Kurian, S. S., & Nair, S. (2011). Gastrointestinal lymphomas: Pattern of distribution and histological subtypes: 10 years experience in a tertiary centre in South India. *Indian Journal of Pathology and Microbiology, 54*, 712–719.

Bautista-Quach, M. A., Ake, C. D., Chen, M., & Wang, J. (2012). Gastrointestinal lymphomas: Morphology, immunophenotype and molecular features. *Journal of Gastrointestinal Oncology, 3*, 209–225.

Bosman, F., Carneiro, F., Hruban, R. H., & Theise, N. D. (Eds.). (2010). *WHO classification of tumours of the digestive system*. Lyon: IARC.

Swerdlow, S. H., Campo, E., Harris, N. L., Jaffe, E. S., Pileri, S. A., Stein, H., Thiele, J., & Vardiman, J. W. (Eds.). (2008). *WHO classification of tumours of haematopoietic and lymphoid tissues* (4th ed.). Lyon: IARC.

Swerdlow, S. H., Campo, E., Pileri, S. A., Harris, N. L., Stein, H., Siebert, R., Advani, R., Ghielmini, M., Salles, G. A., Zelenetz, A. D., & Jaffe, E. S. (2016). The 2016 revision of the World Health Organization (WHO) classification of lymphoid neoplasms. *Blood, 127*, 2391–2405. pii: blood-2016-01-643569. [Epub ahead of print].

Lynch Syndrome

Armagan Gunal
Department of Pathology, Gulhane Military Medical Academy, Etlik, Ankara, Turkey

Synonyms

Hereditary mismatch repair deficiency syndrome; Hereditary nonpolyposis colorectal cancer (HNPCC) syndrome (see the "Definition")

Definition

Lynch syndrome is a hereditary cancer syndrome caused by the germline mutations in DNA mismatch repair (MMR) genes and characterized by an increased risk of colorectal carcinoma and extracolonic cancers.

Historically, this syndrome has been defined as a "probable hereditary cancer syndrome" by A. S. Warthin and H. T. Lynch in the same family in which the members had cancers (predominantly colorectal cancers in the absence of overt polyposis). Compatible with these features, this syndrome has been named and known as "Hereditary nonpolyposis colorectal cancer (HNPCC) syndrome" for years until 1990s. Clinical criteria known as "Amsterdam criteria" have been developed to define these cases. Based on the presence of the germline mutations in MMR genes (see the "Molecular Features"), which have been defined as the cause of at least half of these hereditary cancers, the syndrome is divided into two groups and reclassified as (1) "Lynch syndrome (LS)" caused by MMR gene mutations and (2) "Familial colorectal cancer type X" with no MMR gene mutation/unknown genetic basis. Additional clinical criteria defined as "revised Bethesda criteria" have also been proposed to select cases for genetic screening and final diagnosis.

Clinical Features

- **Incidence**
  LS, as the most common hereditary colorectal cancer syndrome causes about 3% of all colorectal cancers. Patients with LS have 30–74% lifetime cumulative risk for colorectal cancer (lifetime cumulative risk for sporadic colorectal carcinoma has been calculated as 5.5%). The risk rises higher for specific MMR genes (e.g., 80% for MLH1 mutation carriers). Extracolonic cancer occurrence risk is also higher than population (e.g., 39–50% vs. 2% for endometrium and 7–8% vs. 1% for ovary).
- **Age**
  Cancers associated with LS are early onset tumors. Average presentation age ranges from 45 to 60 years for colorectal cancers and from 47 to 60 years for endometrium. Mean age at the diagnosis can be younger for specific mutations, such as 27–46 years for MLH1 mutated patients.
- **Sex**
  Male predominance has been observed for LS associated colorectal cancers (lifetime cumulative risk 73–66% vs. 59–43%).
- **Site**
  Colorectal carcinoma is the most common tumor in LS. Colonic carcinomas are mostly seen in proximal colon. Extracolonic carcinomas can be seen in endometrium, ovary, stomach, renal pelvis/ureter, bile ducts, pancreas, small bowel, brain, and skin, in descending order. Multiple metachronous or synchronous tumors can be observed.
- **Treatment**
  Further genetic testing and consulting is needed for the chosen cases due to clinical revised Bethesda criteria for LS (see the "Molecular Features").

  Surveillance programs have been defined for frequently seen carcinomas (colon, endometrium, and ovary). Relative risk for these carcinomas is 5.8-fold compared with the nonmutated population. Annual colonoscopy/gastroscopy, abdominal ultrasound, and gynaecological examination (transvaginal ultrasound, and if necessary, endometrial sampling) are recommended beginning from the age of 25 (or 10 years before the youngest tumor diagnosis age in the family). Surveillance programs should continue after tumor resections because of metachronous tumor risk. Benefit of prophylactic extended/subtotal colon resection is not greater than surveillance colonoscopy.

  LS associated colon tumors do not benefit from 5-FU including chemotherapy. According to the guidelines, no adjuvant treatment has been advised for stage II MMR deficient colon carcinomas. These tumors have higher survival rates and do not require additional chemotherapy.
- **Outcome**
  Although they can grow larger in sizes and have poorly differentiated histology, MMR

deficient colonic cancers have better prognosis with higher overall survival.

Macroscopy

LS associated colon carcinomas are mostly right sited (located proximal to splenic flexure), macroscopically polypoid as bulky masses, and reaches big dimensions. Endometrial carcinomas are mostly located in lower uterine segment.

Microscopy

Colon cancers associated with LS are poorly differentiated tumors, which may show mucinous histology. Medullary carcinoma, signet-ring cell carcinoma, and mucinous carcinoma are main histological subtypes. Marked lymphocytic host response (intratumoral lymphocytes and Crohn-like lymphocytic reaction around the tumor), lack of dirty necrosis, and pushing margin rather than infiltrating (Fig. 1) are the main microscopic characteristics for these colon carcinomas.

Immunophenotype

Because of the prognostic and predictive values, performing MMR deficiency testing has been advised by expert groups for all colon carcinomas. Immunohistochemical detection of the loss of MMR proteins is both cheap and easy way of testing. Four MMR proteins (MLH1, MSH2, PMS2, and MSH6) are included in the test. Immunohistochemically, the loss of protein expression for at least one of four proteins is enough to diagnose the tumor as "microsatellite instable (MSI) tumor" (see the "Molecular Features"). Because MMR proteins are normally expressed in nonneoplastic epithelial cells and lymphocytes, positive nuclear expression in these cells in the tissue is accepted as perfect internal control during the evaluation of staining (Fig. 2).

Molecular Features

MMR deficiency is the main molecular abnormality underlying LS. Main function of MMR proteins (MLH1, MSH2, PMS2, MSH6, MSH3, and MLH3) is to detect and repair mismatches during DNA replication. Mutation rates on DNA increases when MMR deficiency is present. Microsatellites, the 1–6 base length repetitive DNA segments, are highly prone to these mutations by changes of their length and structure. This kind of mutation is named as "microsatellite instability (MSI)" and causes defective transcription of

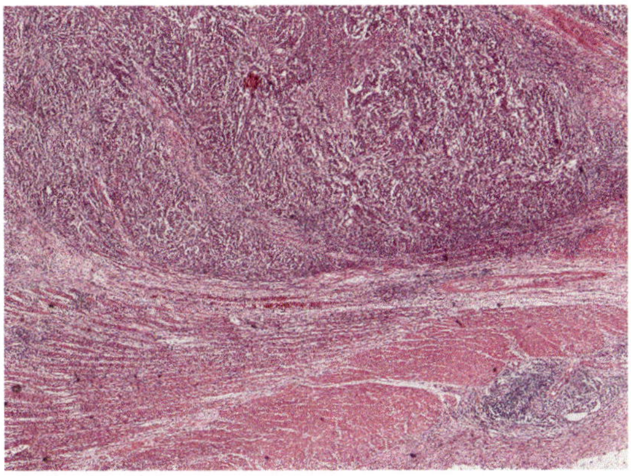

Lynch Syndrome, Fig. 1 Pushing margin in a poorly differentiated tumor is seen (HE×20)

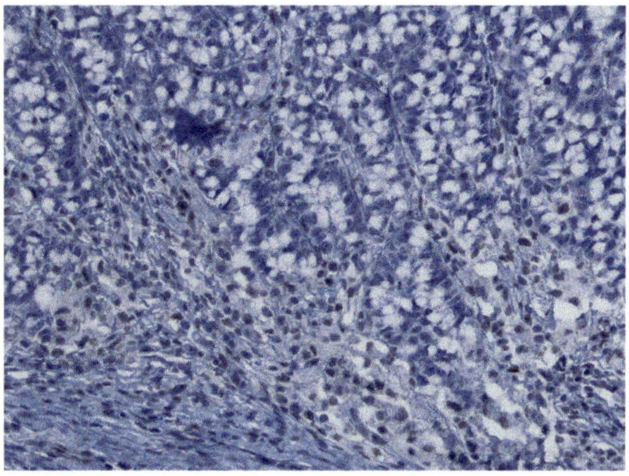

Lynch Syndrome, Fig. 2 Loss of expression for MLH1 in a MSI tumor. Scattered intratumoral lymphocytes are expressing the protein as an internal positive control (MLH1, IHC×40)

tumor suppressor genes as a well-known mechanism of carcinogenesis.

MMR deficiency can cause MSI by two ways: (1) germline mutations on MMR genes and (2) silencing of MMR genes by hypermethylation. The first "genetic" mechanism underlies LS associated tumors. The second "epigenetic" one is the cause of sporadic MSI tumors. Therefore, two questions are needed to be answered for final diagnosis of LS: (1) Whether the tumor is MMR deficient or not and (2) If the MMR deficiency in tumor is caused by a germline mutation (LS associated tumor) or an epigenetic hypermethylation (sporadic tumor).

Flow charts published for the diagnosis of MMR deficiency include tests (1) Mismatch repair immunohistochemistry, (2) microsatellite instability testing, (3) BRAF mutation testing, (4) MLH1 methylation testing, and (5) germline mutation testing.

Differential Diagnosis

Identifying MMR deficient tumors is a prerequisite in determining LS families for further genetic testings. Thereby, genetic consulting, surveillance programs, and prophylactic surgeries can prevent the occurrence of multiple advanced stage tumors in these patients.

References and Further Reading

Geiersbach, K. B., & Samowitz, W. S. (2011). Microsatellite instability and colorectal cancer. *Archives of Pathology and Laboratory Medicine, 135*, 1269–1277.

Peltomaki, P., Offerhaus, G. J. A., & Vasen, H. F. A. (2010). Lynch syndrome. In F. T. Bosman, F. Carneiro, R. H. Hruban, & N. D. Theise (Eds.), *WHO classification of tumours of the digestive system* (pp. 152–155). Lyon: IARC.

Redston, M., & Driman, D. K. (2015). Epithelial neoplasms of the large intestine. In R. D. Odze & J. R. Goldblum (Eds.), *Surgical pathology of the GI tract, liver, biliary tract and pancreas* (pp. 737–778). Philadelphia: Elsevier.

Samowitz, W. S. (2015). Evaluation of colorectal cancers for Lynch syndrome: Practical molecular diagnostic for surgical pathologists. *Modern Pathology, 28*, 109–113.

Schneider, R., Schneider, C., Kloor, M., Fürst, A., & Möslein, G. (2012). Lynch syndrome: Clinical, pathological, and genetic insights. *Langenbeck's Archives of Surgery, 397*, 513–525.

Setaffy, L., & Langner, C. (2015). Microsatellite instability in colon cancer: Clinicopathological significance. *Polish Journal of Pathology, 66*, 203–218.

Shia, J., Holck, S., DePetris, G., Greenson, J. K., & Klimstra, D. S. (2013). Lynch syndrome-associated neoplasms: A discussion on histopathology and immunohistochemistry. *Familial Cancer, 12*, 241–260.

M

Malabsorption Syndrome

Arzu Ensari
Department of Pathology, Ankara University Medical School, Sihhiye, Ankara, Turkey

Synonyms

Insufficient absorption; Maldigestion

Definition

Malabsorption syndrome refers to the clinical picture comprising diarrhea, steatorrhea, malnutrition, weight loss, abdominal pain, and anemia due to maldigestion, mucosal/mural problems, or infections. The small intestine is the part of the gastrointestinal tract where much of the absorption takes place due to high surface area provided by the villous and microvillous architecture and numerous digestive enzymes on its surface actively secreted to optimize uptake of dietary substances. Malabsorption develops when malfunction in any of these components leads to failure of absorption of nutrients resulting from a wide variety of causes which can be classified into three groups: (i) maldigestion which is related to mixing and digestive mediators; (ii) mucosal or mural causes including celiac disease, tropical sprue, autoimmune enteropathy, AIDS enteropathy, and systemic sclerosis; and (iii) microbial causes including bacterial overgrowth, Whipple's disease, and numerous infections mainly seen in immunocompromised hosts (Table 1).

Clinical Features

- **Incidence**
  The incidence of malabsorption varies according to the underlying disorder. While celiac disease has an incidence of 1%, neonatal enteropathies are much rarer.
- **Age**
  Age range depends on the cause of malabsorption.
- **Sex**
  There is no known sex predilection for malabsorption.
- **Site**
  The small intestine, either entirely or segmentally, is affected in malabsorption by the underlying disorder.
- **Treatment**
  Treatment includes replacement of nutrients and vitamins together with the treatment of the underlying cause.
- **Outcome**
  The outcome also depends on the causing illness. Once the cause is determined and appropriate treatment is started, the symptoms subside. However, in the neonatal period, severe malabsorption may result fatally.

F. Carneiro et al. (eds.), *Pathology of the Gastrointestinal Tract*, Encyclopedia of Pathology,
DOI 10.1007/978-3-319-40560-5

Macroscopy

Small intestinal mucosa either may be normal or may show villous abnormalities described as mosaic appearance, scalloping on endoscopy.

Microscopy

Small intestinal biopsy is an indispensable component of the diagnostic work-up of patients with malabsorption and/or chronic diarrhea secondary to mucosal damage. While the majority of disorders causing malabsorption produce mild to moderate villus blunting and crypt hyperplasia, histopathology varies between normal or near-normal mucosa and completely flat mucosa (Table 2). The recognition of mild villous blunting is a difficult task due to biopsy artifacts such as improper orientation of the biopsy, shallow biopsies which lack muscularis mucosae. However, accompanying lamina propria inflammation and/or intraepithelial lymphocytosis should always be looked for before making a diagnosis. The following disorders are those malabsorption syndromes with which a small intestinal biopsy may be diagnostic:

Whipple's disease	Lymphangiectasia
Abetalipoproteinemia	Amyloidosis
Immunodeficiency syndromes	Crohn's disease
Eosinophilic gastroenteritis	Intestinal lymphoma
Systemic mastocytosis	Parasitic infestation

Malabsorption Syndrome, Table 1 Causes of malabsorption

Maldigestion
Inadequate mixing (gastrectomy)
Insufficiency of digestive mediators (brush border enzymes, bile salt deficiencies)
Mucosal/mural problems
Decreased mucosa (bowel resection)
Mucosal disease (GSE, tropical sprue, autoimmune enteropathy, intestinal lymphangiectasia)
Mural disease (neuromuscular disorders, amyloidosis, diverticula)
Immunodeficiencies (congenital ID, AIDS)
Microbial causes
Infections

Immunophenotype

No specific immunophenotypic feature is present for malabsorption.

Molecular Features

No specific molecular feature is present for malabsorption.

Differential Diagnosis

Many disorders can cause malabsorption but classically celiac disease, refractory or collagenous sprue, tropical sprue, small intestinal - bacterial overgrowth, intestinal lymphangiectasia, peptic duodenitis, food allergies, graft versus host disease, immunodeficiencies, neonatal

Malabsorption Syndrome, Table 2 Mucosal pathology in malabsorption

Normal mucosa	IELosis	Villous shortening and crypt hyperplasia	Flat mucosa
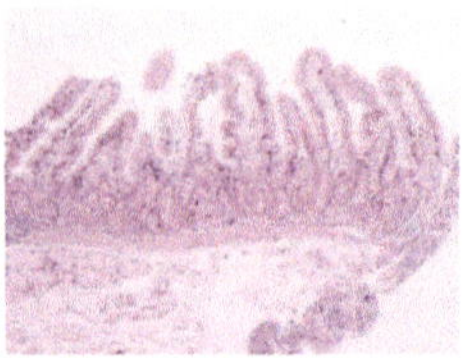	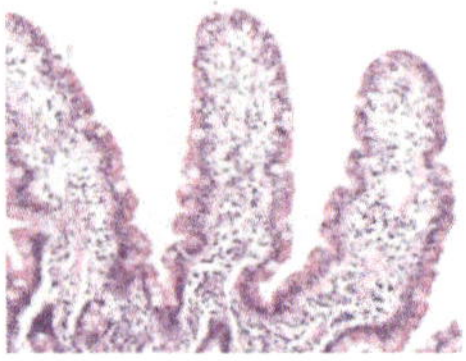	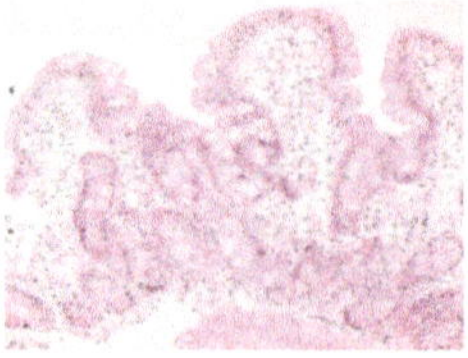	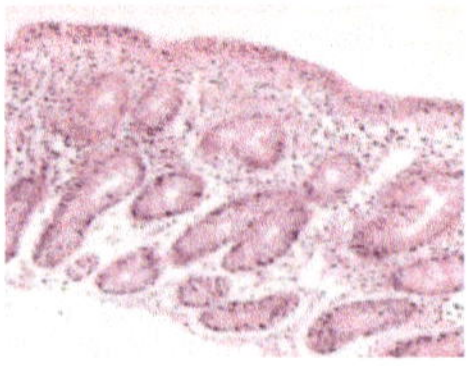

enteropathies, autoimmune enteropathy, inflammatory bowel diseases, and infections such as Whipple's disease, giardiasis, and cryptosporidiosis.

References and Further Reading

Babbin, B. A., Crawford, K., & Sitaraman, S. V. (2006). Malabsorption work-up: Utility of small bowel biopsy. *Clinical Gastroenterology and Hepatology, 4*, 1193–1198.

Fenoglio-Preiser, C. M., Noffsinger, A. E., Stemmermann, G. N., et al. (2008). The nonneoplastic small intestine. In C. M. Fenoglio Preiser (Ed.), *Gastrointestinal pathology. An atlas and text* (3rd ed., pp. 275–470). Philadelphia: Walters Kluwer-Lippincott-Williams and Wilkins.

Murray, J. A., & Rubio-Tapia, A. (2012). Diarrhoea due to small bowel diseases. *Best Practice & Research. Clinical Gastroenterology, 26*, 581–600.

Owens, S. R., & Greenson, J. K. (2007). The pathology of malabsorption: Current concepts. *Histopathology, 50*, 64–82.

Thompson, A. B. R., Keelan, M., Thiesen, A., Clandinin, M. T., Ropeleski, M., & Wild, G. E. (2001). Small bowel review: Disease of the small intestine. *Digestive Diseases and Sciences, 46*, 2555–2566.

Malignant Atrophic Papulosis (Degos' Disease)

Elisabete Rios and Francisco Ferro de Beça
Department of Pathology, Centro Hospitalar de São João, Porto, Portugal
Faculty of Medicine of the University of Porto, Porto, Portugal
IPATIMUP – Institute of Pathology and Molecular Immunology of the University of Porto, Porto, Portugal

Synonyms

Atrophic papulosquamous dermatitis; Degos' disease; Fatal cutaneous-intestinal syndrome; Köhlmeier–Degos disease; Thromboangiitis cutaneointestinalis disseminata

Definition

Malignant atrophic papulosis (MAP) is a rare and often lethal, vaso-occlusive disorder involving small and medium-caliber vessels. It is characterized by narrowing and occlusion of the lumen by intimal proliferation and thrombosis, which leads to ischemia and infarction of the involved organ systems (most commonly the skin, gastrointestinal tract, and central nervous system). It was initially described by Köhlmeier in 1941 as a form of thromboangiitis obliterans, and recognized as a distinct vascular injury syndrome by Degos in 1942, hence the name (Thompson and Rosenbaum 2008).

Two variants have been described (Scheinfeld 2011). A cutaneous or benign variant, that is limited to the skin, with a relatively benign course. A systemic or malignant variant, in which there is a multiorgan involvement, with stereotypical skin lesions frequently associated with infarctive lesions of other organs, particularly the gastrointestinal tract, often with a fatal outcome due to intestinal perforation.

A rare hereditary form has also been described (Magro et al. 2011).

In many cases, the disease may occur in the setting of known autoimmune disease such as lupus erythematosus, dermatomyositis, scleroderma, and certain thrombophilic tendency states, including factor V Leiden mutation and antiphospholipid antibody syndrome (Magro et al. 2011).

The benign and malignant variants are initially clinically indistinguishable but become distinct once systemic manifestations appear. They usually develop from weeks to years after the onset of skin lesions, or, in rare instances, may precede the skin lesions (Ahmadi et al. 2011).

The cutaneous lesions are usually asymptomatic but can cause slight burning or itching.

When gastrointestinal involvement supervenes, patients may present with gastrointestinal bleeding, enterocutaneous fistulae, bowel infarction, and perforation or, most frequently, with nonspecific symptoms (e.g., abdominal pain, fatigue, nausea, vomiting, diarrhea, or constipation).

Involvement of both central and peripheral nervous systems can occur and manifestations include strokes, headaches, epilepsy, or nonspecific neurologic symptoms (e.g., memory loss, altered sensation).

Manifestations from involvement of other organ systems are rare. Pleuritis, bilateral pleural effusions, and constrictive pericarditis may occur with involvement of the lungs and heart. Involvement of the eyes can result in diplopia, blurred vision, and visual field defects.

The underlying pathogenic mechanism remains controversial. Several mechanisms such as viral infection, autoimmune disease, and coagulation defects have been proposed, but there is no convincing evidence to support any single causal factor (Thompson and Rosenbaum 2008).

Some authors hypothesize that MAP is not a distinct disease, but instead an expression of an underlying known autoimmune disease. Others have classified MAP as a vasculitis, a mucinosis, or a thrombotic disorder (Weedon 2010).

Antiphospholipid or anticardiolipin antibodies of uncertain significance have been identified in some patients with MAP, although in most cases, no circulating immune complexes or anti-endothelial cell antibodies have been isolated (Scheinfeld 2011).

Recently, it was found that patients with MAP have high expression of Interferon-α (IFN-α) and prominent vascular complement component 5b-9 (C5b-9), leading to the hypothesis that complement activation may play an important role in the pathogenesis of MAP (Magro et al. 2011). This concept is further supported by the fact that eculizumab, a C5 blocker, can effectively treat systemic MAP. This led Scheinfeld (2011) to reconsider MAP rather as a hematological or endothelial genetic disease and to propose a linkage with paroxysmal nocturnal hemoglobinuria (PNH), since eculizumab has been successfully deployed as its treatment.

Clinical Features

- **Incidence**
  MAP is a very rare disease, with approximately 200 cases reported to date (Weedon 2010).
- **Age**
  The disease predominantly affects young adults, but cases have been described in infants and children with age of onset ranging between 3 weeks of age to 67 years old (Thompson and Rosenbaum 2008).
- **Sex**
  A slight male predominance has been reported but has not been substantiated. The cutaneous-limited variant has been predominantly reported in women (female-to-male ratio of 3:1).
- **Site**
  The three main targeted organ systems are skin, gastrointestinal tract, and central nervous system. The genitourinary tract, peripheral nervous system, cardiopulmonary system, eyes, pancreas, liver, adrenals, and kidneys can also be involved in systemic MAP. The gastrointestinal tract is involved in 50% or more of cases, and neurologic involvement occurs in approximately 20% of patients. The disease is confined to the skin in approximately 15% of cases. Skin lesions tend to affect the trunk and proximal extremities, but the palms, soles, face, scalp, and genitalia tend to be spared, but exceptions have been noted. Although any portion of the intestinal system may be involved, the small bowel is the predominantly affected one.
- **Treatment**
  Medical treatment for MAP, whether cutaneous or systemic, remains to be defined.

  Antiplatelet drugs, such as aspirin and dipyridamole, may reduce the number of new papules in patients with only skin involvement but have not shown any consistent benefit in systemic disease. Many other therapies, such as plasma exchange, intravenous immunoglobulin, interferon 2 alpha, corticosteroids, and other systemic immunosuppressants, have been shown to be ineffective in altering the course of the disease (Weedon 2010).

  Eculizumab, a C5 blocker, which has been approved for PNH, has been recently tested in systemic MAP with promising results (Scheinfeld 2011).

Surgical treatment may be required for patients who develop complications such as gastrointestinal bleeding, intestinal infarction and perforation, or intracranial bleeding.

- **Outcome**
  The cutaneous-limited variant has a relatively benign course with no significant morbidities associated. With systemic involvement, the reported mean survival is approximately 2–3 years, but there is a wide variation, from less than 1 year to more than 20 years (Ahmadi et al. 2011). The main causes of morbidity and mortality are bowel infarction and perforation, CNS infarction and hemorrhage, and pleuropericardial disease. Intestinal perforation is the most severe complication and the most common cause of death.

Macroscopy

Skin lesions arise in crops of asymptomatic, slightly raised, yellowish red papules that are 2–5 mm in diameter. Within a few days, these papules evolve to become umbilicated, with a porcelain-white depressed center covered with a fine scale and surrounded by an erythematous or telangiectatic border; these are the so-called typical atrophic papules. At presentation, most of the papules have reached the atrophic stage (Scheinfeld 2011).

Gastrointestinal involvement may be observed on endoscopy, even in asymptomatic patients. Lesions similar to those on the skin are most often observed in the small bowel but can also be seen in the stomach, esophagus, duodenum, colon, and rectum. Endoscopy of the gastrointestinal tract can also show infarcted lesions or ulcers. Laparoscopy may show typical lesions consisting of white plaques with hyperemic borders on the serosal surface of the bowel and the peritoneum (Thompson and Rosenbaum 2008).

Microscopy

Skin biopsy is usually required for histological diagnosis.

The histopathology observed may vary with the evolution of the lesions.

Early lesions can demonstrate nonspecific findings including a superficial and deep perivascular, periadnexal, and perineural chronic inflammatory cell infiltrate associated with interstitial mucin deposition (highlighted by colloidal iron or Alcian blue stains).

The classic mature lesion shows an atrophic hyperkeratotic epidermis overlying an inverted, cone-shaped area of necrosis in the dermis, with the base parallel to the surface epithelium. This dermal area is uniformly hypereosinophilic and relatively acellular. More common, however, there are edema, extensive mucin deposition, and slight sclerosis, mimicking dermal mucinosis. Typically, vascular damage is noted in the vessels at the edge of the necrotic wedge. Vascular alterations may be subtle and manifest as endothelial swelling, sometimes with obliteration of the lumen. More characteristically, intravascular fibrin thrombi may be noted. There is also some perivascular distribution of fibrin in the dermis. A sparse perivascular lymphocytic infiltrate may be seen, particularly in the middle and lower dermis; however, altered vessels usually lack an inflammatory infiltrate. This feature distinguishes MAP from other vasculitides.

Sometimes the epidermis shows focal infarction or scattered necrotic keratinocytes in addition to the atrophy. There may also be some basal vacuolar changes.

Panniculitis mimicking lupus erythematosus profundus has also been described (Weedon 2010).

Similar changes are observed in the small vessels on histologic examination of other affected organs. Microscopic examination of bowel reveals transmural intestinal inflammation with ulceration and hemorrhage.

A study of ultrathin sections has demonstrated that MAP is a lymphocyte-mediated necrotizing vasculitis (Weedon 2010).

Immunophenotype

Immunofluorescence studies do not yield definitive results. Fibrin is always demonstrated and

M

sometimes immunoglobulins and complement, namely, C5b-9, may be found around dermal vessels or near the basement membrane (Magro et al. 2011).

Differential Diagnosis

Lesions similar to MAP have been noted in several diseases such as systemic lupus erythematosus, scleroderma, polyarteritis nodosa, rheumatoid arthritis, dermatomyositis, Crohn's disease, and tuberculosis. Differential diagnosis is made based on both clinic findings and histomorphologic features. MAP is different from other vasculitides since inflammation is not a prominent component of the disease and no significant immune complexes have been found in the vessel walls. The characteristic finding of an obliterative fibrous and mucinous angiopathy with secondary thrombosis affecting small- and medium-sized vessels defines MAP as a unique vascular injury syndrome.

References and Further Reading

Ahmadi, M., Rafi, S. A., Faham, Z., Azhough, R., Rooy, S. B., & Rahmani, O. (2011). A fatal case of Degos' disease which presented with recurrent intestinal perforation. *World Journal of Gastrointestinal Surgery, 3*, 156–158.

Magro, C. M., Poe, J. C., Kim, C., Shapiro, L., Nuovo, G., Crow, M. K., et al. (2011). Degos disease: A C5b-9/interferon-a-mediated endotheliopathy syndrome. *American Journal of Clinical Pathology, 135*, 599–610.

Scheinfeld, N. (2011). Commentary on 'Degos disease: A C5b-9 interferon-alpha;-mediated endotheliopathy syndrome by Magro et al.: A reconsideration of Degos disease as hematologic or endothelial genetic disease. *Dermatology Online Journal, 17*, 6.

Thompson, O., & Rosenbaum, D. M. (2008). Uncommon causes of stroke. In R. Caplan Louis & J. Bogousslavsky (Eds.), *Kohlmeier-Degos disease (malignat atrophic papulosis)* (pp. 377–380). Cambridge: Cambridge University Press. Books Online. http://dx.doi.org/10.1017/CBO9780511544897.052

Weedon, D. (2010). *Weedon's skin pathology* (3rd ed.). Philadelphia: Churchill Livingstone/Elsevier.

Malignant Melanoma, Anus

Denis Chatelain[1] and Jean-François Fléjou[2]
[1]Service d'Anatomie Pathologique, Centre Hospitalier et Universitaire du Nord, Amiens, France
[2]Faculté de Médecine Pierre et Marie Curie, Service d'Anatomie et Cytologie Pathologiques, Hôpital Saint-Antoine, Paris, France

Synonyms

Anal melanoma

Definition

Anal melanoma is a rare and aggressive mucosal melanocytic malignancy, first described by Moore in 1857.

It constitutes 0.5–2% of all anal malignancies and represents less than 2% of all melanomas. The anus is the third most common site for melanoma after the skin and the eye and is the most common site for primary gastrointestinal melanoma.

Patients usually present with anal bleeding (the most common complaints in 50–90% of patients), anal or perianal mass (30%) or anal pain (10%); they can also complain of tenesmus, change in bowel habits, diarrhea, constipation, or incontinence. If a metastatic disease is present, symptoms may include weight loss, anemia, fatigue, groin masses, or bowel obstruction. The average time between the occurrence of symptoms and a confirmed diagnosis is 5–6 months, because patients tend to delay presentation to their doctors, they cannot see asymptomatic lesions and symptoms of anal melanoma are commonly misdiagnosed as those of other anal lesions such as hemorrhoids (Singer and Mutch 2006).

Because of the delay in diagnosis and the aggressive nature of the disease, patients with anal melanoma frequently present with advanced lesions. At the time of diagnosis, 25–40% of patients will have a metastatic disease present in mesorectal and inguinal lymph nodes, liver, lung, brain, or bones.

Anal melanoma is staged on a clinical basis, focusing on locoregional and distant spread.

Stage I is localized disease, stage II is localized disease with regional lymph nodes, and stage III is distant metastatic disease. The American Joint Commission on Cancer has developed a staging method based on depth of the primary tumor and presence of metastases: T1 $\leq$ 1 mm; T2 1.1–2 mm; T3 2.1–4 mm; T4 > 4 mm, and nodal disease: N1 (single metastatic lymph node); N2 (two to three metastatic lymph nodes); N3 (four or more metastatic lymph nodes).

Clinical Features

- **Incidence**
  The exact incidence of anal malignant melanoma is difficult to assess because of the rarity of the disease and the lack of large published cohorts. A sampling of cancer registries in US cities revealed an incidence of 1.7 cases per 1 million per year.
- **Age**
  The average age for patients with anal malignant melanoma is 55 years, although the range is wide, from 29 to 91 years.
- **Sex**
  The incidence of anorectal malignant melanoma seems to be equal between men and women.

  Although most publications do not suggest significant gender differences, some small series show a discrete female predominance, perhaps with recruitment biases.
- **Site**
  Anal malignant melanoma arises from normal melanocytes present in the transitional mucosa beneath the dentate line. Pathogenesis and etiologic factors are still unknown.

  In contrast to malignant melanomas of the skin, a history of sun exposure does not favor the occurrence of anal melanoma. Other known risk factors for cutaneous melanoma such as dysplastic nevus syndrome or xeroderma pigmentosum have no known association with anal melanoma. Family history of melanoma or ethnicity do not seem to be risk factors There is a strong association with Caucasian race, but most series have a preponderance of Caucasian subjects. There are some data to suggest a role for immune factors in the development of anal melanoma, because a significant rise in the incidence was observed in young men with AIDS in San Francisco between 1988 and 1992, without direct implication of HIV, HHV8, or HPV viruses.
- **Treatment**
  There are still controversies over the therapeutic strategies in anal melanoma (Droesch et al. 2005).

  Surgery remains the mainstay of treatment. Chemotherapy (most frequently consisting of dacarbazine, vincristine, nimustine hydrochloride), immunotherapy (with interferon), and radiation therapy alone have not been shown to be effective but may provide some benefit when used in adjuvant fashion. The most appropriate surgical operation remains questionable: limited wide sphincter-sparing local excision versus radical excision with abdominoperineal resection. Meta-analysis has failed to identify any stage-specific survival advantage of abdominoperineal resection in comparison to sphincter-sparing wide local excision. Abdominoperineal resection carries the theoretical benefit of a wider excision with mesenteric lymphadenectomy. But the majority of patients are diagnosed at a relatively late stage, and curative surgery is not possible for these patients. Wide local excision offers patients a seemingly equivalent opportunity for cure with significantly less surgical mortality and morbidity, and with the avoidance of a permanent colostomy. There are higher local recurrences, but they do not usually cause severe local symptoms. Recurrences can be treated by re-excision (sometimes with abdominoperineal resection). But it is metastatic disease that ultimately causes the death of most patients. Some authors recommend abdominoperineal resection only for patients without evidence of lymph node metastases and with small tumors, less than 2 mm thick. These patients have the best chance of long-term survival, and therefore, more radical surgery would be justified.

For tumors with poor prognostic factors, larger tumors and lymph node or visceral metastasis, local excision may be the most appropriate therapy to maintain local control and to minimize morbidity. Combined sphincter-sparing local excision and radiotherapy is a well-tolerated approach that provides effective local control.

Sentinel lymph node biopsy is technically feasible in patients with anal melanoma. It may detect clinically non-apparent groin adenopathy, and the subsequent inguinal dissection may provide curative resection in a small subset of patients. However, its efficacy remains unknown and its role in the management of patients with anal melanoma is still debated.

- **Outcome**
  Anal melanoma has an extremely poor prognosis (Heeney et al. 2011). The mean survival time of patients is 15–25 months. Survival in patients with recurrent or metastatic disease is less than 10 months. Of all patients with anal melanoma, the 5-year survival rate ranges from 15% to 35%.

  There are very rare reported cases of long-term survivors, but none had metastatic disease at the time of diagnosis. Although approximately 70% of patients present with no detectable metastasis, the vast majority of patients die of distant metastasis within 2–3 years of diagnosis.

Macroscopy

Anal malignant melanoma consists of an ulcerated or polypoid mass, developed in the transitional zone of the anal canal. It ranges in size from 1 to 6 cm. The tumors are generally more than 1 cm thick at diagnosis. They can present as brown-black tumors on gross examination, but 80% of the tumors are whitish and lack obvious pigmentation on macroscopic examination.

Microscopy

The histologic features of anal melanoma resemble those of cutaneous melanomas (Stefanou and Nalamati 2011). The tumors may show variable morphology such as epithelioid, spindle-cell, desmoplastic, lymphocyte-like, or mixed morphology. The tumors have a diffuse or nested architecture. They consist of large or small round or spindle cells (Fig. 1). They have an eosinophilic or clear cytoplasm, which sometimes contains brown-black melanin pigment, stained with the Fontana stain (Fig. 2). Tumors cells have enlarged nuclei, often with marked nuclear pleomorphism, with a vesicular or dense chromatin and often prominent eosinophilic nucleoli. Multinucleated cells can be seen. There is varied mitotic activity with sometimes abnormal mitoses. The stroma may contain numerous lymphocytes. The tumors invade the anal wall and can show tumor necrosis, vascular invasion, and perineural invasion. Most tumors show a junctional component adjacent to the invasive tumor in the anal epithelium with nests of tumor cells or isolated tumor cells migrating into the squamous epithelium.

Very rare cases of anal melanoma have been identified during the routine pathology examination of a hemorrhoidectomy specimen.

The most important histoprognostic factors are perineural invasion and the tumor thickness, which can be identified on the preoperative biopsy and therefore may be useful when deciding the most appropriate surgical therapy. Patients with tumors less than 2-mm thick seem to have a better prognosis. Primary tumor size superior to 10 mm

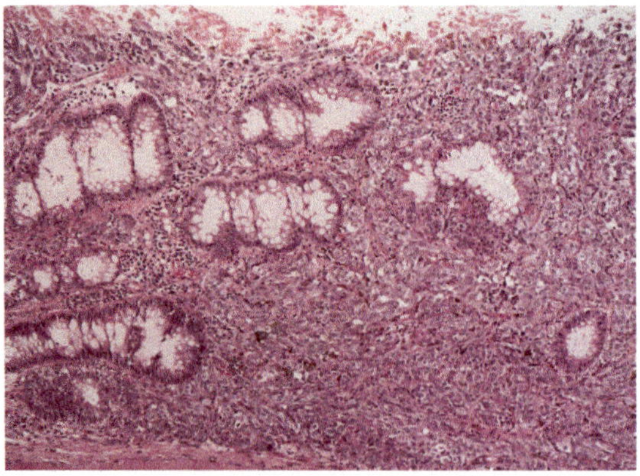

Malignant Melanoma, Anus, Fig. 1 Anal melanoma, invading the glandular anorectal mucosa

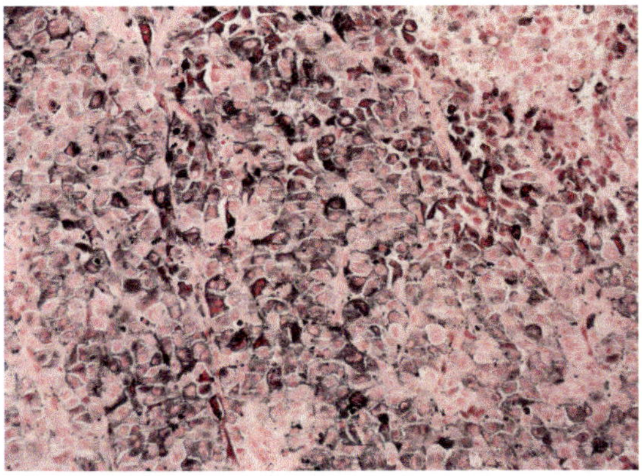

Malignant Melanoma, Anus, Fig. 2 Anal melanoma, with pigment stained on Fontana

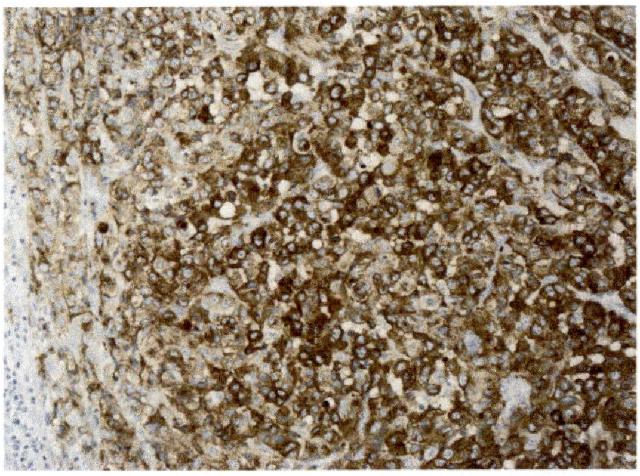

Malignant Melanoma, Anus, Fig. 3 Anal melanoma. Tumor cells strongly express Melan-A

has an association with a shorter disease-specific survival.

Immunophenotype

On immunohistochemistry, tumor cells stain positive for conventional melanoma markers such as S100 protein, HMB-45, Mart-1/Melan-A, and vimentin (Fig. 3). In rare cases, some tumor cells can stain positive for polyclonal CEA, pancytokeratin, and EMA. In 40% of anal melanomas, tumor cells show diffuse and strong CD117 expression, but this positive staining does not correlate with the mutation status of the *KIT* gene.

Molecular Features

Molecular features of anal melanomas are still unclear. Unlike cutaneous melanomas, anal melanomas rarely show *BRAF* mutations. *BRAF* mutations are found only in 5% of cases, and are usually not located in exon 15, where the substitution V600E is found as in cutaneous melanomas. BRAF inhibitors do not seem to be efficient in the treatment of anal melanomas.

In anal melanomas, there is an increased prevalence of activating *KIT* mutation, seen in 15–20% of cases (Ni et al. 2012). The c-kit protein receptor plays an important role in melanocyte development and proliferation. This subset of anal melanomas with activating *KIT* mutations, an uncommon mutation in cutaneous melanomas, could respond to KIT inhibitors. However, there is no correlation between the mutation status and immunohistochemical CD117 expression. The treatment of anal melanomas with tyrosine kinase inhibitors should be based on c-kit mutation status rather than on protein expression level.

Differential Diagnoses

Metastatic melanoma to the anal canal is exceedingly rare. Cutaneous melanoma metastasizes to the gastrointestinal tract in only 2% of cases, and only 2% of these metastases are located in the ano-rectum. However, clinical data and, on microscopic examination, the presence of a junctional component adjacent to the invasive tumor help to confirm the diagnosis of primary malignant melanoma of the anal canal.

Anal malignant melanomas are often amelanotic and on microscopic examination consist of a poorly differentiated tumor, composed of sheets of large round tumor cells with marked nuclear atypia. Immunohistochemistry with positive staining for melanoma markers (S100 protein, HMB-45, and Melan-A) permits to differentiate anal melanoma from other poorly differentiated tumors of the anal canal, such as poorly differentiated basaloid carcinoma or extremely rare anal malignant lymphoma.

References and Further Reading

Droesch, J. T., Flum, D. R., & Mann, G. N. (2005). Wide local excision or abdominoperineal resection as the initial treatment for anorectal melanoma? *American Journal of Surgery, 189*, 446–449.

Heeney, A., Mulsow, J., & Hyland, J. M. (2011). Treatment and outcomes of anorectal melanoma. *The Surgeon, 9*, 27–32.

Ni, S., Huang, D., Chen, X., Huang, J., Kong, Y., Xu, Y., Du, X., & Sheng, W. (2012). c-kit gene mutation and CD117 expression in human anorectal melanomas. *Human Pathology, 43*, 801–807.

Singer, M., & Mutch, M. G. (2006). Anal melanoma. *Clinics in Colon and Rectal Surgery, 19*, 78–87.

Stefanou, A., & Nalamati, S. P. (2011). Anorectal melanoma. *Clinics in Colon and Rectal Surgery, 24*, 171–176.

Mallory Weiss Lacerations, Esophageal

Bruno Pereira[1,2] and António Dias Pereira[1]
[1]Instituto Português de Oncologia de Lisboa Francisco Gentil, E.P.E., Lisbon, Portugal
[2]Servico de Gastrenterologia, Hospital Amato Lusitano, ULS de Castelo Branco, Castelo Branco, Portugal

Synonyms

Gastroesophageal lacerations; Mallory-Weiss tears

Definition

Mallory-Weiss lacerations are mucosal or submucosal longitudinal tears that occur at the gastroesophageal junction or gastric cardia. These lacerations may cause upper gastrointestinal bleeding from submucosal blood vessels (Mallory-Weiss syndrome). They were first described in 15 alcoholic patients with persistent retching and vomiting (Mallory and Weiss 1929).

While the pathogenesis is not completely understood, it appears that any action leading to a sudden rise in intra-abdominal pressure and gastric prolapse or intussusception into the esophagus may cause a Mallory-Weiss laceration. Besides retching and vomiting, other precipitating factors include coughing, straining, convulsions, hiccups, blunt abdominal trauma, and cardiopulmonary resuscitation. Iatrogenic tears can result from procedures like upper gastrointestinal endoscopy and transesophageal echocardiography. Colonoscopic preparation with polyethylene glycol electrolyte solution has also been reported as a risk factor. In some cases, no precipitating event is identified.

The presence of a hiatal hernia and chronic alcoholism seem to be frequent predisposing conditions. Different series have found hiatal hernias in 40–100% of patients with Mallory-Weiss lacerations. During retching or vomiting, the shearing force on the gastroesophageal junction and proximal stomach is maximized by a hiatal hernia, where a higher transmural pressure gradient is generated compared to the rest of the stomach, subsequently increasing the risk for mucosal injury. A history of alcoholism has been described in 40–80% of patients with Mallory-Weiss syndrome. This strong association can be explained not only by the increased occurrence of vomiting episodes but also due to portal hypertension and coagulopathy, which often lead to more severe bleeding and subsequent higher detection rate of the lacerations. Some studies describe the use of antiaggregant or nonsteroidal anti-inflammatory drugs as a potential predisposing factor. Eating disorders have also been associated with Mallory-Weiss lacerations.

Patients with Mallory-Weiss syndrome usually present with hematemesis following retching or non-bloody vomiting. In 25–30% of cases no apparent precipitating factor is recognized. The bleeding is usually self-limited but may be massive in up to 10% of patients. If severe blood loss occurs, patients may present with hematochezia, syncope, and signs of hemodynamic instability like tachycardia, orthostatic changes, hypotension, or shock.

Endoscopy is the procedure of choice for the diagnosis and eventual therapy of Mallory-Weiss lacerations. It also plays an important role in ruling out other causes of upper gastrointestinal bleeding that may coexist, such as peptic ulcer disease or erosive esophagitis. It should be performed early, after assessing the patient's hemodynamic status and initiating volume reposition if necessary. Most patients present a single, red, longitudinal laceration, 2–3 cm in length, located in the gastroesophageal junction, usually extending distally within a hiatal hernia along the lesser curvature of the cardia. The adjacent mucosa is usually normal. Multiple tears can be identified in a minority of patients. A careful inspection of the cardia, including a retroflexed endoscopic view, is essential not to miss any lesions. Mallory-Weiss lacerations can present with diverse bleeding stigmata, including a fibrin crust, adherent clot, oozing, or active spurting. Spontaneous healing can occur in less than 48 h. The diagnosis can be missed if the initial endoscopy is delayed.

Clinical Features

- **Incidence**
  The true incidence of Mallory-Weiss lacerations is hard to establish. The condition accounts for an estimated 1–15% of patients presenting with upper gastrointestinal bleeding. However, patients do not usually seek medical care unless bleeding occurs, leading to a significant proportion of unrecognized lacerations. One study reported an incidence of 0.06% in patients receiving colonoscopic preparation with polyethylene glycol electrolyte solution. A national survey of the American Society for Gastrointestinal Endoscopy estimated an incidence of 0.13% following gastroscopy.
- **Age**
  Mallory-Weiss lacerations can occur at any age. Most series report a median age in the fifth and sixth decades of life, but there have been several case reports of Mallory-Weiss syndrome among infants. There is some evidence suggesting that increasing age might be a predisposing factor due to atrophy of the gastric mucosa and subsequent increased susceptibility to injury.
- **Sex**
  Most series report a higher incidence of Mallory-Weiss syndrome among men, with rates as high as 6:1.
- **Site**
  Mallory-Weiss lacerations occur in the gastroesophageal junction or gastric cardia, more frequently along the lesser curvature of the stomach.
- **Treatment**
  After an initial hemodynamic status evaluation, resuscitative measures should be implemented as appropriate (fluid, blood replacement) and endoscopy performed promptly. Precipitating factors, such as vomiting, should be addressed with specific drugs (e.g., antiemetic drugs). Mallory-Weiss lacerations with a clean base, fibrin crust, or flat spots have a minimal risk of rebleeding and do not require endoscopic treatment. Stigmata like a nonbleeding visible vessel or adherent clot are not usually treated, unless associated with coagulopathy or a rebleeding episode. Endoscopic hemostatic therapy is the first-line treatment of actively bleeding Mallory-Weiss lacerations. Many different methods have been reported to achieve successful hemostasis. No consensus exists as to the best endoscopic treatment for Mallory-Weiss syndrome. The choice depends mainly upon local availability, practice, and experience.

  Injection therapy has been used solely or in combination with other methods. Epinephrine (1:10,000–1:20,000 dilution) causes edema and vasoconstriction and reduces or stops bleeding when injected around the bleeding point. Many authors recommend an association with other therapeutic modalities, such as thermal therapy or hemoclip placement, in order to minimize the risk of rebleeding. Due to potential cardiovascular complications, the use of epinephrine should be avoided in patients with significant cardiovascular risk. Ethanol, polidocanol, and other sclerosants have also been demonstrated to achieve successful hemostasis. Serious complications like tissue necrosis and perforation have been reported, leading to some authors not recommending its use. Sclerotherapy might play a role in the management of Mallory-Weiss lacerations in patients with portal hypertension and esophageal varices.

Among the thermal contact therapies, bipolar or multipolar electrocoagulation is the most widely used. As opposed to peptic ulcer disease, a lower power setting (14–16 W) and shorter pulses (1–2 s) are generally applied due to increased risk of esophagic perforation and smaller artery size. Argon plasma coagulation is a noncontact electrocoagulation method which uses high-frequency energy delivered to tissue through an ionized gas (argon plasma). It has been proved to be safe and effective in achieving hemostasis in acute non-variceal upper gastrointestinal bleeding from different causes, including Mallory-Weiss lacerations. To minimize the risk of esophagic perforation, the power output should not exceed 40–45 W and the gas flow rate 1 L/min.

The efficacy and safety of endoscopic band ligation has been addressed in a small study of 37 patients with Mallory-Weiss syndrome. The technique achieved successful hemostasis in 36 patients with no recurrent bleeding, perforation, or other significant complications occurring in these. One patient with severe liver failure and disseminated intravascular coagulation had a fatal outcome (Higuchi et al. 2006). In another small, randomized, prospective trial, no significant difference was detected in the efficacy or safety of band ligation when compared with epinephrine injection for the treatment of actively bleeding Mallory-Weiss syndrome. Like sclerotherapy, band ligation should be considered in the treatment of Mallory-Weiss lacerations in patients with portal hypertension and esophageal varices.

Endoscopic placement of hemoclips can also achieve hemostasis in actively bleeding Mallory-Weiss lacerations. Hemoclips can target a specific bleeding point or be deployed in order to join the laceration margins, from the distal to the proximal end. A small study of 26 patients with Mallory-Weiss lacerations with active bleeding, visible vessels, or adherent clots treated with endoscopic hemoclipping showed technical success in all cases, with no complications, recurrent bleeding, or deaths occurring. Follow-up endoscopy showed no evidence of hemoclip-induced tissue injury (Yamaguchi et al. 2001).

Most patients with Mallory-Weiss lacerations stop bleeding spontaneously. Those presenting with actively bleeding lacerations on endoscopy usually respond to endoscopic hemostatic therapy. Rare refractory cases might benefit from interventional radiology (selective vasopressin infusion or arterial embolization) or surgery. Some authors do not recommend esophageal balloon tamponade as the radial force it exerts might widen the laceration.

Following the initial endoscopy and eventual hemostatic therapy, it is important to address the risk of rebleeding and the optimal observation or hospitalization period. Portal hypertension, coagulopathy, initial shock, and active bleeding at endoscopy have been identified as major risk factors for rebleeding. Most rebleeding episodes occur during the first 24 h. In the absence of rebleeding risk factors, signs of severe bleeding (e.g., hematochezia, hemodynamic instability), or active bleeding at endoscopy, a brief hospitalization period of 24 h is usually enough in the management of Mallory-Weiss lacerations. Patients with clinical risk factors for rebleeding and nonbleeding endoscopic stigmata should be observed for a longer period, around 48 h. Patients with actively bleeding lesions should be treated with endoscopic therapy and hospitalized for at least 48 h (Bharucha et al. 1994).

Most authors suggest the use of acid-suppressive therapy (e.g., proton pump inhibitors) or cytoprotective agents (e.g., sucralfate) for a few weeks, assuming that it enhances the healing of the laceration by protecting against deleterious factors such as acid and pepsin. However, the benefit of such practice in the prevention of rebleeding in Mallory-Weiss syndrome has never been demonstrated.

- **Outcome**

The Mallory-Weiss syndrome has an excellent prognosis. In 80–90% of patients, lacerations stop bleeding and heal spontaneously. Endoscopic therapy achieves hemostasis in almost every patient presenting with actively bleeding lacerations. However, massive bleeding can occur in up to 10% of patients, and some series report mortality rates as high as 9.7%. Advanced age, shock on arrival, lower hemoglobin level, more prolonged prothrombin time, higher AST and ALT levels, detection of exposed vessels on endoscopy, rebleeding, longer hospital stay, and larger volume of blood transfusion were found to be more common in patients with a fatal outcome (Fujisawa et al. 2011). Recurrence of bleeding is uncommon. Precipitating factors (e.g., alcoholism, eating disorders) should be addressed in order to minimize the risk of rebleeding.

Macroscopy

Mallory-Weiss lacerations usually present as a single, red, longitudinal tear, 2–3 cm in length and few millimeters in width, located in the gastroesophageal junction. It is frequently associated with a hiatal hernia. Unlike other causes of distal esophagic mucosal disruption, like erosive esophagitis, Mallory-Weiss lacerations are usually surrounded by normal appearing mucosa. Some patients may present with multiple tears (Fig. 1).

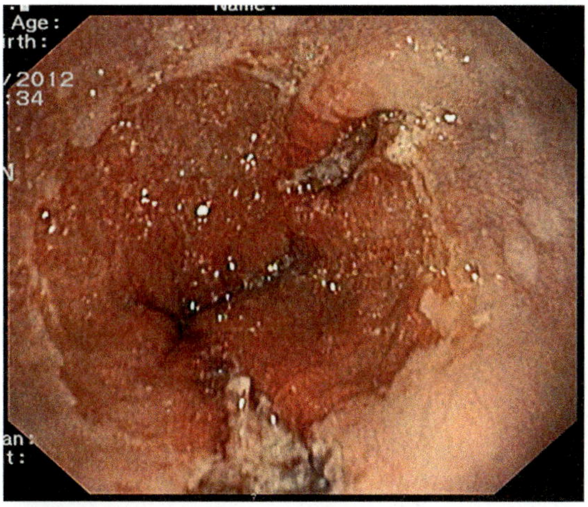

Mallory Weiss Lacerations, Esophageal, Fig. 1 Endoscopic view of two Mallory-Weiss lacerations covered in fibrin in a patient presenting with hematemesis following severe vomiting

Differential Diagnosis

Bleeding from a Mallory-Weiss laceration is usually suspected following a typical presentation, and the diagnosis made upon endoscopy. When atypical features are present, it is important to distinguish it from other esophageal conditions. Spontaneous perforation of the esophagus following severe retching or vomiting (Boerhaave's syndrome) usually presents with intense retrosternal chest and upper abdominal pain. Evidence of mediastinal or free peritoneal air on plain chest radiography suggests the diagnosis which can be confirmed by CT scan. Endoscopy should be avoided due to the increased risk of extending the perforation with the endoscope and air insufflation. Ulcerative diseases of the esophagus, including reflux esophagitis, infectious esophagitis, pill-induced ulcers, or esophageal Crohn's disease, are usually easily distinguished from Mallory-Weiss lacerations due to the different patterns of esophagic involvement.

References and Further Reading

Bharucha, A. E., Gstout, C. J., & Balm, R. K. (1994). Clinical and endoscopic risk factors in the Mallory-Weiss syndrome. *The American Journal of Gastroenterology, 89*, 2147.

Fujisawa, N., Inamori, M., Sekino, Y., et al. (2011). Risk factors for mortality in patients with Mallory-Weiss syndrome. *Hepatogastroenterology, 58*(106), 417–420.

Higuchi, N., Akahoshi, K., Sumida, Y., et al. (2006). Endoscopic band ligation therapy for upper gastrointestinal bleeding related to Mallory-Weiss syndrome. *Surgical Endoscopy, 20*(9), 1431–1434.

Kovacs, T. O., & Jensen, D. M. (1997). Endoscopic diagnosis and treatment of bleeding Mallory-Weiss tears. *The American Journal of Gastroenterology, 92*, 805.

Mallory, G. K., & Weiss, S. W. (1929). Hemorrhages from lacerations of the cardiac orifice of the stomach due to vomiting. *The American Journal of the Medical Sciences, 178*, 506–512.

Sugawa, C., Benishek, D., & Walt, A. J. (1983). Mallory-Weiss syndrome. A study of 224 patients. *American Journal of Surgery, 145*(1), 30–33.

Yamaguchi, Y., Yamato, T., Katsumi, N., et al. (2001). Endoscopic hemoclipping for upper GI bleeding due to Mallory-Weiss syndrome. *Gastrointestinal Endoscopy, 53*(4), 427–430.

Meckel's Diverticulum

Cord Langner
Institute of Pathology, Medical University of Graz, Graz, Austria

Definition

Within the gastrointestinal tract, true diverticula are out-pouchings that contain all layers of the bowel wall. False diverticula (pseudo-diverticula) are out-pouchings of the mucosa and submucosa emerging through the muscularis propria. While true diverticula are mainly congenital, most pseudo-diverticula are acquired.

Meckel's diverticulum is a true congenital diverticulum of the small bowel, caused by the incomplete obliteration of the omphalomesenteric (vitelline) duct. In embryonic life, the omphalomesenteric duct connects the yolk sac to the intestinal tract. It usually obliterates within the 5–7th week of gestation. If the obliteration fails, different congenital anomalies develop, leading to residual fibrous cords, umbilical sinus, omphalomesenteric fistula, and, most commonly, Meckel's diverticulum.

Fabricius Hildanus made the earliest description of the anomaly in 1598. However, it was not until 1809 that the histogenesis of the lesion was correctly identified by the German anatomist Johann Friedrich Meckel, the Younger, (1781–1833; Fig. 1), giving rise to its present name.

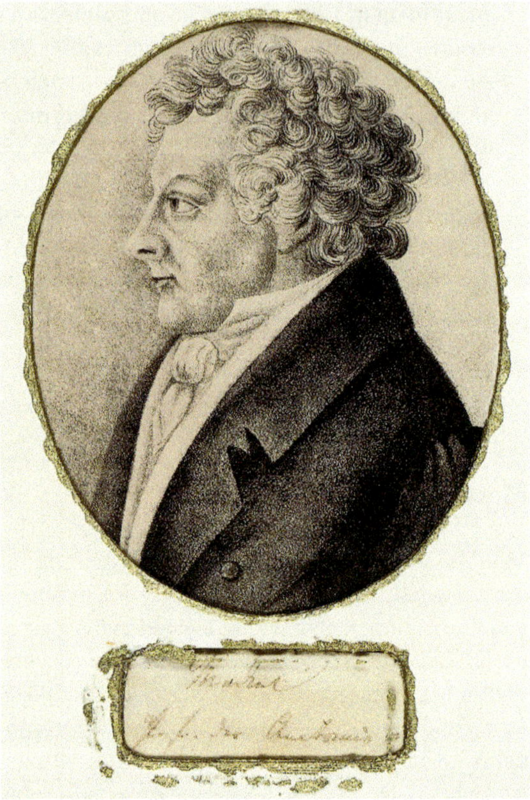

Meckel's Diverticulum, Fig. 1 Johann Friedrich Meckel, the Younger, (1781–1833), from the Archives of the Department of Anatomy and Cell Biology, Martin Luther University Halle-Wittenberg, Germany (with permission; UKH/Norbert Kaltwasser)

Clinical Features

- **Incidence**
  Congenital malformations of the gastrointestinal tract account for approximately 6% of all congenital anomalies. Of these, Meckel's diverticulum is the most common. According to a recent extensive literature review, the prevalence is 1.2%.
- **Sex**
  The occurrence in males and females is equal, but the incidence of complications is higher in males (see Symptoms). In a systematic analysis of the Mayo Clinic experience with the anomaly (based on 1,476 individuals), the male-to-female ratio for symptomatic disease was approximately 3:1 in both the adult (72% vs. 28%) and in the pediatric (72% vs. 28%) population. In asymptomatic cases, the ratio was also approximately 3:1 in the pediatric population (73% vs. 27%), yet lower in the adult population (58% vs. 42%).
- **Site**
  The anomaly is typically located in the terminal ileum, 60–100 cm from the ileocecal valve in adults, and 30–90 cm in children. Rarely, the anomaly has been described to occur in the jejunum, and anecdotally in the rectum.

- **Symptoms**
  In most cases, Meckel's diverticulum is clinically silent and may be detected incidentally during an abdominal procedure. Symptoms occur in 4–6% of cases, the incidence decreasing with age. Clinical and/or anatomical features that have been associated with symptomatic disease generally include younger age, male gender, diverticulum length exceeding 2 cm, and presence of histologically abnormal tissue, particularly gastric heterotopia (see Microscopy).
  In symptomatic cases, the most common presentations are lower gastrointestinal bleeding (ranging from positive fecal occult blood test to massive acute blood loss with hemodynamic compromise), diverticulitis (possibly due to obstruction by enteroliths, parasites, or foreign bodies), and mechanical obstruction of the small bowel. The latter may be due to intussusception or volvulus. Axial torsion with subsequent gangrene has been identified as another possible complication.
  Rarely, neoplastic tumor growth may develop within a Meckel's diverticulum. Neuroendocrine tumors (carcinoids) account for the majority of cases, but conventional adenocarcinomas, mesenchymal tumors such as gastrointestinal stromal tumors (GISTs) and leiomyosarcomas, as well as malignant lymphomas have also been reported. According to a recent analysis of the Surveillance, Epidemiology, and End Results (SEER) database, the adjusted tumor risk is at least 70 times higher compared to any other ileal sites, identifying Meckel's diverticulum to be a "hot-spot" or high-risk area for cancer in the ileum.
- **Treatment**
  A symptomatic Meckel's diverticulum is treated by surgical resection. The management of a Meckel's diverticulum which is incidentally detected during an abdominal procedure is less clear. According to a recent extensive literature review, prophylactic resection of an asymptomatic Meckel's diverticulum during surgery cannot be recommended, because this significantly increases the risk of postoperative complications. In several studies, the long-term outcome of patients with incidentally detected Meckel's diverticulum left in situ has shown no complications. In all, 758 patients would require resection of their asymptomatic diverticulum to prevent 1 death from the anomaly.

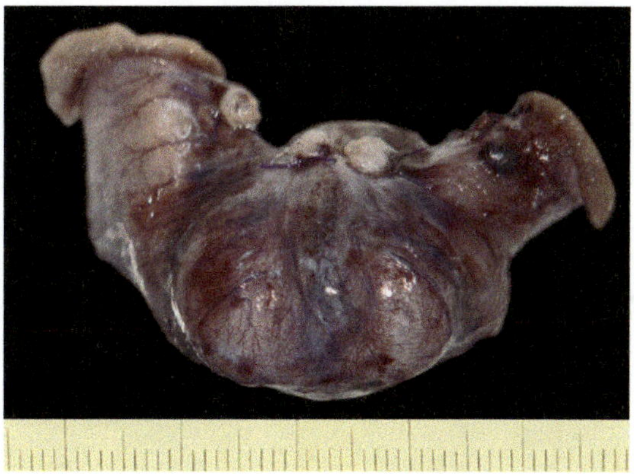

Meckel's Diverticulum, Fig. 2 Operation specimen showing a Meckel's diverticulum at the antimesenteric border of the terminal ileum

Macroscopy

In 90% of cases, Meckel' diverticulum is found at the antimesenteric border of the small bowel (Fig. 2). On average, the anomaly is 2.9 cm long and 1.9 cm wide, but "giant" Meckel's diverticula, their length exceeding 10 cm, have been described. Meckel's diverticulum has its own blood supply, known as the vitelline artery.

Microscopy

As a true diverticulum, Meckel's diverticulum contains all layers of the bowel wall. The lumen is lined by ileal type mucosa as in the adjacent small bowel. In approximately 50% of cases, heterotopic (ectopic) tissue is present, the most common being gastric oxyntic type mucosa (23–50%; Figs. 3 and 4) and pancreatic tissue (5–16%; Figs. 3 and 5). Other heterotopic tissues, such as colonic, duodenal, hepatic, and endometrial mucosa, are rare. In symptomatic cases, acute

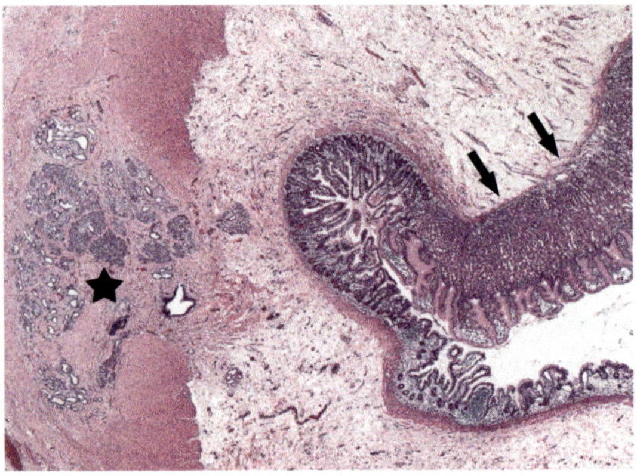

Meckel's Diverticulum, Fig. 3 Histological overview of a Meckel's diverticulum with heterotopic gastric oxyntic type mucosa (*arrows*) and intramural heterotopic pancreatic glands (*asterix*)

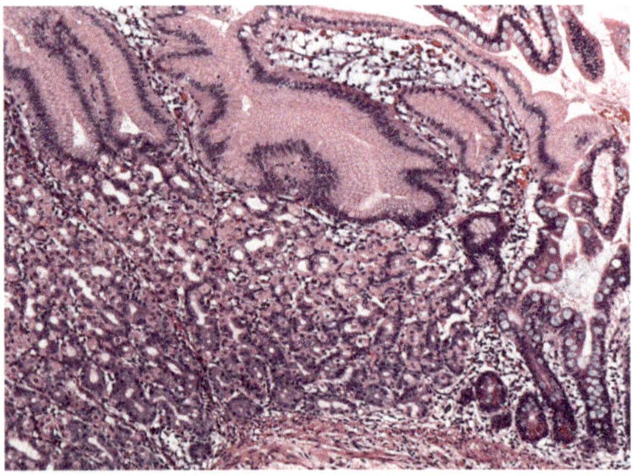

Meckel's Diverticulum, Fig. 4 High magnification of heterotopic gastric oxyntic type mucosa (same case as Fig. 3)

and/or chronic inflammatory changes of varying degree may be observed ("diverticulitis").

Differential Diagnosis

Meckel's diverticulum has to be differentiated from ileal duplication which does not have a separate blood supply and usually lacks communication with the bowel lumen. False diverticula (pseudo-diverticula) are very rare in the small bowel. They mainly occur in the jejunum.

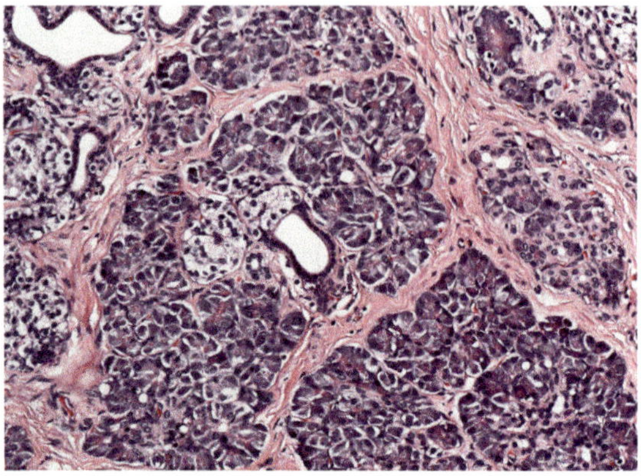

Meckel's Diverticulum, Fig. 5 High magnification of heterotopic pancreatic glands (same case as Fig. 3)

References and Further Reading

Park, J. J., Wolff, B. G., Tollefson, M. K., Walsh, E. E., & Larson, D. R. (2005). Meckel diverticulum. The mayo clinic experience with 1476 patients (1950–2002). *Annals of Surgery, 241*, 529–533.

Sagar, Y., Kumar, V., & Shah, D. K. (2006). Meckel's diverticulum: A systematic review. *Journal of the Royal Society of Medicine, 99*, 501–505.

Thirunavukarasu, P., Sathaiah, M., Sukumar, S., Bartels, C. J., Zeh, H., Lee, K. K. W., & Bartlett, D. L. (2011). Meckel's diverticulum. A high-risk region for malignancy in the ileum. Insights from a population-based epidemiological study and implications in surgical management. *Annals of Surgery, 253*, 223–230.

Uppal, K., Tubbs, R. S., Matusz, P., Shaffer, K., & Lukas, M. (2011). Meckel's diverticulum: A review. *Clinical Anatomy, 24*, 416–422.

Zani, A., Eaton, S., Rees, C. M., & Pierro, A. (2008). Incidentally detected Meckel diverticulum. To resect or not to resect? *Annals of Surgery, 247*, 276–281.

Ménétrier's Disease

Chella R. S. van der Post
and J. Han van Krieken
Department of Pathology, Radboud University Medical Center, Nijmegen, The Netherlands

Synonyms

Giant hypertrophic gastritis; Giant mucosal rugae; Hyperplastic gastropathy; Hyperplastic/Hypertrophic gastritis; Hypoproteinemic hypertrophic gastropathy; Protein-losing gastropathy

Definition

Ménétrier's disease is a rare form of acquired gastropathy involving the gastric fundus and corpus and is characterized by gastric rugal hypertrophy, protein-losing gastropathy, and an increase of gastric luminal pH (hypochlorhydria).

Ménétrier's disease is considered to be a rare acquired disorder of uncertain etiology. It was first described in 1888 by Pierre Ménétrier, a French pathologist who observed enlarged gastric folds during autopsies. Sporadic case reports were described in the following decennia; in most adult cases, an initial pathogenic agent or event could not be determined. A break-through in the pathogenesis was the finding of local overproduction of transforming growth factor-alpha (TGF-α), resulting in enhanced epidermal growth factor receptor (EGFR) signaling in the gastric mucosa. TGF-α is a potent mitogen that binds and activates the tyrosine kinase of EGFR that stimulates gastric growth and inhibits gastric acid secretion. In patients with Ménétrier's disease, enhanced immunoreactivity for TGF-α has been showed in their expanded surface mucous cell compartment and, furthermore, transgenic mice that overproduce TGF-α in the stomach have many features of Ménétrier's disease, including foveolar hyperplasia, increased mucin content, decreased chief cell and parietal cell mass, and reduced acid production. The precise underlying molecular defect resulting in the local gastric upregulation of TGF-α is unknown. The childhood form of Ménétrier's disease has been associated with CMV infection.

Clinical Features

Ménétrier's disease has a progressive clinical course, with typical symptoms being epigastric pain, nausea, vomiting, hematemesis, diarrhea, asthenia, anorexia, and peripheral edema. Biochemical features that are frequently seen include anemia, hypoproteinemia, hypochlorhydria, and increased gastric mucus. The anemia is caused by gastric blood loss. The increase of gastric luminal pH, hypochlorhydria, can be explained by the significant reduction in parietal cells and directly by inhibition of acid secretion in parietal cells through TGF-α signaling. There are usually normal serum gastrin levels. The hypoacidity can also be partly caused by the buffering capacity of the large amount of secreted mucus. Generalized peripheral edema is often seen secondary to protein loss through the gastric mucosa due to wider tight junctions with resultant low serum albumin (<35 g/L). The diagnosis of Ménétrier's disease is based on clinical, endoscopic, and histopathological criteria and may at times be difficult to establish. Familial occurrence of Ménétrier's disease is very rare and has been reported only in few instances. The disease shows similar clinical and pathologic features in children; however, many children have a history of recent respiratory infection, peripheral blood eosinophilia, and cytomegalovirus infection.

- **Incidence**
  Exact incidence is unknown; Ménétrier's disease has been considered a rare disorder, with only a few hundred reported cases in the literature.
- **Age**
  It has been described in children and adults. The average age is around 55 years; most patients are between 30 and 60 years of age.
- **Sex**
  There is sex predominance for men, with a male–female ratio of approximately 3:1.
- **Site**
  Enlarged rugae in Ménétrier's disease characteristically involve the corpus and fundus of the stomach, without involvement of the antrum. However, in rare instances and in children, the antrum may also be involved.
- **Treatment and Outcome**
  The disease course has usually a chronic course, with an unfavorable prognosis. Many patients require primarily supportive care with high-protein diet, intravenous albumin infusions, and sometimes pain

medication. Various treatments reported for adult patients include *Helicobacter pylori* eradication, prednisone, antibiotics, non-steroidal anti-inflammatory drugs, anticholinergic agents, and octreotide therapy; however, the benefits of each treatment are not known and not evaluated in a clinical trial. The only definitive treatment was, until recently, total gastrectomy. Due to the discovery of increased TGF-α production in patients with Ménétrier's disease, a possible treatment has been published using cetuximab, a monoclonal antibody to EGFR, and showed significant and biochemical improvements in patients.

Patients with Ménétrier's disease may have an increased risk of developing gastric carcinoma; however, this is subject to debate. Approximately 15% of cases described in the literature have been associated with carcinoma.

In contrast to adults, in children, CMV infection has been frequently implicated and the disease shows an abrupt onset and a self-limited course, generally lasting only several weeks. In children, CMV should be suspected when presenting with protein-losing gastropathy. Detection of CMV can be best done in a gastric biopsy sample by immunohistochemical staining and PCR for CMV. Most pediatric patients recover spontaneously or with supportive care such as intravenous albumin infusions. Rarely, antiviral-specific therapy is required.

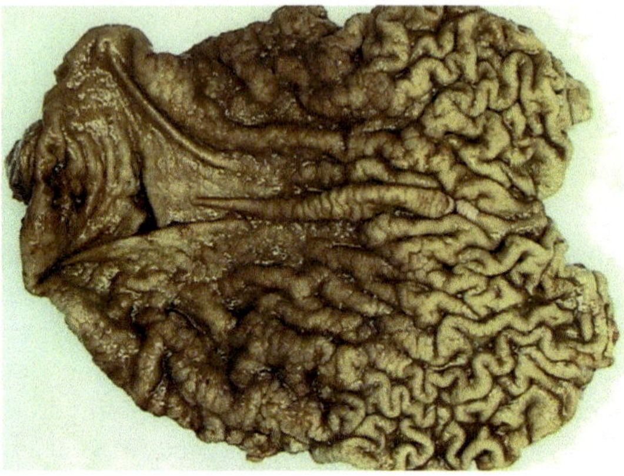

Ménétrier's Disease, Fig. 1 Formalin-fixed gastrectomy resection specimen opened along the greater curvature. Most striking are the giant polypoid mucosal folds in the gastric corpus and fundus resembling cerebral gyri. The antrum has a relatively normal appearance

Macroscopy

At upper endoscopy, large amounts of thick mucus and diffusely enlarged gastric folds are seen (Fig. 1). Most striking are these giant polypoid mucosal folds of 1–3 cm in thickness in the gastric corpus and fundus with typical antral sparing. The large gastric folds resemble spongy, cerebral gyri. In children, the antrum is often involved.

Microscopy

Ménétrier's disease is characterized by expansion of mucous epithelial cells that constitute normally the surface mucous cell compartment. Microscopic features include elongation and tortuosity or a corkscrew appearance of gastric foveolar epithelium lined by mucous cells giving marked thickening of the mucosa. There is often cystic dilatation of the superficial and deeper mucous glands that may resemble gastritis cystica polyposa. The oxyntic glands are usually reduced and replaced by mucous glands (Fig. 2). In normal gastric mucosa, the pit to gland ratio is about 1:4, but in Ménétrier's disease, this ratio can be reversed as the surface mucus cell compartment expands to occupy nearly the entire mucosal thickness. A hypertrophic muscularis mucosa can be seen with smooth muscle bundles extending into the lamina propria. Intestinal metaplasia or dysplasia is usually not encountered. Inflammation can be variable and even absent. There is often some minor, predominantly eosinophilic inflammation in the lamina propria with small clusters of eosinophils. Since the enlarged mucosal folds are subject to erosion, there can be some superficial ulceration with granulation tissue and some influx of neutrophils in the lamina propria. The combination of ulceration with atypical enlarged gastric folds can raise the suspicion of carcinoma to the endoscopist. It may be very difficult or even impossible for pathologists to diagnose Ménétrier's disease at small biopsies of

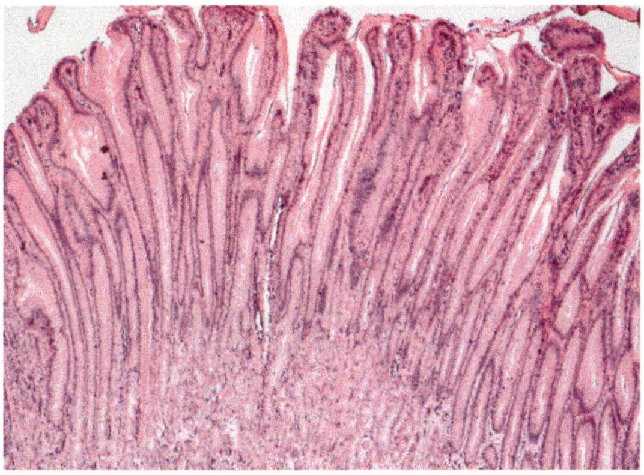

Ménétrier's Disease, Fig. 2 Gastric corpus shows diffuse hyperplasia of foveolar epithelium. There is loss of oxyntic mucosa

the gastric mucosa. Therefore, it is important that the pathologist receives full clinical data and considerations of endoscopy findings with deep or full-thickness gastric mucosal biopsies in order to consider this diagnosis.

Immunophenotype

The foveolar epithelial cells contain diastase-resistant PAS-positive neutral mucin, comparable with normal stomach, and only minor changes in the distribution of the mucin proteins using MUC1-MUC7 are reported. Routine haematoxylin- and eosin-stained slides are sufficient for pathological evaluation and to distinguish Ménétrier's disease from other diseases. Ki-67 may show an increase in the number of proliferating cells in the progenitor zone. In children, immunohistochemical staining for CMV can be performed.

Molecular Features

In children with negative immunohistochemical staining for CMV, PCR in a gastric biopsy sample for CMV can be performed.

Differential Diagnosis

The gross appearance of Ménétrier's disease can mimic Zollinger-Ellison syndrome, hyperplastic polyps, gastric lymphoma, diffusely infiltrative signet ring carcinoma, *H. pylori* lymphocytic gastritis, CMV gastritis, granulomatous gastritis, eosinophilic gastritis, and gastric polyposis such as Cronkhite-Canada syndrome. The histological differential diagnosis includes gastritis cystica polyposa/profunda, hyperplastic chronic active, lymphocytic, or allergic gastroenteritis. Especially on biopsies, the microscopic features are indistinguishable from a gastric hyperplastic polyp and endoscopic correlation is required.

References and Further Reading

Coffey, R. J., Washington, M. K., Corless, C. L., & Heinrich, M. C. (2007). Menetrier disease and gastrointestinal stromal tumors: hyperproliferative disorders of the stomach. *Journal of Clinical Investigation, 117*(1), 70–80.

Dempsey, P. J., Goldenring, J. R., Soroka, C. J., Modlin, I. M., McClure, R. W., Lind, C. D., et al. (1992). Possible role of transforming growth factor alpha in the pathogenesis of Menetrier's disease: supportive evidence form humans and transgenic mice. *Gastroenterology, 103*(6), 1950–1963.

Lambrecht, N. W. (2011). Menetrier's disease of the stomach: A clinical challenge. *Current Gastroenterology Reports, 13*(6), 513–517.

Megged, O., & Schlesinger, Y. (2008). Cytomegalovirus-associated protein-losing gastropathy in childhood. *European Journal of Pediatrics, 167*(11), 1217–1220.

Rich, A., Toro, T. Z., Tanksley, J., Fiske, W. H., Lind, C. D., Ayers, G. D., et al. (2010). Distinguishing Menetrier's disease from its mimics. *Gut, 59*(12), 1617–1624.

Microscopic Colitis

Arzu Ensari
Department of Pathology, Ankara University Medical School, Sihhiye, Ankara, Turkey

Synonyms

Collagenous colitis; Lymphocytic colitis

Definition

Microscopic colitis is an umbrella term for two major entities known as lymphocytic (LC) and collagenous colitis (CC). The term microscopic colitis (MC) describes a clinical pathological entity characterized by three elements: (a) a clinical history of chronic watery (non-bloody) diarrhea, (b) a normal or almost normal endoscopic appearance of the colon, and (c) a distinct histologic pattern. The latter can be either that of collagenous colitis (CC) or that of lymphocytic colitis. Therefore, the term microscopic colitis could be applied only from the endoscopic point of view in the presence of normal or almost normal endoscopic examination. Both LC and CC are clinically characterized by chronic watery diarrhea, while other conditions with normal endoscopy and abnormal histology may have other clinical characteristics. The pathogenesis is still not completely understood and probably multifactorial. It is suggested to represent a specific mucosal response, in susceptible individuals to various noxious luminal agents. These can be drugs, enteric infections, or others.

Clinical Features

- **Incidence**
  The incidence of MC varies between 1 and 3 per 100,000.
- **Age**
  It is common in middle aged or elderly.
- **Sex**
  Though there are reports of female predominance, both sexes are nearly equally affected.
- **Site**
  The entire colon may be involved in MC in a patchy manner. It is important that clinicians submit multiple biopsies from the right and left colon when assessing for the presence of microscopic colitis since left colon may be spared in some cases.
- **Treatment**
  Most patients respond to symptomatic or anti-inflammatory therapy.
- **Outcome**
  MC is a remitting and exacerbating disorder. In some patients spontaneous recovery can be seen, while others may require 5-ASA compounds or immunosuppressants. The overall prognosis is good.

Macroscopy

Endoscopy is normal or near normal with erythema and erosions.

Microscopy

Overlap between CC and LC occurs and has been reported in up to 30% of patients in some series. This overlap may show two patterns: one pattern is the finding of patients who have some biopsies demonstrating lymphocytic colitis and others showing collagenous colitis from the same endoscopic examination. The other pattern of overlap is seen in patients who have had one form of the disease, for example, lymphocytic colitis, for many years and then develop collagenous colitis in subsequent biopsies. Several variants of MC have been described (Table 1). The clinical presentation is usually similar but the histology is different.

Microscopic Colitis with Giant Cells

This is a recently described rare atypical form of microscopic colitis characterized by the presence of multinucleated giant cells in an otherwise classic microscopic colitis. Clinically, all of the reported cases are female patients who presented with persistent watery, bloodless diarrhea. Colonoscopy was macroscopically normal and the

Microscopic Colitis, Table 1 Histopathological variants of microscopic colitis

Variant
Collagenous colitis
Classic CC
Pseudomembranous CC
CC with giant cells
CC with IBD-like features
Lymphocytic colitis
Classic LC
Cryptal LC
Paucicellular LC
LC with giant cells
LC with IBD-like features
Granulomatous microscopic colitis
Microscopic colitis-NOS

biopsies revealed the histopathological features of classic lymphocytic or collagenous colitis with scattered subepithelial multinucleated giant cells. No granulomas were seen and there was no evidence of Crohn's disease. The reason for the giant cell formation is unknown. One plausible hypothesis is that this represents a foreign-body reaction to a luminal agent. The multinucleated giant cells probably arise from fusion of the mucosal macrophages, but it is not clear why this fusion occurs in only a small subset of patients with microscopic colitis.

Microscopic Colitis with Granulomatous Inflammation

This is an atypical form of microscopic colitis with a conspicuous granulomatous reaction. Four such cases have been reported and in all the main symptom was frequent watery diarrhea, all patients were female, and the only endoscopic finding was mild mucosal erythema. In all cases Crohn's disease was excluded on clinical grounds and by radiologic examinations. Histologically, an active chronic inflammatory infiltrate was accompanied by scattered crypt abscesses and non-necrotizing granulomas, often closely associated with crypt epithelium (i.e., cryptolytic or pericryptal granulomas). However, neither epithelial lymphocytosis nor subepithelial collagen deposition was present.

Microscopic Colitis with Inflammatory Bowel Disease-Like Histologic Features

One of the distinguishing features between microscopic colitis and inflammatory bowel disease (IBD) is the lack of architectural distortion in the former. However, it is now well established that several IBD-like histologic features, such as active crypt inflammation, surface erosion or ulceration, Paneth cell metaplasia, and crypt architectural irregularity, may occur in patients with either lymphocytic or collagenous colitis.

Immunophenotype

In LC immunohistochemical analysis shows that the increased IELs retain the normal CD3/CD8-positive T cell phenotype. The predominant cell type in the lamina propria is the CD4-positive T-helper cell. The collagen band consists predominantly of type VI collagen and tenascin, with lesser amounts of collagen type I and III in CC.

Molecular Features

No specific molecular feature has been reported.

Differential Diagnosis

The differential diagnosis comprises of inflammatory bowel disease (ulcerative colitis and Crohn's disease), infective colitis, and drug reactions. Crohn's disease and ulcerative colitis are usually easy to distinguish from microscopic colitis. Patients typically present with a different set of symptoms that include abdominal pain and/or bloody diarrhea. In addition, the majority of patients with Crohn's disease and ulcerative colitis present in the first two to three decades of life, whereas microscopic colitis typically presents after the age of 40. Endoscopic abnormalities are almost always found in Crohn's disease and ulcerative colitis, particularly at initial presentation before the institution of therapy. Finally, the pathology of these idiopathic inflammatory bowel diseases is fairly distinct from that of microscopic colitis. Crohn's disease and ulcerative colitis are characterized by varying degrees of mucosal architectural distortion, with crypt branching, subcryptal plasmacytosis, crypt abscesses, erosions, ulceration, and granulomas in Crohn's disease. Infective colitis can be difficult to distinguish from microscopic colitis on histologic grounds alone. Typically, biopsies from patients with bacterial infections reveal marked neutrophilic infiltrates and crypt abscesses. Resolving infections may have a more subtle pattern of inflammation that resembles lymphocytic colitis. However, infectious diarrhea is usually easily distinguished from microscopic colitis by the self-limited time course and other clinical data, such as stool cultures. Drug toxicity is a category that can be more difficult to distinguish from lymphocytic and collagenous colitis. There are many drugs that have diarrheal side effect. A relatively small subset of these medications are associated with histologic abnormalities in mucosal biopsies. Among these medications, NSAID substances are most commonly associated with gastrointestinal symptoms. Among their many toxic effects, several NSAIDs have been associated with histologic changes identical to lymphocytic and collagenous colitis. Other medications that have been reported to result in lymphocytic or collagenous colitis include carbamazepine and lansoprazole.

References and Further Reading

Fraser, A. G., Warren, B. F., Chandrapala, R., et al. (2002). Microscopic colitis: A clinical and pathological review. *Scandinavian Journal of Gastroenterology, 37*, 1241–1245.

Kingham, J. G. C., Levison, D. A., Ball, J. A., et al. (1982). Microscopic colitis: A cause of chronic watery diarrhoea. *British Medical Journal, 285*, 1601–1604.

Langner C, Aust D, Ensari A, Villanacci V, Becheanu G, Miehlke S, Geboes K, Münch A; Working Group of Digestive Diseases of the European Society of Pathology (ESP) and the European Microscopic Colitis Group (EMCG) (2015) Histology of microscopic colitis-review with a practical approach for pathologists. *Histopathology, 66*(5), 613–626.

Sandmeier, D., & Bouzourene, H. (2004). Microscopic colitis with giant cells: A rare new histopathologic subtype? *International Journal of Surgical Pathology, 12*, 45–48.

Saurine, T. J., Brewer, J. M., & Eckstein, R. P. (2004). Microscopic colitis with granulomatous inflammation. *Histopathology, 45*, 82–86.

Tysk, C., Bohr, J., Nyhlin, N., Wickbom, A., & Eriksson, S. (2008). Diagnosis and management of microscopic colitis. *World Journal of Gastroenterology, 14*(48), 7280–7288.

Microvillous Inclusion Disease

Arzu Ensari
Department of Pathology,
Ankara University Medical School, Sihhiye,
Ankara, Turkey

Synonyms

Congenital microvillous atrophy; Davidson disease; Familial microvillous atrophy; Intestinal microvillous atrophy; Intestinal microvillous dystrophy; Microvillous atrophy

Definition

Microvillous inclusion disease is an uncommon congenital enteropathy characterized by severe, intractable diarrhea within the first weeks of life. The affected infants have a clinical presentation including the presence of diarrhea for more than 2 weeks, severe nutritional malabsorption, and negative stool cultures. The disease was first described by Davidson in 1978 severe secretory diarrhea occurring during the first week of life with villous atrophy in the intestinal biopsy.

Clinical Features

- **Incidence**
  Rare condition. More than 50 cases of MID have been reported so far in the English literature.
- **Age**
  It is a disease of neonates and infants in the first 6 months of life. MID manifests either in the first days (early-onset form) or in the first 2 months (late-onset form) of life. The peak age of onset is the early neonatal period. Although later-onset cases have been described, cases have never been described beyond the first 2–3 months of life.
- **Sex**
  A female preponderance has been observed among the published cases, with a female-to-male ratio of 2:1.
- **Site**
  MID is a disease of the small intestine. There are, however, few reports of colonic involvement in MID.
- **Treatment**
  Currently no treatment is available, and patients with congenital microvillous atrophy are supported by total parenteral nutrition and intravenous fluids for the replacement of their massive intestinal losses. Intestinal

transplantation is the only treatment for the underlying abnormality. Advancements in immunosupressive therapy have allowed the small-bowel transplantation to become a realistic option, with a good survival of both patients and grafts.

- **Outcome**
  This is a life-threatening entity. The outcome is typically poor with most patients requiring intestinal transplantation. The majority of the affected patients eventually die of septic complications or hepatic insufficiency resulting from TPN-induced cholestasis. The survival of patients with typical cases depends on total parenteral nutrition (TPN). Most infants of early series died when aged 3–9 months. The leading causes of death were dehydration, malnutrition, and sepsis. Successful outcomes of small intestinal transplantation have been reported, and evidence suggests that an early transplant might be beneficial. However, the prognosis remains poor, with most patients dying by the second decade of life as a result of complications of parenteral alimentation. Even patients who have undergone small-bowel transplantation have a mean 5-years survival rate of about 50%. Patients with late-onset microvillous atrophy appear to have an improved prognosis.

Macroscopy

Microvillous inclusion disease is usually diagnosed in biopsy specimens rather than gross specimens. No specific gross abnormality has been reported.

Microscopy

Diagnosis rests on light and electron microscopic examination of small intestinal biopsy. Duodenal biopsies show moderate villous blunting, with no active inflammation in the lamina propria or intraepithelial lymphocytosis (Fig. 1). Due to increased crypt cell apoptosis, either crypt hypoplasia or hyperplasia can be observed.

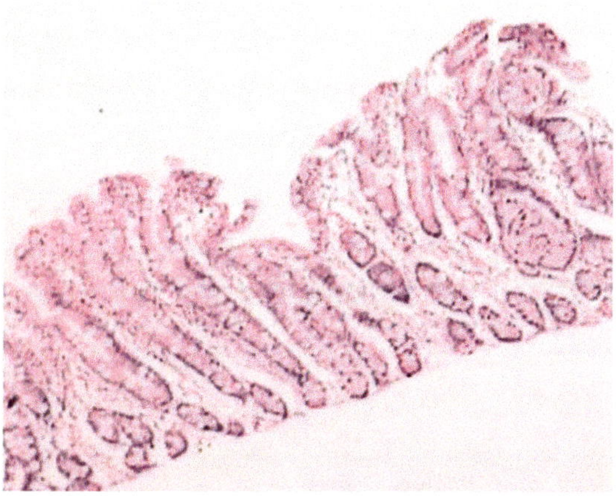

Microvillous Inclusion Disease, Fig. 1 Duodenal mucosa with villous shortening and crypt hyperplasia but no inflammatory infiltrate (H&E; ×100)

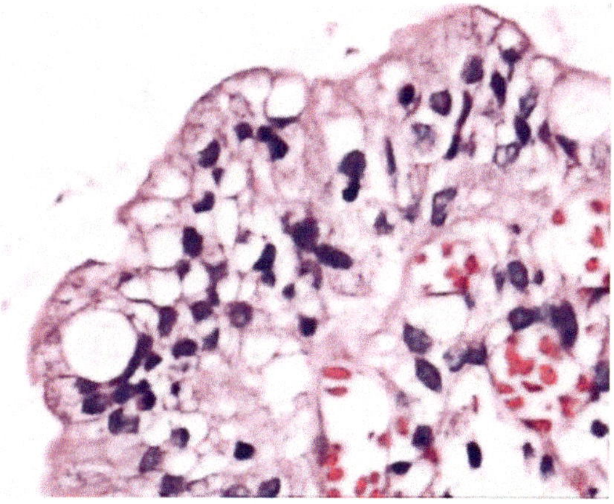

Microvillous Inclusion Disease, Fig. 2 Small apical vacuoles in the enterocyte cytoplasm with no brush border (H&E; ×200)

Changes in the enterocytes are typically found at the villous tips rather than villous bases and crypts where enterocytes appear normal. There is a vacuolated appearance in the apical cytoplasm of the enterocytes with extensive or patchy absence of the brush border (Fig. 2). Light microscopy shows accumulation of PAS-positive granules at the apical pole of immature enterocytes, together with attenuation or absence of brush border indicating microvillous atrophy and, in parallel, an intracellular PAS (Fig. 3) or CD10 positive

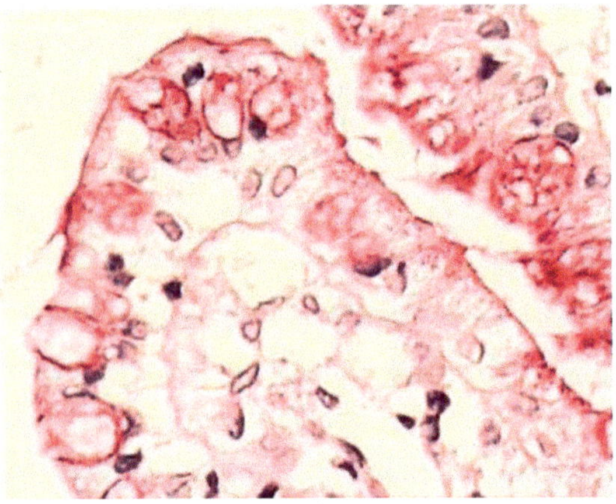

Microvillous Inclusion Disease, Fig. 3 Lack of brush border lining on PAS stain (PAS; ×200)

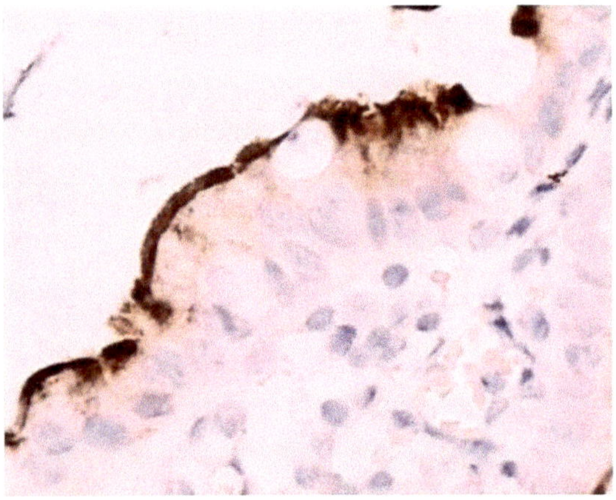

Microvillous Inclusion Disease, Fig. 4 Smudgy staining in the apical cytoplasm with CD10 (IHC; ×200)

(Fig. 4) line (marking the microvillous inclusion bodies seen on electron microscopy). On electron microscopy, the intestinal microvilli are either lacking or short and rudimentary while the apical cytoplasm of the enterocyte reveals microvillous inclusions. Ultrastructural finding of intracytoplasmic inclusions that are lined by intact microvilli is the diagnostic hallmark of the disease. These inclusions are present in the absorptive surface epithelial cells of the small intestine and are associated with poorly developed surface brush border microvilli (Fig. 5). Although

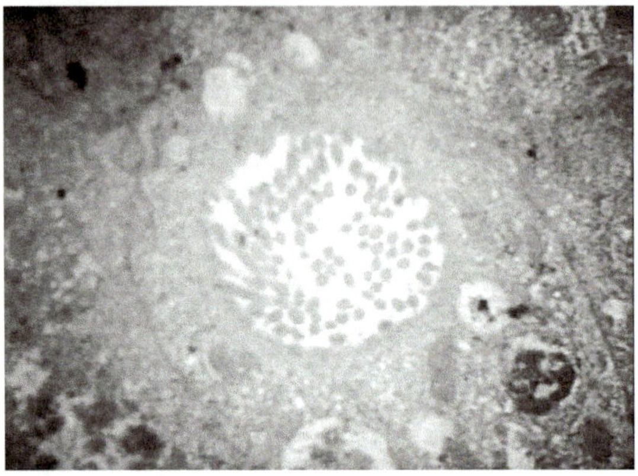

Microvillous Inclusion Disease, Fig. 5 EM picture of a microvillous inclusion in the apical cytoplasm of the enterocyte (EM; ×10000)

ultrastructural detection of pathognomonic microvillous inclusions in the enterocyte cytoplasm is essential for the diagnosis of MID, unusual electron microscopic (EM) features such as intermediate structures between microvillous inclusions and lysosomes, inclusions containing few microvilli, and dense apical granules in the apical cytoplasm can be observed in some cases. Since microvilli on immature crypt cells are most often normal, isolated EM analysis of these cells should not be performed as it could lead to a false negative diagnosis. In addition, the isolated finding of rudimentary or absent microvilli on enterocytes is also not sufficient to diagnose MID with certainty.

Immunophenotype

Immunohistochemically, antibodies to CD10, CEA, alkaline phosphatase, and villain can further help the diagnosis of MID by showing abnormalities in the brush border.

Molecular Features

It was recently discovered that MYO5B gene located on 18q21 encoding myosin Vb which regulates distribution of endosomes in the enterocyte was defective in this disorder.

Differential Diagnosis

The clinical differential diagnosis includes other causes of neonatal diarrhea. These include autoimmune enteropathies, immunodeficiencies, and lesions displaying primary enterocyte abnormalities such as tufting enteropathy.

References and Further Reading

Cutz, E., Sherman, P. M., & Davidson, G. P. (1997). Enteropathies associated with protracted diarrhea of infancy: Clinicopathological features, cellular and molecular mechanisms. *Pediatric Pathology & Laboratory Medicine, 17*(3), 335–368.

Groisman, G. M., Amar, M., & Livne, E. (2002). CD10, a valuable tool for the light microscopic diagnosis of microvillous inclusion disease (familial microvillous atrophy). *The American Journal of Surgical Pathology, 26*(7), 902–907.

Khubchandani, S. R., Vohra, P., Chitale, A. R., & Sidana, P. (2011). Microvillous inclusion disease-an ultrastructural diagnosis: With a review of the literature. *Ultrastructural Pathology, 35*, 87–91.

Shaila, R. K., Pankaj, V., Arun, R. C., & Poonam, S. (2011). Microvillous inclusion disease-an ultrastructural diagnosis: With a review of the literature. *Ultrastructural Pathology, 35*, 87–91.

Szperl, A. M., Golachowska, M. R., Bruinenberg, M., Prekeris, R., Thunnissen, A. M., Karrenbeld, A., Dijkstra, G., Hoekstra, D., Mercer, D., Ksiazyk, J., Wijmenga, C., Wapenaar, M. C., Rings, E. H., & van IJzendoorn, S. C. (2011). Functional characterization of mutations in the myosin Vb gene associated with microvillus inclusion disease. *Journal of Pediatric Gastroenterology and Nutrition, 52*, 307–313.

Mucinous Carcinoma, Upper Gastrointestinal Tract

Chella R. S. van der Post[1] and Fátima Carneiro[2]
[1]Department of Pathology, Radboud University Medical Center, Nijmegen, The Netherlands
[2]Faculty of Medicine of Porto University, Centro Hospitalar São João and Ipatimup/i3S, Porto, Portugal

Synonyms

Colloid carcinoma; Mucinous adenocarcinoma; Mucoid carcinoma

Definition

Mucinous carcinoma is one of the five main types of gastric adenocarcinoma in the World Health Organization (WHO) classification scheme. These adenocarcinomas are characterized by the production of abundant intracellular and extracellular mucus; by convention, more than 50% of the tumor consists of extracellular mucus.

Clinical Features

- **Incidence**
  Gastric carcinoma accounts for the fifth most common form of cancer worldwide. Mucinous gastric carcinoma compromises approximately 2–5% of all gastric carcinomas.
- **Age**
  Incidence increases progressively with age and is not different from other types of gastric carcinoma.
- **Sex**
  Men are more at risk of developing gastric cancer than women. In the study of Choi et al., 77% of patients with mucinous gastric carcinoma were men, while in non-mucinous gastric carcinoma, 67% were men.
- **Site**
  The entire stomach can be involved; most frequently, mucinous gastric carcinomas are located in the lower third of the stomach.
- **Treatment**
  Diagnostic accuracy and adequate preoperative staging of mucinous carcinomas is low, and mucinous gastric carcinoma is mostly detected in an advanced stage. PET imaging seems to have little or no value in the primary detection and preoperative staging of mucinous gastric carcinoma. Calcifications in gastric carcinoma are rare and can serve as a characteristic and diagnostic finding in mucinous gastric carcinoma.

  The recommendations of treatment of mucinous gastric carcinoma are the same compared to other forms of gastric cancer. In curative treatment, (sub-)total gastrectomy is recommended; the extent of surgery depends

M

on the size of tumor, in which an effort is made to obtain free resection margins. There is probably a higher risk of tumor spill during surgery of mucinous carcinomas compared to solid gastric carcinomas.

Chemotherapy, either alone as a perioperative treatment, or in combination with radiation therapy in an adjuvant setting, improves the clinical outcome for patients with resectable tumors. Neoadjuvant chemotherapy leads to downstaging but does not result in a significant improvement in overall survival. Adjuvant chemotherapy alone is currently not standard practice in the treatment of gastric cancer but leads to survival benefits in Asian populations and should be considered in patients at high risk of recurrence who have not received neoadjuvant therapy. Intraperitoneal chemotherapy remains investigational. Palliative chemotherapy can be considered taking into account performance status and patient preference.

- **Outcome**

  Most studies indicate that the overall survival rate for patients with mucinous gastric carcinoma is worse than that for patients with nonmucinous gastric carcinoma. A mucinous histology itself is not considered to be an independent worse prognostic factor, but at initial presentation, mucinous carcinomas are often already in advanced stage with larger tumor size, deeper invasion, more frequent lymphatic invasion, and lymph node metastasis, resulting in poorer prognosis. Possible explanations for the initial presentation of advanced disease may be that mucin interferes with the inflammatory response and the immunologic recognition of tumor cells; furthermore, the mucin may act as an infiltrating medium into surrounding stroma and assists in the penetration of deep invasion by tumor cells.

Macroscopy

The growth pattern of gastric carcinoma is commonly described according to the Borrmann classification, subdividing polypoid, fungating, ulcerative, and infiltrative growth patterns. Mucinous gastric carcinomas more often present as ulcerating lesions with infiltration into the gastric wall (Borrmann type 3) or as diffuse infiltrating tumors (Borrmann type 4). Grossly, mucinous adenocarcinomas have a distinct appearance with a gelatinous aspect and a viscous or glistening cut surface.

Microscopy

Mucinous carcinoma is one of the histologic types of gastric adenocarcinoma in the WHO classification scheme. In the Laurén classification, it depends on the predominance of tubular gland formation or signet ring cell amount whether to classify these tumors as diffuse or intestinal type. In the Ming classification, mucinous carcinoma is considered to be of the "infiltrative type" carcinoma, and in the Japanese classification of gastric carcinoma, it is classified as "undifferentiated type."

Mucinous carcinomas are characterized by a large amount (>50%) of extracellular mucus. Typically, cystic dilated and ruptured carcinomatous glands and/or scattered mucin-containing signet ring cells are floating in large extracellular mucus pools (Figs. 1–3). The glandular structures are either well-defined glands lined by columnar,

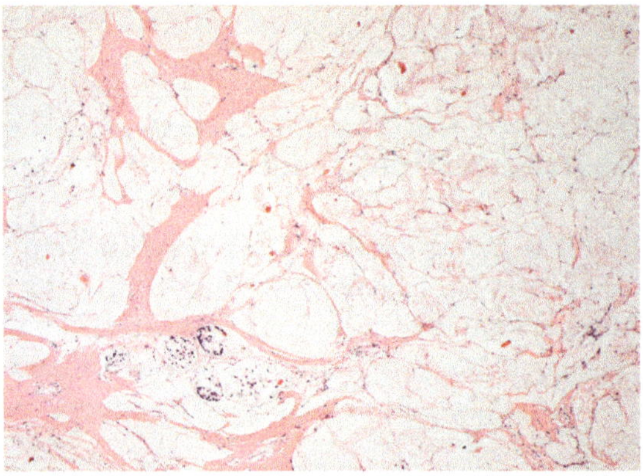

Mucinous Carcinoma, Upper Gastrointestinal Tract, Fig. 1 Low power view shows a large amount of extracellular mucin between bundle strands of muscularis propria. In the mucin lay scattered parts of glands and solitary signet ring cells (Original magnification 25×)

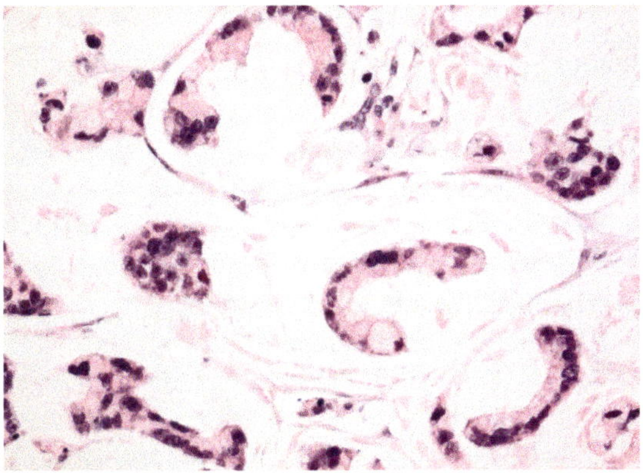

Mucinous Carcinoma, Upper Gastrointestinal Tract, Fig. 2 Higher magnification shows strands of tumor cells lined by attenuated epithelium and occasional goblet cells (Original magnification 200×)

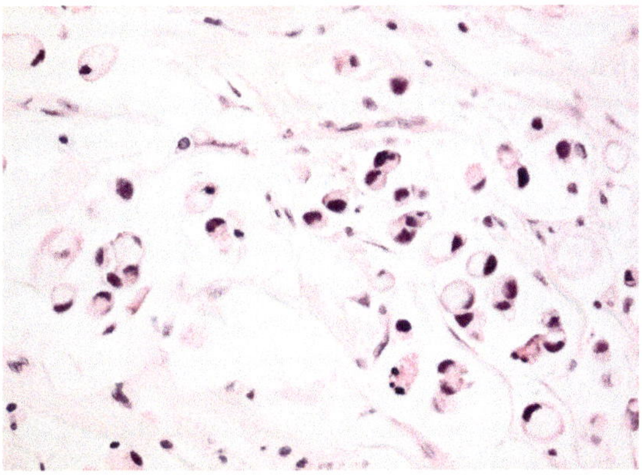

Mucinous Carcinoma, Upper Gastrointestinal Tract, Fig. 3 Intracellular mucin is abundant in solitary tumor cells (Original magnification 200×)

mucus-secreting epithelium or are more irregular structures composed of clusters or chains of mucus producing cells. These are readily identified floating in the abundant mucinous material. Solitary cells with a vacuolated and mucus filled cytoplasm with an eccentric placed flattened nucleus characterize signet ring cells. A predominance of signet ring cells in mucin pools, often designated as poorly differentiated mucinous gastric carcinoma, is associated with poorer disease-specific survival compared to mucinous carcinomas with predominant tubular differentiation.

Mucinous carcinomas are relatively common types of adenocarcinomas in various sites including the gastrointestinal tract, breast, and ovary, and sometimes originate in the lung and genitourinary organs. Despite their diverse anatomic origins, these carcinomas share similar histologic appearances, all characterized by the large amount of mucous. They are not difficult to diagnose when they remain restricted to their primary site of origin. However, specific diagnosis may become challenging or impossible when they metastasize to distant locations.

Immunophenotype

Immunohistochemistry can play an important role in determining the site of origin of metastatic mucinous carcinoma. Gastric mucinous carcinomas are usually positive for CK7, MUC-1, MUC-2, and MUC-6. They can be (focally) positive for CK20 (approximately 50%) and heterogeneously positive for CDX-2. Negative stains are ER, WT-1, and PAX-8, and these can be useful to distinguish gastric origin from breast or ovary.

The mucus stains, Alcian Blue or PAS staining, can be helpful to prove the presence of mucus and to determine the amount of mucus in cases where very minimal epithelial components are present.

Molecular Features

Distinct molecular features of mucinous gastric carcinomas are not reported. The frequency of MSI was reported to be equal to non-mucinous gastric carcinoma (around 9%). MSI was, as in non-mucinous carcinomas, associated with better survival. Probably, mucinous gastric carcinomas have lower incidences of EGFR (5–10%), HER-2 protein overexpression, and/or *HER-2* gene amplification (0.5–1.5%).

Differential Diagnosis

- Mucinous carcinomas are distinguished from mucin-producing adenocarcinomas that are adenocarcinomas with less than 50% mucus production

– Metastasis of a mucinous carcinoma of another primary site is difficult to discriminate from a primary carcinoma. Specific diagnosis may become challenging and immunohistochemical stains play an important role in determining the site of origin of metastatic mucinous carcinoma.

References and Further Reading

Bosman, F. T., Carneiro, F., Hruban, R. H., & Theise, N. D. (2010). *WHO classification of tumours of the digestive system* (4th ed.). Lyon: IARC.

Choi, J. S., Kim, M. A., Lee, H. E., Lee, H. S., & Kim, W. H. (2009). Mucinous gastric carcinomas: Clinicopathologic and molecular analyses. *Cancer, 115*(15), 3581–3590.

Chu, P. G., Chung, L., Weiss, L. M., & Lau, S. K. (2011). Determining the site of origin of mucinous adenocarcinoma: An immunohistochemical study of 175 cases. *The American Journal of Surgical Pathology, 35*(12), 1830–1836.

Sung, C. O., Lee, S. M., Choi, J. S., Kim, K. M., Choi, M. G., Noh, J. H., et al. (2012). Tumor size predicts survival in mucinous gastric carcinoma. *Journal of Surgical Oncology, 106*(6), 757–764.

Mucinous Cystadenocarcinoma, Appendix

Magali Svrcek
Hôpital Saint-Antoine, Service d'Anatomie Pathologique, AP-HP, Hôpitaux Universitaires de l'Est Parisien, Paris, France

Synonyms

High-grade mucinous adenocarcinoma; Well-differentiated mucinous adenocarcinoma

Definition

An appendiceal adenocarcinoma is a malignant epithelial neoplasm of the appendix with invasion beyond the muscularis mucosae.

In the current UICC/AJCC TNM staging (7th edition, 2010), appendiceal adenocarcinomas are separated into mucinous and non-mucinous types (UICC/AJCC TNM staging 2010). Indeed, the 5-year survival of appendiceal mucinous adenocarcinomas with distant metastasis is significantly better than those of non-mucinous carcinomas. This is reflected in the staging considerations for metastatic tumors.

Macroscopically, mucinous adenocarcinomas of the appendix can be cystic or not. The term "mucinous cystadenocarcinoma" may be used for well-differentiated mucinous adenocarcinomas with cystic structures. However, the distinction between a cystic carcinoma (i.e., cystadenocarcinoma) and one that is not cystic has not been shown to be of biologic significance. Therefore, this designation is descriptive and is not meant to designate a separate disease entity.

Other forms of appendiceal adenocarcinomas are signet-ring cell adenocarcinomas and low-grade appendiceal mucinous neoplasm (LAMN) (see Appendiceal Tumors entry).

Clinical Features

- **Incidence**
  Adenocarcinomas of the appendix are rare and heterogeneous. They occur in 0.1–0.2% of appendicectomies, corresponding to an estimated incidence of 0.2 per 100,000 per year, and are accounted for 60% of malignant appendiceal tumors in the United States Surveillance, Epidemiology and End-Results (SEER 1981). Appendiceal mucinous adenocarcinomas and cystadenocarcinomas make up about 50% of appendiceal adenocarcinomas, whereas they represent 10% of colorectal carcinomas.
- **Age**
  The median age at which mucinous and non-mucinous adenocarcinomas occur lies between the sixth or seventh decade of patients' life.

  Patients with familial adenomatous polyposis may develop appendiceal carcinomas at a young age. Appendiceal carcinomas have also been described in patients with underlying inflammatory bowel disease.

- **Sex**
  In the SEER registries (1973–1987), males were more commonly affected than women (Thomas and Sobin 1995). A recent population study in the Netherlands showed however female predominance.
- **Site**
  Clinical presentations include acute appendicitis (also refer to the ▶ Appendicitis, Etiology, Macroscopy, and Histology of entry), the presence of an abdominal or pelvic mass, a widespread peritoneal adenocarcinomatosis or pseudomyxoma peritonei (PP) with sometimes abdominal distension due to the production of large volumes of mucus. PP is defined by the presence of mucinous material on peritoneal surfaces (refer to the Mucocele entry). Mucinous tumors tend to be accompanied by PP, whereas non-mucinous carcinomas are accompanied by appendicitis. In the case of PP in women, the most common symptom is a right-sided ovarian mass. Ovarian masses can be bilateral. Because ovarian involvement is observed in the majority of female patients, an ovarian primary has long been initially suggested as the cause of PP. However, results of several clinical, histopathological, immunohistochemical, and molecular genetic studies show that most cases of PP reflect dissemination of an appendiceal mucinous neoplasms and that ovarian tumor deposits are almost always metastases, even if these lesions are much larger. Nevertheless, other origins have been described, such as colorectum, gallbladder, stomach, pancreas, fallopian tube, urachus, lung, and breast.
- **Treatment**
  Right hemicolectomy and regional lymphadenectomy are required if an adenocarcinoma is diagnosed on an appendicectomy. This surgical resection must be accompanied by a careful surgical exploration of the abdominal cavity in order to detect peritoneal lesions and to remove them.

  Management of a peritoneal dissemination of mucinous appendiceal neoplasms includes cytoreductive surgery (also known as the Sugarbaker procedure), heated intraoperative intraperitoneal chemotherapy, and early postoperative intraperitoneal chemotherapy in established peritoneal treatment centers. The cytoreductive surgery involves a series of visceral resections and peritonectomy procedures (Sugarbaker 2009).

  The extent of peritoneal dissemination by the peritoneal cancer index (PCI) is determined at the time of surgical exploration of the abdomen and pelvis. This index has a significant impact on survival for both high-grade and low-grade disease. Therapeutic decisions for pseudomyxoma peritonei largely depend on the distinction between low- and high-grade peritoneal diseases.
- **Outcome**
  The 5-year survival of appendiceal mucinous carcinomas with distant metastasis is around 40–50% (vs. 10% for other appendiceal carcinomas), which justifies the separation between mucinous and non-mucinous adenocarcinomas. Mucinous adenocarcinomas (also called high-grade mucinous adenocarcinomas in the last UICC/AJCC TNM and WHO classifications), similarly to low-grade appendiceal mucinous neoplasms (LAMN), can spread along the peritoneal surface and can metastasize in the peritoneal cavity, resulting in PP. However, these mucinous adenocarcinomas are more likely to invade the underlying organs and exhibit lymph node metastasis than to produce PP. Although LAMN may spread outside the appendix, LAMNs are associated with a better prognosis than mucinous adenocarcinomas.

  The prognosis is based on the local extent, the presence, and distribution of peritoneal lesions. Only patients with peritoneal dissemination have a very poor prognosis. The presence of an associated perforation is not a pejorative factor, except if the perforation is located within the tumor.

  Starting from the seventh edition of the UICC/AJCC TNM classification, appendiceal carcinomas are staged separately. In the sixth edition, they were in fact included with colorectal carcinoma.

In the last UICC/AJCC TNM classification, T4 and M1 are modified because of the particular nature of mucinous adenocarcinomas. The T4 category is divided into T4a and T4b as for the colon with the exception that T4a denotes both serosal involvement and extra-appendiceal disease limited to the right lower quadrant. Appendiceal mucinous tumors associated with peri-appendiceal lesions or limited to the right lower quadrant are not considered as metastatic (respectively T3 and T4a). Conversely, peritoneal spread beyond the right lower quadrant, including PP, is considered as metastatic and is classified M1a. M1b corresponds to nonperitoneal metastasis.

Histological grading of mucinous tumors as low-grade (corresponding to a diagnosis of LAMN or low-grade PP) or as high-grade (corresponding to a diagnosis of mucinous adenocarcinoma or high- grade PP) is needed for the stage grouping.

The UICC/AJCC TNM classification (7th edition) and anatomic stage/prognostic groups of appendiceal tumors are shown in Tables 1 and 2.

Mucinous Cystadenocarcinoma, Appendix, Table 1 TNM classification of appendiceal carcinomas (7th edition, 2010)

Primary tumor (T)	
Tx	Primary tumor cannot be assessed
T0	No evidence of primary tumor
Tis	Carcinoma in situ: intraepithelial or invasion of lamina propria
T1	Tumor invades submucosa
T2	Tumor invades muscularis propria
T3	Tumor invades through muscularis propria into subserosa or into mesoappendix
T4	Tumor penetrates visceral peritoneum, including mucinous peritoneal tumor within the right lower quadrant and/or directly invades other organs or structures
T4a	Tumor penetrates visceral peritoneum, including mucinous peritoneal tumor within the right lower quadrant
T4b	Tumor directly invades other organs or structures
Regional lymph nodes (N)	
Nx	Regional lymph nodes cannot be assessed
N0	No regional lymph node metastasis
N1	Metastasis in 1–3 regional lymph nodes
N2	Metastasis in four or more regional lymph nodes
Distant metastasis	
M0	No distant metastasis
M1	Distant metastasis
M1a	Intraperitoneal metastasis beyond the right lower quadrant, including pseudomyxoma peritonei
M1b	Nonperitoneal metastasis

Histological examination of a regional lymphadenectomy specimen will ordinarily include 12 or more lymph nodes. If the lymph nodes are negative, but the number ordinarily examined is not met, classify as pN0

Macroscopy

The appendix may be enlarged, deformed, or completely destroyed by a polypoid, ulcerating, or infiltrative mass usually present at the base contrasting with carcinoid tumors that classically develop on the tip of the appendix (see also Tumors, Appendix entry) (Figs. 1 and 2). Tumors may also cause appendiceal intussusception. A mucinous cystadenocarcinoma can display exuberant mucus secretion giving rise to the gross appearance of a mucocele (see also Mucocele entry).

Perforation or diverticula may be present. Perforations of appendiceal adenocarcinomas develop in 50–62% of tumors, and are responsible for the dissemination into the peritoneum.

Cecum can be involved with advanced tumor stages, making it difficult to determine the exact site of origin. If the major part of the tumor lies in the appendix or if microscopic examination reveals a precursor lesion in the appendix, one can consider that the tumor is of appendiceal origin.

During macroscopic examination, margin of the appendix must be individualized. In right hemicolectomy specimens, the ileal and colonic margins are the proximal and distal margins, respectively. In right hemicolectomy specimens, pathologic assessment of the regional lymph node should be performed. Appendices containing mucinous neoplasms should be entirely submitted for histologic examination. In the situation of appendiceal mucinous neoplasms with localized periappendiceal mucin, complete microscopic examination of the entire periappendiceal mucin is also warranted.

Mucinous Cystadenocarcinoma, Appendix, Table 2 Stage grouping (*UICC/AJCC TNM staging system*, 7th edition)

Stage	T	N	M	Histologic grade
Stage 0	Tis	N0	M0	
Stage I	T1	N0	M0	
	T2	N0	M0	
Stage IIA	T3	N0	M0	
Stage IIB	T4a	N0	M0	
Stage IIC	T4b	N0	M0	
Stage IIIA	T1	N1	M0	
	T2	N1	M0	
Stage IIIB	T3	N1	M0	
	T4	N1	M0	
Stage IIIC	Any T	N2	M0	
Stage IVA	Any T	N0	M1a	G1
Stage IVB	Any T	N0	M1a	G2, 3
	Any T	N1	M1a	Any G
	Any T	N2	M1a	Any G
Stage IVC	Any T	Any N	M1b	Any G

Histologic grade (G):
Gx: grade cannot be assessed
G1: well differentiated (mucinous low-grade)
G2: moderately differentiated (mucinous high-grade)
G3: poorly differentiated (mucinous high-grade)
G4: undifferentiated

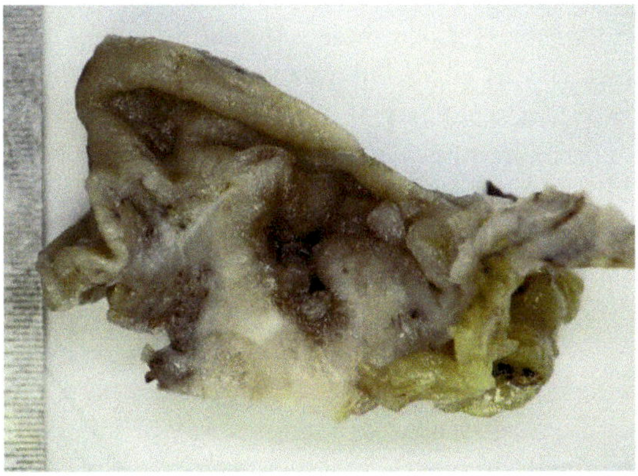

Mucinous Cystadenocarcinoma, Appendix, Fig. 1 Right colectomy after appendicectomy. At the base of the appendix, one notices a residual tumor, with a gelatinous appearance

Microscopy

Mucinous adenocarcinomas are morphologically similar to their colonic counterpart. Mucinous

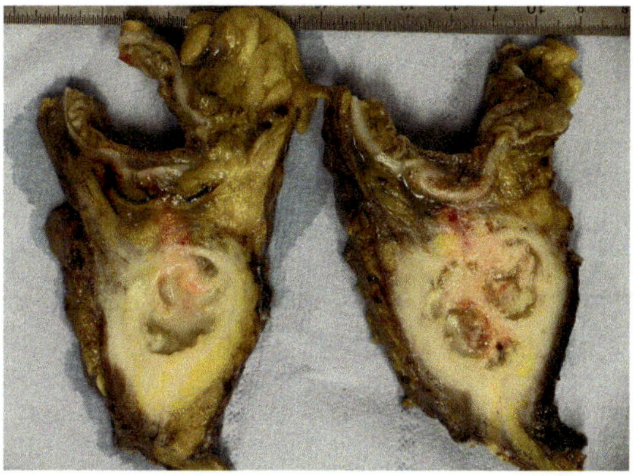

Mucinous Cystadenocarcinoma, Appendix, Fig. 2 Right colectomy with appendicectomy. The appendix is totally destroyed by a necrotic cystadenocarcinoma

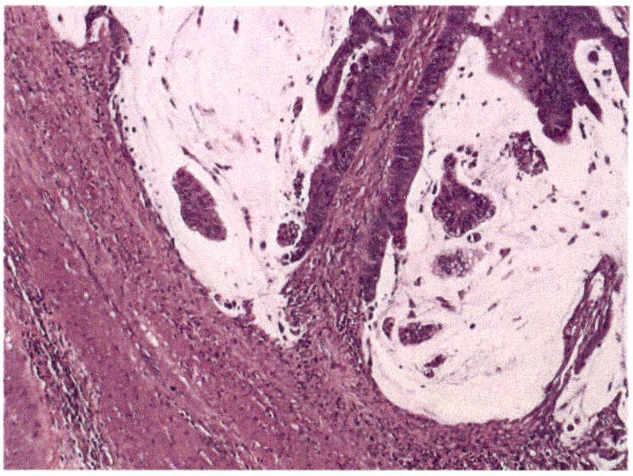

Mucinous Cystadenocarcinoma, Appendix, Fig. 3 Well-differentiated adenocarcinoma of the appendix with large mucin lakes. Large mucus collections extend through the appendix wall

adenocarcinomas are defined as tumors having pools of mucus with either disrupted tubules and/or interstitial mucus in more than 50% of the neoplasm. If signet-ring cells account for more than 50% of the neoplasm, the term "signet-ring cell carcinoma" is more appropriate.

The demonstration of invasion by tumoral cells through the muscularis mucosae into the submucosa is essential to establish malignancy (Fig. 3). Only small infiltrating glands and even single cells may be present. In practice, it can be difficult to determine the extent of invasion. Moreover, the epithelium may be extensively ulcerated.

M

Conversely, in some adenomas, acellular mucin dissecting the appendiceal layers can mimic invasion (see "Differential diagnosis). There is often clear evidence of an origin from a mucinous cystadenoma. In more advanced lesion, the precursor lesion is typically absent and replaced by tumor.

As previously discussed in the entry "▶ Mucinous Cystadenoma, Appendix," the nomenclature of appendiceal mucinous neoplasms is controversial and the terminology used is inconsistent, particularly when they lack overtly malignant features, being associated with extra-appendiceal spread, and not usually displaying high-grade cytological atypia or apparent invasive feature. In the current WHO classification, appendiceal mucinous neoplasms are subdivided into "low-grade appendiceal mucinous neoplasms (LAMN)" and mucinous adenocarcinoma because of differences in behavior and management (Carr and Sobin 2010). This classification is based on architectural and cytologic features. LAMN lack histological evidence of invasion and exhibit a villous or flat proliferation of mucinous epithelium with low-grade atypia, but there is no lamina propria or desmoplasia. Cytologically, neoplastic cells may be columnar, cuboidal, or flattened. Nuclei are small and regular. Low-grade dysplasia may be observed, and mitoses are rare. LAMN generally grow slowly and typically produce the clinical picture of low-grade PP. Lymph node metastasis tends to occur late. This term reconciles the lack of tissue invasion or the frank carcinomatous features of these tumors with their significant morbidity and mortality. Although LAMN may spread outside of the appendix, they have a better prognosis than mucinous adenocarcinomas. In mucinous adenocarcinomas, an invasive pattern with desmoplastic stroma is observed. A residual luminal mucinous tumor resembling LAMN may be present. Cytologically, atypia are marked and mitoses, sometimes atypical, are common.

Immunophenotype

Appendiceal adenocarcinomas express keratin 20, CDX2, and MUC2. Many express keratin 7.

Molecular Features

There are few available data on molecular genetics alterations in appendiceal mucinous because of the limited studied cases. The main molecular alterations are *KRAS* mutations, most are in codon 12 and some in codon 13, and loss of heterozygosity (LOH) at the 18q locus. Mutations of SMAD4/DPC4 have been sometimes described. It is unusual to detect mutations of the beta catenin gene or mutations of TP53. Except in rare cases, tumors mostly have a microsatellite stable phenotype.

Differential Diagnosis

The main differential diagnosis is the pseudo-invasive appendiceal mucinous adenoma. In some cases, displacement of mucin secreting adenomatous lesion into the wall of the appendix as a consequence of raised intraluminal pressure from mucus hypersecretion may be florid, thereby mimicking a well-differentiated mucinous adenocarcinoma. This so-called pseudo-invasion may be especially prominent with inflammation and abscess formation. The displaced adenomatous cells usually retain their surrounding lamina propria. In case of acellular mucin in the appendiceal wall, the diagnosis of adenoma should be made only if the muscularis mucosa is intact. Classically, invasive adenocarcinoma is surrounded by a dense and desmoplastic reaction. However, it should be kept in mind that some well-differentiated adenocarcinomas may invade in a broad, pushing growth pattern, without a desmoplastic response. Moreover, some well-differentiated adenocarcinomas may present only minimal atypical cytologic features. So, low-grade cytology does not exclude a diagnosis of malignancy.

If no conclusive evidence of tissue invasion is found, it seems appropriate to use the term "mucinous tumor of uncertain malignant potential." Those lesions designated as ""mucinous tumor of uncertain malignant potential" are included in the LAMN category of the current version of the WHO. In order not to misdiagnose an invasive lesion of the appendix, sampling of the entire mucinous neoplasm is recommended to rule out invasion.

References and Further Reading

Carr, N. J., & Sobin, L. H. (2010). Tumours of the appendix. In F. T. Bosman, F. Carneiro, R. H. Hruban, & N. D. Theise (Eds.), *WHO classification of tumours of the digestive system* (pp. 122–125). Lyon: IARC Press.

Edge, S. B., Byrd, D. R., Compton, C. C., Fritz, A. G., Greene, F. L., & Trotti, A. (2010). Appendix. In AJCC Cancer Staging Handbook, from *the AJCC cancer staging manuel*, (7th ed., pp. 161–171). New York: Springer.

National Cancer Institute Monograph 57. (1981). *Surveillance, epidemiology, and end results: Incidence and mortality data, 1973–77* (NIH Publication No. 81–2330). Bethesda: US. Department of Health and Human Services.

Sugarbaker, P. H. (2009). Comprehensive management of peritoneal surface malignancy using cytoreductive surgery and perioperative intraperitoneal chemotherapy: The Washington Cancer Institute approach. *Expert Opin Pharmacother, 10*, 1965–1977.

Thomas, R. M., & Sobin, L. H. (1995). Gastrointestinal cancer. *Cancer, 75*, 154–170.

Mucinous Cystadenoma, Appendix

Magali Svrcek
Hôpital Saint-Antoine, Service d'Anatomie Pathologique, AP-HP, Hôpitaux Universitaires de l'Est Parisien, Paris, France

Synonyms

Adenoma of the appendix; Low-grade appendiceal mucinous neoplasm (LAMN); Low-grade appendiceal mucinous tumor

Definition

Appendiceal adenomas are defined as lesions that are confined to the appendix with no evidence of invasion beyond the muscularis mucosae.

Appendiceal adenomas are of two main types. The most common type involves the appendiceal mucosa in a widespread, circumferential fashion. In these, excessive secretion of mucus by neoplastic epithelial cells within the confined appendiceal lumen frequently gives rise to cystic dilatation, creating a mucinous cystadenoma. Less commonly, adenomas of the appendix grow as localized, pedunculated, or sessile lesions.

Some authors recommend not using the term "cystadenoma" anymore, since cystic change does not indicate a separate disease category.

The lesion may contain either low-grade or high-grade dysplasia.

Clinical Features

- **Incidence**
  Appendiceal tumors represent less than 0.4% of all intestinal neoplasms. The most common mucinous neoplasms of the appendix are the mucinous cystadenomas. They account for nearly one-third of all epithelial tumors, but are however detected in only 0.3% of surgically removed appendices.
  Mucinous cystadenomas are usually sporadic, but may sometimes complicate long-standing ulcerative colitis.
- **Age**
  The average age at diagnosis is 53 years, with a median age of 64 years.
- **Sex**
  Mucinous cystadenomas arise in both men and women, with many series reporting female predominance.
- **Site**
  Clinical presentations include acute appendicitis particularly for appendiceal tumors that are located in the base of the appendix. This is due to the obstruction of the appendiceal lumen caused by mucin accumulation. Clinical presentations also include the presence of an abdominal or pelvic mass (usually an ovarian tumor), perforations, or intussusceptions. Cystadenomas can also be discovered during surgery for unrelated conditions.

Because of early luminal obstruction, tumors located at the base and polypoid tumors are expected to have a better prognosis than those located in the distal appendix.

- **Treatment**

  Surgical management of the primary appendiceal neoplasm mainly includes appendectomy. Appendectomy is the treatment of choice for mucinous neoplasm entirely submitted for histologic examination and clearly confined to the appendix without evidence of disease outside of the appendix and with a negative margin of resection. A complete removal of the appendix and surrounding periappendiceal tissue, if grossly involved, is indicated.

  A positive margin on the base of the appendix should not be used as an indication for a right colectomy. Cecectomy can be performed to obtain a negative margin of excision and can save the right colon and ileocecal valve function.

  If a rupture of the appendix is suspected or if the tumor is associated with diverticula, the surgeon must carefully inspect the abdominal cavity in order to eliminate a peritoneal dissemination of the tumor. Prolonged clinical follow-up for these patients for recurrent disease is proposed. If epithelial cells are found within mucin deposits, patients must be referred to an established center for treatment of peritoneal tumors.

- **Outcome**

  Appendiceal adenomas are preinvasive neoplasms with the potential to progress into invasive adenocarcinomas or cystadenocarcinomas.

  Noninvasive appendiceal mucinous neoplasms confined to the mucosa without evidence of disease outside of the appendix and with a negative margin of resection are benign with essentially no risk of recurrence.

  Not infrequently, mucinous tumors of the appendix can be associated with escape of mucus through the appendiceal wall. Mucin is deposited on the appendiceal serosa, within the mesoappendix, or limited to the right lower quadrant, even in the absence of high-grade dysplasia or invasive features. These extra-appendiceal mucin deposits limited to the periappendiceal area are usually acellular, although they may occasionally contain neoplastic cells ("cellular mucin"). Relatively few studies have evaluated the significance of the presence of mucin with or without neoplastic epithelium confined to the immediate vicinity of the appendix. It seems that the most critical prognostic factor in mucinous tumors of the appendix is the presence or absence of mucinous epithelial cells in extra-appendiceal mucin. Patients with appendiceal mucinous neoplasms and acellular periappendiceal mucin are unlikely to develop recurrent disease. However, although quite small, this risk to the patient is not insignificant. In two large series, the risk for developing peritoneal recurrence in cases of localized acellular periappendiceal mucin was 4% (2 of 50 patients) and 8% (one of 12 patients). Importantly, all 3 patients had appendiceal resection specimens that were not entirely submitted for microscopic analysis. By comparison, in the report by Yantiss et al., 33% of patients with neoplastic cells within periappendiceal mucin developed diffuse peritoneal involvement after appendicectomy and 7% died of the disease. Because the risk is not insignificant in patients with low-grade mucinous neoplasms with extra-appendiceal mucin limited to the right lower quadrant, some authors propose these tumors being designated as "low-grade mucinous neoplasms with low grade of recurrence (LG-LR).

  The degree of cellularity of the intraperitoneal mucin deposits also affects prognosis. Cases with acellular peritoneal deposits outside of the right lower quadrant, although limited, seem to be associated with a relatively low risk of recurrence compared with cellular peritoneal mucinous deposits. The number of studied cases with prolonged follow-up is, however, small.

  Generally, peritoneal involvement, carrying the descriptive term "pseudomyxoma peritonei" (PP) complicating low-grade appendiceal mucinous neoplasms, is typically low-grade (see "▶ Mucocele, Appendix" entry). However, in some cases, low-grade appendiceal

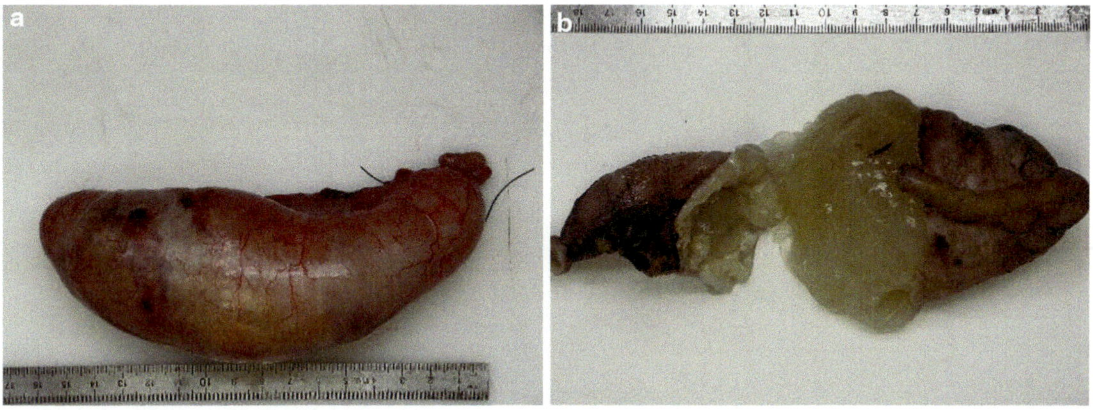

Mucinous Cystadenoma, Appendix, Fig. 1 (**a**) Gross appearance of an unopened appendix. The lumen (particularly the distal portion) is considerably distended, cystic, and the wall is thin. (**b**) The opened specimen showing the presence of an abundant material in the appendiceal lumen

mucinous neoplasms are associated with high-grade PP.

Low-grade PPs are associated with significantly longer survival than high-grade PPs (overall 5-year survival of 63% for low-grade and 23% for high-grade).

Macroscopy

Grossly, mucinous neoplasms are very heterogeneous. They can be cystic, so-called mucinous cystadenoma, or not. In some cases, production of large amounts of mucus may convert the whole appendix into a large, sausage-shaped, cystic or spherical, mucus-filled mass (Fig. 1a, b). Mucus is sometimes calcified, resulting in the formation of calculi. Diverticula can be found and some areas may rupture, leading to mucin discharge on the appendiceal serosa. The appendix can also be grossly unremarkable.

During macroscopic examination, margins of the appendix must be individualized. In right hemicolectomy specimens, the ileal and colonic margins are the proximal and distal margins, respectively. In these cases, pathologic assessment of the regional lymph node should be performed.

Appendices containing mucinous neoplasms should be entirely submitted for histologic examination. In the situation of appendiceal mucinous neoplasms with localized periappendiceal mucin, complete microscopic examination of the entire periappendiceal mucin is required.

Microscopy

Adenomas of the appendix may exhibit tubular, tubulovillous, or villous architectures, with a variable degree of dysplasia.

Microscopic examination shows circumferential replacement of the normal appendiceal epithelium by proliferative mucinous epithelium, with frequent atrophy of the underlying lymphoid tissue (Fig. 2). Most mucinous cystadenomas have a single layer of neoplastic mucinous cells with occasional small epithelial tufts overlying a fibrotic and atrophic lamina propria and submucosa. The neoplastic epithelial cells contain large mucin vacuoles that compress the nuclei. In flat areas, the mucin vacuoles are typically smaller and are confined to the apical portions of the cells.

Most appendiceal adenomas are low-grade (Fig. 3) and some are high-grade (Fig. 4). However, in the latter, one must make sure that the muscularis mucosae is clearly intact. The criteria to determine low-grade dysplasia and high-grade dysplasia are the same as for the large intestine and are based on the cytological and architectural aspect of the neoplastic cells. The nuclei of the

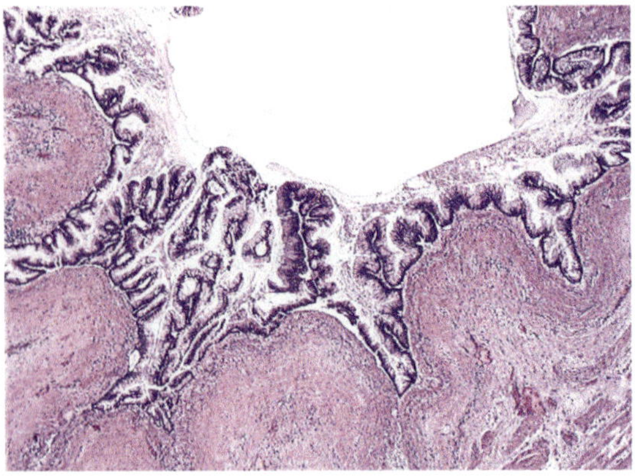

Mucinous Cystadenoma, Appendix, Fig. 2 Low-power histologic features of a mucinous cystadenoma. The lesion is confined to the mucosa

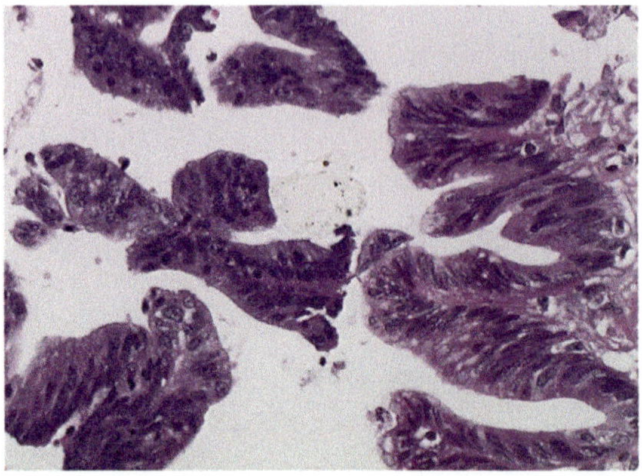

Mucinous Cystadenoma, Appendix, Fig. 4 High-grade dysplasia containing micropapillary tufts of neoplastic cells that show loss of cell polarity, ovoid nuclei with open chromatin and conspicuous nucleoli, and reduction of mucin production (×400 magnification)

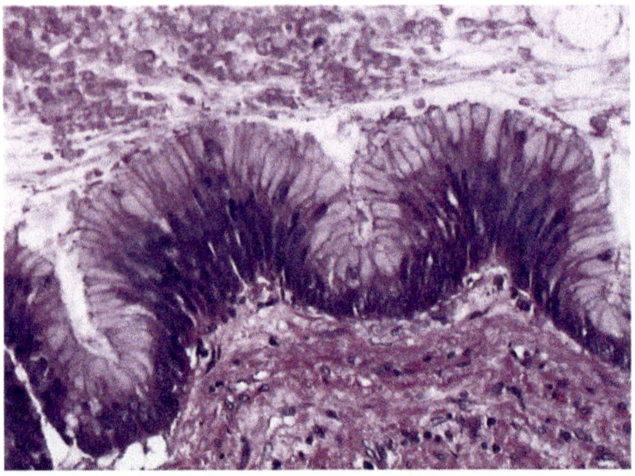

Mucinous Cystadenoma, Appendix, Fig. 3 Low-grade appendiceal mucinous neoplasm. Mucinous epithelium lining a flat region of the tumor shows small apical cytoplasmic mucin droplets, and low-grade cytologic atypia with nuclear enlargement and pseudostratification (×400 magnification)

neoplastic cells are typically elongated, hyperchromatic, lacking prominent nucleoli. Mitotic activity is usually low and limited to the base of the glands. In flat areas, nuclear enlargement is typically more prominent and nuclear stratification more obvious.

Mucosal denudation can be observed. The mucosal ulcers may produce a granulomatous reaction with mural fibrosis. A coexisting appendicitis can be found as well. The wall of the appendix may be perforated, and mucin with or without cells may be present in the perforation and extend to the serosal surface.

The nomenclature of appendiceal mucinous neoplasms is controversial and the terminology used is quite inconsistent, because of the frequent discrepancies between the histological findings and clinical behaviors. Previously, appendiceal mucinous neoplasms were classified as either adenomas or adenocarcinomas based on histological evidence of invasive growth. Although mucinous neoplasms of the appendix confined to the mucosa and tumors with extra-appendiceal spread are histologically identical and may not show high-grade cytological atypia or apparent invasive features, the latter tumors are associated with risk for recurrence and death. For this reason, the term “ruptured adenomas” should be avoided, because it does not adequately reflect the malignant potential of these tumors. Conversely, most of the authors consider that mucinous “cystadenomas” with extra-appendiceal extension should not be called appendiceal adenocarcinomas. The “borderline” terminology is best not applied to the appendix. The term “low-grade appendiceal mucinous neoplasms” (LAMNs), initially suggested by Misdraji in 2003, seems more appropriate and is proposed to replace this non-consensual and confused terminology (Misdraji et al. 2003). This term reconciles the lack of tissue invasion or frank carcinomatous features of these tumors with their significant morbidity and mortality. Moreover, while LAMN may spread outside the appendix, they are associated with a better prognosis than mucinous adenocarcinomas, indicating the prognostic relevance of this classification. Currently, this classification has been adopted by the World Health Organization. In LAMN, the architecture often resembles adenoma, with a villous, serrated, or undulating architecture, but there is no lamina propria and no desmoplasia. Cytologically, neoplastic cells may be columnar, cuboidal, or flattened. Nuclei are small and regular and low-grade dysplasia may be observed. Mitoses are usually rare. Pai and Longacre propose to strictly reserve the term of mucinous adenoma (or mucinous cystadenoma) for cytologically low-grade mucinous neoplasms that are clearly confined to the appendix (i.e., without invasion) without extra-appendiceal mucin or neoplastic epithelium and complete excision with negative surgical margin. In cases in which the mucinous neoplasm seems confined to the appendix but the neoplastic epithelium involves the proximal resection margin and the mucinous neoplasm in which the diagnosis of extra-appendiceal epithelium is dubious, they propose diagnosing these cases as "mucinous tumors of uncertain malignant potential."

Because the risk is not insignificant for patients with low-grade mucinous neoplasms with extra-appendiceal mucin limited to the right lower quadrant, these authors propose to separate low-grade mucinous neoplasms into distinct pathologic entities based on both the presence or not of neoplastic epithelium in the extra-appendiceal mucin deposits and on the risk of recurrence: (i) They propose to call "low-grade mucinous neoplasm with low risk of recurrence" (or LG-LR) low-grade mucinous neoplasms without extra-appendiceal neoplastic epithelium and without invasion, with extra-appendiceal acellular mucin. (ii) They propose the term "low-grade mucinous neoplasm with high risk of recurrence" (LG-HR) for low-grade mucinous neoplasms with the presence of any extra-appendiceal neoplastic epithelium, without extra-appendiceal invasion.

In summary, regardless of the terminology used, the pathology report should indicate the degree of dysplasia, the extend of invasion, the presence of invasive areas, whether neoplastic cells or mucin are seen outside the appendix, the degree of cytologic atypia of the epithelium in the extra-appendiceal mucin or peritoneal implants, and the status of the proximal margin.

Immunophenotype

The mucin-producing cells are stained with diastase-resistant periodic acid-Schiff (PAS) and Alcian blue.

The neoplastic epithelial cells are immunoreactive with keratin 20 and the intestinal mucin marker MUC2.

The proliferative rate can be high.

Molecular Features

Noninvasive lesions with marked cytologic atypia tend to have a higher proliferative rate than low-grade tumors.

Fenoglio-Preiser et al. found that the proliferative rate of the appendiceal tumor as well as its extra-appendiceal extensions is an important prognostic factor and, therefore, propose the use of Ki67 immunostain in the most mitotically active part of the tumor.

Few data about molecular characteristics of low-grade appendiceal mucinous, neoplasms are available. *KRAS* mutations (mostly in codon 12 and some in codon 13) seem to be common and are found in the majority of appendiceal adenomas. Activating *GNAS* mutations are also frequent and constitute a characteristic genetic abnormality of low-grade appendiceal mucinous neoplasm (Nishikawa et al. 2013). *GNAS* mutations often coexist with *KRAS* mutations. Mutant *GNAS* might play a direct role in the prominent mucin production. Microsatellite instability and p53 overexpression are reported to be rare. Appendiceal adenomas frequently display loss of heterozygosity (LOH), in particular LOH at the 5q locus linked to the *APC* tumor suppressor gene.

Differential Diagnosis

Adenomas are defined as lesions that are confined to the appendix with no evidence of invasion. When an adenoma of the appendix is found, the whole lesion must be taken and carefully examined, in order to prevent misdiagnosing an invasive lesion of the appendix. Neoplastic cells can also extend into diverticula, but this does not constitute an invasive carcinoma.

In some cases, displacement of mucin-secreting adenomatous lesion into the wall of the appendix as a consequence of raised intraluminal pressure from mucus hypersecretion may be florid, thereby mimicking a well-differentiated mucinous adenocarcinoma. This so-called pseudo-invasion may be especially prominent if there is inflammation and formation of abscess (refer to Mucinous Cystadenocarcinoma, Appendix entry). In the case of no conclusive evidence of tissue invasion, it seems appropriate to use the term "mucinous tumor of uncertain malignant potential." Those lesions are included in the LAMN category of the last version of the classification provided by the WHO. A diagnosis of low-grade mucinous neoplasm requires rigorous pathologic evaluation of the appendix.

In some cases, mucosal denudation can lead to misdiagnosis of mucinous cystadenoma. Multiple sections should be taken to confirm the diagnosis of mucinous cystadenoma. Staining with PAS or Alcian blue is interesting in that setting.

References and Further Reading

Carr, N. J., McCarthy, W. F., & Sobin, L. H. (1995). Epithelial noncarcinoid tumors and tumor-like lesions of the appendix: A clinicopathologic study of 184 patients with a multivariate analysis of prognostic factors. *Cancer, 75*, 757–768.

Misdraji, J., Yantiss, R. K., Graeme-Cook, F. M., et al. (2003). Appendiceal mucinous neoplasms. A clinicopathologic analysis of 107 cases. *American Journal of Surgical Pathology, 27*, 1089–1103.

Nishikawa, G., Sekine, S., Ogawa, R., et al. (2013). Frequent GNAS mutations in low-grade appendiceal mucinous neoplasms. *British Journal of Cancer, 108*, 951–958.

Pai, R. K., Beck, A. H., Norton, J. A., & Longacre, T. A. (2009). Appendiceal mucinous neoplasms. Clinicopathologic study of 116 cases with analysis of factors predicting recurrence. *American Journal of Surgical Pathology, 33*, 1425–1439.

Yantiss, R. K., Shia, J., Klimstra, D. S., et al. (2009). Prognostic significance of localized extra-appendiceal mucin deposition in appendiceal mucinous neoplasms. *American Journal of Surgical Pathology, 33*, 248–255.

Mucins

Raquel Almeida
Institute of Molecular Pathology and Immunology of the University of Porto (IPATIMUP), Porto, Portugal
Faculty of Medicine, University of Porto, Porto, Portugal

Synonyms

Mucins; MUC

Definition

Mucins (MUC) are high-molecular-weight glycoproteins constituted by a protein backbone (apomucin) and carbohydrate side chains. The vast majority of mucin glycosylation is constituted by *O*-glycans which are linked to serine (Ser) or threonine (Thr) residues on the protein backbone, and, in fact, more than 50% of the mucin molecular mass is composed of carbohydrates. The primary functions of mucins are to hydrate, protect, and lubricate the epithelial surfaces within the human body.

Features

There are two main classes of mucins: membrane-bound mucins, contributing to the composition of the cellular glycocalyx, and secreted mucins, contributing to the composition of the **extracellular matrix** or the mucous barrier that covers all epithelial surfaces in the human body, except the skin. Mucins share a common structural feature which is a **tandem repeat** domain comprising a variable number of tandem repeats (VNTRs) of identical or highly similar sequences rich in serine, threonine, and proline residues, also called the PTS (Pro/Thr/Ser) domains. These domains are highly polymorphic both regarding the number of amino acids in each repeat and the number of repeats. In addition, VNTRs are extensively glycosylated through *N*-acetyl-D-galactosamine (GalNAc) O-linked sugar chains which are enzymatically attached to Ser and Thr residues and further elongated by multiple glycosyltransferases in the Golgi complex (Kufe 2009). Furthermore, mucins have a smaller number of N-linked oligosaccharides that are important for the folding, oligomerization, and surface localization. In addition to the complexity conferred by glycosylation, the secreted mucins form homo-oligomers that are responsible for the viscoelastic properties of the mucous barrier, whose main function is to protect the underlying epithelial cells against chemical, enzymatic, microbial, and mechanical insults and serves as a physical gel to inhibit and entrap microbes. As a consequence of the VNTR polymorphism and glycosylation variations, the size of mucins can differ substantially between individuals, which likely constitute the basis for differences in susceptibility to a number of diseases and particularly to infections (Reis et al. 2010).

Twenty-one distinct mucin genes (MUC1–2, MUC3A, MUC3B, MUC4, MUC5AC, MUC5B, MUC6–9, and MUC12–21) codifying for the protein backbone have been identified to date. In situ hybridization and immunohistochemical studies have shown that mucins have distinct expression patterns with respect to organ, tissue, and cell type as well as developmental stage (Kufe 2009).

In a healthy gastric mucosa, the mucins produced are MUC1, MUC5AC, and MUC6 which are neutral mucins. MUC1 is a membrane-bound mucin, expressed more abundantly in the gastric foveolar epithelium, and to a lesser extent in the mucous glands. MUC1 is known by several other names, the most common being PEM (polymorphic epithelial mucin), but it is also known by episialin, DUPAN-2, DF3, HMFG (human milk fat globule), EMA (epithelial membrane antigen), and CD227. MUC1, like other cell surface mucins, attaches to the membrane through a transmembrane domain and has a short cytoplasmic tail that associates with the cytoskeleton playing a role, not only in protection but also in signal transduction. MUC1 normally attaches to the apical membranes of the gastric epithelial cells, but with malignant transformation and loss of polarity, it becomes expressed over the entire surface of the carcinoma cells (Kufe 2009).

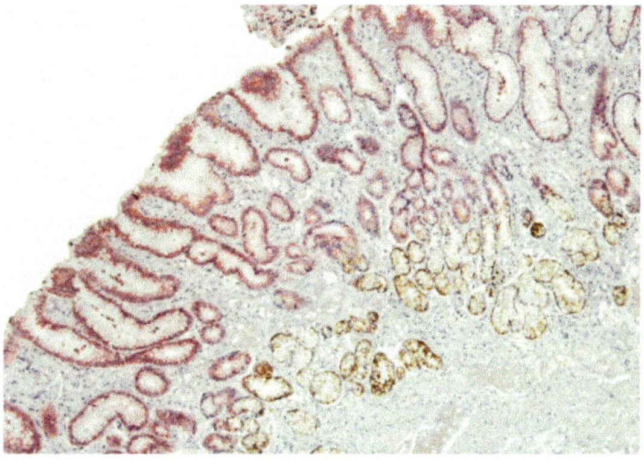

Mucins, Fig. 1 Expression of the soluble mucins MUC5AC (*red*) in the gastric foveolar or superficial epithelium and MUC6 (*brown*) in the deep glands, in a normal gastric mucosa

Gastric mucus, mainly constituted by the secreted mucins MUC5AC and MUC6, forms a protective layer over the surface epithelium against acid and pepsin present in the gastric juice, against deleterious effects of exogenous agents (viz., pathogens and drugs), and against mechanical damage. MUC5AC expression is restricted to the foveolar epithelium of the gastric **antrum** and corpus (Fig. 1). In humans, MUC5AC is encoded by a gene located on the p15 arm of **chromosome** 11 within a cluster of four mucin genes along with MUC2, MUC5B, and MUC6, and all of them share a common ancestor with von Willebrand factor. In the mouse, the organization of the cluster and the structure of the genes are conserved with the cluster being located in the syntenic region (murine chromosome 7) of the human chromosome 11. On the other hand, MUC6 is exclusively expressed in the deep glands of the antrum and in the mucous cells of the neck zone of the body (Fig. 1). Mucin's distribution, in the normal gastric mucosa, is accompanied by a similar distribution of some glycosyltransferases, namely, fucosyltransferases, leading to co-expression of a number of glycan chains with the protein backbone, particularly those related with individual ABO and Lewis blood group phenotypes, which determine the terminal carbohydrate structures that are carried by the mucin backbone proteins (de Bolós et al. 1995). Thus, in the normal gastric mucosa, expression of type 1 antigens, Lewis a (Le^a) and Lewis b (Le^b), is strongly associated with MUC5AC, whereas expression of type 2 antigens, Lewis x (Le^x) and Lewis y (Le^y), is associated with MUC6 (de Bolós et al. 1995). It remains to be fully elucidated whether the amino acid sequence on the protein backbone determines the glycosylation pattern or whether this is due to other external factors.

In the stomach, as well as in other organs, altered mucin expression is seen in precancerous and cancerous lesions, both at the protein and the glycan levels. The first alterations are observed early on in the gastric carcinogenic cascade, triggered by ***Helicobacter pylori*** infection. *H. pylori* causes **inflammation** of the gastric mucosa, which in some individuals will evolve to **intestinal metaplasia** and, in a low percentage of cases, to **gastric carcinoma**. The most common alterations of the mucin gene expression, induced by this bacterium, are MUC5AC underexpression and MUC6 overexpression in gastritis and de novo expression of the intestinal mucin MUC2 in intestinal metaplasia (Fig. 2a) (see section "Table with Examples and Links" for other examples). In fact, the profile of mucin expression has been used to categorize intestinal metaplasia. The oldest classification of intestinal metaplasia, based on the mucin profile, uses histochemical methods that allow the discrimination between the neutral gastric mucins that stain magenta with periodic acid-Schiff (PAS) and the acidic mucins present in IM which stain blue with Alcian blue at pH 2.5. In addition, high-iron diamine staining distinguishes

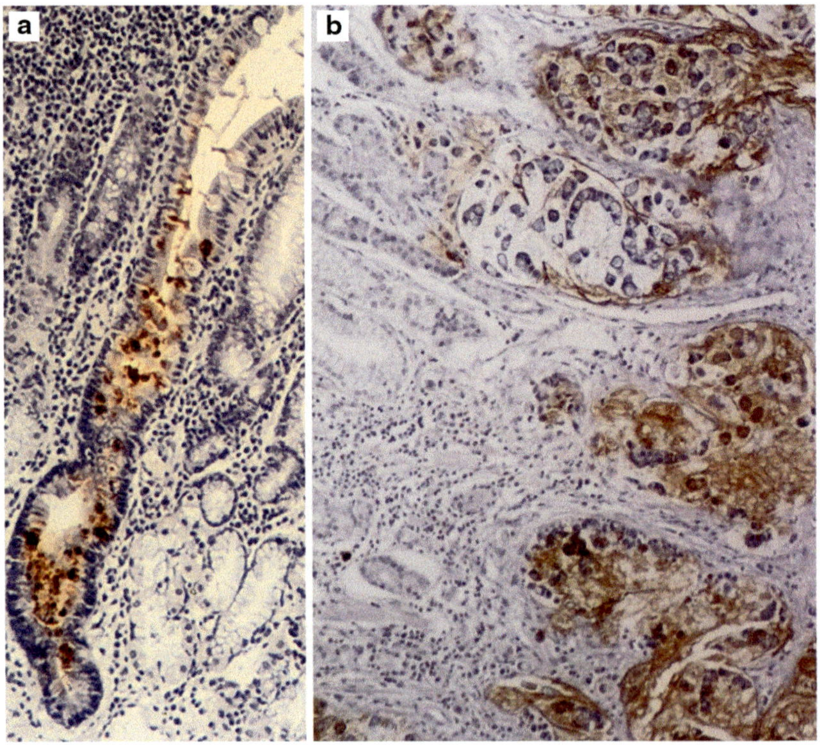

Mucins, Fig. 2 MUC2 expression in the goblet cells of intestinal metaplasia (**a**) and in a gastric carcinoma (**b**)

between acidic mucins that are sulfated from those that are sialylated. With this classification, IM is divided into three distinct types: Type I (complete) when only sialomucins are expressed, Type II (incomplete) when gastric and intestinal mucins (sialylated) are present, and Type III (incomplete) when sulfomucins are present. A more recent classification divides intestinal metaplasia into the complete type, characterized by decreased expression of MUC1, absence of MUC5AC and MUC6, and de novo expression of MUC2, and the incomplete type, characterized by the co-expression of the gastric mucins (MUC5AC and MUC6) with the intestinal mucin (MUC2) (Teixeira et al. 2001). The most relevant aspect of this classification is that incomplete intestinal metaplasia (or Type III) is more strongly associated to gastric carcinoma development although these classifications are not widely used in the clinical practice.

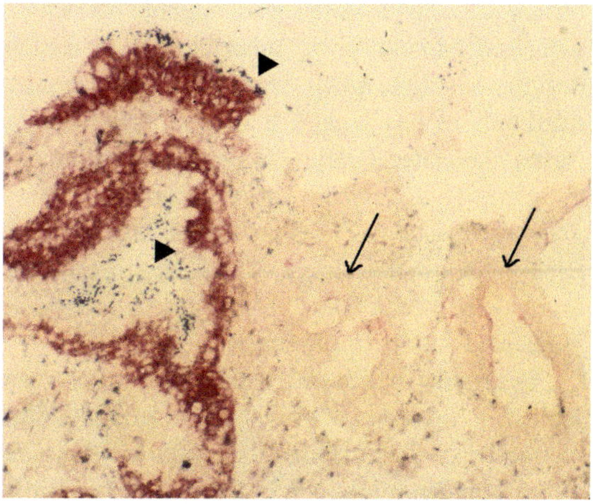

Mucins, Fig. 3 Gastric mucosa with normal foveolar epithelium with MUC5AC expression (*red*) adjacent to complete intestinal metaplasia glands, without MUC5AC expression (*arrows*). *Helicobacter pylori* (*arrowheads*), stained black, is adherent to the normal glands and absent from intestinal metaplasia

In gastric carcinomas, mucin gene expression is also altered being overall highly heterogeneous. Aberrant expression of MUC2 is maintained in about 30% of the gastric carcinomas, particularly in those that are histologically subtyped as **mucinous carcinomas**, characterized by strong expression of mucin proteins that dissociate the extracellular matrix (Fig. 2b). The gastric mucin MUC5AC is mainly expressed (about 65%) in diffuse-type gastric carcinomas (according to Laurén's classification), whereas MUC6 expression is in general low, being present in about 20% of gastric carcinomas, regardless of the histological type. MUC1 expression is detected in the vast majority of the gastric carcinomas, up to 90%, but it has been shown that its detection depends on the glycosylation status and therefore on the antibody that is used (Reis et al. 2010). Though there are conflicting results in the literature, it seems that the pattern of mucin expression in gastric carcinomas does not correlate with clinicopathological parameters that might reflect the behavior of the tumor.

Mucin glycosylation is also dramatically altered in gastric preneoplastic and neoplastic diseases and is also affected by *H. pylori* infection. It is known that binding of *H. pylori* to the gastric mucosa is, at least in part, mediated by mucins and particularly mucin glycans. The initial glycosylation changes induced by this microorganism, the most prominent of which is increased expression of Le^a, favor its adhesion to the gastric mucosa, which is mediated by a variety of bacterial adhesins. Paradoxically, with the course of infection and the concomitant development of more severe lesions namely, intestinal metaplasia, a microenvironment is created that is not favorable to the bacterium and leads to clearing of *H. pylori* from the metaplastic glands (Teixeira et al. 2001). Dramatic alterations of mucin gene expression, namely, absence of gastric mucins (Fig. 3) and de novo MUC2 expression, as well as of the glycosylation pattern, namely, de novo expression of sialylated glycans, particularly sialyl-Le^a, accompany this process (Teixeira et al. 2001). Overexpression of sialyl-Le^a as well as of sialyl-Le^x is also observed in gastric carcinomas (see section "Table with Examples and Links" for other examples) and is associated with increased metastatic potential and poor prognosis. Another common alteration of mucin glycosylation observed along the gastric carcinogenic pathway is increased expression of truncated glycan chains, designated simple mucin-type sugar chains, constituted only by one sugar (Tn antigen) which can be further sialylated (sialyl-Tn) or by two sugars (T antigen). These glycans are pan-carcinoma antigens (see section "Table with Examples and Links" for other examples) and are observed in more than 90% of the gastric carcinomas, also associated with poor prognosis.

As already mentioned, mucins are highly variable in size due to the VNTR **polymorphism** that characterizes them. It has been shown that this polymorphism might confer different susceptibilities to diseases and infections and, in the stomach, it has been demonstrated that "smaller" MUC1 alleles confer increased risk for gastric cancer development as well as chronic atrophic gastritis and incomplete intestinal metaplasia (Carvalho et al. 1997).

Application

Altered expression of carbohydrate and peptide moieties of mucin glycoproteins are thus phenotypic molecular markers of gastric premalignant and malignant lesions. Serological assays based on the detection of the carbohydrate antigens SLe^a (CA19-9) and STn (CA72.4) are currently used to monitor gastric cancer progression, particularly clinical response to therapy and cancer relapse. These are not used for initial screening due to their broad expression by other types of cancer as well as non-neoplastic and inflammatory diseases. Preoperative CA19-9 concentration remains one of the best prognostic factors in gastric carcinoma and is an independent risk factor for cancer recurrence (see section "Table with Examples and Links" for other examples). High CA72-4 expression levels are an independent prognostic factor and are also used to predict gastric tumor recurrence (see section "Table with Examples and Links" for other examples). Numerous studies are still directed at identifying novel biomarkers based on the mucin and glycosylation changes that occur in the gastric carcinogenesis cascade since they are highly expressed and easily accessible in the serum through shedding or cleavage from invading cancer cells (Reis et al. 2010).

Table with Examples and Links

MUC5AC	It is de novo expressed in **Barrett's esophagus** and in **esophageal adenocarcinoma** (**adenocarcinoma, upper gastrointestinal tract**)
MUC6	It is de novo expressed in **Barrett's esophagus** and in **esophageal adenocarcinoma** (**adenocarcinoma, upper gastrointestinal tract**)
MUC2	It is de novo expressed in **Barrett's esophagus** and in **esophageal adenocarcinoma** (**adenocarcinoma, upper gastrointestinal tract**) It is overexpressed in mucinous **colorectal carcinomas**
MUC1	It is decreased in **colorectal carcinomas**
T antigen	It is overexpressed in carcinomas from **breast**, **colon**, **pancreas**, **esophagus**, **bladder**, **ovary**, **endometrium**, and **lung**
Tn antigen	It is overexpressed in carcinomas from **breast**, **colon**, **pancreas**, **esophagus**, **bladder**, **ovary**, **endometrium**, and **lung**
Sialyl-Tn antigen (CA72-4)	It is overexpressed in carcinomas from **breast**, **colon**, **pancreas**, **esophagus**, **bladder**, **ovary**, **endometrium**, and **lung**
	Serological levels are raised in **colorectal** and **pancreatic cancer**, and it is an independent prognostic factor in pancreatic cancer
Sialyl-Le^a (CA19-9)	It is overexpressed in carcinomas from **pancreas**, **colon**, and **lung** where it is associated with increased metastatic potential and poor survival
	It is used to monitor clinical response to therapy in **pancreatic**, **biliary**, and **colorectal** cancer
Sialyl-Le^x	It is overexpressed in carcinomas from **pancreas**, **colon**, and **lung** where it is associated with increased metastatic potential and poor survival

References and Further Reading

de Bolós, C., Garrido, M., & Real, F. X. (1995). MUC6 apomucin shows a distinct normal tissue distribution that correlates with Lewis antigen expression in the human stomach. *Gastroenterology, 109*, 723–734.

Carvalho, F., Seruca, R., David, L., Amorim, A., Seixas, M., Bennett, E., Clausen, H., & Sobrinho-Simões, M. (1997). MUC1 gene polymorphism and gastric cancer – An epidemiological study. *Glycoconjugate Journal, 14*, 107–111.

Kufe, D. W. (2009). Mucins in cancer: Function, prognosis and therapy. *Nature Reviews. Cancer, 9*, 874–885.

Reis, C. A., Osorio, H., Silva, L., Gomes, C., & David, L. (2010). Alterations in glycosylation as biomarkers for cancer detection. *Journal of Clinical Pathology, 63*, 322–329.

Teixeira, A., David, L., Reis, C. A., Costa, J., & Sobrinho-Simões, M. (2002). Expression of mucins (MUC1, MUC2, MUC5AC, and MUC6) and type 1 Lewis antigens in cases with and without *Helicobacter pylori* colonization in metaplastic glands of the human stomach. *The Journal of Pathology, 197*, 37–43.

Mucocele, Appendix

Magali Svrcek
Hôpital Saint-Antoine, Service d'Anatomie Pathologique, AP-HP, Hôpitaux Universitaires de l'Est Parisien, Paris, France

Synonyms

Appendiceal mucinous cystadenoma; Low-grade appendiceal mucinous neoplasm (LAMN); Low-grade appendiceal mucinous tumor; Mucosal hyperplasia; Retention cyst; Retention mucocele

Definition

Appendiceal mucocele is an obstructive dilatation of the appendix caused by intraluminal accumulation of mucoid material (Fig. 1a, b). This purely descriptive term was first coined by Rokitansky in 1855, and does not constitute a pathological diagnosis. The density of goblet cells is far greater within the epithelium of the appendix than within the colon. As a result, the most frequent appendiceal epithelial tumors are mucinous and begin as mucoceles.

The term "appendiceal mucocele" includes traditionally four histological groups: (i) simple mucocele (also called retention cyst or retention mucocele); (ii) mucosal hyperplasia; (iii) mucinous cystadenoma; (iv) mucinous cystadenocarcinoma (Higa et al. 1973). Some authors, however, recommend the use of the term "mucocele" to be reserved solely for appendices that are dilated and contain inspissated mucin and devoid of mucin-secreting neoplasms.

Simple mucoceles (also called retention cysts or retention mucoceles) usually follow acute appendicitis with postinflammatory fibrosis, obstruction by fecalith, and progressive mucin accumulations. Appendiceal endometriosis is also known to cause mucoceles.

Mucinous cystadenomas and mucinous cystadenocarcinomas are not fully discussed in this chapter (for a more detailed description, refer to "▶ Mucinous Cystadenoma, Appendix" entry, and "▶ Mucinous Cystadenocarcinoma, Appendix" entry).

One rare variant of appendiceal mucocele is called myxoglobulosis. The mucin forms small occasionally calcified spheres. The distinctive features of the globules give rise to terms such as "fish-egg" or "caviar" appendix.

Clinical Features

- **Incidence**
  Appendiceal mucocele is rare. It represents only 0.2–0.7% of all appendectomy specimens and 8% of appendiceal tumors.

  Simple mucoceles and mucosal hyperplasia each represent approximately 20% of all mucoceles. Mucinous cystadenomas and mucinous cystadenocarcinomas represent, in average, 50% and less than 10% of all mucoceles, respectively.

  Finally, myxoglobulosis constitute roughly 0.35–8% of all mucoceles.
- **Age**
  The incidence of appendiceal mucoceles is mostly prevalent in the fifth and sixth

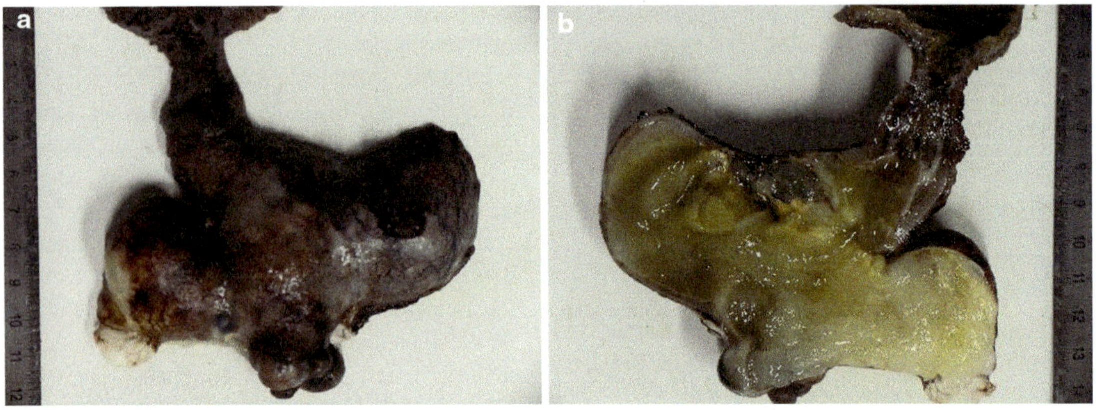

Mucocele, Appendix, Fig. 1 (**a**) The appendix is dilated and thin walled. The distal portion of the appendix is more dilated than the proximal portion. There is no perforation. (**b**) The appendix is opened lengthwise: a gelatinous material is present in the lumen

decades of life, although they may be diagnosed at any age.

- **Sex**
  Discrepancies exist between various reports. However, female predominance is more frequently described.
- **Site**
  The clinical flow of the disease does not have a specific picture. The mucocele of the appendix may be symptomatic or asymptomatic, being discovered, in about 50% of cases, incidentally in a radiological or endoscopic test or at laparotomy performed for other reasons. Acute abdominal pain is the main clinical manifestation of mucocele. Acute or chronic pain in right iliac fossa is the most frequent symptom, sometimes with a palpable abdominal mass. An ovarian mass can also be observed sometimes. Unusual manifestations are low gastrointestinal bleeding associated with intussusception of the mucocele (Fig. 2).

  Clinical presentations also include the presence of mucus outside of the appendix, with sometimes abdominal distension and ascites.
- **Treatment**
  Mucocele of the appendix may correspond to a benign or malignant process, pushing toward an individualized treatment in each case. Because it is impossible to say at the time of surgery if an appendiceal mucocele is benign or malignant, the prudent surgical approach is to regard every mucocele of the appendix as potentially malignant.

  Sugarbaker has proposed an algorithm for the selection of the type of surgery. It includes several factors, which are: (i) whether or not a mucocele is perforated; (ii) whether the base of the appendix (margins of resection) is involved in the process; (iii) whether there are positive mesoappendiceal and ileocolic lymph nodes; and (iv) whether or not there are mucin deposits outside of the appendix.

  Intact mucoceles are not a threat for patients, and appendectomy is the treatment of choice. The right colectomy may not be necessary in the management of appendiceal mucinous

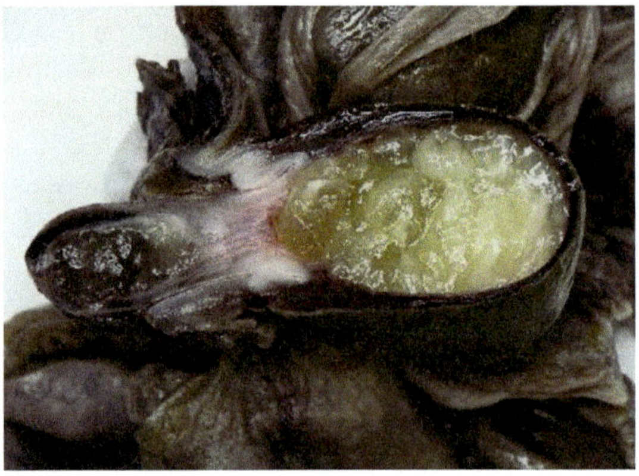

Mucocele, Appendix, Fig. 2 Intussusception of the appendix secondary to a mucinous cystadenoma

neoplasms, particularly when the initial surgical resection margins are not affected by neoplasia.

If treated improperly, the mucocele may progress, epithelial cells may escape into the peritoneal cavity, and pseudomyxoma peritonei (refer to the section "Outcome") may develop. Thus, proper surgical management of an appendiceal mucocele is essential and special care in resection must be taken to avoid trauma and possible rupture of the appendix while being removed.

The peritoneal spaces surrounding the appendix must be carefully inspected, and a complete removal of the appendix and surrounding periappendiceal tissues, if grossly involved, is required. In the same way, if the surgeon suspects a ruptured appendix or if the tumor is associated with diverticula, a careful examination of the abdominal cavity must be performed in order to eliminate a peritoneal dissemination of the tumor. In this case, a prolonged clinical follow-up for these patients for recurrent disease is proposed. Aspiration of fluid from beneath the right liver within the right retrohepatic space and from the pelvis is recommended. The inspection of the abdominal cavity must also include the ovaries. Any fluid or mucus and any tumor nodules outside of the appendix must be sampled for histological examination. If epithelial cells are found in the mucin deposits, the patient must be referred to an established peritoneal treatment center.

Management of peritoneal dissemination of mucinous appendiceal neoplasms includes cytoreductive surgery (known as the Sugarbaker procedure), heated intraoperative intraperitoneal chemotherapy, and early postoperative intraperitoneal chemotherapy. The cytoreductive surgery involves a series of visceral resections and peritonectomy procedures.

The extent of peritoneal dissemination is determined by the peritoneal cancer index (PCI) at the time of surgical exploration of the abdomen and pelvis. This index has a significant impact on survival for both high-grade and low-grade diseases. Therapeutic decisions for pseudomyxoma peritonei largely depend on the distinction between low-grade and high-grade peritoneal diseases.

Various authors have observed an association between mucocele of the appendix and other colorectal neoplasms, with a frequency of ∼20%. It is therefore recommended to perform a complete colonic examination intra and/or postoperatively

In summary, appendectomy is the treatment of choice. It is important to keep a mucocele intact during surgery, to avoid dissemination of mucoid material into the peritoneal cavity. A correct diagnosis before surgery is very important for selecting the appropriate surgical technique.

- **Outcome**

A great majority of appendiceal mucoceles removed by appendectomy are benign. The outcome of simple mucocele, mucosal hyperplasia, and mucinous cystadenoma after appendectomy is excellent, reaching a 10-year survival of about 91%.

When the appendix bursts due to internal pressure from the mucus-producing neoplasm, mucus and mucinous tumoral cells are released into the free peritoneal cavity. Free tumor cells are spread throughout the peritoneal cavity following a distribution pattern dependent on the peritoneal fluid flow and gravity. Once perforation occurs and epithelial cells escape into the peritoneal cavity, the mucocele becomes a potentially lethal entity. The growth of neoplastic mucin-secreting cells within the peritoneal cavity causes a slow but relentless accumulation of mucin, resulting ultimately in peritoneal implants and mucinous ascites called pseudomyxoma peritonei (PP). The hallmark of the PP is the large accumulation of mucinous tumoral cells within the greater and lesser omentum. Around 10–15% of mucoceles progress to PP. The incidence of perforation is much lower in simple mucocele and mucosal hyperplasia than in mucinous cystadenoma and cystadenocarcinoma.

A rupture of a retention mucocele is sometimes possible and may produce mucin accumulation in the environment, potentially mimicking a PP. However, these mucin deposits remain localized in the peri-appendiceal region, do not contain epithelial cells, and do not reaccumulate after appendectomy.

PP lesions are defined by two main parameters: their topography and their pathologic features. Mucin deposits can be localized (located on the appendiceal serosa, within the mesoappendix, or limited to the right lower quadrant), or more generalized to the abdominal cavity where peritoneal fluids mostly accumulate (greater and lesser omentum, the pelvis, when entrapped within the cul-de-sac, the ligament de Treitz, the undersurface of the diaphragms, and the left paracolic sulcus). Mucin deposits in these cases may be acellular and may contain neoplastic cells ("cellular mucin"). The most critical factor predicting behavior of PPs is the cytological grade. In 2010, the World Health Organization published a classification that divides PPs into low- and high-grade (Carr and Sobin 2010). In low-grade lesions, cells form strips or small islands. Typically, mucin deposits are abundant, dissect peritoneal tissue, are separated by collageneous bands, and contain scanty cells. The mucin may sometimes appear acellular. Papillary tufting can occur. These lesions are characterized by low-grade cytological atypia and by small and regularly shaped nuclei. Mitoses are rare (Fig. 3). Nodal metastasis is unusual. In contrast, high-grade PPs show, at least focally, high-grade cytological atypia. Cells are numerous and may form strips, small islands, or cribriform structures. Mitoses are more common and may be atypical. Lesions are accompanied by a desmoplastic stroma. Signet ring cell morphology classifies a lesion as high-grade. Interestingly, the categorization as either low-grade or high-grade correlates with prognosis (Carr et al. 2012). The grade of the PPs is generally consistent with the grade of the primary neoplasm, but discordant cases can still occur. Low-grade appendiceal mucinous neoplasm (LAMN) may be associated with high-grade PPs. In these cases, it is admitted that even if the appendiceal lesion is of low-grade, the patient must be treated the same way a patient with high-grade PP is treated.

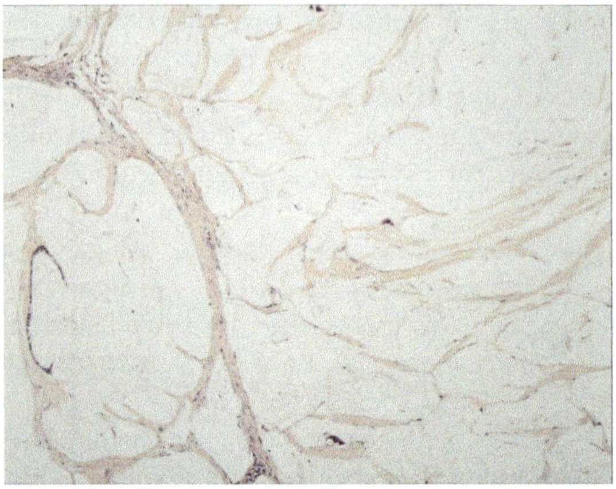

Mucocele, Appendix, Fig. 3 Low-grade pseudomyxoma peritonei

Previously, low-grade PPs, considered to represent passive spread of adenomatous epithelium into the peritoneum, secondary to a mucocele rupture, were called by Ronnett et al. "disseminated peritoneal adenomucinosis." Actual high-grade PPs were designated "peritoneal mucinous carcinomatosis," and cases with both low- and high-grade features were designated "peritoneal mucinous carcinomatosis, intermediate grade."

The overall 10-year survival rates of PPs have reported to be around 21–45%, but a recent study reported a rate of 63% for patients treated with cytoreductive surgery and hyperthermic intraperitoneal chemotherapy. Patients with a complete cytoreduction and low-grade tumors have an 80% survival at 20 years. The most important indicator is the completeness of cytoreduction. Low-grade PPs are associated with significantly longer survival than high-grade PPs.

Macroscopy

Appendiceal mucoceles result from luminal obstruction with distension of part or all of the appendiceal lumen by a large amount of mucus (Fig. 1a, b). They most typically affect distal part

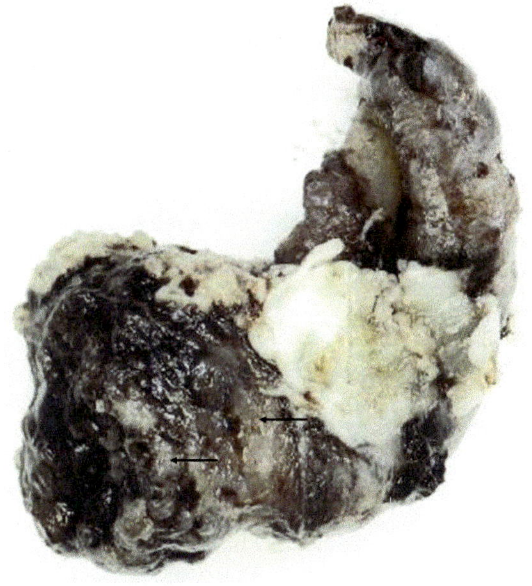

Mucocele, Appendix, Fig. 4 Low-grade appendiceal mucinous neoplasm (LAMN). Mucin extruding from a rupture site are marked by arrows. Considerable vascular engorgement is noticeable and an abundant fibropurulent exudate covers the appendix

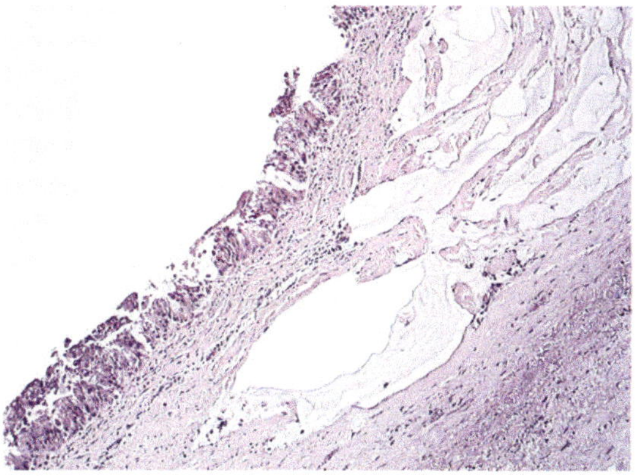

Mucocele, Appendix, Fig. 5 The appendiceal lumen is lined by epithelioid histiocytes. The wall appears fibrotic

of the appendix. An appendiceal mucocele may also cause appendiceal intussusception (Fig. 2).

Most appendiceal tumors begin as a mucocele. An appendix of more than 1 or 2 cm in diameter suggests the existence of an underlying neoplasm. These large mucoceles must be well sampled to rule out the presence of a tumor. When a mucocele is found, it is very important to determine whether the appendiceal wall of that structure is intact or has been breached (Fig. 4).

Given the prognostic implications of the extent of mucin and neoplastic epithelium, it is recommended that appendices containing mucinous neoplasms be entirely submitted for histological examination. In the situation of appendiceal mucinous neoplasms with localized periappendiceal mucin, complete microscopic examination of the entire periappendiceal mucin is also warranted.

When a tumor is found by histological analysis, the pathologist should carefully re-examine the appendix for areas of perforation, serosal mucin accumulations, and invasive carcinoma. The entire tumor should be submitted this examination in order to rule out invasion.

Margins in a simple appendectomy specimen include the proximal and radial margins. It is recommended that the proximal margin on a single appendectomy specimen be taken en face in order to evaluate the entire appendiceal mucosa and muscularis circumferentially. In right hemicolectomy specimens, the ileal and colonic margins are the proximal and distal margins, respectively. In right hemicolectomy specimens, pathological assessment of the regional lymph node must be performed.

M

Microscopy

Simple mucoceles are usually unilocular, thin walled, and characterized by degenerative epithelial changes caused by obstruction, such as flattened, atrophic epithelium, but still often prominent Peyer's patches. There are no proliferative changes. Mucosal denudation is possible. The appendiceal wall may appear fibrotic and chronically inflamed. Granulomatous response may be observed (Fig. 5).

Mucosal hyperplasia is histologically similar to a hyperplastic polyp. The glands have serrated lumens lined by benign epithelium. Cytologic atypia is absent.

The microscopic features of mucinous cystadenoma and mucinous cystadenocarcinomas are described in two specific chapters.

Immunophenotype

The mucin-producing cells are stained with diastase-resistant periodic acid-Schiff (PAS) and Alcian blue. The neoplastic epithelial cells are immunoreactive with keratin-20 and intestinal mucin marker MUC2.

Proliferative rates can be high.

Molecular Features

Molecular features are described in the two chapters "Mucinous Cystadenoma" and "Mucinous cystadenocarcinoma."

Differential Diagnosis

When a mucinous cystadenoma gives rise to a mucocele, the distension of the appendiceal lumen by mucus compresses the neoplastic epithelial cells, flattening it to a single cell and rendering it hardly recognizable as being neoplastic. In some cases, mucosal denudation can be observed, and may lead to misdiagnosis of mucinous cystadenoma. Multiple sections should be taken to confirm the diagnosis of mucinous cystadenoma. Staining with PAS or Alcian blue can be of interest in that setting.

Other differential diagnoses are discussed in the chapters "Mucinous Cystadenoma" and "Mucinous cystadenocarcinoma."

References and Further Reading

Carr, N. J., & Sobin, L. H. (2010). Tumours of the appendix. In F. T. Bosman, F. Carneiro, R. H. Hruban, & N. D. Theise (Eds.), *WHO classification of tumours of the digestive system* (pp. 122–125). Lyon: IARC Press.

Carr, N. J., Finch, J., Ilesley, I. C., et al. (2012). Pathology and prognosis in pseudomyxoma peritonei: A review of 274 cases. *Journal of Clinical Pathology, 65*, 919–923.

Chua, T. C., Moran, B. J., Sugarbaker, P. H., et al. (2012). Early- and long-term outcome data of patients with pseudomyxoma peritone from appendiceal origin treated by a strategy of cytoreductive surgery and hyperthermic intraperitoneal chemotherapy. *Journal of Clinical Oncology, 20*, 2449–2456.

Higa, E., Rosai, J., & Pizzimbono, C. A. (1973). Mucosal hyperplasia, mucinous cystadenoma and mucinous cystadenocarcinoma of the appendix: A re-evaluation of appendiceal "mucocele". *Cancer, 32*, 1525–1541.

Smeenk, R. M., van Velthuysen, M. L., Verwaal, V. J., & Zoetmulder, F. A. (2008). Appendiceal neoplasms and pseudomyxoma peritonei: A population-based study. *European Journal of Surgical Oncology, 34*, 196–201.

Mucoepidermoid Carcinoma, Esophageal

Isabel Fonseca
Serviço de Anatomia Patológica, Instituto Português de Oncologia Francisco Gentil – Lisboa, Lisbon, Portugal
Faculdade de Medicina de Lisboa, Instituto de Anatomia Patológica, Lisbon, Portugal

Synonyms

Adenosquamous carcinoma; Mucoepidermoid tumor; Squamous cell carcinoma with mucin-secreting component

Definition

Mucoepidermoid carcinoma is a malignant epithelial glandular tumor characterized by the presence, in variable proportions, of mucin-producing, intermediate, and squamoid cells that can undergo columnar, clear, and oncocytic change.

Clinical Features

- **Incidence**
  Mucoepidermoid carcinoma is a very rare esophageal neoplasm, accounting for less than 1% of malignant neoplasms.
- **Age**
  Most cases of mucoepidermoid carcinoma of the esophagus are reported in patients in their sixth to seventh decades.

- **Sex**
  Most cases occur in men, with an M/F ratio between 2:1 and 3:1.
- **Site**
  Most mucoepidermoid carcinomas arise in the lower two-thirds of the esophagus.
- **Treatment**
  Surgery is the treatment of choice for mucoepidermoid carcinoma, following the guidelines for the treatment of esophageal squamous cell carcinoma. Positive margins and high histological grade warrant postoperative radiotherapy. There is no demonstration that combined chemoradiotherapy is effective in mucoepidermoid carcinoma.
- **Outcome**
  Prognosis of mucoepidermoid carcinoma of the esophagus is unclear, but most reports show that it has worse prognosis than the salivary counterpart. The 5-year survival is fewer than 40% since most patients present in advanced clinical stages. Disease progression occurs both locally and to distant sites. There is no consistent information on the impact of histological grade in tumor progression.

Macroscopy

Mucoepidermoid carcinomas present as solid, firm submucosal tumors. They can grow to be intraluminal, polypoid masses. Ulceration of the overlying mucosa is frequent.

Microscopy

Mucoepidermoid carcinoma can be cystic or solid or show a mixed architectural pattern. Cystic tumors are usually low grade. It is morphologically characterized by the presence of three cell types, mucin-producing cells, intermediate cells, and squamous cells, in variable proportions. Mucin-producing cells are large, have eccentric nuclei, and have intracytoplasmatic mucin that can be highlighted with PAS, *mucicarmine*, or *Alcian blue* histochemical stains. Intermediate cells are cuboidal, with central nuclei and eosinophilic cytoplasms. They can undergo clear and oncocytic change. Polygonal squamous cells are present but, by definition, no keratinization is present. In mucosal sites, the presence of epithelial dysplasia warrants the differential diagnosis with other tumor types (see below) (Figs. 1 and 2).

Histological grading is based on the systems used for salivary mucoepidermoid carcinoma.

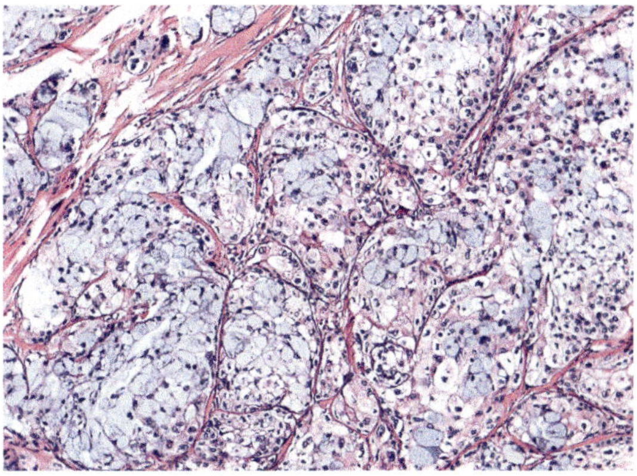

Mucoepidermoid Carcinoma, Esophageal, Fig. 1 Mucoepidermoid carcinoma, grade II. Mucin-producing cells are admixed with intermediate and squamous cells, forming solid aggregates. There is no keratinization. Atypia is mild in any of the cell types (H&E)

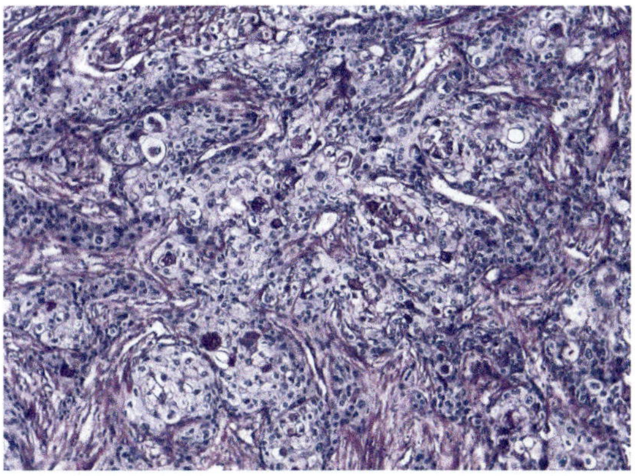

Mucoepidermoid Carcinoma, Esophageal, Fig. 2 Mucoepidermoid carcinoma. PAS highlights the mucin-producing component and can be very useful in the differential diagnosis with squamous cell carcinoma (PAS)

Immunophenotype

Immunohistochemistry is not useful for the diagnosis of mucoepidermoid carcinoma.

Molecular Features

Mucoepidermoid carcinoma has been found to harbor, in around 70% of the cases, the t(11;19) (q21;p13) balanced translocation as the sole genetic abnormality that leads to a fusion gene involving the *MAML2* gene and *CRTC1* gene or, in around 5% of the cases, *CRTC3* gene as chromosomal partner. Currently, there is no data in the literature of similar findings in esophageal mucoepidermoid carcinoma.

Differential Diagnosis

Extensive keratinization and the presence of intercellular bridges favor the diagnosis of *squamous cell carcinoma* or *adenosquamous carcinoma*. Dysplasia of the overlying epithelium almost invariable excluded mucoepidermoid carcinoma. In adenosquamous carcinoma the glandular component is clearly demarcated from the squamous component.

CK7 is present in mucoepidermoid carcinoma and not in squamous cell carcinoma. The most important tool to diagnose mucoepidermoid carcinoma is the search for intermediate cells. The usefulness of the determination of the *CRTC1/3-MAML2* fusion status in the differential diagnosis remains to be established, but there is mounting evidence that points to its routine clinical use.

References and Further Reading

Chen, S., Chen, Y., Yang, J., Yang, W., Weng, H., Li, H., & Liu, D. (2011). Primary mucoepidermoid carcinoma of the esophagus. *Journal of Thoracic Oncology, 6*, 1426–1431.

Huang, Q., Shi, J., Sun, Q., Fan, X., Feng, A., Wu, H., Zhou, Q., Yu, C., Mashimo, H., & Lauwers, G. Y. (2012). Distal esophageal carcinomas in Chinese patients vary widely in histopathology, but adenocarcinomas remain rare. *Human Pathology*. http://dx.doi.org/10.1016/j.humpath.2012.02.018

Lieberman, M. D., Franceschi, D., Marsan, B., & Burt, M. (1994). Esophageal carcinoma. The unusual variants. *The Journal of Thoracic and Cardiovascular Surgery, 108*, 1138–1146.

Tonon, G., Modi, S., Wu, L., Kubo, A., Coxon, A. B., Komiya, T., O'Neil, K., Stover, K., El-Naggar, A., Griffin, J. D., Kirsh, I. R., & Kaye, F. J. (2003). t(11:19)(q21:p13) translocation in mucoepidermoid carcinoma creates a novel fusion product that disrupts a NOTCH signalling pathway. *Nature Genetics, 33*, 208–213.

Mucosal Prolapse Syndrome

Andrzej Mróz
Department of Gastroenterology and Hepatology, Histopathology Unit, Medical Center for Postgraduate Education, Warsaw, Poland

Synonyms

Inflammatory cloacogenic polyp/rectal mucosal prolapse; Rectal prolapse syndrome; Solitary rectal ulcer syndrome/rectal mucosal prolapse

Definition

Mucosal prolapse includes different abnormalities of anorectal region: rectal prolapse, *solitary rectal ulcer syndrome*, inflammatory cloacogenic polyp, inflammatory cap polyp, and proctitis cystica profunda.

These somewhat overlapping entities represent the spectrum of pathologies resulting from ischemic mucosal changes and injury followed by inflammation, repair, and regenerative changes. Mucosal prolapse syndrome is observed in patients with acute diarrhea, chronic constipation, connective tissue diseases, history of radiation or previous surgery, rectal polyps, rectal neoplasia, or hemorrhoids. Substantial number of patients with cystic fibrosis develop mucosal prolapse syndrome.

The primary clinical feature is related to bowel habit abnormalities, usually in the form of constipation. Straining at defecation with secondary muscular spasm causes mucosal shears and ulcerations. Clinical features of rectal bleeding, pain, tenesmus, and fecal incontinence belong to the most commonly reported symptoms in patients with mucosal prolapse.

Rectal prolapse may be complete and graded from first degree (full thickness of the rectum is protruded including mucocutaneous junction), to second degree (complete prolapse without mucocutaneous junction involvement), to third degree (concealed prolapse with rectum wall intussusception in anal canal). Additionally, anatomic abnormalities are present including deep rectovaginal or rectovesical pouch, atonic musculature of pelvic floor, abnormal rectal fixation with elongated mesorectum, redundant rectosigmoid colon, and abnormal sphincter function.

Clinical Features

- **Incidence**
  General incidence is not known; solitary ulcer rectal syndrome affects 1–3 in 100,000.
- **Age**
  At any age starting from childhood (rectal prolapse), with peak incidence in third and fourth decades (SRUS), to older patients (prolapsing mucosal polypoid folds). Eighty percent of patients are younger than 50 years.
- **Sex**
  For SURS patients, females predominate males by several times; inflammatory cap polyps are also more common in women. No evident sex predilection is seen in cases of inflammatory cloacogenic polyps.
- **Site**
  Anterior rectum in SURS, anterior anorectal junction in inflammatory cloacogenic polyps, rectum, and anal canal for proctitis cystica profunda
- **Treatment**
  Medical therapy includes changes in dietary habits (increased fiber consumption, stool softeners), biofeedback, psychological counseling, and pelvic floor exercises. Surgical treatment (rectopexy with rectal resection) in severe cases. Rectal prolapse in children usually corrects without intervention; sclerotherapy may also be used.
- **Outcome (Prognosis)**
  Recurrence rate after surgical treatment reaches 15%. Recurrence of clinical symptoms after medical treatment is common (up to 40–50%; expected results of biofeedback, psychological counseling, and bowel movements training are seen usually no sooner then 9–12 months.

Macroscopy

Rectal prolapse includes all layers of the rectum, which leads to rectal wall intussusception. Mucosa may be erythematous or ulcerated; polypoid lesions often develop. In SURS polypoid lesion may be single or multiple – see section on SURS. Inflammatory cap polyps are usually umbilicated and form red areas of granulation. Areas of protruding fibrin collections are often the feature. Similarly in inflammatory cloacogenic polyps, sessile or pedunculated lesions with surface erosion, ulceration, and fibrin exudates are seen. They range from 1 to 2 cm in diameter. In patients with proctitis cystica profunda mucosal edema, erythema and mucosal irregularity with pronounced lumpy folds are grossly found. Polypoid formations, mucosal friability, ulcers, and cauliflower-shaped mass may also be the case. The cysts may be macroscopically seen within intestinal wall. These cysts contain mucous or mucous-like secretions.

Microscopy

Early histological features include mucosal erosions and ulcers with nonspecific reactive inflammation. Collagenous band beneath surface epithelium thickens; vessels are dilated and congested. Ulcers are superficial. Later on lamina propria is replaced by smooth muscle cells and fibroblasts which are arranged perpendicularly to muscularis mucosae. The glands may become dilated, regenerative, mucin depleted, and hyperplastic.

Microscopic variants of mucosal prolapse syndrome:

- Inflammatory cap polyp – clinically associated with mucus diarrhea, tenesmus, or rectal bleeding consisting of tortuous, hyperplastic crypts, fibromuscular hypertrophy, and goblet cells hypertrophy. The glands have serrated morphology resembling hyperplastic polyps. The lesion is often covered with the cap of granulation tissue and fibrin.
- Inflammatory cloacogenic polyp – a small polyp at anorectal junction, usually on the anterior wall of the rectum. Mucosa is of transitional type and the hypertrophic polypoid glandular epithelium may be mixed with squamous epithelium. Strands of muscles radiate from muscularis mucosae to inflamed lamina propria. Regenerative changes of the epithelium may simulate dysplasia, in addition glands may be displaced in submucosa mimicking carcinoma invasion.

Two abovementioned microscopical manifestations of mucosal prolapse have generally two components – surface erosion with reactive inflammatory and reparative changes and glandular hyperplasia. The degree of superficial pseudovillous mucosal remodeling may be substantial. Glandular pseudoatypia and pseudoinvasion should not be mistaken for dysplasia or neoplastic invasion – see differential diagnosis.

- Solitary rectal ulcer syndrome – see in section on SURS.
- Proctitis cystica profunda – in this condition mucosa is displaced into the stroma and continues to produce mucus. Cysts lined with glandular epithelium are found in submucosa; additional features of mucosal prolapse syndrome may be shown. More superficial changes of inflammatory cloacogenic or cap polyp may be seen.

Immunophenotype

No specific feature is reported.

Molecular Features

No specific feature is reported.

Differential Diagnosis

The mucosal prolapse syndrome with its subtypes may be erroneously diagnosed as IBD – particularly when the ulcers, fistulas, and mucosal inflammation dominate in histological picture. Early stages with collagen bundle thickening are sometimes taken for collagenous colitis.

Fibromuscular proliferation may resemble Peutz-Jeghers polyp, but it is organized in perpendicular fashion. Furthermore inflammatory cloacogenic polyps are usually isolated, while Peutz-Jeghers polyps are multiple in most of the cases.

Proctitis cystica profunda must be differentiated from endometriosis – analysis of epithelium with immunohistochemical stains for estrogen receptors and CD10 may be useful.

The most important risk is confusing mucosal prolapse cases from neoplastic lesion. Tubulovillous growth pattern and regenerative atypia may recall neoplastic process. However, fibromuscular proliferation and the absence of desmoplastic stromal reaction are against the diagnosis of neoplasia. In proctitis cystica profunda, invasive mucinous carcinoma must be ruled out.

References and Further Reading

Iacobuzio-Donahue, C. A., & Montgomery, E. (2005). *Gastrointestinal and liver pathology*. Philadelphia: Elsevier.

Noffsinger, A., et al. (2007). *Gastrointestinal diseases*. Washington, DC: The American Registry of Pathology.

N

Necrotizing Enterocolitis

Erdener Özer
Department of Pathology, Dokuz Eylül University School of Medicine, Izmir, Turkey

Synonyms

NEC; Neonatal necrotizing enterocolitis

Definition

Necrotizing enterocolitis (NEC) is a common distinctive disease of premature infants characterized by coagulative necrosis and inflammation of the small and large intestine. It is the most common gastrointestinal medical and surgical emergency in the neonatal period.

The pathogenesis of NEC is still incompletely understood and is likely attributable to a complex mechanism. Hypoxia-ischemia is less postulated nowadays and there is an increasing evidence of relation between altered mucosal integrity and prematurity itself. Many factors potentially predispose the premature intestine to injury. These include an inadequate intestinal barrier, incomplete microvasculature development or an immature regulation of the intestinal vascular perfusion, an inflammatory response triggered by abnormal bacterial colonization and an immature immune response leading to inefficient killing of microbes that then translocate through the intestinal epithelium.

Immaturities of several pathways that regulate inflammation may predispose premature infants to inflammation, and a large number of inflammatory mediators have been associated with NEC. One particular mediator, platelet-activating factor (PAF), has been implicated in increasing mucosal permeability by promoting enterocyte apoptosis. In addition, inflammatory mediators are induced by the presence of bacterial toxins and play an important role in the pathophysiology of tissue distraction in NEC. Besides prematurity, most cases are associated with enteral feeding, suggesting that some postnatal insult (such as introduction of bacteria) is involved in the pathogenesis. Feeding of milk formulas can cause bacterial colonization and therefore NEC, because they do not contain secretory immunoglobulin A, which binds to the intestinal luminal cells and prevents bacterial transmural translocation. To be noted, while infectious agents are likely to play a role in NEC pathogenesis, no single bacterial pathogen has been linked to the disease.

The etiology of NEC in term and near-term infants may be different than that addressed in the premature infants and may be related to the entities such as cow's milk protein–induced enterocolitis and glucose-6-phosphate dehydrogenase deficiency.

Although various clinical and radiographic signs and symptoms are used to make the

F. Carneiro et al. (eds.), *Pathology of the Gastrointestinal Tract*, Encyclopedia of Pathology,
DOI 10.1007/978-3-319-40560-5

diagnosis, the classic clinical triad consists of abdominal distension, bloody stools, and pneumatosis intestinalis. The latter is the radiological hallmark of the condition. Occasionally, signs and symptoms include temperature instability, lethargy, or other nonspecific findings of sepsis. NEC, in severe cases, can cause profound impairment of multiple organ systems.

Clinical Features

- **Incidence**
  As neonatal intensive care has progressed and premature newborns have become to survive long enough for the development of disease, the incidence of NEC has increased. It is more prevalent in premature infants with incidence inversely related to the birth weight and gestational age. NEC occurs in 1–3 per 1,000 live births and is seen predominately in premature infants with an incidence of about 6–7% in very low birth weight (VLBW) babies (birth weight <1,500 g). Similarly, rates significantly decrease for infants born after 35–36 week postconceptional age.
- **Age**
  NEC typically occurs in the second to third week of life in the infant who is premature and has been formula fed. The average age of onset in premature infants seems to be related to postconceptional age, with babies born earlier developing NEC at a later chronologic age. The average age of onset has been reported to be 20.2 days for babies born at less than 30 weeks of estimated gestational age (EGA), 13.8 days for babies born at 31–33 weeks of EGA, and 5.4 days for babies born after 34 weeks of gestation. However, up to 10% of infants with NEC are born at term, and the disease may develop early with the average age of onset within the first week of life or, sometimes, within the first 1–2 days of life.
- **Sex**
  Studies investigating the relationship between sex and NEC have had inconsistent findings. Therefore, whether gender is a risk factor for NEC remains unclear.
- **Site**
  The small intestine or colon may be also affected alone, whereas the entire tract is involved in the severe cases. In the majority of cases, the most severely affected portions are the terminal ileum and cecum (80%) and the ascending colon, although any part of the gastrointestinal tract may be involved.
- **Treatment**
  The management of NEC depends upon the severity of illness as classified by the Bell staging criteria. Medical management including cessation of oral feedings, administration of antibiotics is appropriate in most cases. Long-term parenteral nutrition is required in many cases. However, infants with advanced NEC and bowel perforation require surgical intervention.
- **Outcome**
  With early recognition and improved supportive intensive care, the survival of infants with NEC has steadily improved. However, NEC accounts for substantial long-term morbidity in survivors of neonatal intensive care, particularly in VLBW infants. Of the patients who survive, 50% develop a long-term complication. The two most common complications are intestinal stricture and short-gut syndrome. Other complications include peritonitis, sepsis, and compromised nutrition. Prolonged hyperalimentation and the absence of enteral nutrition can cause cholestasis, direct hyperbilirubinemia, and other metabolic complications. Infants who survive NEC are at increased risk for neurodevelopmental disorders. Recurrent NEC is an uncommon complication that can occur after management of NEC.

Macroscopy

On gross examination the finding in most of the cases is that of a patchy segmental necrosis with

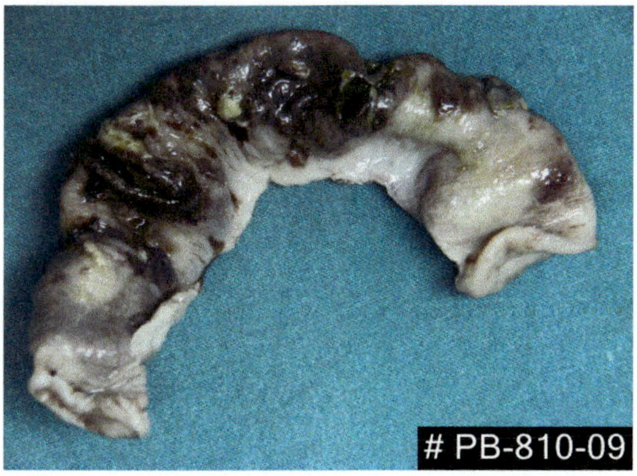

Necrotizing Enterocolitis, Fig. 1 In this resected specimen, scattered and discontinuous areas of necrotic bowel (*yellow-tan areas*) are apparent and demarcated from areas of viable bowel (Courtesy of Dr Diclehan Orhan, Hacettepe University, Ankara, Turkey)

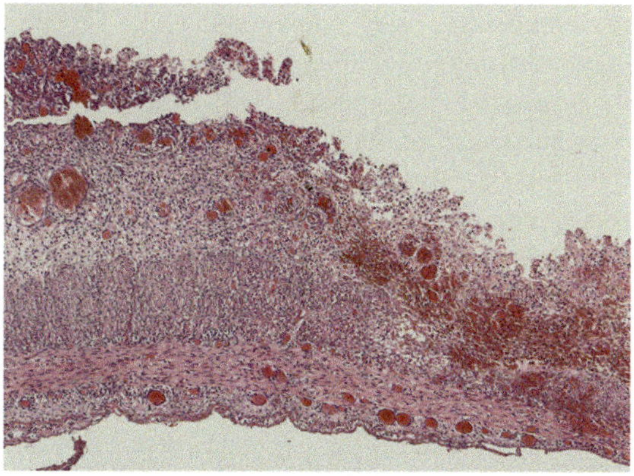

Necrotizing Enterocolitis, Fig. 2 In this medium power H&E stained micrograph, the mucosa is diffusely necrotic, while the mucosa is entirely necrotic on the right side, the basal epithelium appears preserved on the left. The inner layer of the muscular wall on the right is undergoing necrosis and dissolution

intervening spared areas (Fig. 1); half of the cases show a continuous segment of intestine with circumferential necrosis, dilation, and friability. Subserosal collections of gas occasionally are present along the mesenteric border. Gangrenous necrosis occurs on the antimesenteric border, and perforation may be present. If perforation occurs, peritonitis is evident. As the gut heals, thickening of the bowel wall, fibrinous adhesions, and areas of stenosis appear.

Microscopy

Overall microscopic features are similar in most cases of NEC, but the findings vary considerably from one microscopic field to another. The mucosa shows a combination of coagulative necrosis, inflammation, and hemorrhage (Fig. 2). The pathology is limited to the mucosa in the early stages but at least focally transmural in the surgical or autopsy cases. Inflammation and coagulative necrosis often occur together in a given segment, but in some instances, one or the other may predominate. Focal necrotic pseudomembrane formation is seen in approximately 10% of cases. Mixed intestinal bacteria are often visible in the lumen or within the necrotic superficial mucosa. Pneumatosis intestinalis is found in approximately one-half of surgical specimens with NEC, usually limited to the submucosa. These gas bubbles have been shown to contain hydrogen, a product of bacterial fermentation. More than half of the cases undergoing laparotomy show focal reparative epithelial changes and other evidence of healing, such as the formation of granulation tissue and crypt distortion. Villous atrophy may be observed. Intestine compromised by NEC, but not resected during the acute phase of the disease, may develop progressive circumferential submucosal fibrosis during healing, causing intestinal stricture.

Immunophenotype

Immunologic immaturity and immunological dysfunction may play a role in the etiology of the disease.

Molecular Features

Cellular protective mechanisms such as epidermal growth factor, transforming growth factor β1, and erythropoietin are downregulated, further compromising the infant's ability to mount a protective response. Twin studies have suggested susceptibility to NEC may be affected by a genetic component. Animal models have focused on single-nucleotide polymorphisms that negatively affect innate immune responses to bacterial antigens. Infants with distinct genotypes of various cytokines have also been associated with higher frequencies of NEC.

Differential Diagnosis

The histologic findings of neonatal NEC are similar to those of ischemic bowel disease in older children and adults. However, it differs from ordinary ischemic bowel disease in its microscopic features of prominent bacterial colonies and pneumatosis intestinalis. Epidemiologic observations suggest that infection may play a primary role in some cases. Occasional epidemics have been documented to be associated with specific enteric organisms, such as *E. coli, Klebsiella pneumoniae, C. difficile*, and rotavirus. However, most cases of neonatal NEC are sporadic, and in neither the sporadic cases nor in most epidemics is a specific pathogen found.

References and Further Reading

Berman, L., & Moss, R. L. (2011). Necrotizing enterocolitis: An update. *Seminars in Fetal and Neonatal Medicine, 16*, 145–150.

Hunter, C. J., Chokshi, N., & Ford, H. R. (2008). Evidence vs experience in the surgical management of necrotizing enterocolitis and focal intestinal perforation. *Journal of Perinatology, 28*(Suppl 1), S14–S17.

Morgan, J. A., Young, L., & McGuire, W. (2011). Pathogenesis and prevention of necrotizing enterocolitis. *Current Opinion in Infectious Diseases, 24*, 183–189.

Petrosyan, M., Guner, Y. S., Williams, M., Grishin, A., & Ford, H. R. (2009). Current concepts regarding the pathogenesis of necrotizing enterocolitis. *Pediatric Surgery International, 25*, 309–318.

Young, C. M., Kingma, S. D., & Neu, J. (2011). Ischemia-reperfusion and neonatal intestinal injury. *Journal of Pediatrics, 158*(2 Suppl), e25–e28.

Neuroendocrine Neoplasms of the Anus

Denis Chatelain[1] and Jean-François Fléjou[2]
[1]Service d'Anatomie Pathologique, Centre Hospitalier et Universitaire du Nord, Amiens, France
[2]Faculté de Médecine Pierre et Marie Curie, Service d'Anatomie et Cytologie Pathologiques, Hôpital Saint-Antoine, Paris, France

Synonyms

Neuroendocrine carcinoma; Neuroendocrine tumors; Small cell carcinoma

Definition

Neuroendocrine neoplasms very rarely occur in the anus. There is no case of anal carcinoid tumor described in the literature, but some cases have perhaps been assimilated to rectal tumors. There are only rare isolated case reports of anal neuroendocrine carcinoma, small cell neuroendocrine carcinoma, and composite neuroendocrine carcinoma – in situ squamous cell carcinoma or adenocarcinoma published in the literature.

Clinical Features

Patients complain of anal pain, rectal bleeding, and the presence of a perianal mass.

- **Site**
  The neuroendocrine tumors probably arise from neuroendocrine cells residing in colorectal type mucosa or in the anal transitional zone mucosa.
- **Incidence, age, sex**
  Due to the rarity of these tumors, it is difficult to assess the prevalence of this entity, the sex ratio, and the age of patients.

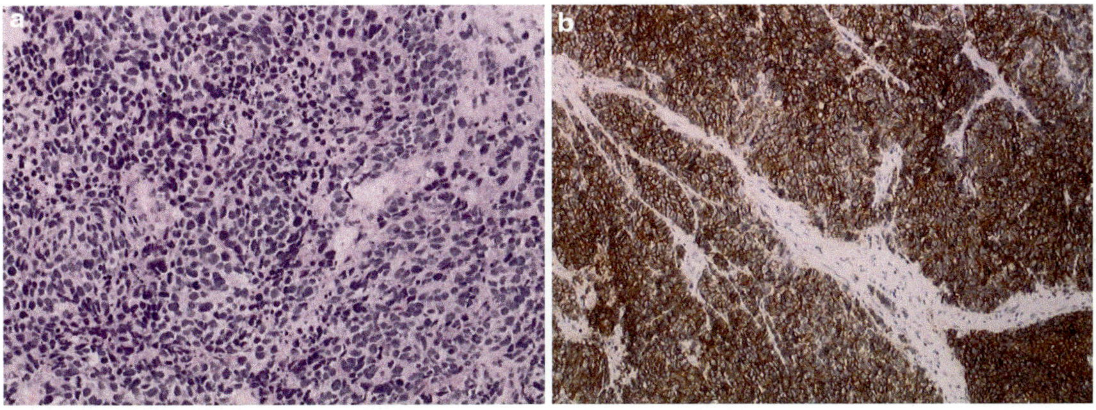

Neuroendocrine Neoplasms of the Anus, Fig. 1 High-grade neuroendocrine carcinoma of the anus (**a**), strongly positive for CD56 – NCAM (**b**)

- **Treatment**
  There is no standard treatment for this rare tumor. A few patients have limited or curative surgical resection such as abdominoperineal resection, but it does not significantly impact the progression of the disease. Chemotherapy consisting of cisplatin and etoposide is often used as palliative therapy.
- **Outcome**
  Well-differentiated neuroendocrine tumors (carcinoid tumors) of the anorectum are usually small, benign tumors, with an indolent clinical course.

  High-grade neuroendocrine carcinomas, small cell or non-small cell type, have an aggressive course and a poor prognosis. Half of the patients have metastases at diagnosis. Some patients develop recurrence, metastases, and die few months after diagnosis or surgery.

Macroscopy

Tumors present as polypoid and or ulcerated, firm, whitish or yellowish masses.

Microscopy

Carcinoid tumors appear as nests, cords with sometimes pseudo-acini in hyaline stroma. They consist of round or cylindrical cells with an eosinophilic cytoplasm having round or oval regular nuclei with no or low mitotic activity.

Cases of anal neuroendocrine carcinoma reported in the literature are usually grade 2 (with 2–20 mitoses per 10 high power fields, and a Ki67 index estimated at 2–20%) or grade 3 (with more than 20 mitoses per 10 HPF and a Ki67 index superior to 20%).

High-grade neuroendocrine carcinoma consists of nests or sheets of round or cylindrical cells with nuclear pleomorphism, a high mitotic activity, and often foci of necrosis (Fig. 1a). It is often a small cell neuroendocrine carcinoma, consisting of small round cells with scant cytoplasm, a markedly high nuclear cytoplasmic ratio, and hyperchromatic nuclei with finely granular chromatin and inconspicuous or rarely conspicuous nucleoli. Mitoses are numerous, and there are foci of necrosis.

Immunohistochemical Features

Neuroendocrine tumors show positive staining for pan-cytokeratin, EMA and neuroendocrine markers: chromogranin A, synaptophysin, and CD56 (Fig. 1b). Ki67 is useful to determine the proliferative index. Small cell carcinoma of the anus may show immunoreactivity for thyroid transcription factor-1 (TTF-1).

Differential Diagnosis

Anorectal carcinoid tumors with a tubular pattern may be confused with conventional adenocarcinoma. High-grade neuroendocrine carcinoma may be confused with poorly differentiated adenocarcinoma, basaloid squamous cell carcinoma, or melanoma.

This may be particularly problematic in biopsy samples so that immunohistochemical neuroendocrine markers are helpful to confirm the diagnosis of neuroendocrine neoplasm.

Cross-References

▶ Paget's Disease of the Anus
▶ Squamous Cell Carcinoma, Anus

References and Further Reading

Eberhardt, J. M., Brown, K., Lo, S., Nagda, S., & Yong, S. (2012). Extrapulmonary small cell carcinoma of the anal canal: A case report and review of the literature. *Case Reports in Medicine, 2012*, 341432.

Shia, J. (2010). An update on tumors of the anal canal. *Archives of Pathology & Laboratory Medicine, 134*, 1601–1611.

Neuroendocrine Tumor, Colon and Rectum

Ozgul Sagol
Department of Pathology, Dokuz Eylul University Medical School, Inciralti, Izmir, Turkey

Synonyms

Carcinoid tumor; Endocrine neoplasm; Neuroendocrine carcinoma; Neuroendocrine neoplasm

Definition

Neuroendocrine neoplasia (NEN) is a general term including broad family of neoplasms originating in neural and endocrine structures. NEN may be localized in pure endocrine organs (thyroid, parathyroid, and adrenal glands), nerve plexuses, extraadrenal paraganglia (paragangliomas), and diffuse endocrine system in different organs including gastrointestinal tract. Fourteen different cell types, producing variety of hormones, have been described as components of diffuse endocrine system. Neuroendocrine cells of diffuse endocrine system that give rise to gastrointestinal NENs are endodermally derived and originate from gastrointestinal stem cells. Neuroendocrine cells and their neoplastic counterparts secrete peptide hormones and biogenic amines. Besides, with electron microscopy, typical large neurosecretory granules and small synaptic like vesicles are shown in their cytoplasm. These structures are also observed in neurons. NENs are composed of one or more of these neuroendocrine cell types. Neuroendocrine nature of tumor cells is revealed by identification of general markers of neuroendocrine differentiation by immunohistochemistry. Additionally these tumors have some histologic patterns enabling them to be recognized as neuroendocrine tumors.

Specific hormones can also be detected in tumor cells by immunohistochemistry. NENs of the colon and rectum are either of enterochromaffin (EC) cell type or L cell type. EC cell NENs occur mainly in the right colon and are characterized by serotonin production. Functioning tumors in the colon and rectum are extremely rare.

NENs of the colon and rectum are classified and graded according to WHO 2010. Three types of entities are recognized: neuroendocrine tumor (NET, G1, and G2), neuroendocrine carcinoma (NEC, G3), and mixed adenoneuroendocrine carcinoma (MANEC). These categories are distinguished by tumor grading which is based on the detection of the proliferative capacity of tumors as well as morphology. Rectal NENs are commonly small and generally low to intermediate grade (Grades 1 or 2), whereas colonic NENs are often aggressive, poorly differentiated, and higher grade (G3), although well differentiated NETs occur in colon as well. Rectal NETs are more frequent than small intestinal NETs. The incidence of multicentric NETs of the colon is low.

NECs primarily occur in the cecum. They usually present in advanced stage and have high capacity of lymph node and distant metastasis.

Clinical Features

- **Incidence**
  The incidence of colonic NETs in the US SEER database is approximately 0.2 per 100,000. In Europe, the reported incidence is 0.06 per 100,000. Colonic NETs account for 7.5% of all NETs in US series while 4–7% in European series and 8% in Asian series.
  NETs of the rectum have been increasing in incidence. The latest SEER report revealed an incidence of 0.86 per 100,000. Rectal NETs account for 18% of all NETs and 27% of all gastrointestinal NETs. Rectal NETs reported in Europe is 5–14% of all NETs. In Asia, rectal NETS accounted for 60–89% of all gastrointestinal carcinoids.
  NECs comprise approximately 0.6% of all carcinomas of large bowel.
- **Age**
  For colonic NETs the mean age of diagnosis is approximately 55–65 years. Rectal NETs are diagnosed in relatively younger patients, with a mean age at diagnosis of 56.2 years.
- **Sex**
  Rectal NETs are more common in women in US population.
- **Site**
  NETs are more common in rectum (54%) followed by cecum (20%), sigmoid colon (7.5%), rectosigmoid (5.5%), and ascending colon (5%). NECs are located either in the right colon or rectosigmoid.
- **Treatment**
  Rectal NETS (<2 cm) are treated by endoscopic resection techniques (simple polypectomy, endoscopic mucosal resection with modified EMR-band ligation, endoscopic submucosal dissection, and transanal endoscopic microsurgery). Rectal tumors (>2 cm), T3 or T4 stage, with G3 grading or rectal tumors with lymph node involvement, are treated like adenocarcinomas. Colonic tumors >2 cm, tumors with muscular invasion, and G3 tumors are also treated like adenocarcinomas.
  Chemotherapy is appropriate for G3 NECs but has little role in G1 and G2 colorectal NETs.
- **Outcome**
  NETs of rectum and cecum are likely to have metastasized to regional lymph nodes or cause distant metastasis if they are larger than 2 cm and have invaded muscularis propria. Rectal tumors less than 1 cm have a very low risk of metastasis. Between 1 and 2 cm, the risk of metastasis is 5%. Endoscopic transanal excision is curative. 5-year survival rate was reported as 100% for rectal NETs less than 2 cm and did not invade the muscular mucosa. Larger rectal tumors carry a higher malignant potential with subsequent metastases to bone, lymph nodes, and liver. Overall, distant metastases from rectal NETs occur in only 2.3% of cases.
  About 40% of colonic NETs have metastases at the time of diagnosis. Metastases are frequently found in the liver, lymph nodes, mesentery, or peritoneum and patients have a 5-year survival rate of about 43–50%.

Macroscopy

Well-differentiated rectal tumors are mostly found incidentally during endoscopy as small (50% <1 cm) moveable submucosal tumors. In the majority of cases, the neoplasm is found 4–13 cm above the dentate line and on the anterior and lateral wall. NETs of the colon are usually located in the cecum. They are usually larger than tumors in small intestine, appendix, and rectum (average size: 4.9 cm). In cases of ulcerative colitis, NETs occur throughout the colon. Colonic NETs can also be found together with Crohn's disease, polypous colonic adenomas, and colorectal carcinomas. Their appearance is of yellowish polypoid or flat doughnut-shaped lesion but there may be central ulceration especially in tumors larger than 2 cm.

Colorectal NECs are grossly similar to adenocarcinomas. They may be polypoid if associated with adenoma or they may be infiltrative.

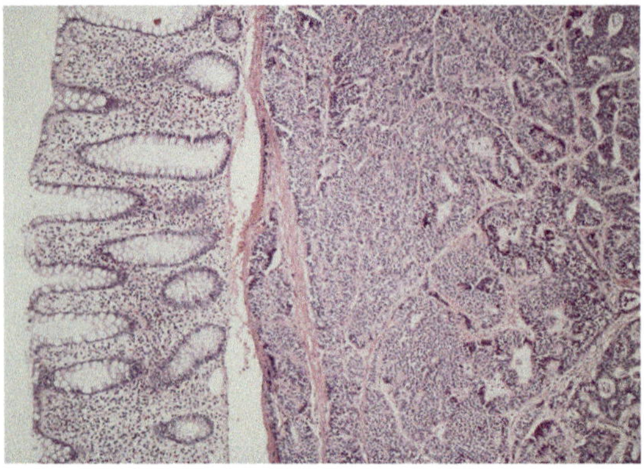

Neuroendocrine Tumor, Colon and Rectum, Fig. 1 Rectal polypoid NET (Grade 1) (100×, H&E)

Microscopy

The microscopic features are related to tumor differentiation and tumor grade. Well-differentiated NETs with low to intermediate proliferative rate are composed of monomorphic, medium sized cells with abundant, eosinophilic, finely granular cytoplasm. The nuclei of tumor cells are regular and have clumped chromatin pattern. Mitoses are rare. In colonic NETs, tumor cells grow as solid nests with peripheral palisading, sometimes with formation of rosettes and cribriform patterns. A prominent desmoplastic stroma frequently surrounds tumor cell nests. NETs of rectum are characterized by a trabecular pattern sometimes with rosettes and tubular structures. The stromal reaction is minimal. Most of these tumors belong to grade G1 category (Fig. 1).

Poorly differentiated NECs (PDNECs) with high proliferative rate are mostly located in cecum and classified as small and large cell types according to cell size and nuclear characteristics. The nuclei of small cell type are usually fusiform and show hyperchromasia, finely granular chromatin pattern, inconspicuous or absent nucleoli, and frequent mitosis. The cytoplasm is sometimes evident, narrow, and eosinophilic. These tumors have a more diffuse architecture. There is usually single cell or geographic necrosis. Large cell NECs more typically demonstrate a nested architecture and prominent nucleoli. In colon and rectum, 75% of NECs are large cell type but in anal region small cell type predominates. In colon, NECs are frequently (61%) associated with adenocarcinoma (Fig. 2). If one of the components exceeds 30%, it qualifies for the diagnosis of MANEC. At least 2 neuroendocrine markers must be diffusely positive in order to establish a diagnosis of large cell NEC.

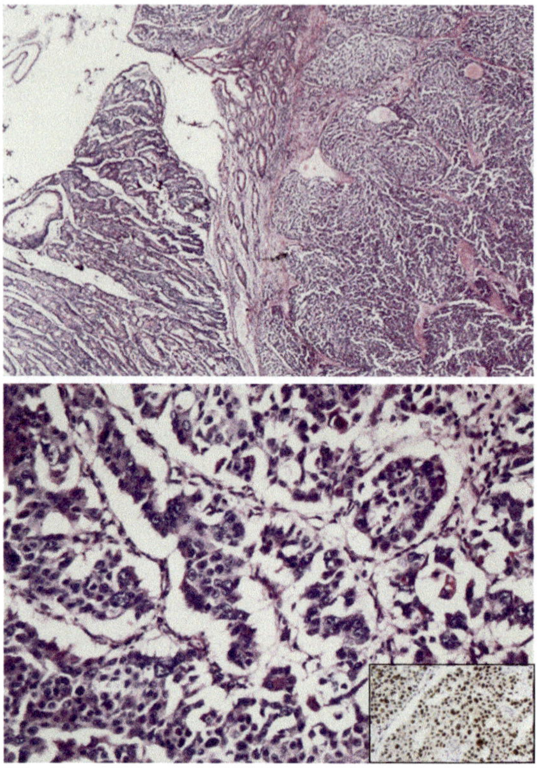

Neuroendocrine Tumor, Colon and Rectum, Fig. 2 Colonic NEC with focal (<30%) adenocarcinoma component (20×, H&E). NEC component large cell type (100×, H&E) with high Ki-67 index

The grading and staging of colorectal NENs are similar to their small intestinal counterparts.

Immunophenotype

NETs of rectum are positive for synaptophysin, glucagon, glicentin, and pancreatic polypeptide, whereas they are usually negative for chromogranin A. Cecal NETs are positive with serotonin, synaptophysin, and chromogranin A.

Prostatic acid phosphatase is positive in most of colorectal NETs.

Molecular Features

Loss of heterozygosity at the MEN-1 gene locus is rare in colorectal NETs. Colorectal NECs display abnormalities in p53 and CDKN2/Rb pathways, FHIT (3p), DCC/SMAD 4(18q), and MEN 1. NECs of small cell type often show loss of expression of RB gene product.

Differential Diagnosis

NETs must be differentiated from low grade adenocarcinomas especially in endoscopic biopsies. NECs especially of large cell type must be differentiated from poorly differentiated carcinomas.

References and Further Reading

Caplin, M., Sundin, A., Nillson, O., Baum, R. P., Klose, K. J., Kelestimur, F., Plöckinger, U., Papotti, M., Salazar, R., Pascher, A., all other Barcelona Consensus Conference participants. (2012). ENETS consensus guidelines for the management of patients with digestive neuroendocrine neoplasms: Colorectal neuroendocrine neoplasms. *Neuroendocrinology, 95*, 88–97.

Klimstra, D. S. (2016). Pathologic classification of neuroendocrine neoplasms. *Hematology/Oncology Clinics of North America, 30*, 1–19.

Klimstra, D. S., Arnold, R., Capella, C., Kloppel, G., Komminoth, P., Solcia, E., & Rind, G. (2010). Neuroendocrine neoplasms of the colon and rectum. In T. F. Bosman, F. Carneiro, R. H. Hruban, & N. D. Theise (Eds.), *WHO classification of tumors of the digestive system* (pp. 174–177). Lyon: International Agency for Research on Cancer.

Kloppel, G. (2011). Classification and pathology of gastroenteropancreatic neuroendocrine neoplasms. *Endocrine-Related Cancer, 18*, S1–S16.

Kloppel, G., Rindi, G., Anlauf, M., Perren, A., & Komminoth, P. (2007). Site specific biology and pathology of gastroenteropancreatic neuroendocrine tumors. *Virchows Archiv, 451*(suppl 1), S9–S27.

Rindi, G., & Wiedenmann, B. (2012). Neuroendocrine neoplasms of the gut and pancreas: New insights. *Nature Reviews Endrocrinology, 8*, 54–64.

Neuroendocrine Tumor, Esophagus

José Manuel Lopes
Faculty of Medicine of the University of Porto and Institute of Molecular Pathology and Immunology of the University of Porto, Porto, Portugal

Synonyms

Mixed adenoneuroendocrine carcinomas (MANECs); Neuroendocrine carcinoma (NECs); Neuroendocrine tumors (NETs)

Definition

Neuroendocrine neoplasms of the digestive system (Rindi et al. 2010), namely, in the esophagus, include (1) Neuroendocrine tumors (***NETs***) – carcinoids and well-differentiated endocrine tumors/carcinomas; (2) Neuroendocrine carcinomas (***NECs***) – poorly differentiated endocrine carcinomas, high-grade neuroendocrine carcinomas, and small-cell and large-cell endocrine carcinomas; and (3) Mixed adenoneuroendocrine carcinomas (***MANECs***) (Arnold et al. 2010); there are also hyperplastic and preneoplastic neuroendocrine lesions. **NETs** are well-differentiated neuroendocrine neoplasms comprising cells with similar features to those of the normal gut endocrine cells, expressing markers of neuroendocrine differentiation (e.g., diffuse and intense chromogranin A and synaptophysin) and hormones, with mild-to-moderate nuclear atypia and low mitotic index and/or low Ki67(proliferation-related antigen) index, including the following: (1) ***NET G1*** (grade 1) displays <2/10 high power field (HPF) mitotic index and/or ≤2% Ki67 index (this is the only situation where the use of the term *carcinoid* may be accepted) and (2) ***NET G2*** (grade 2) displays 2–20/10 high power field mitotic index and/or 3–20% Ki67 index. **NECs** are poorly differentiated malignant neoplasms comprising small, intermediate to large cells, sometimes resembling neuroendocrine tumor, expressing markers of neuroendocrine differentiation (e.g., diffuse synaptophysin and focal chromogranin A), with marked nuclear atypia, multifocal necrosis, and >20/10 high power field mitotic index and/or >20% Ki67 index (grade 3 (G3)). **MANECs** are malignant neoplasms comprising both epithelial gland (rarely squamous) and neuroendocrine components, with at least 30% of either component, that should be graded separately. Grading of neuroendocrine neoplasms of the digestive system is mandatory for their classification (Rindi et al. 2006, 2007).

Clinical Features

- **Incidence**
  Neuroendocrine neoplasms of esophagus are very rare (<0.1%) and most reported cases are neuroendocrine carcinomas or mixed adenoneuroendocrine carcinomas.
- **Age**
  Most reported cases occur in the sixth/seventh decades.
- **Sex**
  The male/female ratio is 6:1 or higher.
- **Site**
  Most neuroendocrine neoplasms occur in the distal (lower third of the) esophagus. Neuroendocrine carcinomas associate with Barrett esophagus. Neuroendocrine tumors are often incidental findings in Barrett esophagus, heterotopic oxyntic mucosa, and esophagus adenocarcinoma.
- **Treatment**
  Safe treatment of small (<1.5 cm) neuroendocrine tumors aiming R0 margin status may be accomplished with endoscopic resection (Arnold et al. 2010). Due to the rarity of neuroendocrine carcinomas and mixed adenoneuroendocrine carcinomas, there are no established guidelines for their treatment. Surgery (subtotal esophagectomy or subtotal variants), neoadjuvant, and other therapies should be personalized based on several parameters, including the histological subtype, grade, and tumor node metastasis (TNM)/stage of each primary, recurrent/metastatic neuroendocrine neoplasm.
- **Outcome**
  The prognosis of patients with neuroendocrine esophagus neoplasms seems to associate with histologic subtype, grade, and stage. The tumor node metastasis and residual tumor (TNMR)/stage system for these neoplasms is the same used for other carcinomas of the esophagus. The limited data available indicates that neuroendocrine carcinomas and mixed adenoneuroendocrine carcinomas bear poor (may give <1 year overall survival) and neuroendocrine tumors better (possible clinical remission after surgical/endoscopic R0 resection of localized neoplasms) prognosis, depending on grade/stage (Arnold et al. 2010).

Macroscopy

Neuroendocrine tumors are small and polypoid (***NET G1***) or may be large ulcerous-infiltrative masses (***NET G2***). Neuroendocrine carcinomas and mixed adenoneuroendocrine carcinomas are usually large (>4 cm), exophytic, and/or ulcerated masses that extend along and infiltrate the esophagus wall (Arnold et al. 2010).

Microscopy

Neuroendocrine tumors (see section “Definitions”) comprise tumor cells with small, rounded, uniform nuclei and moderate cytoplasm, with variable insular, solid nest, acinar, trabecular, and cribriform patterns. Most are found incidentally in association with Barrett esophagus and adenocarcinomas. Neuroendocrine carcinomas (see section definition) associate also with Barrett esophagus; comprise small round to spindle tumor cells with scant or more cytoplasm (intermediate cells), ill-defined cell borders, round or oval hyperchromatic finely granular nuclei with molding, absent or inconspicuous nucleolus; and form solid sheets and nests (small-cell neuroendocrine carcinomas) (Fig. 1); foci of squamous and/or mucoepidermoid differentiation may be

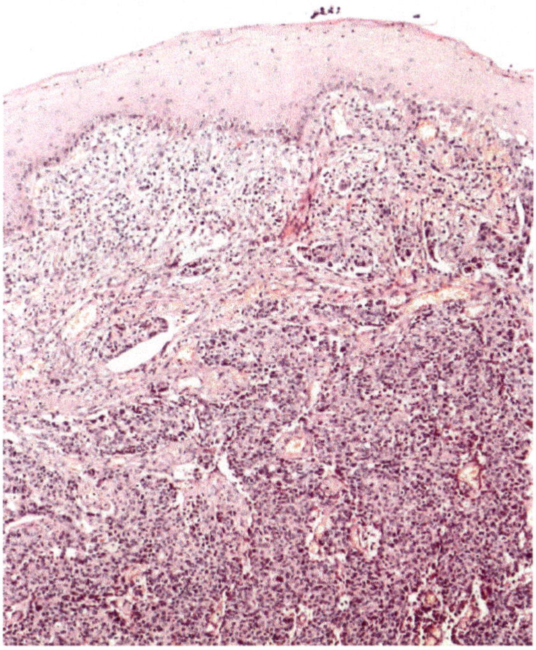

Neuroendocrine Tumor, Esophagus, Fig. 1 Esophagus neuroendocrine carcinoma. Note the absence of intraepithelial neoplasia

observed. Large-cell neuroendocrine carcinomas comprise large to intermediate cells, with low nucleus/cytoplasm ratio, eosinophilic cytoplasm, and vesicular nuclei with evident nucleoli and display organoid pattern with solid nests or acinar structures. Mixed adenoneuroendocrine carcinomas (see definitions) may combine a neuroendocrine carcinoma (very rarely a neuroendocrine tumor) with (mostly) adenocarcinoma or squamous carcinoma (Arnold et al. 2010).

Immunophenotype

See definitions. Neuroendocrine neoplasms express low-molecular-weight keratins. Neuroendocrine tumors may express vesicular monoamine transporter, indicating enterochromaffin phenotype. Neuroendocrine carcinomas/mixed adenoneuroendocrine carcinomas express CD56 (cluster differentiation molecule 56), CD57 (cluster differentiation antigen 57 (Leu-7)), NSE (neuron-specific enolase), and rarely TTF1 (transcription termination factor 1), calcitonin, ACTH (adrenocorticotrophic hormone), and other hormones.

Molecular Features

There are no consistent available molecular data for neuroendocrine esophagus neoplasms.

Differential Diagnosis

The diagnosis of neuroendocrine neoplasms is usually straightforward based on adequate clinical/imaging evaluation, sampling, histology, and immunohistochemistry studies. Small-cell neuroendocrine carcinomas should be distinguished from poorly differentiated squamous cell carcinoma, basaloid squamous carcinoma, malignant lymphoma, and secondary invasion of primary small-cell carcinoma of the lung.

References and Further Reading

Arnold, R., Capella, C., Klimstra, D. S., Kloppel, G., Kominoth, P., Solcia, E., & Rindi, G. (2010). Neuroendocrine neoplasms of the esophagus. In F. T. Bosman, F. Carneiro, R. H. Hruban, & N. E. Theise (Eds.), *WHO classification of tumours of the digestive system* (pp. 32–34). Lyon: International Agency for Research on Cancer (IARC).

Rindi, G., Kloppel, G., Alhman, H., Caplin, M., Couvelard, A., de Herder, W. W., Erikssson, B., Falchetti, A., Falconi, M., Komminoth, P., Korner, M., Lopes, J. M., McNicol, A. M., Nilsson, O., Perren, A., Scarpa, A., Scoazec, J. Y., Wiedenmann, B., & Frascati Consensus Conference P. (2006). TNM staging of foregut (neuro) endocrine tumors: A consensus proposal including a grading system. *Virchows Archiv, 449*, 395–401.

Rindi, G., Kloppel, G., Couvelard, A., Kommonoth, P., Korner, M., Lopes, J. M., NcNicol, A. M., Nilsson, O., Perren, A., Scarpa, A., Scoazec, J. Y., & Wiedenmann, B. (2007). TNM staging of midgut and hindgut (neuro) endocrine tumors: A consensus proposal including a grading system. *Virchows Archiv, 451*, 757–762.

Rindi, G., Arnold, R., Bosman, F. T., Capella, C., Klimstra, D. S., Kloppel, G., & Solcia, E. (2010). Nomenclature and classification of neuroendocrine neoplasms of the digestive system. In F. T. Bosman, F. Carneiro, R. H. Hruban, & N. E. Theise (Eds.), *WHO classification of tumours of the digestive system* (pp. 13–14). Lyon: International Agency for Research on Cancer (IARC).

Neuroendocrine Tumor, Gastric

José Manuel Lopes
Faculty of Medicine of the University of Porto and Institute of Molecular Pathology and Immunology of the University of Porto, Porto, Portugal

Synonyms

Mixed adenoneuroendocrine carcinomas (MANECs); Neuroendocrine carcinomas (NECs); Neuroendocrine tumors (NETs)

Definition

Neuroendocrine neoplasms of the digestive system (Rindi et al. 2010), namely, in the stomach (g-NENs), include (1) Neuroendocrine tumors (NETs) – carcinoids and well-differentiated endocrine tumors/carcinomas; (2) Neuroendocrine carcinomas (NECs): poorly differentiated endocrine carcinomas, high-grade neuroendocrine carcinomas, small-cell and large-cell endocrine carcinomas; and (3) Mixed adenoneuroendocrine carcinomas (MANECs) (Solcia et al. 2010); there are also hyperplastic and preneoplastic neuroendocrine lesions. **Precursor neuroendocrine lesions** of the stomach that occur in hypergastrinemic conditions (autoimmune chronic atrophic gastritis, multiple endocrine neoplasia type 1, and Zollinger-Ellison syndrome) include (a) enterochromaffin-like cell *(ECL) hyperplasia* (linear, micronodular <150 μm, and adenomatoid) and (b) *dysplasia* (enlarged micronodules >150 μm, fused micronodules, microinfiltration of lamina propria, association with new stroma). **Micro-NETs** are neuroendocrine neoplasms >0.5 mm or with invasion of submucosa, but <0.5 cm in largest dimension. **NETs** are well-differentiated neuroendocrine neoplasms ≥0.5 cm largest dimension, comprising cells with similar features to those of the normal gut endocrine cells, expressing markers of neuroendocrine differentiation (e.g., diffuse and intense chromogranin A and synaptophysin) and hormones, with mild-to-moderate nuclear atypia and low mitotic index and/or low Ki67(proliferation-related antigen) index: (a) ***NET G1*** (grade 1) displays <2/10 high power field mitotic index and/or ≤ 2% Ki67 index (this is the only situation where the use of the term *carcinoid* may be accepted), and (b) ***NET G2*** (grade 2) displays 2–20/10 high power field mitotic index and/or 3–20% Ki67 index. Most **g-NENs** comprise non-functioning enterochromaffin-like (ECL) cells and encompass three distinct types: (1*) **type I*** (often NET G1), associated with achlorhydria secondary to autoimmune atrophic fundic gastritis (A-CAG); (2) ***type II*** (NET G1-G2), associated with hypergastrinemia resulting from neoplastic secretion from gastrinomas (Zollinger-Ellison syndrome – ZES), mostly in patients with multiple endocrine neoplasia type 1 (MEN1); and (3) ***type III*** (mostly NEC G3) (Fave et al. 2012), sporadic, not associated with autoimmune atrophic fundic gastritis or MEN1-ZES. **NECs** are poorly differentiated malignant neoplasms comprising small, intermediate to large cells, sometimes resembling neuroendocrine tumor, expressing markers of neuroendocrine differentiation (e.g., diffuse synaptophysin and focal chromogranin A), with marked nuclear atypia, multifocal necrosis, and >20/10 high power field mitotic index and/or >20% Ki67 index (G3). **MANECs** are malignant neoplasms comprising both epithelial gland (rarely squamous) and neuroendocrine components, with at least 30% of either component, that should be graded separately. Grading of neuroendocrine neoplasms of the digestive system is mandatory for their classification (Rindi et al. 2006, 2007).

Clinical Features

- **Incidence**
  Neuroendocrine tumors show an incremental trend incidence up to 0.18–0.24/100 000 Caucasians/year, higher in African Americans, reaching 11–41% of the digestive neuroendocrine neoplasms (Solcia et al. 2010). Gastric neuroendocrine neoplasias (g-NENs) include

type I neoplasms (50–75%), type II (25–50%), type III (mostly G3), and neuroendocrine carcinomas (<1–3%); enterochromaffin, gastrin, and ghrelin cell tumors comprise < 1% of g-NENs (Fave et al. 2012). Neuroendocrine carcinomas and mixed adenoneuroendocrine carcinomas account for 6–12% g-NENs (Solcia et al. 2010).

- **Age**
  NETs type I, mean age 63 years (range, 15–88); type II, mean age 50 years (range, 28–67); type III, mean age 55 years (range, 21–38). NECs/MANECs: mean age 63 years (range, 41–61) (Solcia et al. 2010).
- **Sex**
  Male/Female ratio: NETs type I (1:2.5), type II (1:1), and type III (2.8:1); NECs/MANECs (2:1) (Solcia et al. 2010).
- **Site**
  Type I, type II, and type III g-NENs: gastric body-fundus or body-antrum border; gastrin cell neuroendocrine tumors in antropyloric region, EC cell tumors in any gastric region, and the only reported ghrelin cell tumor in the corpus; gastrin cell neuroendocrine tumors in the antropyloric region; neuroendocrine carcinomas; and mixed adenoneuroendocrine carcinomas in any gastric site (Solcia et al. 2010).
- **Treatment**
  NETs type 1: conservative based on endoscopic follow-up and/or polypectomy of tumors; endoscopic ultrasound evaluation particularly if tumor >1 cm and when there is neither evidence of involvement beyond submucosa nor evidence of lymph node involvement, polypectomy/endoscopic mucosal resection; safe surgical resection (local resection, antrectomy, and total gastrectomy) should be based on surgical margin status, location, and stage for NET types I and II. For NETs type III, neuroendocrine carcinomas, and mixed adenoneuroendocrine carcinomas, surgical treatment should follow the same principles as for gastric adenocarcinomas.
- **Outcome**
  NETs type I usually have an excellent prognosis (80–100% survival) (Solcia et al. 2010; Fave et al. 2012) when managed by endoscopic follow-up and tumor resection; there is a median recurrence-free survival of 24 months and 3% develop neuroendocrine carcinoma (Fave et al. 2012); 5% develop lymph node metastases (Solcia et al. 2010). NETs type II have a metastatic rate of 10–30% (Solcia et al. 2010) mostly in lymph nodes (30%) (Solcia et al. 2010) and liver (Fave et al. 2012); mortality rate is <10%. NETs type III have a metastatic rate of 50–100% and a mortality of 25–30% (Fave et al. 2012). Neuroendocrine carcinomas have usually poor prognosis and short survival (Solcia et al. 2010).

Macroscopy

NETs type I: small (most <1 cm, often <1–2 cm), multiple (65%), and polypoid (78%) in the mucosa; less often in the submucosa; and 7% involving the muscularis propria. NETS type II: often <1–2 cm, 75% <1.5 cm, multiple, and polypoid mucosal-submucosal tumors associated with thickened gastric wall. NETs type III: single, >2 cm (33%), polypoid, and ulcerated, with infiltration of the muscularis propria (76%) and the serosa (53%). Neuroendocrine carcinomas and mixed adenoneuroendocrine carcinomas present features similar to gastric adenocarcinomas (Solcia et al. 2010).

Microscopy

NETs (see definitions) comprise tumor cells with regular uniform nuclei, usually unapparent nucleoli, and moderate eosinophilic cytoplasm, with variable microlobular-tabecular (Figs. 1 and 2), mosaic-like, solid nests, and gyriform patterns. NETs type I associate with complete or near-complete (type A) gastric atrophy with extensive intestinal metaplasia of the gastric body-fundus; ECL cell (diffuse, linear, and micronodular) hyperplasia may be observed in up to 30% of the cases, and dysplasia in 6% (see definitions). NETs type II associate with hypertrophic-hypersecretory-type gastropathy. NETs type III display solid or large trabecular patterns comprising round to spindle and polyedric tumor cells with large vesicular nuclei

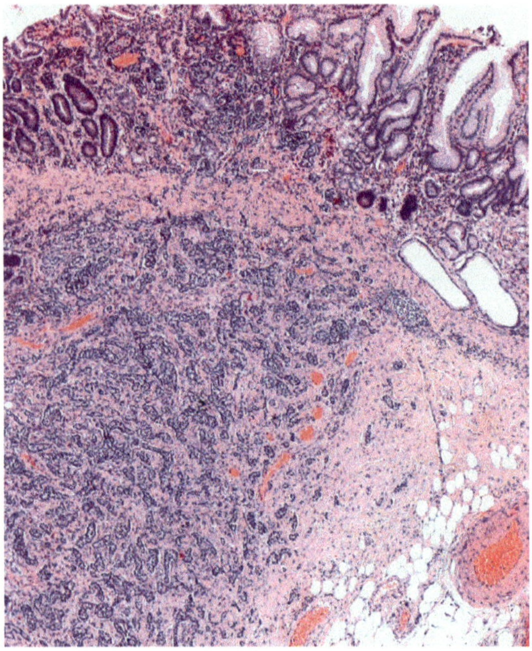

Neuroendocrine Tumor, Gastric, Fig. 1 Low power features of gastric NET

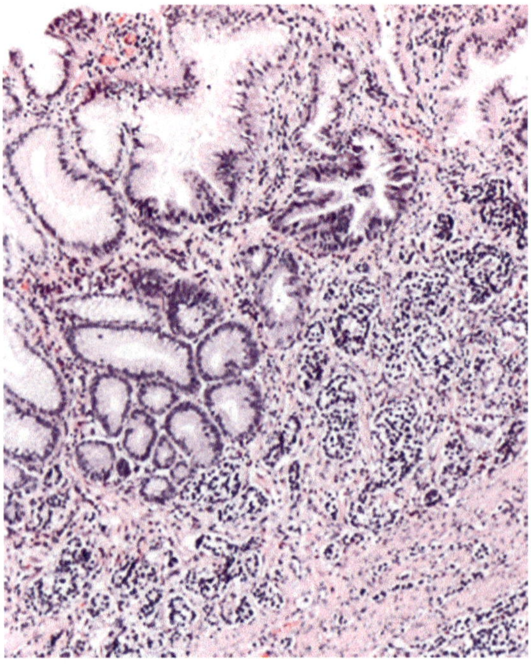

Neuroendocrine Tumor, Gastric, Fig. 2 High power view of monotonous neoplastic cells of gastric neuroendocrine tumor

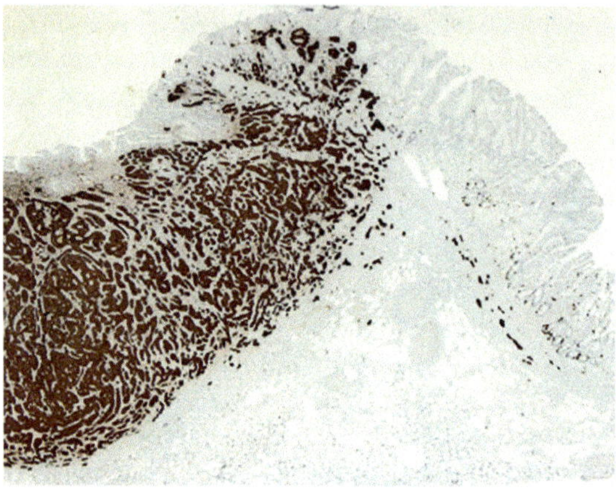

Neuroendocrine Tumor, Gastric, Fig. 3 Low power features of diffuse chromogranin A expression in gastric NET

and prominent nucleoli or small hyperchromatic nuclei with chromatin clumps and small nucleoli. NECs (see definitions) comprise small round to spindle tumor cells with scant or more cytoplasm (intermediate cells), ill-defined cell borders, and round or oval hyperchromatic finely granular nuclei with molding, absent, or inconspicuous nucleolus and form solid sheets and nests (small-cell NECs). Large cell NECs comprise large to intermediate cells, with low nucleus/cytoplasm ratio, eosinophilic cytoplasm, vesicular nuclei with evident nucleoli, and organoid pattern. MANECs (see definitions) may combine a NEC (often of large-cell type) with (usually) adenocarcinoma (Solcia et al. 2010).

Immunophenotype

See definitions. Neuroendocrine neoplasms express low-molecular-weight keratins, chromogranin A (Fig. 3), and synaptophysin. NETs may express vesicular monoamine transporter (ECL cells), serotonin, ghrelin, gastrin, somatostatin, pancreatic polypeptide, and alpha-human chorionic gonadotrophin. NETs type III express (tumor suppressor protein 53) p53 (60%). NECs/MANECs express CD56 (cluster differentiation molecule 56) and NSE (neuron-specific enolase).

Molecular Features

NETs type II: LOH (loss of heterozygosity) at 11q13 in patients with MEN1 (multiple endocrine neoplasia type 1); differences in deletion size from multiple NETs in the same stomach suggest their multiclonal origin. Less than half of non-MEN 1 NETs display LOH at 11q13 and 11q14. Mutation of *MEN1* is rare in sporadic g-NENs. Mutations of *REG1A* (*regenerating islet-derived 1 gene*) occur in ECL NETs type I. Minimal deletion region restricted to Xq25 and Xq26 occurs in NETs and NECs. *TP53* (*tumor suppressor protein 53), FHIT* (*fragile histidine triad), DCC* (*deleted in colorectal cancer), SMAD4/dpc4* (*deleted in pancreatic carcinoma, locus 4)*, and *MEN1* gene alterations are more frequent in NECs than in NETs. Mixed adenoneuroendocrine carcinomas seem to display higher frequency of chromosomal alterations than neuroendocrine carcinomas.

Differential Diagnosis

The diagnosis of neuroendocrine neoplasms is usually straightforward based on adequate clinical/imaging evaluation, sampling, histology, and immunohistochemistry studies. Small-cell neuroendocrine carcinomas should be distinguished from basaloid squamous carcinoma, malignant lymphoma, and secondary involvement of primary small-cell carcinoma from other location.

References and Further Reading

Fave, G. D., Kwekkeboom, D. K., Cutsem, E. V., Rindi, G., Kos-Kudla, B., Knigge, U., Sasano, H., Tomasseti, P., Salazar, R., Ruszniewski, P., & Barcelona Consensus Conference participants. (2012). ENETS consensus guidelines for the management of patients with gastroduodenal neoplasms. *Neuroendocrinology, 95*, 74–87.

Rindi, G., Kloppel, G., Alhman, H., Caplin, M., Couvelard, A., de Herder, W. W., Erikssson, B., Falchetti, A., Falconi, M., Komminoth, P., Korner, M., Lopes, J. M., McNicol, A. M., Nilsson, O., Perren, A., Scarpa, A., Scoazec, J. Y., Wiedenmann, B., & Frascati Consensus Conference Participants. (2006). TNM staging of foregut (neuro)endocrine tumors: A consensus proposal including a grading system. *Virchows Archiv, 449*, 395–401.

Rindi, G., Kloppel, G., Couvelard, A., Kommonoth, P., Korner, M., Lopes, J. M., NcNicol, A. M., Nilsson, O., Perren, A., Scarpa, A., Scoazec, J. Y., & Wiedenmann, B. (2007). TNM staging of midgut and hindgut (neuro) endocrine tumors: A consensus proposal including a grading system. *Virchows Archiv, 451*, 757–762.

Rindi, G., Arnold, R., Bosman, F. T., Capella, C., Klimstra, D. S., Kloppel, G., & Solcia, E. (2010). Nomenclature and classification of neuroendocrine neoplasms of the digestive system. In F. T. Bosman, F. Carneiro, R. H. Hruban, & N. E. Theise (Eds.), *WHO classification of tumours of the digestive system* (pp. 13–14). Lyon: International Agency for Research on Cancer (IARC).

Solcia, E., Arnold, R., Capella, C., Klimstra, D. S., Kloppel, G., Kominoth, P., & Rindi, G. (2010). Neuroendocrine neoplasms of Stomach. In F. T. Bosman, F. Carneiro, R. H. Hruban, & N. E. Theise (Eds.), *WHO classification of tumours of the digestive system* (pp. 64–68). Lyon: International Agency for Research on Cancer (IARC).

Neuroendocrine Tumor, Small Intestine

Ozgul Sagol
Department of Pathology, Dokuz Eylul University Medical School, Inciralti, Izmir, Turkey

N

Synonyms

Carcinoid tumor; Endocrine neoplasm; Neuroendocrine carcinoma; Neuroendocrine neoplasm

Definition

Neuroendocrine neoplasm (NEN) is a general term including a broad family of neoplasms with neural and endocrine features. NENs may be localized in pure endocrine organs (tyroid, parathyroid and adrenal glands), nerve plexuses, extraadrenal paraganglia (paragangliomas) and diffuse endocrine system in different organs including gastrointestinal tract. Fourteen different cell types, producing variety of hormones have been described as components of diffuse endocrine system. Neuroendocrine cells of diffuse endocrine system that give rise to small intestinal

NENs are endodermally derived and originate from gastrointestinal stem cells. Neuroendocrine cells and their neoplastic counterparts, secrete peptide hormones and biogenic amines. On electron microscopy, typical large neurosecretory granules and small synaptic like vesicles are found in their cytoplasm. These structures are also observed in neurons. NENs are composed of one or more of these neuroendocrine cell types. Neuroendocrine nature of tumor cells is based on the identification of general markers of neuroendocrine differentiation. Additionally, these tumors have some histologic patterns enabling them to be recognized as neuroendocrine tumors.

Specific hormones (Somatostatin, gastrin, glucagon, etc.) can also be detected in tumor cells by immunohistochemistry. Tumors causing a clinical syndrome (functional tumors) by excess production of a specific hormone are named by adding -oma to that specific hormone (gastrinoma, glucagonoma etc.).

In the current classification of neuroendocrine tumors, first proposed by the European Neuroendocrine Tumor Society (ENETS) and then adopted by the World Health Organization (WHO), there are two main neuroendocrine tumor groups with completely different clinical courses: well-differentiated neuroendocrine tumor (WD-NET) and poorly-differentiated neuroendocrine carcinoma (PD-NEC). WD-NETs closely resemble non-neoplastic neuroendocrine cells, while PD-NECs are high-grade carcinomas. These two entities are distinguished by tumor grading which is based on the detection of the proliferative capacity of tumors as well as the morphology. Majority of small intestinal tumors are WD-NETs with low to intermediate proliferative activity. All NETs of small intestine are considered as potentially malignant neoplasms and shouldn't be reported as benign neoplasms. They differ in their metastasizing capacity. NETs of the small intestine are difficult to diagnose and account for a substantial number of "unknown primary" NETs.

Neuroendocrine tumors of small intestine may be associated with a clinical syndrome (functioning) or may be non-functioning. In small intestine, on the basis of their clinical, morphological and hormonal features the following types of neuroendocrine tumors have been described:

Gastrin producing NETs with Zollinger Ellison Syndrome (Gastrinomas): Gastrinomas are sporadic or occur in the setting of MEN1 syndrome in 20–30% of cases. They are most frequently seen in the first part of the duodenum. They are usually small (less than 2 cms). In the setting of MEN 1 syndrome the tumors tend to be multiple and very tiny. Gastrinomas are found to have regional lymph node metastasis at the time of diagnosis in 50–90% of cases.

Non-functioning duodenal NETs: These tumors are also localized in the proximal duodenum. They are small and limited to mucosa-submucosa like gastrinomas. When compared with gastrinomas, their lymph node and distant metastasis are rare (5–10% of cases). They are not associated with a clinical syndrome but hormons like gastrin, serotonin or calcitonin are often demonstrated within the tumors by immunohistochemistry.

Somatostatin producing NETs with or without Neurofibromatosis type 1: Somatostatin producing NETs account for 20% of all duodenal NETS and occur predominantly in the ampullary and periampullary region. About 20–30% of tumors are associated with NF1. They are non-functional unlike pancreatic somatostatinomas. Their mean size is reported as 2.3 cms.

Gangliocytic paragangliomas are discussed separately.

Neuroendocrine carcinomas (Poorly differentiated, grade 3 NECs): NECs account for less than 1–3% of duodenal neuroendocrine neoplasia and primarily occur in or close to ampulla of Vater. They usually present in advanced stages and have high capacity of lymph node and distant metastasis.

In studies reporting five types of duodenal NENs, duodenal gastrinomas are the most frequent, followed by somatostatinomas, non-functional serotonin-containing tumors, non-functional calcitonin-containing NETs (mean 9 8 2.5%, 4 series) and finally rare gangliocytic paragangliomas or NE carcinomas.

Jejunal/Ileal NETS: Tumors originating from small intestine outside duodenum are located in ileum, jejenum and Meckel diverticulum. They usually present in the distal part of the ileum close to the ileocecal valve. NETS of ileum are not associated with inherited syndromes like MEN1 or NF1, but they are sometimes familial. Twenty six to 30% of cases are multiple. Ileal NETs are well differentiated serotonin secreting neoplasms usually with low proliferation index. Though grade 3 tumors are exceptional, metastasis to regional lymph nodes and liver are frequently seen at the time of diagnosis. Ileal NETs may cause hormonal (carcinoid) syndrome (5–7.7% of cases with serotonin producing NETs) due to serotonin hypersecretion. The carcinoid syndrome is most frequently (95%) seen in patients with liver metastasis and characterized by chronic diarhoea, flushing, bronchial constriction, tricuspid valve sclerosis and regurgitation and right sided heart failure.

Neuroendocrine tumors of the jejunum are rare and poorly characterized. The prognostic difference of proximal and distal tumors were reported recently. Upper jejunal neuroendocrine tumors are considered as a small subset of duodenal-like tumors, which are larger, locally invasive and usually metastatic tumors with good prognosis. In contrast, lower jejunal neuroendocrine tumors form a homogeneous group of enterochromaffin cell tumors, similar to their ileal counterparts.

Clinical Features

- **Incidence**
  Neuroendocrine neoplasms originating in the small intestine are rare. The current ENETS guideline on small intestinal tumors reports their incidence as 0.32/100,000 in England, 0.33/100,000 in Japan, 0.67/100,000 in the USA, 0.81/100,000 in Norway and 1.12/100,000 in Sweden according to the most recent literature. Duodenal neuroendocrine neoplasias comprise 1.8–3.8% of all NE tumors, they occur in 0.03–0.05% of all autopsies and comprise 1–3% of all primary duodenal tumors.

  Duodenal and jejunal NETs account for 22% of all gastrointestinal NETs. Ileal NETs account for 25% of all gastrointestinal NETs.
- **Age**
  Duodenal and jejunal NETs are usually seen in the 5th and 6th decades. Ileal NETs are seen between 3rd and 10th decades with a peak in sixth decade.
- **Sex**
  Duodenal and jejunal NETs are seen more frequently in men (Male/Female = 1.5/1) while ileal NETs are seen equally in both sexes.
- **Site**
  Neuroendocrine tumors can occur in all parts of small intestine but proximal duodenum, papilla of Vater and terminal ileum are preferred sites. More than 90% of all duodenal -NENs arise in the first and second part of the duodenum. Approximately 20% of duodenal -NENs occur in the periampullary region.
- **Treatment**
  Duodenal neuroendocrine neoplasias should be completely excised unless there are distant metastases or limiting medical conditions. Endoscopic mucosal resection is applied to small duodenal tumors (<1 cm). For tumors in the periampullary region, surgical resection with lymphadenectomy is recommended. Larger tumors (i.e., 1–2 cm) or tumors of any size with lymph node metastases should be treated surgically.

  For patients with functional hormonal syndromes, specific therapy for the state of excess hormone should be instituted (somatostatin analogs -SSA for carcinoid syndrome, and treatment of ectopic Cushing's syndrome medically or by adrenalectomy).

  For jejunoileal NETs surgery of the primary tumor should be performed by segmental resection with wide lymphadenectomy. After curative surgery, there is no indication for specific medical treatment and there is no proven role for neoadjuvant or adjuvant medical treatment in small intestinal NEN.

  In patients who has hepatic metastases that are potentially resectable surgical resection and/or ablative therapy should be considered.

Medical therapy options for anti-proliferative purposes include SSA and peptide receptor radionuclide therapy (PRRT). SSA are preferred for G1 tumors. Chemotherapy is recommended to treat G3 tumors, with combinations of cisplatin and etoposide.

- **Outcome**

  Despite their small size, gastrinomas are found to have regional lymph node metastasis at the time of diagnosis in 50–90% of cases. Liver metastasis are seen in 10% of cases. Non-functioning gastrin producing NETs rarely metastasize (in 5–10% of cases) to lymph nodes and liver. Somatostatin producing NETs show paraduodenal lymph node metastasis in >50% of cases especially when larger than 2 cms, and involving the muscularis propria. It has been reported that 30% of ileal NETs with a diameter of 1 cm and 100% of ileal NETs larger than 2 cm have lymph node metastasis.

  The 5-year survival with different tumor extent with duodenal neuroendocrine neoplasia is 80–95% for local disease, 65–75% with regional metastasis only, and 20–40% for the 5–10% of patients with liver or distant metastatic disease. Invasion of duodenal neuroendocrine neoplasia into the muscularis mucosa, large primary tumor size, and increased mitotic activity correlate with the occurrence of metastatic disease or aggressive growth.

  In jejunoileal neuroendocrine neoplasia, survival rates depend on tumor grade and TNM-stage: 5-year overall survival rates for all stages are between 50% and 60%. Five year survival is between 80% and 100% for locally-advanced disease, 70–80% for cases with regional lymph node involvement (stages I–IIIa) and 35–80% for stage IV disease.

Macroscopy

Gastrinomas are usually small (<2 cm, mean: 0.8 cm) polypoid lesions located in the first part of duodenum. The overlying mucosa may be intact or ulcerated. In the setting of MEN 1 syndrome the tumors may be multiple and very tiny. The lymph node metastasis of gastrinomas may be larger than their primaries. Well differentiated NETs of lower jejunum and the ileum present as small sessile nodules with a diameter of 1–2 cm. They are multiple in 30% of cases. Their cut surface is yellow-gray. Deep infiltration of muscular wall and peritoneum is frequent. Involvement of mesentery may cause desmoplastic reaction with subsequent angulation and luminal obstruction.

Microscopy

The microscopic features of neuroendocrine neoplasia are related to tumor differentiation and tumor grade. Well differentiated neuroendocrine tumors with low to intermediate proliferative rate, are composed of monomorphic, medium sized cells with abundant, eosinophilic, finely granular cytoplasm. The nuclei of tumor cells are regular and have clumped chromatin pattern. Mitoses are rare (Fig. 1). Oncocytic and clear cell features have also been described. Cytologic atypia of varying degrees can be seen especially in tumors with large size. In well differentiated NETs, the cells are arranged in various combination of insular, trabecular, gyriform or glandular patterns enabling them to be recognized as NETs. Histologic patterns may sometimes be associated with specific localizations and cell types. Somatostatin producing NETs in ampulla have a glandular pattern frequently with psammoma bodies in the lumina. Ileal NETs show cells with insular pattern embedded in sclerotic hypocellular stroma (Fig. 2) and may cause bowel obstruction. Gastrinomas are well differentiated tumors with trabecular and pseudoglandular pattern.

On the other hand, poorly differentiated NECs (PDNECs) with high proliferative rate are classified as small and large cell types according to cell size and nuclear characteristics. The nuclei of small cell type is usually fusiform and show hyperchromasia, finelly granular chromatin pattern, inconspicuous or absent nucleoli and frequent mitosis (Fig. 3). The cytoplasm is sometimes prominent, narrow and eosinophilic. These tumors have a more diffuse architecture. There is

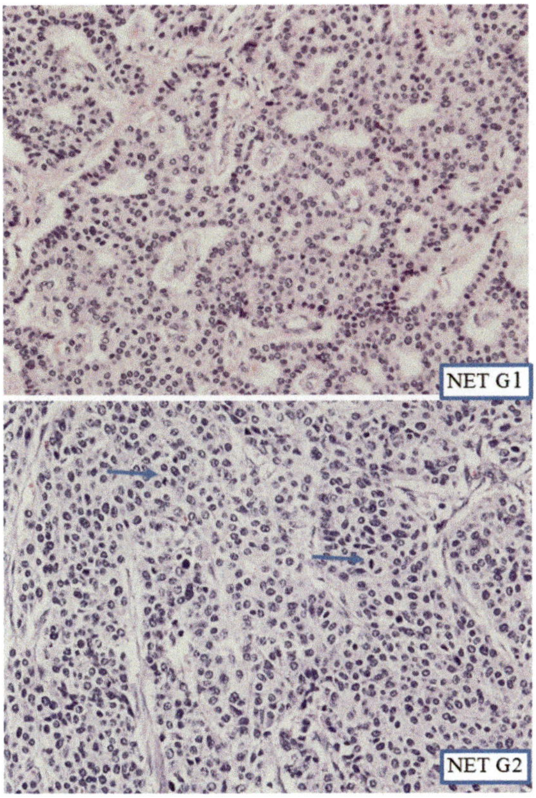

Neuroendocrine Tumor, Small Intestine, Fig. 1 NET (Grade 1 and 2). Note more prominent mitotic activity and nuclear atypia in G2 tumor when compared with G1 tumor (*Arrows* show mitosis)

usually single cell or geographic necrosis. Large cell NECs more typically demonstrate a nested architecture and prominent nucleoli.

The distinction of well differentiated from poorly differentiated tumors is probably one of the most important pathologic assessments related to these neoplasms. The introduction of grading and staging with WHO 2010 classification enabled patient stratification and management in these tumors. The grade of NETs has been found to be a fundamental predictor of outcome. A three-tiered grading system of gastroenteropancreatic neuroendocrine neoplasms was proposed by European Neuroendocrine Society (ENETS) and World Health Organization (WHO). The system is based on assessment of the proliferative capacity of tumors by counting mitosis and calculating the Ki-67 index of tumor cells. ENETS and WHO recommend counting mitosis and Ki-67 stained cells in the most proliferative regions (hot spots). Mitosis should be counted in hematoxylin and eosin stained slides in at least 40 HPFs and expressed as the number of mitosis in 10 HPFs (2 mm). The Ki-67 index should be assessed in 2000 tumor cells and expressed as percentage.

In WHO 2010 classification, the terminology of gastroenteropancreatic neuroendocrine tumors reflects their grade and differentiation: Grade 1 (<2 mitosis per 10 HPFs and/or Ki-67 index $\leq$ 2%) and Grade 2 (2–20 mitosis per 10 HPFs and/or Ki-67 index between 3% and 20%) tumors correspond to well differentiated NETs and Grade 3 (>20 mitosis per 10 HPFs and Ki-67 index > 20%) indicates a poorly differentiated "neuroendocrine carcinoma" (NEC).

One of the issues to be considered in this grading system is that mitotic rate and Ki-67 index are not always concordant. When they are discordant, it is the Ki-67 index that points to a higher rate. In that situation it is recommended that the tumor should be defined according to the higher grade.

Tumor stage is the other factor predicting prognosis in NETs. AJCC and ENETs staging systems use the same parameters for intestinal NETs as for the staging of exocrine intestinal carcinomas. For all NETs, size of the tumor, depth of maximal invasion through the intestinal wall, number of metastatic lymph nodes (together with the total number of nodes examined) must be reported for proper staging.

Immunophenotype

Neuroendocrine cells and their neoplastic counterparts stain with general neuroendocrine markers which include Chromogranin A, Synaptophysin, NSE, PGP-9.5, CD57 and CD-56. Additionally, specific hormons like gastrin, serotonin, calcitonin, pancreatic polypeptide, ACTH and somatostatin can be shown in tumor cells by immunohistochemistry.

The minimal immunohistochemical tests recommended by ENETs guidelines are Chromogranin A, Synaphtophysin and Ki-67. Ki67 is useful to classify patients according to WHO classification 2010 (G1-G3, NET or

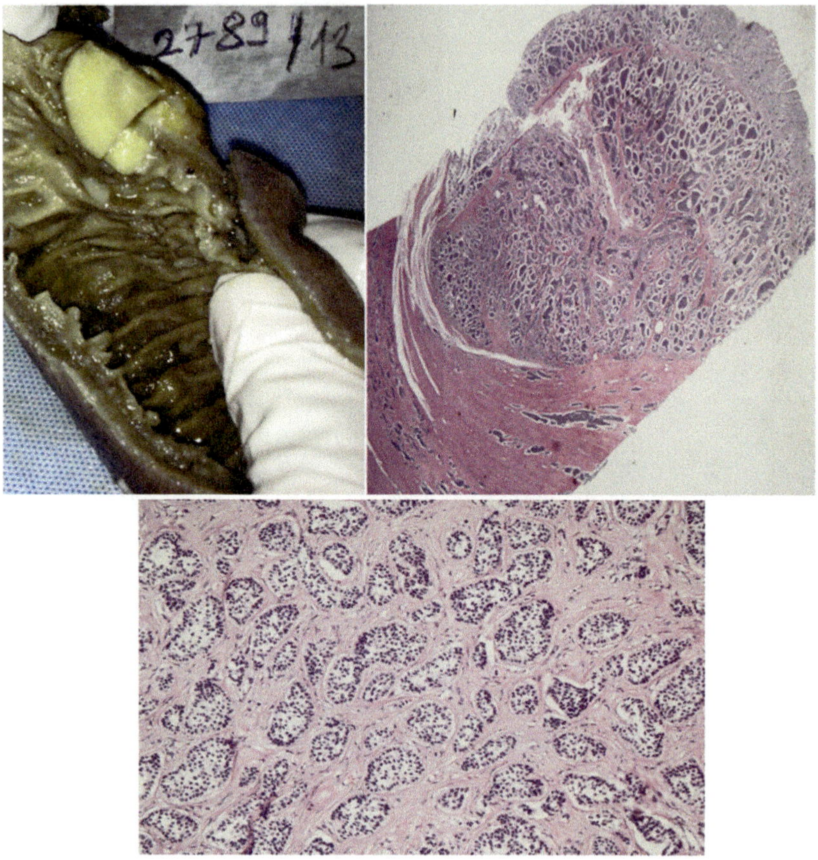

Neuroendocrine Tumor, Small Intestine, Fig. 2 Ileal NET (Grade 2) with muscularis propria invasion. Typical organoid pattern and desmoplastic stroma is seen (H&E, 20X, 100X)

NEC). Chromogranin A and Synaptophysin reactivity is generally diffuse, but the intensity varies. In NECs Chromogranin staining may be focal or absent, whereas Synapthophysin staining is diffuse and intense.

Fifty percent of the gastrinoma cases stains with CDX2 while one-half of the somatostatin producing NETs lack Chromogranin A expression although they stain with synaphtophysin and somatostatin.

Immunohistochemical staining for somatostatin receptor subtype 2 (SSR-2) has been suggested by several studies as indicative of a therapeutic response to SSA treatment. However, currently it is considered optional.

In the setting of liver metastases from a neuroendocrine neoplasia of unknown primary, immunohistochemical CDX-2 positivity and/or serotonin with negativity for TTF-1 and ISL-1 is supportive of intestinal, especially jejuno-ileal origin.

Molecular Features

Abnormalities in several cell cycle regulatory pathways have been described in neuroendocrine neoplasias. Abnormalities in chromosome 11 often at the *MEN1* gene locus, has been detected in duodenal neoplasms in both NETs and NECs. LOH at the MEN-1 locus was found in 60% of sporadic duodenal gastrinomas. MEN1 mutations were detected in 10–25% of sporadic gastrinomas. Ileal NETs rarely show MEN 1 gene abnormalities. Comparative genomic hybridization studies of ileal NETs have demonstrated losses of chromosome 9p18p, 18q and gains of chromosome17q and and 19p. LOH of chromosome 18 has been detected in 88% of ileal NETs. Loss of chromosome 18q have been reported to indicate adverse prognosis but currently not tested routinely. APC gene mutations and Homeobox gene HOXC6 upregulation are also detected in ileal NETs.

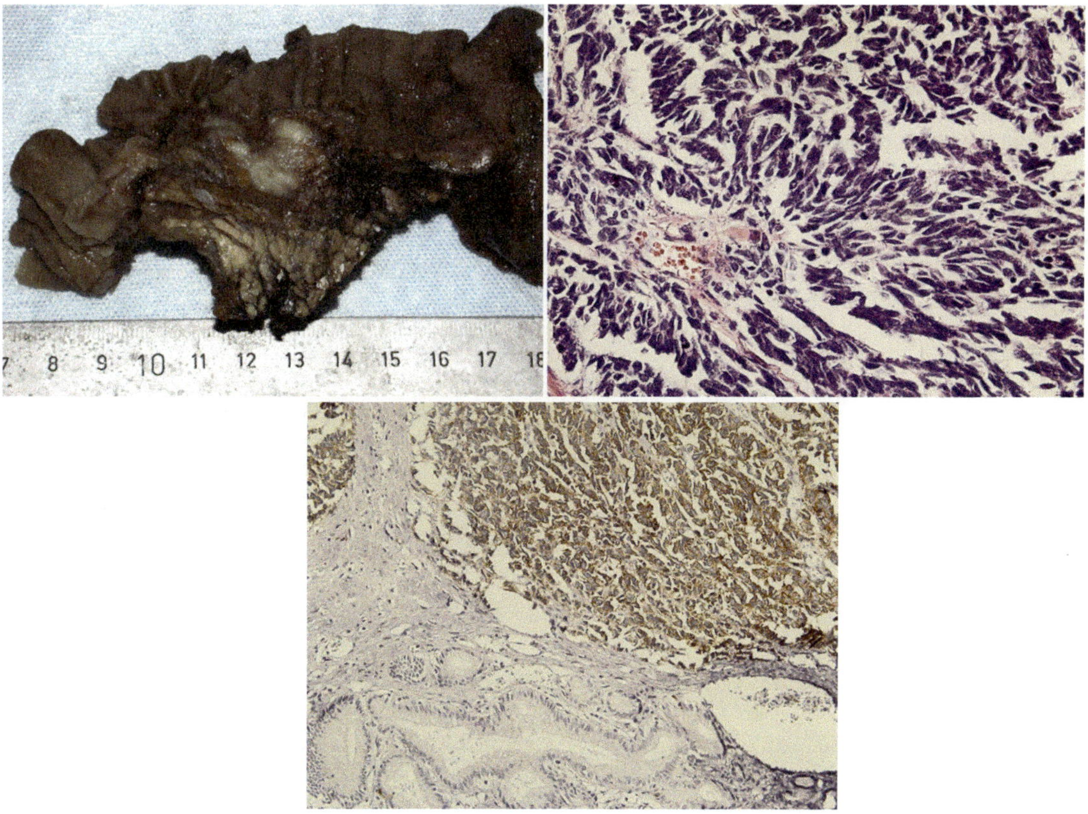

Neuroendocrine Tumor, Small Intestine, Fig. 3 Ampullary NEC. Note small to medium sized cells with hypercromatic nuclei and sparse cytoplasm. Synaptophysin positivity is demonstrated in tumor cells (H%E, Synaptophysin, 100X)

High-grade NECs share gene abnormalities with conventional cancers, *TP53* is the the most frequent abnormality but genetic testing does not have diagnostic relevance.

Germline DNA testing is only recommended in the presence of a positive family history of MEN-1 or if multiple tumors are present. Genetic analysis should also be performed in suspected cases of MEN-1. Somatic (tumor) DNA testing is not recommended.

Differential Diagnosis

Small intestinal NETs, especially somatostatin producing tumors of ampulla must be differentiated from low grade adenocarcinomas. Ampullary NECs which are predominantly large cell type must be differentiated from poorly differentiated adenocarcinomas.

References and Further Reading

Capella, C., Arnold, R., Klimstra, D. S., Kloppel, G., Komminoth, P., Solcia, E., & Rind, G. (2010). Neuroendocrine neoplasms of the small intestine. In T. F. Bosman, F. Carneiro, R. H. Hruban, & N. D. Theise (Eds.), *WHO classification of tumors of the digestive system* (pp. 102–107). Lyon: IARC Press.

Gianfranco, D. F., Kwekkeboom, D. J., Van Cutsem, E., Rindi, G., Kos-Kudla, B., Knigge, U., Sasano, H., Tomassetti, P., Salazar, R., Ruszniewski, P., & all other Barcelona Consensus Conference participants. (2012). ENETS consensus guidelines for the management of patients with gastroduodenal neoplasms. *Neuroendocrinology, 95*, 74–87.

Kloppel, G. (2011). Classification and pathology of gastroenteropancreatic neuroendocrine neoplasms. *Endocrine-Related Cancer, 18*, S1–S16.
Kloppel, G., Rindi, G., Anlauf, M., Perren, A., & Komminoth, P. (2007). Site specific biology and pathology of gastroenteropancreatic neuroendocrine tumors. *Virchows Archiv, 451*(Suppl 1), S9–S27.
Niederle, B., Pape, U. F., Costa, F., Gross, D., Kelestimur, F., Knigge, U., Öberg, K., Pavel, M., Perren, A., Toumpanakis, C., O'Connor, J., O'Toole, D., Krenning, E., Reed, N., Kianmanesh, R., & all other Vienna Consensus Conference participants. (2016). ENETS consensus guidelines update for neuroendocrine neoplasm of the jejunum and ileum. *Neuroendocrinology, 103*, 125–138. 2 Jan 2016 [Epub ahead of print].
Rindi, G., & Wiedenmann, B. (2012). Neuroendocrine neoplasms of the gut and pancreas: New insights. *Nature Reviews. Endocrinology, 8*, 54–64.

Neutropenic Colitis

Ann Driessen
Department of Pathology, University Hospital Antwerp, Edegem, Belgium
Maastricht University Medical Centre, Maastricht, The Netherlands

Synonyms

Agranulocytic colitis; Ileocaecal syndrome; Neutropenic enteropathy; Phlegmonous caecitis; Typhlitis

Definition

Neutropenic enterocolitis is an inflammatory and necrotizing process, predominantly involving the caecum, occurring in neutropenic patients. Because of its caecal localization, the disease is also named typhlitis, deriving from the Greek word typhlon, meaning caecum.

Neutropenic enterocolitis is a life-threatening disease for the first time described in children with leukemia in 1933. It is most commonly observed after chemotherapy for a hematological or a lymphoproliferative malignancy, but it may also found in relationship to a wide variety of solid tumors, e.g., colorectal, breast, lung, and ovarian cancer. It is also reported in patients with an acquired immunodeficiency syndrome (AIDS), aplastic anemia, cyclic neutropenia, after an autologous stem cell transplantation or in those, showing idiosyncratic drug reactions involving antibiotics or immunosuppressives. Neutropenic enterocolitis has been associated with several chemotherapeutics, such as taxanes, 5-fluorouracil, capecitabine, cyclophosphamide, and cisplatin.

The clinical presentation is variable with symptoms such as vomiting, diarrhea, abdominal cramping, abdominal pain, frequently situated in the right lower quadrant, eventually with rebound tenderness, abdominal distension, abdominal guarding, pyrexia, stomatitis, and occult fecal blood loss. Sepsis may develop within hours or a number of days. As these symptoms are not specific, other diseases should be excluded such as infectious colitis, pseudomembranous colitis, inflammatory bowel disease, diverticulitis, appendicitis, or colonic pseudo-obstruction. Neutropenia (peripheral blood absolute neutrophil count $<0.1 \times 10^9$/L) is in the majority of patients diagnosed, but 12% patients show these symptoms without neutropenia.

The pathogenesis of neutropenic enterocolitis is multifactorial. Due to the application of chemotherapeutics, the mucosa becomes injured, causing a destruction of the surface epithelium. Because of the loss of epithelial integrity and the defective immune response due to the neutropenia, patients are at risk to develop an abdominal infection. The intestinal flora may be replaced with opportunistic micro-organisms, such as bacteria and fungi. The flora consists mainly of Gram-positive cocci, Gram-negative bacilli, anaerobes, and less common fungi, in particular *Candida* species. Originally it was thought that *Clostridium septicum*, a rod-shaped, spore-forming, anaerobic, Gram-positive bacterium, is the primary pathogen in neutropenic enterocolitis. Studies however have shown that the bacteremia, occurring in nearly 50% of the patients, is caused by enteric organisms such as *Escherichia coli*, *Pseudomonas aeruginosa*, enterococci, or anaerobes, e.g., *Clostridium* species. Fungi, which are isolated in 53% of the postmortem cases, belong to the *Candida* species in the majority of cases, but other fungi such as *Aspergillus* species have been reported.

Because of the nonspecific symptoms, the diagnosis of neutropenic enterocolitis may be delayed. Early diagnosis and intervention is however necessary to reduce morbidity and mortality. Routine laboratory tests are not specific but are applied to assess the condition of the patient. Routinely used radiological imaging techniques in the diagnosis of neutropenic enterocolitis are abdominal ultrasonography and CT scan. Abdominal plain radiography is of limited utility, because this technique reveals nonspecific findings. Radiological imaging may show features such as dilated loops of bowel with air-fluid levels, mural thumbprinting, and pneumatosis intestinalis. An important feature is the bowel wall thickness. Studies have shown that the mortality rate is significantly higher in patients, having a bowel wall thickness of more than 10 mm (60–80%) than those with a bowel thickness of less than 10 mm (4.2–20%). An increase in bowel wall thickness is however not a diagnostic feature as it is also observed in other conditions such as pseudomembranous colitis, graft versus host disease. Colonoscopy with biopsy sampling is rarely performed in these patients because of the risk of perforation and bleeding.

Clinical Features

- **Incidence**
  The exact incidence of neutropenic enterocolitis is not known. Studies have revealed a variable incidence between 1% and 26%. Originally, the incidence has been determined on postmortem studies in children with a very high incidence of 46%. A large study, performed in 2005, on children with leukemia/lymphoma or solid tumors, shows an incidence between 2.4% and 3.3%. In adults, the reported incidence varies considerably from 0.8% up to 26%. Based on a systematic analysis of 21 studies, a pooled incidence rate of 5.3% is observed in patients hospitalized for hematological malignancies, solid tumors, or with aplastic anemia. In patients treated with antineoplastic chemotherapeutics and presenting with neutropenia, fever, and abdominal pain, nearly 50% of this patient population is affected by the disease.
- **Age**
  Neutropenic enterocolitis may occur at any age, in children as well as in adults.
- **Sex**
  Neutropenic enterocolitis shows no gender predilection.
- **Site**
  Neutropenic enterolitis is mainly situated in the caecum, ileum, and colon ascendens, but it may involve the whole gastrointestinal tract. Occasionally, the appendix is affected. Originally, it was thought that the caecum was predominantly involved because of its thin bowel wall, which distends because of the inflammation, and the diminished vascular supply. A recent study however has shown that this inflammatory and necrotizing process is in only 28% of the patients confined to the caecum, whereas extensive colonic involvement (75%) and small intestinal involvement (66%) is more commonly found.
- **Treatment**
  There is no uniform management strategy for neutropenic enterolitis. As the clinical presentation is highly variable, an individualized approach of the therapy, consisting of a conservative medical treatment or surgery, is necessary. The medical treatment consists of cessation of chemotherapeutics, aggressive hemodynamic support to restore the fluid and electrolyte, total parenteral nutrition, and broad-spectrum antibiotics. Treatment with antifungal agents may significantly reduce the mortality rate. In order to normalize the leukocyte count, recombinant granulocyte colony stimulating factor (G-CSF) is given in a selected group of patients with the greatest degree of neutropenia, multisystem organ failure, and pneumonia with an invasive fungal infection. Surgery is indicated in case of bowel perforation, obstruction, septicemia, or

persistent gastrointestinal bleeding despite resolution of the thrombocytopenia, neutropenia, or hypocoagulability.

- **Outcome**
  Neutropenic enterocolitis has a poor prognosis with a high mortality rate ranging from 40% to 50%. This mortality rate may even increase because of complications, such as intestinal hemorrhage, perforation, peritonitis, and shock. Despite surgical intervention in these circumstances, the mortality rate remains very high, varying between 50% and 70%. An important prognostic feature is the bowel wall thickness, which is associated with a poor prognosis if the thickness is more than 10 mm.

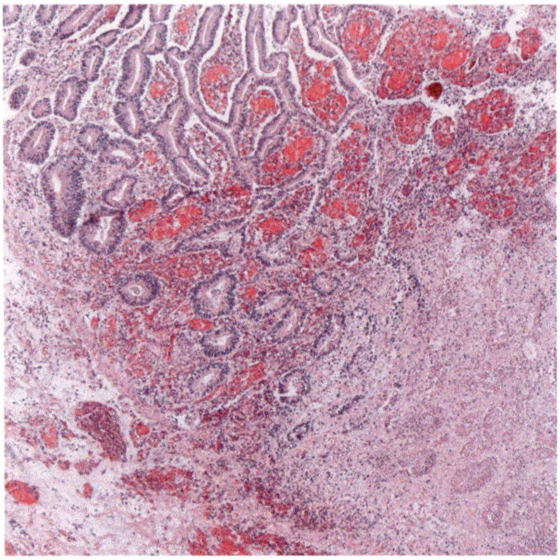

Neutropenic Colitis, Fig. 1 In neutropenic enterocolitis, the mucosa of the small intestine has a hemorrhagic appearance with transition to a complete necrosis of the mucosa (H/E, ×200)

Macroscopy

Gross examination of a resection specimen reveals a bowel with a markedly thickened and dusky wall with scattered serosal ecchymoses. Erosions and ulcerations are found at the level of the mucosa, which is covered by pseudomembranes. These ulcerations may be deeply infiltrating, causing a perforation. Rarely, multiple polypoid and fungiform lesions are seen.

Microscopy

Neutropenic enterocolitis is characterized by mucosal necrosis or full-thickness necrosis. The mucosa becomes eroded or ulcerated with presence of pseudomembranes. These pseudomembranes, covering the mucosal surface, consist of fibrin and necrotic cell debris. At first instance, detachment of the epithelium occurs at the surface, but in time, the epithelial damage extends to the base of the crypts, causing a dropout of crypts. The lamina propria is edematous and hemorrhagic. This edema is more pronounced at the level of the submucosa. The inflammatory infiltrate in the stroma is sparse and consists of lymphocytes, plasmocytes, or macrophages, but without neutrophils (Figs. 1 and 2).

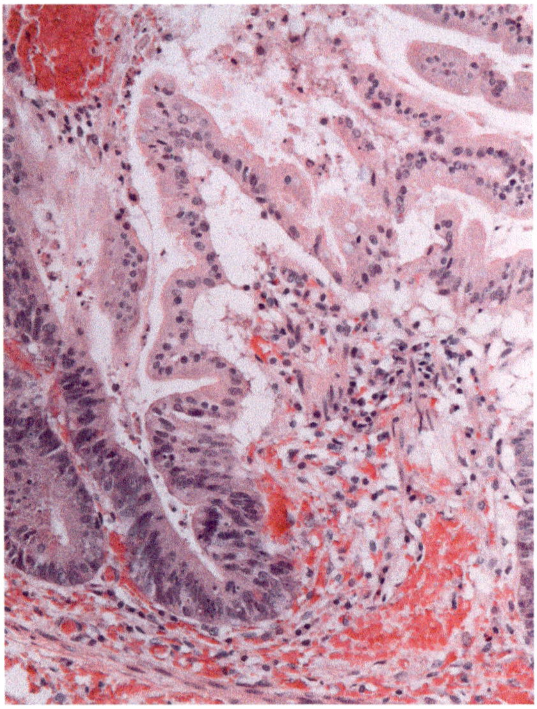

Neutropenic Colitis, Fig. 2 The lack of neutrophils in the hemorrhagic lamina propria is the characteristic of neutropenic enterocolitis (H/E, ×200)

Due to loss of the epithelial integrity, the bowel wall becomes invaded by bacteria. Besides bacteria, fungi, such as *Aspergillus*, may invade blood vessels, causing intravascular thrombosis with secondary necrosis of the mucosa or deeper layers of the wall. Besides thrombi, secondary to a fungal invasion, fibrin thrombi can be found in the submucosa. These thrombi will lead to an ischemic appearance to the mucosa, eventually with disintegration of the muscularis propria.

Although the microscopical features are not pathognomonic, the discrepancy between the severity of the cell injury and the absence of neutrophils points toward neutropenic enterocolitis.

Differential Diagnosis

Microscopic features are not diagnostic but give rise to a differential diagnostic problem with pseudomembranous colitis and ischemic colitis. Pseudomembranous colitis and ischemic colitis have both a different clinical presentation. Pseudomembranous colitis is due to a *Clostridium difficile* infection, occurring in patients treated with antibiotics. Similar to neutropenic enterocolitis, the surface of the mucosa is covered with pseudomembranes. However, in contrast to neutropenic enterocolitis, the mucosal inflammatory infiltrate and pseudomembranes contain numerous neutrophils. The lack of neutrophils is a specific diagnostic feature, not present in ischemic colitis, which is characterized by a hyalinized lamina propria.

References and Further Reading

Cloutier, R. L. (2009). Neutropenic enterocolitis. *Emergency Medicine Clinics of North America, 27*, 415–422.

Ebert, E. C., & Hagspiel, K. D. (2012). Gastrointestinal manifestations of leukemia. *Journal of Gastroenterology and Hepatology, 27*, 458–463.

Fenoglio-Preiser, C. M., Noffsinger, A. E., Stemmermann, G. N., Lantz, P. E., & Isaacson, P. G. (2008). *Gastrointestinal pathology. An atlas and text* (3rd ed., pp. 838–841). Philadelphia: Lippincott, Williams & Wilkins.

Gil, L., Poplawski, D., Mol, A., Nowicki, A., Schneider, A., & Komarnicki, M. (2012). Neutropenic enterocolitis after high-dose chemotherapy and autologous stem cell transplantation: Incidence, risk factors, and outcome. *Transplant Infectious Disease: An Official Journal of the Transplantation Society, 15*(1), 1–7. doi:10.111/j.1399-3062.2012:0:1 7.

Ullery, B. W., Pieracci, F. M., Rodney, J. R., & Barie, P. S. (2009). Neutropenic enterocolitis. *Surgical Infections, 10*, 307–314.

Nonsteroidal Anti-Inflammatory Drug-Induced Gastrointestinal Injury

Liesbeth Ferdinande
Department of Pathology, Ghent University Hospital, Ghent, Belgium

Synonyms

Diaphragm disease

Definition

Nonsteroidal anti-inflammatory drug (NSAID)-induced gastrointestinal injury ranges from erosion and ulceration to more severe complications such as gastrointestinal bleeding, perforation, or bowel strictures. The association between NSAID use and ulceration in the upper gastrointestinal tract was first reported in 1938 by a gastroscopic study of Douthwaite and Lintott. Since then, this type of lesions has been well characterized and documented. Their pathogenesis is related to the inhibitory role of NSAID on cyclo-oxygenase (COX)-1 and -2, resulting in inhibition of prostaglandin synthesis. Beside the intended anti-inflammatory effect, decreased prostaglandin production can also result in gastroduodenal injury, because prostaglandins enhance and stimulate many aspects of mucosal defense. Topical irritant effects of NSAID are described to contribute to the development of erosions and ulcerations in the gastrointestinal tract. For the gastroduodenal injuries, the presence of acid plays a key role: when mucosal defense is weakened through suppression of mucosal prostaglandin synthesis, the

N

tissue is less able to resist the damaging effects of acid. In contrast, the pathogenesis of small intestinal damage is less well understood, involving more complex mechanisms. There does not seem to be a primary role for COX inhibition in the development of NSAID-induced enteropathy. Direct adverse effects of NSAID themselves to intestinal epithelial cells start the initial cellular damage, and these effects are enhanced when NSAID are combined with bile and when they are reabsorbed in the ileum and subsequently secreted back into the duodenum via the enterohepatic circulation. This will lead to increased mucosal permeability, which facilitates entry and actions of luminal factors such as dietary macromolecules, bile acids, or bacteria. Moreover, administration of NSAID can change the numbers and types of enteric bacteria, thereby contributing to the development of small intestinal ulcers.

As most clinical and histological findings in patients with NSAID-induced gastrointestinal injury are not specific, the correct diagnosis of NSAID pathology is often difficult to make, especially if the clinician and/or pathologist is not informed about the NSAID intake. Moreover, NSAID can affect preexisting disease, increasing the diagnostic challenge. Patients on NSAID therapy are reported to have an increased incidence of appendicitis, a more aggressive course of diverticulitis and an increased relapse rate and persisting chronic activity of preexisting inflammatory bowel disease.

Clinical Features

- **Incidence**
  Approximately 20% of regular users of NSAID will develop an ulcer of the stomach or duodenum. The extent of NSAID-induced small intestinal injury was only relatively recently revealed using new imaging and endoscopical techniques that allow better assessment of damage in this part of the gastrointestinal tract. Recent video-capsule endoscopy and other studies demonstrated the high incidence of NSAID-induced enteropathy: 50–60% of patients on long-term NSAID develop NSAID enteropathy, with an annual rate of at least 1% of serious outcomes (perforation, bleeding, and strictures).
- **Age**
  NSAID-induced gastrointestinal injury can occur at any age, but the elderly, of whom one study showed that 70% are taking NSAID at least once a week, have an increased risk of adverse drug reactions. The high risk for the development of NSAID-induced gastrointestinal complications in older patients was demonstrated in several surveys and is probably due to the presence of other associated risk factors.
- **Site**
  NSAID can provoke damage at all levels of the gastrointestinal tract, but gastroduodenal and small intestinal injuries are most common.
- **Treatment**
  The most effective treatment is discontinuation of NSAID ingestion, which will result in resolution of clinical symptoms and histological injury. In patients with severe disease or protracted healing, additional active treatment may be required. Strictures formed in the small or large bowel cannot be reversed, and in these cases, surgery or endoscopic dilatation is sometimes mandatory.

  When cessation of NSAID intake is not an option, preventive measures can be taken. As gastric acid plays a major role in the pathogenesis of gastroduodenal mucosal lesions, cotherapy of NSAID and acid-suppressing drugs such as proton pump inhibitors (PPI) is used to decrease the risk of NSAID-associated injuries. This strategy reduces the incidence and severity of NSAID-induced gastroduodenal damage and accelerates healing of established mucosal damage. However, chronic use of PPI is associated with bacterial overgrowth and significant increase in incidence of various infections (e.g., *Clostridium difficile*). These changes in small intestinal bacterial flora caused by PPI intake may contribute to a significant worsening of NSAID enteropathy. For prevention of small intestinal NSAID-induced injury, cotherapy with probiotics or antibiotics is suggested.

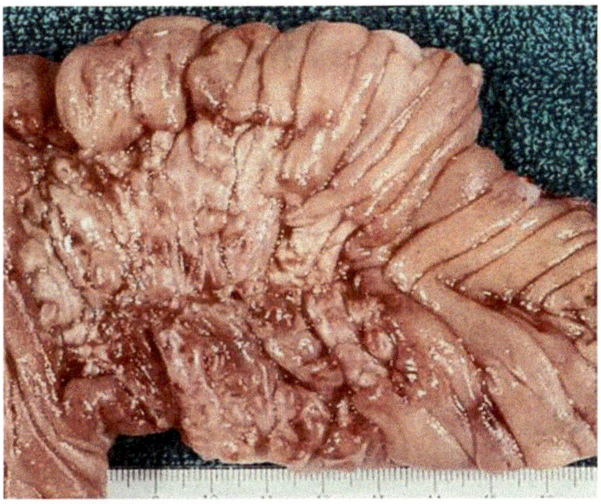

Nonsteroidal Anti-Inflammatory Drug-Induced Gastrointestinal Injury, Fig. 1 Macroscopy of a NSAID-induced ulceration in the colon (courtesy of Karel Geboes)

Other strategies to reduce the risk of NSAID-induced mucosal damage comprise the development of new drug formulations, e.g., enteric-coated preparations, selective COX-2 inhibitors, etc.

Macroscopy

Macroscopy of NSAID-induced injury such as ulcerations is usually not specific (Fig. 1). Rarely, NSAID can induce a specific pathology with a particular macroscopic appearance: diaphragm disease. Diaphragm disease is characterized by multiple, concentric, 2–4-mm-thick septae-like projections of the bowel mucosa that narrow the lumen. It is believed to be pathognomonic for NSAID use and was first described by Lang in 1988 in the small bowel. Later this disease was also reported in the right colon, especially in patients taking sustained release preparations of NSAID. The underlying cause seems to be a scarring reaction secondary to the ulcerative injuries during long-term NSAID use. The clinical presentation is usually nonspecific with obstructive symptoms, gastrointestinal blood loss, or abdominal pain. Biopsies are mostly taken from the mucosa that covers the diaphragm and show also nonspecific findings. Diagnosis is therefore based on macroscopy. The mucosal projections into the lumen should be differentiated from normal plicae circulares, and histologically, they can be recognized by submucosal fibrosis and occasional thickening of the muscularis mucosae. Superficial erosions can occur.

Microscopy

Microscopic findings of NSAID-induced gastrointestinal injury such as erosions and ulcerations are mainly aspecific. Some clues may suggest the iatrogenic origin of the lesions.

Increased apoptosis or an elevated number of eosinophils can alert the pathologist that a drug-induced etiology, including NSAID-induced pathology, should be considered. The observation of ulcerations surrounded by normal mucosa at either side of the lesion can also point to drug pathology (Fig. 2).

In the esophagus, NSAID pills are one of the most frequent causes of pill esophagitis. Histologically, this is characterized by acute inflammation with or without prominent eosinophilic infiltrate, erosions or ulcers, but the presence of polarizable crystalline material may be an important clue to the diagnosis in these cases (cfr. ► Drug-Induced Esophagitis).

In the stomach, the injury pattern of reactive gastropathy is often attributed to NSAID (cfr. Gastropathy, Reactive (Chemical)). Up to 45% of NSAID users will develop reactive gastropathy. NSAID erosions are mainly located in the gastric body and heal within days, whereas NSAID ulcers that are often large and multiple and located in the gastric antrum tend to be chronic and more susceptible for complications such as bleeding and perforation. The relationship between *Helicobacter pylori* infection and NSAID-induced gastric injury remains controversial, with some studies suggesting an increased risk of NSAID injury in *Helicobacter pylori* negative patients and other studies suggesting an increased risk in *Helicobacter pylori* infected patients.

In the colon, different types of NSAID-induced injury are described: (focal) active colitis, ► microscopic colitis (lymphocytic and collagenous colitis), ischemic colitis, or ► inflammatory bowel disease–like pattern.

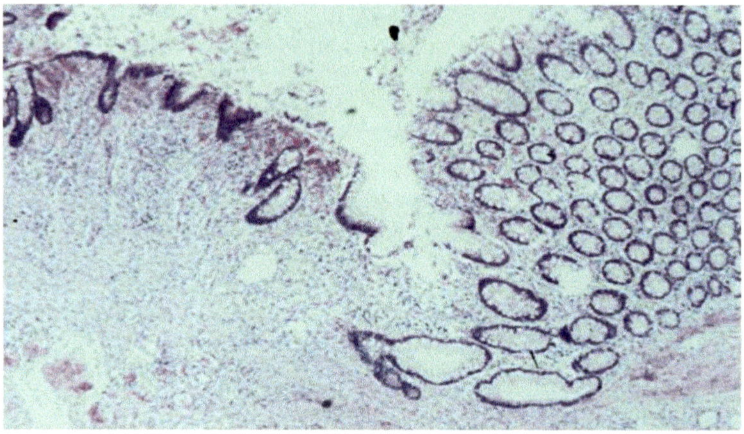

Nonsteroidal Anti-Inflammatory Drug-Induced Gastrointestinal Injury, Fig. 2 Microscopy of the border of the NSAID-induced ulceration seen in Fig. 1: the adjacent mucosa shows normal histology, which may suggest a drug-induced etiology (courtesy of Karel Geboes)

Differential Diagnosis

Since microscopic findings in gastrointestinal biopsies from NSAID-induced damage are not specific, the diagnosis of NSAID-induced pathology is difficult to make based on morphology alone. However, these injuries are reversible when NSAID intake is stopped and therefore, a timely and correct diagnosis of this entity is important. Certain histological clues can draw the pathologist's attention to the possibility of NSAID-induced gastrointestinal injury, but without clinical information including drug use, a definite diagnosis cannot be made.

The finding of reactive gastropathy in gastric biopsies is suggestive for NSAID use, but is entirely not specific and other etiologies such as bile reflux should be taken into account.

The differential diagnosis between NSAID-induced injury and inflammatory bowel disease can be very challenging, especially in biopsies of the terminal ileum. A history of NSAID use, older age, and less inflamed mucosa in biopsies adjacent to the ulceration favor NSAID-induced pathology.

NSAID-induced colonic damage can present as many different injury patterns (cfr. section "Microscopy") and clinicopathological correlation can help in distinguishing between these entities.

Diaphragm disease should be differentiated from other causes of strictures. ► Crohn's disease can inflict strictures. However, mucosal inflammation and disturbances in crypt architecture are usually more prominent in these cases. Strictures can be found in ► radiation colitis, a clinical history of radiotherapy can rule out this differential diagnosis. Potassium chloride, a drug that is used to replenish potassium in patients with hypokalemia, may cause ulcers and strictures throughout the gastrointestinal tract. The luminal projections are usually broader than the typical NSAID-associated diaphragms. Pancreatic enzyme replacement in children with cystic fibrosis can be associated with fibrosing colonopathy, mostly in the right colon with localized strictures, but stenosing fibrosis of the entire colon can occur. Methacrylic acid within the enzyme preparations was suggested to be the offending agent.

References and Further Reading

Geboes, K., De Hertogh, G., & Ectors, N. (2006). Drug-induced pathology in the large intestine. *Current Diagnostic Pathology, 12*, 239–247.

Lang, J., Price, A. B., Levi, A. J., Burke, M., Gumpel, J. M., & Bjarnason, I. (1988). Diaphragm disease: pathology of disease of the small intestine induced by non-steroidal anti-inflammatory drugs. *Journal of Clinical Pathology, 41*, 516–526.

Price, A. B. (2003). Pathology of drug-associated gastrointestinal disease. *British Journal of Clinical Pharmacology, 56*, 477–482.

Wallace, J. L. (2012). NSAID gastropathy and enteropathy: distinct pathogenesis likely necessitates distinct prevention strategies. *British Journal of Pharmacology, 165*, 67–74.

Nonsteroidal Anti-Inflammatory Drugs (NSAIDs)

Alexandra Thiel and Ari Ristimäki
Division of Pathology, Haartman Institute and Genome-Scale Biology, Research Programs Unit, HUSLAB/Helsinki University Central Hospital and University of Helsinki, Helsinki, Finland

Synonyms

Acetylsalicylic acid; Analgesics; Antipyretics; Aspirin; Cancer; Coxibs; Cyclooxygenase (COX); Diseases; Drugs; Duodenal ulcer; Eicosanoids; Enzymes; Erosion; Gastric ulcer; *Helicobacter (H.) pylori* infection; Ibuprofen; Mediators; Mucosal injury peptic ulcer disease; Naproxen; Nonselective COX inhibitors; Nonsteroidal anti-inflammatory drugs (NSAIDs); Painkillers; Prostacyclin (PGI_2); Prostaglandin-endoperoxide synthase; Prostaglandins (PGs); Prostanoids, thromboxane (TXA_2); Selective COX-2 inhibitors

Definition

Eicosanoids are locally acting signal transducers that are synthesized by oxidation of 20 carbon essential fatty acids, of which arachidonic acid is the most important one. Two distinct enzyme systems produce eicosanoids, of which cyclooxygenase enzymes (COX, also known as prostaglandin-endoperoxide synthase) and subsequent action of prostaglandin synthases produce prostanoids, i.e., prostaglandins (PGs), prostacyclin (PGI_2), and thromboxane (TXA_2). Synthesis of prostanoids is inhibited by the use of nonsteroidal anti-inflammatory drugs (NSAIDs) that act by inhibiting COX enzymes. Peptic ulcer disease is an injury of the lining of the stomach or duodenum. The most common causes of peptic ulcers are *H. pylori* infection or the use of NSAIDs or a combination of these two. Selective COX-2 inhibitors (coxibs) have been developed to obtain beneficial pharmacological effects with minimal side effect profile. Since COX-2 is also overexpressed in gastrointestinal adenocarcinomas and in their precursor lesion, it has been suggested that inhibition of COX-2 could be chemopreventive.

Molecule Type and Chemical Structure (Optional)

See above (section "Definition").

Physiological Relevance and Function

Prostanoids mediate their effects through specific cell membrane receptors and regulate a wide diversity of physiological functions, including inflammation and immunity, smooth muscle contraction, aggregation of platelets, and several reproductive functions. COX enzymes are the rate-limiting step in production of prostanoids, namely, PGE_2, PGD_2, $PGF_{2\alpha}$, PGI_2, and TXA_2. COX inhibitors, i.e., NSAIDs (e.g., aspirin, ibuprofen, and naproxen), are pharmacologically used as analgesics and antipyretics and thus are generally called painkillers or fever medicines. They also have modest anti-inflammatory effects. Aspirin is also used in secondary prevention of myocardial infarction. The most common side effect of NSAIDs is mucosal injury of the gastrointestinal tract.

There are two COX enzymes, of which COX-1 isoform is in most tissues constitutionally expressed and functions as a housekeeping gene. It has been hypothesized that COX-1-derived prostanoids are primarily responsible for production of prostanoids responsible for cytoprotection of the gastrointestinal tract. NSAIDs may interfere with this by reducing mucosal blood flow, impairing barrier properties and buffering capacity of the mucosa, and injuring the surface epithelium. In contrast to COX-1, COX-2 is usually expressed only after induction by agents that are related to inflammation and carcinogenesis, such as cytokines, growth factors, and hormones. To this end, it was hypothesized that selective COX-2 drugs might not cause the gastrointestinal side effects related to nonselective COX inhibitors, namely, peptic ulcer disease, observed for nonselective NSAIDs, but would be effective anti-inflammatory drugs.

Relevance for Pathology

NSAIDs are clinically widely used as analgesics and in the treatment of arthritis and other musculoskeletal disorders. They can be divided into different groups, based on their selectivity for COX-1 or COX-2. Aspirin (acetylsalicylic acid), one of the longest-used NSAIDs, has more than 10 times greater selectivity for COX-1 than COX-2. When used in low doses, aspirin exhibits an antiplatelet and antithrombotic effect through inhibition of COX-1 and subsequent TXA_2 inhibition of the platelets. At high doses, aspirin inhibits both COX isoforms and is used as pain reliever and anti-inflammatory agent. The use of aspirin and other NSAIDs is associated with adverse events in the upper gastrointestinal tract that include mucosal injury, peptic ulcer disease that can lead to life-threatening bleeding, and perforation. Especially vulnerable are those individuals with high age, previous history of NSAID-related injury, and use of certain co-medication (anticoagulants or corticosteroids and naturally the use of other NSAIDs including low-dose aspirin). Although NSAID-induced side effects are more common when high doses are used, it is important to remember that even low-dose aspirin alone can induce significant gastrointestinal complications. In addition, *H. pylori* infection increases the risk of NSAID-related gastrointestinal complications. Therefore, testing for and treatment of *H. pylori* is indicated especially when long-term NSAID therapy is considered. Several studies have shown that the use of selective COX-2 inhibitors is associated with lower incidence of gastric and duodenal ulcers when compared to patients treated with nonselective NSAIDs. However, this beneficial effect was not evident in patients taking also low-dose aspirin.

Gastrointestinal side effects of COX inhibitors can be reduced by the use of misoprostol, a prostaglandin E1 analog, but its use has been limited by gastrointestinal side effects, namely, diarrhea and cramping. These side effects have been shown to be reduced without the loss of the protective effect by lowering the dose of the drug. Proton pump inhibitors are another means to reduce gastric and duodenal ulcers in patients taking NSAIDs or COX-2 inhibitors. Cardiovascular side effects were initially found to be related to the use of selective COX-2 inhibitors, but it has been later recognized that also nonselective NSAIDs, with the possible exception of naproxen (and obviously low-dose aspirin), increase the cardiovascular risk. Thus, for patients with cardiovascular disease risk who need NSAID treatment, naproxen is recommended combined with misoprostol or a proton pump inhibitor.

Epidemiological studies have demonstrated that long-term use of NSAIDs reduces the risk of gastrointestinal cancer, including adenocarcinoma of the stomach and the colorectum. This effect may be facilitated by the inhibition of COX-2 that has been shown to be overexpressed by these tumor types. Thus, it has been hypothesized that COX-2 inhibitors could be used as chemopreventive agents against gastrointestinal carcinogenesis. Several studies have been performed, mainly in Asian populations, in which the effect of selective COX-2 inhibitors on progression of precancerous gastric lesions has been studied. Indeed, there is some evidence supporting the role of celecoxib, a selective COX-2 inhibitor, in regression of precancerous gastric lesions, namely, intestinal metaplasia. However, the data are contradictory, and that could be due to small trial sizes and heterogeneous study populations. To this end, the use of NSAIDs of any form cannot be currently recommended as an approach to decrease the risk of gastric cancer. Further prospective clinical trials are needed to address the effects of both selective and nonselective NSAIDs on the development and progression of gastrointestinal precancerous lesions.

References and Further Reading

Dinis-Ribeiro, M., Areia, M., de Vries, A. C., Marcos-Pinto, R., Monteiro-Soares, M., O'Connor, A.,

Pereira, C., Pimentel-Nunes, P., Correia, R., Ensari, A., Dumonceau, J. M., Machado, J. C., Macedo, G., Malfertheiner, P., Matysiak-Budnik, T., Megraud, F., Miki, K., O'Morain, C., Peek, R. M., Ponchon, T., Ristimaki, A., Rembacken, B., Carneiro, F., Kuipers, E. J., MAPS Participants, European Society of Gastrointestinal Endoscopy, European Helicobacter Study Group, European Society of Pathology & Sociedade Portuguesa de Endoscopia Digestiva. (2012). Management of precancerous conditions and lesions in the stomach (MAPS): Guideline from the European Society of Gastrointestinal Endoscopy (ESGE), European Helicobacter Study Group (EHSG), European Society of Pathology (ESP), and the Sociedade Portuguesa de Endoscopia Digestiva (SPED). *Virchows Archiv, 460*, 19–46.

Lanza, F. L., Chan, F. K., Quigley, E. M., & Practice Parameters Committee of the American College of Gastroenterology. (2009). Guidelines for prevention of NSAID-related ulcer complications. *The American Journal of Gastroenterology, 104*, 728–738.

Malfertheiner, P., Megraud, F., O'Morain, C. A., Atherton, J., Axon, A. T., Bazzoli, F., Gensini, G. F., Gisbert, J. P., Graham, D. Y., Rokkas, T., El-Omar, E. M., Kuipers, E. J. & European Helicobacter Study Group. (2012). Management of *Helicobacter pylori* infection–the Maastricht IV/Florence Consensus Report. *Gut, 61*, 646–664.

Sostres, C., & Lanas, A. (2011). Gastrointestinal effects of aspirin. *Nature Reviews. Gastroenterology & Hepatology, 8*, 385–394.

Thiel, A., Mrena, J., & Ristimäki, A. (2011). Cyclooxygenase-2 and gastric cancer. *Cancer Metastasis Reviews, 30*, 387–395.

Normal Appendix and Tumoral Appendix

Magali Svrcek
Hôpital Saint-Antoine, Service d'Anatomie Pathologique, AP-HP, Hôpitaux Universitaires de l'Est Parisien, Paris, France

Synonyms

Vermiform appendix

Anatomy

The appendix is a derivative of the cecum and matures in the second trimester of the embryonic life. As the appendix lengthens, the junction between the appendix and the cecum becomes increasingly more distinct. The appendix usually arises from the posteromedial cecal wall, at a point about 2.5–3 cm below the ileocecal valve, with its orifice opening into the cecum. However, four types of ceco-appendiceal junction are possible. The appendix arises at the junction of three of the taenia coli present at the surface of the cecum. The appendix is suspended from the mesoappendix, which is a mesenteric extension from the ileum; the base of the appendix is attached to the posterior abdominal wall and its tip is free. The position of the appendix varies considerably; most commonly, the appendix lies behind the cecum and ascending colon. It may also lie beside the ascending colon, in front of or behind the terminal ileum, lying on the psoas muscle, or in the subhepatic region. The appendix is vascularized by a branch of the posterior cecal artery which runs in the mesentery, and its venous drainage is to the portal system. The lymphatics first drain into nodes in the mesoappendix, then to the right pericolic lymph nodes, and then to those of the ileocecal angle.

Function

In humans, the function of the appendix is not clear. The appendix may be vestigial. Besides it is not observed in many mammals, except herbivorous animals. While its exact function in humans has been debated by physicians, it is known that there is immune system tissue in the appendix and the appendix may play an immunological role: it could be implicated in the recognition of foreign protein and bacteria in the bowel and the formation of IgA immunoglobulins. Moreover, the gut is populated with different microbes that help the digestive system breakdown the food. It is now believed that the immune system cells found in the appendix are there to protect the commensal bacteria. It is obvious that the appendix contains many goblet cells, and, consequently, its exocrine production of mucus is abundant. The density of these goblet cells is far greater within the epithelium of the appendix than within the colon. Thus the role of the appendix in mucus production and lubrification of the fecal contents within the right colon is important.

Size, Weight

The adult appendix averages 6–7 cm in length, though variations between 5 and 12 cm are common. Lengths up to 20 cm have been reported. The appendix is correspondingly shorter in children.

Its external diameter ranges from 0.3 to 0.8 cm. The appendiceal lumen normally varies from 1 to 2 mm.

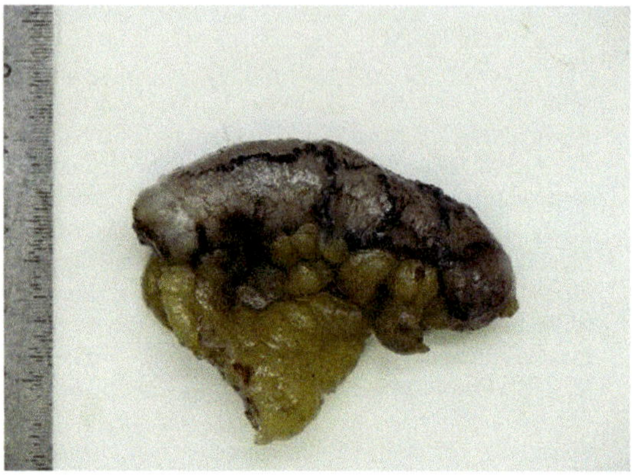

Normal Appendix and Tumoral Appendix, Fig. 1 Macroscopic view of a normal appendix. Note the hyperemia of surface vessels related to surgical trauma

Macroscopy

The appendix, which is a tubular structure, is composed of:

- The base.
- The body.
- The tip. Obliteration of the tip of the appendix is a frequent finding.

The serosa is smooth and transparent. Its surface can be hyperemied, related then to surgical trauma. The mesoappendix, largely made of adipose tissue, contains the appendiceal vessels (Fig. 1).

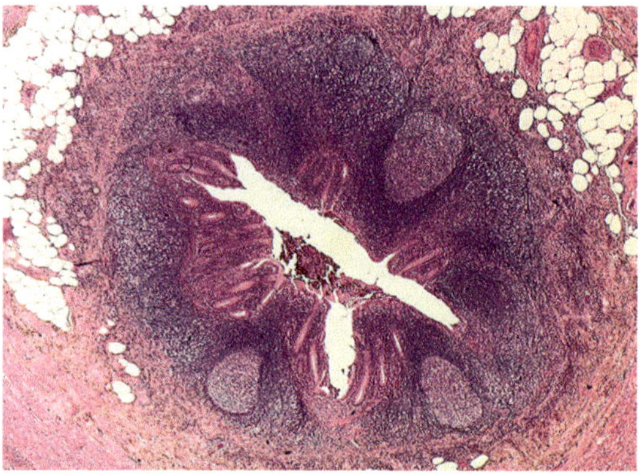

Normal Appendix and Tumoral Appendix, Fig. 2 Low-power magnification showing numerous lymphoid follicles

Microscopy

The appendix has the same four layers as the remainder of the gut and possesses a colonic-type mucosa, but is thinner than that lining the colon or rectum. A distinguishing feature of this organ is the extremely rich lymphoid tissue of the mucosa and submucosa, characterized by a prominent circumferential arrangement of lymphoid follicles known as Peyer patches (Fig. 2). The surface epithelial cells over the dome of each lymphoid follicle are modified to form M cells which transmit potentially antigenic protein similarly to that seen in the small intestine. A well-defined lymphatic sinus surrounds both the lateral and basal parts of the follicle and empties into the submucosal-collecting lymphatics.

Non-branching crypts are lined predominantly by mucus-secreting columnar cells that extend from the luminal surface down to the muscularis mucosae and by absorptive cells. The density of goblet cells is far greater within the epithelium of the appendix than within the colon. As in the colon, the proliferative zone is located in the basal portion of the crypts. The two types of differentiated cells (absorptive and goblet cells) come from immature cells migrating upward to the luminal surface.

The crypts also contain endocrine cells, Paneth cells in small numbers, and intraepithelial lymphocytes. Endocrine cells are present at the base of the crypts and occur individually or in small clusters. These endocrine cells can harbor bright eosinophilic cytoplasmic granules which may lead to some confusion with those of Paneth cells. These endocrine cells are more prominent in the distal than in the proximal appendix. Additionally, in about 50% of cases, endocrine cells can be detected within the lamina propria, non-attached to crypt epithelium and in close association with nerves, in a structure termed "the enterochromaffin cell-nerve fiber complex." These endocrine cells are mainly EC (enterochromaffin) cells (secreting serotonin), the most numerous endocrine cell populations in the gut. ECL cells (enterochromaffin-like cells, secreting histamine), D cells (secreting somatostatin), L cells (secreting enteroglucagon and pancreatic polypeptide-like peptide), and N cells (secreting neurotensin) can also be observed.

The muscularis mucosae is poorly developed and can be absent in places, rendering sometimes difficult the determination of the mucosal-submucosal boundary (Fig. 3).

The submucosa is constituted by connective and fat tissues and contains nerve plexus consisting only of a few scattered ganglion cells.

The muscularis propria, thin, contains two layers of smooth muscle (a circular and a longitudinal muscle coat) in which the cells of the myenteric plexus are also scattered diffusely instead of having a plexiform arrangement. There is a well-defined serosa also called the mesoappendix.

The histological structure of the appendix varies with age. Peyer patches are most prominent in young individuals and undergo progressive atrophy during life to the point of complete disappearance in the elderly. In the elderly, it is frequent to observe an atrophy of the epithelial elements of the mucosa and an increase of the fibrous and fat tissues of the submucosa, tending to the obliteration of the lumen, particularly at the distal tip.

Immunophenotype

Appendiceal epithelial cells express keratin 20, CDX2, and MUC2. Many express keratin 7. Endocrine cells express immunologic markers of neuroendocrine differentiation such as neuron-specific enolase (NSE), synaptophysin, and chromogranin (Fig. 4). Both crypt and lamina propria endocrine cells contain serotonin, somatostatin, enteroglucagon, vasoactive intestinal polypeptide, and substance P.

N

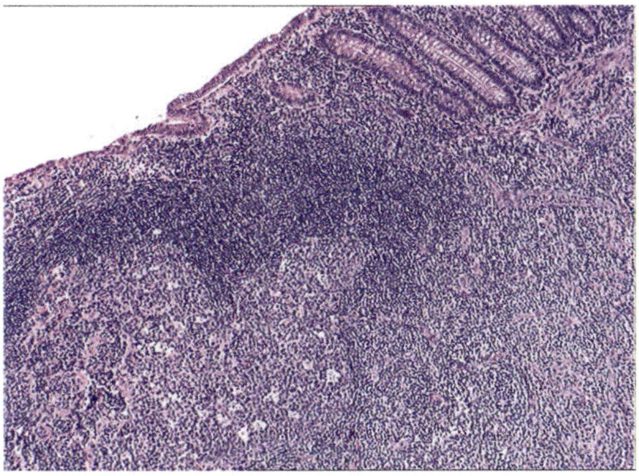

Normal Appendix and Tumoral Appendix, Fig. 3 The lymphoid cells are within both the mucosa and submucosa. Note the discontinuation of the muscularis mucosae

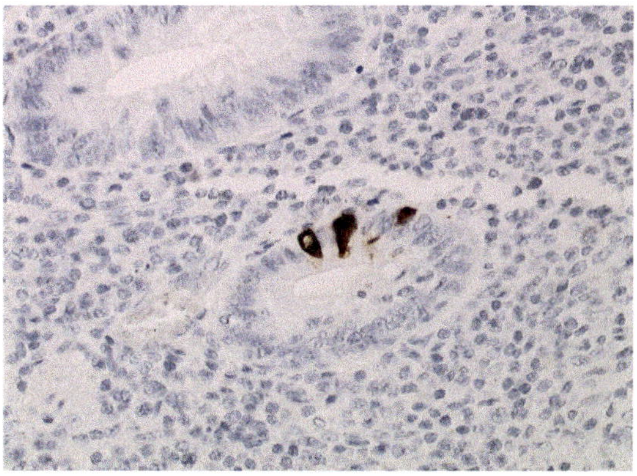

Normal Appendix and Tumoral Appendix, Fig. 4 Appendiceal endocrine cells are present within the appendiceal crypts. These endocrine cells are stained by chromogranin (×400 magnification)

Tables with Important Diseases

Important Diseases of the Appendix
Developmental abnormalities:
Duplications, diverticula, and cysts
Absence of the appendix
Malpositions
Heterotopias
Hamartomas
Inflammatory disorders (see also ► Appendicitis, Etiology, Macroscopy, and Histology of entry):
Acute nonspecific appendicitis
Chronic atrophic appendicitis
"Specific" appendicitis
Tumors:
Benign and malignant epithelial tumors: neuroendocrine tumors (see also ► Appendiceal Tumors entry), adenomas, and adenocarcinomas (see also ► Mucinous Cystadenoma, Appendix entry, ► Mucinous Cystadenocarcinoma, Appendix entry)
Miscellaneous (or non-epithelial tumors)
Metastatic tumors
Miscellaneous conditions:
Acquired diverticular disease
Intussusception
Torsion
Endometriosis
Malakoplakia

References and Further Reading

Gramlich, T. L., & Petras, R. E. (2007). Vermiform appendix. In S. E. Mills (Ed.), *Histology for pathologists* (3rd ed., pp. 649–662). Philadelphia: Lippincott Williams and Wilkins.

Guidry, S. P., & Poole, G. V. (1994). The anatomy of appendicitis. *American Surgeon, 60*, 68–71.

Randal Bollinger, R., Barbas, A. S., Bush, E. L., Lin, S. S., & Parker, W. (2007). Biofilms in the large bowel suggest an apparent function of the human vermiform appendix. *Journal of Theoretical Biology, 249*, 826–831.

Wakeley, C. P. G., & Gladstone, R. F. (1928). The relative frequency of the various positions of the vermiform appendix as ascertained by an analysis of 5000 cases. *Lancet, 1*, 178.

P

Paget's Disease of the Anus

Denis Chatelain[1] and Jean-François Fléjou[2]
[1]Service d'Anatomie Pathologique, Centre Hospitalier et Universitaire du Nord, Amiens, France
[2]Faculté de Médecine Pierre et Marie Curie, Service d'Anatomie et Cytologie Pathologiques, Hôpital Saint-Antoine, Paris, France

Definition

Paget's disease is a rare intraepithelial adenocarcinoma that may occur in the perianal skin. Its histogenesis is not completely understood. Paget's disease could represent the epidermotropic spread of tumor cells from cancers of regional organs and from adenocarcinoma of skin adnexa such as eccrine or apocrine glands. It could also originate from an intraepidermal ectopic sweat gland or Bartholin's glands' epithelial cells or could originate from an in situ transformation of a pluripotential stem cell within the epidermis.

Perianal Paget's disease was first reported in 1893 by Darier and Coulillaud. It encompasses two entities: primary and secondary Paget's disease.

Secondary perianal Paget's disease represents half of the cases. It results from the epidermotropic spread of an underlying neoplasm such as adnexal adenocarcinoma or an internal malignancy mainly gastrointestinal carcinoma (usually anal or rectal cancer) or genitourinary carcinoma (mainly urethral carcinoma). The visceral malignancy may be synchronous or metachronous.

The other half of perianal Paget's disease are primary and are not associated with internal malignancy. However, they may become invasive and may progress from an in situ intraepidermal neoplasia to a dermally invasive adenocarcinoma, which may in turn, metastasize to local lymph nodes and distant sites.

Clinical Features

Perianal Paget's disease presents as a pruritic, red or white, crusted patch in anal skin (Fig. 1). Symptoms are usually nonspecific such as perianal itching, burning sensation, oozing, and bleeding. The diagnosis is often delayed, because the disease is frequently treated initially as a benign dermatologic condition (notably eczema) and the diagnosis is often made 2–8 years after the beginning of the symptoms.

- **Frequency**
  The true incidence of the disease is difficult to assess due to its rarity. Perianal Paget's disease represents less than 1% of anal disease and 6.5% of all cases of Paget's disease (mammary and extramammary).

F. Carneiro et al. (eds.), *Pathology of the Gastrointestinal Tract*, Encyclopedia of Pathology,
DOI 10.1007/978-3-319-40560-5

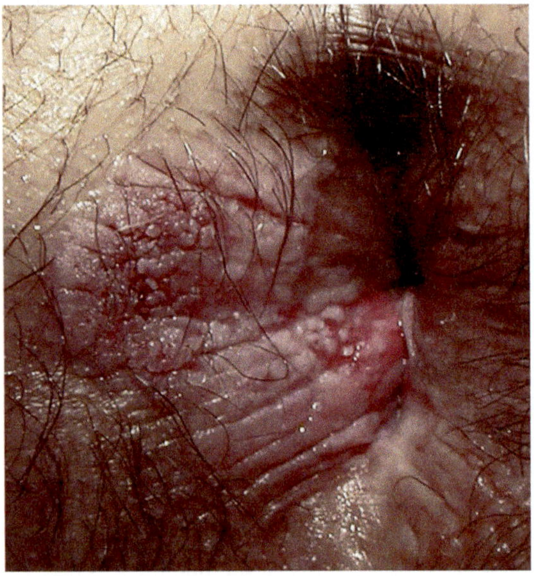

Paget's Disease of the Anus, Fig. 1 Clinical aspect of perianal Paget's disease

- **Sex**
  Perianal Paget's disease is most commonly detected in postmenopausal Caucasian females.
- **Age**
  Perianal Paget's disease is usually diagnosed in the sixth and seventh decades.
- **Treatment**
  Therapeutic management depends on the local extent and depth of invasion of the Paget's disease, regional lymph node involvement, and systemic extent of the disease.

  The treatment of Paget's disease is essentially surgical. Wide surgical excision, with a sphincter-saving technique, and a circumferential split-thickness skin graft, often with diverting stoma, is proposed as treatment of choice. A margin more than 1–3 cm should be obtained (due to a high post-resection local recurrence rate 40–50%). An intraoperative frozen section analysis of resection margins has been proposed to reduce the local recurrence rate.

  The role of adjuvant therapies is controversial. However, noninvasive modalities such as radiotherapy, photodynamic therapy, topical chemotherapeutic agent (5FU, bleomycin or imiquimod), systemic chemotherapy, argon beam laser therapy, or cryotherapy may be reasonable alternatives to surgery in selected cases, such as those patients who are medically unfit for surgery, those who wish to avoid radical and mutilating surgery, and those who have a multifocal widespread disease. Radiotherapy may be used as an adjunct to surgery to reduce long-term local recurrence or to treat postoperative local recurrence.
- **Outcome**
  The overall and disease-free survival rate of perianal Paget's disease at 5 years after treatment is 59% and 64%, and decreases to 33% and 39% at 10 years.

  There is a high rate of recurrence after excision exceeding 40–60% at 5 years. Progression from in situ to invasive carcinoma has been reported to be as high as 40% in untreated lesions of primary Paget's disease. Metastases can involve lymph nodes (inguinal, perirectal, retroperitoneal, iliac, and para-aortic), the liver, bones, the lungs and adrenal glands. Survival outcome in patients with Paget's disease is often dictated by the presence or absence of underlying malignancy and the presence and stage of an invasive component. Patients with intraepidermal neoplasia have a better prognosis than patients with dermal invasion. Patients who have perianal Paget's disease and underlying malignancy have a poorer prognosis.

Macroscopy

Perianal Paget's disease presents as a slowly spreading erythematous plaque, moist and reddish, scaling or macerated, with an eczematous surface and well-defined borders. It can extend to the anal canal, up to the dentate line.

Microscopy

Perianal Paget's disease is microscopically characterized by the presence of specific tumor cells called Paget's cells. These are large cells with pale clear or eosinophilic cytoplasm, and large round

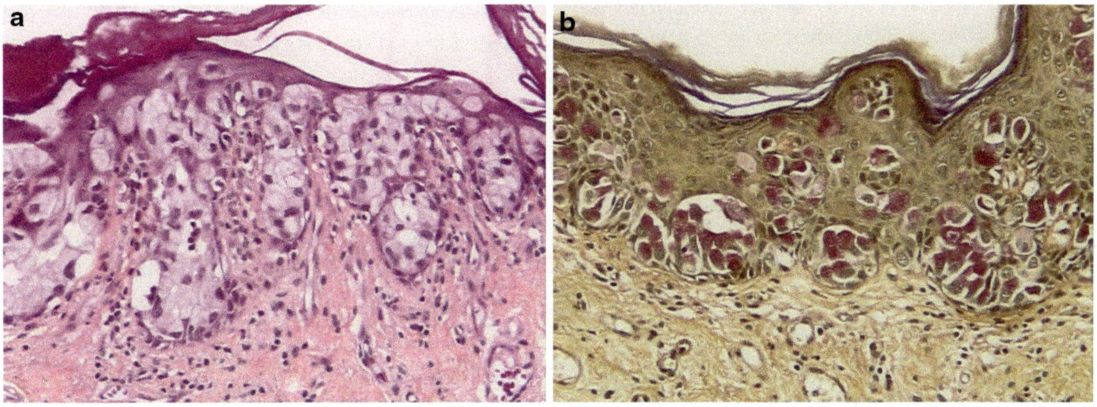

Paget's Disease of the Anus, Fig. 2 Anal Paget's disease. (**a**) H&E, (**b**) PAS

hyperchromatic nuclei (Fig. 2a). They tend to form clusters, solid nests, or tubules, or can migrate solely in the whole epidermis in a pagetoid pattern. Some cells can have the appearance of signet ring cells. In some cases, dirty necrosis can be identified in intraluminal gland formations.

Paget's disease can be categorized as noninvasive (tumor confined onto epidermis) or as invasive disease (tumor penetrating the basement membrane and entering into underlying stroma). Minimally invasive Paget's disease is defined as groups of Paget's cells protruding no more than 1 mm below the basement membrane in the underlying dermis.

Histochemistry and Immunohistochemistry

Paget cells invariably react positively for mucin stains (Alcian blue, PAS) (Fig. 2b). In primary Paget's disease, tumor cells stain positive for CK7, GCDFP15, and MUC5AC. In secondary Paget's disease associated with rectal adenocarcinoma, tumor cells are positive for CK20 and MUC2 and do not express CK7, GCDFP15, and MUC5AC.

Molecular Features

The molecular features of perianal Paget's disease are still unknown.

Differential Diagnosis

Perianal Paget's disease can be differentiated from a clear cell variant of Bowen's disease by the positivity of tumor cells with PAS that identify sialomucins, in contrast to Bowen's disease that does not display positive PAS staining.

Primary Paget's disease can be distinguished from secondary Paget's disease linked to rectal adenocarcinoma by its morphological features and immunohistochemical profile.

The presence of signet ring Paget's cells and the presence of intraepithelial glands with intraluminal dirty necrosis appear to be morphological markers of an underlying rectal adenocarcinoma. Tumor cells of Paget's disease associated with rectal adenocarcinoma often show a CK20+/CK7-/GCDFP15-/MUC2+/MUC5AC+ phenotype. Tumor cells of primary Paget's disease more often show a CK20-/CK7+/GCDFP15+/MUC2-/MUC5AC+ phenotype.

Cross-References

▶ Paget's Disease of the Anus
▶ Squamous Cell Carcinoma, Anus

References and Further Reading

Goldblum, J. R., & Hart, W. R. (1998). Perianal Paget's disease: A histologic and immunohistochemical study

P

of 11 cases with and without associated rectal adenocarcinoma. *The American Journal of Surgical Pathology, 22*, 170–179.
Shia, J. (2010). An update on tumors of the anal canal. *Archives of Pathology & Laboratory Medicine, 134*, 1601–1611.

Pancreatic Heterotopia

Berna Savaş
Department of Pathology, Ankara University Medical School, Ankara, Turkey

Synonyms

Aberrant pancreas; Accessory pancreas; Ectopic pancreas

Definition

Pancreatic heterotopia (PH), a congenital anomaly of the exocrine pancreas, is defined as the existence of the pancreatic tissue in topographic anomaly, with no anatomic, neural, or vascular connection to the main pancreas.

The exact etiology of ectopic pancreas remains unclear. Different theories have been proposed to explain its appearance, the transplantation of embryonic pancreatic cells to adjacent structures during axial rotation of the intestine being one of them. Moreover, embryonic buds that remain adhered to the primitive duodenum could be taken to proximal or distal sites during the growth and development of the gastrointestinal tract. The incidence of pancreatic tissue in distant organs should deserve further explanation, remembering the possibility of having been originated by multipotent cell endodermic metaplasia or teratomas.

Heterotopic pancreatic tissue is susceptible to many of the same inflammatory pathologies that may affect the normal pancreas, such as acute and chronic pancreatitis, and cancer, although the latter complication is extremely rare. Depending on the localization, PH may present with various symptoms. Abdominal pain and bleeding are frequent for gastric PHs. Also there may be symptoms due to mechanical obstructions, such as when PH is the lead point in intussusceptions, or when PH in the antrum of the stomach, or in the gall bladder, obstructs the outflow from the respective organ. PH may manifest some symptoms of carcinoid syndrome, and surgical treatment may eliminate such symptoms.

Clinical Features

- **Incidence**
  The incidence of PH is 0.55–15% of autopsy specimens, and the mean frequency is between 1% and 2%.
- **Age**
  PH has been found in all age groups including pediatric patients, the average age is 45 years, despite the fact that most of the cases are diagnosed in adulthood and are not suspected before surgery.
- **Sex**
  In adults, the incidence is higher in males, while in pediatric patients, the female gender is more common.
- **Site**
  In approximately 70% of cases, PH tissue is located in the upper GI tract. It is found mainly in the stomach, duodenum, and jejunum, in much smaller proportions in the ileum and Meckel's diverticulum, and it is rarely found in the esophagus, liver, gallbladder, omentum, lungs, mediastinum, fallopian tubes, and umbilicus.
- **Treatment**
  Benign asymptomatic lesions generally do not require surgical intervention. Symptomatic tumors, with the typical appearance and localization, should be operated on using minimally invasive techniques, laparoscopic, endoscopic or endoscopic-guided laparoscopy in selected cases. Preoperative biopsy is recommended. In the absence of endoscopic biopsy confirmation, surgical exploration and frozen section histopathologic study for all symptomatic patients are recommended. Limited local

excision has been shown to be a safe and adequate procedure for patients. Endoscopy should be performed whenever epigastric pain is the presenting symptom.

- **Outcome**
  The prognosis of benign PH is excellent. The outcome of PH cases with malignant transformation may show differences depending on the histological type. Review of the literature reveals adenocarcinomas arising within heterotopic pancreas to have a somewhat better prognosis than patients with adenocarcinoma of the pancreas. The difference in survival between adenocarcinoma arising in ectopic and normally situated pancreas may be due to earlier presentation of carcinoma in ectopic pancreas.

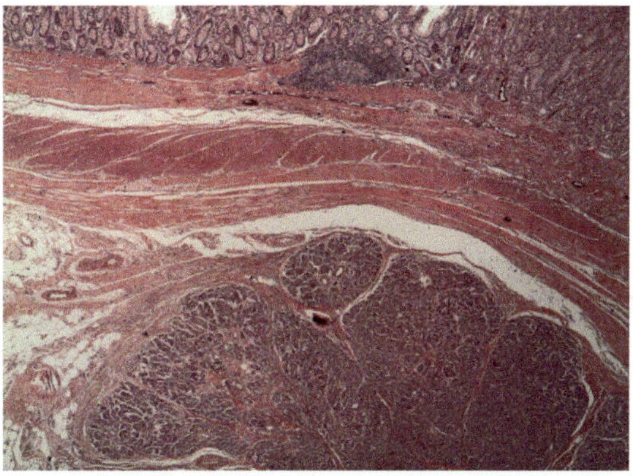

Pancreatic Heterotopia, Fig. 1 Heterotopic pancreatic tissue in Meckel's diverticulum. Mural heterotopia consist of lobules of pancreatic acini (H&E, ×25)

Macroscopy

Commonly, PH tissue present in the form of small yellowish nodules, ranging from 1 to 5 cm, typically covered by intact mucosa, and often exhibits a central hole (larger lesions). In this umbilication, there is exteriorization of the usually rudimentary pancreatic duct, which can be detected by endoscopic study or barium contrast. Gastroduodenal lesions are usually larger than those of other locations.

Microscopy

The heterotrophic pancreatic tissue is detected more frequently in the submucosa and muscularis propria layers of the gastrointestinal tract and may be observed in the sub-serosa or even in the serosa of the affected segment (Fig. 1). Histologically, the normal pancreatic lobular architecture, with acinar and ductal components, may all be present. Up to 84% of cases contain islets of Langerhans. Rare cases may have only neuroendocrine cell elements.

Immunophenotype

The cytologic distribution and staining percentages of immunohistochemical staining are similar to those of the normal pancreas. The immunohistochemical findings support the histologic impression of heterotopic pancreas. Pan-epithelial markers such as CAM 5.2, CK8, and CK18 are expressed in the pancreatic acini and ducts. Acinar cells are generally negative with AE1/AE3 and CK19, whereas ductal cells are strongly positive. Both acini and ducts are typically negative for CK20. Islets of Langerhans stain strongly positively with chromogranin. A large percentage of the cells express insulin, mainly in the central portion of the nodules, while fewer cells show somatostatin positivity in the periphery.

P

Molecular Features

No specific molecular feature was defined for PH. The molecular features of normal pancreas are summarized somewhere else.

Differential Diagnosis

It is often impossible to distinguish PH from primary or metastatic cancer as endoscopic biopsies are often negative. This often leads to operative treatment. Therefore, frozen sections should be taken rapidly and routinely so as to confirm the diagnosis and avoid unwanted radical surgery such as Whipple's procedure or subtotal gastrectomy. PH should be considered in the differential diagnosis of *GIST*. Purely endocrine PH may mimic a *neuroendocrine tumor*. The scattered nature of the lesion, the small size of the nests, and the lack of stromal reaction strongly favored PH. Immunohistochemical characterization helps to confirm the histologic impression of PH.

References and Further Reading

Dabbs, D. J. (2010). Diagnostic immunohistochemistry. Theranostic and genomic applications. In O. Basturk, A. B. Farris, & N. V. Adsay (Eds.), *Immunohistology of the pancreas, biliary tract and liver* (pp. 541–592). Philapdelphia: Saunders/Elsevier.

Emerson, L., Layfield, L. J., Rohr, L. R., & Dayton, M. T. (2004). Adenocarcinoma arising in association with gastric heterotopic pancreas: A case report and review of the literature. *Journal of Surgical Oncology, 87*, 53–57.

Lai, E. C., & Tompkins, R. K. (1986). Heterotopic pancreas. Review of a 26 year experience. *American Journal of Surgery, 151*, 697–700.

Solcia, E., Capella, C., & Kloppel, G. (1997). *Tumors of the pancreas* (pp. 146–148, 231–232). Washington, DC: Armed Forces Institute of Pathology. *Atlas of tumor pathology*; 3rd series, fascicle 20.

Parasitic Colitis

Gert De Hertogh
Department of Pathology, Pathologische Ontleedkunde, UZ Leuven, Leuven, Belgium

Definition

Human intestinal parasites can be classified into four different groups: the protozoa and the nematodes (roundworms), cestodes (tapeworms), and trematodes (flukes). Many of these organisms pass cysts or eggs in the feces, which forms the basis for diagnostic tests. About 12 protozoan species and at least 15 helminthic species can lead to gastrointestinal (GI) pathology, representing a significant disease burden worldwide. In the past, these infections were mainly seen in developing countries. This geographic pattern is quickly changing under the influence of increasing world travel, globalized economy, and the growing number of chronically immunosuppressed patients in western countries. With helminthic infections, the additional problems arise that some worms can survive in the host for decades and that infection may remain asymptomatic until complications develop (e.g., occult *Strongyloides stercoralis* infection until treatment with glucocorticoids causes fulminant disease, occult *Schistosoma mansoni* until development of portal hypertension and bleeding of esophageal varices). Hence, a basic knowledge of histopathological aspects of the most common parasitic GI diseases benefits pathologists worldwide. Although many parasites can infect the GI tract, relatively few of them will actually be encountered in the colon. The following discussion is therefore limited to the following species: (1) protozoa, *Entamoeba histolytica* and *Cryptosporidium* species; (2) nematodes, *Strongyloides stercoralis*, *Enterobius vermicularis*, and *Anisakis simplex*; (3) cestodes, *Taenia saginata* and *Taenia solium*; and (4) trematodes, *Schistosoma* species.

Clinical Features

Entamoeba histolytica is found worldwide, but especially in Central and South America, Africa, and India. It causes up to 50 million symptomatic infections per year, resulting in up to 100,000 deaths annually. This protozoon has a simple life cycle consisting of the infectious cyst and the amoeboid motile trophozoite. Infection occurs after ingestion of cysts present in fecally contaminated food or water. Cysts give rise to trophozoites in the small bowel. In about 10% of infected persons, these trophozoites will invade the colonic epithelium leading to amoebic colitis and possibly spread to distant organs (e.g., amoebic liver abscess). Persons most at risk for amoebic colitis are travelers to endemic regions, male homosexuals, and institutionalized persons. Most patients present with slowly worsening diarrhea, which can be bloody. Other symptoms such as abdominal pain, tenesmus, and fever are variable.

A fulminant course can be seen in elderly or malnourished people, infants, pregnant women, and those on glucocorticoids. Clinically, the main differential diagnoses are bacillary dysentery, inflammatory bowel diseases (IBD), and ischemic colitis. Treatment of all patients (also the asymptomatic ones) is with a luminal or a tissue amebicide, e.g., paromomycin and metronidazole, respectively. Most patients respond quickly and outcome is generally good.

Cryptosporidia are small, 2–5 μm large intracellular protozoal parasites related to *Plasmodium* species (malaria) and *Toxoplasma gondii* (toxoplasmosis). Although first described in the early twentieth century, *Cryptosporidia* only came to the forefront in the 1980s with the peak of the AIDS epidemic. They cause watery diarrhea which may range from mild and self-limited in immunocompetent persons to catastrophic and protracted (cholera-like) in immunosuppressed individuals such as AIDS patients, persons with immunoglobulin deficiencies, and those with hematologic malignancies. The life cycle of the parasite is complex with successive stages of infectious oocysts and sporozoites which are engulfed by host cell microvilli and locate in vacuoles beneath the brush border, asexually replicating merozoites and sexual gametocytes. The infection can be treated with nitazoxanide. In AIDS patients, the restoration of normal CD4 counts is most important in controlling the disease.

Strongyloides stercoralis is endemic in tropical and semitropical areas and in Europe also in Northern Italy. This worm does not require a host to replicate. It ordinarily lives in the soil and lays eggs that develop into rhabditiform and then filariform larvae. These can penetrate the skin of a host in contact with the soil. The larvae then travel to the lungs via the veins, break through the alveolar wall, and ascend in the airways and are swallowed. They embed in the jejunum where they mature to adult worms. Eggs hatch in the small intestine and develop into rhabditiform larvae, which are passed in the stools. A minority of the rhabditiform larvae also develop into infectious filariform larvae within the intestine, thus continuing the infection for decades. Patients are usually asymptomatic. However, any Disruption of normal immunity (e.g., by immunosuppression or glucocorticoid therapy) may cause a fulminant, often fatal disease due to massive autoinfection. Treatment is with ivermectin and must be repeated after 2 weeks to be successful.

Enterobius vermicularis, also called the pinworm, is the most commonly encountered helminthic parasite both by clinicians and pathologists in western countries of temperate climate. The worm is acquired by ingesting eggs upon close contact with infected persons (e.g., among school-age children and in their families). Eggs are quite resistant to environmental conditions and can be passed via the hands or even via the air. They hatch in the duodenum, releasing larvae that migrate to the cecum, appendix, and ascending colon and mature on their way. Adult males measure up to 5 mm and females 8–13 mm. Gravid females reside in the rectum and migrate out of the anus to the perianal skin during the night to lay eggs. The maturing eggs cause itching and scratching by the patient, which promotes reinfection and transmission to others. Usually there are no other symptoms, so that pinworm is an example of an extremely well-adapted parasite (Human infection has been documented for thousands of years). The infection is however always treated since it is so highly transmissible. One dose of mebendazole repeated after 2 weeks for the index case and all contacts, with a washing of all clothes and bed linens in between, is sufficient.

Anisakis simplex is actually a parasite of marine mammals. Eggs are passed in the feces and develop into infective larvae which infest crustaceans. When these are eaten by saltwater fish, the larvae migrate to the fish musculature. When the initial intermediary host, or a predator fish, is eaten by a marine mammal, the larvae develop into adult intestinal worms. Humans become infected accidentally when eating raw or pickled fish (e.g., herring, mackerel, and salmon). Infections are becoming more common with the increased popularity of some eastern food practices (e.g., sushi). Humans are no suitable hosts; thus, the larvae do not develop into adult worms and lay no eggs. They may however invade the gastric or intestinal, appendiceal, or colonic wall, causing an intense inflammatory reaction and sometimes an allergic reaction. The typical symptom of anisakidosis is severe epigastric pain within 3 days of consuming raw fish. With lower GI tract infection, a symptom complex mimicking acute appendicitis or Crohn's disease can develop. Endoscopic removal of the parasite alleviates symptoms. Since the worms do not survive in humans, treatment with an anthelmintic is not needed. Some patients may present with intestinal obstruction or peritonitis, necessitating surgery.

Taenia saginata and *Taenia solium* (beef and pork tapeworm, respectively) colonize an estimated 80 million people worldwide. In Europe, mainly beef tapeworm is encountered. The transmission cycle requires exposure of livestock to untreated human waste and subsequent human consumption of raw or undercooked meat. Adult tapeworms release gravid proglottids containing eggs. Both are passed in the stool. Proglottids of *Taenia saginata* are up to 2 cm long and remain motile for a while. They may "crawl" out of the feces and "swim" in the toilet, alarming the patient. Eggs ingested by cattle or pork release an embryo, a so-called onchosphere, that penetrates the intestinal wall and is carried by the bloodstream to several organs developing into cysticerci, awaiting human consumption. When a human ingests a cysticercus, this releases a scolex which attaches itself to the bowel wall in the proximal jejunum. The worm lengthens over several months by forming maturing proglottids in a chain behind the scolex. The worms may live in the small intestine for up to 25 years. They feed by absorption of nutrients through their surface. Usually there are no symptoms or only vague abdominal complaints. Therapy is with a single dose of niclosamide. An alternative and feared disease course is (neuro)cysticercosis in *Taenia solium* infestation. This must be treated with a longer course of albendazole to kill the cysticerci.

The most important intestinal parasitic trematodes are the blood flukes *Schistosoma mansoni* and *japonicum*. These are typical for tropical countries, with *S. mansoni* being common in Africa, the Middle East, and the Americas, while *S. japonicum* is endemic in China, Indonesia, the Philippines, and Thailand. More than 200 million people are infected worldwide. Schistosomes live in tropical snails for part of their life cycle. People acquire the parasite by moving about in contaminated fresh water containing the larval form (cercariae). Upon penetrating the skin, these transform into schistosomules that are carried to the lungs with the venous blood. They pass the lung circulation and eventually reach the liver, where they mature and mate. Adult worms swim countercurrent into the portal vein and take up residence in the mesenteric veins (usually the inferior mesenteric vein for *S. mansoni* and the superior for *S. japonicum*). There the worms consume blood and nutrients and lay eggs. About half of these eggs will pass through the intestinal wall and enter the bowel lumen. When deposited in fresh water, they release ciliated miracidia which swim off to infect a tropical snail. Within the snails, miracidia transform in sporocysts which give rise to cercariae that exit the snail in search for a suitable mammalian host. In humans, larval and adult worms are protected from immune attack by their tegument. The worms themselves cause few symptoms and may live for up to 5 years in their host. The eggs however cause a strong immune reaction which is first acute and possibly symptomatic (Katayama fever) and then enters a chronic phase. The classical response of the body to the presence of eggs is by forming a granuloma of mixed composition around it. This may actually benefit the parasite, by allowing it to exit blood vessels and penetrating the mucosa into the lumen (a process that may take up to 2 weeks). Passage of *S. mansoni* eggs through the bowel wall causes colitis with tenesmus, tenderness over the sigmoid, and bloody stools. Other eggs remain buried in the intestinal wall or lodge in the veins of the portal system. The ensuing granulomas will gradually involute to leave fibrotic scars. Eventually, hepatic and portal vessels will show widespread fibrosis with the development of portal hypertension due to presinusoidal venous obstruction. This is the characteristic of hepatosplenic schistosomiasis. All forms of the disease can be treated with praziquantel given once or twice.

Macroscopy

In amoebic colitis, the cecum and ascending colon are most commonly affected. The bowel wall is thickened with multiple 2–10 mm large, punctate ulcers which remain superficial and undermine the intervening mucosa, thus acquiring a characteristic flask shape. The number of neutrophils is variable and higher in early lesions. The amoebae attach to the lateral walls of the ulcers. Occasionally, large inflammatory masses ("amoebomas") may form. In contrast, Cryptosporidiosis causes no specific endoscopic lesions in the colon.

Strongyloidiasis can cause colonic inflammation that resembles ulcerative colitis but is frequently right sided; features resembling pseudomembranous colitis have also been reported. The gravid female forms of *Enterobius vermicularis* can sometimes be seen during colonoscopy as motile thread-like 1 cm long pale worms in the rectum or more proximal in the colon. Anisakidosis can be diagnosed on endoscopy when finding the larvae burying into the bowel wall. The adult form of *Taenia saginata* can become 4–10 m long and may be encountered by the endoscopist in the colon. Patients with schistosomiasis may come to the attention of the gastroenterologist for mild anemia, positive fecal occult blood tests, or unexpected variceal hemorrhage. Colonoscopy may show multiple inflammatory polyps or small pale excrescences containing eggs on biopsy.

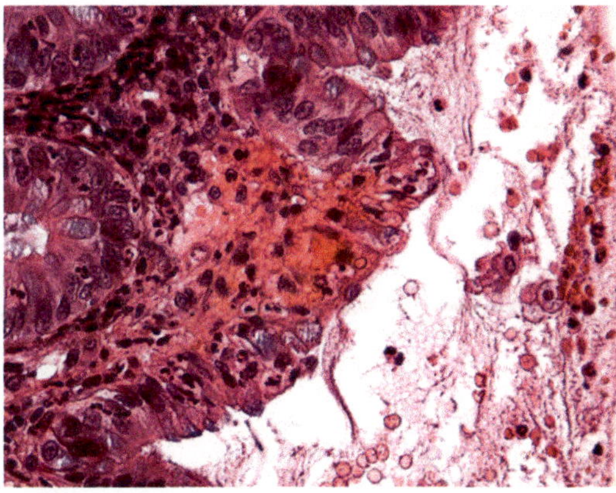

Parasitic Colitis, Fig. 1 Colonic mucosal biopsy, HE high power view. *Entamoeba histolytica* trophozoites

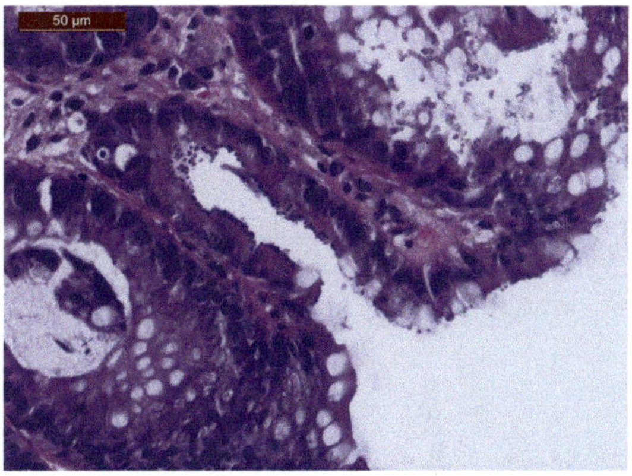

Parasitic Colitis, Fig. 2 Colonic mucosal biopsy, HE high power view. *Cryptosporidia* at the apex of crypt and surface epithelial cells

Microscopy

The gold standard for the diagnosis of *Entamoeba histolytica* colitis is colonoscopy with mucosal biopsies. These should be taken from the ulcers' edges, where the amoebic trophozoites intermingle with neutrophils. The amoebae are relatively large and may be confused with histiocytes. They have a central or eccentric nucleus with a prominent karyosome and contain ingested red blood cells (erythrophagocytosis) (Fig. 1). Their detection can be facilitated by PAS staining, with which the trophozoites stain magenta. A CD68 stain may help in the differentiation with histiocytes.

A high index of suspicion is of great importance for the diagnosis of cryptosporidiosis. Any epidemic outbreak of watery diarrhea lasting longer than a week, or chronic watery diarrhea in an immunocompromised person, should trigger microscopic investigation of the stools for oocysts. *Cryptosporidia* are only occasionally seen in colonic biopsies. They can be recognized as small basophilic spherical bodies protruding from the apex of the enterocytes, both in crypts or at the surface (Fig. 2). Neutrophils may be present in the lamina propria. Giemsa stains may help with the diagnosis.

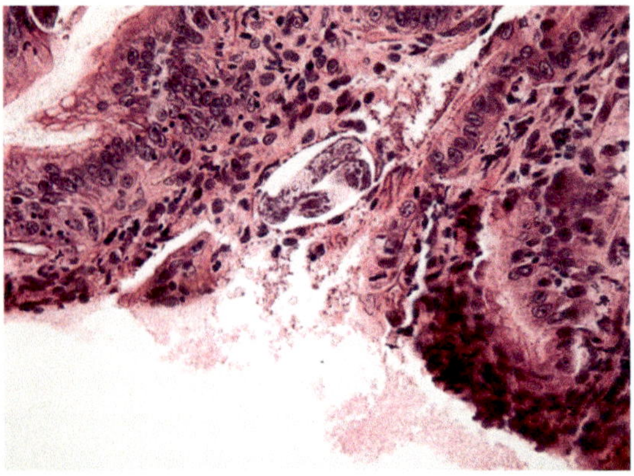

Parasitic Colitis, Fig. 3 Gastric mucosal biopsy, HE high power view. *Strongyloides stercoralis* filariform larva embedded in the mucosa

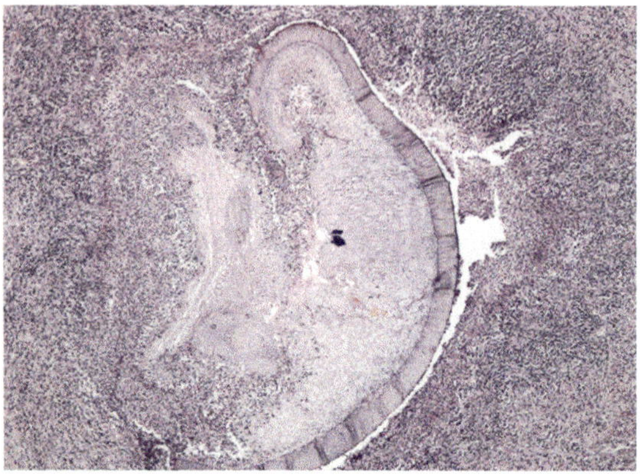

Parasitic Colitis, Fig. 5 Jejunum surgically removed for intestinal obstruction, HE low power view. *Anisakis simplex*, larval form penetrating the bowel wall

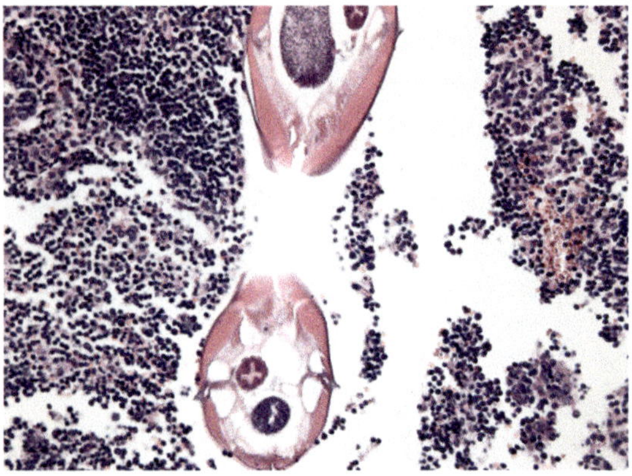

Parasitic Colitis, Fig. 4 Appendix removed for acute appendicitis, HE high power view. *Enterobius vermicularis*, adult form on cross-section

The preferred diagnostic test for *Strongyloides stercoralis* infection is serology, while colonic mucosal biopsy is insensitive at best. One may see edema, ulcers, a mixed infiltrate which also contains many eosinophils, and adult and larval worms (Fig. 3). Granulomas may be present.

Pinworm infection is usually diagnosed with the cellophane tape test. Clear tape is applied to the perianal skin in the morning before washing. The tape is then pushed on a glass slide and examined for eggs. This is repeated every day during 1 week. *Enterobius vermicularis* is occasionally seen in the lumen of appendices removed for acute appendicitis or en passant (Fig. 4). It is unclear whether they can cause appendicitis by themselves. Even when they become invasive, which happens rarely, there is usually little or no inflammatory reaction. There may be a somewhat increased tissue eosinophilia. Granulomas, sometimes with necrosis, can be seen around degenerating worms and eggs. These lesions have been described in the appendix, colon, anus and even in the cervix, the endometrium, the fallopian tubes, the peritoneum, and the omentum, which testifies to the migratory effect of the female worms.

When biopsies are taken in a case of anisakidosis, histologic findings include a dense inflammatory infiltrate rich in eosinophils, eosinophilic microabscesses, solitary giant cells, and granulomas. The infiltrate is commonly transmural and concentrated around the 0.5–3 cm long larvae which may be seen in the bowel wall (Fig. 5).

Beef and pork tapeworms are diagnosed by detection of proglottids and eggs in feces. The proglottids may occasionally be submitted for histology (Fig. 6). They are 1–2 cm large, with a thick wall, and contain 10–12 uterine branches full of eggs.

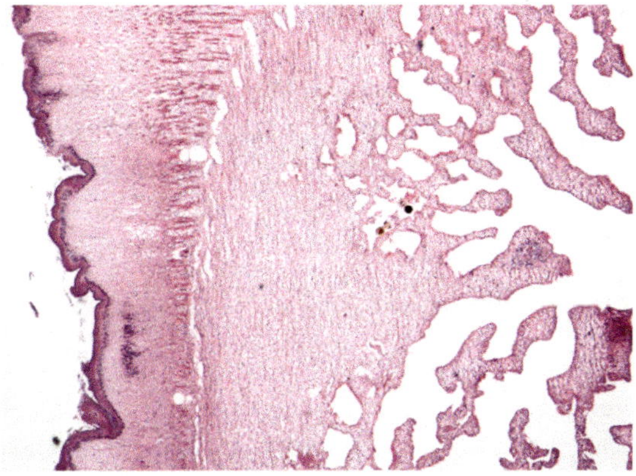

Parasitic Colitis, Fig. 6 HE, low power view. Gravid proglottid of *Taenia saginata* passed with the stools and submitted for microscopic examination

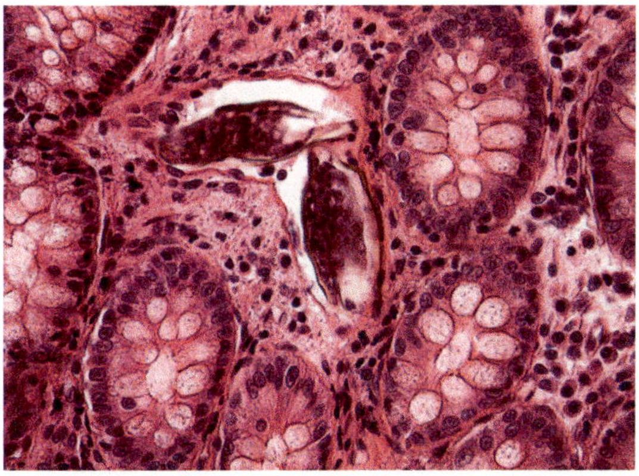

Parasitic Colitis, Fig. 7 Colonic mucosal biopsy, HE high power view. Eggs of *Schistosoma mansoni* embedded in the lamina propria

Schistosoma infection can be diagnosed by identification of eggs in the stools, or better in crushed tissue specimens, or via serology. Eggs and surrounding granulomas may be detected in colonic mucosal biopsies (Fig. 7). The granulomas are composed of a mixed infiltrate of macrophages, lymphocytes, and eosinophils, which account for 50% of the cell population. When they degranulate and deposit their major basic protein, an eosinophilic halo may develop around the degenerating egg (so-called Splendore-Hoeppli phenomenon). Worms are occasionally seen within submucosal veins.

Immunophenotype, Molecular Features

These tests are not used for routine histological diagnosis of parasitic colitis.

Differential Diagnosis

Many forms of parasitic colitis may resemble IBD, both in its acute and chronic presentations. The differential diagnosis rests on awareness of the clinical context, a high index of suspicion, and an appropriate handling of the biopsies to maximize the chance of finding representative forms of the pathogens. Multiple sections at additional levels may be required. Amoebic colitis especially must be differentiated from IBD, because an erroneous treatment with glucocorticoids may lead to a fulminant disease course with a high mortality.

References and Further Reading

Arca, M. J., Gates, R. L., Groner, J. I., et al. (2004). Clinical manifestations of appendiceal pinworms in children: An institutional experience and a review of the literature. *Pediatric Surgery International, 20*, 372–375.

Deng, M., Rutherford, M. S., & Abrahamsen, M. S. (2004). Host intestinal epithelial response to *Cryptosporidium parvum*. *Advanced Drug Delivery Reviews, 56*, 869–884.

Geboes, K., el-Dosoky, I., el-Wahab, A., et al. (1990). The immunopathology of *Schistosoma mansoni* granulomas in human colonic schistosomiasis. *Virchows Archiv A, Pathological Anatomy and Histopathology, 416*, 527–534.

Marcus, V. A., Ward, B. J., & Jutras, P. (2001). Intestinal amebiasis: A diagnosis not to be missed. *Pathology Research and Practice, 197*, 271–274.

Qu, Z., Kundu, U. R., Abadeer, R. A., et al. (2009). Strongyloides colitis is a lethal mimic of ulcerative colitis: The key morphologic differential diagnosis. *Human Pathology, 40*, 572–577.

Takei, H., & Powell, S. Z. (2007). Intestinal anisakidosis (anisakiosis). *Annals of Diagnostic Pathology, 11*, 350–352.

Pemphigoid, Bullous, Esophageal

Ana Afonso[1] and Joaninha Costa Rosa[2]
[1]Serviço de Anatomia Patológica, Hospital Cuf Descobertas e IPOLFG, E.P.E Parque das Nações, Lisbon, Portugal
[2]Serviço de Anatomia Patológica, Instituto Português de Oncologia de Lisboa Francisco Gentil, Lisbon, Portugal

Synonyms

Anti-epiligrin cicatricial pemphigoid; Anti-laminin 5 cicatricial pemphigoid; Bullous pemphigoid; Cicatricial pemphigoid; Mucous membrane pemphigoid

Definition

Esophageal pemphigoid is an uncommon disorder belonging to a group of autoimmune blistering diseases that can affect the mucosa, hence the designation of mucous membrane pemphigoid (MMP). It was formerly named cicatricial pemphigoid because, in the majority of the patients, the lesions have a tendency to heel with a scar. Bullous pemphigoid (BP) is nowadays the preferred term for the bullous disease limited to the skin, where it may initially start as an urticarial eruption that progressively evolves to large and tense bullae. BP rarely affects mucosal membranes. Skin involvement in MMP is seen in 20–25% of patients (Sallout et al. 2000); in 10% of the cases, skin lesions are the first sign of the disease, but they are usually less severe than in BP. MMP has the singular quality of healing with scar formation, and this is the most important characteristic, contributing to morbidity and mortality of this disease.

MMP is characterized by linear deposition of immunoglobulins and/or complement components along the epithelial basement membrane zone (BMZ). The result of this alteration is a subepithelial loss of cohesion, vesicle formation, and epithelial detachment.

MMP may occur simultaneously with thymoma; pancreatic, gastric, and lung carcinoma; acquired hemophilia; celiac disease; and other autoimmune diseases (rheumatoid arthritis, systemic lupus erythematosus) (Bernard and Borradori 2012; Sallout et al. 2000).

Clinical Features

The patients may present with odynophagia, dysphagia, and weight loss and usually have involvement of the oral or conjunctival mucosa. There is one exceptional report of MMP with exclusive esophageal disease at initial presentation (Sallout et al. 2000). Sometimes the initial symptoms are related to the formation of erosions and webs. Later, strictures and even complete occlusion of the esophagus may occur. The disease runs a chronic, relapsing course and rarely remits spontaneously. Scarring and esophageal stenosis are the major sequelae. The diagnosis of esophageal pemphigoid needs a high level of clinical suspicion and combined clinical, histological, and immunopathological results.

- **Incidence**
  The incidence of mucous membrane pemphigoid varies from 1:12,000 to 1:20,000, per year, 4% of these patients having esophageal disease (Calonje et al. 2012).
- **Age**
  There is some variation in age of presentation. Mucous membrane pemphigoid is a disease of elderly people that typically begins in the fifth or sixth decade of life (Bruch-Gerharz et al. 2007), although there are reports in children and young adults.
- **Sex**
  There is a female predominance (1,5–2:1) (Bruch-Gerharz et al. 2007). There are no known ethnic or racial preferences.
- **Site**
  Esophageal involvement in mucous membrane pemphigoid is rare and usually limited to the patients with multiorgan disease.

- **Treatment**
  To control the symptoms and prevent the complications of esophageal stenosis, systemic treatment with corticosteroids is indicated.
  Prednisone is the most useful drug since it is simultaneously anti-inflammatory and immunosuppressive; dapsone may be used as a steroid-sparing adjuvant.
  More aggressive cases may require additional treatment with cyclophosphamide. Other therapeutic options are intravenous immunoglobulin, mycophenolate mofetil, thalidomide, dexamethasone, cyclophosphamide pulse therapy, etanercept, and infliximab.
  Surgical dilation of the esophagus is the last choice in severe stenosis, but it should be remembered that every surgical manipulation may exacerbate disease.
- **Outcome**
  The prognosis of MMP is quite variable and is related to the involved site, esophageal location being associated with medical treatment resistance and a worse prognosis (Chan et al. 2002). Progressive disease from the onset, frequent relapses in the first years and the permanent involvement of other organs, as ocular mucosa, are predictive of poor outcome. Severe complications related to infection and malnutrition may shorten life and cause death.

Macroscopy

Endoscopic findings include bullae, ulcerations, webs, and stenosis (Sallout et al. 2000).

Microscopy

The characteristic microscopic feature in MMP is a subepithelial blister with different types of inflammatory cells related to the evolution of the lesion (Fig. 1). In a recent lesion, less than 48 h' duration, there are neutrophil microabscesses in the subepithelial corion; in the next phase, the inflammatory infiltrate will have a growing number of eosinophils; later in the evolution of the lesion, the predominant cells will be lymphocytes and plasma cells. The number of eosinophils is always lower than in bullous pemphigoid.

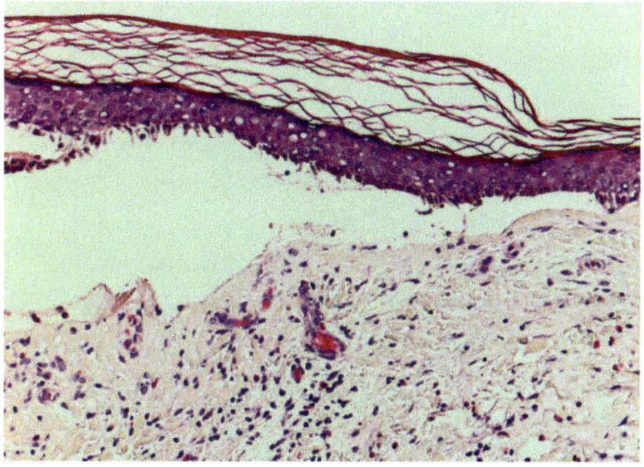

Pemphigoid, Bullous, Esophageal, Fig. 1 Mucosal lesions, similarly to the skin ones, show subepithelial detachment with polymorphous inflammatory infiltrate

If an old lesion is sampled, the histological picture will show an erosion with less intense inflammation and important fibroblast proliferation, with new collagen bundles parallel to the surface. A new vesicle may supervene in an old, scarred lesion, so a given sample may show simultaneously scarring and blistering formation with polymorphous infiltrate.

Immunophenotype

Direct immunofluorescence is a specific and sensitive test, the best results being obtained from perilesional mucosa (Bruch-Gerharz et al. 2007; Sallout et al. 2000). These studies are more frequently positive (50–90%) in mucosa than in skin (20–50%). A positive test displays a continuous, fine, linear band of IgG and C3 along the basement membrane. IgA and other immunoglobulins may also be present, but only rarely is IgA the single immunoglobulin present. However, false-negative results may justify the need to repeat the biopsy in some doubtful cases.

Indirect immunofluorescence for serum circulating antibodies is a less sensitive method as it is positive in only 20–30% of MMP patients. However, the use of multiple substrates, including salt-split skin, and/or the use of concentrated serum samples may increase the number of positive results. Antibody titers are usually very low. The levels of these circulating antibodies correlate with disease activity, and the presence of both IgG and IgA antibodies may be associated with more severe and persistent disease (Chan et al. 2002).

Electron microscopy studies are useful in patients in whom tissue immunocomplexes cannot be demonstrated by conventional immunofluorescence, but being expensive and time consuming, this technique is not indicated as a first-line diagnostic method.

On a recent blister, electron microscopy demonstrates that the dermal–epidermal cleavage forms within the lamina lucida.

By direct immunoelectron microscopy, immune deposits are distributed either in the lower lamina lucida or over the lamina densa; they may alternatively be located on and around hemidesmosomes, below the cell membrane. By indirect electron microscopy, autoantibodies typically bind to the lower lamina lucida near by the lamina densa (Bernard and Borradori 2012).

Molecular Features

Mucous membrane pemphigoid belongs to a group of immunological diseases traditionally classified together. They result from the binding of autoantibodies to the BMZ of stratified epithelia, which recognize distinct structural components of the hemidesmosomal adhesion complex that bind to extracellular antigenic sites within the anchoring filament zone. Immunochemical techniques have identified the most frequently involved antigens: laminin 332 (previously designated laminin 5) or epiligrin is an adhesion molecule, component of the anchoring filaments, within the lamina lucida; bullous pemphigoid antigen 2 (BP 180) that also appears to function as an adhesion molecule, sharing the anchoring filament complex together with laminin 332; and the β4 integrin subunit that takes part in the epidermal hemidesmosome.

Recent demonstration of these autoimmune reactions enabled the separation of these groups of diseases into four distinct subgroups on the basis of the reactivity outline of patients' autoantibodies. Nevertheless, for practical purposes, the mucosal cases are considered together, as they share the same clinical phenotype (Chan et al. 2002).

The first subgroup, known as anti-laminin 332 cicatricial pemphigoid or anti-epiligrin cicatricial pemphigoid (AECP), includes patients with autoantibodies directed against laminin 332. The patients have circulating IgG autoantibodies that bind to the dermal side of salt-split skin and react with the α3 chain (G domain) or, less frequently, the β3 and/or γ2 chain of laminin 5 (α3β3γ2).

Recent studies have shown that patients with this form of mucous membrane pemphigoid have an increased relative risk for malignant tumors. The mechanism underlying this association of AECP and cancer is unknown, but there is accumulating evidence that laminin 5 plays a central role. These patients with anti-laminin 332 autoantibodies cannot be distinguished clinically from those with other variants of mucous membrane pemphigoid. The second subgroup has pure or predominant ocular disease. The patients have autoantibodies that bind to the β4 subunit of α6β4 integrin, a transmembrane hemidesmosomal component that interacts with laminin 332. These patients have a lower risk of cancer than controls and a better prognosis. The third subgroup encompasses patients with mucosal and skin lesions and has tissue-bound and circulating IgG antibodies that react with the same target antigens as for bullous pemphigoid, especially BP180. These patients should be classified as having anti-BP180 antigen mucous membrane pemphigoid. The fourth group includes patients who have variable involvement of mucosae without involvement of the skin. In these patients, it is unclear if damage occurs as a result of an autoantibody-mediated response to proteins of the epithelial basement membrane (Bernard and Borradori 2012).

Some studies mention the possibility that genetic factors may influence the susceptibility to MMP. Some major histocompatibility complex class II markers and extended haplotypes have been linked to several clinical forms of MMP. The allele HLA-DQB1*0301, initially described in patients with pure ocular disease, was further associated with other locations and related with a more aggressive clinical course (Bruch-Gerharz et al. 2007). The higher association of MMP with other autoimmune disorders provides good evidence to the importance of genetic factors.

Differential Diagnosis

Differential diagnosis must include the autoimmune diseases group: pemphigus vulgaris, bullous pemphigoid, epidermolysis bullosa acquisita, linear IgA bullous disease, and bullous systemic lupus erythematosus. If a non-bullous or cicatricial lesion is sampled, non-autoimmune diseases must be considered, such as lichen planus, erythema multiforme, scleroderma, chronic graft-versus-host disease, and congenital esophageal stenosis.

Distinction from bullous pemphigoid, epidermolysis bullosa acquisita, and linear IgA bullous dermatosis may be very difficult, requiring the use of sophisticated immunopathological techniques.

Pemphigus vulgaris and non-autoimmune diseases may be distinguished by conventional and immunofluorescence microscopy combined with adequate clinical context.

References and Further Reading

Bernard, P., & Borradori, L. (2012). Pemphigoid group. In J. L. Bolognia, J. L. Jorizzo, & J. V. Schaffer (Eds.), *Dermatology* (pp. 475–490). Philadelphia: Elsevier/Saunders.

Bruch-Gerharz, D., Hertl, M., & Ruzicka, T. (2007). Mucous membrane pemphigoid: Clinical aspects, immunopathological features and therapy. *European Journal of Dermatology, 17*, 191–200.

Calonje, E., Brenn, T., Lazar, A., & McKee, P. H. (2012). Inherited and autoimmune subepidermal blistering diseases. In E. Calonje, T. Brenn, A. Lazar, & P. H. McKee (Eds.), *MacKee's pathology of the skin* (pp. 133–137). Edinburgh: Elsevier Limited.

Chan, L. S., Ahmed, R. A., Anhalt, G. J., Bernauer, W., Cooper, K. D., Elder, M. J., Fine, J. D., Foster, S., Ghohestani, R., Hashimoto, T., Hoang-Shuan, T., Kirtschig, G., Korman, N. J., Lightman, S., Lozada-Nur, F., Marinkovich, P., Mondino, B. J., Prost-Squarcioni, C., Rogers, R. S., Setterfield, J. F., West, D. P., Wojnarowska, F., Woodley, D. T., Yancey, K. B., Zillikens, D., & Zone, J. J. (2002). The first international consensus on mucous membrane pemphigoid. Definition, diagnostic criteria, pathogenic factors, medical treatment and prognostic indicators. *Archives of Dermatology, 138*, 370–379.

Sallout, H., Anhalt, G., & Al-Kawas, F. (2000). Mucous membrane pemphigoid presenting with isolated esophageal involvement: A case report. *Gastrointestinal Endoscopy, 52*, 429–433.

Pemphigus Vulgaris, Esophageal

Joaninha Costa Rosa[1] and Ana Afonso[2]
[1]Serviço de Anatomia Patológica, Instituto Português de Oncologia de Lisboa Francisco Gentil, Lisbon, Portugal
[2]Serviço de Anatomia Patológica, Hospital Cuf Descobertas e IPOLFG, E.P.E Parque das Nações, Lisbon, Portugal

Synonyms

Pemphigus vulgaris

Definition

Pemphigus vulgaris (PV) is a rare, chronic, life-threatening, autoimmune, blistering disease of the skin and mucosal membranes. It results from the loss of integrity of normal intercellular attachments within epithelia, producing suprabasal acantholytic blisters. The separation of the epithelial cells at their desmosomal junctions is due to the production of autoantibodies targeting epithelial adhesion molecules.

The disorder may have a complex etiology involving genetic and environmental factors. The susceptibility to pemphigus is described as being related to several human leukocyte antigen (HLA) alleles and to ethnic groups.

The disease is commonly associated with other immune disorders and with an increase in the incidence of neoplasia, but it is distinct from the variant paraneoplastic pemphigus.

P

In a majority of cases, *pemphigus vulgaris* starts in the oral mucosa, but it may also occur in a variety of other mucosal sites. After the onset of the disease in the oral mucosa, blistering may spread to involve the skin.

Esophageal lesions are known to occur in a large number of cases, and the esophagus may be the only site of involvement (Faias et al. 2004). The symptoms of esophageal involvement may include dysphagia, odynophagia, and retrosternal burning. PV has even been reported as a cause of *esophagitis dissecans superficialis* (Hokama et al. 2010), a condition that is characterized by sloughing of large fragments of esophageal mucosa.

The clinical phenotype of this disease may be dominated by mucosal lesions or by mucocutaneous lesions. The pathogenesis of the disorder depends on the formation of antibodies against autoantigens that, in *pemphigus vulgaris*, are desmoglein 3 (Dsg3) and desmoglein 1 (Dsg1). Autoantibodies reactive to other antigens such as acetylcholine receptor are also produced in PV, but they have not shown to directly mediate blister formation (Stanley and Amagai 2006). The clinical picture – the mucosal dominant type versus the mucocutaneous involvement pattern – has been related to the normal distribution of desmoglein 3 and 1 proteins in skin and mucosal epithelium, as well as to the type of antibody(ies) that is(are) produced (anti-Dsg3/anti-Dsg1) (Stanley and Amagai 2006; Hokama et al. 2010).

The examination of a skin or mucosal biopsy will reveal the presence of a suprabasal acantholytic cleft or bulla. Direct and indirect immunofluorescence techniques are used for the final diagnosis. Immunohistochemistry for IgG4, the predominant subclass present in these patients, is also a specific test for diagnosing pemphigus (Zhang et al. 2012).

Serum from patients with *pemphigus vulgaris* contains IgG antibodies and not infrequently IgA antibodies (Calonje et al. 2012). The circulating autoantibodies may be detected in serum by enzyme-linked immunosorbent assay (ELISA). This sensitive technique may be used for the initial diagnosis and for monitoring the disease (Hokama et al. 2010), as circulating antibody levels and type (IgG1 and IgG4 subclasses) are related to the clinical phase of the disease (Calonje et al. 2012).

Clinical Features

- **Incidence**
  Pemphigus is a rare disorder whose annual incidence ranges from 0.1 to 0.7 per 100,000. *Pemphigus vulgaris* is the most common form of the disease, accounting 80% of the cases (Calonje et al. 2012). Recent data has shown that the incidence of esophageal involvement is higher – 46–87% (Hokama et al. 2010) – than it was previously thought.
- **Age**
  Pemphigus vulgaris usually develops in middle-aged adults (40–60 years). It may also occur up to 2.6% in children and even in newborns (Calonje et al. 2012).
- **Sex**
  Male to female ratio of *pemphigus vulgaris* is 1:1 (Calonje et al. 2012).
- **Site**
  The clinical picture of PV may be dominated by mucosal lesions with minimal skin involvement or by a mucocutaneous pattern of involvement. The esophagus is often involved and may be the only site of involvement (Faias et al. 2004). The disease is rarely confined to the skin (Calonje et al. 2012).
- **Treatment**
  Oral corticoids are considered the first-line option for treatment of *pemphigus vulgaris*. Other therapeutic options include megadose pulse steroids, immunosuppressants, intravenous immunoglobulins, plasmapheresis, and anti-CD20 monoclonal antibody (Hokama et al. 2010).
- **Outcome (Prognosis)**
  Nowadays, the mortality rate in *pemphigus vulgaris* is 5–15% (Calonje et al. 2012). The clinical course is variable and spontaneous remission has been reported in some patients. Most morbidity and mortality events depend on the side effects of therapy.

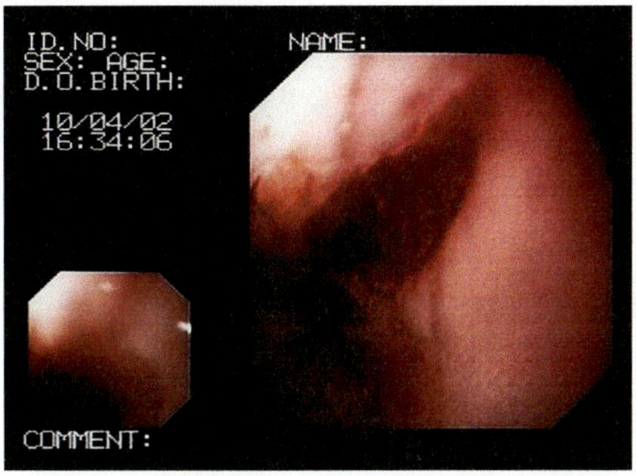

Pemphigus Vulgaris, Esophageal, Fig. 1 On withdrawal of endoscope, areas of sloughed mucosa are seen

Macroscopy

Clinically, vesicles, bullae, or erosions may be seen on the skin or mucosal surfaces. Esophageal local erythema, red erythematous longitudinal lines, erosions, ulcers, blisters (Fig. 1), and *esophagitis dissecans superficialis* were described in esophageal *pemphigus vulgaris* (Hokama et al. 2010).

The biopsy specimen, usually small and obtained from the periphery of the lesions, has no particular gross features.

Microscopy

Histologically, the disease is characterized by the presence of acantholysis. When the cells lose their attachments, a cleft appears in a suprabasal position and a suprabasal acantholytic blister develops (Fig. 2). The basal layer of the epidermis, which remains attached to the basal membrane, looks like a "row of tombstones." In some cases dermal papillae protrude into the blister cavity as villi. Acantholytic cells and some inflammatory cells, particularly eosinophils, may be seen inside the bullae. The acantholytic epidermal cells are rounded; they have eosinophilic cytoplasm and picnotic nuclei, surrounded by a perinuclear halo. As the bullae are fragile, in some biopsy specimens, a naked bulla without roof may be obtained, and the characteristic "tombstone" appearance of the basal cells may be the only histological finding.

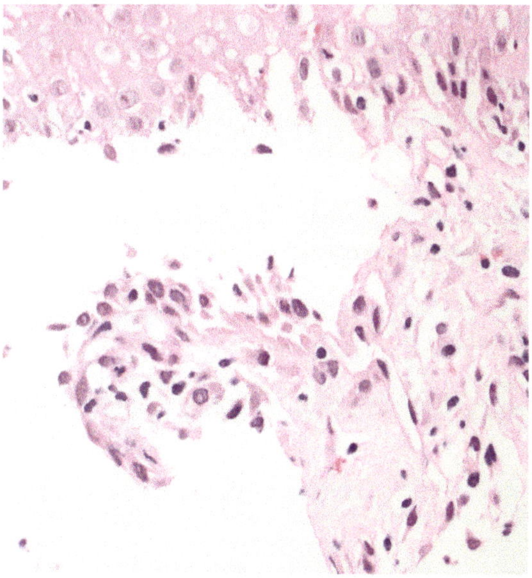

Pemphigus Vulgaris, Esophageal, Fig. 2 Photomicrograph from an esophageal biopsy showing a suprabasal acantholytic cleft and some acantholytic cells

Eosinophilic spongiosis and a slight to intense chronic perivascular inflammatory infiltrate with eosinophils may also be seen.

Immunophenotype

Direct immunofluorescence performed on fresh-frozen tissue is a quite specific and sensitive morphological test. A fine granular band – which corresponds to autoantibodies and complement components attached to the epithelial cells – is seen in the intercellular junctions. Immunohistochemistry for IgG4 performed on paraffin sections is also a sensitive test for diagnosing pemphigus (Zhang et al. 2012).

Molecular Features

Desmogleins and desmocollins are desmosomal cadherins, which means that they contribute to modulate cell-cell adhesion and tissue integrity. It explains why antibody production against desmogleins 3 and 1 results on mucosal and skin blistering. Some studies have suggested that inactivation of desmoglein by antibodies may not be sufficient to explain blistering phenomena. Complex signaling mechanisms leading to internalization of desmoglein 3, reorganization of the cytoskeleton, and apoptosis of the keratinocytes have also been proposed to explain blister formation (Stanley and Amagai 2006).

Differential Diagnosis

Pemphigus vulgaris may be mimicked by other forms of *pemphigus*, including paraneoplastic and drug-induced *pemphigus*, and by other dermatologic diseases involving the esophagus, such as *benign mucous membrane pemphigoid*, *Darier's disease*, *Halley-Halley disease*, *dermatitis herpetiformis*, *epidermolysis bullosa acquisita*, and erythema multiforme. If a picture of eosinophilic spongiosis is the dominant morphological feature, the differential diagnosis may include eosinophilic esophagitis.

References and Further Reading

Calonje, E., Brenn, T., Lazar, A., & McKee, P. H. (2012). Acantholytic disorders. In E. Calonje, T. Brenn, A. Lazar, & P. H. McKee (Eds.), *McKee's pathology of the skin* (pp. 151–179). Edinburgh: Elsevier.

Faias, S., Lage, P., Sachse, F., Pinto, A., Fidalgo, P., Fonseca, I., & Nobre-Leitão, C. (2004). Pemphigus vulgaris with exclusive involvement of the esophagus: Case report and review. *Gastrointestinal Endoscopy, 60*(2), 312–315.

Hokama, A., Yamamoto, Y., Taira, K., Nakamura, M., Kobashigawa, C., Nakamoto, M., Hirata, T., Kinjo, N., Kinjo, F., Takahashi, K., & Fujita, J. (2010). Esophagitis dissecans superficialis and autoimmune bullous dermatosis: A review. *World Journal of Gastrointestinal Endoscopy, 2*(7), 252–256.

Stanley, J. R., & Amagai, M. (2006). Pemphigus, bullous impetigo and the staphylococcal scalded- skin syndrome. *The New England Journal of Medicine, 355*, 1800–1810.

Zhang, X., Hyjek, E., Soltani, K., Petronic-Rosic, V., & Shea, C. R. (2012). Immunohistochemistry for immunoglobulin g4 on paraffin sections for the diagnosis of pemphigus. *Archives of Pathology and Laboratory Medicine, 136*(11), 1402–1407.

Peptic Duodenal Disease

Arzu Ensari
Department of Pathology, Ankara University Medical School, Sihhiye, Ankara, Turkey

Synonyms

Chronic (peptic) duodenitis; Chronic active duodenitis; Chronic nonspecific duodenitis; *H. pylori*-associated chronic duodenitis; Peptic ulcer disease

Definition

Peptic duodenal disease represents a continuum of the same disease process of acute and chronic inflammation of the duodenal mucosa resulting from the toxic effects of excess gastric acid. In the setting of increased gastric acid secretion, such as in antral predominant *H. pylori* gastritis, duodenal inflammation and ulceration may occur. Chronic *H. pylori* infection is highly associated with peptic disease of the duodenum in more than 80% of the cases. It is also commonly seen in patients who smoke, take NSAIDs chronically for other conditions, have renal insufficiency, or have duodenal immobility. The clinical picture is characterized by burning epigastric pain relieved with food ingestion. In severe cases the pain may be accompanied by nausea and vomiting.

Clinical Features

- **Incidence**
  It is estimated to affect up to 10% of the population in Westernized countries.
- **Age**
  The prevalence of *H. pylori*-associated duodenitis increases with age, and peptic disease is more common in patients older than 40 years.
- **Sex**
  It is more common in males than in females.

- **Site**
  Peptic duodenitis is most commonly seen in the duodenal bulb.
- **Treatment**
  Eradication of *H. pylori* and use of acid inhibitors improve symptoms of the patients. Medical therapy includes small meals, antacids, proton-pump inhibitors, and antibiotics.
- **Outcome**
  Up to 5% of the patients may have upper gastrointestinal bleeding. In elderly, rebleeding may occur in up to one third. Refractory ulcers heal slowly or follow a remitting course. Though rare, perforation may be seen in the elderly due to NSAIDs.

Macroscopy

Duodenal bulb appears nodular, friable, deformed, or scarred on endoscopy. Ulcers resemble ulcers in other sites of the gastrointestinal tract. Most duodenal ulcers are circular and less than 3 cm in diameter.

Microscopy

The microscopic findings include one or more of the following: inflammatory cells, namely, plasma cells and neutrophils in the epithelium, and/or lamina propria, damaged reactive epithelium with or without gastric foveolar metaplasia, villus blunting, mucosal hemorrhage and edema, and Brunner's gland hyperplasia with prominent ingrowth towards the mucosae (Figs. 1–4). Gastric foveolar metaplasia is not an absolute criterion for the diagnosis of peptic duodenitis in the absence of mucosal inflammation while it represents an adaptive process to chronic hyperacidic state. *H. pylori* may be present within the metaplastic surface. A combined PAS/alcian blue stain may be performed to highlight neutral mucin present in the metaplastic gastric epithelium. The changes are usually patchy and thus can be missed due to sampling error. Peptic injury may also cause increased IELs in duodenal bulb mucosa causing a major diagnostic confusion with GSE.

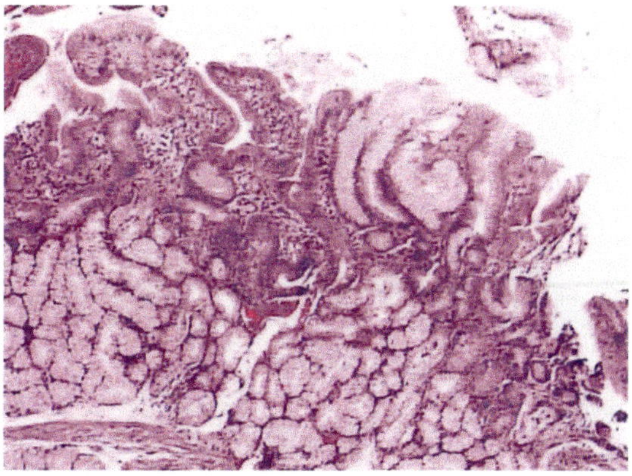

Peptic Duodenal Disease, Fig. 1 Duodenal mucosa showing gastric foveolar metaplasia (H&E; ×100)

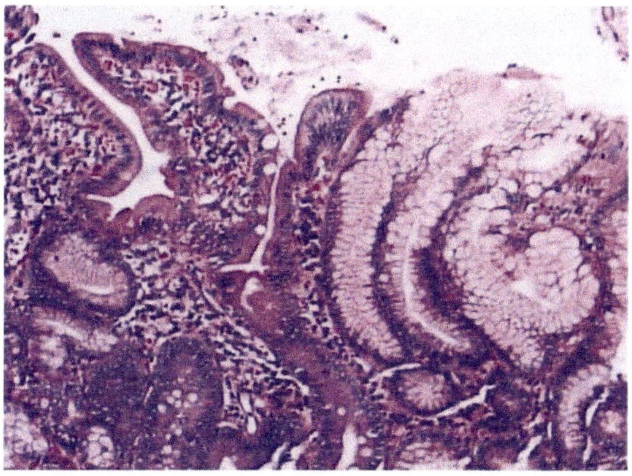

Peptic Duodenal Disease, Fig. 2 Gastric foveolar metaplastic area in inflamed duodenal mucosa (H&E; ×200)

This is, particularly, a problem when distal duodenum is not biopsied since it is usually normal in *H. pylori* infection. In severe cases surface erosions and ulcerations may be seen.

Immunophenotype

There is no specific immunophenotypic feature of peptic duodenal disease.

Molecular Features

There is no specific molecular feature of peptic duodenal disease.

P

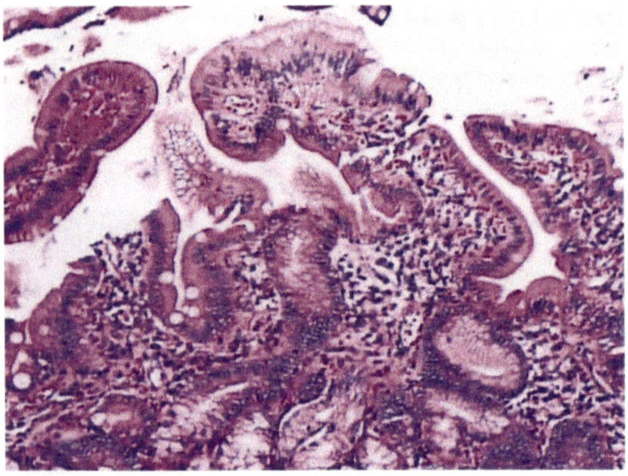

Peptic Duodenal Disease, Fig. 3 Damaged surface epithelium with gastric metaplasia and mixed cellular inflammatory infiltrate in the lamina propria (H&E; ×200)

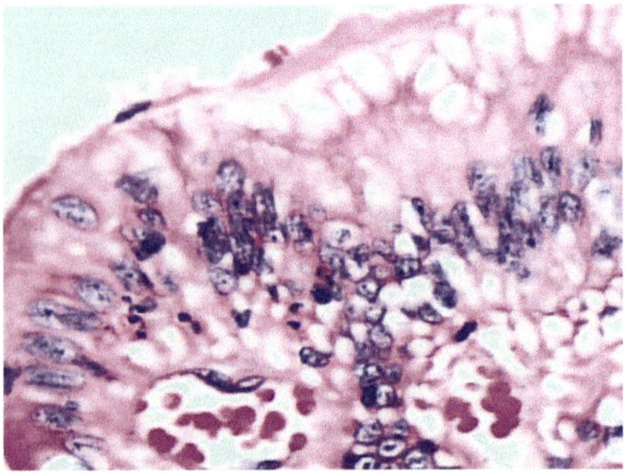

Peptic Duodenal Disease, Fig. 4 Neutrophils and IELs in the surface epithelium showing gastric metaplasia (H&E; ×400)

Differential Diagnosis

Since pathologic changes are usually nonspecific in peptic duodenal disease, NSAID injury, Crohn's disease, coeliac disease, and infections with similar histology should be considered in the differential diagnosis. Clinical correlation and special stains for microorganisms may help to differentiate between these conditions. Features useful in distinguishing this condition from coeliac disease are the heavy neutrophilic infiltration of the lamina propria, as well as the surface epithelium, relatively less architectural damage in terms of villous shortening, and the presence of foveolar metaplasia, though the latter may also be seen in coeliac disease if the biopsy is taken from the bulbus affected by *H. pylori*. Specific features to aid in the diagnosis of Crohn's disease are the presence of granulomas and evidence of lower GI tract involvement and the patchy nature of the inflammatory changes. Gastric heterotopy may also be included in the differential diagnosis as there is prominent gastric epithelium in this condition. However, unlike peptic duodenitis, oxyntic glands are present in heterotopic gastric mucosa.

References and Further Reading

Dixon, M. F. (2000). Patterns of inflammation linked to ulcer disease. *Baillière's Best Practice & Research. Clinical Gastroenterology, 14*(1), 27–40.

Suriani, R., Venturini, I., Actis, G. C., Rocca, G., Rizzetto, M., Cerutti, E., Mazzucco, D., Cardesi, E., & Zeneroli, M. L. (2004). Effect of *Helicobacter pylori* eradication on bulbitis and duodenal gastric metaplasia. *Hepato-Gastroenterology, 51*(55), 176–180.

Voutilainen, M., Juhola, M., Farkkila, M., & Sipponen, P. (2003). Gastric metaplasia and chronic inflammation at the duodenal bulb mucosa. *Digestive and Liver Disease, 35*, 94–98.

Walker, M. M., & Dixon, M. F. (1996). Gastric metaplasia: Its role in duodenal ulceration. *Alimentary Pharmacology and Therapeutics, 10*, 119–128.

Wyatt, J. I., Rathbone, B. J., Sobala, G. M., Shallcross, T., Heatley, R. V., Axon, A. T. R., & Dixon, M. F. (1990). Gastric epithelium in the duodenum: Its association with *H. pylori* and inflammation. *Journal of Clinical Pathology, 43*, 981–986.

Peptic Ulcer

Pedro Pimentel-Nunes[1,2], Ricardo Marcos-Pinto[1,3] and Mário Dinis-Ribeiro[1,2]
[1]Serviço de Gastrenterologia, Portuguese Oncology Institute, Porto, Portugal
[2]Instituto Português de Oncologia (IPO - Porto), Cintesis (FMUP-UP), Porto, Portugal
[3]Centro Hospitalar do Porto, Instituto de Ciências Biomédicas Abel Salazar (ICBAS-UP), Cintesis (FMUP-UP), Porto, Portugal

Synonyms

Duodenal ulcer; Gastric ulcer; Gastroduodenal ulcers; Peptic erosions; Peptic ulcer disease

Definition

Peptic ulcers are the most common form of gastroduodenal ulcerations caused by the combined effect of acid and gastric pepsin. They are clinically defined as a mucosal break equal to or greater than 5 mm that extend through the muscularis mucosa, in the stomach or duodenum, organs that are normally exposed to acidic environment. As many as 70–80% of the cases of peptic ulcers are associated with *Helicobacter pylori* gastric infection, and 20–30% associated with the use of nonsteroidal anti-inflammatory drugs (NSAIDs), with 10% being idiopathic. Peptic ulcers are most commonly caused by a decrease in mucosal defense mechanisms that can be related to Helicobacter infection and/or NSAIDs use, allowing the action of acid and pepsin on an unprotected gastroduodenal mucosa. Uncommonly, they are associated with hypersecretory states like gastrinomas (Zollinger-Ellison syndrome). Epigastric pain is the most common symptom of peptic ulcers.

Clinical Features

- **Incidence**
  Although the incidence of peptic ulcers has declined (in parallel with the decline in *Helicobacter pylori* infection), the lifetime risk for developing a peptic ulcer is calculated to be approximately 10–15%. Population-based studies suggest that in developed countries the 10-year cumulative incidence of peptic ulcer is about 2–5%, with almost equal incidence of gastric and duodenal ulcers. However, in countries with a high prevalence of *Helicobacter pylori* infection, the 2-year incidence is about 2–3%, with 70–80% of the ulcers being duodenal.
- **Age**
  Peptic ulcers can occur at any age, although they are more commonly diagnosed at older ages (>40 years). Complications of peptic ulcers are more common at ages older than 60–65.
- **Sex**
  Historically, the prevalence of peptic ulcer is higher in men than in women. However, recent reports suggest that the prevalence has shifted to almost equal prevalence's in both genders (slightly more common in men).
- **Site**
  Most gastric ulcers tend to occur at the junction of the corpus and antrum (incisura) along the lesser curvature; however, they may occur at any gastric location. More than 95% of the duodenal ulcers are found in the first part of the duodenum, either at the posterior or anterior wall of the duodenum bulb.
- **Treatment**
  Peptic ulcers almost always heal with 8–12 weeks of therapy with proton pump inhibitors (PPIs); however, if the baseline condition (*Helicobacter pylori* or NSAIDs use) is not resolved, the risk of recurrence is high when PPIs are stopped. So, for peptic ulcers related to *Helicobacter pylori* gastritis, the recommended treatment is PPI-based triple therapy (14 days of PPI with two antibiotics, twice daily), resulting in ulcer healing in 85–90% of cases. The risk of recurrence is high in the absence of successful H. pylori eradication, and, so, confirmation of eradication is recommended. In patients with NSAID-associated ulcer disease, if it is clinically feasible, NSAIDs should be discontinued. For patients who must continue NSAIDs, PPI maintenance therapy is recommended as well as H. pylori eradication. Other antisecretory medications like H2 blockers may also heal peptic ulcers, however, with worse results than PPIs. Surgery is only needed for complications of peptic ulcers like perforation or bleeding.
- **Outcome**
  When diagnosed in the uncomplicated phase, the prognosis is excellent, with almost all patients obtaining total healing of the ulcers. Recurrence is possible if the underlying cause of the ulcer is not adequately managed (see "Treatment"). However, although the incidence of ulcers may be decreasing, the

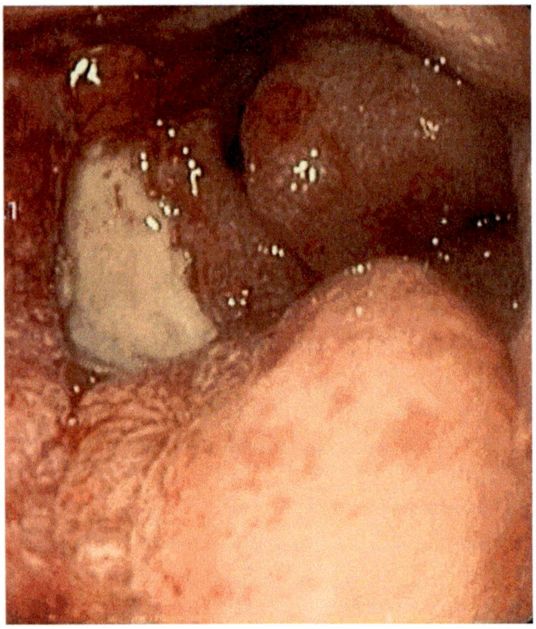

Peptic Ulcer, Fig. 1 Duodenal ulcer

incidence of complicated ulcers has remained the same, with a combined risk of complications (bleeding, perforation, obstruction) of 1–2% per ulcer per year. The mortality rate is approximately 1 death per 100,000 cases with the mortality rate due to ulcer hemorrhage being 5–10%.

Macroscopy

Upper gastrointestinal endoscopy is the diagnostic test of choice. At endoscopy the ulcer appears as a round to oval parietal defect ("hole"), generally with 0.5–2 cm diameter and with a smooth base which often presents some whitish fibrinoid exudate and perpendicular borders (Fig. 1). These borders are not elevated or irregular in the acute form of peptic ulcer, but they may be regular with elevated borders and inflammatory surrounding in the chronic form. Surrounding mucosa may present radial folds, as a consequence of the parietal scarring. In the ulcerative form of gastric cancer, the borders are irregular and there is generally some nodular or mass component in the lesion. Nevertheless, at least 5% of apparently benign gastric ulcers are in fact malignant, and for this reason, biopsy and confirmation of ulcer healing is generally recommended.

Microscopy

A peptic ulcer is a mucosal defect, which penetrates the muscularis mucosae and sometimes also the muscularis propria particularly in the duodenum, produced by acid-pepsin aggression. The histology depends on its chronicity. Ulcer margins are perpendicular and present chronic gastritis. During the active phase, the base of the ulcer shows four zones: inflammatory exudate with neutrophilic infiltration, fibrinoid necrosis, granulation tissue, and fibrous tissue. The fibrous base of the ulcer may contain vessels with thickened wall or with thrombosis.

Differential Diagnosis

Clinical: Cholecystitis; Cholelithiasis; Biliary colic; Gastroesophageal reflux disease; Cholangitis; Hepatitis; Gastritis/gastroenteritis; Acute coronary syndrome; Abdominal aneurysm; Mesenteric ischemic disease; Diverticulitis.

Endoscopic: Malignant ulcer (adenocarcinoma, lymphoma); Peptic erosions; Esophagitis; Infectious ulcer (tuberculosis, fungus, virus); Ischemic ulcer; Ulcer caused by inflammatory bowel disease.

References and Further Reading

Cryer, B., & Spechler, S. J. (2010). Peptic ulcer disease. In M. Feldman, L. S. Friedman, & L. J. Brandt (Eds.) *Sleisenger & Fordtran's gastrointestinal and liver disease* (9th ed.). Philadelphia: Saunders, Elsevier.

Malfertheiner, P., Megraud, F., O'Morain, C., et al. (2012). Management of *Helicobacter pylori* infection – The Maastricht IV/Florence Consensus Report. *Gut, 61*, 646–664.

Tytgat, G. N. (2011). Etiopathogenetic principles and peptic ulcer disease classification. *Digestive Diseases, 29*(5), 454–458.

Peutz-Jeghers Syndrome

Armagan Gunal
Department of Pathology, Gulhane Military Medical Academy, Etlik, Ankara, Turkey

Synonyms

Periorificial lentiginosis; Polyps and spots syndrome

Definition

Peutz-Jeghers polyposis is a hereditary cancer syndrome which belongs to hamartomatous polyposis syndromes. It is characterized by mucocutaneous melanotic hyperpigmentation and hamartomatous polyps in gastrointestinal tract with an increased risk of intestinal and also extra-intestinal malignancies.

Hamartoma defines an overgrowth of normal tissues in their own native localisations. Hamartomatous polyps in gastrointestinal tract can be seen sporadically, but multiple polyps can occur as a component of genetically inherited or acquired hamartomatous polyposis syndromes. Hamartomatous polyposis syndromes include: (1) Juvenile polyposis, (2) Peutz-Jeghers polyposis (PJP), (3) Cowden syndrome and Bannayan-Ruvalcaba-Riley syndrome (these two are also called as "PTEN hamartoma tumor syndrome" because of the same affected gene locus), (4) Cronkhite-Canada syndrome (the latter is different from the former three because of its inflammatory basis rather than genetic).

Diagnostic criteria for defining hamartomatous polyps in gastrointestinal tract as PJP are: (1) three or more morphologically defined Peutz-Jeghers polyps; or (2) any number of Peutz-Jeghers polyps with a family history of PJP; or (3) characteristic mucocutaneous hyperpigmentation with a family history of PJP; or (4) any number of Peutz-Jeghers polyps with characteristic mucocutaneous hyperpigmentation.

Clinical Features

- **Incidence**
  The prevalence of PJP has been estimated between 1 per 50,000 birth to 1 per 200,000 births. This rate corresponds to approximately one tenth of familial adenomatous polyposis.
- **Age**
  PJP is generally diagnosed in the first and second decades although the first presentation has been reported with an age range of 2–62 years.
- **Sex**
  No sex predilection has been defined for PJP.
- **Site**
  Peutz-Jeghers polyps in PJP are most commonly found in small intestine (95%), particularly upper jejunum followed by colon (60%) and stomach (50%). Peutz-Jeghers polyps have also been detected outside the gastrointestinal tract, such as gallbladder, bladder and nasopharynx, bronchi and ureter.

  Mucocutaneous melanotic hyperpigmentations are seen on the lips (characteristically vermilion borders), nostrils, buccal mucosa, palmar surfaces, genitalia and perianal region. Malignancies occur in the entire gastrointestinal tract (including pancreas) in PJP. Extra-gastrointestinal malignancies have been reported in breast, ovary, testis, and uterus.
- **Treatment**
  Surgery is required when intussusception causing ileus occurs. Endoscopic polypectomy of pedinculated polyps is important to prevent such complications.

  The most important point in PJP is the surveillance programs for the early diagnosis and prevention for gastrointestinal and extra-intestinal malignancies. Proposed surveillance programs comprise of (1) colonoscopy, gastroscopy and appropriate small intestine screening method in every 2–3 years beginning from the age of 18 (or eight as more rigidly), (2) Ultrasound examination for pancreas and ovary in every 1–2 years, (3) breast self-examination annually and mammography in every 2–3 years, (4) Cervicovaginal smears and pelvic examination in every 3 years, and

P

(5) Testicular examination beginning from the birth.

- **Outcome**

Intussusception is the main nonneoplastic presentation of PJP and is the major cause of mortality during childhood. Abdominal pain and bleeding are usually related to this complication. It mainly occurs in the small intestine. Rectal prolapse of the polyps may also be seen in childhood.

The most warrisome complication of PJP is malignancy. Overall relative risk of malignancy at any site has been reported as 15-fold for PJP. Cumulative risk for any malignancy has been calculated as 93% in PJP patients between 15 and 64 year old age group. This rate is also higher for some organs: 39% for colorectal carcinoma, 36% for pancreatic carcinoma, 29% for gastric carcinoma and 54% for breast carcinoma.

Macroscopy

Typically, hamartomatous polyps in PJP are coarsely lobulated with a short peduncle. Multilobulated architecture and eroded smooth surface of juvenile polyps or the characteristic velvety texture of adenomatous polyps are not seen. The size of polyps changes from millimetres to several centimetres.

Mucocutaneous hyperpigmented lesions are millimetric macules on areas described above. They are present 95% of patients in childhood and may disappear after puberty.

Microscopy

The distinctive microscopic view of PJP polyps is prominent tree branch-like smooth muscle proliferation between mucosal epithelial components (Fig. 1). These arborizing smooth muscle fibers derives from the muscularis mucosa. Mucosal component consists of cysticly dilated glands with condensed mucin in their lumen. Lamina propria can be inflamed and fibrotic. This specific pattern may be indistinct for small polyps and the polyps in gastric localisation. Ischemic change and pseudoinvasion pattern may complicate the diagnosis in pedunculated polyps of PJP. Dysplasia of the epithelium has been rarely reported in PJP polyps.

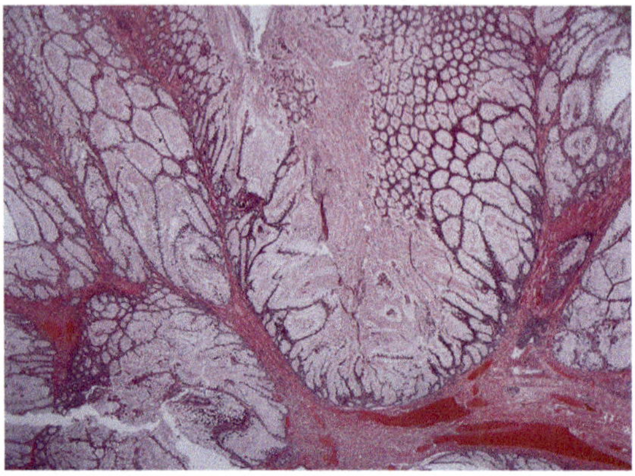

Peutz-Jeghers Syndrome, Fig. 1 Tree branch-like smooth muscle bundles are seen in between mucosal glands (HEx100)

Immunophenotype

No specific immunophenotypic feature has been reported for PJP.

Molecular Features

PJP is a genetically inherited syndrome with autosomal dominant trait. Germline mutation is seen in LKB1/STK11 gene, locused in 19p13.3. Serine/threonine kinase, the product of this pleiotropic tumor suppressor gene, is responsible from many regulatory activities including cell growth and inhibits some anabolic metabolism activities.

Differential Diagnosis

Hyperplastic polyps, other types of hamartomatous polyps and even adenomas are in the differential diagnosis group for PJP polyps. Arborizing smooth muscle proliferation and absence of diffuse dysplasia are helpful diagnostic features. Foveolar hyperplastic features without arborizing smooth muscle fibers may be seen in gastric polyps. Clinical correlation is needed in such situations.

Epithelial misplacement (pseudoinvasion) may be problematic in pedunculated polyps of PJP, causing confusion for adenocarcinoma. Thorough evaluation of the fundamental features of epithelial misplacement may prevent a misdiagnosis of adenocarcinoma.

References and Further Reading

Cauchin, E., Touchefeu, Y., & Matysiak-Budnik, T. (2015). Hamartomatous tumors in gastrointestinal tract. *Gastrointestinal Tumors, 2*, 65–74.

Hornick, J. L., & Odze, R. D. (2015). Polyps of the large intestine. In R. D. Odze & J. R. Goldblum (Eds.), *Surgical pathology of the GI tract, liver, biliary tract and pancreas* (pp. 607–655). Philadelphia: Elsevier.

Jung, I., Gurzu, S., & Turdean, G. S. (2015). Current status of familial gastrointestinal polyposis syndromes. *World Journal of Gastrointestinal Oncology, 7*, 347–355.

Offerhaus, G. J. A., Billaud, M., & Gruber, S. B. (2010). Peutz-Jeghers syndrome. In F. T. Bosman, F. Carneiro, R. H. Hruban, & N. D. Theise (Eds.), *WHO classification of tumours of the digestive system* (pp. 168–170). Lyon: IARC.

Shaco-Levy, R., Jasperson, K. W., Martin, K., Samadder, N. J., Burt, R. W., Ying, J., & Bronner, M. P. (2016). Morphologic characterization of hamartomatous gastrointestinal polyps in Cowden syndrome, Peutz-Jeghers syndrome and juvenile polyposis syndrome. *Human Pathology, 49*, 39–48.

Turner, J. R. (2015). The gastrointestinal tract. In V. Kumar, A. K. Abbas, & J. C. Aster (Eds.), *Pathologic basis of disease* (pp. 750–817). Philadelphia: Elsevier.

Plummer-Vinson Syndrome

Isadora Rosa and António Dias Pereira
Instituto Português de Oncologia de Lisboa
Francisco Gentil, E.P.E., Lisboa, Portugal

Synonyms

Paterson-Brown-Kelly syndrome; Paterson-Kelly syndrome; Sideropenic dysphagia; Waldenström and Kjellberg syndrome

Definition

Plummer-Vinson syndrome is the most common name attributed to the association of dysphagia, upper esophageal webs, and iron-deficiency anemia. Henry Stanley Plummer and Porter Paisley Vinson were the American physicians who first reported clinical cases of patients with this entity. However, its full description was done later by the British laryngologists Donald Ross Paterson and Adam Brown-Kelly. Waldenström and Kjellberg later documented cases of the syndrome also occurring with sideropenia without anemia.

The pathogenesis of Plummer-Vinson syndrome (PVS) remains unknown, but the main purposed theories are based on nutritional deficiencies (mainly of iron) or autoimmune phenomenon. The syndrome's diagnosis implies iron deficiency, with or without anemia, and this deficiency is proposed to lead both to atrophy of the esophageal mucosa, with formation of webs, and to changes in muscles involved in swallowing. These alterations would mainly be due to the depletion of iron-dependent enzymes. The fact that PVS can be improved, and sometimes cured, with iron supplementation supports this theory, but the vast majority of patients with iron deficiency do not develop the syndrome and esophageal webs are found without it. This could be explained by a genetic predisposition, which might also explain the fact that while in some populations the decline of PVS's incidence paralleled the nutritional status improvement, in others it remains rare even with chronic iron deficiency.

The fact that PVS has been associated with some autoimmune diseases, such as celiac disease, rheumatoid arthritis, or thyroiditis, led to the autoimmune theory of its etiology, but it has also never been demonstrated.

Finally, it has been proposed that the syndrome originates from a patch of heterotopic gastric mucosa in the upper esophagus that ulcerates, causing bleeding and iron deficiency, and then leads to scaring, with web formation. Again, this has never been demonstrated.

Clinically, patients usually report intermittent, sometimes progressive, painless dysphagia. The dysphagia in PVS is usually limited to solids and may be associated with weight loss. All other symptoms and signs that may be present, namely, fatigue, pallor, tachycardia, glossitis, angular cheilitis, koilonychia, and hepatosplenomegaly, result from anemia and iron deficiency.

The diagnosis of PVS is done after documenting iron deficiency, with or without anemia (and usually with no other laboratory alterations) and postcricoid upper esophageal webs. The webs (single or multiple) are usually limited to the first centimeters of the esophagus and start from its anterior wall, extending laterally and rarely encircling the lumen. They may be seen at endoscopy, but they are easily ruptured and missed, which makes videofluoroscopy the best diagnostic exam. Occasionally, the webs can also be demonstrated by barium swallow X-ray.

Manometric studies are not used for diagnosis, but some authors have described low pharyngeal swallowing pressures and low amplitude contractions in the esophagus that are typically corrected by iron supplementation.

Clinical Features

- **Incidence**
  The exact incidence and prevalence of PVS are unknown, but the syndrome seems to be extremely rare nowadays, with only a few case reports being published. In the beginning of the twentieth century, PVS was apparently common in northern European countries, but it rapidly declined, in parallel with the improvement of the population's nutritional status.
- **Age**
  The syndrome has typically been described between the fourth and seventh decades of life, but there are case reports at younger ages.
- **Sex**
  PVS has been more commonly described in women, with a clear female predominance in the early high incidence studies from Scandinavia.
- **Site**
  The characteristic webs are typically limited to the proximal third of the esophagus.

  The syndrome may have systemic manifestations, secondary to the anemia and/or iron deficiency.
- **Treatment**
  Iron replacement therapy is the cornerstone of treatment and sometimes, by itself, leads to complete resolution of the syndrome. The cause of the iron deficiency should be clarified and corrected whenever possible.

  When the dysphagia persists after iron supplementation, dilation and/or incision of the web should be performed. Usually, one session of endoscopic therapy is enough, but multiple procedures may be required.
- **Outcome (Prognosis)**
  If the iron deficiency is corrected, the syndrome does not seem to reoccur after therapy. The main concern is the description of cases of hypopharynx or upper esophagus squamous cell carcinomas complicating PVS. The syndrome is therefore considered a premalignant condition, and yearly surveillance by upper gastrointestinal endoscopy is recommended, although the effectiveness of this strategy is unproven.

Macroscopy (Gross)

The esophageal webs in PVS are thin membranes (1–2 mm) that emerge from the anterior wall, just below the cricopharyngeal muscle, and are rarely circumferential but may be multiple.

Microscopy

Webs are composed of mucosa and submucosa layers and, by definition, have no muscular layer. They are usually covered, on both sides, by normal squamous epithelium and have a subepithelial layer of connective tissue. Occasionally, mucosal atrophy, chronic submucosal inflammation, and atrophy or degeneration of the muscularis mucosa may be seen.

Immunophenotype

Thyroid cytoplasmic autoimmune antibodies have been found in a higher proportion of patients with PVS, when compared to other iron-deficient patients. No other antibodies have been associated with the syndrome.

Molecular Features

The molecular basis of the syndrome is unknown. The proposed depletion of iron-dependent enzymes has never been demonstrated.

Differential Diagnosis

The main differential diagnosis to be made is that of the cause of dysphagia, which has to include all mechanical (especially malignant tumors) and motor causes. It is also essential to diagnose the cause of the iron deficiency, which may imply specific treatment.

References and Further Reading

Geerlings, S. F., & van Eps, L. W. S. (1992). Pathogenesis and consequences of Plummer-Vinson syndrome. *The Clinical Investigator, 70*, 629–630.

Hoffman, R. M., & Jaffe, P. E. (1995). Plummer-Vinson syndrome. A case report and literature review. *Archives of Internal Medicine, 155*, 2008–2011.

Novacek, G. (2006). Plummer-Vinson syndrome. *Orphanet Journal of Rare Diseases, 1*, 36.

Popescu, C. R., Bertesteanu, S. V. G., Mirea, D., Grigore, R., Ionescu, D., & Popescu, B. (2010). The epidemiology of hypopharynx and cervical esophagus cancer. *Journal of Medicine and Life, 3*, 396–401.

Polyp, Gastrointestinal

Arzu Ensari
Department of Pathology, Ankara University Medical School, Sihhiye, Ankara, Turkey

Synonyms

Benign neoplasia; Growth; Protuberance

Definition

The term polyp refers to any overgrowth of tissue from the surface of the mucous membranes. Gastrointestinal polyp is any mass of tissue that arises from the bowel wall and protrudes into the lumen. Gastrointestinal polyp is a common form of benign neoplastic growth.

Polyps show a great variation in shape and size. They may have round, shiny smooth surfaces or may be eroded/ulcerated depending on the size of the polyp.

All gastrointestinal polyps arise from the mucosa. Majority of these polyps are asymptomatic and may be discovered accidentally at endoscopy performed for other reasons. The main concern is malignant transformation; most colon cancers arise in a previously benign adenomatous polyp.

Clinical Features

- **Incidence**
  Incidence of polyps ranges from 7% to 50%; the higher figure includes very small polyps (usually hyperplastic polyps or microadenomas) found at autopsy. About one third of the general population will develop intestinal polyps at some point in life.
- **Age**
  The incidence of preneoplastic polyps such as adenomas increase with age. In general, however, hamartomatous or nonneoplastic polyps may be found starting from the first decades of life.
- **Sex**
  There is no sex predilection in gastrointestinal polyps.
- **Site**
  Gastrointestinal polyps, often multiple, occur most commonly in the rectum and sigmoid and decrease in frequency toward the cecum. Stomach and small intestine are the sites where isolated or multiple polyps of various types may also be observed.

- **Treatment**
- **Outcome**

Macroscopy

Polyps may be sessile or pedunculated and vary considerably in size from a few millimeters to a few centimeters.

Microscopy

Gastrointestinal polyps comprise of adenomatous polyps or adenomas, hyperplastic, serrated polyps, hamartomatous polyps, namely juvenile polyp, Peutz-Jeghers type polyps, lymphoid, lipomatous, leiomyomatous, and ganglioneuromatous polyps. The classification of gastrointestinal polyps is presented in Table 1.

Immunophenotype

No specific immunophenotype is present in gastrointestinal polyps.

Polyp, Gastrointestinal, Table 1 Classification of gastrointestinal polyps

Site	Neoplastic	Nonneoplastic
Stomach	Adenoma Gastric type Intestinal type Pyloric gland adenoma Fundic gland polyp associated with FAP Traditional serrated adenoma	Hyperplastic polyp Inflammatory fibroid polyp Hamartomatous polyp
Small intestine	Adenoma Traditional serrated adenoma	Hamartomatous polyp
Colorectum	Adenoma Sessile serrated adenoma Traditional serrated adenoma	Hyperplastic polyp Hamartomatous polyp

Molecular Features

Sporadic gastrointestinal polyps do not usually possess the molecular aberrations as their polyposis counterparts. However, conventional adenomas show somatic APC mutations while hyperplastic/serrated polyps show BRAF mutations.

Differential Diagnosis

All polyps arising in gastrointestinal tract come into the differential diagnosis grossly. However, microscopy reveals specific features that characterize each one of these polyps.

References and Further Reading

Burgart, L. J. (2002). Colorectal polyps and other precursor lesions. Need for an expanded view. *Gastroenterology Clinics of North America, 31*, 959–970.
Geboes, K. C., Ectors, N., & Geboes, K. P. (2005). Pathology of early lower GI cancer. *Best Practice & Research Clinical Gastroenterology, 19*(6), 963–978.

Polyposis Syndromes

Arzu Ensari
Department of Pathology, Ankara University Medical School, Sihhiye, Ankara, Turkey

Synonyms

Gastrointestinal polyposis syndromes; Hereditary polyposis syndromes

Definition

Gastrointestinal polyposis syndrome is characterized by the presence of at least 15 polyps dispersed throughout the gastrointestinal tract. Most polyposis syndromes however present with hundreds of polyps in the gastrointestinal tract. These are rare, autosomal dominant syndromes characterized by multiple polyps and a high risk for gastrointestinal and extraintestinal cancer. Polyposis syndromes are classified by the polyp type, age of presentation, gastrointestinal distribution, number of polyps, presence of extraintestinal findings, and the underlying germline genetic abnormality. They are characterized and named by the predominant polyp type (e.g., juvenile polyp and juvenile polyposis syndrome). Extraintestinal findings include congenital retinal hypertrophy, osteomas, perioral pigmentation, epidermoid cysts, subcutaneous lipomas, sebaceous gland tumors, medulloblastoma, and hepatoblastoma. Types of gastrointestinal polyps that are found in polyposis syndromes vary from conventional adenoma to hamartomatous, juvenile, hyperplastic, serrated, inflammatory, ganglioneuromatous, and lipomatous polyps. The classification of gastrointestinal polyposis syndromes is presented in Table 1.

Polyposis Syndromes, Table 1 Classification of gastrointestinal polyposis syndromes

Hereditary polyposis syndromes		Nonhereditary polyposis syndromes
Adenomatous polyposis syndromes	**Hamartomatous polyposis syndromes**	Serrated polyposis syndrome
Familial adenomatous polyposis (FAP) **Classical FAP** **Gardner's syndrome** **Turcot's syndrome** **Attenuated FAP** **MUTYH (MYH)-associated polyposis syndrome (MAP)** **Lynch syndrome** **Muir-Torre syndrome**	Juvenile polyposis syndrome Peutz-Jeghers syndrome PTEN-hamartoma tumor syndrome Cowden syndrome Bannayan-Riley-Ruvalcaba syndrome Proteus syndrome Hereditary hemorrhagic telangiectasia	Cronkhite-Canada syndrome Inflammatory "cap" polyposis Lymphomatoid polyposis Nodular lymphoid hyperplasia Pneumatosis cystoides intestinalis
	Other: Neurofibromatosis type 1, multiple endocrine neoplasia type 2, Birt-Hogg-Dube syndrome	

Clinical Features

- **Incidence**
  The incidences of polyposis syndromes vary between 1: 10,000 and 1: 200,000 and even lower in the rarer forms of polyposis.
- **Age**
  Polyposis syndromes arise in a background of germline mutations of associated genes, and therefore present at young ages ranging from the first decade to the fourth-fifth decade of life depending on the type of polyposis syndrome. Juvenile polyposis may present in the first decade while adenomas in familial adenomatous polyposis may be diagnosed in second or third decade. Polyps increase in size and number with age. Neoplastic progression of adenomas leading to colorectal carcinoma may be detected at the age of 40.
- **Sex**
  There is no known sex predilection in gastrointestinal polyposis syndromes. An equal distribution between men and women is expected.
- **Site**
  The majority of gastrointestinal polyposis syndromes involve the entire gastrointestinal tract with a predominance of polyps in the colon. However, the polyps of Peutz-Jeghers syndrome show a predilection to the small intestine, while proximal involvement is very common in MUTYH-associated polyposis in comparison to familial adenomatous polyposis. Therefore, the site of involvement is determined by the type of polyposis syndrome.
- **Treatment**
  Treatment of gastrointestinal polyposis syndromes focuses on prophylactic surgery before the development of malignancy. In most cases, surgery is delayed until the patient completes secondary education with annual surveillance. Polyp number and size determine the need for early surgery. Surveillance should be continued following surgery.

Polyposis Syndromes, Table 2 Histopathologic and molecular features of gastrointestinal polyposis syndromes

Polyposis syndrome	GI involvement	Polyp type	Aberrant gene
Classical FAP	Mainly colorectum + entire GI	Conventional adenoma	APC
MAP	Colorectum + extensive upper GI polyposis	Conventional adenoma, serrated polyp	MUTYH (MYH)
Juvenile polyposis	Entire GI	Juvenile polyp	SMAD4 or BMPR1A
Peutz-Jeghers syndrome	Entire GI, predominantly small intestine	Peutz-Jeghers polyp	LKB1 (STK11)
Cowden syndrome	Entire GI	Hamartoma	PTEN

- **Outcome**
  Early diagnosis of the polyposis syndrome together with prophylactic surgery and appropriate surveillance usually result in favorable outcome. The reverse is true however for cases whose initial presentation is with malignancy.

Macroscopy

Macroscopically gastrointestinal polyposis syndromes are characterized with the presence of numerous polyps distributed throughout the gastrointestinal tract. The gross features of the polyps and the polyposis syndromes may differ depending on the predominant polyp type. Carpeting with millimetric sessile polyps is a frequent finding in familial adenomatous polyposis while hamartomatous polyposis syndromes are characterized by the presence of protruding, large polyps fewer in number.

Microscopy

Microscopy of the polyposis syndromes varies according to the predominant polyp type. Conventional adenomas, serrated polyps, hyperplastic polyps, hamartomatous polyps, juvenile polyps, ganglioneuromatous, and lipomatous polyps can be found in gastrointestinal polyposis syndromes.

Immunophenotype

No specific immunophenotype is present.

Molecular Features

Molecular abnormalities underlying the polyposis syndromes are presented in Table 2.

Differential Diagnosis

Though initial presentation may be similar, gastrointestinal polyposis syndromes can be differentiated according to the predominant polyp type, number, distribution of the polyps, age of the patient, and the underlying molecular abnormality (see Table 2).

References and Further Reading

Bronner, M. P. (2003). Gastrointestinal inherited polyposis syndromes. *Modern Pathology, 16*(4), 359–365.

Brosens, L. A. A., van Hattem, W. A., Marnix, J., Jansen, M., Wendy, W. J., de Leng, W. W. J., Giardiello, F. M., & Offerhaus, G. J. A. (2007). Gastrointestinal polyposis syndromes. *Current Molecular Medicine, 7*, 29.

Jelsig, A. M., Qvist, N., Brusgaard, K., Nielsen, C. B., Hansen, T. P., & Ousager, L. B. (2014). Hamartomatous polyposis syndromes: A review. *Orphanet Journal of Rare Diseases, 9*, 101–111.

Kastrinos, F., & Syngal, S. (2011). Inherited colorectal cancer syndromes. *Cancer Journal, 17*(6), 405–415.

Lynch, H. T., Lynch, J. F., & Shaw, T. G. (2011). Hereditary gastrointestinal cancer syndromes. *Gastrointestinal Cancer Research, 4*(Suppl 1), S9–S17.

Pseudodiverticulum (Pseudodiverticula), Esophageal

Catarina Fidalgo and Sandra Faias
Instituto Português de Oncologia de Lisboa
Francisco Gentil, E.P.E., Lisbon, Portugal

Synonyms

Esophageal traction or pulsion diverticula; Pseudodiverticula of the esophageal body

Definition

Pseudodiverticula of the esophageal body are outpouchings of the esophageal lumen containing mucosa and submucosa, through a defect in the muscular layer. The term pseudodiverticulum implies that congenital diverticula are excluded as the latter are "true" diverticula, meaning that they contain all layers of esophageal wall. Pseudodiverticula can also be classified according to their pathogenesis as pulsion or traction diverticula, the former resulting from high intraluminal pressure (a mechanism shared by Zenker's and epiphrenic diverticula) and the latter from a mechanism of traction from the outside of the esophagus. Pulsion diverticula can also be associated with motility disorders of the esophagus such as achalasia, diffuse esophageal spasm, or hypertensive lower esophageal sphincter, although this causal relationship is more established in the case of epiphrenic diverticula. Traction diverticula are a consequence of mediastinal inflammation, occurring in the setting of tuberculosis, histoplasmosis, or sarcoidosis. This traction mechanism can also take place in the setting of malignant disease with enlarged mediastinal lymph nodes. These outpouchings can occur anywhere in the esophagus but are usually located in the middle or lower third. When the diverticulum is located near the diaphragmatic hiatus, it is called epiphrenic diverticulum. The etiology of this

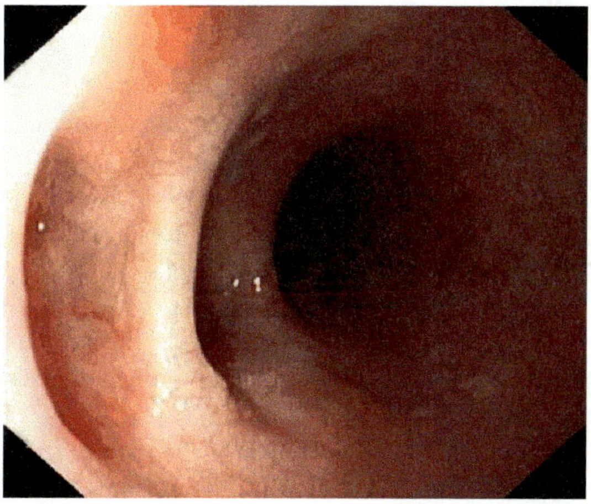

Pseudodiverticulum (Pseudodiverticula), Esophageal, Fig. 1 Endoscopic view of an esophageal pseudodiverticulum

anatomic alteration is usually inflammatory but can also be traumatic. Pseudodiverticula of the esophagus can occur as a complication of sclerotherapy for esophageal varices or as a consequence of thoracic surgery. Esophageal pseudodiverticula are usually asymptomatic, being an incidental finding in barium esophagogram or upper endoscopy (Fig. 1) performed for unrelated symptoms. When symptomatic, the most common symptoms are dysphagia, regurgitation, and, rarely, weight loss and chest discomfort. A special type of pseudodiverticulum, known as esophageal intramural pseudodiverticulosis, refers to the finding of multiple, small outpouchings of the esophageal wall that can be seen on contrast esophagogram. These are dilatations of the excretory ducts of submucosal mucus glands, forming tiny outpouchings or pseudodiverticula. Sometimes intramural tracks bridge between two or more pseudodiverticula, a process called intramural tracking. It sometimes progresses to benign stricture, resulting in variable degrees of dysphagia. The definite etiology remains unknown, although it has been associated with gastroesophageal reflux, fungal infection, diabetes, and alcohol abuse. There have been case reports of pseudodiverticular perforation leading to mediastinitis.

P

Clinical Features

- **Incidence**
  Esophageal pseudodiverticula are extremely rare. In fact they correspond to less than 10% of all pharyngoesophageal diverticula (Zenker's prevalence, the most frequent pseudodiverticulum, is 0.1%).
- **Age**
  As the diagnosis is almost always accidental, there is no knowledge about a typical age at diagnosis.
- **Sex**
  There is no known gender difference in terms of prevalence.
- **Site**
  Esophageal diverticula are usually located in the middle or lower third of the esophagus. This designation excludes epiphrenic diverticula (addressed in another chapter).
- **Treatment**
  Only symptomatic esophageal pseudodiverticula merit any treatment. If serious symptoms are attributable to the diverticulum and the patient is fit to undergo surgery, a correction may be considered. Both open surgery and thoracoscopical/laparoscopical options can be used. It is advisable to perform a motility study by manometry to exclude associated motility disorder, prior to treatment.
- **Outcome**
  The majority of these diverticula are asymptomatic and do not become symptomatic over time.

Macroscopy

Pseudodiverticula are outpouchings of the esophageal wall anywhere in the esophagus.

Microscopy

These outpouchings contain mucosal and submucosal layers protruding through a defect in the muscular layer. In the particular case of intramural pseudodiverticulosis, the outpouchings correspond to dilated mucus glands in the submucosal layer.

Immunophenotype

No immunophenotypic features have been identified as associated with esophageal pseudodiverticula.

Molecular Features

No distinctive molecular features have been proposed in this condition.

Differential Diagnosis

Epiphrenic diverticulum, esophageal intramural pseudodiverticula

References and Further Reading

Canon, C., Levine, M., Cherukuri, R., et al. (2000). Intramural tracking: a feature of esophageal intramural pseudodiverticulosis. *American Journal of Roentgenology, 175*, 371–374.

Chiba, T., Lijima, K., Koike, T., et al. (2012). A case of severe esophageal intramural pseudodiverticulosis whose symptoms were amiliorated by oral administration of anti-fungal medicine. *Case Reports in Gastroenterology, 6*, 103–110.

Harford, W., & Jeyarajah, D. (2010). Diverticula of the pharynx, esophagus, stomach, and small intestine. In *Sleisenger and Fordtran's Gastrointestinal and liver disease* (9th ed., pp. 371–378). Philadelphia: Saunders.

Pseudoepitheliomatous Hyperplasia, Esophageal

Ricardo Fonseca[1] and Paula Chaves[2,3]
[1]Serviço de Anatomia Patológica, Instituto Português de Oncologia de Lisboa Francisco Gentil, Lisboa, Portugal
[2]Serviço de Anatomia Patológica, Instituto Português de Oncologia de Lisboa de Francisco Gentil, Lisbon, Portugal
[3]Faculdade de Ciências da Saúde, Universidade da Beira Interior, Covilhã, Portugal

Synonyms

Atypical regenerative hyperplasia; Reactive hyperplasia

Definition

Pseudoepitheliomatous hyperplasia (PEH) is a morphologic pattern of reactive squamous epithelial proliferation that occurs in response to underlying infections, inflammations, or neoplasms (Kune 2012; Noffsinger 2007). It is characterized by parallel, elongated, and occasionally irregular columns of highly reactive squamous cells, with prominent nucleoli and abundant mitoses that may extend deep into the lamina propria. Its appearance may simulate invasive squamous cell carcinoma. On occasion, this reaction may be endoscopically visible, and this may cause diagnostic confusion with a malignant lesion (Odze 2009).

Clinical Features

As PEH is a reactive epithelial proliferation, and so its clinical features (incidence, age, sex, site, or macroscopic features) are mostly dependent on the underlying infectious, inflammatory, or neoplastic conditions.

- **Treatment**
  No specific treatment for this condition is required, if the correct diagnosis is rendered. Treatment is aimed at the underlying condition.
- **Outcome**
  PEH is a benign condition that does not require surveillance. An endoscopy should be used only when the appearance is atypical and/or the clinical suspicion of an underlying esophageal disease is high.

Microscopy

Histologically, PEH is characterized by proliferating strands of thin, markedly elongated, anastomosing epithelium, and heavy infiltration of inflammatory cells as well as varying degrees of hyperkeratosis and papillomatosis (Kune 2012). PEH corresponds to an extensive acantosis (Noffsinger 2007). Histologically, PEH does not demonstrate cytological features of malignancy such as nuclear pleomorphism, maturation atypia, mitosis, and stromal invasion, although it may show reactive atypia (Bouquot 2001).

It may be primary, as described in primary gingival PEH, or secondary, when associated with granular cell tumor or chronic irritation processes (Bouquot 2001).

Regenerating basal esophageal epithelium is characterized by nuclear enlargement, hyperchromasia, and rare mitotic figures in the basal cell layers. When the epithelium becomes very hyperplastic, *acanthosis* occurs (extension of elongated epithelial pegs into the underlying lamina propria).

Hyperplasia of basal cells observed in squamous epithelial regeneration can be present in acute or chronic damage. This hyperplasia is a consequence of an increase in cell turnover, contributing to an expansion of the basal proliferative zone.

Molecular Features

The molecular features studied in this condition besides those mentioned for specific differential diagnosis.

Differential Diagnosis

It is sometimes difficult to distinguish PEH from invasive squamous cell carcinoma, in some tissue samples. Many times the problem is partially due to small tissue size, dense inflammation, and poor orientation.

Various morphologic features may help differentiate these two entities. The reactive cells generally maintain their normal polarity, the nuclei do not overlap, and there is no abnormal mitosis. The more superficial layers have squamous cell maturation, and there is no individual cell keratinization (characteristic of high-grade dysplasia) (Noffsinger 2007). The epithelial-stromal boundary appears smooth, with an obvious basement membrane, if no inflammation is present. The lamina propria and submucosa can become inflamed, but there should not be any desmoplasia, surrounding the epithelial cells (Noffsinger 2007).

In contrast to squamous cell carcinoma, hyperplastic cells have no signs of malignancy, having possible signs of reactive atypia.

Several markers have been identified as aiding on the differential diagnosis with squamous cell carcinoma (SCC) of the esophagus, like p53, matrix metalloproteinase 1, and E-cadherin (Zarovnaya 2005).

The p53 tumor suppressor gene has been found in the mucosa from patients with PEH, although with a different pattern from that found in tumor samples.

Zarovnaya E. et al (Zarovnaya 2005) observed an increased reactivity for p53 within the nuclei of invasive tumor cells, but on PEH cells the surface mucosa showed nuclear staining limited to the basal cells and, occasionally, the cells immediately adjacent in a linear pattern. The staining decreased or disappeared as the squamous cells matured (Bouquot 2001).

In contrast, the same authors observed that the invasive SCC showed nuclear reactivity for p53, with staining of nuclei throughout the full thickness of the epithelium rather than just the basal area as in the benign tissues (Bouquot 2001).

Matrix metalloproteinase 1 showed an increased reactivity within the invasive tumor cells. In contrast, PEH basal cells and the cells immediately adjacent were the ones that stained most strongly (Bouquot 2001).

E-cadherin can also be used in the differential diagnosis of PEH from malignant transformation, showing a decreased staining in invasive cells (Bouquot 2001).

It is important to assure adequate samples for diagnosis, since small or poorly oriented biopsies may be difficult to interpret.

Differential Diagnosis

Squamous Cell Carcinoma of the Esophagus

Unlike squamous cell carcinoma of the esophagus, PEH lacks "paradoxical maturation" and characteristically has an intact basal layer (Zarovnaya 2005). Antibodies like p53, matrix metalloproteinase 1, and E-cadherin can help in the differential diagnosis.

Squamous Dysplasia

Unlike squamous dysplasia, the PEH is adjacent to a healing ulcer or overlying granular cell tumors. It often shows abundant inflammatory cells and surface erosion. There is neither significant nuclear pleomorphism nor loss of polarity present.

References and Further Reading

Bouquot, J. E. (2001). *Diagnostic surgical pathology of the head and neck* (pp. 205–207). Philadelphia: WB Saunders.

Kune, Y. T. (2012). *The Korean Journal of Pathology, 46*(4), 331–340.

Lamps, L. (2010). *Diagnostic pathology: Gastrointestinal.* Salt Lake City, UT: Amirsys.

Noffsinger, A. (2007). *Gastrointestinal diseases. Atlas of non tumour pathology.* Washington, DC: American Registry of Pathology.

Odze, R. (2009). *Surgical pathology of the GI tract, liver, biliary tract, and pancreas.* Philadelphia, PA: Saunders Elsevier.

Zarovnaya, E. (2005). Distinguishing pseudoepitheliomatous hyperplasia from squamous cell carcinoma in mucosal biopsy specimens from the head and neck. *Archives of Pathology & Laboratory Medicine, 129*, 1032–1036.

Pseudogoblet Cells

Namrata Setia[1] and Gregory Y. Lauwers[2]

[1]Department of Pathology, Massachusetts General Hospital, Boston, MA, USA

[2]Department of Pathology, Massachusetts General Hospital, Harvard Medical School, Boston, MA, USA

Overview

Pseudogoblet cells are distended columnar epithelial cells that mimic goblet cells. They are commonly detected in columnar-lined esophagus. These cells are important to recognize, since they are indicators of intestinal metaplasia in the esophagus and a diagnostic criterion of the Barrett esophagus according to the American College of Gastroenterology. The recognition of goblet cells guides the surveillance protocol, although the clinical validity has been debated, and thus it is vital to appreciate the histology and histochemical staining properties of pseudogoblet cells in order to differentiate them from goblet cells.

Histology of Goblet Cells Versus Pseudogoblet Cells

Goblet cells are mucin-producing cells normally present in the intestine (small and large), respiratory tract, and conjunctiva. They result from the accumulation of tightly packed large mucin granules at the cellular apex and consequently have a distinctive flask or wine goblet shape. The basal portion of the cell is narrow, as it lacks mucin granules. Notably, the nucleus of a goblet cell is indented or cup-shaped and pushed to the basal area of the cell. The cytoplasm characteristically displays a pale blue hue on H&E due to acidic high molecular weight glycoproteins. In the Barrett epithelium, goblet cells are randomly distributed between the surface and crypt foveolar-type epithelial cells; however, they are more frequently detected in the proximal segment of BE.

Pseudogoblet cells also display a distended apex, but the nucleus is not commonly compressed against the base of the cells. Furthermore, the cytoplasm of these cells is homogenously pink instead of pale blue on H&E (Fig. 1). Frequently, pseudogoblet cells are present as rows of cells in linear stretches amidst surface foveolar cells and, rarely, in deeper crypts (Figs. 2 and 3).

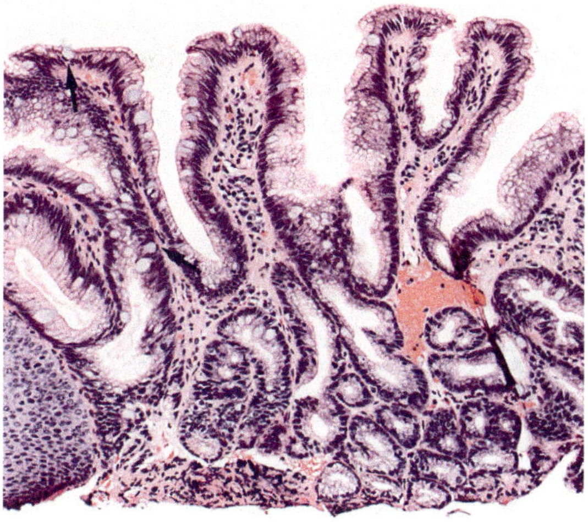

Pseudogoblet Cells, Fig. 1 Goblet cells (*arrows*) in the Barrett esophagus. The cells are seen randomly distributed between the surface and crypt foveolar-type epithelial cells. Note that the apex is distended and the nucleus compressed against the base of the cells. The cytoplasm is *pale blue* instead of *pink*

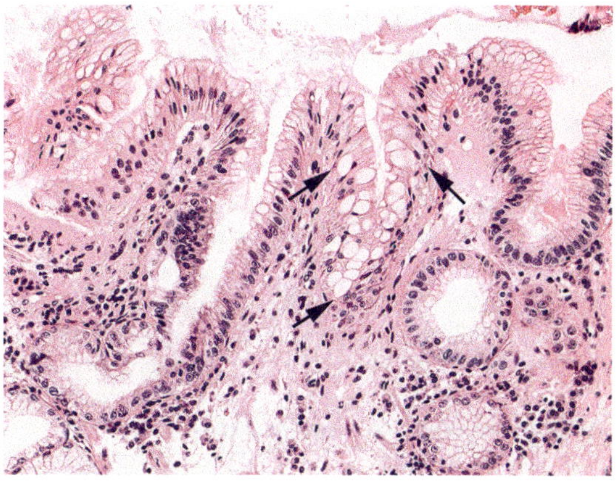

Pseudogoblet Cells, Fig. 2 Pseudogoblet cells (*arrows*) present as rows of cells in linear stretches in surface foveolar epithelial cells

Histochemical Staining Properties of Goblet Versus Pseudogoblet Cells

It is important to be aware of the staining characteristics, but in practice, they are not recommended for identification of goblet cells and differentiation from pseudogoblet cells, since they add cost. Pseudogoblet cells either are negative or display a light blue blush when stained by Alcian Blue at pH 2.5, which detects acidic mucin; goblet cells are strongly positive (dark blue) instead. Furthermore, goblet cells exhibit brown reactivity when high iron diamine is applied, detecting sulfomucins while pseudogoblet cells are negative.

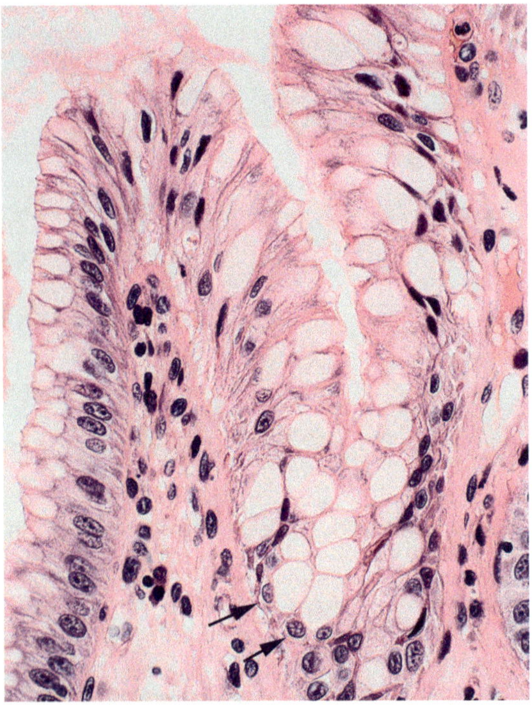

Pseudogoblet Cells, Fig. 3 Pseudogoblet cells (higher magnification) display a distended apex, but the nucleus is not compressed against the base of the cells (*arrows*), and the cytoplasm is homogenously pink

References and Further Reading

Bronner, M. P. (2004). Inflammatory disorders of the GI tract: Inflammatory disorders of the esophagus. In R. D. Odze, J. R. Goldblum, & J. M. Crawford (Eds.), *Surgical pathology of the GI tract, liver, biliary tract, and pancreas* (1st ed., pp. 121–1423). Philadelphia: Saunders.

Ovalle, W. K., & Nahirney, P. C. (2013). Lower digestive system. In W. K. Ovalle & P. C. Nahirney (Eds.), *Netter's essential histology* (2nd ed., pp. 285–309). Philadelphia: Saunders.

Weinstein, W. M., & Ippoliti, A. F. (1996). The diagnosis of Barrett's esophagus: Goblets, goblets, goblets. *Gastrointestinal Endoscopy, 44*(1), 91–95.

Younes, M., Ertan, A., Ergun, G., Verm, R., Bridges, M., Woods, K., Meriano, F., Schmulen, A. C., Colman, R., Johnson, C., Barroso, A., Schwartz, J., McKechnie, J., Lechago, J., et al. (2007). Goblet cell mimickers in esophageal biopsies are not associated with an increased risk for dysplasia. *Archives of Pathology & Laboratory Medicine, 131*(4), 571–575.

Pyloric Gland Adenoma

Helena Baldaia
Serviço de Anatomia Patológica, Centro Hospitalar de São João, Porto, Portugal

Synonyms

Gastric-type adenoma

Definition

Pyloric gland adenomas (PGAs) are localized epithelial neoplastic growths with pyloric differentiation (Park et al. 2012). They were first described in 1976 by Elster but misinterpreted as adenoma-like hyperplasia of mucous glands. In 1990, Borchard et al. published the first characterization of two cases with mucin analysis. Although 85% are found in the stomach, 15% are found in extra-gastric locations (Vieth et al. 2003). Like intestinal-type adenomas, pyloric gland adenomas can arise in a background of autoimmune gastritis and *Helicobacter pylori* infection (Lash et al. 2011). Even if rare, PGAs are precancerous lesions and frequently associated with high-grade dysplasia and adenocarcinoma (Kushima et al. 2006; Vieth et al. 2003).

Clinical Features

- **Incidence**
  In one study, in a period of 10 years, pyloric gland adenomas corresponded to 2.7% of all gastric polyps (Vieth et al. 2003).
- **Age**
  The peak age at diagnosis is in the seventh decade (73 ± 12.8 years) (Kushima et al. 2006).
- **Sex**
  There is a threefold predominance in women (Lash et al. 2011). This finding, together with

the age range, can probably be explained by the fact that autoimmune gastritis is also more commonly found in women of advanced age, and this is the usual background in which PGAs are diagnosed (Vieth et al. 2003).

- **Site**
  Gastric PGAs are more commonly encountered in the corpus/fundic mucosa (64%) (Vieth et al. 2003). Pyloric gland adenomas have also been described in the gallbladder, duodenum, pancreas, bile duct, and even in the uterine cervix (Lash et al. 2011) (Vieth et al. 2003). In these locations, there is frequently associated gastric heterotopia and it is presumed that the lesion is originated from the heterotopic tissue. More recently, there have been reports of PGAs arising in the esophagus and in gastric heterotopia of the rectum (Kushima et al. 2006).
- **Treatment**
  Although further studies are necessary, excision therapy is guided by the presence or absence of associated malignancy. In the presence of PGA, careful searching for malignancy in the surrounding non-affected mucosa is prudent (Park et al. 2012). At the present, polipectomy and complete surgical excision by endoscopic submucosal resection or gastrectomy (if adenocarcinoma is present) is curative (Park et al. 2012).
- **Outcome**
  At the present, limited follow-up data are available. The outcome is associated with the presence of malignancy. In two case series, 30–47% of pyloric gland adenomas were associated with gastric-type adenocarcinoma (Vieth et al. 2003; Vieth et al. 2010). In one study, a slightly higher frequency of malignant transformation was observed in the extragastric lesions (Vieth et al. 2010). These were well-differentiated lesions confined to the mucosa. Follow-up data on three patients with deeply invasive adenocarcinomas arising in PGAs found a 10-year survival with local recurrence in one patient and that the other two patients were alive and well 2 and 10 months since surgery (Chen et al. 2009).

Macroscopy

Endoscopically, these lesions usually appear as nodular, dome-like protrusions of the mucosa (Fig. 1) (Kushima et al. 2006). The mean size at diagnosis is approximately 16 mm (16 ± 9 mm) (Vieth et al. 2003; Park et al. 2012).

P

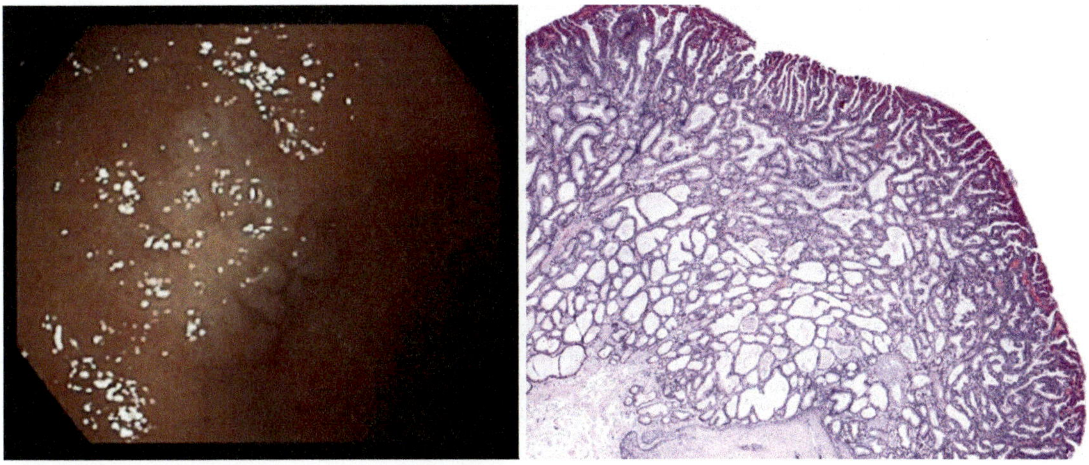

Pyloric Gland Adenoma, Fig. 1 Pyloric gland adenoma, histologic aspect with of closely packed pyloric gland tubules

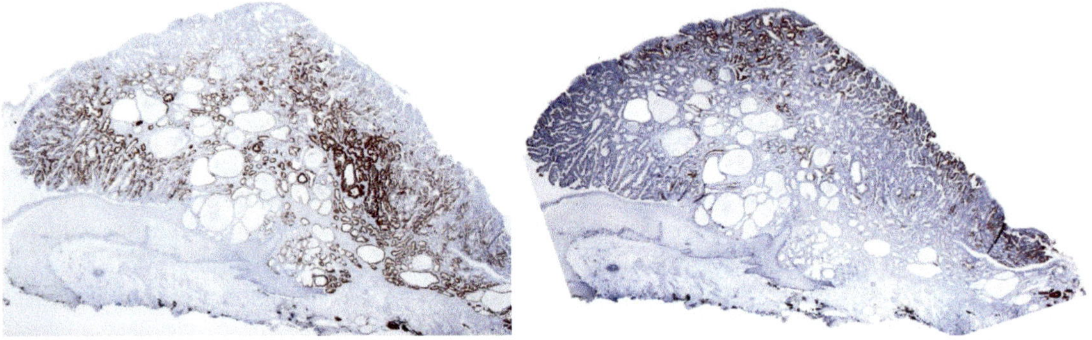

Pyloric Gland Adenoma, Fig. 2 Immunoreactivity with MUC6 and MUC5AC (left and right, respectively)

Microscopy

Histologically, pyloric gland adenomas are composed of closely packed pyloric gland tubules composed by a monolayer of cuboidal to low columnar epithelial cells containing pale to eosinophilic cytoplasm, with a ground glass appearance (Chen et al. 2009) (Fig. 1). In contrast with gastric foveolar adenomas, these lesions do not show an apical mucin cap (Lash et al. 2011). The nuclei are usually round without prominent nucleoli (Chen et al. 2009).

In low-grade dysplastic lesions, the nuclei remain round with only slight enlargement or elongation. Tubule architecture is somewhat irregular. In high-grade dysplastic lesions, however, there is nuclear pseudostratification and pleomorphism, with complex, cribriform structures. In view of the continuum and variability of these lesions, some authors have used a three-tier classification of dysplasia (none; low grade; high grade) (Lash et al. 2011; Chen et al. 2009). Nonetheless, even lesions named "without dysplasia" are still neoplastic (Park et al. 2012).

The unaffected gastric mucosa usually shows atrophic autoimmune gastritis and intestinal metaplasia. In one study, autoimmune gastritis was found in 34% of cases, while *H. pylori* gastritis was found in 30% of gastric samples studied. Chemical gastritis was found in 20%. Only 3.8% of cases had a normal mucosa (Vieth et al. 2003).

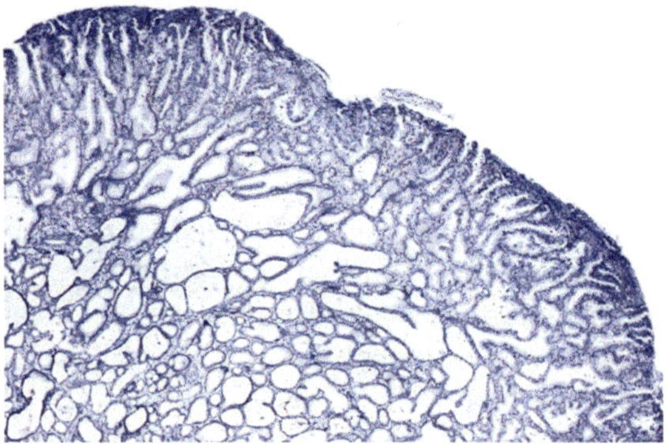

Pyloric Gland Adenoma, Fig. 3 Absence of MUC2 expression

Immunophenotype

Pyloric gland adenomas express MUC6 universally and MUC5AC variably (Fig. 2). Some studies have shown a multifocal variable expression of MUC2 and CD10 (large bowel and small bowel type mucins, respectively) in these lesions (Fig. 3). For those authors, these findings indicate that a relatively large proportion of early gastric carcinomas arise as adenocarcinomas of the gastric type and secondarily convert into gastric carcinomas of the intestinal type (Vieth et al. 2010).

Molecular Features

The molecular features of pyloric gland adenomas are yet to be well characterized. A study using microdissection and CGH analysis found some chromosomal abnormalities common to invasive gastric adenocarcinoma such as gains of 17pq and 20q (Kushima et al. 2006). At present, no study revealed significant molecular differences between intestinal-type gastric adenomas and pyloric gland adenomas (Park et al. 2012).

Differential Diagnosis

The main differential diagnosis is with gastric foveolar type adenoma and reactive epithelial changes. The round, bland-appearing and basally located nuclei of pyloric adenomas, the absence of a mucin cap and immunolabeling with MUC6 may permit a differential diagnosis (Chen et al. 2009).

Furthermore, although PGA arise in the setting of gastritis, the fact that they appear as polyps and the tightly packed pyloric glands without nucleoli prominence allow a differential diagnosis with reactive alterations.

References and Further Reading

Chen, Z. M., Scudiere, J. R., Abraham, S. C., & Montgomery, E. (2009). Pyloric gland adenoma: An entity distinct from gastric foveolar type adenoma. *American Journal of Surgical Pathology, 33*(2), 186–193.

Kushima, R., Vieth, M., Borchard, F., et al. (2006). Gastric-type well-differentiated adenocarcinoma and pyloric gland adenoma of the stomach. *Gastric Cancer, 9*(3), 177–184.

Lash, R. H., Kinsey, S., Genta, R. M., & Lauwers, G. Y. (2011). Gastric polyps. In D. Tan & G. Y. Lauwers (Eds.), *Advances in surgical pathology gastric cancer* (pp. 308–309). Philadelphia: Lippincott Williams & Wilkins.

Park, J. Y., Fenton, H., Lewin, M., & Dilworth, H. (2012). Epithelial neoplasms of the stomach. In C. A. Iacobuzio-Donahue, E. Montgomary, & J. R. Golblum (Eds.), *Gastrointestinal and liver pathology* (pp. 148–150). Philadelphia: Saunders.

Vieth, M., Kushima, R., Borchard, F., & Stolte, M. (2003). Pyloric gland adenoma: A clinico-pathological analysis of 90 cases. *Virchows Archiv, 442*(4), 317–321.

Vieth, M., Kushima, R., Mukaisho, K., Sakai, R., et al. (2010). Immunohistochemical analysis of pyloric gland adenomas using a series of Mucin 2, Mucin 5AC, Mucin 6, CD10, Ki67 and p53. *Virchows Archiv, 457*(5), 529–536.

Pyloric Stenosis

Filipe Vilas-Boas[1], Francisco Baldaque-Silva[1], Fátima Carneiro[2] and Guilherme Macedo[1]
[1]Centro Hospitalar de São João, Alameda Professor Hernani Monteiro, Porto, Portugal
[2]Faculty of Medicine of Porto University, Centro Hospitalar São João and Ipatimup/i3S, Porto, Portugal

Synonyms

Congenital hypertrophic pyloric stenosis; Idiopathic pyloric stenosis; Juvenile hypertrophic pyloric stenosis; Primary pyloric stenosis

Definition

Infantile hypertrophic pyloric stenosis (IHPS) is a form of gastric outlet obstruction, usually presenting with projectile nonbilious vomiting in infants in the first 3–12 weeks of life. It is caused by an acquired stenosis of the pylorus, not present at birth, but developing in the first weeks of life.

On the contrary, adult pyloric obstruction is usually secondary to local diseases such as peptic ulcers or carcinomas near the pylorus, lymphomas, Crohn's disease, or adjacent carcinoma of the pancreas. There are few reports of primary adult forms with unknown etiology, which are probably missed infantile cases that had a milder course. In these cases, the treatment of choice has been distal gastrectomy and the diagnosis usually relies on the pathological examination of surgical specimens showing total or segmental hypertrophy of the smooth muscle without any underlying disease.

IHPS etiology and pathogenesis is largely unknown but is probably multifactorial involving interaction of genetic and environmental factors. Predisposition is conferred by several susceptible interacting loci and complex molecular pathways.

Abnormalities of various components of the pyloric muscle such as smooth muscle cells, extracellular matrix elements, nerve and ganglion cells, synapses, nerve supporting cells, neurotransmitters and interstitial cells of Cajal have been reported.

Familial aggregation with autosomal dominant forms is recognized, and is associated with two loci, IHPS2 and IHPS5.

NOS1 (IHPS1) encodes neuronal nitric oxide synthase and is implicated in the lack of nitric oxide, affecting pyloric smooth muscle relaxation. In fact, abnormal pyloric innervation has been reported in IHPS and is associated with decreased muscle neurofilaments, nerve terminals, synaptic vesicle protein, and neural cell adhesion molecules.

IHPS is associated with several genetic syndromes involving neuromuscular, connective tissue, and metabolic disorders, such as Smith-Lemli-Opitz syndrome and Cornelia de Lange. Suspected environmental factors include postnatal exposure to macrolides, bottle-feeding, and prone sleeping position.

Clinical Features

- **Incidence**
  Wide variations have been observed with geographic location, season, and ethnic origin. IPHS incidence has been stable over time and varies from 1 to 8 in 1,000 live births according to ethnic groups and regions. It is highest in white males and lowest among Asians.
- **Age**
  Almost all patients are diagnosed between 3 and 12 weeks of age. Symptoms usually begin between 3 and 5 weeks of age and rarely after 12 weeks.
- **Sex**
  It is more common in males than females, with a male/female ratio of 4:1 to 6:1.
- **Site**
  IHPS produces gastric outlet obstruction due to involvement of the pylorus/pyloric channel.
- **Treatment**
  Pyloromyotomy, either open or laparoscopic, is the treatment of choice and involves longitudinal incision of the hypertrophic pylorus with muscular layer disruption. Surgery should be performed after correction of dehydration and electrolyte disturbances that are common in these patients.

  The laparoscopic procedure is associated with lower incidence of postoperative emesis and shorter hospital stay.

  The use of oral and intravenous atropine has been described in several reports from Asian countries as effective and safe but should be reserved for patients with contraindication for surgery. In these patients, endoscopic balloon dilation has been described.
- **Outcome**
  IHPS was associated with high mortality rates in the past, but the advances in pediatric anesthesia and surgical care result, nowadays, in a very low rate of complications with minimal mortality and morbidity.

Macroscopy

The resected specimens from adults with idiopathic hypertrophic stenosis show thickening of the muscularis layer in the pylorus.

Microscopy

Full thickness pyloric muscle biopsy specimens show that hypertrophy and hyperplasia of the muscularis propria and muscularis mucosae are responsible for the increased smooth muscle mass, resulting in pyloric stenosis in IHPS patients. Increase in extracellular matrix components is also frequently reported. Various degrees of inflammatory infiltrate and degenerative changes in the ganglion cells of the myenteric plexus are also described in histological specimens.

Interstitial cells of Cajal (ICC) play a major role on motility coordination and are found on the muscular layer of the gastrointestinal (GI) tract. Specimens from IHPS patients show, under electron microscopy, a smaller number of ICC both in the myenteric plexus and in the circular muscle layer compared with biopsies from normal individuals.

Immunophenotype

Immunohistochemistry is being used by some investigators to study the etiopathogenesis of IHPS. Some authors (Okazaki et al. 1994) found abnormal nerve terminals and neurofilaments numbers and distribution in IHPS specimens using monoclonal antibodies 171B5 and 2F11 compared with normal controls. Other reports (Guarino et al. 2000; Gentile et al. 1998) show that extracellular matrix and cytoskeletal elements (e.g., desmin, vinculin) of pyloric smooth muscle cells are altered in IHPS.

Molecular Features

Molecular studies have concluded that there is a reduced expression of neuronal nitric oxide synthase (nNOS) in the pylorus of patients with IHPS. Also, growth factors such as EGF, IGF-I, PDGF, and TGF-B-1 were shown to be markedly increased in hypertrophic pyloric muscle in IHPS.

Differential Diagnosis

The typical presentation of IHPS is the development of forceful or projectile nonbilious, nonbloody vomiting immediately after every feeding in an infant in the second to third week of life, which usually shows a voracious appetite.

Depending on the duration of symptoms, dehydration and electrolyte disturbances may ensue. The loss of acid content, sodium, and potassium from continuous vomiting, usually results in hypokalemic, hypochloremic metabolic alkalosis.

Gastroesophageal reflux disease and food allergy are the most frequent conditions usually considered in the differential diagnosis of IHPS. In premature infants and babies with concomitant medical problems such as neurological deficits or cleft palate, vomiting may be less vigorous and lethargy may ensue.

On examination of the abdomen, there may be visible peristalsis and a firm, ovoid ("olive shape") palpable mass in the right upper quadrant, corresponding to exaggerated gastric peristalsis and hypertrophied pylorus, respectively. The "olive" is most easily felt immediately after emesis.

Ultrasonography is, nowadays, the standard diagnostic procedure. It is highly sensitive but operator-dependent. Pyloric muscle thickening and pyloric muscle length are the most frequently used parameters to define IHPS. The pyloric volume and ratio are rarely used. The finding of a pyloric muscle with a thickness of 3 mm or more and 15 mm or more of extension is diagnostic of IHPS.

Gastrointestinal contrast studies are less frequently used because they are time consuming and involve radiation exposure. The "string" sign that corresponds to the elongated pylorus is the most frequent sign of barium meal studies in IHPS.

When ultrasonography and barium studies fail to show the typical features of IHPS and diagnosis is in doubt, upper endoscopy should be performed and may be helpful in confirming the diagnosis. The "cervix sign" consisting of a cervix-like look in the pyloric area is a frequent but nonspecific endoscopic feature of IHPS. Additionally, upper endoscopy may be useful in excluding conditions like esophagitis, gastritis, or pyloric web, which may be the cause of persistent infantile vomiting.

In the case of the adult forms of primary hypertrophic pyloric stenosis, symptoms include nausea, vomiting, early saciety and epigastric pain. Physical examination may not be helpful because the hypertrophic pylorus is not generally palpated. Upper endoscopy is mandatory to exclude secondary causes of gastric outlet obstruction.

References and Further Reading

MacMahon, B. (2006). The continuing enigma of pyloric stenosis of infancy: A review. *Epidemiology, 17*(2), 195–201.

Panteli, C. (2009). New insights into the pathogenesis of infantile pyloric stenosis. *Pediatric Surgery International, 25*, 1043–1052.

Ranells, J. D., Carver, J. D., & Kirby, R. S. (2011). Infantile hypertrophic pyloric stenosis: epidemiology, genetics, and clinical update. *Advances in Pediatrics, 58*(1), 195–206.

Semrin, M. G., & Russo, M. A. (2010). Anatomy, histology, embryology, and developmental anomalies of the stomach and duodenum. In M. Feldman, L. S. Friedman, & L. J. Brandt (Eds.), *Sleisenger & Fordtran's gastrointestinal and liver disease: Pathophysiology, diagnosis, management* (pp. 773–785). Philadelphia: Saunders.

Okazaki, T., et al. (1994). Abnormal distribution of nerve terminals in infantile hypertrophic pyloric stenosis. *Journal of Pediatric Surgery, 29*, 655–658.

Guarino, N., Shima, H., Oue, T., & Puri, P. (2000) Glial-derived growth factor signaling pathway in infantile hypertrophic pyloric stenosis. *Journal of Pediatric Surgery, 35*(6), 835–839.

Gentile, C., Romeo, C., Impellizzeri, P., Turiaco, N., Esposito, M., Di Mauro, D., & Mondello, M. R. (1998). A possible role of the plasmalemmal cytoskeleton, nitric oxide synthase, and innervation in infantile hypertrophic pyloric stenosis. A confocal laser scanning microscopic study. *Pediatric Surgery International*, 14(1–2), 45–50.

R

Radiation Colitis

Liesbeth Ferdinande
Department of Pathology, Ghent University Hospital, Ghent, Belgium

Synonyms

Radiation-associated colitis; Radiation proctitis

Definition

Radiation colitis results from exposure to ionizing radiation in the treatment of malignancies where the colon is localized in the path of the radiation beam. Tissues containing numerous actively dividing cells such as intestinal epithelial cells are more at risk for the development of radiation-induced injury. An acute and chronic type of radiation colitis is described. The *acute* changes develop very early within hours to several days after exposure. In this phase, the radiosensitive actively dividing cells of the intestinal epithelium are affected, and histologic changes are mainly observed in the mucosa. This acute syndrome, characterized by nausea, vomiting, and diarrhea, is usually transient and does not require further diagnostic or therapeutic action. *Chronic* radiation colitis develops after a symptom-free interval of 6 months to 30 years after radiation. The pathogenesis of this type of injury is based on (1) impaired vascular function due to radiation injury of blood vessels and (2) late effects of ionizing radiation by damage to slow proliferating parenchymal and connective tissue cells. The characteristic histologic features are mostly found in the submucosa in this phase. Vascular changes and fibrosis will give rise to stenoses, obstruction, or perforation.

Clinical Features

- **Incidence**
  Acute radiation colitis is very common causing transient diarrhea, cramps, and tenesmus. Mostly these symptoms disappear shortly after discontinuation of radiotherapy, and the lesions are usually not documented by biopsy and histologic examination. The incidence of chronic radiation-induced injury to the rectum is approximately 10% after doses above 60 Gy and increases to 50% as doses reach 80 Gy, leading to complications such as ulcerations, stenoses, and rectovaginal fistulae. Incidence rates of intestinal toxicity are lower using new radiotherapeutic modalities like intensity-modulated radiotherapy (IMRT). Reduction in radiation dose and field size are the most important factors in the prevention of acute and chronic radiation-induced intestinal damage.

F. Carneiro et al. (eds.), *Pathology of the Gastrointestinal Tract*, Encyclopedia of Pathology,
DOI 10.1007/978-3-319-40560-5

Predisposing factors in the development of radiation colitis include coexisting vascular changes secondary to diabetes or hypertension, previous abdominal surgery, and treatment with chemotherapy.

The relationship between the presence and severity of acute radiation colitis and the incidence of chronic radiation colitis is not well understood.

- **Site**
  The sigmoid and rectum are segments of the gut that are frequently damaged by radiation as they are anatomically in close proximity to commonly radiated organs like uterus and prostate. Moreover, the relative immobility of this part of the bowel implicates that it is constantly localized in the path of the radiation beam.
- **Treatment and Outcome**
  The finding of acute radiation colitis in biopsies should not lead to further diagnostic or therapeutic procedures. A study comparing histopathologic findings in resection specimens of rectal cancer after radiation therapy showed significantly less mucosal inflammation in patients that underwent surgery 3–4 weeks after the end of the irradiation versus patients with a 2–5-day interval between radiation therapy and surgery, indicating resolution of histologic changes in this period. Therefore, conservative treatment is preferred for radiation-induced colitis. When severe adverse effects such as perforation or obstruction occur, surgical intervention may be needed. In these cases, however, vascular insufficiency, which is considered to be an important factor in the pathogenesis of radiation-induced injury, can also contribute to postoperative complications.

Macroscopy

Acute radiation colitis will present with erosions, ulcerations, edema, or bleeding of the mucosa.

Chronic radiation colitis is macroscopically characterized by the presence of fibrosis with adhesions or areas of stenosis. The mucosa may appear pale and telangiectatic with focal ulcerations. Perforation or fistulization can occur.

Microscopy

Acute radiation colitis mainly affects the mucosa, featuring inflammatory changes and epithelial atypia. The lamina propria shows an increase in cellularity with often prominent infiltration of eosinophils. Eosinophilic crypt abscesses may be present. The surface epithelium is commonly damaged with reactive cytological atypia of surviving cells. Loss of nuclear polarity and hyperchromatic and enlarged nuclei can be observed, mimicking dysplasia in cases of marked nuclear abnormalities. The submucosa typically shows edema with a few eosinophils and other leukocytes in the stroma.

In chronic radiation colitis, the mucosa may appear normal, may be ulcerated, or may show atrophy, mucosal fibrosis or inflammation, crypt branching, loss of goblet cells, cuboidal or flattened surface epithelium, or mild atypia of cells with nuclear enlargement and loss of polarity. The most apparent alterations are seen in the mesenchymal tissue in the submucosa. Stromal fibroblasts are often prominent, probably more because of increase in size than increase in number. The atypical fibroblasts have multiple cytoplasmic projections and large hyperchromatic and irregular nuclei (Fig. 1). The cells increase in size, but their nuclear-cytoplasmic ratio remains within the normal range. Collagen proliferation results in fibrosis of the submucosa, causing strictures when extensive. Radiation injury to blood vessels manifests as several types of lesions. Capillaries often show telangiectatic dilations (Fig. 2). Hyalinization of the media by replacement with an acidophilic amorphous material is often found in arteries and arterioles (Fig. 3).

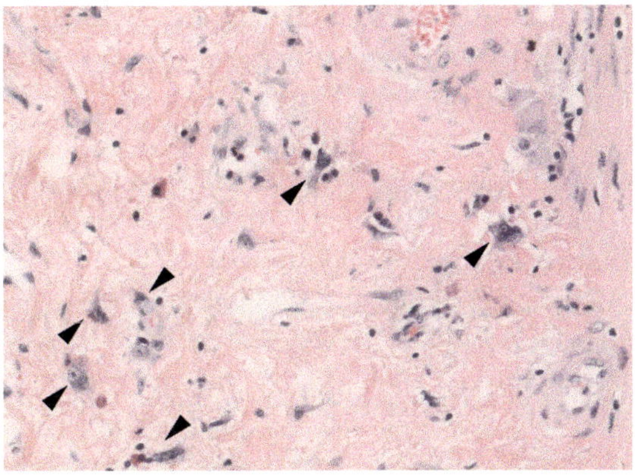

Radiation Colitis, Fig. 1 Atypical "radiation" fibroblasts (*arrowheads*) in the submucosa

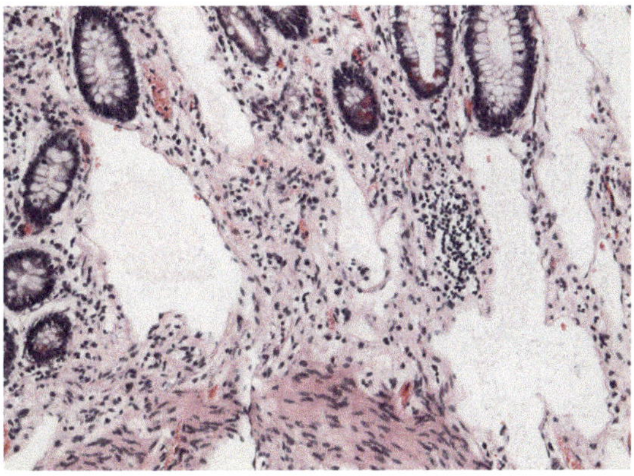

Radiation Colitis, Fig. 2 Radiation-induced vascular changes: telangiectatic blood vessels in the mucosa

Myointimal proliferation or accumulation of foamy cells in the intima can narrow the lumen (Fig. 4). Endothelial cells may be prominent and protrude into the lumen. Also the muscular layer may display fibrosis and vascular changes. Case reports in literature illustrate the appearance of colitis cystica profunda in radiation-induced colonic strictures. This condition is characterized by "invasion" of mucosal glands or glandular cysts in the submucosa and muscularis propria. In radiation colitis, these lesions are assumed to result from healing of deeply fissured ulcers, where failure of the muscularis mucosae to regenerate allows regenerating epithelium to herniate into the submucosal and muscular layer. This particular finding should be differentiated from invasive mucinous adenocarcinoma.

Differential Diagnosis

With correct clinical information including a reference to recent radiotherapy, the diagnosis of acute radiation colitis is usually not problematic. However, without a complete clinical history, a broad differential diagnosis may be considered: infectious colitis, ▶ ischemic colitis, ▶ drug-induced intestinal injury, or

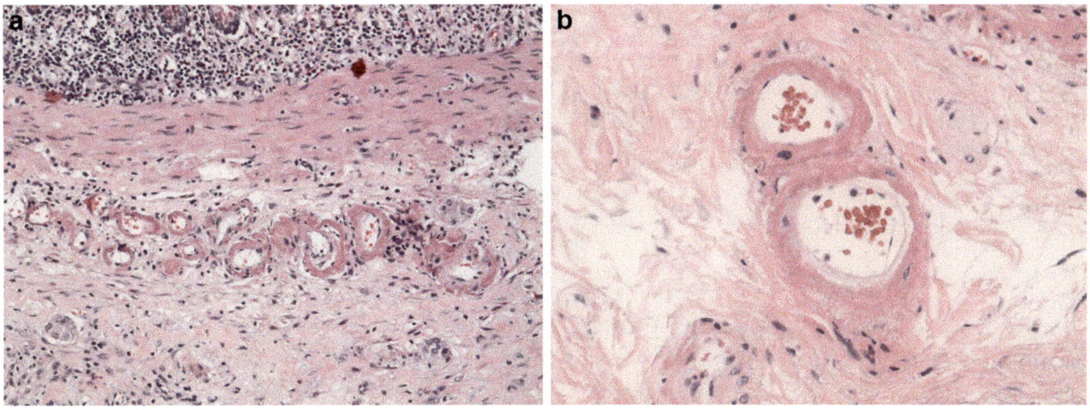

Radiation Colitis, Fig. 3 Radiation-induced vascular changes: hyalinization of the arteriolar wall

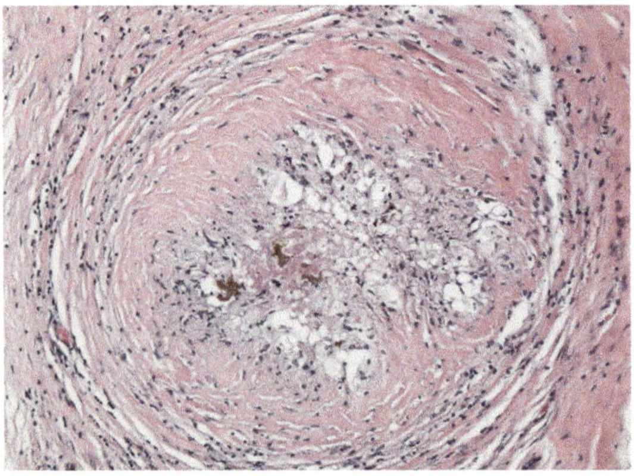

Radiation Colitis, Fig. 4 Radiation-induced vascular changes: accumulation of foamy macrophages in the vascular wall

▶ inflammatory bowel disease. Reactive cytological atypia in epithelial cells should be differentiated from true dysplasia.

Stenoses in chronic radiation colitis should be differentiated from other causes of strictures such as ▶ Crohn's disease, ▶ nonsteroidal anti-inflammatory drug injury, or potassium chloride. The characteristic vasculopathy and the presence of atypical fibroblasts suggest the radiation-induced etiology even in cases with unknown clinical history.

References and Further Reading

Berthrong, M., & Fajardo, L. F. (1981). Radiation injury in surgical pathology. Part II. Alimentary tract. *American Journal of Surgical Pathology, 5*, 153–178.

Coia, L. R., Myerson, R. J., & Tepper, J. E. (1995). Late effects of radiation therapy on the gastrointestinal tract. *International Journal of Radiation Oncology, Biology, Physics, 31*, 1213–1236.

Gardiner, G. W., McAuliffe, N., & Murray, D. (1984). Colitis cystica profunda occurring in a radiation-induced colonic stricture. *Human Pathology, 15*, 295–298.

Leupin, N., Curschmann, J., Kranzbühler, H., Maurer, C. A., Laissue, J. A., & Mazzucchelli, L. (2002). Acute radiation colitis in patients treated with short-term preoperative radiotherapy for rectal cancer. *American Journal of Surgical Pathology, 26*, 498–504.

Novak, J. M., Collins, J. T., Donowitz, M., Farman, J., Sheahan, D. G., & Spiro, H. M. (1979). Effects of radiation on the human gastrointestinal tract. *Journal of Clinical Gastroenterology, 1*, 9–39.

Radiation Therapy Injury, Upper Gastrointestinal Tract

Wen-Yih Liang[1] and Gregory Y. Lauwers[2]
[1]Department of Pathology, Taipei Veterans General Hospital, Taipei, Taiwan
[2]Department of Pathology, Massachusetts General Hospital, Harvard Medical School, Boston, MA, USA

Definition

Radiation therapy injury represents the sum of injuries to the gastric mucosa caused by ionizing radiation. This type of iatrogenic injury is associated with either external beam therapy or brachytherapy utilized as part of the treatment of various cancers (e.g., esophagus, lung, liver) or as part of induction therapy of future bone marrow transplant (BMT) recipients.

No definite minimal dosage is associated with a diagnosis of radiation injury, but symptoms start to occur at doses in the range of 40–50 Gy. Major complications tend to develop with increasing dosage. Gastric ulcers occur in approximately 15% of patients who received a cumulative dose of 50 Gy and gastric perforation in 6% of patients who accumulated 40–50 Gy, 10% of those irradiated to 50–60 Gy, and 38% of a small cohort of patients irradiated to over 60 Gy.

Clinical Features

The patients usually complain of nausea shortly after the delivery of the radiation. The symptoms are generally transient and will often last for a few hours, to abate rapidly after completion of the radiation course. Other symptoms include dyspepsia, which can present 6 months to 4 years after irradiation. Gastritis can be detected 1–12 months after completion of the therapy and can be accompanied by spasm or stenosis of the antrum; gastroscopy usually reveals smoothed mucosal folds and mucosal atrophy. If acute ulceration occurs, it usually develops shortly after the completion of the course of radiation; it rarely perforates. Late ulceration typically presents 5 months after irradiation and is indistinguishable from an ordinary ulcer. It can heal spontaneously, but may be accompanied by submucosal fibrosis. Hemorrhage has been seen primarily in situations where there is neoplastic gastric involvement or as a secondary effect of gastric ulcer. In rare cases of irradiation of primary gastric neoplasms, primarily gastric lymphoma, catastrophic complications such as perforation and hemorrhage have been observed.

Incidence

A month after completion of the radiotherapeutic course, about 53% of patients display endoscopic evidence of radiation-induced complications. Gastritis is the most common alteration, found in 41% of patients, followed by radiation-induced ulcer, seen in 26% of patients. Bleeding is less common (11% of patients). Serious gastroduodenal complications occurred in about 15% of patients and are more common in debilitated individuals (e.g., cirrhotic patients).

Treatment

Generally, the acute symptomology subsides quickly. Decreasing the radiation dose per fraction can be effective in ameliorating nausea and vomiting. Standard antiemetics also can be useful. A light meal prior to radiation therapy, rather than treatment on either a full or an empty stomach, can be helpful as well. Various antiulcer medications are commonly prescribed (proton pump inhibitors, histamine H2 receptor antagonists such as ranitidine, or coating agents such as sucralfate). Surgery is usually necessary for severe complications such as perforation, severe hemorrhage, and gastric outlet obstruction.

Outcome

While acute changes are self-limited or require only supportive care, changes often remain lifelong problems. Between 1% and 12% of patients may develop chronic severe complications including radionecrotic ulceration with stenosis, obstruction, internal fistula, perforation, and hemorrhage.

Macroscopy

The gastric mucosa is diffusely erythematous and friable. Contact bleeding and erosions are frequent. Ultimately, ulceration, stricture, fistula formation, and even perforation may be seen at different stages.

Microscopy

Early changes (8–10 days after irradiation) consist of nuclear karyorrhexis and cytoplasmic eosinophilia of the gastric pit epithelium (Fig. 1). Over

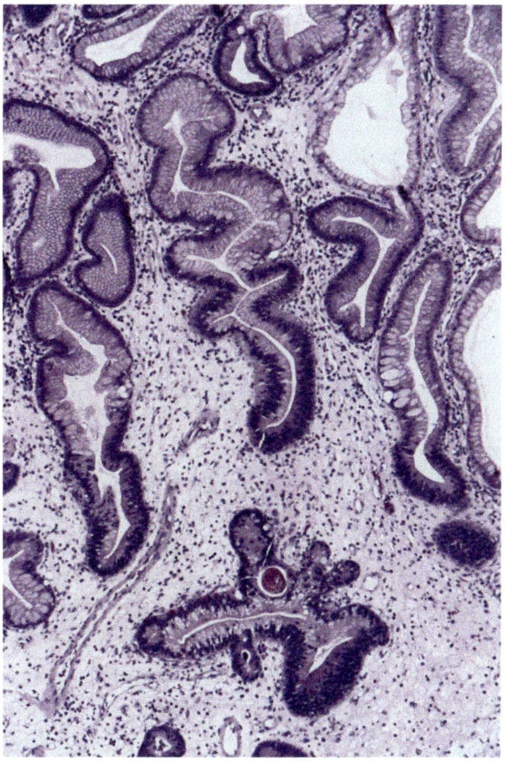

Radiation Therapy Injury, Upper Gastrointestinal Tract, Fig. 1 Gastric mucosal changes within a week of radiation therapy injury. The mucosa is edematous and the surface epithelium eroded. Inflammation is minimal and mucin depletion of the epithelium is present

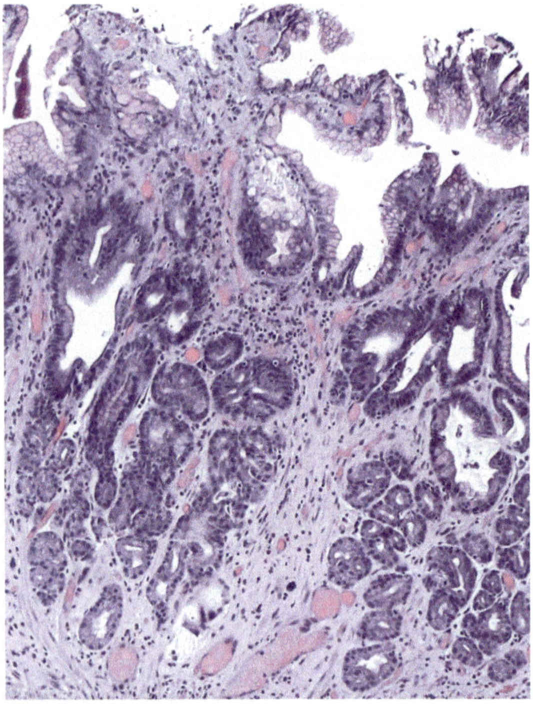

Radiation Therapy Injury, Upper Gastrointestinal Tract, Fig. 2 Healed radiation gastritis. The mucosa is characterized by its architectural disarray and paucicellular lamina propria. The surface epithelium is restored. Fibrosis is not present in this case

the next few days, mucosal edema and congestion ensue and are accompanied by swelling of submucosal collagen bundles, fibrin deposition, and telangiectasia. Inflammation is usually minimal. Glandular necrosis with characteristic radiation-induced nuclear atypia follows. Vessel walls are swollen. In cases of selective internal radiation, eosinophilic microspheres of yttrium-90 may be detected in the microscopic sections. Over time, late radiation effects may ensue, including endothelial proliferation and fibrinoid necrosis of the vessel walls. Healing usually begins during the third week and is complete within 2–3 months. When the mucosa is restored, architectural disarray and fibrosis of the lamina propria are commonly recognized (Fig. 2). Chronic ulceration also may eventually develop, characterized by atypical fibroblasts and endothelial cells. The fibrous bed may be exuberant, with hyalinized changes including the vessel walls.

Differential Diagnosis

Drug-induced mucosal changes, particularly those associated with chemotherapy and graft versus host disease, share similar histologic features with radiation gastritis. To determine the respective roles of radiation and of chemotherapy agents may be difficult, given the overlap.

References and Further Reading

Chon, Y. E., Seong, J., Kim, B. K., Cha, J., Kim, S. U., Park, J. Y., Ahn, S. H., Han, K. H., Chon, C. Y., Shin, S. K., & do Kim, Y. (2011). Gastroduodenal complications after concurrent chemoradiation therapy in patients with hepatocellular carcinoma: Endoscopic findings and risk factors. *International Journal of Radiation Oncology, Biology, Physics, 81*(5), 1343–1351.

Coia, L. R., Myerson, R. J., & Tepper, J. E. (1995). Late effects of radiation therapy on the gastrointestinal tract. *International Journal of Radiation Oncology, Biology, Physics, 31*(5), 1213–1236.

Fajardo, L. F. (2005). The pathology of ionizing radiation as defined by morphologic patterns. *Acta Oncologica, 44*(1), 13–22.

Ogawa, F., Mino-Kenudson, M., Shimizu, M., Ligato, S., & Lauwers, G. Y. (2008). Gastroduodenitis associated with yttrium 90-microsphere selective internal radiation: An iatrogenic complication in need of recognition. *Archives of Pathology and Laboratory Medicine, 132*(11), 1734–1738.

Radiation-Induced Esophagitis

Ricardo Fonseca[1] and Paula Chaves[2,3]
[1]Serviço de Anatomia Patológica, Instituto Português de Oncologia de Lisboa Francisco Gentil, Lisboa, Portugal
[2]Serviço de Anatomia Patológica, Instituto Português de Oncologia de Lisboa de Francisco Gentil, Lisbon, Portugal
[3]Faculdade de Ciências da Saúde, Universidade da Beira Interior, Covilhã, Portugal

Definition

Radiation therapy for thoracic malignancies is often complicated by radiation-induced esophagitis.

Radiation esophagitis corresponds to esophageal damage secondary to radiation or chemotherapy.

Gastrointestinal toxicity occurring after radiation therapy can occur early on, after the treatment being acute, or later, months, or even years after radiotherapy.

Acute radiation esophagitis is primarily due to effects on the basal epithelial layer. This causes a thinning of the mucosa, which can progress to denudation.

Incidence and Location

It is not infrequent as a result of the high incidence of pulmonary and mediastinal neoplasms. A radiation dose of 5,000 cGy or more to the mediastinum may cause severe injury to the esophagus. Acute radiation-induced esophagitis usually occurs 2–4 weeks after the initiation of radiation therapy. The technique used for radiotherapy administration, the radiation dose to the esophagus, and the use of concurrent chemotherapy all influence the likelihood of esophageal complications.

It affects both sexes and occurs mainly in adults and the elderly.

Clinical Features

The manifestations of radiation esophagitis are characterized by dysphagia, odynophagia, or symptoms suggestive of dysmotility. Hematemesis and melena may occur.

Dysphagia occurring during radiotherapy is probably secondary to epithelial damage and disordered motility. The occurrence of esophagitis depends on the dose intensity of radiation. Most cases of acute radiation esophagitis are self-limited, but some patients may have progressive dysphagia due to the development of radiation strictures 4–8 months after completion of radiation therapy.

In those cases, dysphagia can be secondary to stricture or altered motility caused by fibrosis/muscular damage or nerve injury. Chronic ulceration appears to be related to the total dose of radiation. In rare cases, there can be fistula formation.

Patients receiving radiation therapy are also at risk for infectious esophagitis, which can be indistinguishable clinically from radiation-induced esophagitis.

Because the clinical presentation of radiation and infectious esophagitis is very similar, the correct diagnosis is important since treatment approaches are different.

Pathologic Features

Gross Findings

The mucosa typically has a granular appearance because of edema and inflammation of the irradiated segment; in acute cases, esophagitis presents on endoscopy with a friable mucosa with edema and mucositis (lesions appear ulcerative, hyperplastic, or both). Acute confluent ulcers may also be seen.

In chronic cases, there may be strictures up to 13–21 months after therapy (characteristic).

Microscopic Findings

Histologic examination reveals significant cellular atypia in epithelium and stromal cells. All these changes result from ischemia due to vascular lesions. Cytological findings include: bizarre cytomegaly of epithelial and stromal cells, large pale nuclei, and abundant vacuolated cytoplasm. It is possible to see multinucleated cells. In more chronic cases, there is usually the presence of acanthosis, parakeratosis, hyalinized blood vessels, submucosal fibrosis, and muscular degeneration (Fig. 1).

So the most common microscopic findings include:

- Bizarre cytomegaly in epithelial and stromal cells
- Large pale nuclei and abundant vacuolated cytoplasm
- Multinucleation

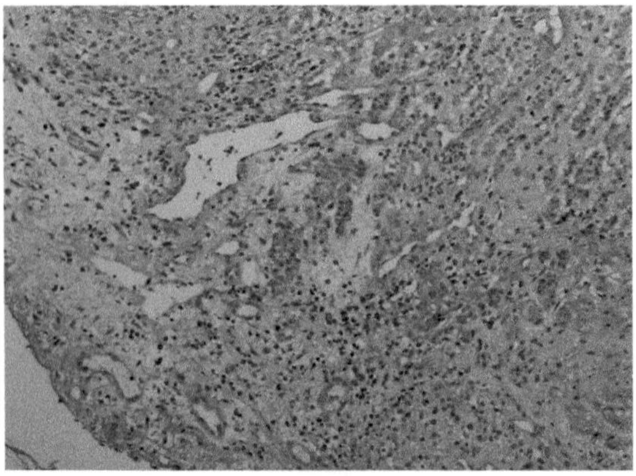

Radiation-Induced Esophagitis, Fig. 1 Ectatic and hyalinized blood vessels in a chronic radiation esophagitis

- Parakeratosis, acanthosis, and blood vessel hyalinization in chronic cases

Differential Diagnosis

It is important to differentiate radiation esophagitis from malignancy and viral esophagitis. Malignant epithelial cells as well as chemotherapy may mimic radiation-induced changes on esophageal mucosae.

Radiation-induced damage is characterized by uniform enlargement of the cells (cytomegaly), large pale nuclei, and abundant vacuolated cytoplasm. In chronic cases, acanthosis, parakeratosis, hyalinized blood vessels, submucosal fibrosis, and muscular degeneration can occur.

In contrast, in malignancy, there is usually an increased nuclear/cytoplasmic ratio with hyperchromatic nuclei and condensed chromatin. Mitotic activity is usually present. Multinucleation can also be present in certain viral infections like herpes virus, but in those cases the chromatin is normal. In some cases immunostains for herpes virus may be needed to differentiate the two.

So in the differential diagnosis, we must consider:

- Neoplasia and viral infections
  - Neoplasia has a high nucleus/cytoplasmic ratio, mitosis, and hyperchromatism.
  - Sometimes neoplasia and radiation coexist in the same patient – immunostains are recommended.
  - Multinucleation may be confused with HSV infection.
  - Immunoperoxidase stains for HSV and CMV are recommended in difficult cases.

Prognosis and Therapy

Prognosis is dependent on the doses of radiation. If less than 6,000 rads, the damage can be reversible. In cases of significant stricture, esophageal dilation may be indicated.

Treatment will be different for acute or later esophagitis.

Acute Esophagitis Treatment

The management of acute esophagitis is symptomatic. In some cases, interruption of radiotherapy treatment may be necessary, although this measure should be avoided since it can compromise the treatment of the primary illness.

Treatment for acute esophagitis includes:

1. Topical anesthetics, analgesics (anti-inflammatory agents, narcotics), antacid therapy (proton-pump inhibitors, H2 receptor blockers), and promotility agents.
2. Dietary modification (bland, pureed, or soft foods, soups), to help a patient maintain adequate caloric and liquid intake. Eating more frequent, smaller meals and avoiding foods that are very hot or very cold may also be useful. Avoidance of smoking, alcohol, coffee, spicy or acidic foods or liquids, chips, crackers, and fatty and indigestible foods can be helpful.
3. Treatment of any superimposed *Candida* infection.

In the case of esophageal strictures, management may need endoscopic dilation that may result in symptomatic relief. A possible complication of esophageal dilation is the esophageal rupture. Surgical intervention may be required for patients developing esophageal fistula.

References and Further Reading

Iacobuzio-Donahue, C. A., & Montgomery, E. A. (2005). *Gastrointestinal and liver pathology*. Philadelphia: Elsevier.

Levine, M. S. M.D., & Rubesin, S. E. M.D. (2005). Diseases of the esophagus: Diagnosis with esophagography. *Radiology, 237*, 414–427.

Noffsinger, A., Fenoglio-Preiser, C., Maru, D., & Glinsky, N. (2007). *Atlas of non tumour pathology – Gastrointestinal diseases*. Washington, DC: American Registry of Pathology.

Perez, R. A., & Early, D. S. (2002). Endoscopy in patients receiving radiation therapy to the thorax. *Digestive Diseases and Science, 47*(1), 79–83.

Rectum

Cevriye Cansiz Ersöz
Department of Pathology, Ankara University Medical School, Sihhiye, Ankara, Turkey

Synonyms

Distal part of the large intestine; The pelvic part of the alimentary tract

Anatomy (Macroscopy)

Begins at the rectosigmoid junction- at the level of third sacral vertebra and ends at the anorectal junction- 2–3 cm in front of and a little below the coccyx. The median sacral vessels and the roots of the sacral nerve plexus lie posterior to the rectum. Anteriorly; in women, the rectum is closely related to the uterine cervix and posterior vaginal wall, in men, it lies behind the bladder, vas deferens, seminal vesicles, and prostate. The non-mobilized rectum has three lateral curves: the upper and the lower are convex to the right and the middle is convex to the left. These curves correspond intraluminally to the folds or valves of Houston (Fig. 1). The middle valve is the most consistent in presence and location (also known as Kohlrausch's plica) and corresponds to the level of the anterior peritoneal reflection. The rectum is characterized by the absence of taeniae, epiploic appendices, haustra, or a well-defined mesentery. Superior 1/3rd of rectum is covered by peritoneum on the anterior and lateral surfaces. Middle 1/3rd is covered by peritoneum on the anterior surface, but inferior 1/3rd is subperitoneal- devoid of peritoneum (Fig. 2).

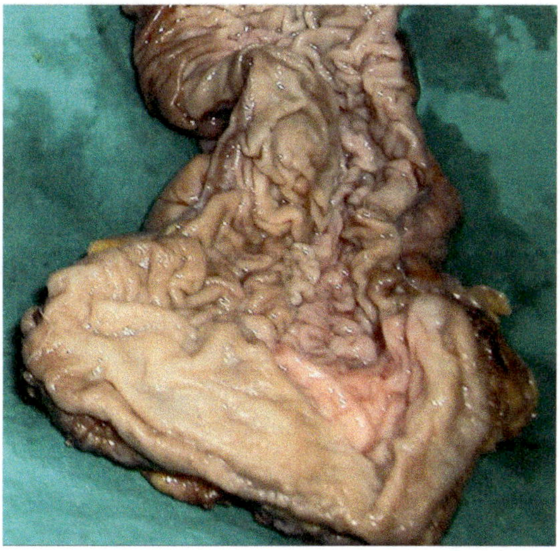

Rectum, Fig. 1 The gross picture from the mucosal aspect of rectum. There are three transverse folds (superior, middle and inferior folds)

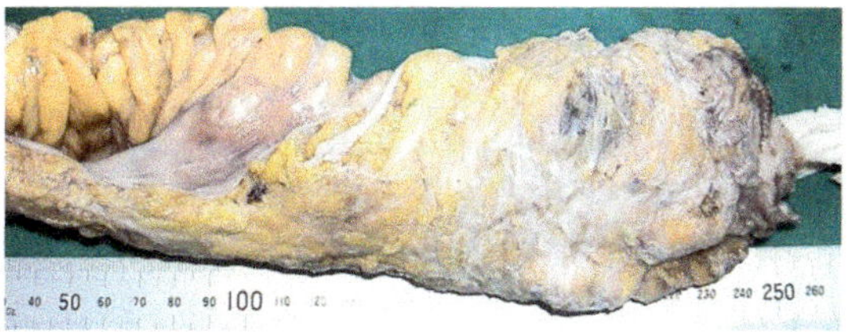

Rectum, Fig. 2 Macroscopic feature of the inferior, non-peritonealized part of the rectum

Arterial supply is from superior, middle and inferior rectal artery and median sacral artery. The venous drainage of the rectum basically follows its arterial supply. The submucosal venous plexus above the pectinate line drains into the superior rectal veins (portal system). The submucosal plexus below the pectinate line drains into the inferior rectal veins. The unions of the superior with the middle and inferior rectal veins are important portal-systemic anastomoses. Lymph from the upper two thirds of the rectum drains exclusively upward to the inferior mesenteric nodes and then to the paraaortic nodes. Lymphatic drainage from the lower third of the rectum occurs, not only cephalad along the superior hemorrhoidal and inferior mesentery arteries but also laterally, along the middle hemorrhoidal vessels to the internal iliac nodes. The sympathetic supply arises from L1, L2, and L3. The parasympathetic supply derives from S2, S3, and S4.

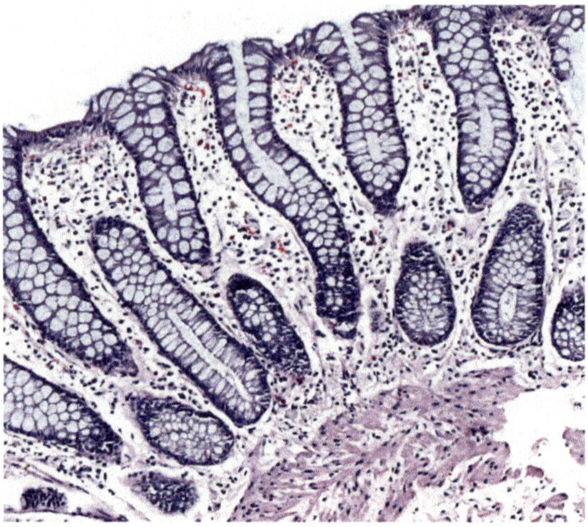

Rectum, Fig. 3 Normal histology of the rectum, showing mild crypt distortion (H&E; x100)

Function

The key role of rectal ampulla is to act as a temporary storehouse for feces.

Size, Weight

The rectum is believed to be 12–15 cm in length. Its diameter is approximately 4 cm in the upper part. However; it becomes larger near the anus, where it forms the rectal ampulla.

Microscopy (Histology)

The discontinuous tinea coli converge, unite, and again constitute a complete outer longitudinal smooth muscle layer of the muscularis propria. Where the rectum exits the peritoneal cavity to enter the anal canal, it is completely invested by both inner and outer smooth muscle coats of the muscularis propria, and acquires an adventitia rather than a serosal covering.

Mucosa, submucosa and muscularis propria is overlying the perimuscular tissue in rectum.

Mucosa:

The mucosa is composed of epitehelium, lamina propria and muscularis mucosa. There are subtle differences in the normal histology of the distal rectal mucosa. Compared with non-rectal colonic mucosa, distal rectal mucosa exhibits crypts that are not as closely spaced and are slightly shorter. Unlike the rest of the colon, the crypts do not extend directly down to the muscularis mucosae. The crypts may be slightly dilated or tortuous, and somewhat less numerous (Fig. 3). The surface epithelium may be slightly cuboidal rather than tall columnar. The rectal mucosa has a higher ratio of goblet cells to absorbtive cells, with a less dense lamina propria and more easily identified muciphages. Paneth's cells are not normally seen within the rectum. The rectum contains the same endocrine cell types as the colon, namely serotonin, peptide YY (PYY), pancreatic polypeptide (PP),oxyntomodulin, and somatostatin-cells, predominantly located in the crypts,and rarely scattered within the lamina propria. The lamina propria of the large intestine contains solitary lymphoid follicules extending into the submucosa, and these follicules are more developed in the rectum and decrease in number with age. It is important to recognize the simplified and somewhat distorted mucosal architecture of the distal rectal columnar mucosa as normal, and not indicative of true "architectural distortion" characteristic of chronic inflammatory bowel disease. The muscularis mucosa is a thin layer of muscle, located outside the lamina propria mucosae and separating it from the submucosa.

Submucosa:

In the submucosa, there is loose connective tissue with submucosal plexus of Meissner-composed of nonmyelinated, postganglionic sympathetic fibers, and parasympathetic ganglion cells-, and minimal inflammatory cells.

Muscularis propria:

The muscularis propria is composed of inner circular layer, myenteric plexus of Auerbach, and outer longitudinal layer.

Immunohistochemistry

Like the other parts of the colon, the epithelium is characterized by a CK7 negative and CK20 positive immunophenotype. There is also nuclear CDX2 positivity in the epithelium.

References and Further Reading

Adler, D. G., Crawford, J. M., & Farraye, F. A. (2015). GI tract endoscopic and tissue processing techniques and normal histology. In R. D. Odze & J. R. Goldblum (Eds.), *Surgical pathology of the GI tract, liver, biliary tract and pancreas* (pp. 4–33). Philadelphia: Elsevier.

Bass, L. M., & Wershil, B. K. (2016). Small and large intestine. In M. Feldman, L. S. Friedman, & L. J. Brandt (Eds.), *Sleisenger & Fordtran's gastrointestinal and liver disease* (pp. 1649–1678). Philadelphia: Elsevier.

Garza, A., & Beart, R. W. (2013). Anatomy and embryology of the anus, rectum, and colon. In M. L. Corman (Ed.), *Corman's colon and rectal surgery* (pp. 1–26). Philadelphia: Lippincott.

Katzin, W. E., & Petras, R. E. (2012). Small intestine. In S. E. Millis (Ed.), *Histology for pathologists* (pp. 673–696). Philadelphia: Lippincott.

S

Salmonellosis

Anne Jouret-Mourin
Department of Pathology, Cliniques Universitaires St. Luc, UCL, Brussels, Belgium

Synonyms

Typhoid fever

Definition

Salmonella is a gram-negative bacteria which invades the epithelium of the ileum and colon and is divided into two forms of disease affecting the gastrointestinal tract: typhoid and non-typhoid species. *Salmonella typhi* is the most common cause agent of typhoid fever; *S. paratyphi* can cause similar clinical symptoms. Non-typhoid species including *S. enteritidis*, *S. typhimurium*, *S. javania*, *S muenchen*, *S. anatum*, *S. Newport*, *S. oranienburg* are generally associated with self-limited gastroenteritis or enterocolitis. The infective dose is relatively low; approximately 10^2–10^3 organisms may cause human disease.

Salmonella infection is a global health problem. It is transmitted through contaminated food and water and is prevalent in the developing countries. *Salmonella* infection is also an important cause of sporadic food poisoning in developed countries and traveler's diarrhea. It has been steadily increasing steadily during the past decade. More than 95% of *Salmonella* infections are food-borne causing sporadic food poisoning. *Salmonella* can be present in eggs and egg products, fish, dry cereal, ice cream, fresh sprouts, juice, vegetables, or fruits. Poultry represents the main source of non-typhoidal *Salmonella* strains. They may survive partial cooking, freezing, and drying. Infection can be acquired from animals.

Salmonella typhi originates from a human reservoir and is transmitted by secondary fecal contamination of food and water.

The pathogenic mechanism is an invasion. *Salmonella* are intracellular parasites that enter the host by penetrating intestinal epithelial barriers. They adhere to different epithelial cells including M cells as well as enterocytes. The invasive process begins when the *Salmonella* in proximity of the microvilli cause degeneration of the microvilli and apical site of the intestinal epithelial cells. *Salmonella* sp. invade epithelial cells by inducing extensive cytoskeletal rearrangements and destroy these cells, causing a defect in the epithelial layer, and eventual ulcerations and deeper infection. Replication also occurs in macrophages of the lymphoid follicles, leading to bacteremia.

Salmonella produce different clinical syndromes such as gastroenteritis, enterocolitis, typhoid fever, and localized infections in joints or bones. Some patients can be asymptomatic carriers.

The incubation period is generally 1 week, followed by a 2–3 weeks of illness.

F. Carneiro et al. (eds.), *Pathology of the Gastrointestinal Tract*, Encyclopedia of Pathology,
DOI 10.1007/978-3-319-40560-5

Patients with typhoid fever present with fever that rises over several days, abdominal pain and headache. Abdominal rash, delirium, and hepatosplenomegaly are also common. Typhoidal disease is not truly an intestinal disease but is characterized by a systemic involvement. The diarrhea which begins in the second or third week of infection is initially watery but may progress to complications including massive intestinal hemorrhage and perforation often in the terminal ileum.

Non-typhoid species usually cause a less severe illness corresponding to a self-limited disease that develops 8–48 h after ingestion of contaminated food and usually resolves over 2–12 days. Symptoms of *Salmonella* gastroenteritis vary widely. Symptoms include nausea, abdominal cramps, vomiting followed by watery or bloody diarrhea and fever.

Rarely, *Salmonella* cause severe bloody diarrhea or toxic megacolon. Infections are particularly virulent in individuals with HIV and may be complicated by perforation.

Cultures from stool or eventually blood (if bacteremia) are the mainstay for *Salmonella* diagnosis.

Clinical Features

- **Incidence**
  The incidence is estimated as 20 cases per 100,000 population in the USA.
- **Age**
  The peak of incidence occurs in extremes of age (infancy <1 year old and elderly >70 year old). There is no difference between male and female. Patients with low gastric acidity, immunosuppressed, and AIDS patients have a greater risk of *Salmonella* as well.
- **Site**
  Any level of the gastrointestinal tract may be involved, but the most prominent pathology is in the ileum, appendix, and right colon. After reaching the small bowel, *Salmonella* penetrates the mucosa predominantly in the ileocaecal area and multiplies within the intestinal lymphoid follicles.
- **Prognosis**
  Although most *Salmonella* infections resolve with antibiotics and supportive care, intestinal infection may progress to septicemia and death particularly in the elderly, the very young, neonates, and immunocompromised patients or those with comorbidities like prosthesis, artificial cardiac valves, etc. Typhoid fever is a systemic illness with a mortality rate of 15% in untreated patients.
- **Treatment**
  Most cases of non-typhoidal *Salmonella* enterocolitis are self-limiting and do not require treatment other than supportive care.

  Antimicrobial therapy should be instituted in patients with severe gastroenteritis or in those at risk for developing disseminated disease.

  Typhoid fever is a systemic illness with a high rate of mortality. Fluoroquinolones are the most effective drugs for treatment of typhoid fever. Quinolone-resistant *Salmonella* strains have emerged and are often resistant to multiple drugs. They are usually treated with azithromycin or cephalosporins.

Macroscopic Features

In the typhoid fever, findings are prominent in the ileum, right colon, and appendix. Classically, the bowel wall is thickened with raised nodules corresponding to hyperplastic Peyer's patches. There are ulcerations over the button-like protrusions of the enlarged Peyer's patches. Typically, the ulcers are long, oval, or linear. There are usually parallel with the longitudinal axis of the terminal ileum. Smaller punctate ulcers overlying lymphoid follicles are found in the caecum. The lesions can be deeper with necrosis leading to perforation. Toxic megacolon may complicate typhoid fever. Suppurate mesenteric lymphadenitis may be present. Rarely, the mucosa can be normal or mildly inflamed.

In the non-typhoid *Salmonella*, the ileum and colon manifest focal and latter diffuse lesions. The lesions are often milder including mucosal erythema, hemorrhage, friability of the mucosa and surface erosions, ulcerations, or deep fissures with segmental involvement of the colon. Sometimes the mucosa is grossly normal or edematous.

Microscopic Findings

The hallmark lesion of typhoid fever is an ulceration overlying the hyperplastic Peyer's patches, causing ulcerated lymphoid follicles. In the adjacent right colon, lymphoid follicles are infiltrated by mononuclear cells, and an abundance of macrophages in the floor and edges of the ulcer are observed. These cells are actively phagocytic and contain erythrocytes and other cellular debris. Neutrophils are usually inconspicuous. The ulcers are typically very deep at the level or into the muscularis propria, with a transmural inflammation.

Typhoid fever is sometimes associated with marked architectural distortions that mimic chronic IBD.

Non-typhoid infection features are usually like nonspecific acute infectious type such as edema, congestion, and focal inflammation in the lamina propria. Areas of hemorrhage and ulcerations are also present. Rarely, they show cryptitis, severe inflammation, fibrinous exudates, and small thrombi. Occasionally, significant crypt distortions and branching can be observed, especially in case with persistent diarrhea.

A significant overlap between pathologic features of typhoid and non-typhoid species exists. Some patients with typhoid fever may lack the classic ulcer overlying a Peyer's patch and may show acute self-limited colitis similar to non-typhoid species. Conversely, patients with non-typhoid salmonellosis may have severe colitis, with deep ulceration and transmural involvement.

Differential Diagnosis

The differential diagnosis includes other enteric bacterial pathogens such as *Yersinia*, ulcerative colitis, and Crohn's disease (Fig. 1). Clinical presentation and stool cultures may be very helpful in resolving the differential diagnosis.

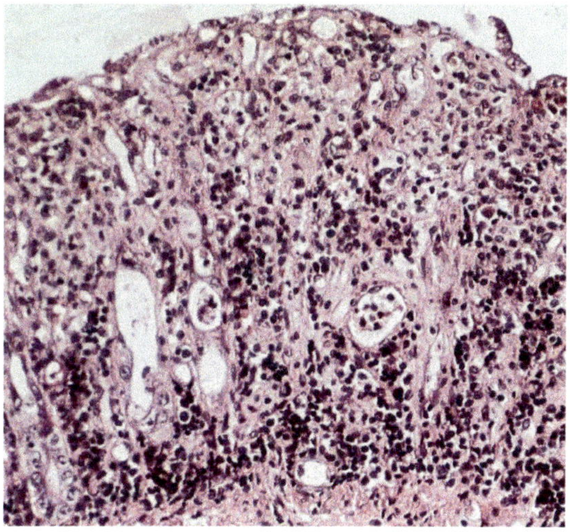

Salmonellosis, Fig. 1 Non-typhoid salmonellosis: surface epithelial damage, inflammatory infiltrate with mononuclear cells and crypt abscesses can mimic IBD (Courtesy Dr P. van Eycken)

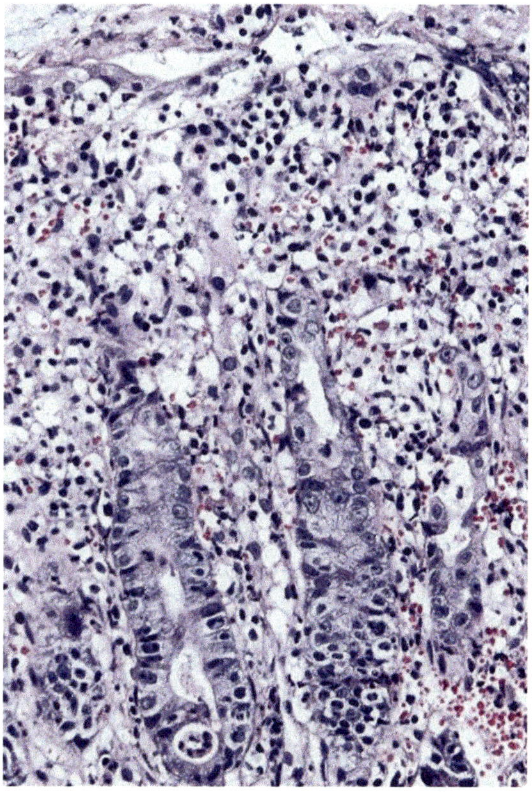

Salmonellosis, Fig. 2 Non-typhoid salmonellosis: pattern of acute infectious colitis: Mucosal edema, cryptitis, and a mixed infiltrate in the lamina

S

Clinically, the incubation period of *Salmonella* infection is longer than that of other enteric pathogens.

Histologically, *Salmonella* infection shows a more intense infiltration of neutrophils in the lamina propria than in the epithelial glands (Fig. 2). When crypt distortion is present, a significant overlap between salmonellosis and IBD may exist, but crypt distortion is generally more pronounced in ulcerative colitis and there is a relative scarcity of chronic inflammatory cells in *Salmonella* infection.

In severe forms, giant cells or histiocytic aggregates are present and they may coexist with a transmural inflammation. In such cases, a diagnosis of Crohn's disease may be confusedly proposed. However, it is very uncommon that giant cells form compact granulomas.

References and Further Reading

Boyd, J. F. (1985). Pathology of the alimentary tract in *Salmonella typhimurium* food poisoning. *Gut, 26*, 935–944.

Dagash, M., et al. (1997). Transient radiological and colonoscopic features of IBD in a patient with severe *Salmonella gastroenteritis*. *The American Journal of Gastroenterology, 92*, 349–351.

Lamps, L. W. (2007). Infective disorders of the gastrointestinal tract. *Histopathology, 50*, 55–63.

McGovern, V. J., et al. (1979). Pathology of *Salmonella* colitis. *The American Journal of Surgical Pathology, 3*, 483–490.

Lamps, L. W. (2009). *Salmonella species in surgical pathology of the gastrointestinal system: Bacterial, fungal, viral and parasitic infections* (pp. 27–31). New York: Springer.

Sarcoidosis, Gastrointestinal

Susana Rodrigues
Serviço de Gastrenterologia, Centro Hospitalar de São João, Alameda Professor Hernani Monteiro, Porto, Portugal

Synonyms

Abdominal sarcoidosis; Gastrointestinal manifestations of sarcoidosis; Granulomatous gastroenteritis

Definition

Sarcoidosis is a noncaseating granulomatous disease, likely of autoimmune etiology, that causes inflammation and tissue damage in multiple organs, most commonly the lung, but also skin, and lymph nodes, characterized by the formation of noncaseating granulomas. The infiltration of CD4 + −activated T-cells represents the immunological hallmark of sarcoidosis. If persistent, this inflammatory process is followed by the formation of granulomas. The accumulated inflammatory cells and granulomas result in distortion of the architecture of the affected tissue and, ultimately, organ dysfunction. Constitutional symptoms include weight loss, myalgias, night sweats, and fever and are most frequent early in the disease. A common acute presentation is erythema nodosum with arthralgias and hilar adenopathy (Lofgren's syndrome). Over 90% of patients have lung involvement. The diagnosis of sarcoidosis is based on the following criteria: (1) a compatible clinical and/or radiological picture, (2) histological evidence of noncaseating granulomas, and (3) exclusion of other diseases capable of producing a similar histological or clinical picture. Sarcoidosis of the gastrointestinal (GI) tract is rare, and clinical features are related to the location.

Diagnosis of sarcoidosis is generally based upon a compatible history, demonstration of granulomas in biopsies with negative staining and culture for acid-fast bacilli, absence of occupational or domestic exposure to toxins, and lack of drug-induced disease. ACE levels are elevated in 60% of patients and have been shown to correlate with the level of disease activity.

Esophageal involvement of sarcoidosis is exceedingly rare. The most frequent clinical manifestations are dysphagia and weight loss. These are related to the granulomatous infiltration of the wall which leads to dysmotility which may be attributed to neuropathy and myopathy or mechanical obstruction. The macroscopic features at endoscopy vary from aphthous lesions, plaque-like protrusions, long distorted, ulcerated strictures, and narrowing of the distal esophagus.

The stomach, particularly the antrum, is the most frequent GI organ affected in sarcoidosis. Epigastric pain is the most common symptom. Abdominal pain is characteristically dull, burning, or cramping in nature and is often postprandial. Heartburn, early satiety, nausea, vomiting, weight loss, generalized abdominal discomfort, and diarrhea may also be reported. The diagnosis is histological, but gastric aspirate ACE levels may be higher than in the serum, and in some patients, a pernicious anemia-type picture has also been described.

The small bowel is the least common location of sarcoidosis. Patients present with diarrhea, malabsorption, protein-losing enteropathy, colicky, epigastric and periumbilical abdominal pain, and bleeding. Weight loss, anorexia, low-grade fever, and weakness may be present. Intestinal granulomatosis of other etiologies such as Crohn's disease, tuberculous enteritis, and Histoplasma enteritis must be excluded.

Sarcoidosis rarely involves the colon and rectum. In these patients, abdominal pain was the most common symptom with rare reports of bleeding. External compression by lymphadenopathy is the most common cause of intestinal obstruction.

Patients with appendiceal sarcoidosis may present with acute right lower quadrant abdominal pain or subacute to chronic pain in association with a right lower quadrant mass. Appendiceal abscesses are unusual.

As many as 40% of patients with sarcoidosis have serological evidence of gastric autoimmunity and gluten-associated immune reactivity; however, the incidence of pernicious anemia or celiac disease in patients with sarcoidosis remains low. On the contrary, sarcoidosis is more frequently reported in association with either Crohn's disease or ulcerative colitis.

Clinical Features

- **Incidence**
  Sarcoidosis of the GI tract is exceptionally rare. While several autopsy studies did not detect GI involvement, one study reported intestinal and gastric disease in 3.4% and 2.5%, respectively. GI involvement is generally subclinical, but clinically detectable disease is found in 0.1–0.9% of patients with sarcoidosis.
- **Age**
  Sarcoidosis affects predominantly individuals in the 20–40-year-old range.
- **Sex**
  There is no clear gender predominance in sarcoidosis. On the other hand, the incidence of sarcoidosis in African Americans is at least threefold higher than in Caucasians.
- **Site**
  Sarcoidosis may involve the peritoneum and various intra-abdominal organs such as the liver, gallbladder, pancreas, esophagus, stomach, small bowel, appendix, colon, and rectum. The stomach is the most commonly involved organ in the GI tract, and gastric sarcoidosis, particularly occurring in the antrum, may affect around 10% of patients with systemic disease.
- **Treatment**
  The decision to treat GI sarcoidosis is based upon the activity and extent of disease. The role of therapy in GI sarcoidosis is unclear. Patients generally do not require treatment and are merely monitored. For symptomatic patients with granulomatous inflammation on tissue biopsy, glucocorticoids are the elected treatment. The therapy initiated is prednisone 0.5 mg/kg per day. This dose is maintained during a 6–8 week course until a positive response is noted and then gradually tapered over a period of approximately 6 months, to a low to moderate maintenance dose (10–15 mg). Treatment with corticosteroids results in symptomatic improvement in 66% of patients although normalization of the radiological changes does not necessarily occur

  Antacids and prokinetic drugs have been used for symptomatic relief of delayed gastric emptying and abdominal pain. Patients with pyloric structuring or severe GI bleeding may require surgery. Gastrointestinal sarcoidosis is monitored clinically and radiographically. The role of serum angiotensin converting enzyme levels in monitoring gastrointestinal sarcoidosis is unknown. Repeat endoscopy is performed when the response to therapy remains absent or unclear, particularly when change of therapy is being considered for persistent symptoms.

- **Outcome**
  The overall prognosis is good, although most patients will manifest some permanent organ impairment. Risk factors for poor prognosis in sarcoidosis include African ethnicity, disease onset after 40 years, and stage III pulmonary involvement. Mortality is related to heart and lung involvement.

Macroscopy

Upper GI endoscopy may show gastritis, ulcerations and diffusely erythematous, friable, and elevated mucosa. In gastric sarcoidosis, four principal categories of lesions have been distinguished: subclinical (the commonest), ulcerative, infiltrative, and polypous. Ulcerations may lead to bleeding. Mucosal enlargements such as polyps, nodules, or enlarged Menetrier-like folds may develop and lead to gastric outlet obstruction. Segmental mucosal thickening and nondistensibility resembling linitis plastica is the most common finding at gastroscopy. Changes may be mistaken for a gastric carcinoma although endoscopic ultrasound may aid in the diagnosis. Colonoscopy may reveal multiple nodules, polyps, strictures, aphthous ulcers, and small punctuate bleeding sites.

Microscopy

The diagnosis of GI sarcoidosis is based on the presence of noncaseating granulomas with multinucleated giant cells and macrophages in the biopsy specimens with negative staining and culture for acid-fast bacilli and fungi and in the absence of particulate foreign material (Figs. 1 and 2). There is an overall scarcity of acute inflammation and mucosal architectural distortion. Several types of cytoplasmic inclusion bodies can accompany granulomatous inflammation including laminated calcific Schaumann bodies, stellate asteroid bodies, and small oval brown Hamazaki-Wesenberg bodies located in the mucosa. These inclusion bodies are common in sarcoidosis but are nonspecific. In cases where resolution is incomplete, granulomas become enclosed by fibrous rims and later replaced by collagenous fibrous tissue.

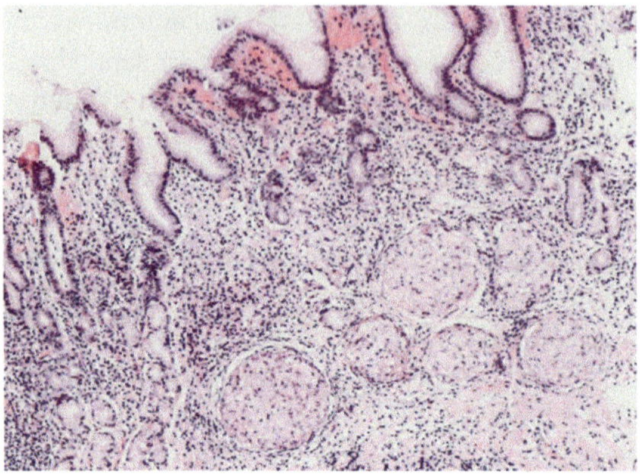

Sarcoidosis, Gastrointestinal, Fig. 1 Low-power H&E stain demonstrates gastric mucosa with noncaseating granulomas with multinucleated giant cells and macrophages

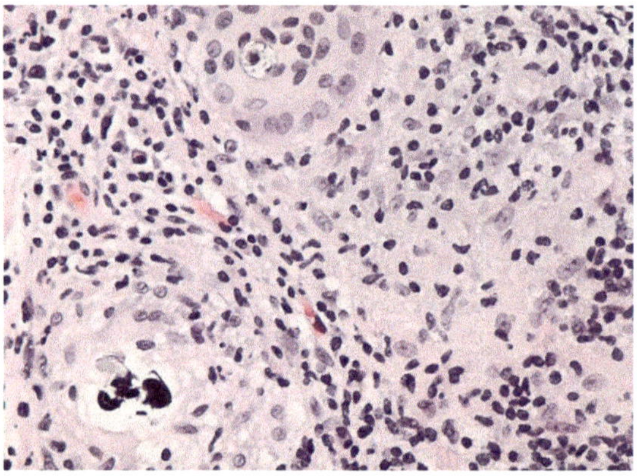

Sarcoidosis, Gastrointestinal, Fig. 2 Medium power H&E shows aggregates of epithelioid histiocytes and Langhans-type giant cells surrounded by lymphocytes. No central necrosis is present. Schaumann bodies are visible in the giant cells in the lower left hand corner

Immunophenotype

Although immunophenotyping of the bronchoalveolar lavage lymphocytes with the CD4/CD8 ratio and the CD103/CD4 ratio is possible, immunophenotyping of the gastrointestinal mucosa is not used.

Molecular Features

Several alleles on the short arm of chromosome 6 confer susceptibility to disease (HLA DR 11, 12, 14, 15, 17). Regarding gastrointestinal involvement of sarcoidosis, the relevance of molecular analysis is limited.

Differential Diagnosis

Exclusion of other diseases is not always as rigorous as necessary. It is sometimes unclear whether symptomatic GI disease is truly due to sarcoidosis or to another process with granulomas discovered as an incidental finding.

Tuberculosis, fungal infections, vasculitis, foreign body reactions, radiation injury, Crohn's disease, microscopic colitis, Whipple's disease, schistosomiasis, enterobiasis, lymphoma, and carcinoma are all associated with gastrointestinal granulomas.

Histological examination with staining and culture for fungi and acid-fast bacilli helps to distinguish between fungal infections such as *histoplasmosis* and the presence of *tuberculosis*.

Sarcoidosis of the colon and terminal ileum (TI) can mimic *Crohn's disease* with moderate fibrosis and narrowing of the terminal ileum. It is differentiated from CD by the presence of (Schaumann bodies), prominent intramucosal rather than sparse submucosal granulomas, and the lack of fistulas. Serum angiotensin converting enzyme may help to differentiate these entities. Resolution of granulomatous inflammation and significant clinical improvement with corticosteroid therapy favors the diagnosis of sarcoidosis.

References and Further Reading

1. Akdogan, M., Ulas, M., Kayhan, B., Orug, T., & Aydog, G. (2008). Gastrointestinal sarcoidosis mimicking colonic cancer. *Turkish Journal of Gastroenterology, 19*(2), 136–138.
2. Kchaou Ouakaa, A., Kochlef, A., Kilani, A., Kharrat, J., Romani, M., Gargouri, D., Belhadj, N., Ghorbel, A., Khayat, O., & Ben Ayed, M. (2003). Gastric and colonic sarcoidosis. A case report. *La Tunisie Médicale, 81*(11), 902–906.
3. Maàmouri, N., Guellouz, S., Ben Hariz, F., Ketari, S., Belkahla, N., Ouerghi, H., Chelly-Enneifer, I., Chouaib, S., Moncef Zitouna, M., & Ben Mami, N. (2010). Gastrointestinal sarcoidosis. *La Revue de Médecine Interne, 31*(4), 262–267.
4. Vahid, B., Spodik, M., Braun, K. N., Ghazi, L. J., & Esmaili, A. (2007). Sarcoidosis of gastrointestinal tract: a rare disease. *Digestive Diseases and Sciences, 52*(12), 3316–3320.
5. Ushiki, A., Koizumi, T., Kubo, K., Suzawa, K., Arakura, N., & Suzawa, H. (2009). Colonic sarcoidosis presenting multiple submucosal tumor-like lesions. *Internal Medicine, 48*(20), 1813–1816.

Scleroderma, Esophageal

J. Alberto Pereira da Silva
Serviço de Reumatologia, Hospital de S. Maria, Lisbon, Portugal

Synonyms

Esophageal; Esophagus in progressive systemic sclerosis (PSP); Esophagus in systemic sclerosis (SSc); Scleroderma

Definition

Esophageal disease in scleroderma is the result of dysmotility and lower esophageal sphincter dysfunction.

Both neurogenic impairment and microvascular insufficiency lead to smooth muscular atrophy and fibrosis. Endothelial activation is followed by the production of autoantibodies. Autoantibodies against enteric neurons and anti-muscarinic antibodies have been described in some patients.

Dysmotility is a consequence of smooth muscle involvement in the distal two-thirds of the esophagus. Esophageal sphincter dysfunction with reduced pressure leads to gastroesophageal reflux.

Involvement of the upper esophagus is the result of inflammation of striated muscle and should raise the possibility of other diagnosis (overlap syndromes or dermatomyositis).

Symptoms consist of retrosternal pain, dysphagia, heartburn, and regurgitation. Delayed gastric emptying, loss of secondary peristalsis, and impaired salivary bicarbonate secretion may further aggravate gastroesophageal reflux.

Structural disorders may occur such as Barrett's metaplasia, hiatal hernia, and esophageal strictures. Strictures have been found in up to 29% and are the consequence of reflux and other factors such as candidal esophagitis. Barrett's esophagus was described up to 37%; it remains controversial however if there is an increased incidence of esophageal malignancy and even if Barrett's esophagus is more frequent than in the general population. Some Authors suggest that the use of proton pump inhibitors may have decreased the prevalence of these conditions.

Several studies suggested that gastroesophageal reflux may contribute to interstitial lung disease (ILD) in consequence of microaspiration and bronchoconstriction; it has been found that ILD is correlated with acid and nonacid reflux. It is not yet sure that treatment of reflux has a positive effect in ILD.

Clinical Features

- **Incidence**
  In scleroderma, the esophagus is the most frequently involved organ of the gastrointestinal tract, with more than 50% of patients having clinical esophageal involvement; dysmotility is found in 90% by manometry, even in the 30–40% asymptomatic patients.

  Gastrointestinal involvement which occurs in up to 90% may appear in both diffuse and limited forms of scleroderma although other visceral involvement is more frequent in diffuse forms.

  Scleroderma is a rare disease with a worldwide distribution. The incidence of scleroderma varies from 9 to 19 new cases per million per year, and the prevalence is 100–286 per million population. It is more prevalent in African-American and black Africans (about two-fold increase).
- **Age**
  The most common age of disease onset is between 30 and 50 years, the mean age being 42–44 years.
- **Sex**
  Scleroderma is more common in females (3–5:1), in particular in African-Americans.
- **Site**
  The esophageal involvement in scleroderma is limited to the two inferior thirds. The dysmotility of the superior third should raise suspicion of other diagnosis (mixed connective tissue disease or polymyositis/dermatomyositis).
- **Treatment**
  The treatment of scleroderma esophageal disorders should include lifestyle measures, as in other cases of reflux, and antiacid therapy with PPI or histamine-2-receptor antagonists.

  The head of the bed should be taken during the 3 hours before sleep; alcohol, caffeine, nicotine, chocolate, tomatoes, and drugs that relax the lower esophageal sphincter should be avoided.

  The use of PPI is recommended for treatment and prevention of strictures and ulcers.

  Prokinetic drugs such as metoclopramide, domperidone, and erythromycin are often used in spite of the lack of strong evidence of their benefits.

  Surgery of gastroesophageal reflux in scleroderma is associated with dysphagia and achalasia. In consequence surgery is generally avoided and reserved for cases where medical therapy could not achieve any relieve of the symptoms.

  General therapies for control of scleroderma with immunosuppressors or stem-cell transplantation did not improve gastrointestinal involvement.
- **Outcome**
  In SSc the outcome is determined by the involvement of internal organs, in particular of the lungs. There is not any proven disease-modifying drug.

Risk factors for decreased survival are male sex, proteinuria, elevated sedimentation rate, pulmonary arterial hypertension, restrictive pulmonary disease, dyspnea, decreased pulmonary diffusion capacity, higher age at onset of Raynaud's phenomenon, anti-Scl-70 and anti-U3 RNP antibodies, and greater modified Rodnan skin score.

African-Americans have higher mortality; the presence of anti-Scl-70 and anti U3 RNP is greater in this ethnic group.

Macroscopy

Autopsy studies showed atrophy in 94% without fibrosis, and esophageal thickening was found in a study using endoscopic ultrasound.

Microscopy

Early lesions are seen in arterioles consisting of a disruption of the internal elastic lamina, a thickened capillary basement membrane, swollen endothelial cells, and vessel sclerosis. Initially muscle atrophy and fibrosis are scattered, but eventually, collagen infiltration in the lamina propria, submucosa, and smooth muscle occurs. Inflammatory cells are seen around vessels.

Metaplasia of the normal squamous epithelium into columnar epithelium (Barrett's esophagus) is found in about one-third of patients.

Immunophenotype

Anti-topoisomerase I (Scl 70) and anti-centromere are present in the serum of scleroderma patients and are very specific of this disease.

Patients with anti-topoisomerase I antibodies present the diffuse subset of scleroderma and are in greater risk of interstitial lung disease. Anti-centromere antibodies are associated with the limited forms of the disease, digital ischemia, and pulmonary hypertension.

The anti-RNA polymerase antibodies are associated with scleroderma renal crisis.

Other autoantibodies have been described in scleroderma with putative pathogenic effects (anti-endothelial cell, anti-fibroblast, anti-fibrillin, anti-matrix metalloproteinases 1 and 3, anti-platelet-derived growth factor receptor, and anti-muscarinic receptor).

It has been purposed that anti-M3 muscarinic receptor antibodies could be involved in the pathogenesis of gastrointestinal dysmotility.

Differential Diagnosis

Impaired motility, chronic use of antiacids and immunosuppressors, and the use of antibiotics may predispose to candidal esophagitis which may contribute to stricture formation.

References and Further Reading

Clarke, J. O., & Hirano, I. (2012). Upper gastrointestinal tract. In J. Varga et al. (Eds.), *Scleroderma: From pathogenesis to comprehensive management* (pp. 471–484). New York: Springer.

Doma, S., Wo, J. M., & Parkman, H. P. (2012). Esophageal involvement in systemic diseases. In J. E. Richter & D. O. Castell (Eds.), *The esophagus* (pp. 367–382). Chichester: Wiley-Blackwell.

Sjogren, R. W. (1994). Gastrointestinal motility disorders in scleroderma. *Arthritis and Rheumatism, 37*, 1265–1282.

Serrated Polyposis Syndrome

Arzu Ensari
Department of Pathology, Ankara University Medical School, Sihhiye, Ankara, Turkey

S

Synonyms

Hyperplastic polyposis syndrome; Serrated adenomatous polyposis syndrome

Definition

Serrated polyposis syndrome is a clinically defined syndrome characterized by the occurrence of multiple serrated polyps in the large intestine. The definition of serrated polyposis syndrome (SPS) includes (1) at least 5 serrated polyps proximal to the sigmoid with two or more being larger than 10 mm, (2) any number of serrated polyps proximal to sigmoid in an individual who has a first-degree relative with serrated polyposis, and (3) more than 20 serrated polyps of any size distributed throughout the colon. SPS is usually asymptomatic with no associated extracolonic manifestations. Two clinical forms have been described, namely, type 1 characterized by larger and proximally located serrated polyps commonly showing BRAF mutations and/or MMR gene methylation and MSI and a high risk of cancer, whereas type 2 is characterized by numerous small hyperplastic polyps which show KRAS mutations and carry a low risk, if any, for colorectal cancer.

Clinical Features

- **Incidence**
  Approximately 200 cases have been published so far.
- **Age**
  SPS can occur at any age but is more common in middle-aged and elderly.
- **Sex**
  Females and males are affected equally.
- **Site**
  SPS affects the entire colon.
- **Treatment**
  Polyps should be removed by colonoscopy in SPS as they carry a risk of progression to cancer. The interval for colonoscopy is longer for small polyps, while those larger than 1 cm in diameter should be controlled annually. When colonoscopy is technically ineffective as for right-sided large polyps, then total colectomy is recommended.
- **Outcome**
  SPS patients usually have good prognosis if they receive appropriate treatment. Individuals with SPS and their first-degree relatives are at increased risk of colorectal cancer. Follow-up of patients with SPS with repeated colonoscopies is necessary to lower the risk of carcinoma.

Macroscopy

Macroscopically polyps in the context of SPS are mostly sessile, round to oval, flat or slightly elevated lesions located over the mucosal plicae. They possess the same color as the surrounding mucosa (Fig. 1). There may be some pedunculated polyps. They are usually larger than 5 mm in diameter.

Microscopy

The majority of polyps in SPS are sessile serrated adenomas/polyps (SSA/Ps), though there are some microvesicular hyperplastic polyps. As SSA/Ps progress, they become dysplastic and

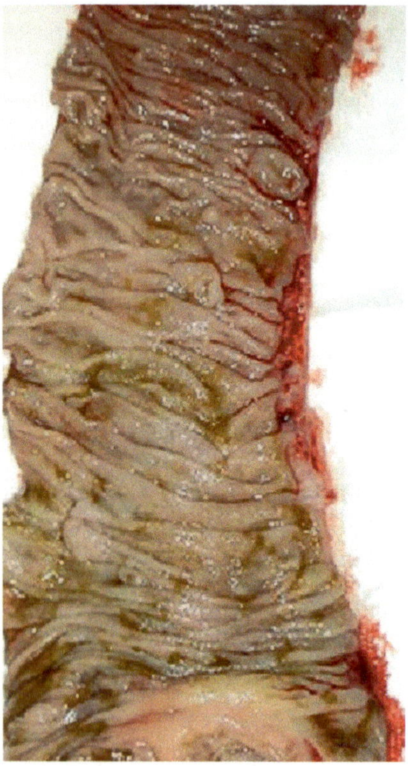

Serrated Polyposis Syndrome, Fig. 1 Gross picture of a case with SPS

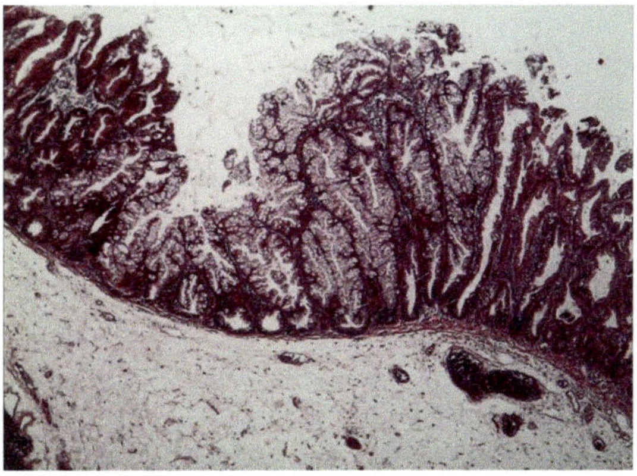

Serrated Polyposis Syndrome, Fig. 2 A dysplastic SSA/P (H&E; ×100)

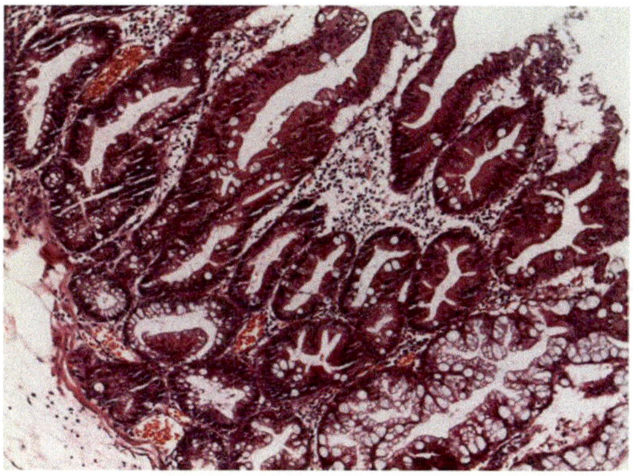

Serrated Polyposis Syndrome, Fig. 3 Dysplastic area of an SSA/P (H&E; ×200)

may be mistaken for adenomatous polyps. Despite earlier reports on SPS, conventional adenomas are not found in the context of SPS. SSA/Ps have distinct architectural features such as dilated, horizontal crypts and T- or L-shaped crypts with exaggerated serration in their epithelium (Fig. 2). The basally located crypts have different cell types comprising goblet cells, gastric foveolar cells, and undifferentiated cells. When dysplasia develops in SSA/Ps, nuclei become vesicular with prominent nucleoli and frequent mitoses are observed (Fig. 3).

Immunophenotype

No specific immunophenotypic feature is reported for SPS.

Molecular Features

The genetic abnormality in SPS is not known. The serrated pathway for sporadic serrated polyps may also be involved in SPS. BRAF and KRAS mutations are the most common molecular abnormalities observed in the polyps in SPS. There are also some reports for methylation of MMR genes in some polyps of SPS. However, no consistent data is available on the molecular features of SPS.

Differential Diagnosis

The differential diagnosis of SPS includes all polyposis syndromes affecting the colon. Among these are FAP, MUTYH-associated polyposis, and hamartomatous polyposis syndromes. The histopathologic features of the dominant polyp type allow distinction between these polyposis syndromes. FAP and associated polyposis syndromes including MUTYH-associated polyposis are characterized by conventional adenomas, while hyperplastic and/or hamartomatous polyps are found in hamartomatous polyposis syndromes.

References and Further Reading

Crowder, C. D., Sweet, K., Lehman, A., & Frankel, W. L. (2012). Serrated polyposis is an underdiagnosed and unclear syndrome: The surgical pathologist has a role in improving detection. *The American Journal of Surgical Pathology, 36*(8), 1178–1185.

Guarinos, C., Sánchez-Fortún, C., Rodríguez-Soler, M., Alenda, C., Payá, A., & Jover, R. (2012). Serrated polyposis syndrome: Molecular, pathological and clinical aspects. *World Journal of Gastroenterology, 18*(20), 2452–2461.

Kalady, M. F., Jarrar, A., Leach, B., Laguardia, L., O'malley, M., Eng, C., & Church, J. M. (2011). Defining phenotypes and cancer risk in hyperplastic polyposis syndrome. *Diseases of the Colon and Rectum, 54*(2), 164–170.

Snover, D. C. (2011). Update on the serrated pathway to colorectal carcinoma. *Human Pathology, 42*(1), 1–10, Epub 2010 Sep 24.

S

Snover, D. C., Ahnen, D. J., Burt, R. W., & Odze, R. D. (2010). Serrated polyps of the colon and rectum and serrated polyposis. In F. T. Bosman, F. Carneiro, R. H. Hruban, & N. D. Theise (Eds.), *WHO classification of tumours of the digestive system* (4th ed.). Lyon: IARC.

Shigellosis

Gert De Hertogh
Department of Pathology, Pathologische Ontleedkunde, UZ Leuven, Leuven, Belgium

Synonyms

Shiga bacillus dysentery; *Shigella* dysentery

Definition

Before defining shigellosis, it is necessary to clarify the meaning of a few terms commonly employed in the gastroenterology clinic. Diarrhea means the passage of three or more unformed stools per day. It can be a symptom of colitis, which is a disease characterized by the presence of a histological lesion: colonic inflammation. The inflammatory process may be limited to the mucosa or extend to the deeper layers of the bowel wall. The diagnosis of colitis can be established when, in a patient with diarrhea, one or more of the following features are present: (1) passage of multiple small-volume stools containing blood and mucus (this symptom is called "dysentery"), (2) positive markers for colonic inflammation in the stools (leukocytes adherent to the mucus on microscopic examination, positive fecal lactoferrin or calprotectin test), and (3) colonoscopy showing mucosal inflammation. Colitis is classified as acute when it develops within 14 days of onset of diarrhea and chronic when arising later than 30 days. In infectious colitis, there is a strong reason to believe, or positive proof, that the disease is caused by an infectious agent. The arguments for this diagnosis may be epidemiological evidence (a cluster of cases with similar symptoms, spreading around a well-characterized index patient) or a positive microbiological test. *Shigella* species are a common cause of acute dysentery requiring hospital admission.

Clinical Features

- **Presentation**
  Every patient presenting with acute diarrhea must get a thorough anamnesis and a clinical evaluation. Diarrhea should initially be classified as one of two syndromes: noninflammatory and inflammatory.

  Noninflammatory diarrhea is usually of large volume and watery, without blood or pus. The patient may have severe abdominal pain, but systemic symptoms and fever are absent. The most likely causative agents are viruses (rotavirus, norovirus), enterotoxigenic *Escherichia coli*, *Vibrio cholerae*, staphylococcal and clostridial food poisoning, and *Giardia* and *Cryptosporidium* infections. Usually the small intestine is the only seat of the disease, there is no damage to the mucosa, and rehydration is the first therapeutic action.

  Inflammatory diarrhea is dysenteric, and systemic signs such as a toxic appearance and fever may be present. With such symptoms, there is typically tissue damage in the colon. This consists of a disruption of the epithelial integrity and a disturbance of the mucosal microcirculation which may be due to the action of cytotoxins produced by infectious microorganisms. Common causative agents include *Shigella*, *Campylobacter*, enterohemorrhagic *Escherichia coli*, *Clostridium difficile*, *Salmonella*, *Yersinia*, and *Entamoeba histolytica*. Fecal examination for neutrophils or their products lactoferrin or calprotectin may be positive although results depend on the type of microorganism. With shigellosis, the stools are typically mixed with large numbers of neutrophils and erythrocytes. Clinically, one should consider *Shigella* infection especially when acute dysenteric diarrhea or colitis develops in an international traveler. The incidence of community-acquired infections is typically low in developed countries. Shigellosis may also present with a proctitis syndrome, where the patient has prominent tenesmus with rectal pain.

There are several different *Shigella* species, which are all gram-negative enteric organisms resembling *E. coli*, but with the following differences: they are nonmotile, they do not produce gas from glucose, and they are usually lactose negative. The four major subgroups are *Shigella dysenteriae*, *S. flexneri*, *S. boydii*, and *S. sonnei*. In developed countries, *S. sonnei* is the most common causative agent of bacillary dysentery.

During infection, *Shigella* organisms are present in the stools in large numbers. Transmission is via the fecal-oral route. Although the bacteria are sensitive to heat and drying and prefer an alkaline milieu, they can survive under relatively acidic conditions. This may explain the small infectious dose and the rapid spreading typical for this disease. The diagnosis requires routine stool culture, which also differentiates from *Salmonella* and *Campylobacter* infections.

- **Treatment**
  The initial therapy for every patient is oral rehydration or intravenous fluid replacement when indicated. Antidiarrheal medication is not commonly employed. Antimicrobial agents are given in moderate or severe dysentery. One should consider this when the culture report returns positive. Any patient with diarrhea for longer than a week should also receive antibiotics. The drugs of choice are quinolone antibiotics, e.g., ciprofloxacin. Alternatively, a neomacrolide such as azithromycin may be used.
- **Outcome**
  The outcome is generally good. Deaths are rare in healthy persons, especially in adults. Most lethal cases have occurred in young malnourished children in developing countries or in elderly or immunodeficient patients. Chronic carriage is rare and self-limited. It also responds to antibiotic treatment. About 10% of patients with well-treated shigellosis may suffer from prolonged mild diarrhea and cramps (so-called postinfectious irritable bowel syndrome).

Macroscopy

Sigmoidoscopy can confirm the diagnosis of colitis, but will not usually be employed in the setting of acute dysentery because it may then be very painful. The usual colonoscopic picture consists of reddened edematous mucosa with erosions and ulcers, limited to the rectum or the colon and rarely extending into the terminal ileum. With severe illness or in cases left untreated for a long period (2–4 weeks), the endoscopic picture may be undistinguishable from that observed in idiopathic chronic ulcerative colitis.

Microscopy

There are few descriptions in the literature of the histologic picture of acute bacillary dysentery due to shigellosis. This may relate to the large number of clinically mild cases, the limited access to colonoscopy for many patients in developing countries, and the satisfactory use of other diagnostic tests in moderate and severe cases.

The typical case presents with a spectrum of histopathological findings which vary in function of the natural history of the disease. In the peak activity stage (0–4 days after the onset of bloody diarrhea), mucosal biopsies show a preserved architecture, edema, and an increased number of inflammatory cells (Fig. 1). This infiltrate is mixed lymphoplasmacytic and neutrophilic in most cases. A predominance of neutrophils is associated with *S. dysenteriae* infection and acute presentation. Other findings are cryptitis, crypt abscesses, loss of integrity of surface and crypt epithelium, and erosions and ulceration (Figs. 2 and 3). There may be mild crypt distortion, but branching crypts are rare. Epithelial damage manifests most clearly as loss of goblet cells, especially after 48 h. At the time of resolution (within 6–9 days of onset of bloody diarrhea),

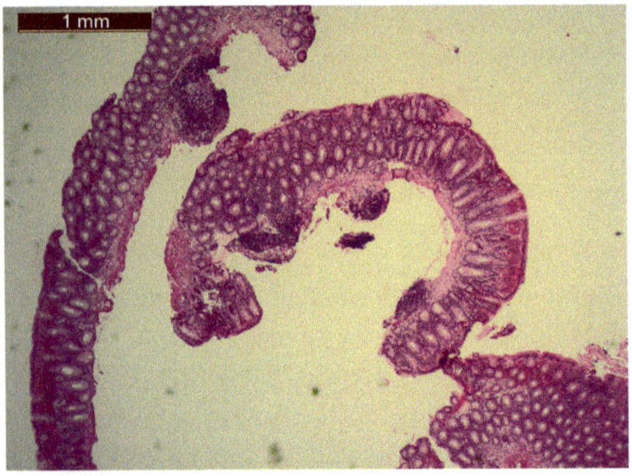

Shigellosis, Fig. 1 Low-power H&E stain shows colon mucosa with a preserved architecture and an increased inflammatory cell infiltrate. This is a case of culture-proven *Shigella colitis*

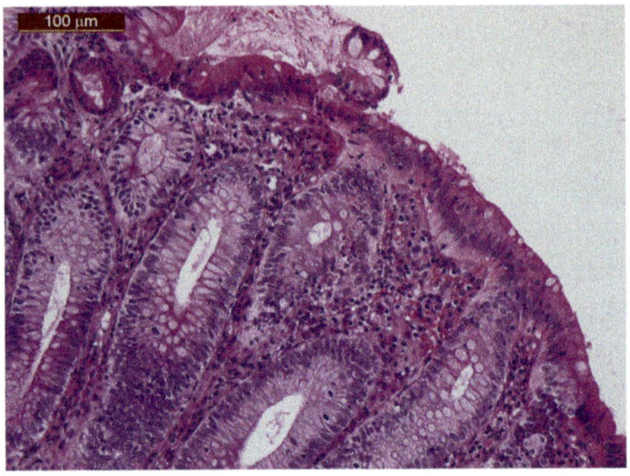

Shigellosis, Fig. 2 Medium-power H&E stain. Regenerative epithelial changes and a mixed infiltrate with cryptitis

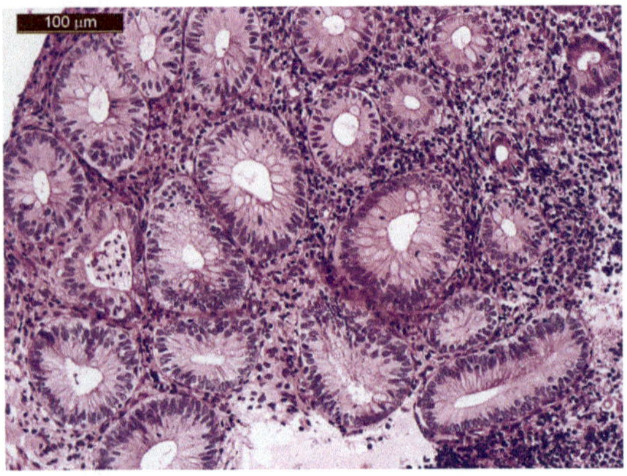

Shigellosis, Fig. 3 Medium-power H&E. Mixed infiltrate with a crypt abscess

the neutrophils become more scarce and the epithelium shows regenerative changes. A few foci of cryptitis may still be present. In the late stage, the number of intraepithelial lymphocytes may be increased in a limited number of crypts. This succession of patterns corresponds to the entity "acute self-limited colitis" for which *Shigella*, *Campylobacter*, and *Salmonella* species are the most common causative agents.

As described earlier, a problem may arise when patients have not been treated for a long period of time. Typically, the endoscopic aspect may then be difficult to distinguish from chronic idiopathic ulcerative colitis. Features pointing to ulcerative colitis are extensive crypt branching and well-developed basal plasmacytosis. Clinically, the major differences between shigellosis and idiopathic ulcerative colitis are a positive stool culture and a dramatic improvement in symptoms after appropriate antimicrobial treatment. When in doubt, treatment for shigellosis is recommended.

Immunophenotype: Molecular Features

Immunohistochemical or molecular pathologic tests are not employed for the diagnosis.

Differential Diagnosis

Endoscopy with biopsies may be indicated in patients with acute proctitis syndrome to aid in the differential diagnosis with sexually transmitted diseases (herpes simplex virus infection, gonorrhea, syphilis, lymphogranuloma venereum) or noninfectious causes such as ulcerative colitis, Crohn's disease, radiation proctitis, and solitary rectal ulcer syndrome. Sigmoidoscopy may also point to *Clostridium difficile* colitis by revealing the characteristic pseudomembranes; biopsies in this situation may be helpful. In HIV-infected patients, biopsies can be taken of ulcer bases to reveal *Cytomegalovirus* inclusions in stromal cells.

References and Further Reading

Anand, B. S., Malhotra, V., Bhattacharya, S. K., et al. (1986). Rectal histology in acute bacillary dysentery. *Gastroenterology, 90*, 654–660.

DuPont, H. L. (2012). Approach to the patient with infectious colitis. *Current Opinion in Gastroenterology, 28*, 39–46.

Kumar, N. B., Nostrant, T. T., & Appelman, H. D. (1982). The histopathologic spectrum of acute self-limited colitis (acute infectious-type colitis). *The American Journal of Surgical Pathology, 6*, 523–529.

Sachdev, H. P., Chadha, V., Malhotra, V., et al. (1993). Rectal histopathology in endemic Shigella and Salmonella diarrhea. *Journal of Pediatric Gastroenterology and Nutrition, 16*, 33–38.

Talan, D., Moran, G. J., Newdow, M., et al. (2001). Etiology of bloody diarrhea among patients presenting to United States emergency departments: Prevalence of Escherichia coli O157:H7 and other enteropathogens. *Clinical Infectious Diseases, 32*, 573–580.

Short Gut Syndrome

Arzu Ensari
Department of Pathology, Ankara University Medical School, Sihhiye, Ankara, Turkey

Synonyms

Small intestinal insufficiency

Definition

Short bowel syndrome (SBS) refers to the clinical consequences including malabsorption resulting from loss of small bowel absorptive surface area either due to congenital defect or surgical resection or bypass. The syndrome is characterized by maldigestion, malabsorption, and malnutrition. SBS occurs when more than one half of the bowel is removed or missing, especially if terminal ileum and ileocecal valves are removed. After removal of a large portion of the small intestine, the remaining small intestine goes through a process of adaptation that increases its ability to absorb nutrients. The inner lining grows, increasing its absorptive surface area. Intestinal adaptation can take up to 2 years to occur. Clinical symptoms of SBS include diarrhea, fatigue, steatorrhea, weight loss, and edema. The diagnosis rests on the clinical history and routine laboratory tests revealing the deficiency of nutrients.

Clinical Features

- **Incidence**
  True incidence of SBS is not known.
- **Age**
  The congenital form affects the infants,while adults can develop SBS after bowel surgery.
- **Sex**
  There is no sex predilection for SBS.
- **Site**
  Congenital defect or removal of more than half of the small intestine may cause SBS.
- **Treatment**
  Treatment may involve use of oral rehydration solutions, parenteral nutrition, enteral nutrition, and medications. Having an intestinal transplant may be an option for some patients. Antisecretory and antidiarrheal medications are prescribed to slow intestinal transit times and optimize fluid and nutrient absorption. Based on postsurgical anatomy, enteral feedings, parenteral infusions, complex diet plans, and vitamin and mineral supplementation are used in various combinations to nourish patients with SBS. Diet education and discharge planning are also important factors in the treatment.
- **Outcome**
  Survival of patients with SBS is dependent on adaptation in the remaining bowel and a combination of pharmacologic and nutrition therapies. Individual plans of care are developed based on the length and sites of remaining bowel, the degree of intestinal adaptation, and the patient's ability to adhere to the medication and dietary regimens. The condition may improve over time if it occurs as a result of surgery. There may be a gradual improvement in nutrient absorption. Survival rate ranges

from 80% to 94%, and the presence or absence of the ileal cecal valve does not appear to impact the mortality rate, but does significantly affect the length of time on total parenteral nutrition TPN. The most common morbidities remain sepsis, both central line related and bacterial overgrowth, and TPN cholestasis. Long-term recovery of these children often is remarkably normal, but there is a 10–15% incidence of neurologic and developmental defects.

Macroscopy

Small intestinal biopsy is not included in the diagnostic workup of patients with SBS.

Microscopy

The histopathologic changes in SBS can either be related to the adaptation process of the bowel or be associated with the effects of TPN on the bowel mucosa. Adaptive process involves epithelial hyperplasia in the small intestinal mucosa in the form of crypt hyperplasia, increased mitotic activity in the crypt epithelium, and lack of maturation in the villus epithelium, while long-term TPN causes focal or diffuse villus blunting and mucosal atrophy.

Immunophenotype

No specific immunophenotypic feature is reported.

Molecular Features

No specific molecular feature is reported.

Differential Diagnosis

The differential diagnosis of SBS involves active Crohn's disease, celiac disease, small intestinal bacterial overgrowth (SIBO), and malignancy of the small intestine. Though symptoms may be similar in all of these conditions, endoscopy and clinical history may aid in the diagnosis. SIBO may occur in the context of SBS.

References and Further Reading

Rossi, T. M., Lee, P. C., Young, C., & Tjota, A. (1993). Small intestinal mucosa changes, including epithelial cell proliferative activity, of children receiving total parenteral nutrition (TPN). *Digestive Diseases and Sciences, 38*(9), 1608–1613.

Sigalet, D. L. (2001). Short bowel syndrome in infants and children: An overview. *Seminars in Pediatric Surgery, 10*(2), 49–55.

Wall, E. A. (2013). An overview of short bowel syndrome management: Adherence, adaptation, and practical recommendations. *Journal of the Academy of Nutrition and Dietetics, 113*(9), S2212–S2672.

Wilmore, D. W., & Robinson, M. K. (2000). Short bowel syndrome. *World Journal of Surgery, 24*(12), 1486–1492.

Wood, S. J., Khalil, B., Fusaro, F., Folaranmi, S. E., Sparks, S. A., & Morabito, A. (2013). Early structured surgical management plan for neonates with short bowel syndrome may improve outcomes. *World Journal of Surgery, 37*(7), 1714–1717.

Signet Ring Cell Carcinoma

Chella R. S. van der Post[1] and Fátima Carneiro[2]
[1]Department of Pathology, Radboud University Medical Center, Nijmegen, The Netherlands
[2]Faculty of Medicine of Porto University, Centro Hospitalar São João and Ipatimup/i3S, Porto, Portugal

Synonyms

Diffuse carcinoma; Poorly cohesive carcinoma

Definition

Signet ring cell carcinoma is defined as a tumor composed predominantly (more than 50%) or exclusively of signet ring cells, characterized histologically by cells with a large vacuolated mucinous cytoplasm and an eccentrically placed flattened nucleus.

Various classification schemes for gastric cancer have been proposed; the Laurén and the World Health Organization (WHO) classification systems are the most widely used. Gastric adenocarcinomas are subtyped in the WHO classification based on the predominant morphologic component of the tumor. These subtypes include tubular, papillary, mucinous, poorly cohesive (including signet-ring cell type), and mixed carcinomas. The Laurén scheme separates gastric adenocarcinomas into intestinal, diffuse, and mixed or indeterminate subtypes. Signet ring cell carcinomas are categorized into the diffuse type in the Laurén scheme.

Clinical Features

- **Incidence**
  Gastric adenocarcinoma is the fifth most common cancer worldwide and is the third leading cause of cancer death with about 700,000 patients dying each year. Signet ring cell carcinomas are classified as diffuse type carcinoma in the classification of Laurén. The diffuse type is relatively more common in low-incidence areas (defined as <15 gastric cancers per 100 000) including North America, northern Europe, and most countries in Africa and southeastern Asia, while the intestinal type of adenocarcinoma predominates in high-incidence countries (defined as >60 gastric cancers per 100 000), including eastern Asia, eastern Europe, and central and Latin America. Reported incidences of signet ring cell carcinomas of all gastrectomies performed range from 3.4% in Japan to 39% in the Unites States. Incidences are different geographically, in time, in different age groups, and in sex. However, also problems with definitions of the different subtypes of gastric cancer play a role, so not all reported numbers may be representative. A higher incidence of early signet ring cell carcinomas was reported in high-incidence countries, of up to 20%.
- **Age**
  Incidence of gastric cancer increases progressively with age and is rare in persons younger than 30 years. Signet ring cell carcinoma occurs more frequently in younger patients compared to other subtypes of gastric adenocarcinoma. One rare presentation of signet ring cell carcinoma occurs in the setting of hereditary diffuse gastric cancer. Signet ring cell carcinoma and distinct premalignant lesions characterize this autosomal-dominant cancer-susceptibility syndrome, and gastric cancer can occur at already young age. For more about this topic, the reader is referred to the chapter concerning ▶ E-cadherin gastric carcinoma or hereditary diffuse gastric cancer.
- **Sex**
  Signet ring cell carcinoma has a higher predilection for women.
- **Site**
  Signet ring cell carcinoma can occur throughout the stomach, but most often, the lower antro-pyloric region and/or corpus is involved and in approximately 10% the entire stomach is involved.
- **Treatment**
  The therapy regimen of gastric cancer depends on characteristics, stage, location, and genetics (for instance *HER2* status) (Allum et al. 2011). Diagnostics should lead to accurate initial staging and assessment of treatment response. Imaging techniques, including multidetector CT, gastroduodenoscopy, and PET-CT, should provide staging assessment according to the TNM classification. The incidences of lymph node metastases and distant metastasis are high; therefore, initial assessment must establish the presence or absence of distant disease.

  Radical surgery represents the standard form of curative therapy aiming to excise the primary tumor with clear longitudinal and circumferential margins. Advanced carcinomas should be treated according to the location, distally by subtotal gastrectomy and proximally by total gastrectomy. Cardia tumors should be treated by trans-hiatal extended total gastrectomy or esophageo-gastrectomy. The extent of lymphadenectomy should be tailored to the age and fitness of the patient together with the location and stage of the cancer. The distal pancreas, spleen, and splenic nodes should be removed only when there is direct invasion and still a chance of a curative procedure in patients with carcinoma of the proximal stomach. Limited gastric resections should only be used for palliation or in the very elderly and may improve survival and quality of life. If patients present with gastric outlet obstruction and a curative intent is impossible, the use of a stent can be considered.

Chemotherapy, either alone as a perioperative treatment, or in combination with radiation therapy in an adjuvant setting, improves the clinical outcome for patients with resectable gastric cancer. However, it is unclear whether pre- or perioperative chemotherapy leads to improved survival in patients with signet ring cell carcinoma and further research is needed (Heger et al. 2014; Messager et al. 2011).

- **Outcome**
  Asian reports indicate that signet ring carcinoma has better 5-year survival rates than other gastric cancers. The better prognosis is related in these countries to a higher prevalence of mucosa-confined carcinomas and early detection of signet ring cell carcinoma. When corrected for disease stage, the histologic type does not seem to be an independent predictor of outcome. Advanced gastric carcinoma (independent of histologic type) presents in advanced stage with larger tumors, lower curative rate, serosal invasion, and peritoneal dissemination and is associated with poor prognosis with reported 1-year and 5-year survival rates of 42% and 24%, respectively.

Macroscopy

The growth pattern of gastric carcinoma is commonly described according to the Borrmann classification, subdividing polypoid, fungating, ulcerative, and infiltrative growth patterns. Signet ring cell carcinomas more often present as ulcerating lesions with infiltration into the gastric wall (Borrmann type 3) or as diffuse infiltrating tumors (Borrmann type 4). Tumor cells spread superficially and produce flat, plaque-like lesions with or without shallow ulcerations. With extensive infiltration, linitis plastica may develop characterized by a thickened, firm, fibrotic, and leathery appearance of the gastric wall. In contrast to intestinal-type carcinoma, the mucosa appears relatively normal.

Microscopy

The WHO classification scheme describes five main types of gastric adenocarcinoma including tubular adenocarcinoma, papillary adenocarcinoma, mucinous adenocarcinoma, poorly cohesive carcinoma, and mixed carcinoma. Signet ring cell type is a distinct type of poorly cohesive carcinoma, defined as a tumor composed predominantly or exclusively of signet ring cells. Other cellular variants of poorly cohesive carcinoma include tumors composed of neoplastic cells resembling histiocytes, lymphocytes, or pleomorphic poorly cohesive cells with irregular and bizarre nuclei. A mixture of different cell types can be present, including few signet ring cells. Signet ring cell carcinomas have been classified as "diffuse type" by Laurén, 'infiltrative type' by Ming, and 'undifferentiated type' in the Japanese classification system. The largest part of all signet ring cell carcinomas (presumably >90%) occur in the stomach, breast, and colorectum, with the remaining arising in several other organs, including the gallbladder, pancreas, urinary bladder, prostate, and lung.

Signet ring cell carcinoma is characterized by cells with a central optically clear, globoid droplet of cytoplasmic mucin with a flattened or crescent-shaped nucleus (Figs. 1 and 2). These cells are called "signet ring cells" since the intracytoplasmic vacuole of mucin compresses the nucleus against the periphery of the cell, giving it its typical signet ring appearance. The tumor cells exhibit hyperchromatic, pleomorphic nuclei with mitosis, and there is infiltration of cells into and beyond the lamina propria. Signet ring cells

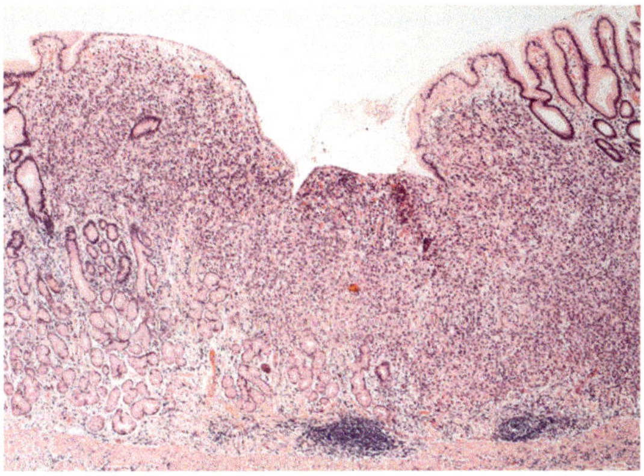

Signet Ring Cell Carcinoma, Fig. 1 Low-power view of a poorly cohesive/diffuse gastric adenocarcinoma. No well-formed glands are identified (Original magnification 25×)

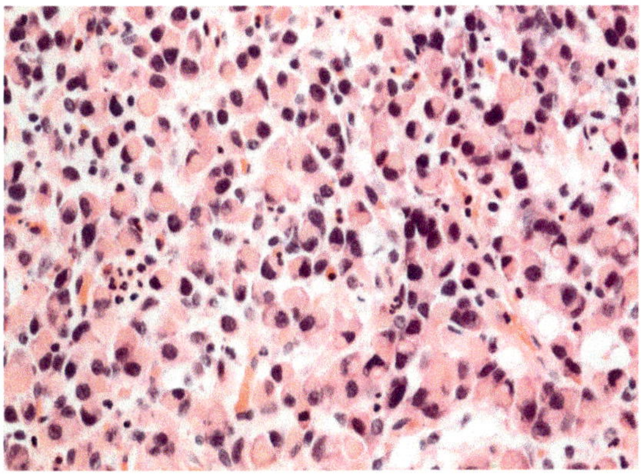

Signet Ring Cell Carcinoma, Fig. 2 Typical signet ring cells with peripheral nuclei and intracytoplasmic mucin (Original magnification 200×)

may form a lace-like gland or delicate micro-trabecular pattern in the mucosa or be accompanied by marked desmoplasia in deeper levels of the stomach wall with formation of Indian-files. In some cases, signet ring cells may be restricted to the mucosa, while other variants of poorly cohesive cells extend into the deeper levels of the gastric wall. There can also be an admixture of glandular or solid elements especially in deeper portions of the tumor. When signet ring cells infiltrate the submucosa and deeper tissues, they often provoke a dense fibrous desmoplastic reaction that frequently results in a markedly thickened leather bottle-like stomach (linitis plastica). However, this lesion is not unique to signet ring cell carcinomas and can be seen with other (diffuse) adenocarcinomas and sometimes with metastatic tumors, especially breast tumors.

Immunophenotype

Gastric signet ring cell carcinomas are positive for pankeratin staining with varying degrees of CK7 and CK20 positivity. CK18 or CAM5.2 is most often negative. Gastric signet ring cell carcinomas may express Hep Par 1, heterogeneous CDX-2, MUC2, and MUC5AC.

The type and amount of intracytoplasmic mucus vary in signet ring cells; they can be filled with acid mucin, with secretory granules containing acid or neutral mucin, with eosinophilic granules containing neutral mucin or they contain almost no mucin. The detection of signet ring cells within the mucosa is sometimes subtle and easily missed as they may occur in rather normal looking mucosa. The PAS with diastase stain, mucicarmine, or Alcian blue are often useful histochemical stains for highlighting signet ring cells. The recognition of cytoplasmic mucin is of utmost importance to prove that these cells are indeed signet ring cells and to exclude 'pseudo-signet ring cells' or 'glassy cells' that are cells with vacuoles sometimes resembling mucosal signet ring cell carcinoma. These glassy cells contain eccentric bland nuclei and a cytoplasmic clear or glassy appearance and can simulate signet ring cell carcinoma, especially in small gastric biopsies. Signet ring cells are positive on mucin staining, but they need to be distinguished from goblet cells and foamy macrophages (mucophages) that also contain mucin. In biopsies, a negative keratin stain and positive CD68 stain can be used to prove macrophages. Other conditions that can be confused with signet ring cell carcinoma include signet ring cell lymphoma, characterized by lymphoid cells distended with immunoglobulin and metastasis of other primary signet ring cell carcinomas.

Mucins are high-molecular-weight heavily O-glycosylated glycoproteins produced by secretory epithelial cells. Specific types of mucin are individually referred to as MUC and designated with a number representing the order in which the mucin was described. Mucin expression profiles may be useful in some cases to help determine the primary origin of metastatic signet ring cell carcinoma. However, signet ring cell carcinoma originating in the stomach has variable expression patterns of MUC1, MUC2, MUC4, MUC5AC, and MUC6 and is therefore not specific. Signet ring cell carcinoma of the breast shows strong staining for MUC1 and colorectal signet ring cell carcinoma is consistently strongly positive for MUC2 and MUC4.

Molecular Features

Gastric cancers are characterized by genetic and epigenetic changes that affect tumor suppressor genes, oncogenes, and mismatch repair genes. Consequently, deregulation of cellular proliferation, adhesion, differentiation, signal transduction, telomerase activity, and DNA repair has been reported. The most important described genetic pathway for diffuse gastric cancer is the loss of function of E-cadherin. Diffuse-type or signet ring cell carcinomas have been considered to start developing through the loss of function of the *CDH1* gene encoding for E-cadherin. In sporadic diffuse carcinomas, genetic and epigenetic alterations are described in the *CDH1* gene, and in hereditary diffuse gastric cancer, germline mutations in the *CDH1* gene have been identified in up to 40% of cases. E-cadherin is a transmembrane glycoprotein that is primarily expressed in the epithelium, and is a key player in the induction of cell-cell adhesion and in the organization of epithelial structures by establishing calcium-dependent homophilic binding at the zonula adherens. E-cadherin has also been shown to play important roles in tumorigenesis, cancer progression, and metastasis. Downregulation of E-cadherin has been demonstrated to decrease the strength of cellular adhesion within a tissue, resulting in an increase in cellular motility, which allows cancer cells to cross the basement membrane and to thereby invade surrounding tissues. Mouse studies revealed that inactivation of E-cadherin strongly affected gastric epithelial cell polarity, growth, and differentiation. However, the loss of E-cadherin is not sufficient for gastric tumor formation, and loss of other tumor suppressor genes such as *p53* is necessary for the development of diffuse gastric cancer.

Recent and upcoming high-throughput genomic analysis studies have been revealing many new mutations and pathways involved in gastric cancer, and this will result in potential targets for personalized therapy. Identified genes involved in gastric tumorigenesis are *PIK3CA, P53, APC, STK11, CTNNB1, CDKN2A, ERBB2, EGFR,* and *FGFR2.* These studies generally do not distinguish between different histological subtypes of gastric cancer.

Differential Diagnosis

- Hereditary diffuse gastric cancer: advanced gastric carcinomas of *CDH1* mutation carriers present as diffuse carcinomas and are indistinguishable from diffuse sporadic gastric cancers. Patient and family history are important to suspect a genetic cause. The typical pagetoid-spread of signet ring cells and in situ lesions have only been observed in patients with germline *CDH1* mutations.
- Conditions that can be confused with signet ring cell carcinoma include lymphomas, because of its diffuse growth pattern and round cell morphology.
- Metastases of malignancies of other organs are uncommon, but especially metastases from lobular breast cancer are a pitfall that is easily missed and mistaken for primary gastric cancer. Even though metastases from breast cancer to the gastrointestinal tract are rare, the stomach is the organ most often involved with incidences varying from 0.1% in retrospective series up to 10% in autopsy series. Possible immunohistochemical antibodies with varying sensitivities and specificities include the breast markers ER, PR, mammaglobulin, and BRST-2 or GCDFP-15. Immunohistochemical stainings favoring gastric cancer include

CDX-2, MUC5AC, MUC6, CK20, and HNFA. The marker hepatocyte nuclear factor 4A (HNF4A) was identified as especially specific in discriminating a breast cancer metastasis (negative) from a primary gastric adenocarcinoma (positive staining).
- Clear cell carcinoid: these present often as small yellow nodules, immunohistochemistry for chromogranin and synaptophysin is positive in carcinoids.
- Diffuse-type carcinomas may also be mistaken for a variety of benign processes including gastritis, reactive endothelial cells, and xanthomas. Gastric xanthomas consist of a cluster of lipid-laden macrophages in the lamina propria. The macrophages show foamy cytoplasm and contain neutral fats. They stain positive with Sudan Black and CD68. Negative stains include PAS and cytokeratins.

References and Further Reading

Allum, W. H., Blazeby, J. M., Griffin, S. M., Cunningham, D., Jankowski, J. A., & Wong, R. (2011). Guidelines for the management of oesophageal and gastric cancer. *Gut, 60*(11), 1449–1472.

Bosman, F. T., Carneiro, F., Hruban, R. H., & Theise, N. D. (2010). *WHO classification of tumours of the digestive system* (4th ed.). Lyon: IARC.

Heger, U., Blank, S., Wiecha, C., Langer, R., Weichert, W., Lordick, F., Bruckner, T., Dobritz, M., Burian, M., Springfeld, C., Grenacher, L., Siewert, J. R., Büchler, M., & Ott, K. (2014). Is preoperative chemotherapy followed by surgery the appropriate treatment for signet ring cell containing adenocarcinomas of the esophagogastric junction and stomach?

Jiang, C. G., Wang, Z. N., Sun, Z., Liu, F. N., Yu, M., & Xu, H. M. (2011). Clinicopathologic characteristics and prognosis of signet ring cell carcinoma of the stomach: Results from a Chinese mono-institutional study. *Journal of Surgical Oncology, 103*(7), 700–703.

Koyama, T., Sekine, S., Taniguchi, H., Tsuda, H., Ikegami, M., Hano, H., & Kushima, R. (2011). Hepatocyte nuclear factor 4A expression discriminates gastric involvement by metastatic breast carcinomas from primary gastric adenocarcinomas. *Human Pathology, 42*(11), 1777–1784.

Lauren, P. (1965). The two histological main types of gastric carcinoma: Diffuse and so-calles intestinal-type carcinoma. An attempt at a histo-clinical classification. *Acta Pathologica et Microbiologica Scandinavica, 64*, 31–49.

Messager, M., Lefevre, J. H., Pichot-Delahaye, V., Souadka, A., Piessen, G., & Mariette, C. (2011). The impact of perioperative chemotherapy on survival in patients with gastric signet ring cell adenocarcinoma: a multicenter comparative study. *Ann Surg, 254*, 684–693.

Mimata, A., Fukamachi, H., Eishi, Y., & Yuasa, Y. (2011). Loss of E-cadherin in mouse gastric epithelial cells induces signet ring-like cells, a possible precursor lesion of diffuse gastric cancer. *Cancer Science, 102*(5), 942–950.

Small Intestine, Anatomy and Histology

Ayca Kirmizi
Department of Pathology, Ankara University Medical School, Sihhiye, Ankara, Turkey

Synonyms

Small bowel

Anatomy (Macroscopy)

The small intestine is a specialized tubular structure within the abdominal cavity in continuity with the stomach proximally and the colon distally. The small bowel is about 6 m in the adult. Three subdivisions; "the duodenum, jejunum, and ileum"are defined and characterized by various anatomic relationships. The first 25 cm of small intestine, *the duodenum*; excluding the most proximal several centimeters, is a fixed, retroperitoneal structure that forms a C- or U-shape around the head of the pancreas. Four subdivisions of the duodenum have been described: (a) the first portion, the duodenal bulb, is the most proximal and superior segment; (b) the descending or second portion, which the common bile duct and major and minor pancreatic ducts empty into the papillae; (c) the horizontal or third portion; and (d) the ascending or fourth portion. Duodenum ends at the ligament of Treitz, where it turns to the peritoneal cavity. The remainder of the small intestine is intraperitoneal, until it enters the colon at the

S

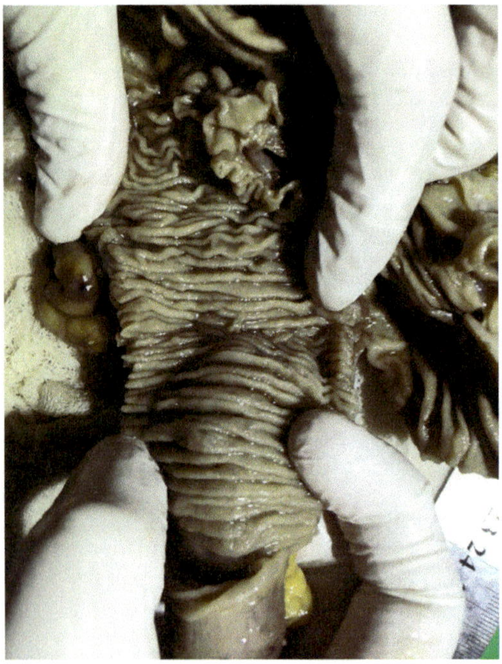

Small Intestine, Anatomy and Histology, Fig. 1 A macroscopic example of small intestine showing mucosal folds (the plicae circulares)

ileocecal valve. *Jejenum* and *ileum* are suspended by a thin, broad-based mesentery in the abdominal cavity that allows free movement of the small intestine. No distinct anatomic demarcation exists between jejunum and ileum. The proximal 40% of the mobile small intestine is the jejunum, and the remaining 60% is the ileum. The jejunum occupies the left upper portion of the abdomen, and the ileum is positioned in the right lower portion of the abdomen and upper part of the pelvis.

Visual examination of the luminal surface of the small intestine reveals mucosal folds, the *plicae circulares* (Fig. 1). More numerous in the proximal jejunum, the plicae circulares decrease in number in the distal small bowel and are absent in the terminal ileum. The small bowel is in continuity with the colon at the ileocecal valve, which comprises two semilunar lips that protrude into the cecum. The ileocecal valve provides a barrier to the retrograde flow of colonic contents into the small intestine. This barrier appears to be a function of the angulation between the ileum and cecum that is maintained by the superior and inferior ileoceal ligaments, and a true tonic, sphincter-type pressure does not appear to be present in this region.

The superior mesenteric artery delivers oxygenated blood to the distal duodenum, the entire jejunum and ileum. Veins follow the arterial distribution. The superior mesenteric vein join the splenic vein to form the portal vein. The lymphatic drainage of the small bowel follows their respective blood supplies to lymph nodes in the celiac, superior preaortic, and inferior preaortic regions. Lymphatic drainage proceeds to the cisterna chyli and then via the thoracic duct into the left subclavian vein. Sympathetic neural input to the small bowel is carried by the celiac and superior mesenteric plexuses, whereas the parasympathetic supply is derived from distal branches of the vagus nerve; these both closely follow the arterial paths into the bowel wall.

Function

Small intestine has important roles at chemical digestion, absorption of nutrients and as a mucosal immune barier.

Microscopy (Hystology)

The wall of the small intestine is composed of four layers: mucosa, submucosa, muscularis propria and serosa.

Mucosa

The mucosa is the innermost layer formed by glandular epithelium, lamina propria, and muscularis mucosa. The most distinctive feature of the small intestine is its mucosal lining, which is designed to provide maximal surface area for the purpose of food absorption. It is studded with innumerable villi. These extend into the lumen as finger-like projections. Between the bases of the villi are the pitlike crypts of Lieberkühn (intestinal crypts), which contain stem cells that replenish and regenerate the epithelium (Fig. 2). The crypts extend down to the muscularis mucosae. The

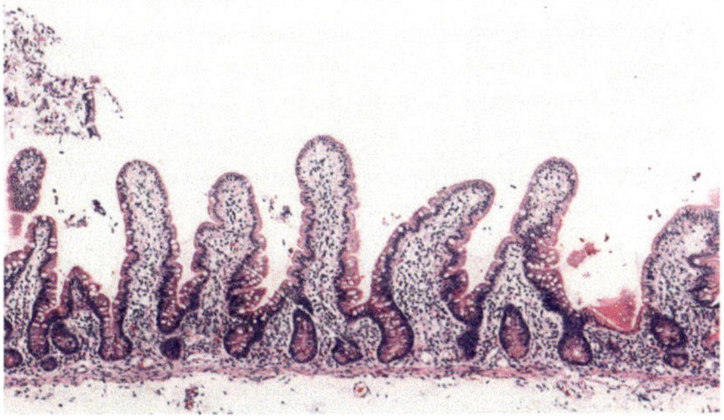

Small Intestine, Anatomy and Histology, Fig. 2 A mucosal example of small intestine showing the intestinal villi and crypts of Lieberkühn (H&E; x100)

villus-to-crypt height ratio is about 4 : 1 to 5 : 1, but this is variable. For instance at the proximal duodenum, the villus-to-crypt height ratio may reach only 2 : 1 to 3 : 1. The lamina propria, which supports the epithelium, is a layer of reticular connective tissue with elastin, reticulin, and collagen fibers, lymphocytes, plasma cells containing primarily IgA, eosinophils, mast cells, scattered fibroblasts, as well as lymphatics and capillaries. Smooth muscle is found in the lamina propria, extending from the muscularis mucosa vertically. Aggregates of lymphoid follicles are scattered throughout the small intestine but are found in highest concentration within the ileum, where they are designated *Peyer's patches*. Peyer's patches normally are more prominent during infancy and childhood. The muscularis mucosa consists of a thin layer of smooth muscle at the boundary of the mucosa and submucosa.

The surface epithelium of the small intestinal villi contains three principal cell types. *Columnar absorptive cells* are recognized by the dense array of microvilli on their luminal surface (the "brush border"), interspersed regularly between absorptive cells are mucin secreting *goblet cells*, and a few *endocrine cells*. Within the crypts reside stem cells, goblet cells, more abundant endocrine cells, and scattered *Paneth cells*. Paneth cells contain apically oriented, bright eosinophilic granules that contain growth factors and a variety of antimicrobial proteins. A certain number of $CD3^+$ intraepithelial T lymphoctes (30 per 100 epithelial cells) normally are present in the villi.

Submucosa

The submucosa is a fibrous connective tissue layer that contains fibroblasts, mast cells, blood and lymphatic vessels, and a nerve fiber plexus (Meissner's plexus); composed of nonmyelinated, postganglionic sympathetic fibers, and parasympathetic ganglion cells. Within the duodenum; immediately distal to the pyloric channel are abundant submucosal mucous glands, termed Brunner's glands. Brunner's glands open into the intestinal crypts and morphologically resemble pyloric glands. These glands secrete bicarbonate ions, glycoproteins and pepsinogen II.

Muscularis Propria

The muscularis propria, mainly responsible for contractility, consists of two layers of smooth muscle: an inner circular coat and an outer longitudinal coat arranged in a helicoidal pattern. A prominent nerve fiber plexus called the myenteric plexus, or Auerbach's plexus, is found between these two muscle layers.

Serosa

The serosa is the outermost layer of connective tissue and covered by a single layer of mesothelial cells.

Immunohistochemistry

Normal small intestinal mucosa is diffusely positive for cytokeratin 20 and completely negative for cytokeratin 7.

References and Further Reading

Adler, D. G., Crawford, J. M., & Farraye, F. A. (2015). GI tract endoscopic and tissue processing techniques and normal histology. In R. D. Odze & J. R. Goldblum (Eds.), *Surgical pathology of the GI tract, liver, biliary tract and pancreas* (pp. 4–33). Philadelphia: Elsevier.

Bass, L. M., & Wershil, B. K. (2016). Small and large intestine. In M. Feldman, L. S. Friedman, & L. J. Brandt (Eds.), *Sleisenger & Fordtran's gastrointestinal and liver disease* (pp. 1649–1678). Philadelphia: Elsevier.

Chen, Z. M., & Wang, H. L. (2004). Alteration of cytokeratin 7 and cytokeratin 20 expression profile is uniquely associated with tumorigenesis of primary adenocarcinoma of the small intestine. *Am J Surg Pathol, 28*(10), 1352–1359.

Katzin, W. E., & Petras, R. E. (2012). Small intestine. In S. E. Millis (Ed.), *Histology for pathologists* (pp. 647–672). Philadelphia: Lippincott.

Solitary Rectal Ulcer Syndrome

Andrzej Mróz
Department of Gastroenterology and Hepatology, Histopathology Unit, Medical Center for Postgraduate Education, Warsaw, Poland

Synonyms

Mucosal prolapse syndrome – part of; SRUS

Definition

Solitary rectal ulcer syndrome (SRUS) is the part of the spectrum of mucosal prolapse syndrome. It affects mainly young females with defecation problems and changed bowel habits. Excessive and prolonged straining on defecation leads to rectal mucosal prolapse with secondary ulceration and polypoid lesions development. Anterior wall of the rectum is particularly vulnerable to prolapse on straining, since it is physiologically redundant. Most of SRUS cases locate at the anterior wall of the rectum. While the mucosa is impacted to anal canal, it may become ischemic due to obliteration of mucosal vessels. Patients with SRUS have rectal bleeding, diarrhea, anorectal pain, pruritus, abdominal pain, and difficulty in defecating. These include constipation, straining, increased laxative use, and incomplete rectal evacuation.

SRUS is a misnomer – patients may have no ulceration and the lesions may be multiple.

Clinical Features

- **Incidence**
  1–3, 6 per 100,000.
- **Age**
  Young adults in third and fourth decades of life.
- **Sex**
  Females predominate in patients with SRUS.
- **Site**
  Anterior rectal wall – 4–10 cm from anal verge, rarely at posterior rectal wall.
- **Treatment**
  Appropriate diet with bulk laxatives and stool softeners. Regulation of defecation habits with some psychological consultation. In severe cases, surgery is required – rectopexy.
- **Outcome (Prognosis)**
  Fifteen percent rate of recurrence after surgical operation is observed.

Macroscopy

Reddening of mucosa may be the earliest feature of SRUS syndrome. Then the mucosa becomes granular and ulcerated. The ulcers may be multiple or isolated. Polypoid lesions develop which endoscopically cannot be distinguished from adenomas, hyperplastic polyps, or can mimic elevated lesions of inflammatory bowel disease.

Endoscopic picture of SRUS is shown in Fig. 1.

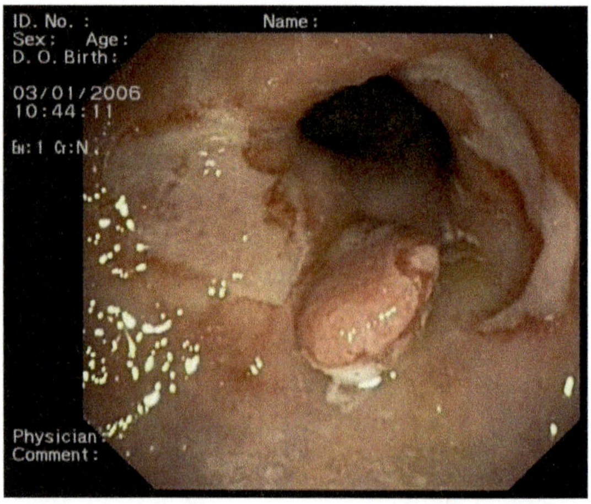

Solitary Rectal Ulcer Syndrome, Fig. 1 Ulceration and polypoid lesion in SRUS (Courtesy of Dr. J. Pachlewski)

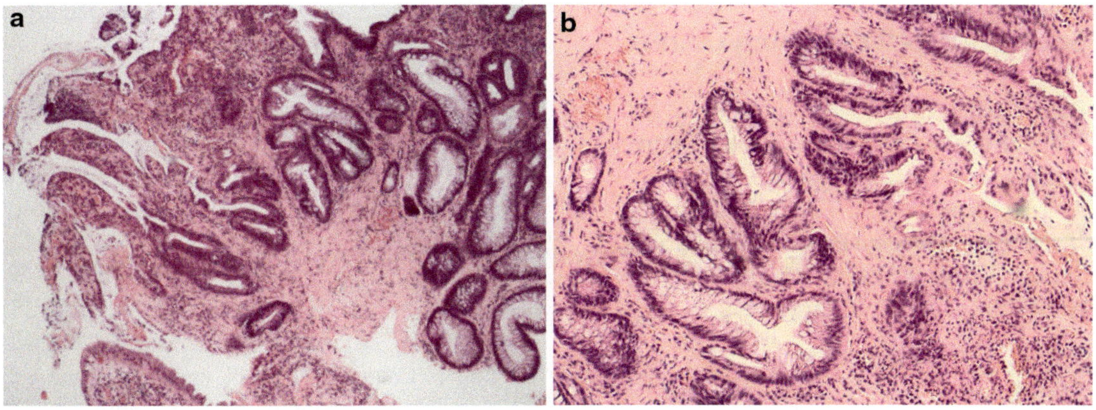

Solitary Rectal Ulcer Syndrome, Fig. 2 (**a**) Histology of SRUS. Superficial villiform part is eroded, crypts are distorted. (**b**) Proliferating muscularis mucosae penetrates between distorted crypts

Microscopy

The diagnostic feature of SRUS is fibromuscular proliferation, which replace lamina propria of rectal mucosa. Smooth muscle strands are situated perpendicularly to muscularis mucosae. Their nature is confirmed by histochemical stains (e.g., trichrome stain) and immunohistochemical stains (desmin). Obliteration of the mucosa by proliferating muscularis mucosae results in elongation and dilation of crypts which are lined with immature basophilic epithelium. Architectural distortion may be significant. The mucosa becomes hyperplastic, polypoid, and ulcerated. The superficial part of mucosa acquires villous configuration, resembling adenomas.

Mucosal changes include also reactive inflammation, hemosiderin depositions around congested blood vessels, pronounced epithelial inflammation, and reaction resembling dysplastic epithelial changes.

Typical histological pictures of SRUS are presented in Fig. 2.

Immunophenotype

Desmin stain for proliferating smooth muscles fibers in lamina propria.

Differential Diagnosis

The solitary rectal ulcer syndrome may be misinterpreted as rectal adenoma or even invasive carcinoma with dramatic consequences for patient. Tubulovillous growth pattern and regenerative atypia may recall neoplastic process. However, fibromuscular proliferation and the absence of desmoplastic stromal reaction are against the diagnosis of neoplasia. The epithelial changes are of hyperplastic/regenerative type, which should be critically judged.

SRUS may be erroneously diagnosed as IBD – particularly when the ulcers are the case and the superficial layer of the mucosa is available. Fibromuscular proliferation may not be evident in these specimens, and the additional stains are of value.

Fibromuscular proliferation may resemble Peutz-Jeghers, but it is organized in perpendicular fashion rather than displaying arborizing architecture characteristic for Peutz-Jeghers polyps.

S

References and Further Reading

Iacobuzio-Donahue, C. A., & Montgomery, E. (2005). *Gastrointestinal and liver pathology*. Philadelphia: Elsevier.

Noffsinger, A., et al. (2007). *Gastrointestinal diseases*. Washington, DC: The American Registry of Pathology.

Squamous Cell Carcinoma, Anus

Denis Chatelain[1] and Jean-François Fléjou[2]
[1]Service d'Anatomie Pathologique, Centre Hospitalier et Universitaire du Nord, Amiens, France
[2]Faculté de Médecine Pierre et Marie Curie, Service d'Anatomie et Cytologie Pathologiques, Hôpital Saint-Antoine, Paris, France

Synonyms

Epidermoid carcinoma

Definition

Anal squamous cell carcinoma is a malignant epithelial tumor of the anal canal, composed of squamous-type epithelium, showing keratinization and/or intercellular bridges.

Clinical Features

Most patients present with anorectal bleeding. Other symptoms include anorectal pain and mass sensation. Tenesmus and fecal incontinence can suggest tumor invasion into the anal sphincters. Weight loss, inguinal adenopathy, and rectovaginal fistula are indicators of an advanced disease. At presentation, 30–50% of patients have a locally advanced disease with a mean tumor size of 3–4 cm. Clinically suspicious inguinal adenopathy can be found in 10–20% patients during physical examination, and this increases to 30–60% when the tumor is larger than 5 cm. Misdiagnosis and delay in diagnosis are common, because presenting symptoms are often nonspecific and similar to the symptoms of benign anal diseases such as hemorrhoids or fissures.

- **Incidence**
  Anal squamous cell carcinoma is a rare disease with an incidence of 1.5 per 100,000 people in Western industrialized countries. Its incidence has increased in recent years. The incidence rate of squamous cell carcinoma in the USA has increased by approximately 1.9 fold for men (notably for men having sex with men) and 1.5 fold for women, from 1973–1979 to 1994–2000. There is a marked increase in the male homosexual population, with incidence rates reported as high as 37 per 100,000 men.
- **Etiology**
  Various etiologies are implicated in squamous cell carcinoma development, the most significant being human papilloma virus. HPV infection is found in 80–90% anal squamous cell carcinomas, predominantly oncogenic type 16 (detected in approximately 70% cases) and type 18. But other high-risk HPV subtypes can also be found such as HPV 31, 33, 35, 39, 45, 50, 51, 53, 56, 58, 59, 68. Anal intercourse is among the presumed mechanisms by which HPV is introduced into the anal canal. Other risk factors for the occurrence of squamous cell carcinoma include an increasing number of sexual partners, a history of anogenital warts, previous lower genital tract dysplasia or carcinoma, a history of smoking, HIV seropositivity, low CD4 count, and immunosuppression following solid organ transplant and immune disorders. Benign lesions of the anal canal such as fissures, fistulae, abscesses, and hemorrhoids have been hypothesized to increase the risk of anal squamous cell carcinoma due to chronic irritation of the tissues; however, this hypothesis has never been confirmed. In HIV-positive patients, highly active antiretroviral therapy (HAART) has no protective effect on the development of anal squamous cell carcinoma, contrary to what is observed in other HIV-associated tumors.
- **Age**
  Squamous cell carcinoma usually occurs in the sixth or seventh decade of life. It can occur in younger patients when they are immunocompromised.
- **Sex**
  Anal squamous cell carcinoma occurs more frequently in women than in men. But the incidence is much higher in men who practice anoreceptive intercourse and in those with HIV seropositivity.

- **Site**
  Anal squamous cell carcinoma originates from the squamous epithelium of the lower part of the anal canal, of the anal transitional zone, or of the hair-bearing perianal skin.
- **Treatment**
  Treatment of anal squamous cell carcinoma relies on chemotherapy (5 fluorouracil and mitomycin) associated with radiation therapy (45–59 Gy, with the total dose delivered and the irradiation fields determined by tumor stage) (Cacheux et al. 2012). Abdomino-perineal resection is nowadays reserved as salvage therapy for those individuals with persistent disease, with biopsy-proven evidence of locoregional progressive or recurrent disease, after combined chemoradiation.

  For patients with metastatic disease at presentation, the standard treatment is exclusive chemotherapy (cisplatin-based chemotherapy with 5FU) or clinical trials. Colostomy is sometimes indicated in the case of sphincter destruction by the tumor with severe incontinence.

  HIV-positive patients may be treated with the same regimen as HIV-negative patients. However, dosage adjustment has to be performed in some cases due to more frequent complications and toxicity.

  Trials are underway with agents targeting the EGF receptor, anti-angiogenic agents, tyrosine kinase inhibitors, or molecules targeting other intracellular signaling pathways (PI3 kinase or mTOR inhibitors).

  Sentinel lymph node biopsy is a feasible technique in the management of anal squamous cell carcinoma. It could improve disease staging and may be useful to select patients for inguinal radiation. However, further prospective studies are needed to assess the clinical impact of this procedure.

  The efficacy of HPV prophylactic vaccines in preventing anal squamous cell carcinoma still has to be assessed.

  Recommendations for the primary treatment of anal margin cancer are similar. The exception is for small well-differentiated anal margin squamous cell carcinomas which can be treated with margin-negative local excision alone.
- **Outcome**
  With the chemoradiotherapy regimen, complete response is obtained in 70% patients (64–86%) and the 5-year overall survival rate is 75% (66–92%). Locoregional failures rates vary between 16% and 42%. One half of patients with locoregional failure are considered to have persistent disease after chemoradiotherapy and the other half to have true local recurrences.

  Persistent disease is defined as a tumor which remains evident after maximal treatment response or a tumor that recurs within 6 months of a complete response. Recurrent disease is defined as lesions that reappear 6 months or longer after a complete clinical response. Approximately 80% true local recurrences occur in a 2-year follow-up.

  The 5-year survival following salvage surgery for persistent squamous cell carcinoma following chemoradiation is 31–33% compared with 30–82% in patients operated for a true recurrence. Predictors of a poor outcome following surgery are positive surgical margins, inguinal lymph node status, tumor size larger than 5 cm, adjacent organ involvement, male gender, and comorbidities. In the era of highly active antiretroviral therapy, the outcome after chemoradiotherapy for HIV-related cancers is comparable to that for patients without HIV, although there may be significant toxicity.

  The incidence of lymph node metastasis is approximately 10% at diagnosis but can increase to 20–60% for T4 lesions. Metastatic disease develops in 10–17% of patients treated with chemoradiation therapy. The most common sites of distant metastases are the liver and the lungs. Only 10% patients with distant metastases survive 2 years after the diagnosis.

Macroscopy

Squamous cell carcinoma presents as an ulcerated or polypoid, exophytic, firm, and whitish mass

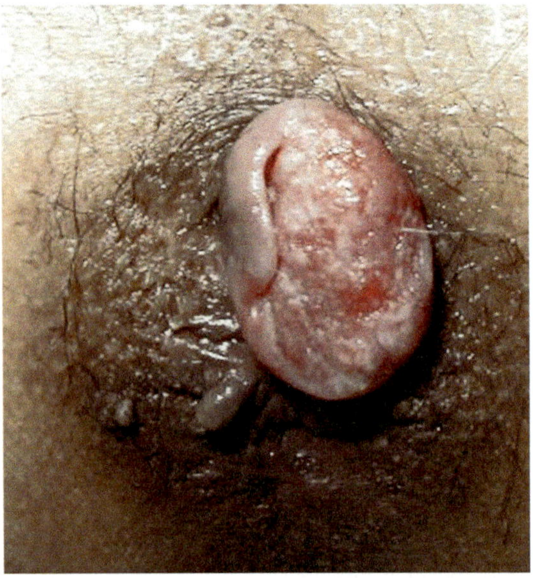

Squamous Cell Carcinoma, Anus, Fig. 1 Anal squamous cell carcinoma, presenting as a large fungating lesion

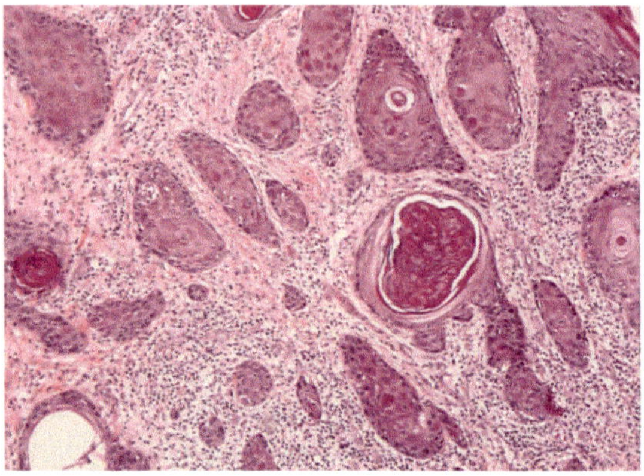

Squamous Cell Carcinoma, Anus, Fig. 2 Well-differentiated keratinizing squamous cell carcinoma of the anus

(Fig. 1). It usually measures from 1 to 5 cm in diameter at diagnosis. Extension to the vagina, bladder, or prostate affects 20% of patients.

Microscopy

Histologic subtyping of anal squamous cell carcinoma was recommended in the past and included large-cell keratinizing squamous cell carcinoma, large-cell nonkeratinizing squamous cell carcinoma, and basaloid carcinoma (also referred to cloacogenic carcinoma). In practice, very commonly a single tumor shows mixtures of areas with different histological features. The histologic subtyping is difficult for pathologists, with a poor diagnostic reproducibility, and finally lacks prognostic significance. Histological features do not correlate with HPV type, although some studies have shown that the presence of HPV16 and 18 was more frequently associated with squamous cell carcinoma with basaloid features and absent keratinization.

The WHO now recommends that the generic term "squamous cell carcinoma" be used for all these variants, accompanied by a comment describing those histopathological features that may possibly affect the prognosis: degree of differentiation and keratinization, basaloid features, presence of mucinous microcysts, and size of predominant neoplastic cells.

Keratinizing squamous cell carcinoma consists of nests of round or polygonal medium or large cells surrounded by desmoplastic and sometimes inflammatory stroma (Fig. 2). Tumor cells have eosinophilic or clear cytoplasm. Nuclei are enlarged, with irregular shapes and hyperchromatic or vesicular chromatin, with often prominent nucleoli. Mitoses are often scanty. Tumor cells often show discernible intercellular junctions, and there is central keratinization in the tumor nests, with lamellar keratin pearls.

Nonkeratinizing squamous cell carcinoma accounts for 80% anal carcinomas. Transitional cell variant resembles transitional cell carcinomas of the urinary bladder, and consists of larger elongated cells with clear or slightly eosinophilic cytoplasm, arranged in anastomosing cords and islands, sharply demarcated from the surrounding stroma. The basaloid or cloacogenic variant consists of nested and trabecular growth of small cells, with basophilic cytoplasm and without the intercellular bridges typical of conventional squamous cell carcinoma. Inconsistently tumor cells show a peripheral palisading, similar to that observed in cutaneous basal cell carcinoma with retraction artifact (Fig. 3). Central eosinophilic

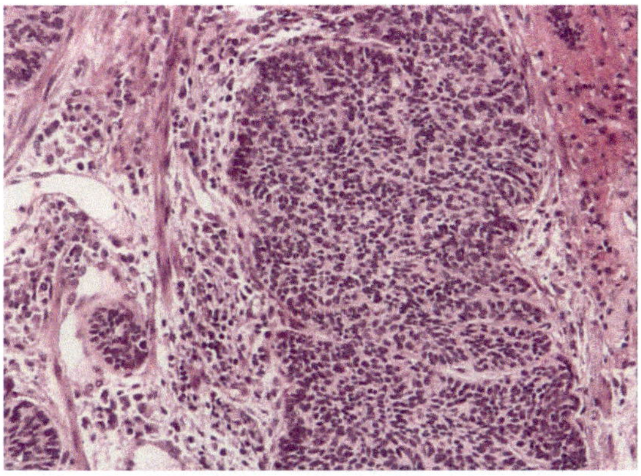

Squamous Cell Carcinoma, Anus, Fig. 3 Basaloid type squamous cell carcinoma of the anus

necrosis and mitotic features may be prominent, but cellular pleomorphism is not typical. Small foci of more conventional squamous differentiation are frequent. Some tumors may grow in lobules and contain prominent eosinophilic hyaline paucicellular basement membrane-like material around and within tumor nests, resulting in an appearance simulating that of an adenoid cystic carcinoma. Tumors can also have small cystic foci lined by mucin-producing cells, similar to mucoepidermoid carcinoma, microscopic features of which seem to be correlated with a poorer prognosis.

The small cell/anaplastic variant consists of nests and compact masses of small cells with high mitotic activity and diffuse infiltration of the surrounding stroma, without expression of neuroendocrine markers. This entity is distinct from small "oat" cell carcinoma or poorly differentiated neuroendocrine carcinoma but seems to have a poorer prognosis.

The sarcomatoid pattern is very rare with a polypoid tumor in the anal canal, poorly differentiated and consists of sheets of atypical round and spindle cells, that may show evidence of neuroendocrine and rhabdomyoblastic differentiation.

Differentiation of squamous cell carcinoma is based mainly on the extent of keratin production and cell cohesion. Well-differentiated squamous cell carcinomas have a close resemblance to normal squamous epithelium and contain round or polygonal cells with intercellular bridges and full keratinization, mitoses are scanty. Moderately differentiated squamous cell carcinomas have less keratinization and more nuclear pleomorphism, with more numerous mitoses including abnormal mitoses. Keratinization and intercellular bridges are minimal and barely discernible in poorly differentiated carcinomas, with a higher nuclear pleomorphism, numerous mitoses, central necrosis, and basaloid features.

Verrucous carcinoma/giant condyloma of Buschke and Löwenstein is a particular variant of anal and perianal squamous cell carcinoma, described in a specific entry.

Immunophenotype

Squamous cell carcinoma expresses cytokeratin 5/6 and p63 protein (a p53 protein homologue) (Fig. 4). Poorly differentiated squamous cell carcinoma expresses cytokeratins such as CK7, CK8, CK18, and CK19. With increasing degrees of differentiation, squamous cell carcinoma stains positive with keratin subtypes associated with stratification and cornification, such as CK1, CK4, CK10, CK13, and CK16. Most squamous cell carcinomas of the anal canal show a diffuse nuclear and cytoplasmic stain for p16, due to an associated high-risk HPV infection.

Molecular Features

Carcinogenesis of squamous cell carcinoma of the anal canal is principally linked to HPV infection. The viral DNA integration leads to the overexpression of viral oncoproteins E6 and E7 that silence important tumor-suppressor proteins in normal cells, implicated in the normal cell cycle regulation, namely, p53 and Rb, and overexpression of other proteins, notably p16. Specific gene mutations or translocation have not yet been identified. EGFR mutations are absent or rare in squamous cell carcinoma of the anus.

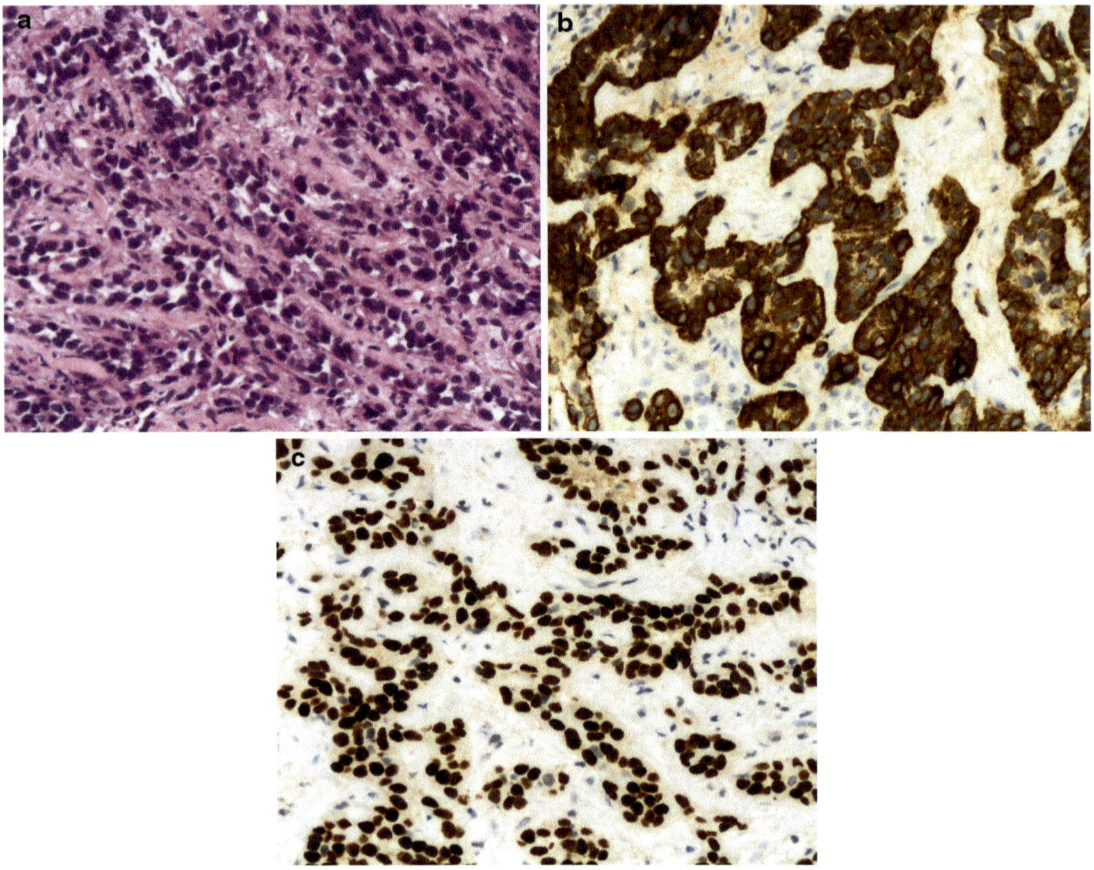

Squamous Cell Carcinoma, Anus, Fig. 4 Poorly differentiated squamous cell carcinoma of the anus (**a**), showing strong expression of cytokeratin 5/6 (**b**) and p63 protein (**c**)

Differential Diagnosis

The main differential diagnoses of poorly differentiated squamous cell carcinoma of the anal canal include neuroendocrine carcinoma, poorly differentiated adenocarcinoma, and malignant melanoma.

Morphologic diagnostic clues are the presence of keratin pearl formation in squamous cell carcinoma, gland formation in adenocarcinoma, and brown-black melanin pigment in the cytoplasm of tumor cells in melanoma. However, poorly differentiated tumors can look similar in small biopsies and a panel of immunostains is often useful for differential diagnosis.

Squamous cell carcinoma expresses cytokeratins 5/6 (but poorly differentiated squamous cell carcinoma can lose cytokeratin 5/6 expression) and p63 (Fig. 4). They sometimes focally express cytokeratin 7. They stain negative for neuroendocrine markers, synaptophysin and chromogranin A, and melanoma markers, S100 protein, HMB-45, and melan-A.

Anal adenocarcinoma stains positive for cytokeratin 7 and/or cytokeratin 20. In some cases, they can express cytokeratin 5/6 focally and rarely p63. But immunohistochemical staining for p63 is a highly specific and useful tool in the diagnosis of squamous cell carcinoma of the anal canal, with a specificity of 98%. PAS and mucicarmine stains may also highlight intra- and extracellular pools of mucin in adenocarcinoma.

References and Further Reading

Cacheux, W., Lievre, A., De La Rochefordiere, A., Dieumegard, B., Cvitkovic, F., Labib, A., Mitry, E., & Buecher, B. (2012). Chemotherapy in the treatment of anal canal carcinoma. *Digestive and Liver Disease, 44*, 803–811.

Rousseau, D. L., Jr., Thomas, C. R., Jr., Petrelli, N. J., & Kahlenberg, M. S. (2005). Squamous cell carcinoma of the anal canal. *Surgical Oncology, 14*, 121–132.

Shia, J. (2010). An update on tumors of the anal canal. *Archives of Pathology & Laboratory Medicine, 134*, 1601–1611.

Uronis, H. E., & Bendell, J. C. (2007). Anal cancer: An overview. *The Oncologist, 12*, 524–534.

Squamous Papilloma, Upper Gastrointestinal Tract

Rita Canas Marques[1] and Paula Chaves[2,3]
[1]Serviço de Anatomia Patológica, Instituto Português de Oncologia de Lisboa de Francisco Gentil and Faculdade de Ciências Médicas, Universidade Nova de Lisboa, Lisbon, Portugal
[2]Serviço de Anatomia Patológica, Instituto Português de Oncologia de Lisboa de Francisco Gentil, Lisbon, Portugal
[3]Faculdade de Ciências da Saúde, Universidade da Beira Interior, Covilhã, Portugal

Synonyms

Benign papillomata; Malpighian papilloma

Definition

The upper gastrointestinal tract squamous papilloma described in this section will address exclusively the esophageal squamous papilloma. Anatomically, one could argue if pharyngeal squamous papilloma could also be included in this section, but it will be discussed in the squamous papilloma of the upper respiratory tractsection.

Esophageal squamous papilloma is a benign polypoid lesion that usually presents with a wart-like configuration at upper endoscopy. In general, the microscopic appearance of esophageal squamous papilloma is composed of a stromal core of lamina propria lined by mature stratified squamous epithelium.

Clinical Features

- **Incidence**
  Esophageal squamous papilloma is an uncommon lesion with less than 200 cases described in the worldwide literature.

  The estimated incidence varies between 0.01% and 0.45%, in endoscopic series, while studies based on autopsies series reveal a prevalence of 0.006–0.04% of the general population (Brandt 2011; Odze et al. 1993).

  Esophageal squamous papilloma is usually a rare incidental finding at autopsy or at upper gastrointestinal endoscopy in asymptomatic patients with no characteristic symptoms.

  There are no specific symptoms associated with esophageal squamous papilloma. The nonspecific described symptoms include dysphagia, dyspepsia, heartburn, gastro-esophageal reflux, which are not directly connected with the papillomatous lesion and are usually the reason for endoscopy. Therefore, the endoscopic resection of the lesion, usually, does not relieve the symptoms.

  Esophageal squamous papilloma underlying etiology is unknown. There are two proposed theories regarding different etiologic mechanisms for squamous papilloma, which include a hyper-regenerative response to mucosal irritations (probably trauma, esophagitis, chemicals, or gastro-esophageal reflux disease), and alternatively, a viral etiology related to human papilloma virus (HPV) infection (Kanth and Go 2011; Odze et al. 1993). Some authors defend a multistep mechanism in which these etiologic factors could act synergically in squamous papilloma pathogenesis.
- **Age**
  Typically squamous papilloma occurs in adults over 50 years old, although the reported cases have a wide range of age at presentation,

S

varying between 10 and 90 years old (Rebeuh et al. 2011; Gomez et al. 1997).

- **Sex**
  Males are more commonly affected than females with a ratio of 1.8:1. Women have usually older age than men (Lewin and Appelman 1995).
  These data regarding age and gender is probably related to the profile of the population submitted to gastro-esophageal endoscopy.
- **Site**
  The lower segments of the esophagus (middle and distal thirds) are the more frequently involved.
- **Treatment**
  Treatment options include endoscopic resection with diathermic snare or conservative approach with periodic endoscopic and observation.
- **Outcome**
  Squamous papilloma is a benign lesion with no proven malignant potential and there are, currently, no guidelines for its management (Kanth and Go 2011).
  Only very rarely, large squamous papillomas have been associated with malignant transformation (Attila et al. 2009). However, whether these lesions represent *de novo* carcinomas from the onset or true malignant transformation of a squamous papilloma is still a matter of discussion.

Macroscopy

Usually, esophageal squamous papilloma appears as a single esophageal mucosa lesion.

The endoscopic (macroscopic) appearance of this lesion is usually of a round lesion with well-defined outlines that tell apart from the surrounding tissue.

Three morphologic variants have been described. The exophytic variant has an endoscopic picture of an elevated sessile polypoid formation, with a warty-like outline, while the endophytic and spiked variants have the appearance of non-polypoid flat lesions, with a smooth surface in the former and a verrucous covering in the latter (Mosca et al. 2001).

Papillomas are usually of small dimension (less than 0.6 cm) but cases of giant papillomas up to 6.8 cm have been reported (Tabatabaei et al. 2009).

Some of the reported cases exhibited multiple lesions, which has been described with the designation of esophageal papillomatosis (Attila et al. 2009; Waterfall et al. 1978).

Microscopy

Histologically, esophageal squamous papilloma has a branched fibro-vascular core of lamina propria covered by a benign acanthotic squamous epithelium with a well-defined basal layer and a mature appearance toward the surface.

The three different forms of squamous papilloma described in the literature are divided according to their different growth patterns: exophytic, endophytic, and spiked (Odze et al. 1993; Lewin and Appelman 1995; Odze and Goldblum 2009).

The *exophytic* type is the more common one. At endoscopy, these lesions appear as cauliflower-like polypoid lesions arising in the esophageal mucosa (Fig. 1). Histologically, the exophytic type has a branching core of lamina propria producing fronds lined by squamous epithelium giving a finger-like acuminate configuration (Fig. 2). Sometimes squamous papilloma exophytic type appears to have a narrow stalk by which the polyp

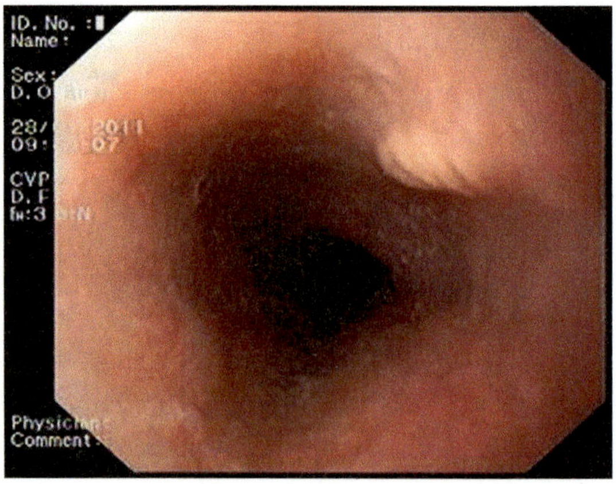

Squamous Papilloma, Upper Gastrointestinal Tract, Fig. 1 Exophytic squamous papilloma – the endoscopic appearance of a polypoid, wart-like mucosal lesion

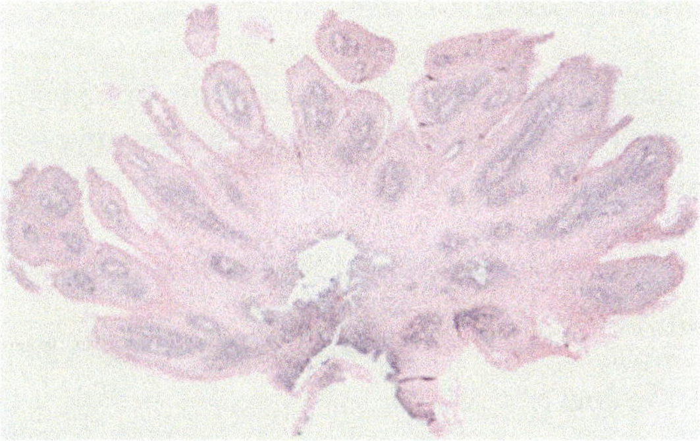

Squamous Papilloma, Upper Gastrointestinal Tract, Fig. 2 Exophytic squamous papilloma – microscopic appearance (5×). This lesion is composed of a branching core of lamina propria producing fronds lined by squamous epithelium giving a finger-like acuminate configuration

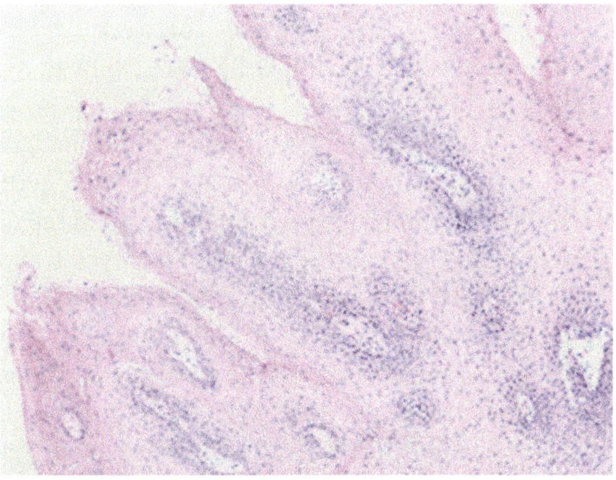

Squamous Papilloma, Upper Gastrointestinal Tract, Fig. 3 Exophytic squamous papilloma – microscopic appearance (10×). Narrow branching fibro-vascular stalks are covered by squamous epithelium of variable thickness that is usually normal or slightly diminished

is attached to the mucosa. The squamous epithelium may be of any thickness, but it is usually normal or slightly diminished. The number of branches varies with some polyps having two to three and others a complex branching system (Fig. 3). Exophytic squamous papillomas occur most frequently in the distal esophagus, but they also can occur in the middle and upper esophagus as well.

In the *endophytic* type of papilloma, the lamina propria has a bulbous round configuration covered by squamous epithelium with an inverted

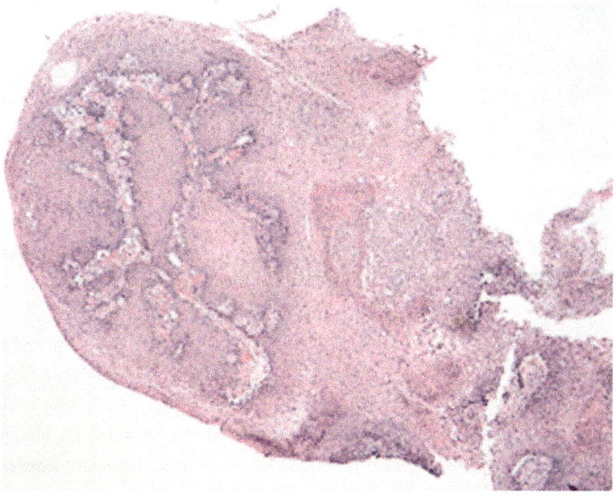

Squamous Papilloma, Upper Gastrointestinal Tract, Fig. 4 Endophytic squamous papilloma – microscopic appearance (5×). This lesion is composed of a lamina propria with bulbous round configuration covered by squamous epithelium with an inverted papillomatous growth pattern

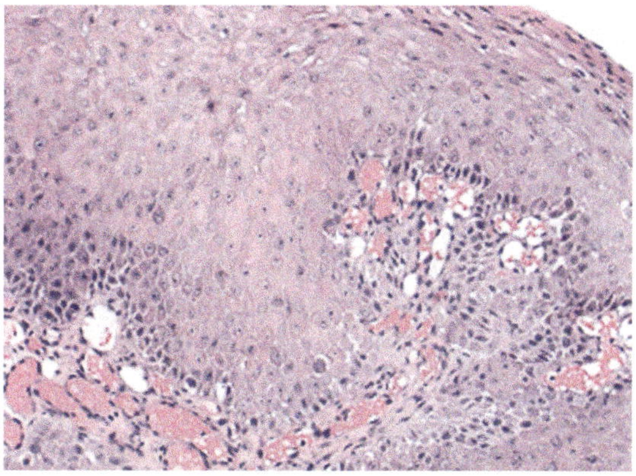

Squamous Papilloma, Upper Gastrointestinal Tract, Fig. 5 Endophytic squamous papilloma – microscopic appearance (20×). The lesion is composed of non-branching fibro-vascular stroma lined by squamous epithelium

papillomatous growth pattern (Figs. 4 and 5). The endoscopic appearance of this variant is usually of a non-polypoid lesion with a round, smooth surface contour similar to that of an inverted papilloma (Fig. 6). Some investigators believe these represent an inflammatory or fibroepithelial polyp.

The third variant is the least common, called *spiked* squamous papilloma, which has a lamina

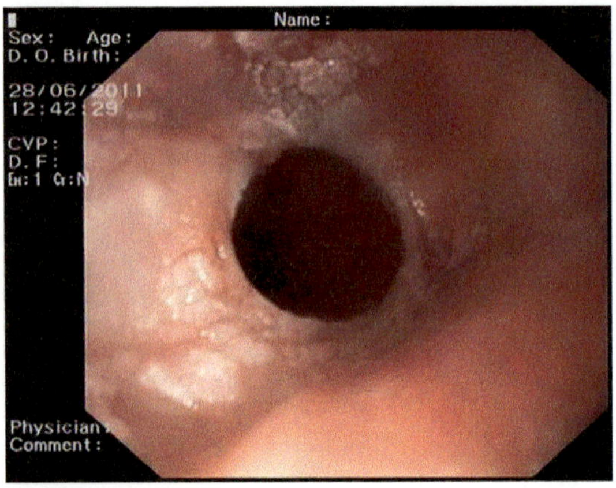

Squamous Papilloma, Upper Gastrointestinal Tract, Fig. 6 Endophytic squamous papilloma – the endoscopic appearance is of a round smooth contour, non-polypoid mucosal lesion

propria that forms stromal spikes covered by hyperplastic squamous epithelium with hyperkeratosis and a prominent granular cell layer, giving an endoscopic verrucoid non-polypoid appearance.

Squamous epithelium of esophageal squamous papilloma may have koilocytic-like features, and sometimes even binucleated cells can be observed. These features overlap with the ones that are so typical of the HPV-infected squamous cells, although one should refer that in esophageal squamous papilloma, the squamous cells usually lack the large hyperchromatic nuclei otherwise seen in the HPV-infected squamous cells. (Odze et al. 1993; Lewin et al. 1995). These koilocytic-like features of the squamous cells have not been described in the spiked type of esophageal squamous papilloma.

Inflammation of the lamina propria is another feature that can be observed in esophageal squamous papillomas; usually, the inflammatory infiltrate is composed mainly of neutrophils with occasional lymphocytes or eosinophils. This inflammatory component is mainly observed in the exophytic and endophytic variants, in which the inflammatory intensity may vary from mild to severe with a variable involvement of the surface epithelium.

Immunophenotype

Immunohistochemical studies performed in esophageal squamous papilloma lesions revealed that there is a basal and focal expression of p53 in about 90% of cases. Positive expression of p16 was present in less than 45% of cases and the Ki67 proliferative index was found to be usually between 10% and 30% (Bohn et al. 2008; Takeshita et al. 2006).

Molecular Features

Supporting a viral etiology, studies to detect HPV DNA (using Polymerase Chain Reaction (PCR) or Southern Blot methods) in upper gastrointestinal tract squamous papillomas showed a variable percentage of HPV positive cases, between 10.5% (Takeshita et al. 2006) and 87.5% (Bohn et al. 2008).

Most of esophageal squamous papillomas are HPV 16 type positive. A combination of HPV type 16 and HPV type 18 positivity is observed in fewer cases and only very rarely are both HPV type 6 and HPV type 11b detected (Odze et al. 1993).

Features associated with a higher probability of HPV positivity in esophageal squamous papillomas include: exophytic growth pattern, location in the upper or mid esophagus, younger age at presentation, and female gender, while esophageal squamous papilloma presented in patients with gastro-esophagic reflux disease is usually associated with a lower prevalence of HPV positivity (Odze et al. 1993; Bohn et al. 2008; Takeshita et al. 2006).

Differential Diagnosis

The differential diagnosis that should be considered would include dysplastic squamous epithelium or squamous cell carcinoma. It is mandatory to exclude the latter entities since they could arise in the same anatomic location as esophageal squamous papilloma, although one should remember that squamous cell carcinoma of the esophagus tends to arise in older patients, with a mean age of incidence of about 10 years older (Lewin and Appelman 1995).

References and Further Reading

Attila, T., et al. (2009). Esophageal papillomatosis complicated by squamous cell carcinoma. *Canadian Journal of Gastroenterology, 23*, 415–419.

Bohn, O. L., et al. (2008). Identification of human papillomavirus in esophageal squamous papillomas. *World Journal of Gastroenterology, 14*, 7107–7111.

Brandt, L. J. (2011). Esophageal squamous papilloma. *Gastrointestinal Endoscopy, 73*, 1035.

Gomez, N. A., et al. (1997). Esophageal squamous papilloma: A case report and a review of the literature. *Acta Gastroenterologica Latinoamericana, 27*, 131–133.

Kanth, P., & Go, F. (2011). Squamous papilloma: An unusual esophageal entity. *Endoscopy, 53*, E405–E406.

Lewin, K. J., & Appelman, H. D. (1995). Tumors of theesophagus & stomach: Atlas of tumor pathology. In *American registry of pathology* (pp. 31–32). Washington, DC: Armed Forced Institute of Pathology.

Mosca, S., et al. (2001). Squamous papilloma of the esophagus: Long-term follow up. *Journal of Gastroenterology and Hepatology, 16*, 857–861.

Odze, R., & Goldblum, J. (2009). *Surgical pathology of the GU tract, liver, billiary tract and pancreas* (pp. 406–407). Philadelphia: Saunders Elsevier.

Odze, R., et al. (1993). Esophageal squamous papillomas: A clinicopathological study of 38 lesions and analysis for human papillomavirus by the polymerase chain reaction. *American Journal of Surgical Pathology, 17*, 803–812.

Rebeuh, J., et al. (2011). Esophageal squamous papilloma in children. *Endoscopy, 43*, E256.

Tabatabaei, S. A., et al. (2009). Giant esophageal squamous papilloma: A case report. *Journal of Digestive Diseases, 10*, 228–230.

Takeshita, K., et al. (2006). Clinicopathological characteristics of esophageal squamous papillomas in japonese patients – With comparison of findings from western countries. *Acta Hitochemistry Cytochemistry, 39*, 23–30.

Waterfall, W. E., et al. (1978). Benign oesophagealpapillomatosis. A case report with a review of the literature. *Journal of Clinical Pathology, 31*, 111–115.

S

T

Tropical Sprue

Arzu Ensari
Department of Pathology, Ankara University Medical School, Sihhiye, Ankara, Turkey

Synonyms

Non-celiac sprue; Postinfectious sprue; Post-infective tropical malabsorption

Definition

Tropical sprue (TS) is a rare acquired enteropathy of unknown etiology, characterized by malabsorption, multiple nutritional deficiencies, and mucosal abnormalities in the small bowel mainly occurring among the individuals living in or visiting the tropical countries. Tropical sprue results from a nutritional deficiency, or a transmissible microorganism and/or a toxin. Malabsorption is usually initiated by an infection followed by colonization of the small bowel by enterotoxigenic bacteria. Several microorganisms have been suspected, but none are common to all patients. Genetic or ethnic predispositions have also been suggested. Symptoms of TS include chronic non-bloody diarrhea, weight loss, bloating, and abdominal cramps. Physical examination may reveal pallor, angular stomatitis, glossitis, mouth ulcers, and peripheral edema due to protein deficiency. Anemia related to B_{12} and folic acid deficiencies is common.

Clinical Features

- **Incidence**
  The incidence varies considerably with geography. It occurs mostly in Southeast Asia and the Caribbean accounting for 40% of cases of diarrhea.
- **Age**
  It tends to affect adults but can also occur in children.
- **Sex**
  There is no predilection for either gender.
- **Site**
  The entire small bowel including the terminal ileum is affected in tropical sprue.
- **Treatment**
  Management involves restoration of fluid and electrolytes and repleting vitamin deficiencies. A quick and dramatic response to folate therapy is frequently observed in TS which is considered to be diagnostic. Antibiotics, including tetracycline and doxycycline, are commonly used.
- **Outcome**
  Untreated disease runs a chronic, relapsing course. However, treatment is associated with a good prognosis. Travelers returning to nontropical regions will generally recover

F. Carneiro et al. (eds.), *Pathology of the Gastrointestinal Tract*, Encyclopedia of Pathology,
DOI 10.1007/978-3-319-40560-5

completely after treatment. Relapse rates of 20–50% are seen in people living in endemic areas.

Macroscopy

The endoscopy is usually normal except in a small percentage of cases showing villous abnormalities such as fusing and broadening of the villi, all reminiscent of celiac disease.

Microscopy

The mucosal lesion is similar to CD with varying degree of villous blunting, though completely flat mucosa is rare. Crypt hyperplasia together with an increase in lamina propria lymphocytes, plasma cells, neutrophils, and eosinophils as well as intraepithelial lymphocyte (IEL) (Figs. 1 and 2) which are more prominent in the crypts than the surface epithelium is usually present. In severe cases, decreased mitotic activity is combined with a lack of epithelial maturation. The cells become cuboidal and mucin-depleted and accumulate fat droplets in their cytoplasm. Megaloblastic change can be seen due to B_{12} and folate deficiencies. In some cases, features of chronicity such as mucin cell metaplasia and crypt distortion may be seen.

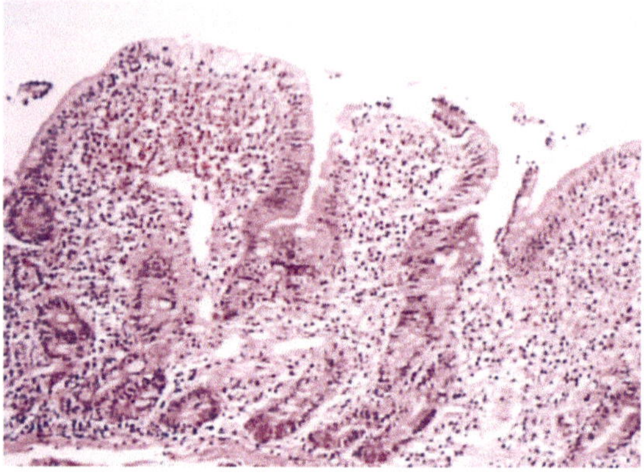

Tropical Sprue, Fig. 1 Villus blunting and crypt hyperplasia with increased inflammatory cells in the lamina propria (H&E; ×100)

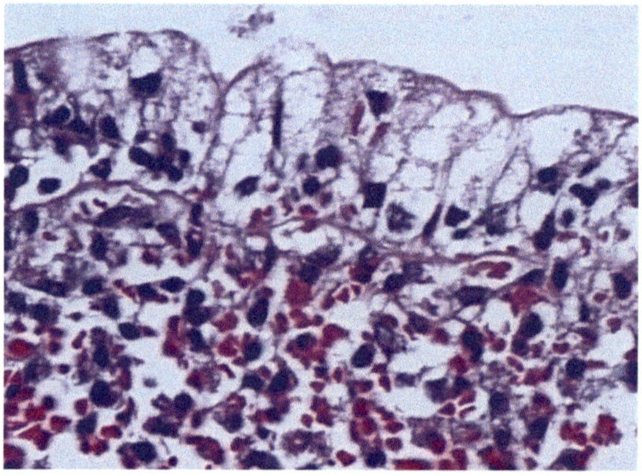

Tropical Sprue, Fig. 2 Increased IELs and neutrophils in the villus epithelium (H&E; ×400)

Immunophenotype

There is no specific immunophenotypic feature.

Molecular Features

There is no specific molecular feature.

Differential Diagnosis

The histologic changes in TS are nonspecific and can be seen in a variety of conditions causing malabsorption. Therefore, the differential diagnosis of TS includes secondary malabsorption due to protozoal (e.g., giardial), helminthic, bacterial, or viral infections, celiac disease, especially when children are affected, Crohn's disease, tuberculosis of the gut without pulmonary manifestations, diseases of the pancreas, and AIDS enteropathy.

References and Further Reading

Batheja, M. J., Leighton, J., Azueta, A., & Heigh, R. (2010). The face of tropical sprue in 2010. *Case Reports in Gastroenterology, 19*, 168–172.

Ghoshal, U. C., & Ranjan, P. (2011). Post-infectious irritable bowel syndrome: The past, the present and

the future. *Journal of Gastroenterology and Hepatology, 26*(Suppl 3), 94–101.
Ghoshal, U. C., Ghoshal, U., Ayyagari, A., et al. (2003). Tropical sprue is associated with contamination of small bowel with aerobic bacteria and reversible prolongation of orocecal transit time. *Journal of Gastroenterology and Hepatology, 18*, 540–7.
Ramakrishna, B. S., Venkataraman, S., & Mukhopadhya, A. (2006). Tropical malabsorption. *Postgraduate Medical Journal, 82*, 779–787.
Veitch, A. M., Kelly, P., Zulu, I. S., et al. (2001). Tropical enteropathy: A T-cell-mediated crypt hyperplastic enteropathy. *European Journal of Gastroenterology and Hepatology, 13*, 1175–81.

Tubular Adenocarcinoma

Chella R. S. van der Post[1] and Fátima Carneiro[2]
[1]Department of Pathology, Radboud University Medical Center, Nijmegen, The Netherlands
[2]Faculty of Medicine of Porto University, Centro Hospitalar São João and Ipatimup/i3S, Porto, Portugal

Synonyms

Intestinal-type adenocarcinoma

Definition

Tubular adenocarcinoma is one of the five main types of gastric adenocarcinoma in the WHO classification scheme and represents the most common type of gastric adenocarcinoma. Together with papillary carcinoma and (part of) mucinous carcinoma, tubular carcinoma represents intestinal-type adenocarcinoma in the Laurén classification. Tubular adenocarcinomas are made up of simple or branching tubules resembling colorectal carcinoma and less commonly small, acinar structures sometimes resembling antral glands.

Gastric cancer has a complex pathogenesis, in which several factors are involved including a familial risk and environmental factors, with the strongest known risk factor being chronic gastritis induced by *H. pylori* infection. In 1994, the WHO classified *H. pylori* as a class I carcinogen based mainly on epidemiological evidence for its role in the pathogenesis of gastric adenocarcinoma. Several bacterial virulence factors define the malignant potential of each *H. pylori* strain. Host genetic factors contribute to the regulation of the inflammatory response and in the aggravation of mucosal damage. Other identified harmful environmental factors include high salt intake and smoking of tobacco. Ingestion of fruit and vegetables possibly has some protective effect.

Clinical Features

The clinical history of tumor-related symptoms is usually of recent date with alarm symptoms including weight loss, anemia, nausea, vomiting, and loss of appetite.

- **Incidence**
  Gastric adenocarcinoma is the fifth most common cancer worldwide and the third leading cause of cancer death with about 700,000 patients dying each year. The incidence shows an impressive decrease in certain areas in the world. The intestinal type gastric adenocarcinoma predominates in high-incidence countries (defined as >60 gastric cancers per 100 000), including eastern Asia, Eastern Europe, and central and Latin America, while the diffuse type is relatively more common in low-incidence areas (defined as <15 gastric cancers per 100 000) including North America and northern Europe.
- **Age**
  Incidence of gastric cancer progressively increases with age, with peak incidence occurring at 60–80 years and is rare in persons younger than 30 years.
- **Sex**
  Males are more frequently affected than females.
- **Site**
  The majority (50–60%) of gastric carcinomas is located distally in the antrum and pylorus,

followed by the cardia (25%) and the corpus or fundus (15–25%).

- **Treatment**
  Complete resection remains the only curative therapy with evidence for increased survival with the addition of perioperative chemotherapy. The therapy regimen of gastric cancer depends on characteristics, stage, location, and genetics (for instance, *HER2* status). Diagnostics should lead to accurate initial staging and assessment of treatment response. Imaging techniques, including multidetector CT, EUS, and PET-CT, should provide staging assessment according to the TNM classification. The incidences of lymph node metastases and distant metastasis are high; therefore, initial assessment must establish the presence or absence of distant disease.

  Surgery represents the standard form of curative therapy aiming to excise the primary tumor with clear longitudinal and circumferential margins. Early, limited gastric mucosal cancer can be treated with endoscopic mucosal or submucosal dissection. Advanced carcinomas should be treated according to the location, distally by subtotal gastrectomy and proximally by total gastrectomy. Cardiac tumors should be treated by trans-hiatal extended total gastrectomy or esophageo-gastrectomy. The extent of lymphadenectomy should be tailored to the age and fitness of the patient together with the location and stage of the cancer. The distal pancreas, spleen, and splenic nodes should be removed only when there is direct invasion and still a chance of a curative procedure in patients with carcinoma of the proximal stomach. Limited gastric resections should only be used for palliation or in the very elderly and may improve survival and quality of life. If patients present with gastric outlet obstruction and a curative intent is impossible, the use of a stent can be considered.

  Chemotherapy, either alone as a perioperative treatment, or in combination with radiation therapy in an adjuvant setting, improves the clinical outcome for patients with resectable tumors. Neoadjuvant chemotherapy leads to downstaging but does not result in a significant improvement in overall survival. Adjuvant chemotherapy alone is currently not standard practice in the treatment of gastric cancer but leads to survival benefits in Asian populations and should be considered in patients at high risk of recurrence who have not received neoadjuvant therapy. Intraperitoneal chemotherapy remains investigational. Palliative chemotherapy can be considered taking into account performance status and patient preference.

  In patients suffering from metastatic disease, chemotherapy and targeted therapies play a major role in improving survival and quality of life compared with best supportive care. The *HER-2* proto-oncogene is an important target in the therapeutic approach of gastric adenocarcinoma. *HER-2* encodes a transmembrane tyrosine kinase receptor and is highly expressed in malignant gastrointestinal neoplasias. Trastuzumab, a monoclonal antibody against HER-2, was shown to be beneficial in combination with chemotherapy for first-line treatment of HER-2-positive advanced gastric cancer.
- **Outcome**
  The prognosis of early gastric cancer is good; however, this is predominantly seen in Asian countries, owing to active screening programs. In Western countries, approximately 80–90% of patients are diagnosed at an advanced stage with high recurrence rates after curative intent therapy. The outlook for advanced gastric cancer remains poor, with median overall survival generally under 12 months. The reported 1-year and 5-year survival rates of advanced gastric cancer are 42% and 24% respectively.

Macroscopy

The growth pattern of gastric carcinoma is commonly described according to the Borrmann classification, subdividing polypoid (type I), fungating (type II), ulcerating (type III), and diffusely infiltrating (type IV) growth patterns. Advanced tubular carcinomas commonly appear as well-circumscribed polypoid, fungating masses with or without surface ulceration (Borrmann type I or II).

Microscopy

Tubular adenocarcinoma is one of the five main types of gastric adenocarcinoma in the WHO classification and resembles colorectal adenocarcinoma. The tubular type is composed of dilated and branching tubules (Figs. 1–3). The glands are of varying diameter, may be cystically dilated and may contain mucin and inflammatory debris. Certain tubular adenocarcinomas are made up of mainly small, acinar structures resembling antral glands. Adenocarcinomas containing both glandular and solid structures are included under tubular carcinomas.

The glands of tubular adenocarcinoma are composed of columnar, cuboidal, or flattened tumor cells that contain variable amounts of intracytoplasmic mucin. Occasional psammoma bodies may be found. The degree of cytonuclear atypia varies from low- to high-grade with also various degrees of mitoses. Desmoplastic stroma is surrounding the glands.

A poorly differentiated variant of tubular carcinoma with only few gland-like structures is called solid carcinoma. A clear cell variant has also been recognized. Tumors with prominent lymphoid stroma are sometimes called carcinoma with lymphoid stroma, medullary carcinoma, or lymphoepithelioma-like carcinoma.

Surrounding gastric mucosa often shows features of chronic *Helicobacter pylori* gastritis, with lymphoid inflammatory infiltrate, atrophy, and intestinal metaplasia.

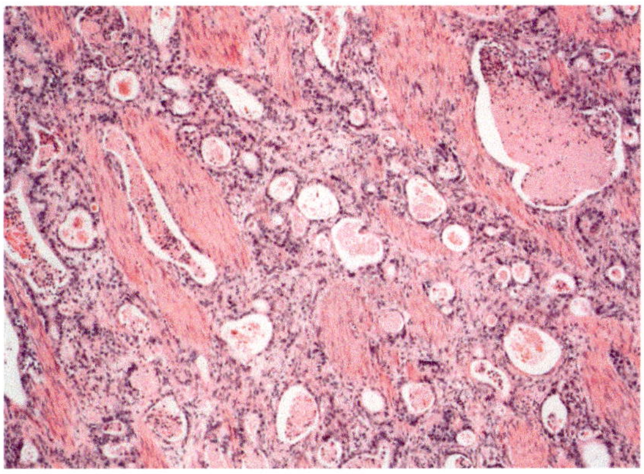

Tubular Adenocarcinoma, Fig. 1 Tubular adenocarcinoma extending into the muscularis propria composed of glands of various sizes with luminal inflammatory debris (Original magnification 50×)

Immunophenotype

Gastric carcinomas are positive for pankeratin staining with varying degrees of CK7 and CK20 positivity. CK18 or CAM5.2 is most often negative. Gastric carcinomas may express Hep Par 1, heterogeneous CDX-2, MUC2, and MUC5AC.

Molecular Features

Gastric cancers are characterized by genetic and epigenetic changes that affect tumor suppressor

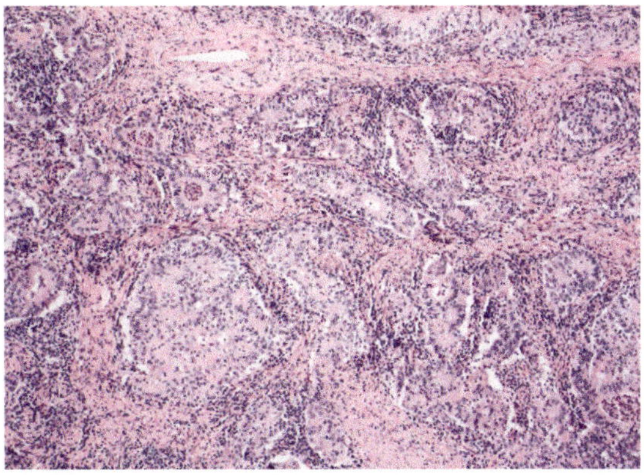

Tubular Adenocarcinoma, Fig. 2 Tubular adenocarcinoma with poorly formed branching glands (Original magnification 50×)

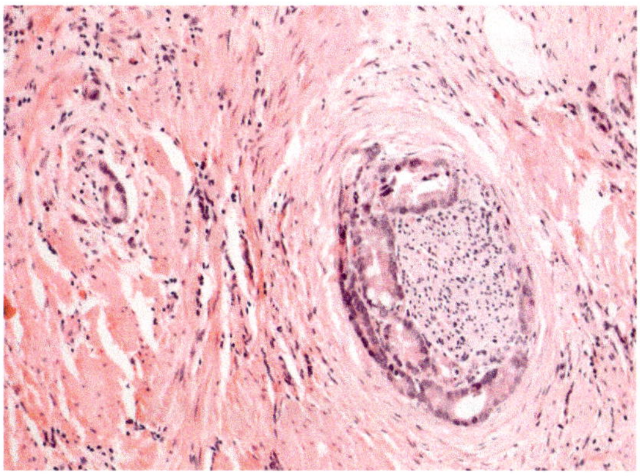

Tubular Adenocarcinoma, Fig. 3 Detail of tubular adenocarcinoma with perineural invasion (Original magnification 100×)

genes, oncogenes, and mismatch repair genes. Consequently, deregulation of cellular proliferation, adhesion, differentiation, signal transduction, telomerase activity, and DNA repair have been reported.

Chromosomal instability may manifest as gain or loss of whole chromosomes (aneuploidy) or parts of chromosomes (loss of heterozygosity, translocations, and amplifications). Comparative genomic hybridization analysis has revealed many DNA copy number variations. Microsatellite instability is seen in 15–20% of gastric cancers, with a higher frequency in familial cases. Mutations in oncogenes include *KRAS* in intestinal-type gastric cancer and overexpression of *HER-2*, a cell surface receptor of the tyrosine kinase family. Tumor suppressor genes *p53, PTEN, RUNX3* are frequently inactivated in gastric carcinomas. Studies applying exon sequencing identified frequent somatic mutations in the *ARID1A* gene which is involved in processes of DNA repair, differentiation, development and has a regulatory role in proliferation. Other identified genes involved in gastric tumorigenesis are *PIK3CA, APC, STK11, CTNNB1, CDKN2A, ERBB2, EGFR,* and *FGFR2*. Tubular adenocarcinomas can be subdivided, depending on the molecular abberations, into Epstein-Barr virus-infected tumors, microsatellite unstable tumors and chromosomally unstable tumors according to the molecular classification of The Cancer Genome Atlas. See more details in the entry "► Adenocarcinoma, Upper Gastrointestinal Tract".

Differential Diagnosis

Early, limited gastric mucosal tubular adenocarcinoma may be difficult to differentiate from high-grade dysplasia.

References and Further Reading

Allum, W. H., Blazeby, J. M., Griffin, S. M., Cunningham, D., Jankowski, J. A., & Wong, R. (2011). Guidelines for the management of oesophageal and gastric cancer. *Gut, 60*(11), 1449–1472.

Bosman, F. T., Carneiro, F., Hruban, R. H., & Theise, N. D. (2010). *WHO classification of tumours of the digestive system* (4th ed.). Lyon: IARC.

Cancer Genome Atlas Research, N. (2014). Comprehensive molecular characterization of gastric adenocarcinoma. *Nature, 513*(7517), 202–209.

Ferlay, J., Soerjomataram, I., Ervik, M., et al. (2013). GLOBOCAN 2012 v1.0, cancer incidence and mortality worldwide. IARC CancerBase 11. International Agency for Research on Cancer (http://globocan.iarc.fr)

Price, T. J., Shapiro, J. D., Segelov, E., Karapetis, C. S., Pavlakis, N., Van Cutsem, E., et al. (2012). Management of advanced gastric cancer. *Expert Review of Gastroenterology & Hepatology, 6*(2), 199–208. quiz 209.

Wong, H., & Yau, T. (2013). Molecular targeted therapies in advanced gastric cancer: Does tumor histology matter? *Therapeutic Advances in Gastroenterology, 6*(1), 15–31.

Zang, Z. J., Cutcutache, I., Poon, S. L., Zhang, S. L., McPherson, J. R., Tao, J., et al. (2012). Exome sequencing of gastric adenocarcinoma identifies recurrent somatic mutations in cell adhesion and chromatin remodeling genes. *Nature Genetics, 44*(5), 570–574.

Tufting Enteropathy

Arzu Ensari
Department of Pathology, Ankara University Medical School, Sihhiye, Ankara, Turkey

Synonyms

Congenital enteropathy; Congenital familial intractable diarrhea with enterocytes assembly abnormalities; Congenital tufting enteropathy; Intestinal epithelial dysplasia

Definition

Tufting enteropathy (TE), also known as intestinal epithelial dysplasia (IED), is a congenital enteropathy presenting with early-onset severe intractable diarrhea and persistent villous atrophy with low or no mononuclear cell infiltration of the lamina propria but specific histological abnormalities involving the epithelium. TE is a rare cause of severe diarrhea in the first week of life accompanied with various dysmorphic features including choanal atresia, oesophageal/rectal atresia in some of the affected infants. Nonspecific punctuated keratitis was reported in more than 60% of patients. TE is characterized by clinical and histological heterogeneity and association with malformations or other epithelial diseases. It is thought to be related to abnormal enterocytes development and/or differentiation. In general, infants with TE develop watery diarrhea within the first days after birth. It is severe in most of the cases. Stool volumes may be as high as 100–200 ml/kg body weight per day, with electrolyte concentrations similar to those seen in small intestinal fluid. In rare cases the diarrhea may be less abundant and sometimes may mislead the diagnosis. The growth is impaired. There is no past history of hydramnios suggesting congenital chloride diarrhea or sodium malabsorption diarrhea. Most patients have consanguineous parents and/or affected siblings, some of whom died during the first months of life from severe diarrhea of unknown origin.

Clinical Features

- **Incidence**
  The prevalence can be estimated at around 1/50,000–100,000 live births in Western Europe. The prevalence seems higher in areas with high degree of consanguinity and in patients of Arabic origin.
- **Age**
  It is common in neonates and infants younger than 6 months of age.
- **Sex**
  No sex predilection has been reported.
- **Site**
  Tufts are not limited to the small intestine and may also involve the colonic mucosa.
- **Treatment**
  The infant is dependent on TPN and intestinal transplantation is the treatment of choice.
- **Outcome**
  Though some infants present with milder forms, most require long-term TPN with a subsequent risk of complications. The long-term prognosis is variable. Most patients with tufting enteropathy have been treated with long-term parenteral nutrition, which can lead to liver failure, sepsis, and the loss of vascular access.

Macroscopy

Microvillous inclusion disease is usually diagnosed in biopsy specimens rather than gross specimens. No specific gross abnormality has been reported.

Microscopy

Histology shows varying degrees of villous atrophy, with low or no mononuclear cell infiltration in the lamina propria (Fig. 1). The epithelium looks disorganized as the surface enterocytes form tufts, buds, or small papillae some of which seem to drop off into the lumen on sections (Fig. 2). Villous atrophy is present in all patients but is variable in severity. In the typical form, abnormalities are localized mainly in the epithelium and include disorganization of surface enterocytes with focal crowding, resembling tufts (Fig. 3). These characteristic "tufts" of extruding epithelium, first described by Reifen et al., are seen towards the villous tip and may affect up to 70% of villi. Focal enterocyte crowding can also be observed in the crypt

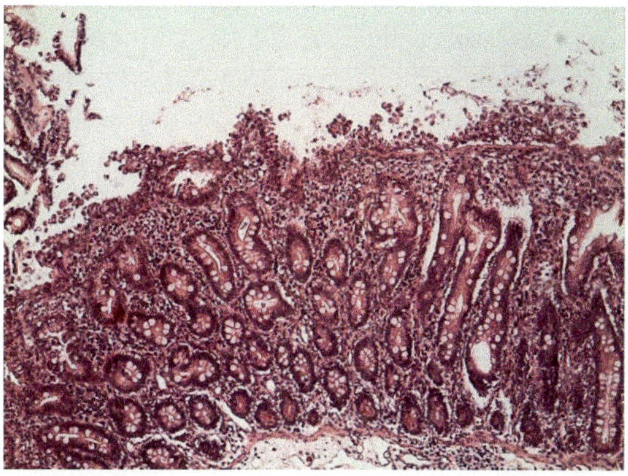

Tufting Enteropathy, Fig. 1 Small intestinal mucosa with irregular surface and villous shortening (H&E; ×100)

T

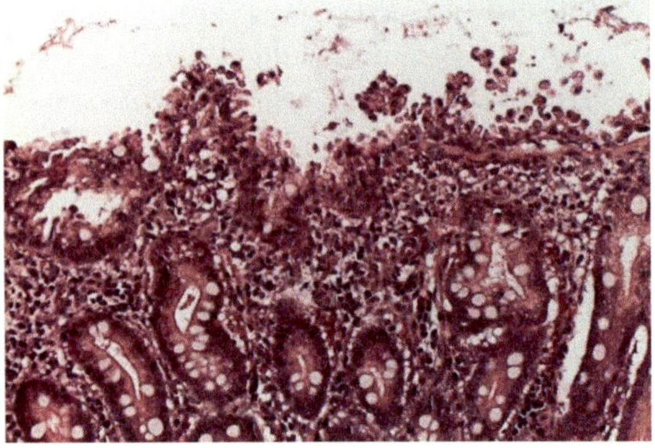

Tufting Enteropathy, Fig. 2 Epithelial tufts floating in the lumen (H&E; ×200)

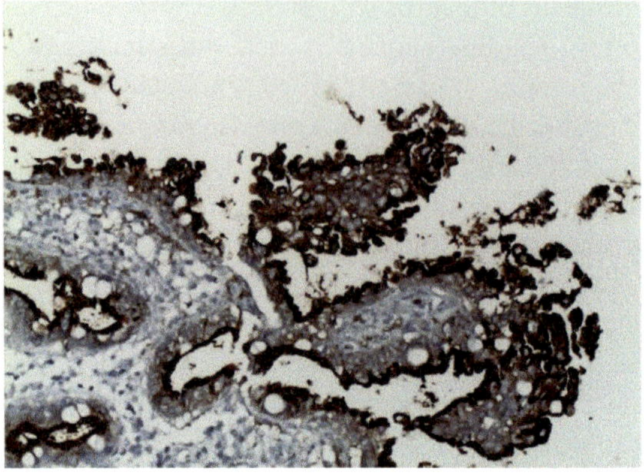

Tufting Enteropathy, Fig. 4 CD10 expression on the irregular surface surrounding the tufts (ICH; ×200)

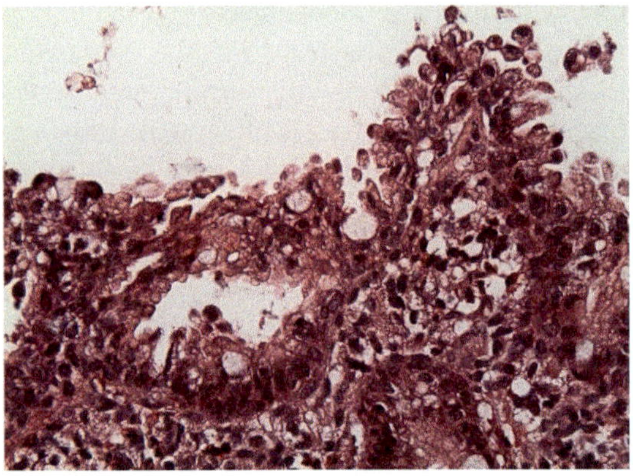

Tufting Enteropathy, Fig. 3 Epithelial tufts formed by desquamated surface enterocytes (H&E; ×400)

epithelium, and in addition, crypts often have an abnormal aspect: they are dilated with abnormal regeneration in the form of branching. The brush border is usually intact and no ultrastructural abnormalities are present. Colonic mucosa may also be involved (Fig. 4). Sometimes, histopathological presentation of TE does not show evidence of tufts. Diagnosis can be made by performing repeated intestinal biopsies. Indeed, biopsies change from being near normal in early life (showing only signs of nonspecific villous atrophy, with or without monocellular cell infiltration of the lamina propria) to revealing the characteristic tufts. In addition, specific abnormalities of basement membrane components (integrins or desmosomes) in parts of mucosa are rare and difficult to detect in the absence of tufts. Ultrastructural changes may be observed in the desmosomes, which are increased in length and number.

Immunophenotype

Deposition of laminin and heparin sulfate proteoglycan in the basement membrane, increased expression of desmoglein, and abnormal distribution of $\alpha 2\beta 1$ integrin adhesion molecules have been described.

Molecular Features

Mutations in the epithelial cell adhesion molecule (EpCAM; CD326) gene on chromosome 2p21 are causal for congenital tufting enteropathy (CTE), a disease characterized by intestinal abnormalities resulting in lethal diarrhea in newborns. Why the different mutations all lead to the same disease is not clear. Most mutations will result in lack of EpCAM's transmembrane domain, whereas two mutations allow transmembrane localization. It was recently found that these mutants are not routed to the plasma membrane and that truncated mutants are secreted or degraded. Thus, all EpCAM mutations lead to loss of cell-surface EpCAM, resulting in CTE.

Differential Diagnosis

The clinical differential diagnosis includes other causes of neonatal diarrhea. These include autoimmune enteropathies, immunodeficiencies, and lesions displaying primary enterocyte abnormalities such as MID.

References and Further Reading

Goulet, O., Salomon, J., Ruemmele, F., de Serres, N. P., & Brousse, N. (2007). Intestinal epithelial dysplasia (tufting enteropathy). *Orphanet Journal of Rare Diseases, 2*, 20.

Lemale, J., Coulomb, A., Dubern, B., Boudjemaa, S., Viola, S., Josset, P., Tounian, P., & Girardet, J. P. (2011). Intractable diarrhea with tufting enteropathy: A favorable outcome is possible. *Journal of Pediatric Gastroenterology and Nutrition, 52*(6), 734–739.

Reifen, R. M., Cutz, E., Griffiths, A. M., Ngan, B. Y., & Sherman, P. M. (1994). Tufting enteropathy: A newly recognized clinicopathological entity associated with refractory diarrhea in infants. *Journal of Pediatric Gastroenterology and Nutrition, 18*, 379–385.

Schnell, U., Kuipers, J., Mueller, J. L., Veenstra-Algra, A., Sivagnanam, M., & Giepmans, B. N. (2013). Absence of cell-surface EpCAM in congenital tufting enteropathy. *Human Molecular Genetics, 22*(13), 2566–2571.

Sivagnanam, M., Mueller, J. L., Lee, H., Chen, Z., Nelson, S. F., Turner, D., Zlotkin, S. H., Pencharz, P. B., Ngan, B. Y., Libiger, O., Schork, N. J., Lavine, J. E., Taylor, S., Newbury, R. O., Kolodner, R. D., & Hoffman, H. M. (2008). Identification of EpCAM as the gene for congenital tufting enteropathy. *Gastroenterology, 135*(2), 429–437.

Typhoid Fever

Karel Geboes
Department of Pathology, N. Goormaghtig Institute, University Gent, Gent, Belgium
Department of Pathology, KU Leuven, Leuven, Belgium

Synonyms

Enteric fever; Gastric fever; Slow fever

Definition

Typhoid fever is a severe systemic bacterial disease caused by *Salmonella enterica* serovar *Typhi*. It is characterized by prolonged fever, persistent bacteremia and severe inflammation of the intestines, especially the lymphoid tissue. *Salmonella typhi* has been a human pathogen for thousands of years thriving in conditions of poor sanitation and crowding. The name is derived from the ancient Greek "typhos" which means "cloud" or "smoke" and refers to the level of consciousness of the patients in the advanced stage of the disease. The classic presentation includes fever, malaise, diffuse abdominal pain, and diarrhea or constipation (in up to 38% of the patients). Untreated disease progresses through different stages. Incubation lasts 5–21 days depending on the health and immune status of the patient and the virulence of the bacteria. The onset is usually insidious with low-grade fever appearing first. During active invasion of the bacteria, in the second week of infection, daily, stepwise elevations of temperature are noted. In some patients, rose spots may develop on the trunk. Symptoms increase during the third week, and fever becomes continuous with only slight daily fluctuations. Various complications can occur including delirium (typhoid state, nervous fever, or vigil coma), intestinal hemorrhage, bowel perforation, and death within 1 month of onset. During the next stage, symptoms wane and fever slowly fails. Most symptoms resolve by the fourth week of infection, without antimicrobial therapy in approximately 90% of the patients. In convalescence, weakness and fatigue persist for months and some patients may relapse. Survivors may also be left with long-term or permanent neuropsychiatric complications. A less severe, but similar illness is caused by the related *Salmonella paratyphi* bacteria. The latter is usually referred to as paratyphoid fever. The bacteria spread through food, drink, or water contaminated by the feces or urine of infected persons. *S. typhi* has no reservoir other than humans. So the ultimate source of every infection is an infected person, usually a carrier. In carriers, the pathogens colonize diseased gall-bladders.

Clinical Features

- **Incidence**
  Typhoid fever is rare in industrial countries but continues to be a significant public-health issue in developing countries. It is estimated that approximately 21.5 million illnesses and 216,510 deaths worldwide occurred in 2000. Countries have been categorized as having a low incidence (<10 cases per 100,000 per year), a medium incidence (10–100 cases per 100,000 per year), or a high incidence (>100 cases per 100,000 per year). The decline in incidence in low-risk countries is mainly due to improved living conditions and sanitation. Typhoid fever remains nevertheless a common bacterial disease worldwide, with the incidence in developed countries estimated to be 5 cases per 1,000,000 per year but a much higher in some developing countries. In India and Pakistan, the annual incidence is estimated to be 50 and 40 cases per 1,000,000 respectively. As a result, there is a risk for travelers. The incidence of typhoid fever among US travelers to developing countries is approximately 30–300 cases per 1,000,000 per year.
- **Age**
  Children of 12 years or younger carry a bigger risk for the disease in developing countries and areas with poor sanitation. Invasive *Salmonella*-associated gastroenteritis with ileal perforation occurs mainly in children, often under 5 years of age. Overall the incidence is highest in children and young adults between 5 and 19 years. The incidence of carriers increases with age.
- **Sex**
  There is no gender predilection for the disease, but women are three times as likely to become carriers as men. They have a higher prevalence of gall-bladder disease.
- **Site**
  The primary focus of enteric fever is in the ileum and colon.
- **Treatment**
  Typhoid fever is treated with antibiotics. Chloramphenicol has been the treatment of choice for years. It has reduced mortality to 1% and duration of fever to 3–5 days. Because of the serious side effects of this drug, it has now been replaced by other effective antibiotics. The choice of the precise drug depends on the region where the infection occurred and the results of cultures and sensitivity analysis. Ciprofloxacin, ampicillin, and trimethoprim-sulfamethoxasole are frequently used. Oral rehydration is indicated in patients with diarrhea. Surgery is performed when perforation occurs. Carriers need prolonged treatment with antibiotics or surgical removal of the gall-bladder. In order to prevent infection, vaccination is now recommended for travelers only to medium-risk and high-risk countries as classified on the basis of a final risk classification for each destination. In addition, sanitation and hygiene are critical measures.
- **Outcome**
  The outcome is likely good with early appropriate treatment. Symptoms may recur if treatment failed and did not completely cure the infection.

Macroscopy

The macroscopic aspect varies throughout the natural course of the infection. During the invasive stage, the small intestine is dilated and has a light red, mildly injected serosa, rarely with fibrinous exudates. The mucosa is red and edematous. Peyer's patches and small lymphoid aggregates throughout the small and large intestine are enlarged and raise 0.1–0.4 cm above the adjacent mucosa. They are soft and slightly erythematous, often with a necrotic surface in the later stage. The cut surface is reddish. Mesenteric lymph nodes are enlarged and soft. The appendix is frequently involved. The spleen is enlarged, red soft, and congested. The surface can be covered with fibrinous exudates.

Microscopy

Ingested bacteria are able to resist the acidic environment of the stomach and antibacterial substances secreted in the small intestine. They interact with the M cells of Peyer's patches in the ileum, are rapidly internalized, and enter the bloodstream. After multiplication in the blood stream, they are secreted by the liver into the gall-bladder and the intestine. Increasing concentrations of bacteria induce hyperplasia of the lymphoid tissue of Peyer's patches and mesenteric lymphadenitis. The lymphoid tissue becomes infiltrated with large deeply staining macrophages containing intracellular organisms (so-called typhoid cells or Mallory's cells), plasma cells, and lymphocytes. Neutrophils are rare. Endotoxins cause tissue necrosis which can extend toward the muscularis propria, and vascular thrombosis. The entire ileum and colon become inflamed and hyperemic. Ulcerations appear predominantly in the ileum but also in the colon. The lesions can lead to intestinal hemorrhage and single or multiple perforations of the ileum (in up to 3% of the patients), often on the anti-mesenteric surface. Bacteremia originating from the lymphoid tissue can result in liver lesions (swelling and fatty change of hepatocytes), "typhoid nodules" composed of macrophages, and diffuse inflammatory changes with hepatosplenomegaly, splenomegaly, and bone marrow involvement. In the spleen, the red pulp is congested and contains aggregates of macrophages. The white pulp may be hyperplastic. Other organ systems such as the lungs, central nervous system, and skin may also develop significant lesions. Mild interstitial pneumonitis, "ring" hemorrhages in the brain, and capillary microthrombi can be seen. Skin lesions are characterized by a perivascular mononuclear cell infiltrate. The heart can be dilated, and cardiac myocytes may contain lipid vacuoles. Zenker's degeneration of skeletal muscle may be severe in untreated patients and is most prominent in muscles of the chest, diaphragm, abdomen, and thigh. Nephritis, orchitis, osteitis, and arthritis have also been reported. Bacteria will be discharged from the liver into the biliary tract, thereby infecting the gall-bladder and duodenum. Pancreatitis is rarely observed. During the late phases, oval ulcers are seen in the intestine, oriented along the long axis of the bowel. The ulcer base consists of granulation tissue. Ultimately, the intestine returns to normal with minimal scarring of the mucosa. Adhesions are rarely formed.

Immunophenotype

In humans, attenuated strains of *Salmonella* induce a variety of cell-mediated immune responses, resulting in long-lasting immunological memory. Serum and mucosal responses are directed toward a broad spectrum of antigens including "Vi (for virulence), a heat labile antigen which renders the strain non-agglutinable in the presence of the "O" specific antigen, porins, outer membrane proteins, lipoproteins, heat-shock proteins, flagella, and fimbriae". Cellular responses are of Th1 type. Class Ib CD8+ T cells capable of lysing *Salmonella*-infected target cells also appear after oral vaccination. T-cell responses are directed toward several antigens, including protein antigens, porins, flagellar epitomes, pilin, and to the Vi antigen. T cells modulate humoral responses during immunization with live attenuated *Salmonella* vaccines.

Molecular Features

Salmonella enterica serovar Typhi are gram-negative bacteria that utilize glucose, maltose, and mannitol in culture. The molecular mechanisms of pathogenicity are complex. Pathogenic *Salmonella* are distinguished from their non-pathogenic relatives by the presence of specific pathogenicity genes, often organized in so-called pathogenicity islands (PIs). The type III secretion system (T3SS) proteins encoded by two *Salmonella* PIs (SPIs) are associated with pathogenicity at the molecular level. The T3SS encoded by SPI-1 contains invasion genes, while SPI-2 is probably responsible for intracellular survival and has a crucial role for systemic infections.

Differential Diagnosis

The diagnosis of typhoid fever is made by isolating the pathogen in blood cultures, stool cultures (which are often negative in the first week), or bone marrow cultures. The Widal test measuring antibodies against the O and H antigens is more time consuming. A polymerase chain reaction on blood samples can provide an early diagnosis. Differential diagnosis includes malaria, bacterial endocarditis, appendicitis, relapsing fever, military tuberculosis, trichinosis, and meningitis as well as intestinal bacterial infections caused by *S. choleraesuis*, *Yersinia*, and *Campylobacter*.

References and Further Reading

Anita, S., Amir, K. M., Fadzilah, K., Ahamad, J., Noorhaida, U., Marina, K., Paid, M. Y., & Hanif, Z. (2012). Risk factors for typhoid outbreak in Sungai Congkak Recreational park, Selangor 2009. *The Medical Journal of Malaysia, 67*, 12–16.

Geboes, K. (2013). Inflammatory disorders of the small intestine. In N. A. Shepherd, B. F. Warren, G. T. Williams, J. K. Greenson, G. Y. Lauwers, & M. R. Novelli (Eds.), *Morson and Dawson's gastrointestinal pathology* (pp. 315–372). Oxford: Wiley-Blackwell.

Johnson, K. J. (2012). CDC updates recommendations for typhoid vaccination. *Clinical Infectious Diseases, 54*, 5–6.

Kaur, J., & Jain, S. K. (2012). Role of antigens and virulence factors of Salmonella enteric serovar Typhi in its pathogenesis. *Microbiological Research, 167*, 199–210.

Khan, M. I., Sajid Bashir Soofi, R., Ochiai, L., Khan, M. J., Sahito, S. M., Habib, M. A., Puri, M. K., von Seidlein, L., Park, J. K., You, Y. A., Ali, M., Nizami, Q., Acosta, C. J., Sack, R. B., Clemens, J. D., & Bhutta, Z. A. (2012). Epidemiology, clinical presentation, and patterns of drug resistance of *Salmonella typhi* in Karachi, Pakistan. *Journal of Infection in Developing Countries, 6*, 704–714.

Sabitha, P., Prabha Adhikari, M. R., Chowdary, A., Prabhu, M., Soofi, M., Shetty, M., Kamath, A., Lokaranjan, S. S., & Bangera, S. S. (2004). Comparison of the immunogenicity and safety of two different brands of *Salmonella typhi* VI capsular polysaccharide vaccine. *Indian Journal of Medical Sciences, 58*, 141–149.

Smith, J. H. (1976). Typhoid fever. In C. H. Binford & D. H. Connor (Eds.), *Pathology of tropical and extraordinary diseases* (pp. 123–129). Washington, DC: Armed Forces Institute of Pathology.

U

Ulcerative Colitis

Ann Driessen
Department of Pathology, University Hospital Antwerp, Edegem, Belgium
Maastricht University Medical Centre, Maastricht, The Netherlands

Synonyms

Colitis ulcerosa

Definition

Ulcerative colitis is a chronic inflammatory process of the colon, beginning in the rectum and extending proximally in the colon. This inflammatory process is continuous and normally limited to the mucosa. In case of pancolitis, the inflammation may involve the first centimeters of the ileum, the so-called backwash ileitis. Rarely, a left-sided colitis is associated with an area of inflammation in the caecum, named the caecal patch.

The pathogenesis of ulcerative colitis is not fully elucidated. It is a multifactorial process, in which besides genetic factors, other factors such as the innate immune system and environmental factors, in particular the intestinal flora, play a role. Genome-wide association studies have shown that in ulcerative colitis, numerous genes are involved. These genes are responsible for different functions such as the maintenance of epithelial integrity, innate immune function, immune regulatory function, and in cellular homeostasis. In ulcerative colitis, the intestinal epithelial barrier is damaged, leading to an increased permeability with an increased uptake of luminal antigens. The disease is characterized by an aberrant immune response against commensal non-pathogenetic bacteria. This immune response consists of an atypical Th2 response mediated by natural killer T-cells, producing different cytokines, involved in the development of epithelial damage and tissue injury. These cytokines are essential as blocking them prevents the development of ulcerative colitis. Numerous leukocytes, recruited from the systemic circulation by release of chemoattractants, are involved in the inflammatory response, characteristic for this disease.

The natural history of the disease is characterized by periods of remission and relapse. Ulcerative colitis patients present with a variety of symptoms. Classical features are rectal bleeding, diarrhea, urgency, and tenesmus. Patients have a vague abdominal discomfort or abdominal cramping. Abdominal pain is mostly not pronounced except in case of severe inflammation. Moderate fever is only present in patients having severe attacks. Up to 35% patients may show some extra-intestinal manifestations such as

F. Carneiro et al. (eds.), *Pathology of the Gastrointestinal Tract*, Encyclopedia of Pathology,
DOI 10.1007/978-3-319-40560-5

peripheral arthritis, erythema nodosum, or primary sclerosing cholangitis.

As the onset of ulcerative colitis is usually slow and insidious, the diagnosis of the disease is commonly delayed. Less than 10% of the patients have severe symptoms at first presentation. The disease may have an acute begin in patients in which the diagnosis of ulcerative colitis is made after a gastrointestinal infection.

The diagnosis of ulcerative colitis requires a multidisciplinary approach, based on clinical information, laboratory data, endoscopy, and pathological examination. Laboratory tests comprise a stool examination, to exclude an infection, and blood examination, including, e.g., total blood count, blood sedimentation rate, c-reactive protein to evaluate the degree of inflammation and the disease activity. Different imaging modalities are used for diagnosis, evaluation of the disease extent, and severity, and to investigate for possible complications. Computer tomography (CT scan) is considered to be the gold standard for assessment of the disease extent and severity and the detection of complications, such as a perforation or an abscess in the neighborhood of the bowel. Ultrasound and magnetic resonance imaging however are more preferred in young age people, because of the absence of risk of radiation. Plain abdominal radiography is used to determine the extent of the colitis, to exclude the possibility of a toxic megacolon or a perforation. Endoscopy with tissue sampling is performed to exclude other causes of inflammation, to subtype the inflammatory bowel disease, to determine the extent of the disease and to assess its severity, to evaluate the response on medical therapy or to exclude a malignancy. The endoscopic appearance of the mucosa differs in function of the severity of the disease. The mucosa has a granular, erythematous, and friable aspect in mild cases. If the intensity of the inflammation increases, the mucosa shows superficial ulcerations with spontaneous bleeding. The mucosa has numerous pseudopolyps, which are the result of the course of the disease, characterized by remission and relapse.

Clinical Features

- **Incidence**
  Ulcerative colitis is more prevalent than Crohn's disease in Western countries. The highest incidence and prevalence rates are found in North America and Northern Europe, with an incidence between 9 and 20 cases per 100,000 person-years and prevalence between 156 and 291 cases per 100,000 person-years. Recent studies have shown that the incidence and prevalence in Southern Europe is increased to rates similar to as in Northern Europe. Other parts of the world such Asia, Africa, and Latin America have the lowest incidence and prevalence rates. The occurrence of ulcerative colitis is related to some socioeconomic and lifestyle factors, in which this disease is more common in industrialized than in less developed countries, in urban than in rural areas, in people with a high socioeconomic status.

  Genetic factors are also important, in which a family history of inflammatory bowel disease is the most important risk factor: Patients with this disease will have in up to 15% a first-degree relative with the same disease.

  Other environmental factors are cigarette smoking, which has a protective effect, whereas an acute intestinal infection with *Salmonella spp*, *Shigella spp* increases the risk of development of ulcerative colitis.
- **Age**
  The age-distribution of ulcerative colitis has a bimodal pattern, with the highest peak between 15 and 30 years and second smaller peak between 50 and 70 years.
- **Sex**
  Ulcerative colitis has no obvious gender predilection, except in some studies a slight predominance in man.
- **Site**
  Classically, ulcerative colitis is a diffuse and continuous chronic inflammation without skip-areas, which always involves the rectum, spreading proximally. The severity of the inflammatory process gradually decreases

proximally. The inflammation may be confined to the rectum, presenting as proctitis, or extending throughout the colon as a pancolitis. The most common distribution patterns are pancolitis (19%), left-sided colitis (39%), proctosigmoiditis (17%), and proctitis (25%). Involvement of the ileum is uncommon except in case of a pancolitis, in which the inflammation may spread a few centimeters into the ileum, a condition named backwash ileitis.

- **Treatment**

  The treatment of ulcerative colitis consists of medical or surgical therapy. The therapy choice is based on several factors, namely, the severity of the inflammatory process and its extent, the course of the disease during follow-up, complications, and extra-intestinal manifestations.

  The first-line treatment consists of sulfasalazine and 5-aminosalicylates, which may achieve a clinical remission in approximately half of the patients. In case of failure, other drugs such as glucocorticoids or immunosuppressive agents such as azathioprine should be administered. Patients with extensive, severe disease are treated with intravenous glucocorticoids, but in case of unresponsiveness, cyclosporine and especially infliximab is the therapy of choice. In case, remission is achieved, the aim of medical therapy is to maintain this symptom-free condition in the patient. First choice is 5-aminosalicylates and if not effective immunosuppressives, such as azathioprine, or infliximab. Higher rates of remission and improvement on endoscopy, as well as lower rates of colectomy, are achieved with this drug.

  A colectomy, performed in approximately 5–20% of the ulcerative colitis patients, is indicated in different circumstances such as failure of medical therapy, perforation, toxic megacolon, uncontrollable bleeding, strictures, unresectable high-grade or multifocal dysplasia, and cancer. Nowadays, the surgical therapy of choice is a total proctocolectomy with an ileal pouch-anal anastomosis.

- **Outcome**

  The natural history of the disease is characterized by periods of remission and relapse. In function of the pattern of disease activity, the disease has a variable course in time with a complete clinical remission or only mild symptoms. The disease however is characterized by flares and even progression toward a fulminant colitis. In the latter, these patients may be unresponsive to medical therapy and requiring surgery. Several factors determine the risk of relapse such as fever, weight loss, active disease 1 year before relapse, or a short period of less than 2 years between diagnosis and first flare.

  Approximately 20–25% of the patients with distal colitis will show progression, with extension of the disease proximally during the course of their disease. Pancolitis is mostly seen in patients with a severe active disease. The disease extent determines also the risk of a colectomy: Patients with a proctitis have 3–4 times lower risk than those with more extensive disease.

  The overall mortality from UC is not higher than that of the general population. However, the mortality is increased in some subgroups, such as those with extensive disease.

  Patients with long-standing ulcerative colitis are at an increased risk for developing colorectal cancer: A meta-analysis has shown that the risk of CRC is 2% at 10 years, 8% at 20 years, and 18% at 30 years of disease. The incidence of CRC in the UC is approximately 4/1,000 per person year of disease, with an average prevalence of 3.5%. The strongest risk factors for the development of colorectal cancer are the duration of the disease and the extent of the disease. Other risk factors are a family history of colorectal cancer, the onset of colitis at young age, the severity of disease activity, and primary sclerosing cholangitis. Therefore, the American Gastroenterology Association recommends a thorough follow-up with sampling of multiple biopsies starting 8 years after onset of symptoms, repeated every 1–3 years.

Macroscopy

The mucosa in ulcerative colitis has a friable granular appearance with presence of superficial ulcers (Fig. 1). In severe disease, these ulcers may become more extensive, undermining the mucosa, finally resulting in a denudation of the surface. Extensive ulceration with sparing of the remaining islands of mucosa will result in the development of inflammatory pseudopolyps. These inflammatory polyps, which reflect healing of the mucosa, are slightly elevated nodules or occasionally finger-like projections of submucosa, covered with mucosa. They are common in sigmoid and descending colon, and rare in the rectum.

The transition between the involved and normal mucosa is sharp in ulcerative colitis. As the inflammation is normally restricted to the mucosa, no signs of serositis are observed except in case of a fulminant colitis. In fulminant colitis, the macroscopic appearance of the mucosa is not sufficiently distinct to differentiate ulcerative colitis from Crohn's disease. In case of toxic megacolon, the colon has a very thin attenuated bowel with complete loss of the mucosal folding pattern, due to the enormous dilatation.

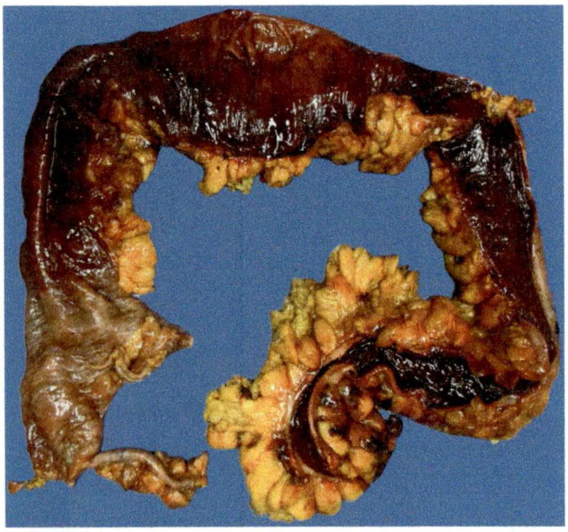

Ulcerative Colitis, Fig. 1 A gross specimen of ulcerative colitis, involving nearly the whole colon with sparing of the caecum

Unusual inflammation patterns are rectal sparring, caecal patch, and backwash ileitis. Rectal sparing is diagnosed in approximately 30% of untreated children with ulcerative colitis, and in adults with fulminant colitis (13%) or in patients (44%), undergoing either topical or systemic treatment. Patchiness is also a therapy-effect, a change from a continuous to a discontinuous inflammation.

In case of a "caecal patch," a left-sided colitis is associated with an inflammation in the caecum, surrounding the appendix. In between, the colonic mucosa is spared. Discontinuous periappendiceal inflammation has been diagnosed in up to 37% and 75% of the histopathological and endoscopic examinations. Awareness of these abnormal distribution patterns is important to avoid a misdiagnosis of Crohn's disease in a patient with ulcerative colitis.

Backwash ileitis is observed in patients with a pancolitis, in which the inflammation is not restricted to the colon, but there is limited involvement of the ileum.

In long-standing ulcerative colitis, tissue repair is associated with fibrosis, restricted to mucosa or submucosa. This fibrosis induces strictures in 3.2% up to 11.2% of cases.

Microscopy

The histological diagnosis of ulcerative colitis is most commonly made on biopsies. In order to improve the accuracy of the diagnosis, it is recommended to perform an ileocolonoscopy with adequate sampling of multiple biopsies of different segments of the bowel. As the topography of the lesions is essential, it is necessary to collect these samples, which are analyzed on semi-serial sections, in separate vials. Endoscopic data and clinical information, such as age, the duration of the disease, and the type of therapy, is important for a reliable diagnosis of ulcerative colitis.

Ulcerative colitis is a diffuse or continuous inflammatory process, restricted to the mucosa with disturbance of the crypt architecture (Fig. 2). Characteristically, the intensity of the

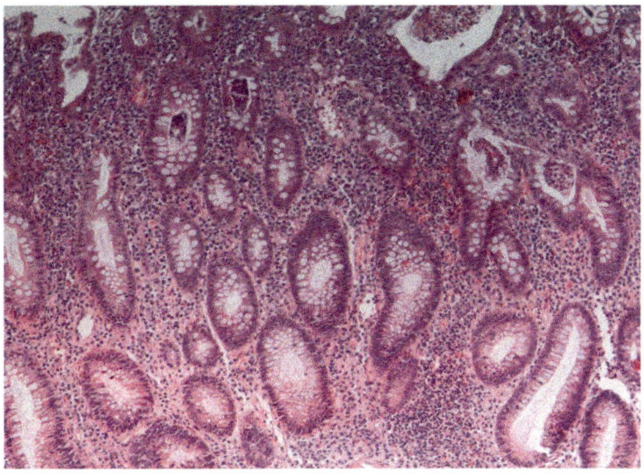

Ulcerative Colitis, Fig. 2 The colon has a disturbed crypt architecture with presence of a diffuse lymphoplasmocytic infiltrate, intermingled with eosinophils and neutrophils. These neutrophils infiltrate some crypts, causing crypt abscesses (H/E, 200×)

inflammation increases toward the rectum. The inflammatory infiltrate is composed of lymphocytes, plasma cells, and neutrophils, of which the latter penetrate into crypts, causing cryptitis and crypt abscesses. The plasma cells are predominantly situated between the base of the crypts and the muscularis mucosae (basal plasmocytosis). At the transition mucosa to submucosa lymphoid aggregates are seen. Due to this chronic inflammatory process the architecture is disturbed, with crypt branching, crypt distortion, crypt atrophy, and an irregular villous mucosal surface. The inflammation may also cause some epithelial changes such as a loss of goblet cells with mucin depletion of the epithelium. Other features of chronicity are Paneth cell metaplasia, inflammatory pseudopolyps, hypertrophy of the muscularis mucosae, and the rarely present (of seldom seen) submucosal fibrosis. Occasionally, pyloric metaplasia is found in the biopsies, but this feature is more common in Crohn's disease.

The morphologic features of ulcerative colitis may change in function of treatment and age. Due to treatment, the normal distribution pattern of the inflammation may change from continuous to discontinuous with patchiness and rectal sparing. Eventually the inflamed mucosa may completely normalize after therapy. Clinical information about the treatment is necessary to avoid misdiagnosis of the subtype of inflammatory bowel disease.

In approximately 15% of the cases, the diagnosis of ulcerative colitis is made below the age of 18 years. The histological diagnosis is however not easy, as biopsies from children under 10 years of age show a colonic mucosa with significantly less crypt branching, plasma cells in the lamina propria, cryptitis, crypt abscesses, and epithelial injury when compared with adults. As children approach adulthood, the morphological features are similar to those found in adults.

In case patients are treated with immunosuppressives because of a flare of their disease, a reactivation of a latent cytomegalovirus infection may occur. A CMV infection in ulcerative colitis patients, of which the prevalence varies between 10% and 56.7%, is possibly due to the Th2-immune response, in which the involved cytokines are inefficient in the control of this viral reactivation. The prevalence is even higher in steroid-refractory (25–30%) versus non-refractory ulcerative colitis patients (0–9.5%). Detection of cytomegalovirus should therefore routinely be performed in case of flares or unresponsiveness to treatment. Although CMV viral inclusions may be detected on H/E-stained slides, immunohistochemistry and molecular techniques, such as semiquantitative PCR, are more accurate diagnostic tests.

Differential Diagnosis

The most important differential diagnosis is Crohn's disease. Distinction is important, as the treatment of the disease, e.g., surgical approach, is different. Whereas ulcerative colitis is a transmucosal, diffuse and continuous inflammatory process, Crohn's disease is a transmural inflammatory process, discontinuous and variable in intensity. The inflammation may spread outside the bowel, inducing the formation of the fissures, sinuses, and fistulous tracts. Granulomas are found in approximately 50% of the biopsies. In ulcerative colitis, granulomas are not found, except in association with a ruptured crypt. Both

U

diseases are characterized by a different distribution pattern. Ulcerative colitis begins at the level of the rectum and extends proximally. The intensity of the inflammation increases toward the rectum. Involvement of the ileum is uncommon except in patients with a pancolitis. Crohn's disease may affect the whole gastrointestinal tract.

The outcome and the therapeutic approach of infectious colitis and ulcerative colitis are different, but distinction can be difficult especially in an early stage ulcerative colitis. In contrast to ulcerative colitis, the crypt architecture is preserved in infectious colitis. The lamina propria is infiltrated by numerous neutrophils, but invasion of the crypts is uncommon. In contrast to ulcerative colitis (63%), basal plasmocytosis is rarely seen in an infectious colitis (6%).

Ischemic colitis may resemble ulcerative colitis with presence of a disturbed crypt architecture and inflammation. The clinical presentation such as age is different. Features in favor of ischemic colitis is the distribution pattern of the lesions, the involvement of the deeper layers of the bowel wall with presence of hemosiderin macrophages in these layers, and the absence of cryptitis or crypt abscesses.

References and Further Reading

Danese, S., & Fiocchi, C. (2011). Ulcerative colitis. *The New England Journal of Medicine, 365*, 1713–1725.

Fenoglio-Preiser, C. M., Noffsinger, A. E., Stemmermann, G. N., Lantz, P. E., & Isaacson, P. G. (2008). *Gastrointestinal pathology. An atlas and text* (3rd ed.). Philadelphia: Lippincott, Williams & Wilkins.

Geboes, K. (2009). What histologic features differentiate Crohn's disease from ulcerative colitis? *Inflammatory Bowel Diseases, 14*, S168–S169.

Magro, F., Langner, C., Driessen, A., Ensari, A., Geboes, K., Mantzaris, G. J., Villanacci, V., Becheanu, G., Nunes, P. B., Cathomas, G., Fries, W., Jouret-Mourin, A., Mescoli, C., de Petris, G., Rubio, C. A., Shepherd, N. A., Vieth, M., & Eliakim, R. (2013). European consensus on the histopathology of inflammatory bowel disease. *Journal of Crohns and Colitis, 7*, 827–851.

Odze, R. D., & Goldblum, J. R. (2009). *Surgical pathology of the GI tract, liver, biliary tract, and pancreas* (2nd ed.). Philadelphia: Saunders/Elsevier.

Ordas, I., Eckmann, L., Talamini, M., Baumgart, D. C., & Sandborn, W. J. (2012). Ulcerative colitis. *Lancet, 380*, 1606–1619.

Uremic Gastropathy

Elisabete Rios and Francisco Ferro de Beça
Department of Pathology, Centro Hospitalar de São João, Porto, Portugal
Faculty of Medicine of the University of Porto, Porto, Portugal
IPATIMUP – Institute of Pathology and Molecular Immunology of the University of Porto, Porto, Portugal

Synonyms

Uremic gastritis

Definition

Uremic gastropathy is a term commonly used to describe the upper gastrointestinal signs and histopathologic changes associated with uremia, secondary to renal failure.

The clinical spectrum of upper gastrointestinal disorders in the uremic patients varies widely, since it might be influenced by several factors, such as the severity of renal function impairment, the stress level of the patients, and the assigned treatment. Gastrointestinal (GI) bleeding and dyspeptic symptoms, such as anorexia, vomiting, heartburn, and postprandial fullness, are common in these patients, although they may have no symptoms (Nardone et al. 2005). Uremic fetor (ammonia or urine-like odor to the breath) also may be present. Endoscopic and histological lesions are more frequent in symptomatic patients but may also be present in asymptomatic subjects (Khazaei et al. 2008). Hemorrhagic gastropathy is the most prevalent lesion, particularly in patients receiving chronic hemodialysis or in the setting of acute renal failure. It is mostly due to mucosal lesions, with gastroduodenal erosions and/or peptic ulcers detected in up to 67% of patients (Walker et al. 2004). Other uncommon disorders such as esophagitis, gastric angiodysplasia, and inflammatory gastric polyps have also been described (Sotoudehmanesh et al. 2003).

Underlying mechanisms and factors contributing to the development of these gastropathies remain unclear. In acute renal failure (ARF), gastropathy is thought to be more likely related to physiologic stress, with additional factors that increase the risk of bleeding such as NSAIDs, liver disease, and other comorbidities (Walker et al. 2004). Hypergastrinemia, gastrointestinal dysmotility, and acid secretion alterations are considered to be key factors in the pathophysiology of gastrointestinal lesions in patients with chronic renal failure (CRF). Possible mechanisms for dysmotility include increased levels of hormones involved in the modulation of gastrointestinal motility (e.g., cholecystokinin, gastrin, and neurotensin) and other humoral disorders (hypercalcemia, hypokalemia, and acidosis), that are mainly ascribed to the reduced renal clearance as well as autonomic nervous system dysfunction. The mechanisms that lead to hypergastrinemia are commonly attributed to reduced renal clearance but may also be due to a feedback mechanism from gastric acid neutralization with gastric ammonia, a breakdown product of urea that is higher in gastric mucus among patients with advanced renal failure (Nardone et al. 2005).

This concept has been used as substrate by several investigators (Khazaei et al. 2008) to explain the high susceptibility of these patients to colonization of *Helicobacter pylori* (HP). These linkage stems from the notion that HP possesses a powerful urease, which converts urea to ammonia and, thus, provides protection against the low pH of the gastric environment. Since uremic patients have an increased level of gastric urea in gastric mucus, they might be more susceptible to HP infection. However, the reported prevalence of HP infection and its relationship to upper GI pathologic changes in uremic patients have been controversial. While some studies have demonstrated a higher prevalence of HP infection in uremic patients (Khazaei et al. 2008), others have determined that the prevalence of the infection is less than in the general population (Day et al. 2003).

Clinical Features

- **Incidence**
  The reported prevalence of uremic gastropathy in the uremic patients is quite varied, there being a wide range of between 7% and 100% (Nardone et al. 2005; Khazaei et al. 2008).
- **Age**
  Prevalence of uremia and subsequently uremic gastropathy among different age groups is largely unknown. Several reports demonstrate it can affect both adults and children, being more prevalent in older adults (Khazaei et al. 2008).
- **Sex**
  Uremia is slightly more prevalent in men than in women (male-to-female ratio, 1.2:1). Sotoudehmanesh et al. (2003) reported that male gender had higher risk of uremic gastropathy.
- **Site**
  Up to 67% of uremic patients lesions occur in the stomach and duodenum, with gastric lesions predominantly in the antrum (approx. 50%).
- **Treatment**
  Treatment of uremic gastropathy relies on the resolution of uremia, which can be accomplished by medical treatment for associated metabolic and electrolyte abnormalities, such as anemia, hyperkalemia, hypocalcaemia, hyperparathyroidism, and iron deficiency. When these treatments fail, renal replacement therapy with hemodialysis, peritoneal dialysis, or renal transplantation is the treatment of choice.

  Other therapeutic interventions include dietary changes and hemostatic procedures, in case of uremic bleeding.
- **Outcome**
  Uremic gastropathy can be a significant cause of morbidity and mortality, likely due to the considerable risk of complicated upper GI lesion in uremic patients, namely, acute upper GI bleeding, despite its rarity. Increased prevalence of peptic ulcers after renal transplantation is reported historically, having accounted for approximately 4% of deaths (Walker et al.

2004). However, the use of acid-suppression therapies and corticosteroid-sparing immunosuppressive regimens has reduced the frequency of this complication.

Macroscopy

Upper gastrointestinal endoscopy features are variable and include erythema, multiple small petechial hemorrhages, erosions, ulcerations, and nodularity in either the stomach or duodenum or, less frequently, in the esophagus (Walker et al. 2004; Khazaei et al. 2008). Gastric and duodenal angiodysplastic lesions as well as gastric polyps have also been reported (Sotoudehmanesh et al. 2003). Hypertrophic folds in mucosa of the corpus may frequently be associated with successful kidney transplantation (Day et al. 2003). Normal findings on endoscopy can occur with uremic gastropathy; nevertheless, histological evaluation of blindly collected biopsies can identify epithelial lesions within normal-appearing mucosa.

Microscopy

Characteristic findings of uremic gastropathy include foveolar hyperplasia, multinucleated parietal cells with vacuolation and fragmentation of the cytoplasm, and extension of parietal cells into the antrum and even the duodenum. This may be related to long-term steroid therapy and the trophic effects of hypergastrinemia. In addition, heterotopic calcification within the gastric mucosa may occur. *Helicobacter pylori* organisms may be seen on H&E staining in some cases; identification is enhanced with special stains (Giemsa, Diff-Quik, immunohistochemistry, or silver stain). The increased incidence of CMV infection should be considered in patients receiving immunosuppression therapy (Day et al. 2003).

Differential Diagnosis

The main disease to consider in establishing a differential diagnosis, especially based on biopsy specimens, is chronic gastritis. A firm diagnosis can only be made when supportive clinical data (such as known history of uremia) are available.

References and Further Reading

Day, D. W., Jass, J. R., Price, A. B., Shepherd, N. A., Sloan, J. M., Talbot, I. C., Warren, B. F., Williams, G. T., et al. (2003). *Morson and Dawson's gastrointestinal pathology* (4th ed.). Malden: Blackwell Science.

Khazaei, M. R., Imanieh, M. H., & Hosseini Al-Hashemi, G. (2008). Gastrointestinal evaluation in pediatric kidney transplantation candidates. *Iranian Journal of Kidney Diseases, 2*, 40–45.

Nardone, G., Rocco, A., Fiorillo, M., Del Pezzo, M., Autiero, G., Cuomo, R., Sarnelli, G., Lambiase, A., Budillon, G., & Cianciaruso, B. (2005). Gastroduodenal lesions and *Helicobacter pylori* infection in dyspeptic patients with and without chronic renal failure. *Helicobacter, 10*, 53–58.

Sotoudehmanesh, R., Ali Asgari, A., Ansari, R., & Nouraie, M. (2003). Endoscopic findings in end-stage renal disease. *Endoscopy, 35*, 502–505.

Walker, W. A., Durie, P. R., Kleinman, R., & Walker-Smith, J. A. (2004). *Pediatric gastrointestinal disease, pathophysiology, diagnosis and management* (4th ed.). Philadelphia: BC Decker.

V

Varices

Isadora Rosa and António Dias Pereira
Instituto Português de Oncologia de Lisboa
Francisco Gentil, E.P.E., Lisboa, Portugal

Synonyms

Plural of varix

Definition

Varices are pathologically dilated veins. In the digestive system, they are more common in the esophagus or stomach and usually secondary to portal hypertension. They are mostly asymptomatic unless they rupture and bleed.

The portal venous system carries blood from the spleen and digestive system to the liver, where it converges with hepatic artery-derived blood flow in the hepatic sinusoids. If the pressure in these specialized vascular channels increases to 6 mmHg or above, portal hypertension will occur.

Portal hypertension may be due to an increase in portal flow and/or in portal resistance. The increased resistance may be posthepatic, as in Budd-Chiari syndrome; intrahepatic, as in liver cirrhosis; or prehepatic, as in portal vein thrombosis. Cirrhosis is the most common cause of portal hypertension in the western world. Whatever the cause, portal hypertension leads to the expansion of portal vein-systemic collaterals and to reversion of the normal low volume flow in these vessels, with blood flowing out of the portal circulation and into the systemic veins. In the digestive system, the main collaterals are found around the gastroesophageal junction, and their expansion leads to the development of gastroesophageal varices. Varices that occur outside the gastroesophageal junction are called ectopic and include duodenal, colonic, rectal, and stomal varices, among others. When the hepatic venous pressure gradient (HVPG) exceeds 10 mmHg, varices form, but they usually only bleed when it exceeds 12 mmHg.

Clinically, varices usually only manifest when they bleed and the symptoms and signs will depend on their location. Hematemesis and melena are the most common presentations of esophageal, gastric, and duodenal varices bleeding, while rectal varices bleeding presents as hematochezia. Ectopic varices may also manifest with hemobilia, or hemoperitoneum, which may present as increased abdominal volume or abdominal pain. Variceal bleeding is frequently severe and may lead to hypovolemic shock and death.

The diagnosis of varices is usually endoscopic. Ectopic varices in sites not accessible to endoscopy may be diagnosed through angiography. International consensus guidelines state that all cirrhotic patients should be screened for gastroesophageal varices, by endoscopy, at the time of the initial diagnosis of cirrhosis. The initial findings will determine the follow-up (de Franchis and

F. Carneiro et al. (eds.), *Pathology of the Gastrointestinal Tract*, Encyclopedia of Pathology,
DOI 10.1007/978-3-319-40560-5

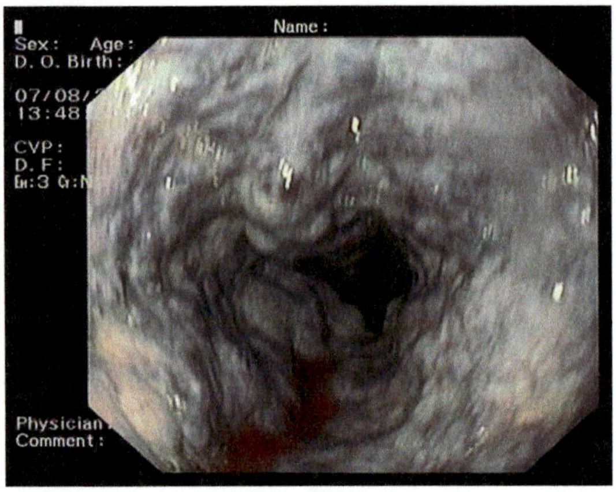

Varices, Fig. 1 Large esophageal varices seen at upper digestive endoscopy

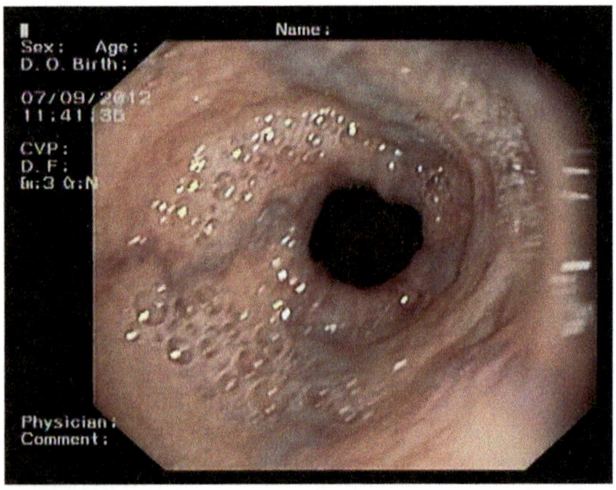

Varices, Fig. 2 Small esophageal varices seen at upper digestive endoscopy

Baveno V Faculty 2010). Esophageal varices are graded as none, small (those that flatten with insufflation or protrude minimally into the esophageal lumen), or large (those that are confluent, protruding into the esophageal lumen and touching each other) (de Franchis et al. 1992) (Figs. 1 and 2). Gastric varices should be described according to the classification by Sarin et al (Sarin et al. 1992). It includes gastroesophageal varices (those in continuity with esophageal varices) type 1 (extending 2–5 cm below the gastroesophageal junction) and type 2 (extending for more than 5 cm into the fundus) and isolated gastric varices type 1 (those that occur in the fundus in the absence of esophageal varices) or type 2 (those that occur in the body, antrum, or pylorus).

Clinical Features

- **Incidence**
  In cirrhosis, esophageal varices develop in 5–15% of patients each year, and therefore, most patients will develop them. About one third of varices will eventually bleed (de Franchis and Primignani 2001; Toubia and Sanyal 2008).
- **Age**
  Varices are usually diagnosed in adults, but may be found in children, in whom extrahepatic portal vein thrombosis is the main cause of portal hypertension.
- **Sex**
  Varices are found in both sexes.
- **Site**
  The esophagus is the most common site for varices. They are more common in the lower third but may extend full length.
- **Treatment**
  The management of varices is usually divided into several stages: prevention of their formation (preprimary prophylaxis), prevention of bleeding (primary prophylaxis), treatment of acute bleeding, and prevention of rebleeding (secondary prophylaxis).

  According to the latest Baveno consensus workshop (Baveno V) (de Franchis and Baveno V Faculty 2010), the only recommendation for preprimary prophylaxis is the treatment of the underlying disease causing portal hypertension.

  Regarding primary prophylaxis, patients with large esophageal varices should be treated by either endoscopic band ligation or nonselective beta-blockers (NSBB). In patients whose endoscopy shows small esophageal varices with red wales or with small varices and Child C class liver disease, NSBB should be used. Data regarding the benefit of NSBB in preventing the first bleeding episode in other patients is still insufficient.

  The management of an acute upper gastrointestinal variceal bleeding episode starts with volume restitution to maintain hemodynamic stability and includes antibiotic prophylaxis instituted from admission; the use of vasoactive drugs, started as soon as possible; and endoscopic therapy. Endoscopy should be performed within the first 12 h. Endoscopic variceal ligation is the recommended therapy for bleeding from esophageal varices and may also be used for GOV1. Sclerotherapy may be used for esophageal varices when ligation is technically difficult, while the use of a tissue adhesive is recommended for GOV2 and IGV. It may also be used for GOV1. Balloon tamponade may be used temporarily in massive bleeding, and an early transjugular intrahepatic portosystemic shunt is an option for high-risk patients.

Finally, for secondary prophylaxis, the use of NSBB associated with variceal ligation is the recommended approach in patients who have bled from esophageal varices. Patients who bled from GOV2 or IGV should be managed with tissue adhesive endoscopic therapy, while this therapy, ligation, or NSBB may be used for GOV1.

- **Outcome (Prognosis)**
  The estimated mortality rate for an episode of esophageal varices bleeding is 20–30% (de Franchis and Primignani 2001). The mortality risk is higher in the first 5 days and then slowly declines, but the rebleeding risk is 70% or larger (Toubia and Sanyal 2008).

  The occurrence of other complications of portal hypertension or of the bleeding episode and the greater severity of the underlying disease worsen the prognosis of patients with gastrointestinal varices.

Macroscopy (Gross)

Endoscopically, varices are seen as dilated vessels that protrude into the lumen, covered by normal appearing mucosa. Active bleeding through a rupture point may be seen. The presence of red signs over the varices signals an increased risk of bleeding, while after recent bleeding adherent clots may be found.

Microscopy

Varices are seen as dilated subepithelial veins. Inflammation and hemorrhage may be seen surrounding a ruptured varix.

Immunophenotype

There are no immunophenotype characteristics specifically associated with the development of varices.

Molecular Features

There are no molecular features specifically associated with the development of varices.

Differential Diagnosis

Varices are usually easily identified by endoscopy, and the differential diagnosis required regards the cause of the varices.

References and Further Reading

de Franchis, R., & Baveno, V. Faculty. (2010). Revising consensus in portal hypertension: Report of the Baveno V consensus workshop on methodology of diagnosis and therapy in portal hypertension. *Journal of Hepatology, 53*, 762–768.

de Franchis, R., & Primignani, M. (2001). Natural history of portal hypertension in patients with cirrhosis. *Clinics in Liver Disease, 5*, 645–663.

de Franchis, R., Pascal, J. P., Ancona, E., Burroughs, A. K., Henderson, M., Fleig, W., Groszmann, R., Bosch, J., Sauerbruch, T., Soederlund, C., et al. (1992). Definitions, methodology and therapeutic strategies in portal hypertension. A Consensus Development Workshop. *Journal of Hepatology, 15*, 256–261.

Sarin, S. K., Lahoti, D., Saxena, S. P., Murthi, N. S., & Makwane, U. K. (1992). Relation between portal pressure response to pharmacotherapy and risk of recurrent variceal haemorrhage in patients with cirrhosis. *Lancet, 346*, 1056–1059.

Toubia, N., & Sanyal, A. J. (2008). Portal hypertension and variceal hemorrhage. *The Medical Clinics of North America, 92*, 551–574.

Vasculitis, Upper Gastrointestinal

Susana Rodrigues
Serviço de Gastrenterologia, Centro Hospitalar de São João, Alameda Professor Hernani Monteiro, Porto, Portugal

Synonyms

Gastrointestinal angiitis; Gastrointestinal manifestations of vasculitis; Localized vasculitis of the gastrointestinal tract; Vasculitides of the gastrointestinal tract

Definition

Vasculitis is a general term for a group of uncommon diseases that are defined by inflammation of the blood vessel walls. Each of the vasculitis diseases has a characteristic distribution of blood vessels, pattern of organ involvement, and laboratory test abnormalities. The actual causes of vasculitides are unknown, but they are generally associated to an immune system abnormality. They are grouped as primary or secondary and localized or systemic. The primary systemic vasculitides are rare and affect blood vessels that may manifest as self-limiting illnesses with a good prognosis (e.g., childhood Henoch-Schonlein purpura) to multi-organ failure with a high rate of mortality if left untreated (e.g., Wegener's granulomatosis). Secondary vasculitides are those caused by underlying rheumatic connective tissue diseases (e.g., rheumatoid arthritis, systemic lupus erythematosus), inflammatory bowel disease, infection (e.g., Hepatitis B, *Neisseria meningitidi*), malignancy (lymphoma), and drugs. Localized vasculitis may affect only the skin or a single-organ system, whereas systemic vasculitides affect multiple organ systems. Vasculitis involving the gastrointestinal (GI) tract often occurs as part of a systemic inflammatory process and is an acknowledged manifestation of small- and medium-sized vessel vasculitides. The distinction between primary and secondary is not absolute because some cases of GI vasculitides that are initially diagnosed as localized may evolve into systemic disease.

GI involvement is frequent in Henoch-Schonlein purpura (HSP) and also often noted in polyarteritis nodosa (PAN), microscopic polyangiitis, Wegener's syndrome, and Churg-Strauss syndrome. Furthermore, GI vasculitis has also been described in giant cell arteritis, Takayasu's disease, Buerger's disease and leucocytoclastic vasculitides as essential mixed cryoglobulinemia, lupus vasculitis, rheumatoid disease, connective tissue diseases, drug-induced vasculitis, and Behçet's disease.

The primary systemic vasculitides are a heterogeneous group of rare disorders with many varying features and presentations. Specific GIT features of each disease reflect the size of vessels involved; large vessel vasculitis predominantly leading to ischemia or infarction of large sections of bowel; medium vessel vasculitides causing bleeding from and infarction of smaller areas; small-vessel vasculitides causing microvascular symptoms of tissue inflammation and patchy infarction with some incidence of bleeding.

Abdominal pain was the most frequent finding, present in almost all patients. The pain was usually intense, and no preferential site could be identified. Other findings were abdominal angina, nausea or vomiting, diarrhea, haematochezia, or melena. Weight loss was present in most patients and some may have fever.

The location, age and gender predominance, disease activity, and the involvement of the GIT vary with the vasculitis in question. Vasculitis may affect any part of the GI tract, but most frequently the appendix, gallbladder, and cecum. Classically, vasculitides are classified according to the size of vessels affected: large, medium, or small sized. Systemic vasculitis may affect various organs, including the GIT, while localized vasculitis is confined to the GIT. Focal single-organ vasculitis tends to have a good prognosis and resection of the vasculitic lesion can be curative, although it may progress to a systemic illness. In both localized and systemic forms, when present, GI complications adversely affect prognosis and are an indicator of disease severity.

Clinical Features

- **Incidence**
  Exclusive GI manifestations as the presenting symptom of vasculitis were found in only 1 of 62 patients from a series of systemic necrotizing vasculitides described by Pagnoux and coworkers. However, earlier series found that 13–16% of their patients had isolated GI involvement. In three series with a total of 351 patients, approximately one-third had gastrointestinal manifestations.
  Systemic vasculitides and the involvement of the GIT vary according to the specific disease in question. A description of the way the GIT is involved in the different systemic vasculitides will be made for each disease.
- **Primary Vasculitides**

Large Vessel Vasculitides

Takayasu's arteritis is a granulomatous disease of the aorta and its primary branches generally affect patients younger than 50 years. It is a rare disease, more common in Asia (Japan) and Mexico. The mesenteric vessels are involved in up to 12% of cases on angiography. Few reports describe major GIT symptoms or bowel ischemia; these include acute intestinal infarction, necrosis and postprandial mesenteric angina with chronic mesenteric and celiac ischemia.

Medium-Sized Vessel Vasculitides

Polyarteritis nodosa (PAN) is defined by necrotizing inflammation of small- and medium-sized vessels without nephritis or arteritis in arterioles, capillaries, or venules. It is frequently associated to hepatitis B virus infection and these patients have a higher risk of GIT complications such as perforation. Positivity to anti-neutrophil cytoplasm antibody (ANCA) may be associated. Patients may present with a variety of symptoms such as fever or weight loss, but 25–60% present with features of GIT vasculitis either at first presentation or during follow-up. Upper GIT features of PAN include: perforation or infarction of stomach or small bowel. The patient may present with nausea and vomiting, diarrhea, melena, or occult GIT bleeding.

Kawasaki's disease is an arteritis involving large, medium-sized, and small arteries, and associated with mucocutaneous lymph node syndrome. Coronary arteries are often involved. It usually occurs in children with a peak at 30 months. Some of the upper GIT features reported include paralytic ileus and hemorrhagic duodenitis.

Small Vessel Vasculitides

Henoch-Schonlein purpura (HSP) is a vasculitis with IgA-dominant immune deposits, affecting small vessels (i.e., capillaries, venules, or arterioles). HSP typically involves skin, gut, and glomeruli, and is associated with arthralgias or arthritis. It is predominantly a childhood disease, more frequent in children of Asian descent, and among males (2.5:1 ratio). The majority of patients develop abdominal angina and around a third may have GIT bleeding. Some GIT features of HSP in children are well documented and include: intussusception, small bowel ischemia and infarction, intestinal perforation, fistula formation, ileal strictures, and massive upper gastrointestinal hemorrhage. Colicky abdominal pain and GIT bleeding (either as melena or positive stool guaiac test) are among the most common manifestations. Individual case reports of GIT involvement in adults resemble cases in children.

ANCA-Associated Small Vessel Vasculitides

Wegener's granulomatosis (WG) is a granulomatous inflammation affecting the respiratory tract and necrotizing vasculitis affecting small- to medium-sized vessels (e.g., capillaries, venules, arterioles, and arteries) commonly associated with necrotizing glomerulonephritis. GI involvement of WG is rare and may include esophageal ulceration and small bowel perforation.

Churg-Strauss syndrome (CSS) is an eosinophil-rich and granulomatous inflammation involving the respiratory tract, and necrotizing vasculitis affecting small- to medium-sized vessels. Necrotizing vasculitis with few or no immune deposits, affecting small- and medium-sized arteries, may be present on histological examination. It is linked to asthma and eosinophilia. CSS can manifest as an upper GI bleed or perforation of the esophagus, stomach, or small intestine (Morgan and Savage 2005). GI symptoms can be present in a third of patients.

Microscopic polyangiitis is a necrotizing vasculitis with few or no immune deposits, affecting small vessels. Necrotizing arteritis affecting small- and medium-sized arteries may be present. The kidney and lung are the organs most frequently involved. GI manifestations are frequently found and include by abdominal pain and GI bleeding. Symptoms of melena and hematemesis may also be present. Regarding upper GI pathology, esophageal reflux has been detected in some patients.

Behcet's disease (BD) is a rare multisystem vasculitis typically characterized by the presence of genital, oral ulcerations and skin lesions. Typically the ileocecal region is the most affected where ulcerations may develop. Ischemia and bowel wall infarction may also arise from BD.

- **Secondary Vasculitides**
  Secondary vasculitides may develop in association to mixed connective tissue diseases, rheumatic diseases, inflammatory bowel disease, infectious diseases, malignancies, or drugs.

Systemic Lupus Erythematosus (SLE)

In patients with SLE who present with nonspecific abdominal pain, the incidence of GI vasculitis may be as high as 35%. Symptoms may include bloating, anorexia, postprandial fullness, diarrhea, upper GI bleeding, or acute abdominal pain. GI manifestations such as gastritis, enteritis, and bowel wall perforation have been described.

Mixed Connective Tissue Disease (MCTD)

MCTD is a combination of disorders, namely, of LES, scleroderma, and polymyositis. Therefore, it is sometimes referred to as an overlap disease and is associated with high titers of ribonucleotide (RNP) antibodies. Dysphagia and heartburn, bowel perforation, and malabsorption syndrome are some of the GI manifestations found. Although rare, there are reports of duodenal bleeding and esophageal dysmotility.

Infectious Disease and Malignancy-Related Vasculitis

Most infectious vasculitides are necrotizing or lymphocytic small-vessel vasculitis. Some of the microbial agents associated to vasculitis include hepatitis B, C, or A; human immunodeficiency virus; cytomegalovirus; and parvovirus B19.

Vasculitis in malignant diseases is generally associated with hematologic disorders rather than solid tumors, such as hairy cell leukemia.

Drugs, such as propylthiouracil and hydroxyurea, have been associated with intestinal vasculitis.

- **Localized Vasculitis**
  Vasculitis of the GI tract may occur in isolation, and may represent a form of single-organ vasculitis (SOV). Isolated vasculitis of the GI tract is a rare entity and tends to have a good prognosis. Its removal can be curative, although SOV may progress to a systemic illness. Isolated vasculitis of the upper GI tract generally manifests itself as gastroduodenal ulcers or bleeding.
- **Treatment**
  GI involvement in the setting of systemic necrotizing vasculitides has a poor prognosis, particularly when surgery is needed. Corticosteroid therapy alone is generally insufficient in the most severe cases and the use of immunosuppressive drugs is mandatory. These include methotrexate, azathioprine, mycophenolate mofetil, cyclophosphamide, and intravenous immunoglobulin Immunosuppressive drugs must not only be considered in steroid refractory

cases but also as first-line therapy for the most severe cases. Vascular intervention, whether angioplasty or surgical, may be necessary in more advanced cases.

- **Outcome**
  When present, GI complications adversely affect prognosis and are an indicator of disease severity.

Macroscopy

The findings at upper endoscopy may reveal small petechiae, multiple, irregular superficial gastric ulcerations without evidence of bleeding, bleeding duodenal ulcers, and ischemic changes in the duodenum and proximal jejunum.

Microscopy

Endoscopic biopsies have a low sensitivity to diagnose GI vasculitis, even though macroscopic endoscopic findings such as the presence of an erythematous hemorrhagic petechial mucosa may be suggestive. Upper GI tract biopsies are rarely helpful, but colon biopsies may contribute to establishing a specific diagnosis of vasculitis. The microscopic findings are variable depending on the etiology of the vasculitis. These may include: acute/chronic inflammation or necrosis of vessel walls, islands of fibrotic tissue and thrombus, necrotizing granulomas, multi-nucleated giant cells, and medial degeneration or hypertrophy.

Differential Diagnosis

The differential diagnosis of upper GI vasculitides comprises any cause of gastroduodenal ulceration, bleeding, or ischemia. Some common differentials are ► peptic ulcers and neoplastic ulceration caused by adenocarcinoma or lymphoma. Infections such as cytomegalovirus gastritis that manifest with multiple ulcers may mimic GI vasculitis. Although rare, gastroduodenal ischemia caused by vascular thrombosis may lead to lesions similar to vasculitis.

References and Further Reading

Ahn, E., Luk, A., Chetty, R., & Butany, J. (2009). Vasculitides of the gastrointestinal tract. *Seminars in Diagnostic Pathology, 26*, 77–88.

Jennette, J. C., Falk, R. J., Andrassy, K., et al. (1994). Nomenclature of systemic vasculitides. Proposal of an international consensus conference. *Arthritis and Rheumatism, 37*, 187–192.

Morgan, M. D., & Savage, O. S. (2005). Vasculitis in the gastrointestinal tract. *Best Practice & Research. Clinical Gastroenterology, 19*, 215–233.

Pagnoux, C., Mahr, A., Cohen, P., & Guillevin, L. (2005). Presentation and outcome of gastrointestinal involvement in systemic necrotizing vasculitides: Analysis of 62 patients with polyarteritis nodosa, microscopic polyangiitis, Wegener granulomatosis, Churg-Strauss syndrome, or rheumatoid arthritis-associated vasculitis. *Medicine, 84*, 115–128.

Salvarani, C., Calamia, K. T., Crowson, C. S., et al. (2010). Localized vasculitis of the gastrointestinal tract: A case series. *Rheumatology, 49*, 1326–1335.

Verrucous Carcinoma/Giant Condyloma of Buschke and Löwenstein

Denis Chatelain[1] and Jean-François Fléjou[2]
[1]Service d'Anatomie Pathologique, Centre Hospitalier et Universitaire du Nord, Amiens, France
[2]Faculté de Médecine Pierre et Marie Curie, Service d'Anatomie et Cytologie Pathologiques, Hôpital Saint-Antoine, Paris, France

Synonyms

Verrucous carcinoma and giant condyloma of Buschke and Löwenstein are identical lesions.

Definition

Verrucous carcinoma is nowadays assimilated by most authors as giant condyloma described by Buschke and Löwenstein. It is a particular variant of anal and perianal squamous cell carcinoma, characterized by its slow growing, and its

V

tendency to form abscesses and fistulae. It is associated with HPV6 and HPV11 infections.

Clinical Features

Patients usually present with a huge perianal oozing mass. The lesion has usually been present for many years and had a slow growth. Patients may also complain of anal pain, bleeding, pruritus, difficulty in walking and defecation, fistula, or perianal abscess.

- **Incidence**
  Anal verrucous carcinoma is a very rare tumor and it is difficult to assess its incidence.
- **Age**
  The mean age at presentation is 42 years (16–82 years).
- **Sex**
  The incidence in males is significantly higher than in females (ratio 3.2:1).
- **Site**
  Verrucous carcinoma often occurs in the perianal region and may extend toward the anal canal.
- **Treatment**
  Wide local excision remains the mainstay of therapy for verrucous carcinoma. It often needs grafts, and left colostomy is usually simultaneously performed in order to facilitate postoperative wound healing without the presence of feces.

  The efficacy of additional or other nonsurgical therapy modalities has not yet been established.

  The use of radiotherapy is controversial as it may favor its transformation into poorly differentiated carcinoma with subsequent metastasis. CO_2 laser therapy has sometimes been applied with success.
- **Outcome**
  Verrucous carcinoma is a slow-growing but locally aggressive and destructive tumor. Distant metastases are rare. This tumor has a high recurrence rate of 60–70% after radical local excision. The rate of malignant transformation to typical invasive squamous cell carcinoma ranges between 30% and 56%. The overall mortality is 20–30% due to mechanical obstruction, fistulas, abscesses, and sepsis.

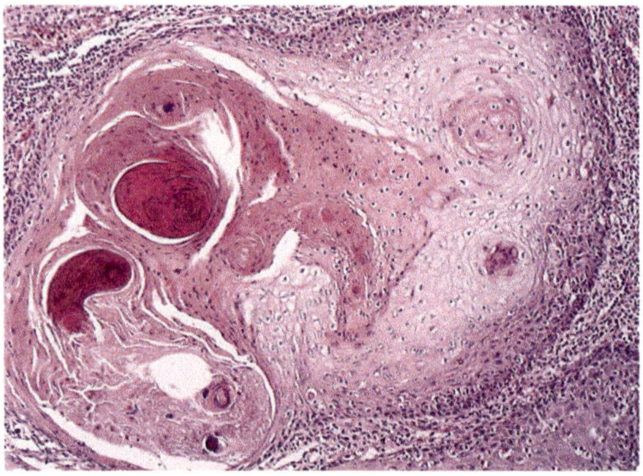

Verrucous Carcinoma/Giant Condyloma of Buschke and Löwenstein, Fig. 2 Verrucous squamous cell carcinoma of the anus, extremely well differentiated

Macroscopy

Verrucous carcinomas present as a unique or multiple confluent, friable masses, measuring several centimeters in diameter, with a cauliflower appearance and reddish, pinkish, or whitish color (Fig. 1). It displays a marked tendency to compress and displace deeper tissues by downward growth rather than infiltrating them. Fistulae and abscesses in the deeper tissues are frequent.

Microscopy

The histological appearance on a biopsy specimen may be identical to that seen in common condyloma acuminatum, with a surface hyperkeratosis, prominent acanthosis, and papillomatosis with orderly arrangement of the epithelial layers. The cells in the superficial and intermediate layers show koilocytotic changes. Hyperplastic epithelium penetrates into the underlying tissues in blunt downward projection and lobules, with keratin-filled cysts, sometimes inflamed with numerous neutrophils, with a pushing rather than an infiltrating pattern (Fig. 2). Diagnosis is difficult on superficial biopsies, and only complete excision

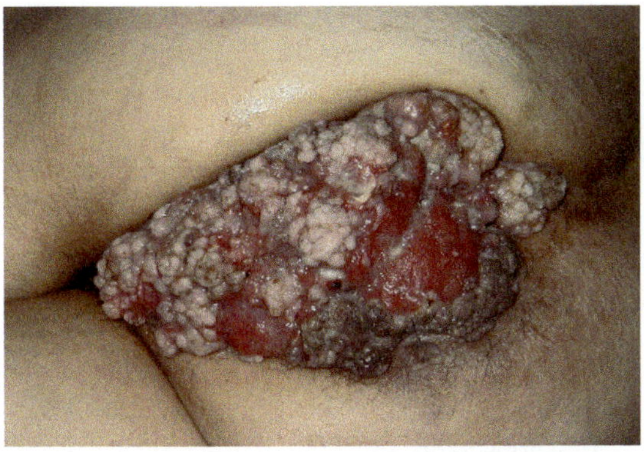

Verrucous Carcinoma/Giant Condyloma of Buschke and Löwenstein, Fig. 1 Verrucous carcinoma of the anus, presenting as a huge cauliflower-like lesion

of the lesions can sometimes provide a final pathological diagnosis.

Immunohistochemistry

In situ hybridization can confirm the presence of HPV6/11 in tumor cells. Tumor cells are positive for pan-cytokeratin and cytokeratin 5/6. Basal cells are positive for Ki67 and p53. They do no express p16 or with a faint focal positivity. No immunohistochemical stain is useful for the diagnosis or to exclude a differential diagnosis.

Molecular Features

Carcinogenesis of perianal verrucous carcinoma is still unclear, but principally linked to HPV 6 and HPV11 infection.

Differential Diagnosis

Verrucous carcinoma has the same microscopic appearance as condyloma acuminatum, notably on microscopic examination of a superficial biopsy. Clinical information about the macroscopic appearance of the tumor is essential for the pathologist in order to give the appropriate diagnosis. Verrucous carcinoma differs from the usual type of invasive squamous cell carcinoma by the lack of typical infiltrative pattern with a desmoplastic reaction surrounding carcinomatous lobules and by the absence of marked nuclear atypia of tumor cells and the lack of high mitotic activity. However, invasive squamous cell carcinoma can be observed in verrucous carcinoma. The diagnosis is sometimes made on macrobiopsy, or more frequently on pathological examination of a surgical specimen. The presence of severe cytologic atypia with stromal invasion in an infiltrative fashion (different from the pushing downward growth) should lead to the diagnosis of invasive squamous cell carcinoma.

References and Further Reading

Longacre, T. A., Kong, C. S., & Welton, M. L. (2008). Diagnostic problems in anal pathology. *Advances in Anatomic Pathology, 15*, 263–278.

Safi, F., Bekdache, O., Al-Salam, S., Alashari, M., Mazen, T., & El-Salhat, H. (2013). Management of peri-anal giant condylomaacuminatum – A case report and literature review. *Asian Journal of Surgery, 36*, 43–52.

Viral Colitis

Xavier Sagaert
Department of Pathology, University Hospitals KU Leuven, Leuven, Belgium

Definition

Viruses such as rotavirus and norovirus can cause colon inflammation, resulting in mild to severe dehydration. Rotavirus is a double-stranded RNA virus belonging to the family of Reoviridae. It is the most common cause of gastroenteritis in infants and young children worldwide. The virus is transmitted by the fecal-oral route. It produces a toxic rotavirus protein that damages the enterocytes of the small intestine and as such causes gastroenteritis (which is often called "stomach flu" despite having no relation to influenza). Symptoms of viral colitis are not

V

much different from colitis from other causes: The infection often starts with vomiting followed by a maximum of 10 days of profuse diarrhea. Dehydration is more common in rotavirus infection than in most of those caused by bacterial pathogens, and is the most common cause of death related to rotavirus infection. As healthy enterocytes secrete lactase into the small intestine, milk intolerance due to lactase deficiency is a symptom of rotavirus infection, which can persist for weeks.

Cytomegalovirus (CMV), a double-stranded DNA virus that is a member of the Herpesviridae family, is another virus that may cause colitis, especially in persons with lower immunity. As such, it is the most common viral cause of diarrhea in AIDS patients and may affect any part of the gastrointestinal tract. It also causes invasive disease in patients who are on long-term immunosuppressive therapy (e.g., solid organ transplants, inflammatory bowel disease), but can also occasionally cause severe infection in immunocompetent individuals. Latent CMV is reactivated in immunocompromised patients, leading to viremia, deposition of viral particles in the vascular endothelium, with subsequent vasculitis, submucosal ischemia, and ulceration. In addition to the symptoms of viral colitis described above, CMV colitis patients will also often present with intestinal bleeding and fever.

Herpetic colitis is another form of viral colitis, caused by the herpes simplex virus (HSV). While most often HSV is associated with cold sores and genital warts, it is also a common cause of proctitis and is usually acquired during anal intercourse. Other possible causes of herpes colitis are associated use of immunosuppressive drugs like Azathioprine, Tacrolimus, Prednisone (and other corticosteroids), methotrexate, and Cyclosporine. Symptoms of HSV proctitis include pruritis ani, tenemus, diarrhea, anorectal burning, constipation, and mucoid or bloody bowel movements, often with bilateral tender inguinal lymphadenopathy. Some patients may also develop symptoms suggestive of lumbosacral radiculopathy, including impotence, inability to urinate, pain localized to the thighs, buttocks, and lower abdomen.

Finally, while very rare, adenovirus-associated colitis is another form of viral colitis that has also been reported in patients with HIV or AIDS.

Clinical Features

- **Incidence, age, and sex**
  By the age of 5, nearly every child in the world has been infected with rotavirus at least once. However, with each infection, immunity develops, and subsequent infections are less severe. As such, adults are rarely affected. In the United States, before initiation of the rotavirus vaccination program, rotavirus caused about 2.7 million cases of severe gastroenteritis in children, almost 60,000 hospitalizations, and around 40 deaths each year. The incidence and severity of rotavirus infections has declined significantly in countries that have added rotavirus vaccine to their routine childhood immunization policy.

  Data on the incidence and prevalence of CMV, HSV, and adenovirus colitis are sparse. In patients with inflammatory bowel disease, CMV colitis has been reported as 5–36%, and higher in patients with disease refractory to steroid therapy.
- **Site**
  While viruses can affect any part of the gastrointestinal tract, rotavirus, CMV, and HSV have a predilection for the small intestine, ileocaecal region, and rectum, respectively.
- **Treatment**
  Viral colitis does not respond to antibiotics. Anti-diarrheal agents may work in mild diarrhea, but in severe diarrhea, use of these medications must be closely monitored, as they can slow down the intestinal motility and cause toxic megacolon, a potentially dangerous complication. Most important in the treatment of rotavirus colitis is the maintenance of hydration as untreated children can die from the resulting severe dehydration. Depending on the severity of diarrhea, treatment consists of oral rehydration, during which the child is given extra water to drink that contains small amounts of salt and sugar.

While treatment of CMV colitis with intravenous antiviral drugs such as ganciclofovir, foscarnet, or cidofovir has improved symptoms, it has not decreased mortality.

HSV colitis is also symptomatically treated including sitz baths, topical anesthetics, and oral pain medication. Acyclovir (first-line treatment), valacyclovir, and famciclovir are potential antiviral treatments.

- **Outcome**

  Rotavirus colitis is usually a self-limited disease in the western world, although it is a major cause of childhood death (up to 500,000 annual deaths) in developing countries.

  The outcome of CMV colitis depends upon the severity of the immunodeficiency and the severity of the infection. People with HIV or AIDS may have a worse outcome than those with a different type of immunodeficiency: In HIV or AIDS patients, CMV infection will typically affect the entire body, even if patients only have gastrointestinal symptoms. Therefore, overall outcome depends on the response to therapy with antiviral drugs. CMV infection in patients with inflammatory bowel disease is associated with poor outcomes, such as the need for colectomy due to perforation.

  HSV colitis has an excellent prognosis, although the disease may relapse from time to time.

Macroscopy

More than one third of individuals affected by CMV colitis have gross disease only proximal to the sigmoid, so colonoscopy rather than flexible sigmoidoscopy may be needed to locate evidence of infection. The appearance of the mucosa on endoscopy may resemble that of ulcerative colitis, with granularity and mucosal friability, and patients may occasionally have mass lesions that may be mistaken for colonic neoplasms. More typical of CMV infection, however, is the presence of colitis alone (defined by edema and hemorrhage), colitis with ulceration, or discrete, variably sized ulcers ranging from 5 to 2 cm in areas of otherwise normal mucosa.

Approximately 1–3 weeks following HSV infection, the perianal skin, anal canal, and rectum will be affected with multiple vesicles, which tend to be localized to the distal 5–10 cm of the rectum, where the initial lesion are seen as small single or grouped coalesce to form aphthous ulcers.

Rotavirus and norovirus, most common causes of viral gastroenteritis, are not known to cause macroscopic changes.

Microscopy

A definite diagnosis of CMV colitis is made by identifying typical inclusion bodies in biopsy specimens, and not by serologic studies or culture of biopsy material. CMV can be identified as the cause of inclusions using immunoperoxidase staining, in situ hybridization, or polymerase chain reaction (PCR). Multiple biopsies from the centers of ulcerations are recommended, as viral inclusions are found most frequently in the endothelial cells of the deeper layers of the gut wall. Besides endothelial cells, these mudgy intranuclear and cytoplasmic inclusions can also be found in fibroblasts and smooth muscle cells (only rarely in epithelial cells) (Fig. 1a). In addition, vasculitis and luminal thrombosis may be observed, typically in the ileocaecal region, and this may be the cause of severe necrotizing gut injury and perforation.

Biopsy of the rectum or anal canal in a patient with HSV infection may reveal typical intranuclear inclusion bodies or multinucleated giant cells (Fig. 1b). In addition, the inflammatory pattern in the rectum may show ulceration with neutrophils within the lamina propria, cryptitis, and crypt abscess formation. HSV is also easily cultured.

In adenovirus-associated colitis, the mucosa will show moderate architectural changes and chronic inflammation. Infected colonic epithelial cells can be seen at the surface, and they have the appearance of dystrophic goblet cells with a crescent-shaped or sickle-shaped amphophilic nucleus that occasionally contains inclusion

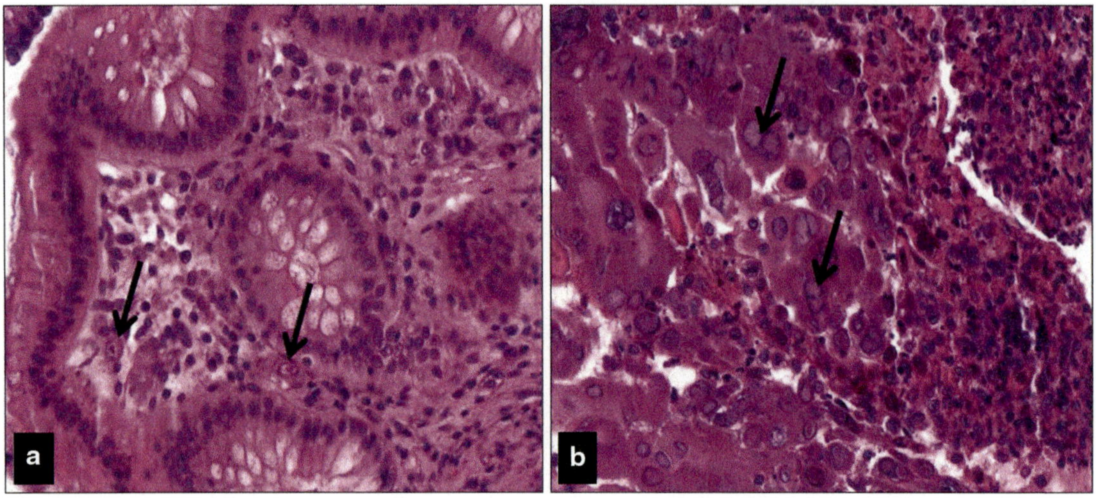

Viral Colitis, Fig. 1 Hematoxylin/eosin stainings of viral colitis subtypes: (**a**) presence of CMV inclusion bodies in endothelial cells in the lamina propria (magnification 400×); (**b**) presence of HSV intranuclear inclusions in the stratified epithelium of the anus (magnification 400×)

bodies. Adenovirus presence can be verified by immunohistochemistry or electron microscopy.

Rotavirus and norovirus, most common causes of viral gastroenteritis, are not known to cause microscopic changes. Diagnosis of infection with rotavirus normally follows diagnosis of gastroenteritis as the cause of severe diarrhea. Most children admitted to hospital with gastroenteritis are tested for rotavirus. A specific diagnosis of infection with rotavirus is made by finding the virus in the child's stool by enzyme immunoassay.

Differential Diagnosis

Viral colitis, especially in an immunosuppressed setting, needs to be differentiated (by means of clinical presentation, blood tests, endoscopic findings, biopsy examination, and/or cultures) from other infections, such as *Campylobacter* infection, *Clostridium difficile* colitis, cryptosporidiosis, and colitis caused by *Mycobacterium Avium-Intracellulare*. In addition, CMV colitis may mimic severe inflammatory bowel disease, so that adequate biopsy sampling (with histologic investigation for presence or absence of CMV in the colonic tissue) in inflammatory bowel disease patients is essential in a diagnostic work-up.

References and Further Reading

Bernstein, D. I. (2009). Rotavirus overview. *Pediatric Infectious Disease Journal, 28*, S50–S53.

Goodgame, R. W. (2001). Viral causes of diarrhea. *Gastroenterology Clinics of North America, 30*, 779–795.

Rafailidis, P. I., Mourtzoukou, E. G., Varbobitis, I. C., & Falagas, M. E. (2008). Severe cytomegalovirus infection in apparently immunocompetent patients: A systematic review. *Virology Journal, 5*, 47.

Rompalo, A. M. (1999). Diagnosis and treatment of sexually acquired proctitis and proctocolitis: An update. *Clinical Infectious Diseases, 28*, S84–S90.

Rotterdam, H., & Tsang, P. (1994). Gastrointestinal-disease in the immunocompromised patient. *Human Pathology, 25*, 1123–1140.

Viral Gastroenteritis

Karel Geboes
Department of Pathology, N. Goormaghtig Institute, University Gent, Gent, Belgium
Department of Pathology, KU Leuven, Leuven, Belgium

Synonyms

Stomach or gastric flu (although the condition is not related to the influenza virus)

Definition

Viral gastroenteritis is an infection caused by a variety of viruses. The most common viruses are rotavirus (so-called because of their wheel-like morphology on electron microscopic examination, belongs to the family of *Reoviridae*), adenoviruses (non-enveloped viruses composed of a nucleocapsid and a double-stranded linear DNA genome), noroviruses (a diverse group of single-stranded RNA viruses, belongs to the family of *Caliciviridae*, so-called because many strains have visible cup shaped depressions on electron microscopy), and picornaviruses (named because they are small and of RNA type). The infection results in inflammation. It involves both the stomach and the small intestine and sometimes the large intestine, resulting in a combination of nausea, vomiting, watery diarrhea, and abdominal pain which may be cramping. The disease may be associated with fever (rotavirus), headache, and muscle pain. Symptoms usually begin 12–72 h after contracting the infection and resolve within 1 week (norovirus: 24–48 h, rotavirus: a few days). In countries with poor hygiene and sanitation and less access to medical services, diarrhea may persist and lead to dehydration. Fatal cases can be observed. Rotavirus is believed to cause an estimated 527,000 deaths among children less than 5 years of age especially in Asia and Africa.

Clinical Features

- **Incidence**
  Infectious diarrhea is a universal health problem that is responsible for extensive morbidity and that accounts for important mortality particularly for children in the developing world. An investigation on more than 30,000 patients hospitalized for diarrhea in the USA found that less than 6% had an identified bacterial pathogen, leaving 94% without a clear pathogen. This diagnostic void was substantially filled in by the introduction of reverse transcription-coupled polymerase chain reaction (RT-PCR) for enteric viral pathogens. Viral gastroenteritis affects people in all parts of the world. Among the viruses, rotaviruses are the leading cause of diarrheal disease in the world. They may affect yearly over 125 million children in developing countries. Norovirus (Norwalk-like virus) is the most common cause of community-acquired diarrhea across all ages, the most common cause of outbreaks of gastroenteritis (40%) and the most common cause of food-borne disease in the USA affecting 23 million patients each year. In adults, norovirus is also the most frequently identified cause of acute gastroenteritis in patients visiting an emergency department with detection of 27% patients for whom stool and serum specimens are available.

  Adenoviruses types 40 and 41 (from species F) cause acute diarrhea, especially as outbreaks in children and can also be detected in the stools of asymptomatic children. The incidence of infection reported for children with gastroenteritis in developed countries has usually been between 4% and 10%. Less common causes are the Picornaviruses (PBVs) which incorporate Enteroviruses (including polio, Coxsackie A and B, and echovirus), Astroviruses, and Coronaviruses. They are detected in sporadic episodes of diarrhea as sole pathogen or coinfection as well as in outbreaks and in immune-compromised patients. However, they can also be found in non-diarrheic healthy hosts.

  Each virus has its own seasonal activity. Rotavirus and astrovirus infections occur more often during the cooler months of the year (October to April), whereas adenovirus infections occur throughout the year. Norovirus infections occur the year round but tend to increase in cooler months. In all age groups, viral gastroenteritis is characteristically associated with epidemics and outbreaks in institutional settings such as schools, child care facilities, and nursing homes, but isolated cases are also well recognized.
- **Age**
  Viruses cause about 70% of episodes of infectious diarrhea in the pediatric age group but. viral gastroenteritis can occur at all ages. However, some viruses tend to cause diarrheal disease primarily in specific age groups. Virtually,

all children have been infected with rotavirus by the time they reach 2–3 years of age. Most symptomatic episodes occur between 7 and 15 months. Children up to the age of 2 year suffer more pronounced symptoms, while neonates and adults are relatively immune from infection and usually have only mild disease. Adenoviruses and astroviruses cause diarrhea mostly in young children, but older children and adults can also be affected. Noroviruses are particularly associated with outbreaks of diarrhea in hospitals and residential facilities for the elderly. Enteroviruses can cause severe gastroenteritis in immune-compromised patients, and they may be found in asymptomatic carriers. Astroviruses are associated with gastroenteritis in children but produce only mild symptoms in adults.

- **Sex**
  There is no gender predilection.
- **Site**
  The effects of viral gastroenteritis are mainly seen in the stomach and small intestine.
- **Treatment**
  Most cases of viral gastroenteritis last only a few days, and therefore, affected persons do not commonly seek or need medical attention. Infants, young children, older persons, and people with unhealthy immune systems (due to cancer, poor nutrition, human immune deficiency virus infection, or other chronic illnesses) may have more severe cases of viral gastroenteritis. Antibiotics or other specific medications are not generally used to treat viral gastroenteritis. Dehydration is the most common complication. Therefore, affected persons should drink plenty of fluids, eventually rehydration solutions. For severe cases, hospitalization and intravenous rehydration may be needed.

  Stopping transmission is the first strategy for prevention. Hand-washing with water and soap, before or after contacting a patient or objects, is essential. Cleaning surfaces and handling raw food with plastic gloves may be useful. Several drugs, such as nitazoxandie, have been tested to treat diarrhea caused by virus gastroenteritis with positive results, and particularly against rotavirus. A vaccine for rotavirus is recommended for infants.

Macroscopy

There is no reliable description of a particular macroscopic pattern as autopsies from fatal cases are rarely performed.

Microscopy

The pathology at the microscopic level is not specific. However, a variety of lesions have been reported. Rotavirus is a lytic virus that causes diarrhea primarily by the reduction of enzymes of the brush-border of enterocytes (disaccharidases, lactase, etc.) and destruction of intestinal villous epithelial cells. Rotaviruses replicate in the gut. The virus can enter the cells by receptor mediated endocytosis. Acute rotavirus (A) gastroenteritis may be associated with variable shortening of the villi, a moderate round cell infiltrate in the lamina propria and elongation of crypts. Early in the infection, supranuclear cytoplasmic vacuolation and shedding of enterocytes from the apical portion of the villi may be observed on routine staining (Figs. 1 and 2). The microscopic aspect in single cells is similar to what can be seen in abetalipoproteinemia (and occasionally in juvenile nutritional megaloblastic anemia), but the distribution of the affected cells is more discontinuous in viral infection. The lamina propria infiltrate looks "top heavy" or denser toward the lumen. Lesions are often patchy in nature. Virus particles, demonstrable by electron microscopy, are present in the villi and crypts. Adenovirus infection is associated with mild mixed mucosal inflammation and slight increase in crypt cell apoptosis. Loss of polarity of surface epithelial cells with dystrophic goblet cells may suggest the infection. Inclusions within the nucleus of surface or crypt epithelial cells are readily demonstrable by immunohistochemical techniques (Fig. 3). Histological changes observed in norovirus infection include villous broadening, blunting and irregularity and vacuolation of the surface enterocytes. The villous changes induce a reduction of the surface area by nearly 50%. In addition, a reactive disarray of surface epithelial cells can be seen. Surface and glandular epithelial

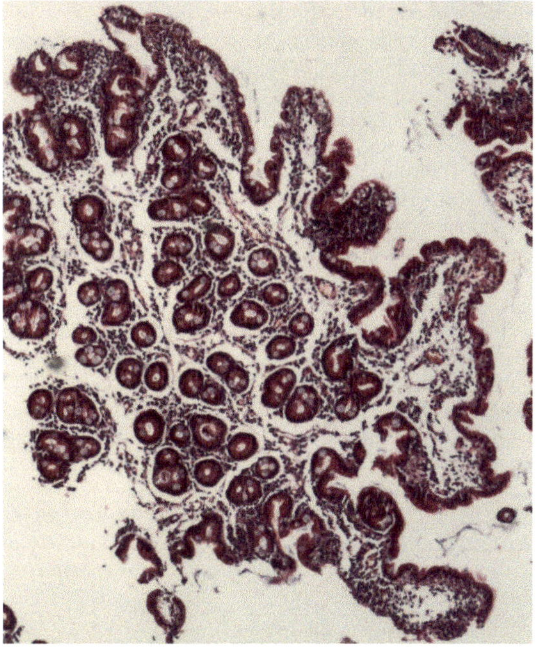

Viral Gastroenteritis, Fig. 1 Rotavirus infection: low power showing variable aspect of the villi with mildly increased cellular infiltrate in the lamina propria

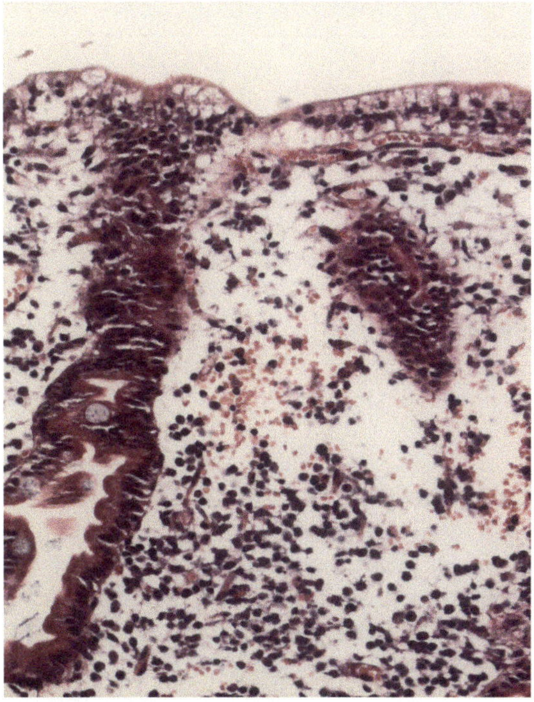

Viral Gastroenteritis, Fig. 2 Rotavirus can induce supranuclear vacuolization in surface epithelial cells

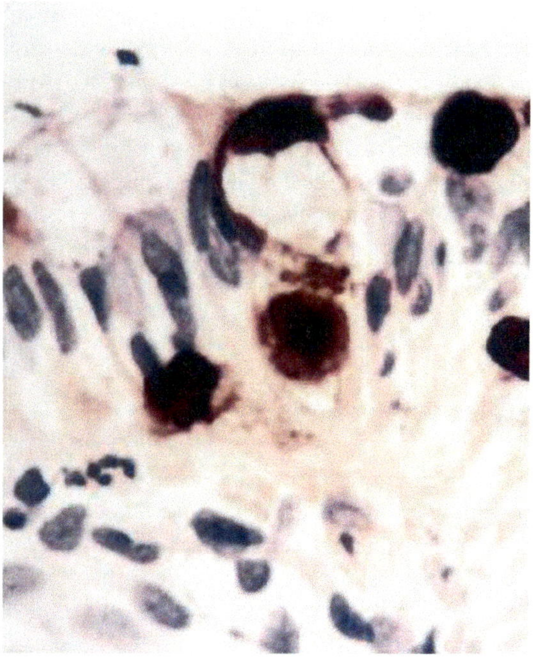

Viral Gastroenteritis, Fig. 3 Immunohistochemistry can demonstrate the presence of adenovirus particles

cells' apoptosis and proliferation of glandular cells are increased. Glandular apoptosis is a feature shared with rejection, and infections in intestinal transplant therefore show features that overlap with allograft rejection. Expression of tight junctional proteins occludin, claudin-4, and claudin-5 is reduced. Intraepithelial lymphocytes are increased (to 60 per 100 enterocytes). In the lamina propria, polymorphonuclear and mononuclear cells are increased in correlation with symptomatic illness. The four major serologically distinct groups of Coronaviruses have been associated with necrotizing enterocolitis in infants.

Immunophenotype

Because of the diversity of the viruses involved in gastroenteritis, there is no specific immunophenotype. Viruses can induce the production of a variety of antibodies. Antibodies can be detected with immunological methods for diagnostic purposes. They show evidence of prior exposure. The exact meaning of antibody positivity remains to be determined. Seroprevalence studies have shown, for instance, that up to 90% individuals develop antibodies against noroviruses by adulthood. However, the humoral protection provided by these antibodies against subsequent exposure remains unclear. In vivo replication of rotaviruses is generally limited to enterocytes. Because of this restriction, most blood circulating rotavirus-specific B cells express the intestinal homing receptor alpha4beta7.

Molecular Features

The different viruses are characterized by a variety of molecular features. These can be used for diagnostic purposes. Molecular DNA-based diagnostics are increasingly used, and real-time PCR provides a dramatic increase in the detection of viruses.

However, overall, there is a problem because of the wide genetic diversity. For rotavirus, for instance, G and P serotypes have been defined by the antigenicity of the outer capsid neutralization proteins, VP7 and VP4, respectively. These serotypes are often are used for molecular assays. Recent genotype classification has been expanded to include all 11 genome segments and in several countries, especially in the developing world, an extensive diversity is identified.

Differential Diagnosis

In the differential diagnosis, bacterial infections by *Campylobacter jejuni*, *Escherichia coli*, *Salmonella*, *Shigella*, and Clostridium difficile, as well as parasitic infections by *Giardia lamblia* and *Cryptosporidium*, must be considered.

References and Further Reading

Braeckman, T., Van Herck, K., Meyer, N., Pirçon, J. Y., Soriano-Gabarro, M., Heylen, E., Zeller, M., Azou, M., Capiau, H., De Koster, J., Maernoudt, A. S., Raes, M., Verdonck, L., Verghote, M., Vergison, A., Matthijnssens, J., Van Ranst, M., & Van Damme, P. (2012). Effectiveness of rotavirus vaccination in prevention of hospital admissions for rotavirus gastroenteritis among young children in Belgium: Case–control study. *BMJ, 345*, e4752.

Bresee, J. S., Marcus, R., Venezia, R. A., Keene, W. E., Morse, D., Thanassi, M., Brunett, P., Bulens, S., Beard, R. S., Dauphin, L. A., Slutkser, L., Bopp, C., Eberhard, M., Hall, A., Vinje, J., Monroe, S. S., & Glass, R. I. (2012). The etiology of severe acute gastroenteritis among adults visiting emergency departments in the United States. *The Journal of Infectious Diseases, 205*, 1374–1381.

Caul, E. O. (1996). Viral gastroenteritis: Small round structured viruses, caliciviruses and astroviruses. Part I. The clinical and diagnostic perspective. *Journal of Clinical Pathology, 49*, 874–880.

Davidson, G. P., & Barnes, G. L. (1979). Structural and functional abnormalities of the small intestine in infants and young children with rotavirus enteritis. *Acta Paediatrica Scandinavica, 68*, 181–186.

Koo, H. L., Ajami, N., Atmar, R. L., & DuPont, H. L. (2010). Noroviruses: The principal cause of foodborne disease worldwide. *Discovery Medicine, 10*, 61–70.

Wolffs, P. F. G., Bruggeman, C. A., Van Well, G. T. J., & Van Loo, I. H. M. (2011). Replacing traditional diagnostics of fecal viral pathogens by a comprehensive panel of real-time PCRs. *Journal of Clinical Microbiology, 49*, 1926–1931.

Volvulus

Gabriel Becheanu
Department of Pathology, Fundeni Clinical Institute, Carola Davila University of Medicine and Pharmacy, Bucharest, Romania

Synonyms

Abnormal torsion; Twisting

Definition

A volvulus is an abnormal twisting of a digestive segment with obstruction of its lumen and/or blood supply. It can occur after birth as a result of a malrotation of a digestive segment or because of the absence of some intraperitoneal visceral ligaments but can be present also in adult life as a consequence of an elongated or abnormally mobile part of the digestive tract or secondary to a local obstacle formed by adhesions, inflammation, or tumors.

Clinical Features

- **Incidence**
  In children, volvulus is related to congenital abnormalities which predispose to a laxity of the segment movements, diaphragm anomalies, or other abdominal defects.

  Gastric volvulus is a rare entity with unknown incidence, usually associated with diaphragmatic congenital anomalies and wandering spleen.

  In pregnancy, volvulus is considered the second most common cause of intestinal obstruction.

  Cecal and sigmoid volvulus was reported more common in India, Africa (Nigeria, Ethiopia, Zimbabwe), and Scandinavian countries, and it appears to be related to high-residue meal or cereal diet which lead to an increased fecal load with elongation of the mesentery.

  Incidence of volvulus is probably underestimated because of the cases with spontaneous reduction.
- **Age**
  Volvulus can occur in early life, usually in the first year, as a consequence of a malrotation or absence of organic ligaments and is unusual in older children.

  Sigmoid volvulus appears to be more frequent in elderly people and patients with diabetes and neuropsychiatric disorders, and cecal volvulus is more common in young patients.
- **Sex**
  Males and females are equally affected in gastric volvulus. In Western countries, sigmoid volvulus usually occurs in elderly males with chronic constipation and some with history of mental diseases.

  Cecal volvulus is more common in younger females according to an American retrospective study.
- **Site**
  The volvulus can involve different segments of the digestive tract, from stomach to sigmoid.

  Some forms of torsion were described especially in stomach such as organo-axial (around of the longitudinal axis), mesentero-axial (around an axis through the middle of the stomach), and combination of both rotations (combined volvulus).

  For the large bowel, the most common sites of volvulus are caecum and sigmoid colon with twisting of the segment around itself and its mesentery. The preponderance of sigmoid involvement is evident in almost all studies with an incidence between 50% and 75% from all episodes of colonic volvulus.
- **Symptoms**
  Clinical symptoms are related to obstruction of the lumen and location of the volvulus. In gastric volvulus, a Borchardt triad (1904) was described: acute epigastric pain, retching without vomiting, and difficulty to pass nasogastric tube in the stomach.

  Midgut volvulus in children can present with biliary vomiting and bloody stools.

  In cecal volvulus, symptoms of intestinal obstruction like nausea, vomiting, lack of fecal material, or flatus are common, but in sigmoid, constipation is the prominent symptom. Clinical examination reveals a distended, sensible abdomen, usually without peritonitis signs.

  Chronic symptoms are nonspecific (widespread abdominal pain), and volvulus can be difficult to diagnose by clinicians, especially in older people.
- **Treatment**
  Acute gastric volvulus is a high digestive occlusion due to torsion with 180 grades of one part around another part of the stomach and is considered a surgical emergency. The procedure usually performed is anterior gastropexy, with fixation of the stomach to the anterior abdominal wall.

  Nonsurgical colonoscopic decompression is usually selected in elderly persons because of different comorbidities but can also be used in clinically stable patients without signs of ischemia or perforation of the bowel. Resective procedures are indicated in cases of necrosis of the intestinal wall. Detorsion with or without fixation techniques is uncommon.

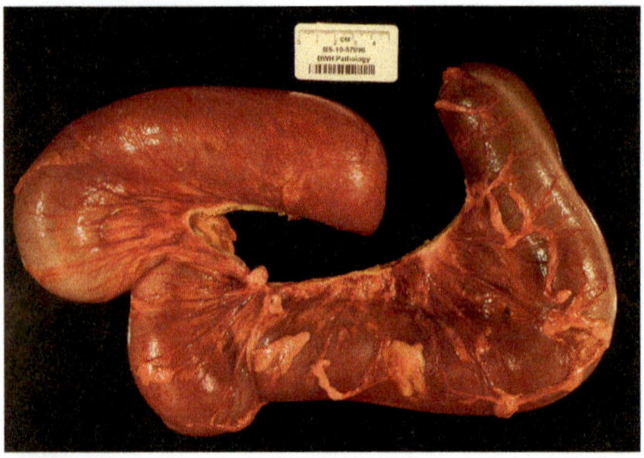

Volvulus, Fig. 1 Gross image of an intestinal volvulus (Courtesy of Dr. Amitabh Srivastava)

- **Outcome**
  Untreated volvulus results in strangulation, with ischemia, necrosis, and finally perforation of the digestive wall with peritonitis. The presence of gangrene and coagulopathy highly predicts mortality, so the prompt diagnosis and management are crucial.

Macroscopy

Features on the resection piece depend on the type of obstruction: complete or partial venous obstruction associated or not with arterial obstruction. The bowel is distended with disappearing of the mucosal folds, with hemorrhagic infarcts and wall necrosis. The serosal surface appears dark red to brown and largely distended (Fig. 1). The obstructed bowel can be long with a thin wall – feature described especially in geographical areas with specific cereal diet, or appears with thickening of muscular wall and fibrous scarring in chronic volvulus with repeated episodes. A rare variant of sigmoid volvulus – ileo-sigmoid knotting – presents when a loop of the ileum knots around the base of a sigmoid volvulus with gangrene of the walls. Lymphatic congestion cad lead to a cyst formation in the mesentery and/or chylous ascites in the peritoneal cavity.

Microscopy

Microscopically, intestinal wall presents subserosal and submucosal venules congestion in mild forms and venous infarction of the obstructive area, ulceration with granulation tissue in the submucosa, and sometimes granulomatous inflammation in acute forms. Reactive hyperplasia in the mesenteric lymph nodes was also noted. Chronic volvulus determines repeated ischemic strangulations of the wall with fibrosis frequently extending into the mesenteric tissue.

Differential Diagnosis

CT scan, MRI examination, and flexible endoscopy are important tools for the positive diagnosis, but in gastric volvulus, barium swallow is considered the gold standard method.

Differential diagnosis includes other causes of digestive obstruction like tumors, chronic active inflammatory bowel diseases, diverticulitis with ileus, intussusception, chronic constipation, and trauma.

References and Further Reading

Ballantyne, G. H., Brandner, M. D., Beart, R. W., Jr., & Ilstrup, D. M. (1985). Volvulus of the colon. Incidence and mortality. *Annals of Surgery, 202*(1), 83–92.

Cirocchi, R., Farinella, E., La Mura, F., Morelli, U., Trastulli, S., Milani, D., Di Patrizi, M. S., Rossetti, B., Spizzirri, A., Galanou, I., Kopanakis, K., Mecarelli, V., & Sciannameo, F. (2010). The sigmoid volvulus: Surgical timing and mortality for different clinical types. *World Journal of Emergency Surgery, 5*, 1. doi:10.1186/1749-7922-5-1.

Halabi, W. J., Jafari, M. D., Kang, C. Y., Nguyen, V. Q., Carmichael, J. C., Mills, S., Pigazzi, A., Stamos, M. J. (2013). Colonic volvulus in the United States: Trends, outcomes and predictors of mortality. *Annals of Surgery.* doi:10.1097/SLA.obo13e31828c88ac.

Mallick, I. H., & Winslet, M. C. (2004). Ileosigmoid knotting. *Colorectal Disease, 6*(4), 220–225.

Türkmen, N., Eren, B., Fedakar, R., & Bulut, M. (2008). Mesenteric volvulus in children: Two autopsy cases and review of the literature. *Journal of Ayub Medical College, Abbottabad, 20*(2), 133–135.

Z

Zenker's Diverticulum

Catarina Fidalgo and Sandra Faias
Instituto Português de Oncologia de Lisboa
Francisco Gentil, E.P.E., Lisboa, Portugal

Synonyms

Cricopharyngeal diverticulum; Hypopharyngeal diverticulum; Pharyngoesophageal diverticulum; Pharyngoesophageal pouch; Posterior pulsion pharyngeal diverticulum; Retropharyngeal diverticulum

Definition

Pharyngoesophageal diverticulum refers to an acquired outpouching of the esophageal mucosa and submucosa, occurring in an area of relative muscular weakness. This area, known as Killian's triangle, corresponds to the zone where the transverse fibers of the cricopharyngeus muscle intersect the oblique fibers of the inferior pharyngeal constrictor muscle. These diverticula are false diverticula as they are a herniation of mucosa and submucosa through the muscular wall. A possible causal mechanism would be an increased luminal pressure caused by impaired upper esophageal sphincter relaxation. Other findings such as achalasia, cricopharyngeal incoordination, or congenital weakness have been implicated, and gastroesophageal reflux could also play a role. Nevertheless the exact etiology remains unclear. The most common presenting symptom is dysphagia (80% of cases). Regurgitation of undigested food is also frequent, mostly nocturnal, and can result in aspiration or even asphyxia. Recurrent aspiration with chronic cough is present in 30–40% of cases and can result in pneumonia. If regurgitation precipitates recurrent vomiting, weight loss can occur. Burdensome symptoms associated with pharyngoesophageal diverticulum are halitosis and dysphonia. A very specific sign is cervical borborygmi. Rarely, bleeding from an ulcerated diverticulum can occur, namely, after corrosive damage by a retained pill. Finally, malignant transformation with squamous cell carcinoma can occur within the pouch (incidence between 0.4% and 1.5%), sometimes signaled by hemoptysis, hematemesis, or a sudden increase in the severity of dysphagia.

Diagnosis of pharyngoesophageal diverticulum can be suspected from clinical history and supported by the findings of a cervical mass with crepitation or borborygmi. Diagnosis is established by a barium esophagogram, which typically shows the diverticulum filled with barium or with an air-fluid level, sometimes blocking the barium passage to the esophageal lumen. Barium swallow can miss small diverticula. An asymptomatic diverticulum can be seen on an upper endoscopy performed for unrelated complaints. It is useful to be aware

F. Carneiro et al. (eds.), *Pathology of the Gastrointestinal Tract*, Encyclopedia of Pathology,
DOI 10.1007/978-3-319-40560-5

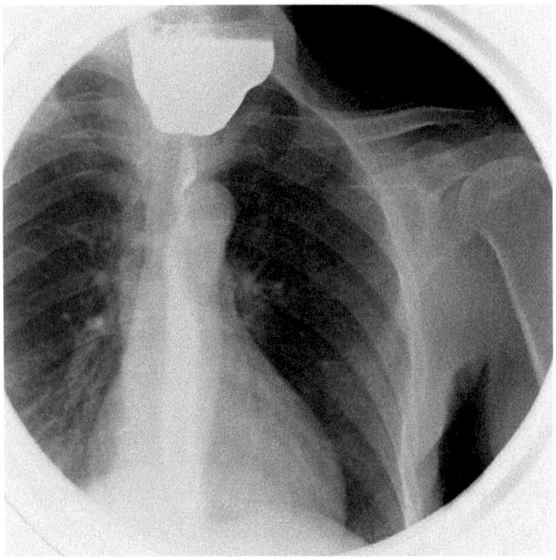

Zenker's Diverticulum, Fig. 1 Barium Esophagogram showing a pharingo-esophageal diverticulum wih an air-fluid level. (Courtesy of António Bettencourt and Daniela Pinto, IPOLFG, EPE)

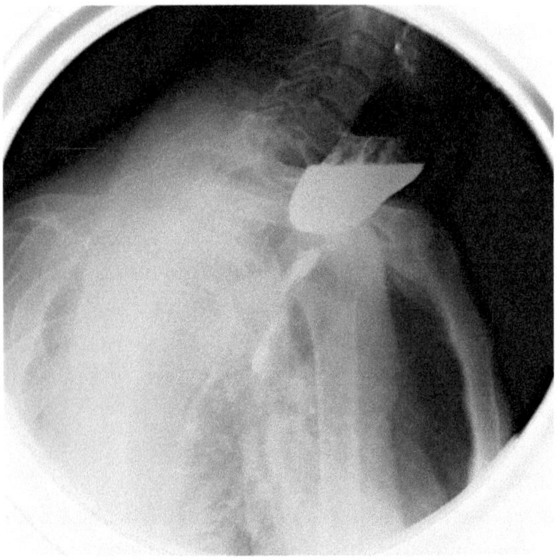

Zenker's Diverticulum, Fig. 2 Barium Esophagogram showing a pharingo-esophageal diverticulum wih an air-fluid level. (Courtesy of António Bettencourt and Daniela Pinto, IPOLFG, EPE)

that a diverticulum exists during esophageal or orotracheal intubation as it can be accidentally perforated during these maneuvers (Figs. 1 and 2).

Clinical Features

- **Incidence**
  Pharyngoesophageal diverticula are the most common diverticula of the upper gastrointestinal tract. The estimated prevalence is between 0.1% and 0.01%. There is considerable geographical incidence variation, which has been attributed to biotype differences. The true incidence is difficult to estimate because there is a proportion of asymptomatic cases.
- **Age**
  Presentation typically occurs in the seventh or eighth decade of life. Anamnesis often reveals that symptoms were present for many years before diagnosis.
- **Sex**
  Gender distribution has a male preponderance, with about 2:1 male/female proportion.
- **Site**
  Pharyngoesophageal diverticulum develops in the cervical esophagus, in an area called Killian's triangle, which is the zone where the transverse fibers of the cricopharyngeus muscle intersect the oblique fibers of the inferior pharyngeal constrictor muscle. It is located on the posterior hypopharyngeal wall, proximally to the upper esophageal sphincter.
- **Treatment**
  There are many treatment options for pharyngoesophageal diverticulum. In asymptomatic patients, with an accidental diagnosis from tests performed for unrelated symptoms (barium swallow or endoscopy), no treatment is the best option. In fact, the majority of these accidentally found diverticula do not become symptomatic over time and follow-up is enough. Minimally symptomatic diverticula or those in patients with high morbidity/surgical risk can be better left untreated with decision made on a case-to-case basis. Symptomatic medically fit patients should be offered treatment in order to end symptoms and prevent complications.

  Open surgery is the advisable treatment option for patients with diverticula larger than 5 cm, especially in young fit candidates. This modality allows optimal exposure while minimizing the risk of damaging thoracic structures. Reported mortality and morbidity are 1–2%. The most common complications are esophago-cutaneous fistula, left vocal cord palsy as a result from recurrent laryngeal nerve lesion and rarely hematoma, wound infection, or respiratory tract infection. By this external approach, a diverticulectomy can be done or instead a diverticulopexy, the latter consisting on the suspension of the diverticulum. Another option is to perform an inversion of the pouch. In any case, upper esophageal sphincter myotomy must be performed to prevent recurrence. More recently, transoral approaches have been developed. Initially using rigid endoscopes, these procedures are performed by ear, nose, and throat surgeons, with the need for neck hyperextension under general anesthesia. These aspects make candidates with severe morbidities or with cervical spine pathology unsuitable for this modality. Later on, flexible endoscopes became popular. With these, general anesthesia and neck hyperextension are not needed and can be performed as an outpatient procedure in most cases. This transoral technique implies the division of the septum between the esophagus and the diverticulum. It obviously includes a cricopharyngeus myotomy as this muscle is contained in the septum. Several endoscopic gadgets have been developed or adapted to perform this (argon plasma coagulation, needle-knife incision, or monopolar coagulation forceps). The downside for this treatment modality is that is not feasible in short diverticula (<3 cm) and may take several sessions for final resolution accomplishment. Nowadays, although formal recommendations still regard transoral route as an alternative for unfit candidates, it is increasingly being offered as a first-line option in many countries, according to local expertise (Figs. 3 and 4).

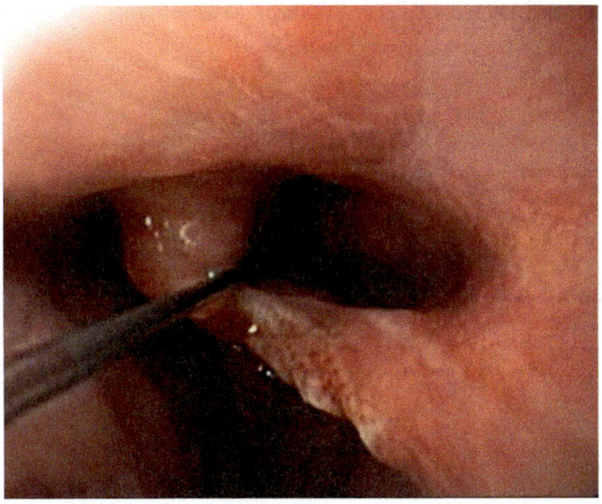

Zenker's Diverticulum, Fig. 3 Endoscopic view of both esophageal and diverticular lumens (above) and pharingo-esophageal diverticulum's *cul de sac* (below). (Courtesy of Pedro Lage, IPOLFG, EPE)

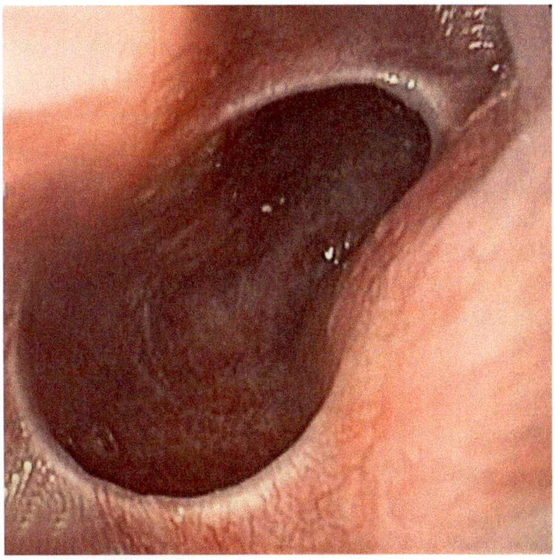

Zenker's Diverticulum, Fig. 4 Endoscopic view of both esophageal and diverticular lumens (above) and pharingo-esophageal diverticulum's *cul de sac* (below). (Courtesy of Pedro Lage, IPOLFG, EPE)

- **Outcome**

  Complications of untreated pharyngoesophageal diverticula include retained foreign body and bezoar, tracheal fistula, vocal cord paralysis, fistula to the prevertebral ligament with cervical osteomyelitis, peptic ulceration, and hemorrhage. Post-open surgery recurrence can be an issue, especially if cricopharyngeal myotomy is not performed and the risks inherent to general anesthesia and surgery should be considered.

Macroscopy

Macroscopically, an outpouching is seen on the posterior esophageal wall in an area called Killian's triangle (where the transverse fibers of the cricopharyngeus muscle intersect the oblique fibers of the inferior pharyngeal constrictor muscle).

Microscopy

Pharyngoesophageal diverticulum is a pseudo-diverticulum, meaning it comprises the mucosal and submucosal layers of the esophageal wall, through a defect in the muscular lining. The histology of the pouch shows a sac lined with stratified squamous epithelium and the submucosa with fibrous tissue surrounding it. Near the neck of the pouch, sparse muscle fibers can be found (Fig. 5). Sometimes erosions or ulcers can be seen due to mucosal damage by retained food or pills. Rarely squamous cell carcinoma may develop inside the diverticulum.

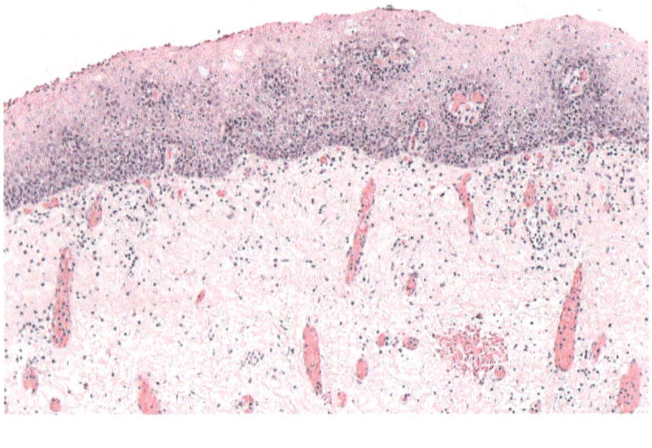

Zenker's Diverticulum, Fig. 5 The pharyngoesophageal pouch is lined by stratified squamous epithelium with inflammatory infiltration. (Courtesy of Isabel Fonseca, IPOLFG, EPE)

Immunophenotype

No immunophenotypic features have been identified as associated with pharyngoesophageal diverticulum. It is thought to be more prevalent in certain regions of the globe, which can be due to variations in individual height. It is postulated that taller individuals have an increased probability of developing pharyngoesophageal diverticula supposedly because, in taller individuals, the Killian's triangle is of greater size.

Molecular Features

No distinctive molecular features have been proposed in this condition.

Differential Diagnosis

Congenital or acquired pharyngeal diverticula (lateral or posterolateral), Killian-Jamieson diverticulum (posterolateral), pharyngoceles (raised intrapharyngeal pressure).

References and Further Reading

Bowdler, D. A. (2008). Pharyngeal pouches. In M. J. Gleeson (Ed.), *Scott Brown's textbook of otorhinolaryngology* (7th ed., pp. 1–22). Oxford.

Case, D. J., & Baron, T. H. (2010). Flexible endoscopic management of Zenker diverticulum: The Mayo Clinic experience. *Mayo Clinic Proceedings, 85*(8), 719–722.

Ferreira, L. E., Simmons, D. T., & Baron, T. H. (2008). Zenker's diverticula: Pathophysiology, clinical presentation, and flexible endoscopic management. *Diseases of the Esophagus, 21*(1), 1–8.

Rizzetto, C., Zaninotto, G., Costantini, M., et al. (2008). Zenker's diverticula: Feasibility of a tailored approach based on diverticulum size. *Journal of Gastrointestinal Surgery, 12*, 2057–2065.

Siddiq, M. A., Sood, S., & Strachan, D. (2001). Pharyngeal pouch (Zenker's diverticulum). *Postgraduate Medical Journal, 77*, 506–511.

Zollinger-Ellison Syndrome

Wen-Yih Liang[1] and Gregory Y. Lauwers[2]
[1]Department of Pathology, Taipei Veterans General Hospital, Taipei, Taiwan
[2]Department of Pathology, Massachusetts General Hospital, Harvard Medical School, Boston, MA, USA

Definition

Zollinger-Ellison syndrome (ZES) is a complex clinicopathologic condition that develops secondary to autonomous production of gastrin and is characterized by massive acid secretion and severe peptic ulcer disease.

Clinical Features

Presentation

The autonomous hypergastrinemia leads to persistent and massive secretion of acid and pepsin, giving rise to multiple refractory peptic ulcers. Abdominal pain, primarily related to the ulcers, is observed in the majority of patients and frequently is accompanied by weight loss. Severe esophagitis and symptoms of gastroesophageal reflux disease, as well as duodenojejunitis and duodenal ulcers, are common findings. In addition, diarrhea is observed in 30–70% of patients, with malabsorption and steatorrhea resulting from concentrated acid entering the small bowel. The presenting symptoms are similar in the 25% of patients with Zollinger-Ellison syndrome who have MEN-1 syndrome, although they may be present at a younger age and more frequent history of nephrolithiasis. Most have a family history of endocrinopathy as well.

Laboratory Tests

An elevated level of fasting serum gastrin level greater than 1,000 pg/mL (a 10× increase) is virtually diagnostic of ZES. Other diagnostic evaluations include a positive secretin test result (secretin injection followed by elevation of gastrin greater than 200 pg/mL, above base level) and a basal acid output greater than 15 mEq/h or resting intragastric pH < 2.0.

Etiology/Pathogenesis

Eighty percent of ZES patients are diagnosed with a sporadic primary gastrin-producing neoplasm. In 20–25% of ZES patients, the gastrinomas are associated with multiple endocrine neoplasia type 1 (MEN-1) syndrome. Primary gastric G cell hyperplasia without the presence of gastrinoma is reported rarely (<5% of patients).

Mechanically, G cell hypersecretion takes place outside the acid feedback loop. Secondarily, gastrin's strong stimulatory and tropic effect on ECL cells and parietal cells results in increased HCl secretion and high basal secretory rates.

- **Incidence**
  ZES has an incidence of 0.1–3 per million population in the United States and comprises 0.1% of all duodenal ulcer patients.
- **Age**
  Zollinger-Ellison can affect adults and children alike, with age range 7–90 years (average age 50 years).
- **Sex**
  There may be a slight male predominance.
- **Site**
  About 50–70% of gastrinomas are located in the duodenum, and 20–40% of cases eventually will be detected in the pancreas. Less than 5% of cases are in other intra-abdominal sites.
- **Treatment**
  Patients with ZES require long-term medical therapy for adequate control of gastric acid hypersecretion with proton pump inhibitors such as omeprazole or lansoprazole. Partial or total gastrectomy may be required for intractable cases. The treatment also should be directed against the gastrin-producing neoplasm. Patients with sporadic gastrinomas that are localized and without metastases are

ideal candidates for surgical removal. Patients with hepatic or distant metastases are managed with chemotherapy, hormonal therapy, or surgical debulking. Achieving surgical cure in ZES patients with MEN-1 is more difficult. Parathyroidectomy in some patients with hyperparathyroidism decreases fasting gastrin levels.

- **Outcome**
  Sixty to ninety percent of gastrinomas are malignant. However, ZES patients who have had a successful tumor resection show a 60–100% survival rate at 10 years. In contrast, patients with unresectable tumors have a 40% survival rate at 5 years; in the absence of liver metastases, 30% of patients have long-term survival. MEN-1 patients have better 5- and 10-year survival rates than do those with sporadic ZES (62–85% vs. 50–70%).

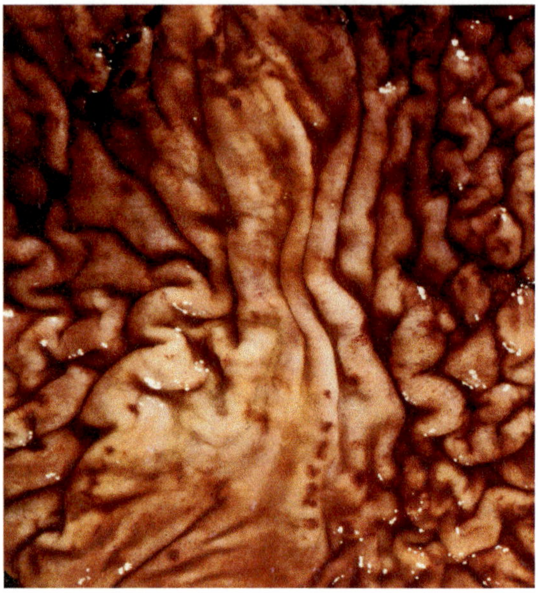

Zollinger-Ellison Syndrome, Fig. 1 Gastrectomy specimen showing the typical enlarged gastric folds of Zollinger-Ellison with a small peptic erosion

Macroscopy

ZES is characterized by massive hypertrophy of gastric rugae in the body and fundus that can range from 0.6 to 4.5 cm in thickness, whereas the antral mucosa often regresses in span (Fig. 1). Duodenal ulcerations are commonly seen as well and most frequently noted in the first part of the duodenum. However, they also can affect the more distal duodenum and jejunum.

Microscopy

The trophic effect of gastrin causes increased thickness of the oxyntic mucosa in Zollinger-Ellison patients. Parietal cells show hypertrophy and hyperplasia and extend up to the foveolar neck region (Figs. 2 and 3). They often extend to the gastric antrum. Gastrin hypersecretion also causes hyperplasia of ECL cells in the oxyntic mucosa, leading to linear and nodular ECL hyperplasia. Eventually, low-grade neuroendocrine tumor (carcinoid tumors) can arise in MEN-1-associated ZES, but not in patients with sporadic ZES. Fundic gland polyps secondary to proton pump inhibitor therapy may be observed.

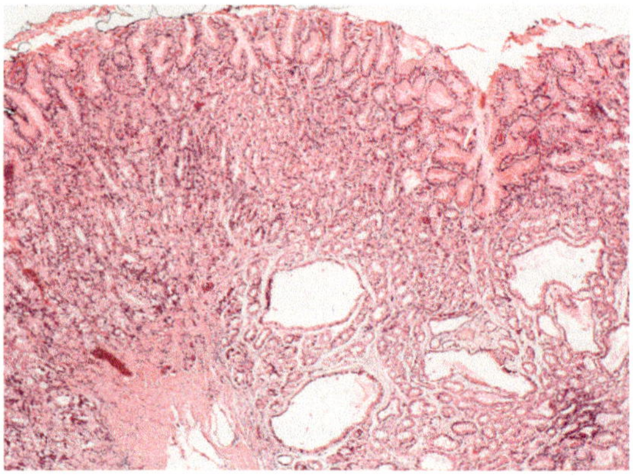

Zollinger-Ellison Syndrome, Fig. 2 Scanning view of hypertrophic oxyntic mucosa. Note the elongation of the glands with parietal cell hyperplasia and cystic glandular changes

Immunohistochemical Evaluation

Gastrinoma will stain with chromogranin, synaptophysin, and gastrin immunostains. ECL hyperplasia and gastric carcinoids stain with chromogranin and vesicular monoamine

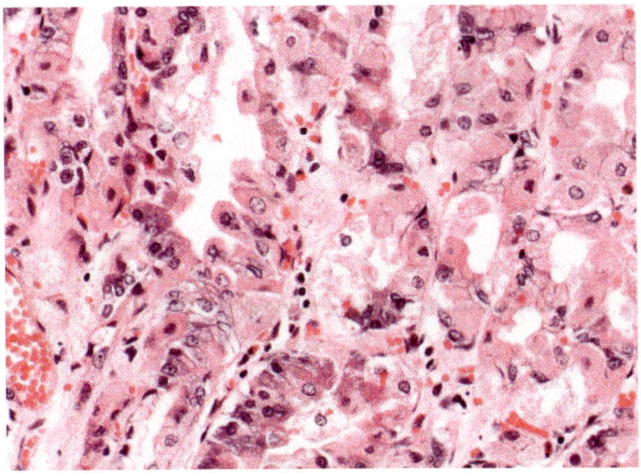

Zollinger-Ellison Syndrome, Fig. 3 Oxyntic fundic mucosa in a Zollinger-Ellison patient. Note the prominent parietal cell hyperplasia

transporter, isoform 2 (VMAT-2). ECL cells are negative for gastrin, somatostatin, and serotonin.

Differential Diagnosis

- Other hypertrophic gastropathy could be considered in the differential diagnosis.
- Ménétrier disease is associated with giant foveolar hyperplasia with cystic formation and mucus glands of the oxyntic mucosa. However, atrophy of the parietal glands is noted.
- Lymphocytic gastritis is characterized by increased intraepithelial lymphocytic exocytosis with foveolar hyperplasia. It can be sporadic, but is also frequently associated with either gluten-sensitive enteropathy or *H. pylori* infection. Pediatric cases have been associated with CMV infection as well.
- In rare cases, chronic active *H. pylori* gastritis can be associated with antral G cell hyperplasia, acid hypersecretion, and peptic ulcer disease. However, the presence of curved bacilli and superficial chronic active gastritis will help distinguish it from ZES.
- Linitis plastica secondary to the infiltrating poorly cohesive adenocarcinoma may be associated with hypertrophic gastric folds. However, neoplastic infiltration reveals the diagnosis. Similarly, infiltrative malignant may present with hypertrophic gastric folds.

References and Further Reading

Berna, M. J., et al. (2008). A prospective study of gastric carcinoids and enterochromaffin-like cell changes in multiple endocrine neoplasia type 1 and Zollinger-Ellison syndrome: Identification of risk factors. *The Journal of Clinical Endocrinology and Metabolism, 93*(5), 1582–1591.

Ellison, E. C., et al. (2009). The Zollinger-Ellison syndrome: A comprehensive review of historical, scientific, and clinical considerations. *Current Problems in Surgery, 46*(1), 13–106.

Jensen, R. T., & Norton, J. A. (2010). Chapter 32: Endocrine tumors of the pancreas and gastrointestinal tract. In *Sleisenger and Fordtran's gastrointestinal and liver disease* (9th ed., Vol. 1, pp. 491–522). Philadelphia: Saunders Elsevier.

Metz, D. C., et al. (2001). Replacement of oral proton pump inhibitors with intravenous pantoprazole to effectively control gastric acid hypersecretion in patients with Zollinger-Ellison syndrome. *The American Journal of Gastroenterology, 96*(12), 3274–3280.

Norton, J. A., et al. (2007). Role of surgery in Zollinger-Ellison syndrome. *Journal of the American College of Surgery, 205*(4 Suppl), S34–S37.